Emery's Elements of Medical Genetics and Genomics

Emery's Elements of Medical Genetics and Genomics

EDITION: 16

Peter D. Turnpenny BSc MB ChB FRCP FRCPCH FRCPath FHEA

Consultant Clinical Geneticist,
Royal Devon and Exeter NHS Foundation Trust,
and
Professor in Clinical Genomics,
University of Exeter Medical School

Sian Ellard OBE BSc PhD FRCPath

Consultant Clinical Scientist,
Royal Devon and Exeter NHS Foundation Trust,
and
Professor of Genomic Medicine,
University of Exeter Medical School

Ruth Cleaver BSc MB ChB PGCert MRCP

Consultant Clinical Geneticist,
Royal Devon and Exeter NHS Foundation Trust

ELSEVIER

EMERY'S ELEMENTS OF MEDICAL GENETICS AND GENOMICS, EDITION: 16
ISBN: 978-0-702-079665

Library of Congress Control Number 2020941978

Content Strategist: Alexandra Mortimer
Content Development Specialist: Deborah Poulson
Publishing Services Manager: Shereen Jameel
Project Manager: Rukmani Krishnan
Design Direction: Amy Buxton

Printed in Poland

Last digit is the print number: 9 8 7 6 5 4 3

Contents

Preface

"Reading maketh a full man; conference a ready man; and writing an exact man."

Francis Bacon (1561–1626)

"To study the phenomena of disease without books is to sail an uncharted sea, while to study books without patients is not to go to sea at all."

William Osler (1849–1919)

In the three years since we last updated *Emery's Elements* the applications of genetic technologies to all medical disciplines have surged forward. Not only is the rich vein of gene discovery in rare disease far from exhausted, but our understanding of broader questions about the nature and function of the human genome have advanced significantly, and there is far more hope for different forms of treatment for genetic disease than ever before. The last few years has seen the dramatic emergence of CRISPR/Cas9 gene editing, not only as a research tool but also as demonstrating treatment potential; cancer genomics is helping to elucidate and manage tumors and malignancy; and non-invasive prenatal testing and diagnosis are becoming embedded in routine fetal medicine practice. On top of this, the often complex process of interpreting and classifying DNA variants is now a well-established discipline, albeit one that is destined to evolve.

All these developments pose huge challenges for clinical practice in terms of the responsible application of the technologies to diagnosis, patient care, and family management. Rolling out the new technologies in healthcare systems and mainstream medicine varies hugely worldwide, but universally relevant issues are those of confidentiality, consent, disclosure, and non-disclosure, all in the context of legal systems that are at best only beginning to understand the implications of the vast amounts of personal data being generated by the "genomics revolution."

The other universally relevant issues relate to "capacity"—both the capacity of healthcare systems to develop the infrastructure to deliver the benefits of genetic knowledge and technologies, and the capacity to inform and educate healthcare professionals. As such, our hope is that this new edition will contribute to the much-needed education and training in this expanding discipline, which has an impact on all the others. We have sought to bring this edition up to date with key developments while maintaining the same tried and tested format. Many chapters have been enriched by case studies that seek to take the reader to problem-solving clinical scenarios, which, after all, are real life. As before, therefore, we hope this text will prove useful to undergraduates and postgraduates alike and help them swim rather than sink when faced with the depth and extent of developments in medical genetics and genomics.

Peter Turnpenny, Sian Ellard, and Ruth Cleaver
Exeter, United Kingdom

Acknowledgments

As always, we feel privileged to be working in an area of healthcare science and service, and research and development, that continues to be exciting and captivating as the technologies and knowledge move forward so inexorably. We work within teams and networks of very talented colleagues who are similarly inspired and, even though unaware, contribute to this volume through their knowledge, professional companionship, and encouragement. We have learned a vast amount of clinical genetics from our patients and we thank those who have agreed for their images to be added to this edition. Particular thanks are due to Dr. Andrew Wood for his assistance with the updating of Chapters 7 and 10. We are grateful to Elsevier, especially Kathleen Nahm, Deborah Poulson, and Alexandra Mortimer, for their help, guidance, and patience throughout the journey during 2019–2020.

*We again dedicate this edition to Alan Emery, a friend, mentor,
and constant source of inspiration and encouragement.*

*Alan E. H. Emery (c. 1983), Emeritus Professor of
Human Genetics & Honorary Fellow, University of Edinburgh,
first established the* Elements of Medical Genetics *in 1968.*

"The book was first conceived and published by the University of California Press in 1968 as Heredity, Disease, and Man: Genetics in Medicine. *However, when appointed Professor of Human Genetics at Edinburgh in 1968, I decided I should prefer the book to be published by Churchill Livingstone under the title* Elements of Medical Genetics, *and made more accessible to UK students with a cheaper paperback edition. This was all achieved and has retained this format ever since. The current 16th edition illustrates very clearly how the subject has advanced so much over the intervening years."*

Alan Emery

1

The History and Impact of Genetics in Medicine

It's just a little trick, but there is a long story connected with it which it would take too long to tell.

Gregor Mendel, in Conversation With C.W. Eichling

It has not escaped our notice that the specific pairing we have postulated immediately suggests a possible copying mechanism for the genetic material.

Watson & Crick (April 1953)

Presenting historical truth is at least as challenging as the pursuit of scientific truth, and our view of human endeavors down the ages is heavily biased in favor of winners—those who have conquered on military, political or, indeed, scientific fields of conflict. The history of genetics in relation to medicine is one of breathtaking discovery from which patients and families have benefitted hugely, and we are privileged to be witnessing such developments at the beginning of what promises to be a dramatic and exciting era. However, success will be measured by ongoing progress in translating discoveries into successful treatment and prevention of disease, while at the same time causing no harm—for the Hippocratic principle of *primum non nocere* applies to this field as any other. It is always inspiring to look back with awe at what our forebears achieved with scarce resources and sheer determination, sometimes aided by serendipity, to lay the foundations of this dynamic science. This perspective can be compared with driving a car: without your eyes on the road ahead, you will crash and make no progress; however, it is also essential to check the rear and side mirrors regularly.

Gregor Mendel and the Laws of Inheritance

Early Beginnings

Developments in genetics during the 20th century have been truly spectacular. In 1900, Mendel's principles were awaiting rediscovery, chromosomes were barely visible, and the science of molecular genetics did not exist. As we write this in 2020, the published sequence of the entire human genome already feels like a piece of history, we are almost a decade into a 'gold rush' era of disease gene discovery, and genomic science is revealing more about humanity (and the entire living world) than most of us ever imagined.

Genetics is relevant and important to almost every medical discipline. Recent discoveries impinge not just on rare genetic diseases and syndromes but increasingly on the common disorders of adult life that may be predisposed by genetic variation, such as cardiovascular disease, cancer, psychiatric illness, and behavior, not to mention influences on obesity, athletic performance, musical ability, longevity, and a host of physiological variations and tolerances. Clearly, a thorough grounding in genetics and genomics should be a fundamental part of any undergraduate medical curriculum.

We start with an overview of some of the most notable milestones in the history of genetics and medical genetics, followed by a review of the overall impact of genetic factors in causing disease. Finally, we mention some new developments of major importance.

It is not known precisely when *Homo sapiens* first appeared on this planet. For a considerable time, estimates based on the finding of fossilized human bones in Ethiopia suggested man was roaming East Africa approximately 200,000 years ago. The finding of skull bones in Morocco, however, suggests the possibility of man's presence on Earth stretching back 300,000 to 350,000 years. It is reasonable to suppose that our early ancestors were as curious as ourselves about matters of inheritance and, just as today, they would have experienced the birth of babies with all manner of physical defects. Engravings in Chaldea in Babylonia (modern-day Iraq) dating back at least 6000 years show pedigrees documenting the transmission of certain characteristics of the horse's mane. However, any early attempts to unravel the mysteries of genetics were severely hampered by a total lack of knowledge and understanding of basic processes such as conception and reproduction, which was not resolved to the satisfaction of modern science until 1875.

Early Greek philosophers and physicians such as Aristotle and Hippocrates concluded, not without a little prejudice, that important human characteristics were determined by semen, using menstrual blood as a culture medium and the uterus as an incubator. Semen was thought to be produced by the whole body; hence, bald-headed fathers would beget bald-headed sons. These ideas prevailed until the 17th century, when Dutch scientists such as Leeuwenhoek and de Graaf recognized the existence of sperm and ova, thus explaining how the female could also transmit characteristics to her offspring.

The blossoming scientific revolution of the 18th and 19th centuries saw a revival of interest in heredity by scientists and physicians, among whom two names stand out. Pierre de Maupertuis, a French naturalist, studied hereditary traits such as extra digits (polydactyly) and lack of pigmentation (albinism) and showed from pedigree studies that these two conditions were inherited in different ways. Joseph Adams (1756–1818), a British doctor, also recognized that different mechanisms of inheritance existed and published *A Treatise on the Supposed Hereditary Properties of Diseases*, which was intended as a basis for genetic counseling. Also

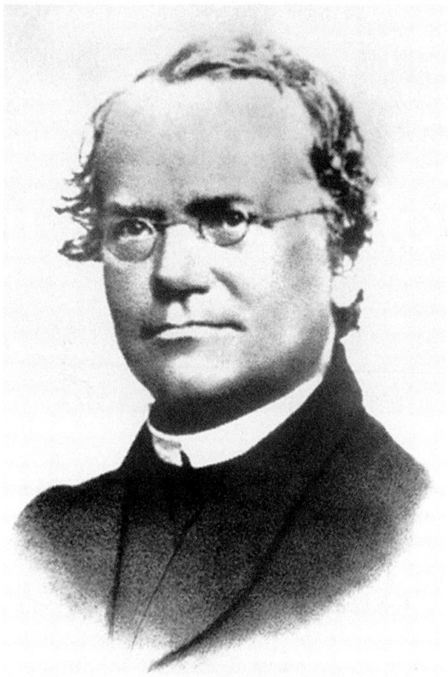

• **Fig. 1.1** Gregor Mendel. (Reproduced with permission from BMJ Books.)

worthy of mention is the English physician Edward Meryon (1809–1880), who in 1851 was the first to provide a systematic clinicopathological study of three boys with the muscular disorder later eponymously attributed to the Frenchman Guillaume Duchenne (1806–1875), who described a larger series in 1868.

The modern scientific era really begins with the work of the Austrian monk Gregor Mendel (1822–1884; Fig. 1.1) who, in 1865, presented the results of his breeding experiments on garden peas to the Natural History Society of Brünn in Bohemia (now Brno in the Czech Republic). Shortly after, Mendel's observations were published in the *Transactions of the Society*, where they remained largely unnoticed until 1900, some 16 years after his death, when their importance was first recognized. In essence, Mendel's work can be considered as the discovery of genes and how they are inherited. The term **gene** was first coined in 1909 by a Danish botanist, Johannsen, and was derived from the term "pangen," introduced by De Vries. This term was itself a derivative of the word "pangenesis," coined by Darwin in 1868. In recognition of Mendel's foundational work, the term **mendelian** is now part of scientific vocabulary, applied both to the different patterns of inheritance and to disorders found to be the result of defects in a single gene.

In his breeding experiments, Mendel studied contrasting characters in the garden pea, using for each experiment varieties that differed in only one characteristic. For example, he noted that when strains bred for a feature such as tallness were crossed with plants bred to be short, all of the offspring in the first filial, or F1, generation were tall. If plants in this F1 generation were interbred, this led to both tall and short plants in a ratio of 3:1 (Fig. 1.2). Characteristics that were manifest in the F1 hybrids were referred to as **dominant**, whereas those that reappeared in the F2 generation were described as being **recessive**. On reanalysis it has been suggested that Mendel's results were "too good to be true" in that the segregation ratios he derived were suspiciously closer to the value of 3:1 than the laws of statistics would predict. One possible explanation is that he may have published only those results

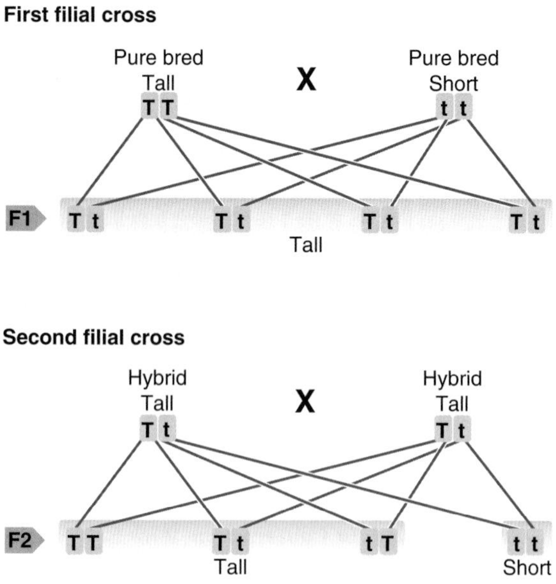

• **Fig. 1.2** An illustration of one of Mendel's breeding experiments and how he correctly interpreted the results.

that best agreed with his preconceived single-gene hypothesis. Whatever the case, events have shown that Mendel's interpretation of his results was entirely correct.

Mendel's proposal was that the plant characteristics being studied were each controlled by a pair of factors, one of which was inherited from each parent. The pure-bred plants with two identical genes used in the initial cross would now be referred to as **homozygous**. The hybrid F1 plants, each of which has one gene for tallness and one for shortness, would be referred to as **heterozygous**. The genes responsible for these contrasting characteristics are referred to as **allelomorphs**, or **alleles** for short.

An alternative method for determining **genotypes** in offspring involves the construction of what is known as a Punnett square (Fig. 1.3). This is used further in Chapter 7 (Fig. 7.1) when considering how genes segregate in large populations, although in reality is seldom referred to nowadays.

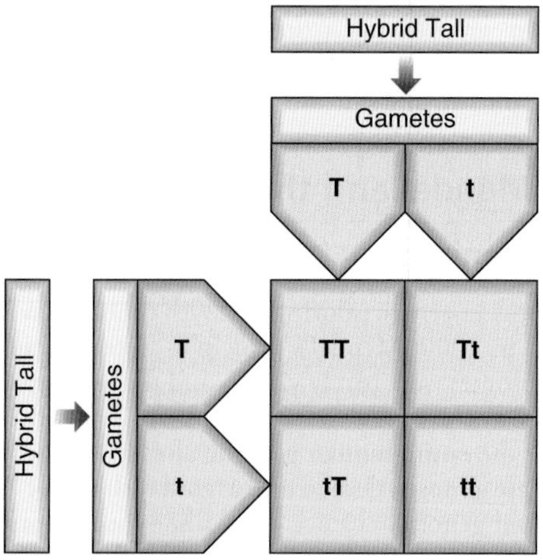

• **Fig. 1.3** A Punnett square showing the different ways in which genes can segregate and combine in the second filial cross from Fig. 1.2. Construction of a Punnett square provides a simple method for showing the possible gamete combinations in different matings.

On the basis of Mendel's plant experiments, three main principles were established, known as the laws of uniformity, segregation, and independent assortment.

The Law of Uniformity

The law of uniformity refers to the fact that, when two homozygotes with different alleles are crossed, all of the offspring in the F1 generation are identical and heterozygous. In other words, the characteristics do not blend, as had been believed previously, and can reappear in later generations.

The Law of Segregation

The law of segregation refers to the observation that each person possesses two genes for a particular characteristic, only one of which can be transmitted at any one time. Rare exceptions to this rule can occur when two allelic genes fail to separate because of chromosome nondisjunction at the first meiotic division (p. 32).

The Law of Independent Assortment

The law of independent assortment refers to the fact that members of different gene pairs segregate to offspring independently of one another. In reality, this is not always true. Genes that are close together on the same chromosome tend to be inherited together because they are "linked" (p. 90). There are a number of other ways by which the laws of mendelian inheritance are breached (see Chapter 6), but overall, they remain foundational to our understanding of the science.

The Chromosomal Basis of Inheritance

As interest in mendelian inheritance grew, there was much speculation as to how it actually occurred. At that time it was also known that each cell contains a nucleus within which there are several threadlike structures known as **chromosomes**, so called because of their affinity for certain stains (*chroma* = color, *soma* = body). Chromosomes had been observed since the second half of the 19th century after development of cytologic staining techniques. Human mitotic figures were observed from the late 1880s, and it was in 1902 that Walter Sutton, an American medical student, and Theodour Boveri, a German biologist, independently proposed that chromosomes could be the bearers of heredity (Fig. 1.4). Subsequently, Thomas Hunt Morgan transformed Sutton's chromosome theory into the theory of the gene (1917), and Alfons Janssens observed the formation of chiasmata between homologous chromosomes at meiosis. During the late 1920s and 1930s, Cyril Darlington helped to clarify chromosome mechanics by the use of tulips collected on expeditions to Persia. It was during the 1920s that the term **genome** entered the scientific vocabulary, being the fusion of *genom* (German for "gene") and *ome* from "chromosome."

When the connection between mendelian inheritance and chromosomes was first made, the normal chromosome number in humans was thought to be 48, although various papers had come up with a range of figures. Key to the number 48 was a paper in 1921 from Theophilus Painter, an American cytologist who had been a student of Boveri. In fact, Painter had some preparations clearly showing 46 chromosomes, even though he finally settled on 48. The discrepancies were probably from the poor quality of the material at that time; even into the early 1950s cytologists were counting 48 chromosomes. It was not until 1956 that the correct number of 46 was established by Tjio and Levan, 3 years after the correct structure of DNA had been proposed. Within a few years, it was shown that some disorders in humans could be caused by loss or gain of a whole chromosome, as well as by an abnormality in a single gene. Chromosome disorders are discussed at length in Chapter 17. Some chromosome aberrations, such as translocations, can run in families (p. 37), and are sometimes said to be segregating in a mendelian fashion.

DNA as the Basis of Inheritance

Although James Watson and Francis Crick are justifiably credited with discovering the structure of DNA in 1953, they were attracted to working on it only because of its key role as the genetic

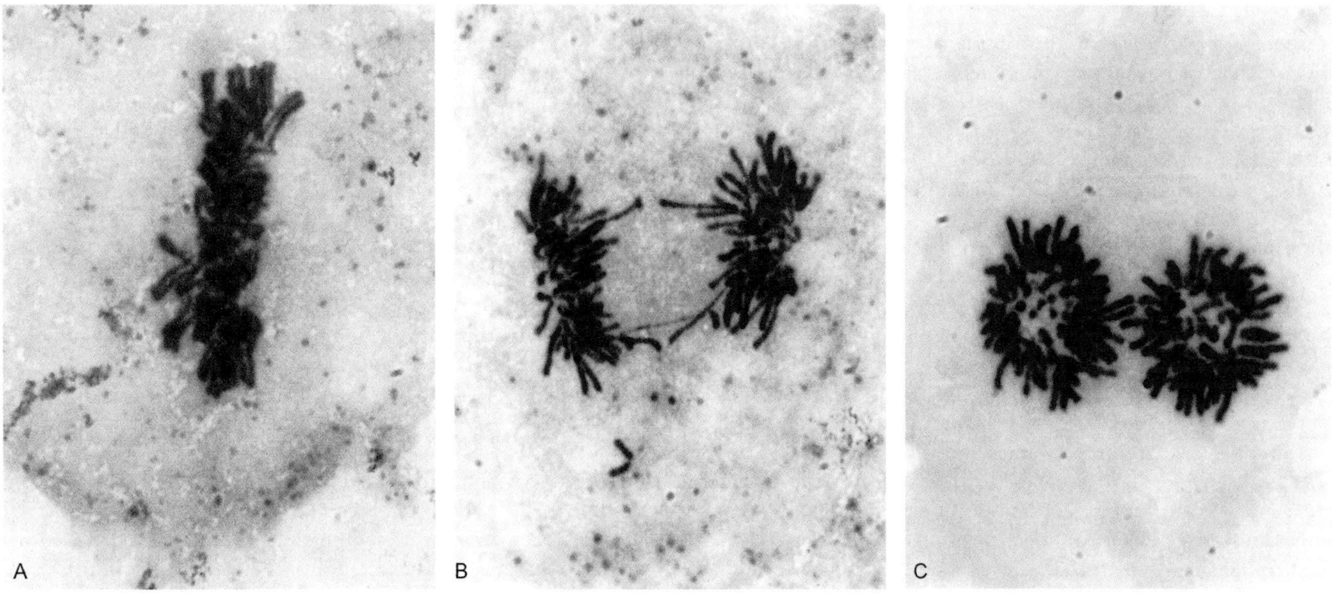

• **Fig. 1.4** Chromosomes dividing into two daughter cells at different stages of cell division. (A) Metaphase; (B) anaphase; (C) telophase. The behavior of chromosomes in cell division (mitosis) is described at length in Chapter 3. (Photographs courtesy Dr. K. Ocraft, City Hospital, Nottingham.)

material, as established in the 1940s. Formerly, many believed that hereditary characteristics were transmitted by proteins, until it was appreciated that their molecular structure was far too cumbersome. Nucleic acids were actually discovered in 1849. In 1928, Fred Griffith, working on two strains of *Streptococcus*, realized that characteristics of one strain could be conferred on the other by something that he called the **transforming principle**. In 1944, at the Rockefeller Institute in New York, Oswald Avery, Maclyn McCarty and Colin MacLeod identified DNA as the genetic material while working on *Streptococcus pneumoniae*. Even then, many in the scientific community were skeptical; DNA was only a simple molecule with lots of repetition of four nucleic acids—very boring! The genius of Watson and Crick, at Cambridge, was to hit on a structure for DNA, the elegant double helix that would explain the very essence of biological reproduction. Crucial to their discovery were the x-ray crystallography images captured by the often-overlooked graduate technician Raymond Gosling, working under the supervision of Maurice Wilkins and Rosalind Franklin in John Randall's laboratory at King's College, London.

This was merely the beginning, for it was necessary to discover the process whereby DNA, in discrete units called genes, issues instructions for the precise assembly of proteins, the building blocks of tissues. The sequence of bases in DNA, and the sequence of amino acids in protein, the **genetic code**, was unraveled in some elegant biochemical experiments in the 1960s, and it became possible to predict the base change in DNA that led to the amino-acid change in the protein. Further experiments involving Francis Crick, Paul Zamecnik, and Mahlon Hoagland identified the molecule transfer RNA (tRNA) (p. 16), which directs genetic instructions via amino acids to intracellular ribosomes, where protein chains are produced. Confirmation of these discoveries came with DNA-sequencing methods and the advent of recombinant DNA techniques. Interestingly, however, the first genetic trait to be characterized at the molecular level had already been identified in 1957 by laborious sequencing of the purified proteins. This was sickle-cell anemia, in which the mutation affects the amino-acid sequence of the blood protein hemoglobin.

The Fruit Fly

It is worth a brief diversion to consider the merits of an unlikely creature that has proved to be of immense value in genetic research. The fruit fly, *Drosophila*, possesses several distinct advantages for the study of genetics:

1. It can be bred easily in a laboratory.
2. It reproduces rapidly and prolifically at a rate of 20 to 25 generations per annum.
3. It has a number of easily recognized characteristics, such as *curly wings* and a *yellow body*, which follow mendelian inheritance.
4. *Drosophila melanogaster*, the species studied most frequently, has only four pairs of chromosomes, each with a distinct appearance.
5. The chromosomes in the salivary glands of *Drosophila* larvae are among the largest known in nature, being at least 100 times bigger than those in other body cells.

Thus fruit flies have been used extensively in early breeding experiments, contributing enormously to developmental biology, where knowledge of gene homology throughout the animal kingdom has enabled scientists to identify families of genes that are important in human embryogenesis (see Chapter 9). Sequencing of the 180 million base pairs of the *Drosophila melanogaster* genome was completed in late 1999.

The Origins of Medical Genetics

In addition to the previously mentioned Pierre de Maupertuis and Joseph Adams, whose curiosity was aroused by polydactyly and albinism, there were other pioneers. John Dalton, of atomic theory fame, observed that some conditions, notably color blindness and hemophilia, show what is now referred to as sex- or X-linked inheritance—color blindness is still occasionally referred to as **daltonism**.

In 1900, Mendel's work resurfaced. His papers were quoted almost simultaneously by three European botanists—De Vries (Holland), Correns (Germany), and Von Tschermak (Austria)—and this marked the real beginning of medical genetics, providing an enormous impetus for the study of inherited disease. Credit for the first recognition of a single-gene trait is shared by William Bateson and Archibald Garrod, who in 1902 proposed that alkaptonuria was a rare recessive disorder. In this relatively benign condition, urine turns dark on standing or on exposure to alkali because of the patient's inability to metabolize homogentisic acid (p. 274). Young children show skin discoloration in the napkin (diaper) area, and affected adults may develop arthritis in large joints. Realising that this was an inherited disorder involving a chemical process, Garrod coined the term **inborn error of metabolism** in 1908, although his work was largely ignored until the mid-20th century when electrophoresis and chromatography revolutionized biochemistry. Hundreds of such disorders have now been identified, giving rise to the field of **biochemical genetics** (see Chapter 18).

During the course of the 20th century, it gradually became clear that hereditary factors were implicated in many conditions and that different genetic mechanisms were involved. Traditionally, hereditary conditions have been considered under the headings of **single-gene**, **chromosomal**, and **multifactorial**. Increasingly, it is becoming clear that the interplay of different genes (**polygenic inheritance**) is important in disease, and that a further category—**acquired somatic genetic disease**—should be included.

Single-Gene Disorders

In addition to alkaptonuria, Garrod suggested that albinism and cystinuria could also be recessive. Other examples followed, leading to an explosion in knowledge and disease delineation. By 1966, almost 1500 single-gene disorders or traits had been identified, prompting the publication by an American physician, Victor McKusick (Fig. 1.5), of a catalog of all known single-gene conditions. By 1998, when the 12th edition of the catalog was published, it contained more than 8500 entries. The growth of "McKusick's Catalog" was exponential, and it became the electronic *Online Mendelian Inheritance in Man* (OMIM) (see Appendix) in 1987. By late 2019, OMIM contained more than 25,000 entries, more than 5500 phenotypes with a known molecular basis, and more than 16,000 gene descriptions.

Chromosome Abnormalities

Improved techniques for studying chromosomes led to the demonstration in 1959 that the presence of an additional number 21 chromosome *(trisomy 21)* results in Down syndrome. Other similar discoveries followed rapidly—Klinefelter and Turner syndromes—also in 1959. Chromosome-banding techniques were developed by 1970 (p. 28), enabling reliable identification of individual chromosomes and confirmation that loss or gain of even

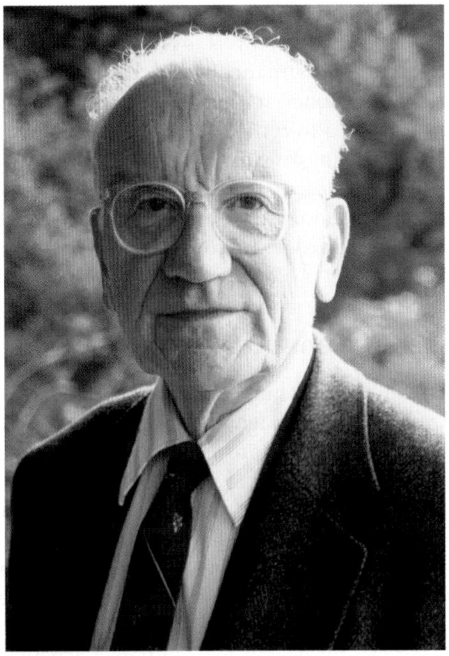

• **Fig. 1.5** Victor McKusick in 1994, whose studies and catalogues have been so important to medical genetics.

a very small segment of a chromosome can have devastating effects on human development (see Chapter 17).

Later it was shown that several rare conditions featuring learning difficulties and abnormal physical features are caused by loss of such a tiny amount of chromosome material that no abnormality can be detected using even the most high-powered light microscope. These conditions are referred to as microdeletion syndromes (see Chapter 17) and can be diagnosed using a technique known as **fluorescence *in situ* hybridization (FISH)**, which combines conventional chromosome analysis (**cytogenetics**) with newer DNA diagnostic technology (**molecular genetics**) (see Chapter 5). Today, the technique of **microarray–comparative genomic hybridization** has revolutionized clinical investigation through the detection of subtle genomic imbalances, that is, microdeletions and microduplications (p. 259), and, where available, is the first-line test of choice.

Multifactorial Disorders

Francis Galton, a cousin of Charles Darwin, had a long-standing interest in human characteristics such as stature, physique, and intelligence. Much of his research was based on the study of identical twins, in whom it was realized that differences in these parameters must be largely the result of environmental influences. Galton introduced to genetics the concept of the **regression coefficient** as a means of estimating the degree of resemblance between various relatives. This concept was later extended to incorporate Mendel's discovery of genes, to try to explain how parameters such as height and skin color could be determined by the interaction of many genes, each exerting a small additive effect. This is in contrast to single-gene characteristics, in which the action of one gene is exerted largely independently, in a non-additive fashion.

The model of **quantitative inheritance** is now widely accepted and has been adapted to explain the pattern of inheritance observed for many relatively common conditions (see Chapter 10). These include congenital malformations such as cleft lip and palate, and late-onset conditions such as hypertension, diabetes mellitus, and Alzheimer disease. In this view, genes at several loci interact to generate a susceptibility to the effects of adverse environmental trigger factors. Recent research has confirmed that many genes are involved in most of these adult-onset disorders, although progress in identifying specific susceptibility loci has been slow. It has also emerged that in some conditions, such as type 1 diabetes mellitus, different genes can exert major or minor effects in determining susceptibility (p. 136). Overall, **multifactorial** or **polygenic** conditions are now known to make a major contribution to chronic illness in adult life (see Chapter 10).

Acquired Somatic Genetic Disease

Not all genetic errors are present from conception. Many billions of cell divisions (**mitoses**) occur in the course of an average human lifetime. During each mitosis there is an opportunity both for single-gene mutations to occur, because of DNA copy errors, and for numerical chromosome abnormalities to arise as a result of errors in chromosome separation. Accumulating somatic mutations and chromosome abnormalities are now known to play a major role in causing cancer (see Chapter 14), and they probably also explain the rising incidence with age of many other serious illnesses, as well as the aging process itself. It is therefore necessary to appreciate that not all disease with a genetic basis is hereditary.

Before considering the impact of hereditary disease, it is helpful to introduce a few definitions.

Incidence

Incidence refers to the rate at which new cases occur. Thus, if the birth incidence of a particular condition equals 1 in 1000, then on average 1 in every 1000 *newborn* infants is affected.

Prevalence

This refers to the proportion of a population affected *at any one time*. The prevalence of a genetic disease is usually less than its birth incidence, either because life expectancy is reduced or because the condition shows a delayed age of onset.

Frequency

Frequency is a general term that lacks scientific specificity, although the word is often taken as being synonymous with incidence when calculating gene "frequencies" (see Chapter 7).

Congenital

Congenital means that a condition is *present at birth*. Thus cleft palate represents an example of a congenital **malformation**. Not all genetic disorders are congenital in terms of age of onset (e.g., Huntington disease), nor are all congenital abnormalities genetic in origin (e.g., fetal disruptions, as discussed in Chapter 16).

DNA Sequencing

The ability to search for mutations in human DNA to identify the causes of genetic disease clearly depended on being able to sequence DNA, which initially was very laborious. The first really practical method was developed by Walter Gilbert, with sequencing based on a cleavage at specific bases after chemical modification of DNA. But it was Frederick Sanger's (Fig. 1.6) ingenious technique (1975), based on dideoxynucleoside chain termination, that proved efficient, reliable, and popular, not least because of low radioactivity. Both men were awarded the Nobel Prize in 1980 for

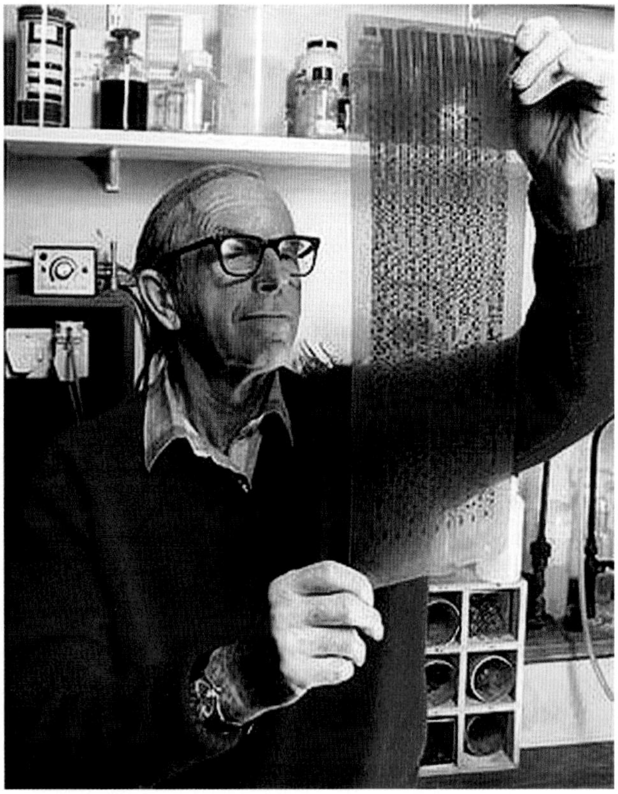

• **Fig. 1.6** Frederick Sanger, inventor of the most widely used method of DNA sequencing, and a double Nobel Laureate. (With permission from Victor A McKusick: *Mendelian Inheritance in Man*, 12th ed. 1998 Johns Hopkins University Press.)

this achievement, which was Sanger's second—he was awarded the Chemistry Prize in 1958 for determining the amino acid sequence of insulin (he remains the only British scientist to have won two Nobel Prizes). **Sanger sequencing** remains central to human molecular genetics, and the term is as prominent in the language of genetics as mendelian inheritance and McKusick's Catalog.

Sequencing techniques formed the basis for embarking on the Human Genome Project (HGP) in the early 1990s. The first genome of a free-living organism to be sequenced was that of *Haemophilus influenzae* in 1995 by Celera Genomics under Craig Venter. Venter's laboratory, together with the HGP under Francis Collins, jointly published the first draft of the human genome in 2001 (Fig. 1.7).

The Impact of Genetic Disease

During the 20th century, huge changes in the patterns of disease have occurred, largely through improvements in public health, programs of vaccination, improved housing and sanitation, and therapeutics. This has resulted in increasing recognition of the role of genetic factors at all ages. For some parameters, such as perinatal mortality, the actual numbers of cases with exclusively genetic causes have probably remained constant, but their **relative** contribution to overall figures has increased as other causes, such as infection, have declined. For other conditions, such as the chronic diseases of adult life, the overall contribution of genetics has almost certainly increased as greater life expectancy has provided more opportunity for adverse genetic and environmental interaction to manifest itself, for example in Alzheimer disease, macular degeneration, cardiomyopathy, diabetes mellitus, and obesity.

Consider the impact of genetic factors in disease at different ages from the following observations.

Spontaneous Miscarriages

A chromosome abnormality is present in 40% to 50% of all recognized first-trimester pregnancy loss. At least one in four pregnancies results in spontaneous miscarriage, so at least 10% of all recognized conceptions are chromosomally abnormal (p. 250). This value would be much higher if unrecognized pregnancies

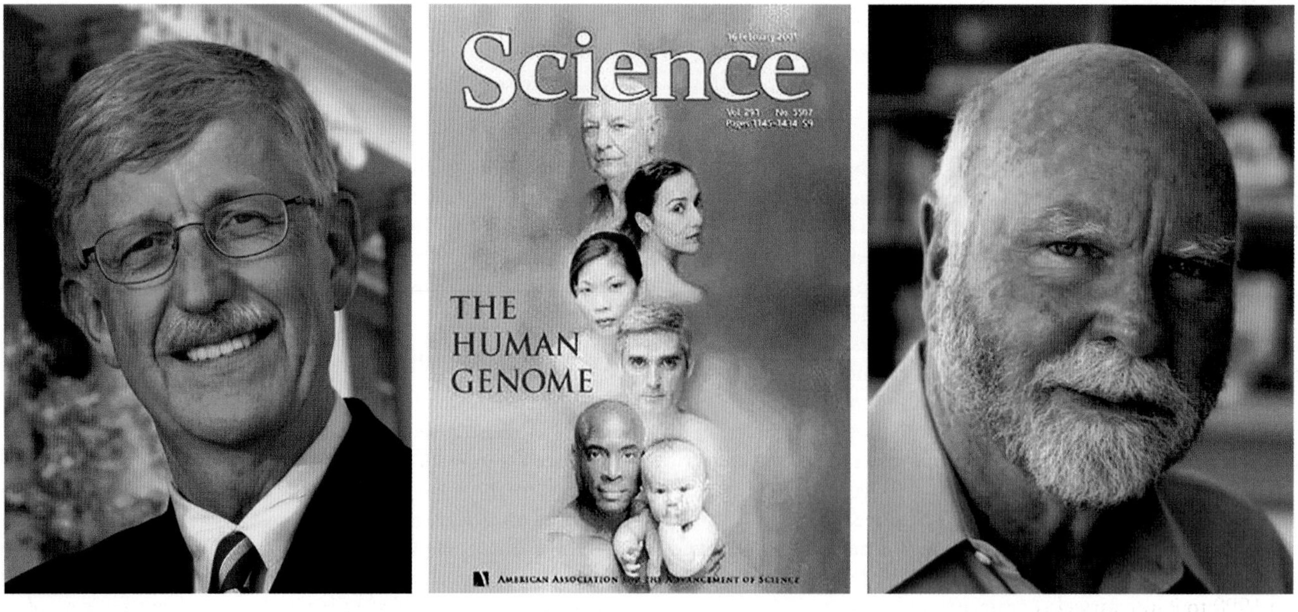

• **Fig. 1.7** Francis Collins (*left*) and Craig Venter (*right*), who published the first draft of the human genome in *Science* in 2001 (center).

could also be included, and it is likely that a significant proportion of miscarriages with normal chromosomes do in fact have catastrophic submicroscopic or DNA sequence genetic errors.

Newborn Infants

Up to 3% of neonates have at least one major congenital abnormality, of which at least 50% are caused exclusively or partially by genetic factors (see Chapter 16), with the incidences of chromosome abnormalities and single-gene disorders in neonates being roughly 1 in 200 and 1 in 100, respectively.

Childhood

By school age, roughly 12% to 14% of children show problems of developmental origin. Genetic disorders account for at least 50% of all childhood visual impairment, at least 50% of all childhood hearing loss, and at least 50% of all cases of severe intellectual disability. In developed countries, genetic disorders and congenital malformations together account for 30% of all childhood hospital admissions and 40% to 50% of all childhood deaths.

Adult Life

Approximately 1% of all malignancies are primarily caused by single-gene inheritance, and between 5% and 10% of common cancers such as those of the breast, colon, and ovary have a strong hereditary component. By the age of 25 years, 5% of the population will have a disorder in which genetic factors play an important role. Taking into account the genetic contribution to cancer and cardiovascular diseases, such as coronary artery occlusion and hypertension, it has been estimated that more than 50% of the older adult population in developed countries will have a genetically determined medical problem.

Major New Developments

The study of genetics and its role in causing human disease is now widely acknowledged as being among the most exciting and influential areas of medical research. Since 1962 when Francis Crick, James Watson, and Maurice Wilkins gained acclaim for their elucidation of the structure of DNA, the Nobel Prize for Medicine and/or Physiology has been won on 28 occasions and the Chemistry Prize on 7 occasions by scientists working in human and molecular genetics or related fields (Table 1.1). These pioneering studies have spawned a thriving molecular technology industry with applications as diverse as the development of genetically modified disease-resistant crops, the use of genetically engineered animals to produce therapeutic drugs, and the possible introduction of DNA-based vaccines for conditions such as malaria, not to mention the growing availability of affordable direct-to-consumer testing for disease susceptibility. Pharmaceutical companies are investing heavily in the DNA-based **pharmacogenomics**—drug therapy tailored to personal genetic makeup (see Chapter 15).

The Human Genome Project

In 1988, a group of visionary scientists in the United States persuaded Congress to fund a coordinated international program to sequence the entire human genome. The program would run from 1990 to 2005, and US$3 billion was initially allocated. Some 5% of the budget was earmarked to study the ethical and social implications of the new knowledge in recognition of the enormous potential to influence public health policies, screening programs, and personal choice. The project was likened to the Apollo moon mission in terms of its complexity, although in practical terms the long-term benefits are likely to be much more tangible. Following publication of the draft DNA sequence of 3 billion base pairs in 2001 (Fig. 1.7), the complete sequence was published ahead of schedule in October 2004. The Sanger Centre at Cambridge made a significant contribution to the HGP under the leadership of Sir John Sulston (Fig. 1.8), sequencing approximately one-third of the genome. Sulston was awarded the Nobel Prize with Sydney Brenner and Robert Horvitz (2002) for elucidating the entire embryonic developmental sequence of the tiny nematode *Caenorhabditis elegans*. However, he also fought with fierce integrity, and successfully, at a time when it was necessary, for genomic data to be openly available to the scientific community, and against commercial exploitation and moves toward patenting of genes and the human genome.

Having previously believed there might be approximately 100,000 coding genes that provide the blueprint for human life, it came as a surprise to many that the number is much lower, now calculated to be around 20,000. However, we have learned that many genes have the capacity to perform multiple functions, thus challenging traditional concepts of disease classification.

The successful HGP gave birth to next generation sequencing—**whole exome sequencing** (WES) and **whole genome sequencing** (WGS)—and the gold rush of disease gene discovery already mentioned. In addition, studies of population groups are taking place on an industrial scale to better understand human variation and associations with health and disease. Alongside has grown the discipline of **bioinformatics**, the science where biology, functional studies, and information technology merge with phenotyping to facilitate interpretation of sequence variation, all of which will continue for the foreseeable future.

The Prospects for Treatment

Most genetic disease is resistant to conventional treatment, so the prospect of successfully modifying the genetic code in a patient's cells is extremely attractive. This is just beginning to become a realistic prospect since the breakthrough known as "gene editing" based on CRISPR (clustered regularly interspaced short palindromic repeats) and Cas9 (CRISPR-associated protein 9) technology (p. 47), in addition to a range of other strategies. Together with increasing optimism for novel (and sometimes old) drug therapies, stem cell treatment (p. 222), cancer therapies that boost the immune system and gene therapy itself (p. 218), there is more hope than ever before for effective management of certain genetic diseases (see Chapter 15).

The Societal Impact of Advances in Genetics

Each new advance in genetic technology has generated fresh ethical concerns about how the science will be applied and used in medicine, at the center of which is the recognition that a person's genetic makeup is fundamental to both their identity and disease susceptibility. These issues are explored in detail in Chapter 22. The most contentious field is prenatal genetics and reproductive choice, although national legal frameworks and cultural practices vary widely worldwide. The controversy surrounding the early ability to perform prenatal karyotyping for Down syndrome in the mid-1960s is mirrored today in the technology that will make it

TABLE 1.1 Genetic discoveries that have led to the award of the Nobel Prize for Medicine or Physiology and/or Chemistry, 1962–2012

Year	Prize Winners	Discovery	Year	Prize Winners	Discovery
1962	Francis Crick James Watson Maurice Wilkins	The molecular structure of DNA	1999	Günter Blobel	Protein transport signaling
1965	François Jacob Jacques Monod André Lwoff	Genetic regulation	2000	Arvid Carlsson Paul Greengard Eric Kandel	Signal transduction in the nervous system
1966	Peyton Rous	Oncogenic viruses	2001	Leland Hartwell Timothy Hunt Paul Nurse	Regulators of the cell cycle
1968	Robert Holley Gobind Khorana Marshall Nireberg	Deciphering of the genetic code	2002	Sydney Brenner Robert Horvitz John Sulston	Genetic regulation in development and programmed cell death (apoptosis)
1972	Christian B. Anfisen Stanford Moore William H. Stein	Ribonuclease	2006	Andrew Fire Craig Mello	RNA interference (Medicine)
1975	David Baltimore Renato Dulbecco Howard Temin	Interaction between tumour viruses and nuclear DNA		Roger D. Kornberg	Eukaryotic transcription (Chemistry)
1978	Werner Arber Daniel Nathans Hamilton Smith	Restriction endonucleases	2007	Mario Capecchi Martin Evans Oliver Smithies	Gene modification by the use of embryonic stem cells
1980	Baruj Benacerraf Jean Dausset George Snell	Genetic control of immunologic responses (Medicine)	2009	Elizabeth Blackburn Carol Greider Jack Szostak	The role of telomerase in protecting chromosome telomeres (Medicine)
	Paul Berg Walter Gilbert Frederick Sanger	Biochemistry of nucleic acids (Chemistry)		Venkatraman Ramakrishnan Thomas A. Steitz Ada E. Yonath	Structure and function of the ribosome (Chemistry)
1983	Barbara McClintock	Mobile genes (transposons)	2010	Robert G. Edwards	*In vitro* fertilization
1985	Michael Brown Joseph Goldstein	Cell receptors in familial hypercholesterolemia	2012	John B. Gurdon Shinya Yamanaka	Mature cells reprogrammed to become pluripotent cells (Medicine)
1987	Susumu Tonegawa	Genetic aspects of antibodies		Robert J. Lefkowitz Brian K. Kobilka	G-protein coupled receptors (Chemistry)
1989	Michael Bishop Harold Varmus	Study of oncogenes (Medicine)	2013	James E. Rothman Randy W. Schekman Thomas C. Südhof	Machinery regulating vesicle traffic, a major transport system in our cells
	Sidney Altman Thomas R. Cech	Catalytic properties of RNA (Chemistry)	2015	Tomas Lindahl Paul Modrich Aziz Sancar	Mechanistic studies of DNA repair (Chemistry)
1993	Richard Roberts Phillip Sharp	"Split genes" (Medicine)	2016	Yoshinori Ohsumi	Mechanisms for autophagy
	Kary B. Mullis Michael Smith	DNA-based chemistry, including the invention of PCR (Chemistry)	2017	Jeffrey C. Hall Michael Rosbash Michael W. Young	Molecular mechanisms controlling the circadian rhythm
1995	Edward Lewis Christiane Nüsslein-Volhard Eric Wieschaus	Homeotic and other developmental genes	2018	James P. Allison Tasuku Honjo	Cancer therapy by inhibition of negative immune regulation
1997	Stanley Prusiner	Prions	2020	Emmanuelle Charpentier Jennifer A. Doudna	Discovery of the technique CRISPR/Cas9 – 'genetic scissors'

possible to perform detailed genetic screening of the unborn baby on cell-free fetal DNA in the maternal circulation, or on embryos created through *in vitro* fertilization. Then there is the possibility of all newborns having their genomes sequenced and screened for disease-causing variants, which is technically feasible and has been seriously mooted at governmental level. Great debate has taken place, and will continue, concerning the disclosure of unexpected but significant "incidental findings" from WES or WGS carried out for specific clinical purposes, and the process of consent that guides decisions, together with the potential availability of

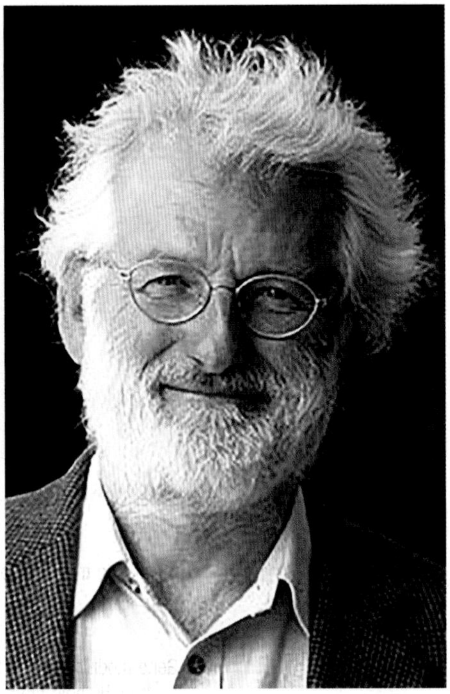

• **Fig. 1.8** Sir John Sulston, who led the British contribution toward sequencing the human genome at the Sanger Centre, Cambridge.

individual DNA sequence data for research and use by the private sector. Many of the questions raised have neither easy nor straightforward answers, which means that there will be a great need for appropriately trained clinicians and counselors to meet the public demands for the foreseeable future.

ELEMENTS

1. Mendel's work on peas laid the foundation for our understanding of single-gene inheritance, and both dominant and recessive patterns.
2. From the rediscovery of Mendel's genetic research to the full sequencing of the human genome, almost exactly 100 years elapsed.
3. The number of human chromosomes was not settled until 1956, 3 years after the structure of DNA was proposed.
4. The success of the Human Genome Project in the early 2000s, and the development of new sequencing techniques, opened the door to a dramatic new phase of disease gene discovery.
5. Advances in genetic science have generated novel issues in medical ethics, and the principle of *primum non nocere* (first do no harm) applies to this discipline as to any other.
6. Molecular genetics and cell biology are at the forefront of medical research, combined with the discipline of bioinformatics, and hold the promise of novel forms of treatment for genetic diseases.

Databases

Online Mendelian Inheritance in Man:
http://www.ncbi.nlm.nih.gov/omim

For Literature:
http://www.ncbi.nlm.nih.gov/PubMed/
http://scholar.google.com/
https://archiveshub.jisc.ac.uk/data/gb1239-609
Genome:
http://www.ncbi.nlm.nih.gov/omim/GenBank
http://www.hgmd.cf.ac.uk (human, Cardiff)
http://www.ensembl.org (human, comparative, European, Cambridge)
http://genome.ucsc.edu (American browser)
http://www.humanvariomeproject.org/

Further Reading

Baird PA, Anderson TW, Newcombe HB, Lowry RB. Genetic disorders in children and young adults: a population study. *Am J Hum Genet.* 1988;42:677–693.

A comprehensive study of the incidence of genetic disease in a large Western urban population.

The first report of the complete sequencing of a human chromosome.

Emery AEH. Portraits in medical genetics—Joseph Adams 1756–1818. *J Med Genet.* 1989;26:116–118.

An account of the life of a London doctor who made remarkable observations about hereditary disease in his patients.

Emery AEH, Emery MLH. *The History of a Genetic Disease: Duchenne Muscular Dystrophy or Meryon's Disease.* 2nd ed. Oxford, UK: Oxford University Press; 2011.

Describes the life and work of Edward Meryon, the first physician to describe Duchenne muscular dystrophy in detail.

Garrod AE. The incidence of alkaptonuria: a study in chemical individuality. *Lancet.* 1902;2:1616–1620.

A landmark paper in which Garrod proposed that alkaptonuria could show mendelian inheritance and also noted that "the mating of first cousins gives exactly the conditions most likely to enable a rare, and usually recessive, character to show itself."

Harper PS. *A Short History of Medical Genetics: 57.* Oxford Monographs on Medical Genetics; 2008.

A well-researched modern account of the development of medical genetics from a century or so before Mendel.

Orel V. *Gregor Mendel: The First Geneticist.* Oxford: Oxford University Press; 1995.

A detailed biography of the life and work of the Moravian monk who was described by his abbot as being "very diligent in the study of the sciences but much less fitted for work as a parish priest."

Sanger F, Coulson AR. A rapid method for determining sequences in DNA by primed synthesis with DNA polymerase. *J Mol Biol.* 1975;94:441–448.

Watson JD, Crick FH. Molecular structure of nucleic acids: a structure for deoxyribose nucleic acid. *Nature.* 1953;171:737–738.

The short, elegant paper proposing the structure of DNA.

Watson J. *The Double Helix.* New York: Atheneum; 1968.

The story of the discovery of the structure of DNA, through the eyes of Watson himself.

2

The Cellular and Molecular Basis of Inheritance

There is nothing, Sir, too little for so little a creature as man.

It is by studying little things that we attain the great art of having as little misery and as much happiness as possible.

Samuel Johnson

The hereditary material is present in the nucleus of the cell, whereas protein synthesis takes place in the cytoplasm. What is the chain of events that leads from the gene to the final product?

This chapter covers basic cellular biology outlining the structure of DNA, the process of DNA replication, the types of DNA sequences, gene structure, the genetic code, the processes of transcription and translation, the various types of mutations, mutagenic agents, and DNA repair.

The Cell

Within each cell of the body, visible with the light microscope, is the **cytoplasm** and a darkly staining body, the **nucleus**, the latter containing the hereditary material in the form of **chromosomes** (Fig. 2.1). The phospholipid bilayer of the plasma membrane protects the interior of the cell but remains selectively permeable and has integral proteins involved in recognition and signaling between cells. The nucleus has a darkly staining area, the **nucleolus**. The nucleus is surrounded by a membrane, the **nuclear envelope**, which separates it from the cytoplasm but still allows communication through **nuclear pores**.

The cytoplasm contains the **cytosol**, which is semifluid in consistency, containing both soluble elements and cytoskeletal structural elements. In addition, in the cytoplasm there is a complex arrangement of very fine, highly convoluted, interconnecting channels, the endoplasmic reticulum. The **endoplasmic reticulum**, in association with the **ribosomes**, is involved in the biosynthesis of proteins and lipids. Also situated within the cytoplasm are other even more minute cellular organelles that can be visualized only with an electron microscope. These include the **Golgi apparatus**, which is responsible for the secretion of cellular products, the **mitochondria**, which are involved in energy production through the oxidative phosphorylation metabolic **pathways** and the **peroxisomes** (p. 284) and **lysosomes**, both of which are involved in the degradation and disposal of cellular waste material and toxic molecules.

DNA: The Hereditary Material

Composition

Nucleic acid is composed of a long polymer of individual molecules called **nucleotides**. Each nucleotide is composed of a nitrogenous base, a sugar molecule, and a phosphate molecule. The nitrogenous bases fall into two types, **purines** and **pyrimidines**. The purines include adenine (A) and guanine (G); the pyrimidines include cytosine (C), thymine (T), and uracil (U).

There are two different types of nucleic acid, **ribonucleic acid (RNA)**, which contains the five-carbon sugar ribose, and **deoxyribonucleic acid (DNA)**, in which the hydroxyl group at the 2 position of the ribose sugar is replaced by a hydrogen (i.e., an oxygen molecule is lost, hence "deoxy"). DNA and RNA both contain the purine bases A and G and the pyrimidine C, but T occurs only in DNA, and U is found only in RNA.

RNA is present in the cytoplasm and in particularly high concentrations in the nucleolus of the nucleus. DNA, on the other hand, is found mainly in the chromosomes.

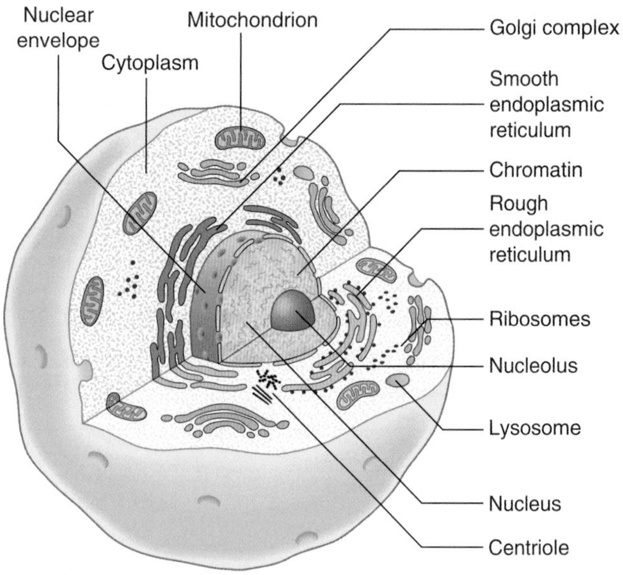

• **Fig. 2.1** Diagrammatic representation of an animal cell.

Structure

For genes to be composed of DNA, it is necessary for the latter to have a structure sufficiently versatile to account for the great variety of different genes and yet, at the same time, be able to reproduce itself in such a manner that an identical replica is formed at each cell division. In 1953, Watson and Crick, based on x-ray diffraction studies by themselves and others, proposed a structure for the DNA molecule that fulfilled all the essential requirements. They suggested that the DNA molecule is composed of two chains of nucleotides arranged in a double helix. The backbone of each chain is formed by phosphodiester bonds between the 3′ and 5′ carbons of adjacent sugars, the two chains being held together by hydrogen bonds between the nitrogenous bases, which point in toward the center of the helix. Each DNA chain has a polarity determined by the orientation of the sugar–phosphate backbone. The asymmetric ends of the DNA chains are called the **5′** and **3′ ends**, with the 5′ end having a terminal phosphate group and the 3′ end a terminal hydroxyl group. In the DNA duplex, the 5′ end of one strand is opposite the 3′ end of the other; that is, they have opposite orientations and are said to be **antiparallel**.

The arrangement of the bases in the DNA molecule is not random. A purine in one chain always pairs with a pyrimidine in the other chain, with specific pairing of the base pairs: G in one chain always pairs with C in the other chain, and A always pairs with T, so that this base pairing forms complementary strands (Fig. 2.2). For their work, Watson and Crick, along with Maurice Wilkins, were awarded the Nobel Prize for Medicine or Physiology in 1962 (p. 8).

Replication

The process of **DNA replication** provides an answer to the question of how genetic information is transmitted from one generation to the next. During nuclear division, the two strands of the DNA double helix separate through the action of enzyme DNA helicase, each DNA strand directing the synthesis of a complementary DNA strand through specific base pairing, resulting in two daughter DNA duplexes that are identical to the original parent molecule. In this way, when cells divide, the genetic information is conserved and transmitted unchanged to each daughter cell. The process of DNA replication is termed **semiconservative**, because only one strand of each resultant daughter molecule is newly synthesized.

DNA replication, through the action of the enzyme DNA polymerase, takes place at multiple points known as **origins of replication**, forming bifurcated Y-shaped structures known as **replication forks**. The synthesis of both complementary antiparallel DNA strands occurs in the 5′ to 3′ direction. One strand, known as the **leading strand**, is synthesized as a continuous process. The other strand, known as the **lagging strand**, is synthesized in pieces called Okazaki fragments, which are then joined together as a continuous strand by the enzyme DNA ligase (Fig. 2.3A).

DNA replication progresses in both directions from these points of origin, forming bubble-shaped structures, or **replication bubbles** (Fig. 2.3B). Neighboring replication origins are approximately 50 to 300 kilobases (kb) apart and occur in clusters or **replication units** of 20 to 80 origins of replication. DNA replication in individual replication units takes place at different times in the

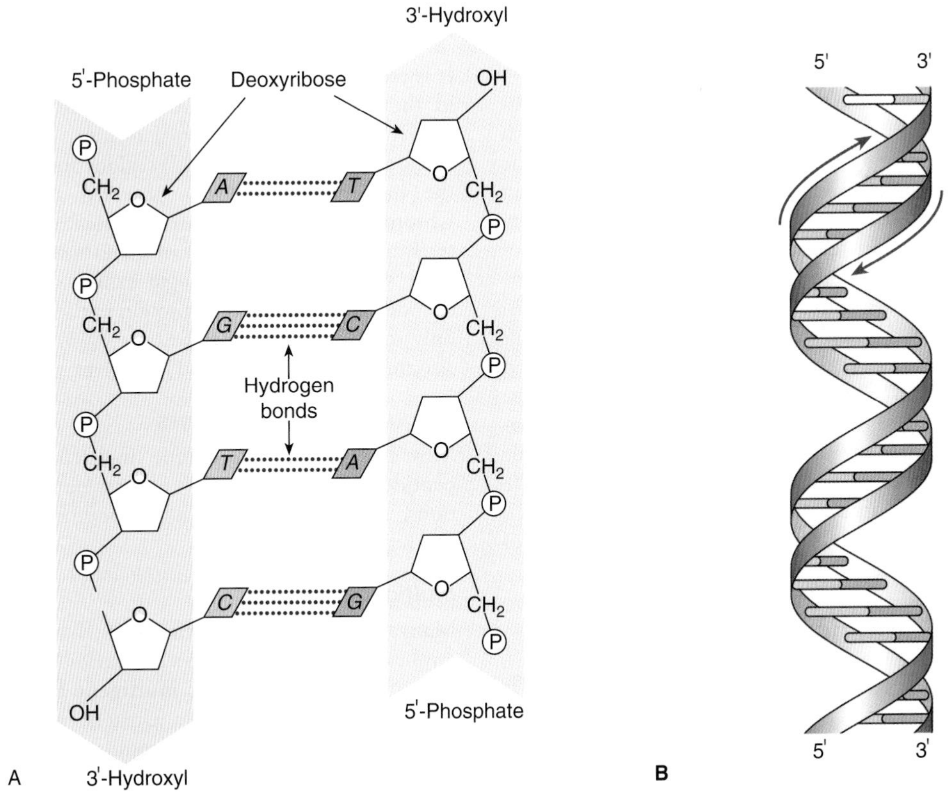

• **Fig. 2.2** DNA double helix. (A) Sugar-phosphate backbone and nucleotide pairing of the DNA double helix (*A*, adenine; *C*, cytosine; *G*, guanine; *P*, phosphate; *T*, thymine). (B) Representation of the DNA double helix.

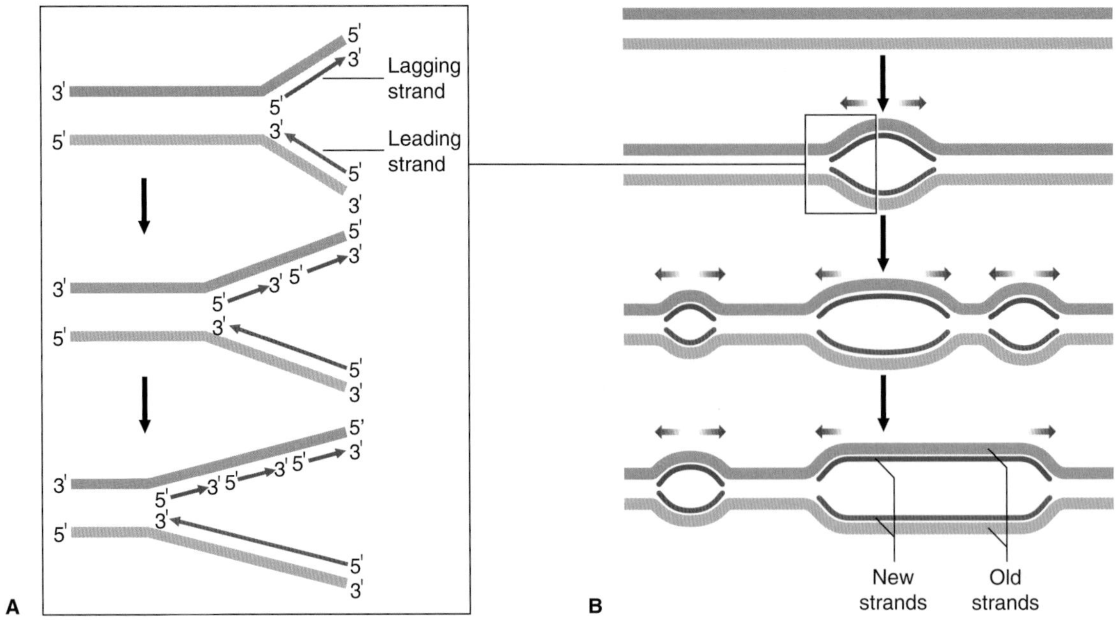

• **Fig. 2.3** DNA replication. (A) Detailed diagram of DNA replication at the site of origin in the replication fork showing asymmetric strand synthesis with the continuous synthesis of the leading strand and the discontinuous synthesis of the lagging strand with ligation of the Okazaki fragments. (B) Multiple points of origin and semiconservative mode of DNA replication.

S phase of the cell cycle (p. 32), adjacent replication units fusing until all the DNA is copied, forming two complete identical daughter molecules.

Chromosome Structure

The idea that each chromosome is composed of a single DNA double helix is an oversimplification. A chromosome is very much wider than the diameter of a DNA double helix. In addition, the amount of DNA in the nucleus of each cell in humans means that the total length of DNA contained in the chromosomes, if fully extended, would be several meters long! In fact, the total length of the human chromosome complement is less than half a millimeter.

The packaging of DNA into chromosomes involves several orders of DNA coiling and folding. In addition to the primary coiling of the DNA double helix, there is secondary coiling around spherical **histone** "beads," forming what are called **nucleosomes**. There is a tertiary coiling of the nucleosomes to form the **chromatin fibers** that form long loops on a scaffold of non-histone acidic proteins, which are further wound in a tight coil to make up the chromosome as visualized under the light microscope (Fig.2.4), the whole structure making up the so-called **solenoid model** of chromosome structure.

Types of DNA Sequence

DNA, if denatured, will reassociate as a duplex at a rate that is dependent on the proportion of unique and repeat sequences present, the latter occurring more rapidly. Analysis of the results of the kinetics of the reassociation of human DNA have shown that approximately 60% to 70% of the human genome consists of single- or low-copy number DNA sequences. The remainder of the genome, 30% to 40%, consists of either moderately or highly **repetitive DNA** sequences that are not transcribed. This latter portion consists of mainly satellite DNA and interspersed DNA sequences (Box 2.1).

Nuclear Genes

It is estimated that there are around 21,000 protein-coding genes in the nuclear genome. The distribution of these genes varies greatly between chromosomal regions. For example, heterochromatic and centromeric (p. 27) regions are mostly non-coding, with the highest gene density observed in subtelomeric regions. Chromosomes 19 and 22 are gene rich, whereas 4 and 18 are relatively gene poor. The size of genes also shows great variability: from small genes with single exons to the *TTN* gene, which encodes the largest known protein in the human body and has not only the largest number of exons (363) in any known gene, but also the single largest exon [17,106 base pairs (bp)].

Unique Single-Copy Genes

Most human genes are unique single-copy genes coding for polypeptides that are involved in or carry out a variety of cellular functions. These include enzymes, hormones, receptors and structural and regulatory proteins.

Multigene Families

Many genes have similar functions, having arisen through gene duplication events with subsequent evolutionary divergence, making up what are known as **multigene families**. Some are found physically close together in clusters, for example, the α- and β-globin gene clusters on chromosomes 16 and 11 (Fig. 2.5), whereas others are widely dispersed throughout the genome, occurring on different chromosomes, such as the *HOX* homeobox gene family (p. 115).

Multigene families can be split into two types, **classic gene families** that show a high degree of sequence homology and **gene**

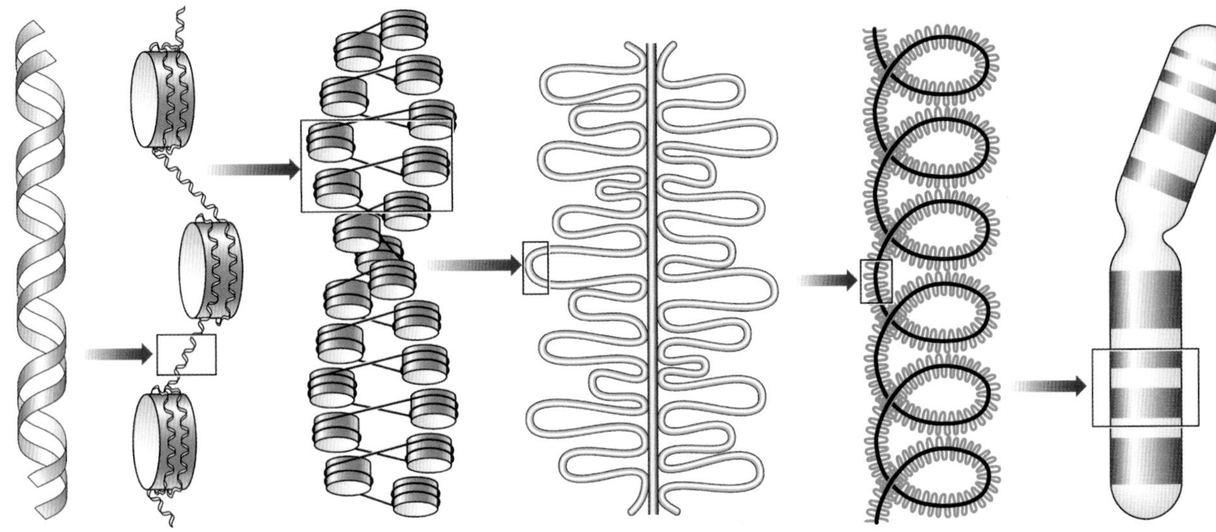

• **Fig. 2.4** Simplified diagram of proposed solenoid model of DNA coiling that leads to the visible structure of the chromosome.

• BOX 2.1 Types of DNA Sequences

Nuclear (~3 × 10⁹ base pairs)

Genes (~20,000)
Unique, single-copy
Multigene families
Classic gene families
Gene superfamilies

Extragenic DNA (unique/low copy number or moderate/highly repetitive)

Tandem repeat
Satellite
Minisatellite
Telomeric
Hypervariable
Microsatellite
Interspersed
Short interspersed nuclear elements
Long interspersed nuclear elements

Mitochondrial (16.6 kilobases, 37 genes)

Two ribosomal RNA genes
22 transfer RNA genes

superfamilies that have limited sequence homology but are functionally related, having similar structural domains.

Classic Gene Families

Examples of classic gene families include the numerous copies of genes coding for the various ribosomal RNAs, which are clustered as tandem arrays at the nucleolar organizing regions on the short arms of the five acrocentric chromosomes (p. 27), and the different transfer RNA [tRNA]; p. 16) gene families, which are dispersed in numerous clusters throughout the human genome.

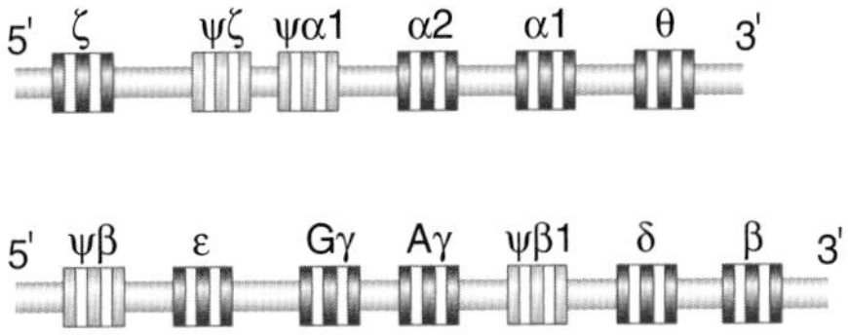

• **Fig. 2.5** Representation of the α- and β-globin regions on chromosomes 16 and 11.

Gene Superfamilies

Examples of gene superfamilies include the human leukocyte antigen (HLA)–encoding genes on chromosome 6 (p. 176) and the T-cell receptor genes, which have structural homology with the immunoglobulin (Ig) genes (p. 176). It is thought that these are almost certainly derived from duplication of a precursor gene, with subsequent evolutionary divergence forming the Ig superfamily.

Gene Structure

The original concept of a gene as a continuous sequence of DNA coding for a protein was turned on its head in the early 1980s by detailed analysis of the structure of the human β-globin gene. It was revealed that the gene was much longer than necessary to code for the β-globin protein, containing non-coding intervening sequences or introns that separate the coding sequences or exons (Fig. 2.6). Most human genes contain introns, but the number and size of both introns and exons is extremely variable. Individual introns can be far larger than the coding sequences, and some have been found to contain coding sequences for other genes (i.e., genes occurring within genes). Genes in humans do not usually overlap, being separated from each other by an average of 30 kb, although there are exceptions, for example some of the genes in the HLA complex (p. 176).

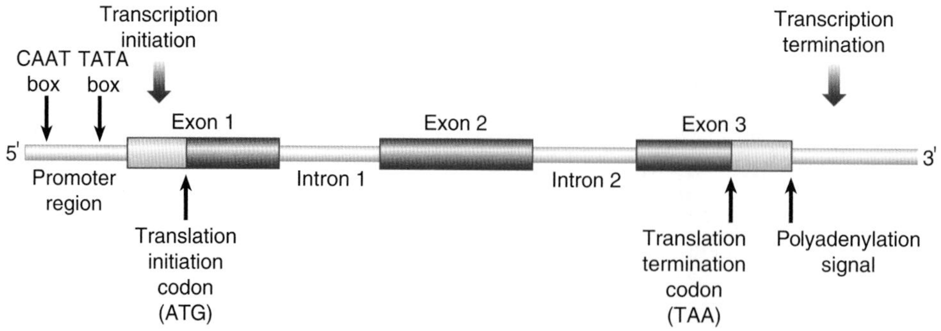

• **Fig. 2.6** Representation of a typical human structural gene.

Pseudogenes

Particularly fascinating is the occurrence of genes that closely resemble known structural genes but which, in general, are not functionally expressed: so-called **pseudogenes**. These are thought to have arisen in two main ways: either by genes undergoing duplication events that were rendered silent through the acquisition of mutations in coding or regulatory elements, or as the result of the insertion of complementary DNA sequences, produced by the action of the enzyme **reverse transcriptase** on a naturally occurring messenger RNA transcript, that lack the promoter sequences necessary for expression.

Extragenic DNA

The estimated 2000 unique single-copy genes that encode proteins represent less than 2% of the human genome. The remainder of the human genome is made up of repetitive DNA sequences that are predominantly transcriptionally inactive. This has been described as **junk** DNA, but some regions show evolutionary conservation and play a critical role in the regulation of temporal and spatial gene expression.

Tandemly Repeated DNA Sequences

Tandemly repeated DNA sequences consist of blocks of tandem repeats of non-coding DNA that can be either highly dispersed or restricted in their location in the genome. Tandemly repeated DNA sequences can be divided into three subgroups: satellite, minisatellite and microsatellite DNA.

Satellite DNA

Satellite DNA accounts for approximately 10% to 15% of the repetitive DNA sequences of the human genome and consists of a very large series of simple or moderately complex, short, tandemly repeated DNA sequences that are transcriptionally inactive and are clustered around the centromeres of certain chromosomes. This class of DNA sequences can be separated on density-gradient centrifugation as a shoulder, or "satellite," to the main peak of genomic DNA, and has therefore been referred to as satellite DNA.

Minisatellite DNA

Minisatellite DNA consists of two families of tandemly repeated short DNA sequences: telomeric and hypervariable minisatellite DNA sequences that are transcriptionally inactive.

Telomeric DNA. The terminal portion of the telomeres of the chromosomes (p. 26) contains 10 to 15 kb of tandem repeats of a 6-bp DNA sequence known as telomeric DNA. The telomeric repeat sequences are necessary for chromosomal integrity in replication and are added to the chromosome by an enzyme known as telomerase (p. 27).

Hypervariable minisatellite DNA. Hypervariable minisatellite DNA is made up of highly polymorphic DNA sequences consisting of short tandem repeats of a common core sequence. The highly variable number of repeat units in different hypervariable minisatellites forms the basis of the DNA fingerprinting technique developed by Professor Sir Alec Jeffreys in 1984 (pp. 53, 343).

Microsatellite DNA

Microsatellite DNA consists of tandem single, di-, tri- and tetranucleotide repeat base-pair sequences located throughout the genome. Microsatellite repeats rarely occur within coding sequences, but trinucleotide repeats in or near genes are associated with certain inherited disorders (Table 2.5). Historically, DNA microsatellites were used for disease gene discovery or for gene tracking in families with a genetic disorder but no identified mutation. They are still used for forensic and paternity tests (pp. 53, 343).

This variation in repeat number is thought to arise by incorrect pairing of the tandem repeats of the two complementary DNA strands during DNA replication, or what is known as **slipped strand mispairing**. Duplications or deletions of longer sequences of tandemly repeated DNA are thought to arise through unequal crossover of non-allelic DNA sequences on chromatids of homologous chromosomes or sister chromatids (p. 27).

Highly Repeated Interspersed Repetitive DNA Sequences

Approximately one-third of the human genome is made up of two main classes of short and long repetitive DNA sequences that are interspersed throughout the genome.

Short Interspersed Nuclear Elements. Approximately 5% of the human genome consists of some 750,000 copies of **short interspersed nuclear elements** (**SINEs**). The most common are DNA sequences of approximately 300 bp that have sequence similarity to a signal recognition particle involved in protein synthesis. They are called **Alu repeats** because they contain an *AluI* restriction enzyme recognition site.

Long Interspersed Nuclear Elements. Approximately 5% of the DNA of the human genome is made up of **long interspersed nuclear elements** (**LINEs**). The most commonly occurring LINE, known as LINE-1 or an L1 element, consists of more than 100,000 copies of a DNA sequence of up to 6000 bp that encodes a reverse transcriptase.

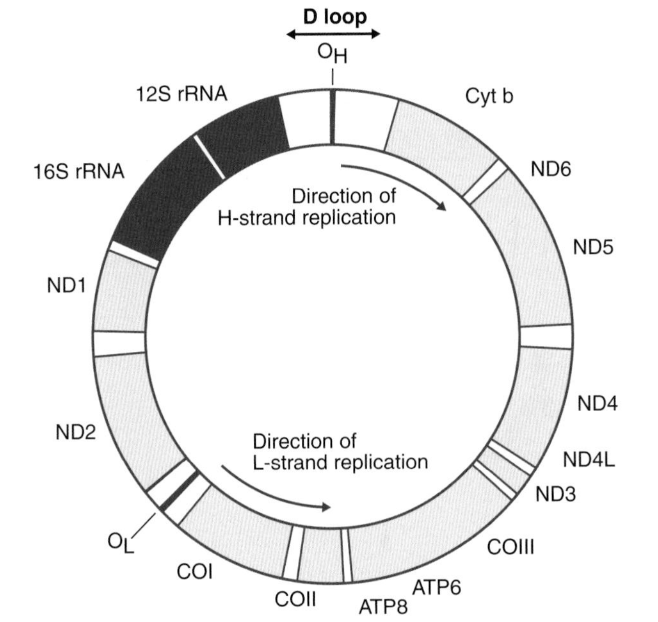

• **Fig. 2.7** The human mitochondrial genome. *H* is the heavy strand and *L* the light strand.

The function of these interspersed repeat sequences is not clear. Members of the Alu repeat family are flanked by short direct repeat sequences, and therefore resemble unstable DNA sequences called transposable elements or **transposons**. Transposons, originally identified in maize by Barbara McClintock (p. 8), move spontaneously throughout the genome from one chromosome location to another and appear to be ubiquitous in the plant and animal kingdoms. It has been postulated that Alu repeats could promote unequal recombination, which could lead to pathogenic mutations (p. 19) or provide selective advantage in evolution by gene duplication. Both Alu and LINE-1 repeat element insertions are reported causes of mutation in inherited human disease.

Mitochondrial DNA

In addition to nuclear DNA, the several thousand mitochondria of each cell possess their own 16.6-kb circular double-stranded DNA, **mitochondrial DNA (mtDNA)** (Fig. 2.7). The mitochondrial genome is very compact, containing little repetitive DNA, and codes for 37 genes, which include two types of ribosomal RNA, 22 transfer RNAs (p. 16) and 13 protein subunits for enzymes, such as cytochrome *b* and cytochrome oxidase, which are involved in the energy-producing oxidative phosphorylation pathways. The genetic code of mtDNA differs slightly from that of nuclear DNA.

The mitochondria of the fertilized zygote are inherited almost exclusively from the oocyte, leading to the maternal pattern of inheritance that characterizes many mitochondrial disorders (p. 286).

Transcription

The process whereby genetic information is transmitted from DNA to RNA is called **transcription**. The information stored in the genetic code is transmitted from the DNA of a gene to **messenger RNA (mRNA)**. Every base in the mRNA molecule is complementary to a corresponding base in the DNA of the gene, but with U replacing T in mRNA. mRNA is single-stranded, being synthesized by the enzyme RNA polymerase II, which adds the appropriate complementary ribonucleotide to the 3′ end of the RNA chain.

In any particular gene, only one DNA strand of the double helix acts as the so-called **template strand**. The transcribed mRNA molecule is a copy of the complementary strand, or what is called the **sense strand** of the DNA double helix. The template strand is sometimes called the **antisense strand**. The particular strand of the DNA double helix used for RNA synthesis appears to differ throughout different regions of the genome.

RNA Processing

Before the primary mRNA molecule leaves the nucleus it undergoes a number of modifications, or what is known as RNA processing. This involves splicing, capping, and polyadenylation.

mRNA Splicing

During and after transcription, the non-coding introns in the precursor mRNA are excised, and the non-contiguous coding exons are spliced together to form a shorter mature mRNA before its transportation to the ribosomes in the cytoplasm for translation. The process is known as **mRNA splicing** (Fig. 2.8). The boundary between the introns and exons consists of a 5′ donor GT dinucleotide and a 3′ acceptor AG dinucleotide. These, along with surrounding short splicing consensus sequences, another intronic sequence known as the branch site, small nuclear RNA molecules and associated proteins, are necessary for the splicing process.

5′ Capping

The **5′ cap** is thought to facilitate transport of the mRNA to the cytoplasm and attachment to the ribosomes, as well as to protect the RNA transcript from degradation by endogenous cellular exonucleases. After 20 to 30 nucleotides have been transcribed, the nascent mRNA is modified by the addition of a G nucleotide to the 5′ end of the molecule by an unusual 5′ to 5′ triphosphate linkage. A methyltransferase enzyme then methylates the N7 position of the G, giving the final 5′ cap.

Polyadenylation

Transcription continues until specific nucleotide sequences are transcribed that cause the mRNA to be cleaved and RNA polymerase II to be released from the DNA template. Approximately 200 **adenylate residues**—the so-called **poly(A) tail**—are added to the mRNA, which facilitates nuclear export and translation.

Translation

Translation is the transmission of the genetic information from mRNA to protein. Newly processed mRNA is transported from the nucleus to the cytoplasm, where it becomes associated with the **ribosomes**, which are the site of protein synthesis. Ribosomes are made up of two different sized subunits, which consist of four different types of **ribosomal RNA (rRNA)** molecules and a large number of ribosome-specific proteins. Groups of ribosomes associated with the same molecule of mRNA are referred to as **polyribosomes** or **polysomes**. In the ribosomes, the mRNA forms the template for producing the specific sequence of amino acids of a particular **polypeptide**.

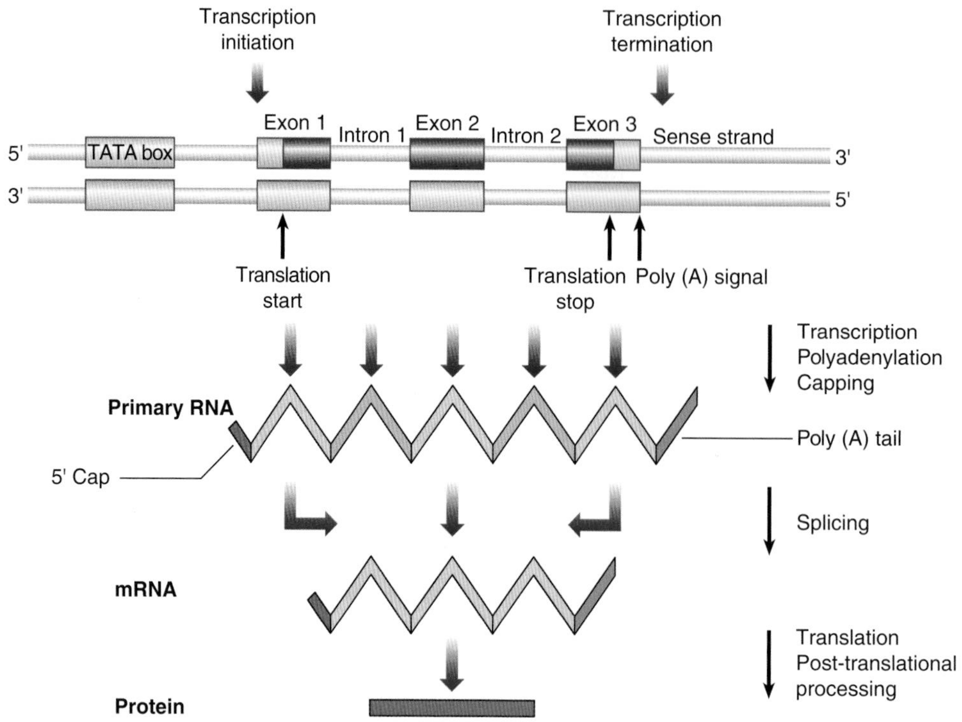

• **Fig. 2.8** Transcription, post-transcriptional processing, translation, and post-translational processing.

Transfer RNA

In the cytoplasm there is another form of RNA called **tRNA**. The incorporation of amino acids into a **polypeptide chain** requires the amino acids to be covalently bound by reacting with adenosine triphosphate (ATP) to the specific tRNA molecule by the activity of the enzyme aminoacyl tRNA synthetase. The ribosome, with its associated rRNAs, moves along the mRNA, the amino acids linking up by the formation of peptide bonds through the action of the enzyme peptidyl transferase to form a polypeptide chain (Fig. 2.9).

Post-translational Modification

Many proteins, before they attain their normal structure or functional activity, undergo **post-translational modification**, which can include chemical modification of amino-acid side chains (e.g., hydroxylation, methylation), the addition of carbohydrate or lipid moieties (e.g., glycosylation) or proteolytic cleavage of polypeptides (e.g., the conversion of proinsulin to insulin).

Thus post-translational modification, along with certain short amino-acid sequences known as **localization sequences** in the newly synthesized proteins, results in transport to specific cellular locations (e.g., the nucleus), or secretion from the cell.

The Genetic Code

Twenty different amino acids are found in proteins; because DNA is composed of four different nitrogenous bases, obviously a single base cannot specify one amino acid. If two bases were to specify one amino acid, there would be only 4^2 or 16 possible combinations. If, however, three bases specified one amino acid then the possible number of combinations of the four bases would be 4^3 or 64. This is more than enough to account for all the 20 known amino acids, and is known as the genetic code.

Triplet Codons

The triplet of nucleotide bases in the mRNA that codes for a particular amino acid is called a **codon**. Each triplet codon in sequence codes for a specific amino acid in sequence, and so the genetic code is non-overlapping. The order of the triplet codons in a gene is known as the translational **reading frame**. However, some amino acids are coded for by more than one triplet, so the code is said to be **degenerate** (Table 2.1). Each tRNA species for a particular amino acid has a specific trinucleotide sequence called the **anticodon**, which is complementary to the codon of the mRNA. Although there are 64 codons, there are only 30 cytoplasmic tRNAs, the anticodons of a number of the tRNAs recognizing codons that differ at the position of the third base, with G being able to pair with U as well as C. Termination of translation of the mRNA is signaled by the presence of one of the three **stop** or **termination codons**.

The genetic code of mtDNA differs from that of the nuclear genome. Of the 22 mitochondrial tRNAs 8 are able to recognize codons with any base in the third position, and 14 can recognize pairs of codons, with either a purine or pyrimidine at the third position. There are four stop codons in the mitochondrial genetic code (Table 2.1).

Regulation of Gene Expression

Many cellular processes, and therefore the genes that are expressed, are common to all cells, for example ribosomal, chromosomal, and cytoskeleton proteins, constituting what are called the **housekeeping genes**. Some cells express large quantities of a specific protein in certain tissues or at specific times in development, such as

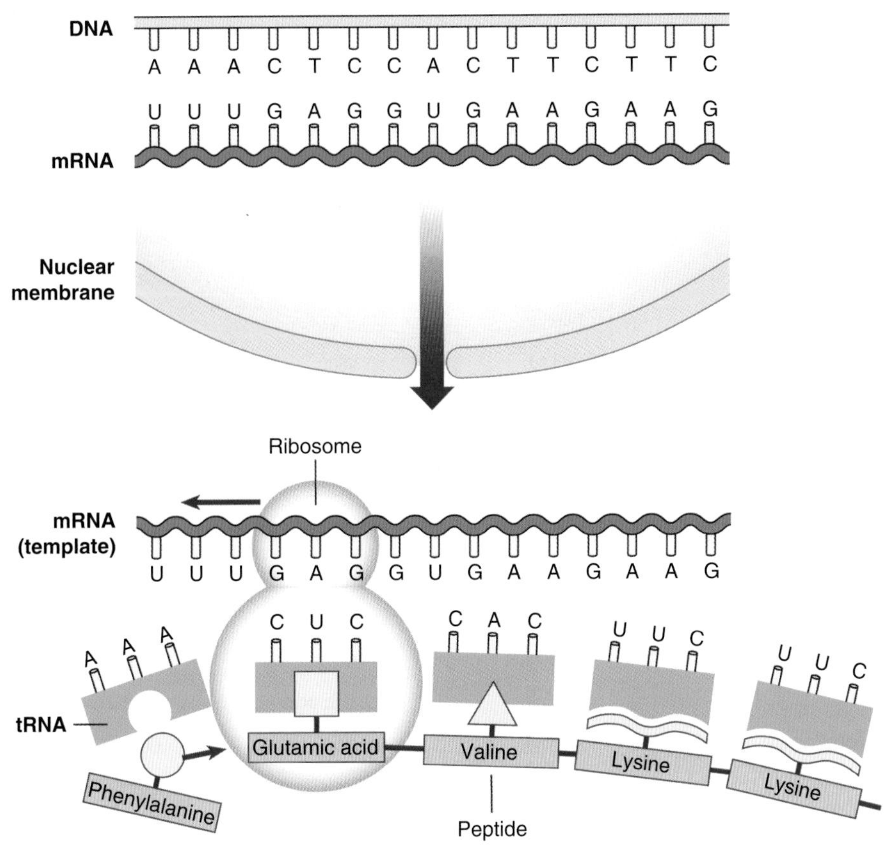

• **Fig. 2.9** Representation of the way in which genetic information is translated into a protein.

hemoglobin in red blood cells (p. 161). This differential control of gene expression can occur at a variety of stages.

Control of Transcription

The control of transcription can be affected permanently or reversibly by a variety of factors, both environmental (e.g., hormones) and genetic (cell signaling). This occurs through a number of different mechanisms that include signaling molecules that bind to regulatory sequences in the DNA known as **response elements**, intracellular receptors known as **hormone nuclear receptors** and receptors for specific ligands on the cell surface involved in the process of **signal transduction**.

All of these mechanisms ultimately affect transcription through the binding of the general transcription factors to short specific DNA promoter elements located within 200 bp 5′ or **upstream** of most eukaryotic genes in the so-called core **promoter region** that leads to activation of RNA polymerase (Figure 2.10). Promoters can be broadly classified into two types, TATA box–containing and GC-rich. The TATA box, which is approximately 25 bp upstream of the transcription start site, is involved in the initiation of transcription at a basal constitutive level and mutations in it can lead to alteration of the transcription start site. The GC box, which is approximately 80 bp upstream, increases the basal level of transcriptional activity of the TATA box.

The regulatory elements in the promoter region are said to be **cisacting**, that is, they affect only the expression of the adjacent gene on the same DNA duplex, whereas the transcription factors are said to be **transacting**, acting on both copies of a gene on each chromosome being synthesized from genes that are located at a distance. DNA sequences that increase transcriptional activity, such as the GC and CAAT boxes, are known as enhancers. There are also negative regulatory elements or **silencers** that inhibit transcription. In addition, there are short sequences of DNA, usually 500 bp to 3 kb in size and known as **boundary elements**, which block or inhibit the influence of regulatory elements of adjacent genes.

Transcription Factors

A number of genes encode proteins involved in the regulation of gene expression. These proteins bind short nucleotide sequences, usually mediated through helical protein motifs, and are known as **transcription factors**. These gene regulatory proteins have a transcriptional activation domain and a DNA-binding domain. There are four types of DNA-binding domains, the most common being the **helix–turn–helix**, made up of two α helices connected by a short chain of amino acids that make up the "turn." The three other types are the **zinc finger**, **leucine zipper** and **helix–loop–helix** motifs, so named as a result of specific structural features.

Post-transcriptional Control of Gene Expression

Regulation of the expression of most genes occurs at the level of transcription, but can also occur at the levels of RNA processing, RNA transport, mRNA degradation and mRNA translation. For example, the G to A variant at position 20,210 in the 3′ untranslated region of the prothrombin-encoding gene increases

TABLE 2.1 **Genetic code of the nuclear and mitochondrial genomes**

	SECOND BASE				
First Base	**U**	**C**	**A**	**G**	**Third Base**
U	Phenylalanine	Serine	Tyrosine	Cysteine	U
	Phenylalanine	Serine	Tyrosine	Cysteine	C
	Leucine	Serine	Stop	Stop (*Tryptophan*)	A
	Leucine	Serine	Stop	Tryptophan	G
C	Leucine	Proline	Histidine	Arginine	U
	Leucine	Proline	Histidine	Arginine	C
	Leucine	Proline	Glutamine	Arginine	A
	Leucine	Proline	Glutamine	Arginine	G
A	Isoleucine	Threonine	Asparagine	Serine	U
	Isoleucine	Threonine	Asparagine	Serine	C
	Isoleucine (*Methionine*)	Threonine	Lysine	Arginine	A
	Methionine	Threonine	Lysine	Arginine (*Stop*)	G
G	Valine	Alanine	Aspartic acid	Glycine	U
	Valine	Alanine	Aspartic acid	Glycine	C
	Valine	Alanine	Glutamic acid	Glycine	A
	Valine	Alanine	Glutamic acid	Glycine	G

Differences in the mitochondrial genetic code are in *italics*.

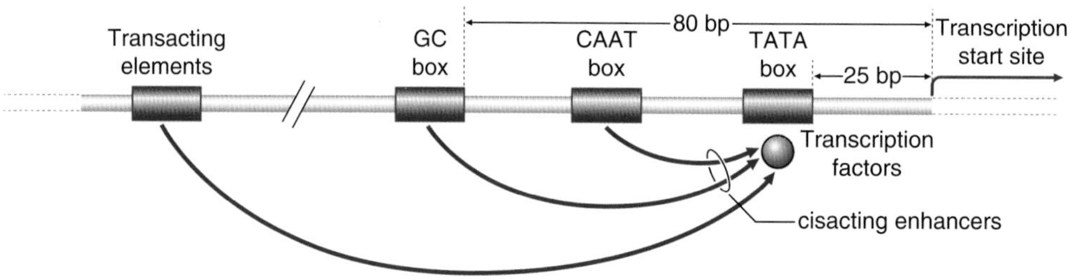

• **Fig. 2.10** Diagrammatic representation of the factors that regulate gene expression.

the stability of the mRNA transcript, resulting in higher plasma prothrombin levels.

RNA-Mediated Control of Gene Expression

RNA-mediated silencing was first described in the early 1990s, but it is only recently that its key role in controlling posttranscriptional gene expression has been both recognized and exploited (see Chapter 15). Small interfering RNAs (siRNAs) were discovered in 1998, and are the effector molecules of the RNA interference pathway. These short double-stranded RNAs (21–23 nucleotides) bind to mRNAs in a sequence-specific manner and result in their degradation via a ribonuclease-containing RNA-induced silencing complex. MicroRNAs (miRNAs) also bind to mRNAs in a sequence-specific manner. They can either cause endonucleolytic cleavage of the mRNA or act by blocking translation.

Alternative Isoforms

Most (~95%) human genes undergo **alternative splicing** and therefore encode more than one protein. **Alternative polyadenylation** generates further diversity. Some genes have more than one promoter, and these **alternative** promoters may result in tissue-specific isoforms. Alternative splicing of exons is also seen with individual exons present in only some isoforms. The extent of alternative splicing in humans may be inferred from the finding that the human genome includes only approximately 20,000 genes, far fewer than the original prediction of more than 100,000.

RNA-Directed DNA Synthesis

The process of the transfer of the genetic information from DNA to RNA to protein has been called the **central dogma**. It was initially believed that genetic information was transferred only from DNA to RNA, and thence translated into protein. However, there is evidence from the study of certain types of virus—retroviruses—that genetic information can occasionally flow in the reverse direction, from RNA to DNA (p. 186). This is referred to as **RNA-directed DNA synthesis**. It has been suggested that regions of DNA in normal cells serve as templates for the synthesis of RNA, which in turn then acts as a template for the synthesis of DNA that later becomes integrated into the nuclear DNA of other cells. Homology between human and retroviral oncogene sequences could reflect this process (Figure 14.3), which could be an important therapeutic approach for the treatment of inherited disease in humans.

Mutations

A **mutation** is defined as a heritable alteration or change in the genetic material. Mutations drive evolution, but can also be pathogenic. Mutations can arise through exposure to mutagenic agents (p. 23), but the vast majority occur spontaneously through errors in DNA replication and repair. Sequence variants with no obvious effect on phenotype may be termed **polymorphisms**.

Somatic mutations may cause adult-onset disease, such as cancer, but cannot be transmitted to offspring. A mutation in **gonadal tissue** or a **gamete** can be transmitted to future generations, unless it affects fertility or survival into adulthood. Harmful alleles of all kinds constitute the so-called genetic load of the population. There are also rare examples of "back mutation" in patients with recessive disorders. For example, reversion of inherited deleterious mutations has been demonstrated in phenotypically normal cells present in a small number of patients with Fanconi anemia.

Types of Mutation

Mutations can range from single base substitutions, through insertions and deletions of single or multiple bases, to loss or gain of entire chromosomes (Table 2.2). Base substitutions are most prevalent (Table 2.3), and missense mutations account for nearly half of all mutations. A standard nomenclature to describe mutations (Table 2.4) has been agreed on (see http://varnomen.hgvs.org/). Examples of chromosome abnormalities are discussed in Chapter 3.

Substitutions

A **substitution** is the replacement of a single nucleotide by another. This is the most common type of mutation. If the substitution involves replacement by the same type of nucleotide—a pyrimidine for a pyrimidine (C for T or *vice versa*) or a purine for a purine (A for G or *vice versa*)—this is termed a **transition**. Substitution of a pyrimidine by a purine or *vice versa* is termed a **transversion**. Transitions occur more frequently than transversions. This may be a result of the relatively high frequency of C to T transitions, which is likely to be the result of the nucleotides C and G occurring together, or what are known as CpG dinucleotides (p represents the phosphate), frequently being methylated in genomic DNA, with spontaneous deamination of methylated C

TABLE 2.2 Main classes, groups and types of mutations and effects on protein products

Class	Group	Type	Effect on Protein Product
Substitution	Synonymous	Silent[a]	Same amino acid
	Non-synonymous	Missense[a]	Altered amino acid—may affect protein function or stability
		Nonsense[a]	Stop codon—loss of function or expression because of degradation of mRNA
		Splice site	Aberrant splicing—exon skipping or intron retention
		Promoter	Altered gene expression
		Enhancer	Altered gene expression
Deletion	Multiple of three (codon)		In-frame deletion of one or more amino acid(s)—may affect protein function or stability
	Not multiple of three	Frameshift	Likely to result in premature termination with loss of function or expression
	Large deletion	Partial gene deletion	May result in premature termination with loss of function or expression
		Whole gene deletion	Loss of expression
Insertion	Multiple of three (codon)		In-frame insertion of one or more amino acid(s)—may affect protein function or stability
	Not multiple of three	Frameshift	Likely to result in premature termination with loss of function or expression
	Large insertion	Partial gene duplication	May result in premature termination with loss of function or expression
		Whole gene duplication	May have an effect because of increased gene dosage
	Expansion of trinucleotide repeat	Dynamic mutation	Altered gene expression or altered protein stability or function

[a]Some have been shown to cause aberrant splicing.

TABLE 2.3 Frequency of different types of mutation

Type of Mutation	Percentage of Total
Missense or nonsense	56
Splicing	9
Regulatory	2
Small deletions, insertions or indels[a]	23
Gross deletions or insertions	9
Other (complex rearrangements or repeat variations)	<1

(From http://www.hgmd.org.)
[a]Indels are mutations that involve both an insertion and a deletion of nucleotides.

converting these residues to T. CpG dinucleotides have been termed "hotspots" for mutation.

Deletions

A deletion involves the loss of one or more nucleotides. If this occurs in coding sequences and involves one, two or more nucleotides that are not a multiple of three, the reading frame will be disrupted. Larger deletions may result in partial or whole gene deletions, and may arise through unequal crossover between repeat sequences (e.g., hereditary neuropathy with liability to pressure palsies; see p. 293).

Insertions

An **insertion** involves the addition of one or more nucleotides to a gene. Again, if an insertion occurs in a coding sequence and involves one, two or more nucleotides that are not a multiple of three, it will disrupt the reading frame. Large insertions can also result from unequal crossover (e.g., hereditary sensory and motor neuropathy type 1a; see p. 292) or the insertion of transposable elements (p. 15).

In 1991, expansion of trinucleotide repeat sequences was identified as a mutational mechanism. A number of single-gene disorders have subsequently been shown to be associated with triplet repeat expansions (Table 2.5). These are described as **dynamic mutations** because the repeat sequence becomes more unstable as it expands in size. The mechanism by which amplification or expansion of the triplet repeat sequence occurs is not clear at present. Triplet repeats below a certain length for each disorder are faithfully and stably transmitted in mitosis and meiosis. Above a certain repeat number for each disorder, they are more likely to be transmitted unstably, usually with an increase or decrease in repeat number. A variety of possible explanations has been offered as to how the increase in triplet repeat number occurs. These include unequal crossover or unequal sister chromatid exchange (p. 268) in non-replicating DNA and slipped-strand mispairing and polymerase slippage in replicating DNA.

Triplet repeat expansions usually take place over a number of generations within a family, providing an explanation for some unusual aspects of patterns of inheritance, as well as possibly being the basis of the previously unexplained phenomenon of anticipation (p. 76).

The exact mechanisms by which repeat expansions cause disease are not completely understood. Unstable trinucleotide repeats may be within coding or non-coding regions of genes, and hence vary in their pathogenic mechanisms. Expansion of the CAG repeat in the coding region of the *HTT* gene and some *SCA* genes results in a protein with an elongated polyglutamine tract that forms toxic aggregates within certain cells, causing Huntington disease or spinocerebellar ataxia. In fragile X syndrome, the CGG repeat expansion in the 5′ untranslated region (UTR) results in methylation of promoter sequences and lack of expression of the FMR1 protein. In myotonic dystrophy (MD) it is thought that a gain-of-function RNA mechanism results from both the CTG expansion in the 3′ UTR of the *DMPK* gene (type 1 MD) and the CCTG expansion within intron 1 of the *CNBP* gene (formerly *ZNF9*; type 2 MD). The expanded transcripts bind splice regulatory proteins to form RNA-protein complexes that accumulate in the nuclei of cells. The disruption of these splice regulators causes abnormal developmental processing where embryonic isoforms of the resulting proteins are expressed in adult myotonic dystrophy tissues. The immature proteins then appear to cause the clinical features common to both diseases (p. 302).

The spectrum of repeat expansion mutations also includes a dodecamer repeat expansion upstream from the cystatin B–encoding gene that causes progressive myoclonus epilepsy (*EPM1*) and a pentanucleotide repeat expansion in intron 9 of the *ATXN10* gene seen in families with spinocerebellar ataxia type 10. Spinocerebellar ataxia is an extremely heterogeneous disorder, and, in addition to the dynamic mutations shown in Table 2.5,

TABLE 2.4 Mutation nomenclature: examples of *CFTR* gene mutations

Type of Mutation	Nucleotide (Ref Seq NM_000492.3)	Protein Designation	Consequence Description
Missense	c.350G > A	p.Arg117His	Arginine to histidine
Nonsense	c.1624G > T	p.Gly542*	Glycine to stop
Splicing	c.489 + 1G > T		Splice donor site mutation
Deletion [1 base pair (bp)]	c.948delT	p.Phe316Leufs*12	Frameshift mutation
Deletion (3 bp)	c.1521_1523delCTT	p.Phe508del	In-frame deletion of phenylalanine
Insertion (1 bp)	c.3767dupC	p.Leu1258Phefs*7	Frameshift mutation

Mutations can be designated according to the genomic or complementary DNA (mRNA) sequence and are prefixed by "g." or "c.," respectively. The first base of the start codon (ATG) is c.1.

TABLE 2.5 Examples of diseases arising from repeat expansions

Disease (Gene)	Repeat Sequence	Normal Range (Repeats)	Pathogenic Range (Repeats)	Repeat Location
Huntington disease (*HTT*)	CAG	9–35	36–100	Coding
Myotonic dystrophy type 1 (*DMPK*)	CTG	5–35	50–4000	3′ UTR
Myotonic dystrophy type 2 (*CNBP*)	CCTG	11–26	75–>11000	Intron 1
Fragile X site A (*FMR1*)	CGG	10–50	200–2000	5′ UTR
Kennedy disease (*AR*)	CAG	13–30	40–62	Coding
Spinocerebellar ataxia 1 (*ATXN1*)	CAG	6–36	39–80	Coding
Spinocerebellar ataxia 2 (*ATXN2*)	CAG	13–31	32–79	Coding
Machado–Joseph disease/Spinocerebellar ataxia 3 (*ATXN3*)	CAG	14–44	52–86	Coding
Spinocerebellar ataxia 6 (*CACNA1A*)	CAG	4–18	19–33	Coding
Spinocerebellar ataxia 7 (*ATXN7*)	CAG	7–17	38–220	Coding
Spinocerebellar ataxia 8 (*ATXN8*)	CTG	15–50	71–1300	3′ UTR
Spinocerebellar ataxia 10 (*ATXN10*)	ATTCT	10–29	400–4500	Intron 9
Spinocerebellar ataxia 12 (*PPP2R2B*)	CAG	7–32	51–78	5′ UTR
Spinocerebellar ataxia 17 (*TBP*)	CAG	25–44	47–63	Coding
Dentatorubral-pallidoluysian atrophy (*ATN1*)	CAG	7–23	53–88	Coding
Friedreich ataxia (*FXN1*)	GAA	5–30	70–>1000	Intron 1
Fragile X site E (*AFF2*)	CCG	6–25	>200	Promoter
Oculopharyngeal muscular dystrophy (*PABPN1*)	GCG	6	8–13	Coding

UTR, Untranslated region.

non-repeat expansion mutations have been reported in four additional genes.

Structural Effects of Mutations on the Protein

Mutations can also be subdivided into two main groups according to the effect on the polypeptide sequence of the encoded protein, being either *synonymous* or *non-synonymous*.

Synonymous or Silent Mutations

If a mutation does not alter the polypeptide product of the gene, it is termed a **synonymous** or **silent mutation**. A single base-pair substitution, particularly if it occurs in the third position of a codon because of the degeneracy of the genetic code, will often result in another triplet that codes for the same amino acid with no alteration in the properties of the resulting protein.

Non-synonymous Mutations

If a mutation leads to an alteration in the encoded polypeptide, it is known as a **non-synonymous mutation**. Non-synonymous mutations are observed to occur less frequently than synonymous mutations. Synonymous mutations are selectively neutral, whereas alteration of the amino-acid sequence of the protein product of a gene is likely to result in abnormal function, which is usually associated with disease, or lethality, which has an obvious selective disadvantage.

Non-synonymous mutations can occur in one of three main ways.

Missense. A single base-pair substitution can result in coding for a different amino acid and the synthesis of an altered protein, a so-called **missense** mutation. If the mutation codes for an amino acid that is chemically dissimilar (e.g., one that has a different charge) the structure of the protein will be altered. This is termed a **non-conservative substitution** and can lead to a gross reduction, or even a complete loss, of biological activity. Single base-pair mutations can lead to qualitative rather than quantitative changes in the function of a protein, such that it retains its normal biological activity (e.g., enzyme activity) but differs in characteristics such as its mobility on electrophoresis, its pH optimum, or its stability so that it is more rapidly broken down *in vivo*. Many of the abnormal hemoglobins (see Chapter 12) are the result of missense mutations.

Some single base-pair substitutions result in the replacement of a different amino acid that is chemically similar, and may have no functional effect. These are termed **conservative** substitutions.

Nonsense. A substitution that leads to the generation of one of the stop codons (see Table 2.1) will result in premature termination of translation of a peptide chain, or what is termed a **nonsense** or **stopgain** mutation. In most cases the shortened chain is unlikely to retain normal biological activity, particularly if the termination codon results in the loss of an important functional domain(s) of the protein. mRNA transcripts containing premature termination codons are frequently degraded by a process known as **nonsense-mediated decay**. This is a form of RNA surveillance that is believed to have evolved to protect the body from the possible consequences of truncated proteins interfering with normal function.

Frameshift. If a mutation involves the insertion or deletion of nucleotides that are not a multiple of three, it will disrupt the reading frame and constitute what is known as a **frameshift** mutation. The amino-acid sequence of the protein subsequent to the mutation bears no resemblance to the normal sequence, and may have an adverse effect on its function. Most frameshift mutations result in a premature stop codon downstream to the mutation. This may lead to expression of a truncated protein, unless the mRNA is degraded by nonsense-mediated decay.

Mutations in Non-coding DNA

Mutations in promoter sequences, enhancers, or other regulatory regions can affect the level of gene expression. With our new knowledge of the role of RNA interference in gene expression, it has become apparent that mutations in miRNA or siRNA binding sites within UTRs can also result in disease.

Splicing Mutations

Mutations of the highly conserved splice donor (GT) and splice acceptor (AG) sites (p. 15) usually result in aberrant splicing. This can result in the loss of coding sequence (exon skipping) or retention of intronic sequence, and may lead to frameshift mutations. **Cryptic splice** sites, which resemble the sequence of an authentic splice site, may be activated when the conserved splice sites are mutated. In addition, base substitutions resulting in apparent silent, missense, and nonsense mutations can cause aberrant splicing through mutation of **exon splicing enhancer** sequences. These purine-rich sequences are required for the correct splicing of exons with weak splice-site consensus sequences.

Functional Effects of Mutations on the Protein

Mutations exert their phenotypic effect in one of two ways, through either loss or gain of function.

Loss-of-Function Mutations

Loss-of-function mutations can result in either reduced activity or complete loss of the gene product. The former can be the result of reduced activity or of decreased stability of the gene product and is known as a **hypomorph**, the latter being known as a **null allele** or **amorph**. Loss-of-function mutations involving enzymes are usually inherited in an autosomal or X-linked recessive manner, because the catalytic activity of the product of the normal allele is more than adequate to carry out the reactions of most metabolic pathways.

Haploinsufficiency. Loss-of-function mutations in the heterozygous state in which half-normal levels of the gene product result in phenotypic effects are termed **haploinsufficiency mutations**. The phenotypic manifestations sensitive to gene dosage are a result of mutations occurring in genes that code for receptors or, more rarely, enzymes with rate-limiting functions; for example, familial hypercholesterolemia (p. 147) and acute intermittent porphyria (p. 282).

In a number of autosomal dominant disorders, the mutational basis of the functional abnormality is the result of haploinsufficiency in which, not surprisingly, homozygous mutations result in more severe phenotypic effects; an example is familial hypercholesterolemia (p. 147).

Gain-of-Function Mutations

Gain-of-function mutations, as the name suggests, result in either increased levels of gene expression or the development of a new function(s) of the gene product. Increased expression levels from activating point mutations or increased gene dosage are responsible for one type of Charcot-Marie-Tooth disease, hereditary motor and sensory neuropathy type I (p. 292). The expanded triplet repeat mutations in the Huntington gene (*HTT*) cause qualitative changes in the gene product that result in its aggregation in the central nervous system, leading to the classic clinical features of the disorder (p. 289).

Mutations that alter the timing or tissue specificity of the expression of a gene can also be considered to be gain-of-function mutations. Examples include the chromosomal rearrangements that result in the combination of sequences from two different genes seen with specific tumors (p. 187). The novel function of the resulting chimeric gene causes the neoplastic process.

Gain-of-function mutations are dominantly inherited, and the rare instances of gain-of-function mutations occurring in the homozygous state are often associated with a much more severe phenotype, which is often a prenatally lethal disorder; for example, homozygous achondroplasia (p. 71).

Dominant-Negative Mutations

A **dominant-negative** mutation is one in which a mutant gene in the heterozygous state results in the loss of protein activity or function as a consequence of the mutant gene product interfering with the function of the normal gene product of the corresponding allele. Dominant-negative mutations are particularly common in proteins that are dimers or multimers; for instance, mutations in genes encoding structural proteins such as the collagens can lead to osteogenesis imperfecta.

Genotype–Phenotype Correlation

Many genetic disorders are well recognized as being very variable in severity, or in the particular features manifested by a person with the disorder (p. 69). Developments in molecular genetics increasingly allow identification of the mutational basis of the specific features that occur in a person with a particular inherited disease, or what is known as the phenotype. This has resulted in attempts to correlate the presence of a particular mutation, which is often called the genotype, with the specific features seen in a person with an inherited disorder, this being referred to as **genotype–phenotype correlation**. This can be important in the management of a patient. One example includes the association of mutations in the *BRCA1* gene with the risk of developing ovarian cancer as well as breast cancer (p. 201). Particularly striking examples are mutations in the receptor tyrosine kinase gene *RET* which, depending on their location, can lead to four different syndromes that differ in functional mechanism and clinical phenotype. Loss-of-function nonsense mutations lead to lack of migration of neural crest–derived cells to form the ganglia of the myenteric plexus of the large bowel, leading to Hirschsprung disease, whereas gain-of-function missense mutations result in familial medullary thyroid carcinoma or one of the two types of multiple endocrine neoplasia type 2 (p. 121). Mutations in the *LMNA* gene are associated with an even broader spectrum of disease (p. 67).

Mutations and Mutagenesis

Naturally occurring mutations are referred to as **spontaneous mutations** and are thought to arise through chance errors in chromosomal division or DNA replication. Environmental agents that cause mutations are known as mutagens. These include natural or artificial ionising radiation and chemical or physical mutagens.

Radiation

Ionising radiation includes electromagnetic waves of very short wavelength (x-rays and γ-rays) and high-energy particles (α particles, β particles and neutrons). X-rays, γ-rays and neutrons have great penetrating power, but α particles can penetrate soft tissues to a depth of only a fraction of a millimeter, and β particles only up to a few millimeters.

Dosimetry is the measurement of radiation. The dose of radiation is expressed in relation to the amount received by the gonads, because it is the effects of radiation on germ cells rather than somatic cells that are important as far as transmission of mutations to future progeny is concerned. The **gonad dose** of radiation is often expressed as the amount received in 30 years. This period has been chosen because it corresponds roughly to the generation time in humans.

The various sources and average annual doses of the different types of natural and artificial ionising radiation are listed in Table 2.6. Natural sources of radiation include cosmic rays, external radiation from radioactive materials in certain rocks and internal radiation from radioactive materials in tissues. Artificial sources include diagnostic and therapeutic radiology, occupational exposure and fallout from nuclear explosions.

The average gonadal dose of ionising radiation from radioactive fallout resulting from the testing of nuclear weapons is less than that from any of the sources of background radiation. However, the possibility of serious accidents involving nuclear reactors, as occurred at Three Mile Island in the United States in 1979 and at Chernobyl in the Soviet Union in 1986, with widespread effects, must always be born in mind.

TABLE 2.6 Approximate average doses of ionising radiation from various sources to the gonads of the general population

Source of Radiation	Average Dose per Year (mSv)	Average Dose per 30 Years (mSv)
Natural		
Cosmic radiation	0.25	7.5
External γ radiation[a]	1.50	45.0
Internal γ radiation	0.30	9.0
Artificial		
Medical radiology	0.30	9.0
Radioactive fallout	0.01	0.3
Occupational and miscellaneous	0.04	1.2
Total	2.40	72.0

(From Clarke RH, Southwood TRE. Risks from ionizing radiation. *Nature.* 1989;338:197–198.)
[a]Including radon in dwellings.

Genetic Effects

Experiments with animals and plants have shown that the number of mutations produced by irradiation is proportional to the dose: the larger the dose, the greater the number of mutations produced. It is believed that there is no threshold below which irradiation has no effect—even the smallest dose of radiation can result in a mutation. The genetic effects of ionizing radiation are also cumulative, so that each time a person is exposed to radiation, the dose received is added to the amount of radiation already received. The total number of radiation-induced mutations is directly proportional to the total gonadal dose.

Unfortunately, in humans there is no easy way to demonstrate genetic damage caused by mutagens. Several agencies throughout the world are responsible for defining what is referred to as the maximum permissible dose of radiation. In the United Kingdom, the Radiation Protection Division of the Health Protection Agency advises that occupational exposure should not exceed 15 mSv in a year. To put this into perspective, 1 mSv is roughly 50 times the dose received in a single chest x-ray and 100 times the dose incurred when flying from the United Kingdom to Spain in a jet aircraft!

There is no doubting the potential dangers, both somatic and germline, of exposure to ionizing radiation. In the case of medical radiology, the dose of radiation resulting from a particular procedure has to be weighed against the ultimate beneficial effect to the patient. In the case of occupational exposure to radiation, the answer lies in defining the risks and introducing and enforcing adequate legislation. With regard to the dangers from fallout from nuclear accidents and explosions, the solution would seem obvious.

Chemical Mutagens

In humans, chemical mutagenesis may be more important than radiation in producing genetic damage. Experiments have shown that certain chemicals, such as mustard gas, formaldehyde, benzene, some basic dyes and food additives, are mutagenic in animals. Exposure to environmental chemicals may result in the formation of DNA adducts, chromosome breaks or aneuploidy. Consequently, all new pharmaceutical products are subject to a battery of mutagenicity tests that include both *in vitro* and *in vivo* studies.

DNA Repair

DNA mutations, if left unrepaired, would have serious consequences for both the individual and subsequent generations. The stability of DNA is dependent upon continuous **DNA repair** by a number of different mechanisms (Table 2.7). Some types of DNA damage can be repaired directly. Examples include the dealkylation of O^6-alkyl G or the removal of T dimers by photoreactivation in bacteria. The majority of DNA repair mechanisms involve cleavage of the DNA strand by an endonuclease, removal of the damaged region by an exonuclease, insertion of new bases by the enzyme DNA polymerase, and sealing of the break by DNA ligase.

Nucleotide excision repair removes T dimers and large chemical adducts. It is a complex process involving more than 30 proteins that remove fragments of approximately 30 nucleotides. Mutations in at least eight of the genes encoding these proteins can cause xeroderma pigmentosum (p. 268), characterized by extreme

TABLE 2.7 DNA repair pathways, genes, and associated disorders

Type of DNA Repair	Mechanism	Genes	Disorders
Base excision repair (BER)	Removal of abnormal bases	*MYH*	Colorectal cancer
Nucleotide excision repair (NER)	Removal of thymine dimers and large chemical adducts	*XP*	Xeroderma pigmentosum
Postreplication repair	Removal of double-strand breaks by homologous recombination or non-homologous end-joining	*NBS*	Nijmegen breakage syndrome
		BLM	Bloom syndrome
		BRCA1/2	Breast cancer
Mismatch repair (MMR)	Corrects mismatched bases caused by mistakes in DNA replication	*MSH* and *MLH*	Colorectal cancer (HNPCC)

HNPCC, Hereditary non-polyposis colorectal cancer.

sensitivity to ultraviolet light and a high frequency of skin cancer. A different set of repair enzymes is used to excise single abnormal bases (**base excision repair**), with mutations in the gene encoding the DNA glycosylase MYH having been shown to cause an autosomal recessive form of colorectal cancer (p. 200).

Naturally occurring reactive oxygen species and ionising radiation induce breakage of DNA strands. Double-strand breaks result in chromosome breaks that can be lethal if not repaired. **Postreplication repair** is required to correct double-strand breaks, and usually involves homologous recombination with a sister DNA molecule. Human genes involved in this pathway include *NBS, BLM* and *BRCA1/2*, which are mutated in Nijmegen breakage syndrome, Bloom syndrome (p. 266), and hereditary breast cancer (p. 201), respectively. Alternatively, the broken ends may be rejoined by non-homologous end-joining, which is an error-prone pathway.

Mismatch repair (MMR) corrects mismatched bases introduced during DNA replication. Cells defective in MMR have very high mutation rates (up to 1000 times higher than normal). Mutations in at least six different MMR genes cause familial colorectal cancer, Lynch syndrome (p. 198).

Although DNA repair pathways have evolved to correct DNA damage and hence protect the cell from the deleterious consequences of mutations, some mutations arise from the cell's attempts to tolerate damage. One example is **translesion DNA synthesis**, in which the DNA replication machinery bypasses sites of DNA damage, allowing normal DNA replication and gene expression to proceed downstream. Human disease may also be caused by defective cellular responses to DNA damage. Cells have complex signaling pathways that allow cell-cycle arrest to provide increased time for DNA repair. If the DNA damage is irreparable, the cell may initiate programmed cell death (**apoptosis**). The ATM protein is involved in sensing DNA damage, and has been described as the "guardian of the genome." Mutations in the *ATM* gene cause ataxia telangiectasia (see p. 181), characterized by hypersensitivity to radiation and a high risk of cancer.

ELEMENTS

1. Genetic information is stored in DNA (deoxyribonucleic acid) as a linear sequence of two types of nucleotide, the purines [adenine (A) and guanine (G)] and the pyrimidines [cytosine (C) and thymine (T)], linked by a sugar–phosphate backbone.
2. A molecule of DNA consists of two antiparallel strands held in a double helix by hydrogen bonds between the complementary G–C and A–T base pairs.
3. DNA replication has multiple sites of origin and is semiconservative, with each strand acting as a template for synthesis of a complementary strand.
4. Genes encoding proteins in higher organisms (eukaryotes) consist of coding (exons) and non-coding (introns) sections.
5. Transcription is the synthesis of a single-stranded complementary copy of one strand of a gene that is known as messenger RNA (mRNA). RNA (ribonucleic acid) differs from DNA in that it contains the sugar ribose instead of deoxyribose and the base uracil instead of thymine.
6. mRNA is processed during transport from the nucleus to the cytoplasm, eliminating the non-coding sections. In the cytoplasm it becomes associated with the ribosomes, where translation (i.e., protein synthesis) occurs.
7. The genetic code is "universal" and consists of triplets (codons) of nucleotides, each of which codes for an amino acid or termination of peptide chain synthesis. The code is degenerate, as all but two amino acids are specified by more than one codon.
8. The major control of gene expression is at the level of transcription by DNA regulatory sequences in the 5′ flanking promoter region of structural genes in eukaryotes. General and specific transcription factors are also involved in the regulation of genes.
9. Mutations occur both spontaneously and as a result of exposure to mutagenic agents such as ionizing radiation. Mutations are continuously corrected by DNA repair enzymes.

Further Reading

Alberts B, Johnson A, Lewis J, et al. *Molecular Biology of the Cell.* 6th ed. London: Garland; 2015.

Very accessible, well written, and lavishly illustrated comprehensive text of molecular biology with more than 170 narrated movies.

Dawkins R. *The Selfish Gene.* 3rd ed. Oxford: Oxford University Press; 1989.

An interesting, controversial concept.

Fire A, Xu S, Montgomery MK, et al. Potent and specific genetic interference by double-stranded RNA in *Caenorhabditis elegans. Nature.* 1998;391:806–811.

Landmark paper describing the discovery of RNAi.

Lewin B. *Genes XII.* 12th ed. Burlington, MA: Jones and Bartlett Publishers; 2014.

The 12th edition of this excellent textbook of molecular biology with color diagrams and figures.

Schull WJ, Neel JV. Radiation and the sex ratio in man. Sex ratio among children of survivors of atomic bombings suggests induced sex-linked lethal mutations. *Science*. 1958;228:434–438.

The original report of possible evidence of the effects of atomic radiation.

Strachan T, Read AP. *Human Molecular Genetics*. 5th ed. London: Garland Science; 2018.

An excellent, comprehensive textbook of molecular aspects of human genetics as it relates to inherited disease in humans.

Watson JD, Crick FHC. Molecular structure of nucleic acids—a structure for deoxyribose nucleic acid. *Nature*. 1953;171:737–738.

The concepts in this paper, presented in just over one page, resulted in the authors receiving the Nobel Prize!

3

Chromosomes and Cell Division

Let us not take it for granted that life exists more fully in what is commonly thought big than in what is commonly thought small.

Virginia Woolf

At the molecular or submicroscopic level, DNA can be regarded as the basic template that provides a blueprint for the formation and maintenance of an organism. DNA is packaged into **chromosomes**, and at a very simple level these can be considered as being made up of tightly coiled long chains of genes. Unlike DNA, chromosomes can be visualized during cell division using a light microscope, under which they appear as threadlike structures or "colored bodies." The word *chromosome* is derived from the Greek *chroma* (=color) and *soma* (=body).

Chromosomes are the factors that distinguish one species from another and that enable the transmission of genetic information from one generation to the next. Their behavior at somatic cell division in mitosis provides a means of ensuring that each daughter cell retains its own complete genetic complement. Similarly, their behavior during gamete formation in meiosis enables each mature ovum and sperm to contain a unique single set of parental genes. Chromosomes are quite literally the vehicles that facilitate reproduction and the maintenance of a species.

The study of chromosomes and cell division is referred to as **cytogenetics**. Before the 1950s it was thought, incorrectly, that each human cell contained 48 chromosomes, and that human sex was determined by the number of X chromosomes present at conception. Following the development in 1956 of more reliable techniques for studying human chromosomes, it was realized that the correct chromosome number in humans is 46 (p. 3) and that maleness is determined by the presence of a Y chromosome regardless of the number of X chromosomes present in each cell. It was also realized that abnormalities of chromosome number and structure could seriously disrupt normal growth and development.

Table 3.1 highlights the methodological developments that have taken place since the 1950s that underpin our current knowledge of human cytogenetics.

Human Chromosomes

Morphology

At the submicroscopic level, chromosomes consist of an extremely elaborate complex, made up of supercoils of DNA, which has been likened to the tightly coiled network of wiring seen in a solenoid (p. 12). Under the electron microscope chromosomes can be seen to have a rounded and rather irregular morphology (Fig. 3.1). However, most of our knowledge of chromosome structure has been gained using light microscopy. Special stains selectively taken up by DNA have enabled each individual chromosome to be identified. These are best seen during cell division, when the chromosomes are maximally contracted and the constituent genes can no longer be transcribed.

At this time each chromosome can be seen to consist of two identical strands known as **chromatids**, or **sister chromatids**, which are the result of DNA replication having taken place during the S (synthesis) phase of the cell cycle (p. 32). These sister chromatids can be seen to be joined at a primary constriction known as the **centromere**. Centromeres consist of several hundred kilobases of repetitive DNA and are responsible for the movement of chromosomes at cell division. Each centromere divides the chromosome into short and long arms, designated p (=petite) and q ("g" = grande), respectively.

The tip of each chromosome arm is known as the **telomere**. Telomeres play a crucial role in sealing the ends of chromosomes and maintaining their structural integrity. Telomeres have been highly conserved throughout evolution, and in humans they consist of many tandem repeats of a TTAGGG sequence. During DNA replication, an

TABLE 3.1 Development of methodologies for cytogenetics

Decade	Development	Examples of Application
1950–1960s	Reliable methods for chromosome preparations	Chromosome number determined to be 46 (1956) and Philadelphia chromosome identified as t(9;22) (1960)
1970s	Giemsa chromosome banding	Mapping of *RB1* gene to chromosome 13q14 by identification of deleted chromosomal region in patients with retinoblastoma (1976)
1990s	Fluorescence *in situ* hybridization (FISH)	Interphase FISH for rapid detection of Down syndrome (1994) Spectral karyotyping for whole genome chromosome analysis (1996)
2000s	Array comparative genomic hybridization (CGH)	Analysis of constitutional rearrangements; e.g., identification of ~5 megabase deletion in a patient with CHARGE syndrome that led to identification of the gene (2004)

CHARGE, coloboma of the eye, heart defects, atresia of the choanae, retardation of growth and/or development, genital and/or urinary abnormalities and ear abnormalities and deafness.

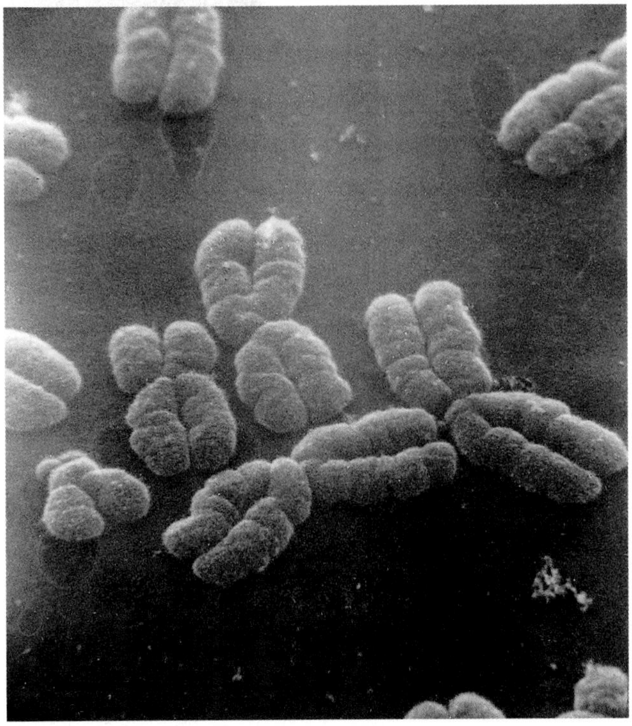

• **Fig. 3.1** Electron micrograph of human chromosomes showing the centromeres and well-defined chromatids. (Courtesy Professor C Harrison. Reproduced from Harrison et al. *Cytogenet Cell Genet*. 1983;35:21–27. With permission of the publisher, S. Karger, Basel.)

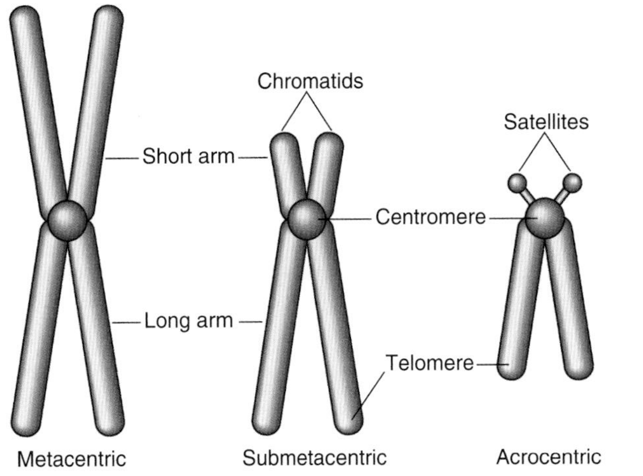

• **Fig. 3.2** Morphologically chromosomes are described as metacentric, submetacentric or acrocentric, depending on the position of the centromere.

enzyme known as **telomerase** replaces the 5′ end of the long strand, which would otherwise become progressively shorter until a critical length was reached when the cell could no longer divide and thus became senescent. This is in fact part of the normal cellular aging process, with most cells being unable to undergo more than 50 to 60 divisions. However, in some tumors, increased telomerase activity has been implicated as a cause of abnormally prolonged cell survival.

Morphologically, chromosomes are classified according to the position of the centromere. If this is located centrally, the chromosome is **metacentric**, if terminal it is **acrocentric**, and if the centromere is in an intermediate position the chromosome is **submetacentric** (Fig. 3.2). Acrocentric chromosomes sometimes have stalk-like appendages called **satellites** that form the nucleolus of the resting interphase cell and contain multiple repeat copies of the genes for ribosomal RNA.

Classification

Individual chromosomes differ not only in the position of the centromere, but also in their overall length. Based on the three parameters of length, position of the centromere and the presence or absence of satellites, early pioneers of cytogenetics were able to identify most individual chromosomes, or at least subdivide them into groups labeled A to G on the basis of overall morphology (A, 1–3; B, 4–5; C, 6–12, X; D, 13–15; E, 16–18; F, 19–20; G, 21–22, Y). In humans the normal cell nucleus contains 46 chromosomes, made up of 22 pairs of **autosomes** and a single pair of sex chromosomes—XX in the female and XY in the male. One member of each of these pairs is derived from each parent. Somatic cells are said to have a **diploid** complement of 46 chromosomes, whereas gametes (ova and sperm) have a **haploid** complement of 23 chromosomes. Members of a pair of chromosomes are known as **homologs**.

The development of chromosome banding (p. 28) enabled very precise recognition of individual chromosomes and detection of subtle chromosome abnormalities. This technique also revealed that **chromatin**, the combination of DNA and histone proteins that comprise chromosomes, exists in two main forms. **Euchromatin** stains lightly and consists of genes that are actively expressed. In contrast, **heterochromatin** stains darkly and is made up largely of inactive, unexpressed, repetitive DNA.

The Sex Chromosomes

The X and Y chromosomes are known as the sex chromosomes because of their crucial role in sex determination. The X chromosome was originally labeled as such because of uncertainty as to its function when it was realized that, in some insects, this chromosome is present in some gametes but not in others. In these insects the male has only one sex chromosome (X), whereas the female has two (XX). In humans, and in most mammals, both the male and the female have two sex chromosomes—XX in the female and XY in the male. The Y chromosome is much smaller than the X and carries only a few genes of functional importance, most notably the gene encoding testis-determining factor, known as *SRY* (p. 128). Other genes on the Y chromosome are known to be important in maintaining spermatogenesis.

In the female each ovum carries an X chromosome, whereas in the male each sperm carries either an X or a Y chromosome. Because there is a roughly equal chance of either an X-bearing sperm or a Y-bearing sperm fertilizing an ovum, the numbers of male and female conceptions are approximately equal (Fig. 3.3). In fact, slightly more male babies are born than females, although during childhood and adult life the sex ratio evens out at 1:1.

The process of sex determination is considered in detail later (p. 127).

Methods of Chromosome Analysis

It was generally believed that each cell contained 48 chromosomes until 1956, when Tjio and Levan correctly concluded on the basis

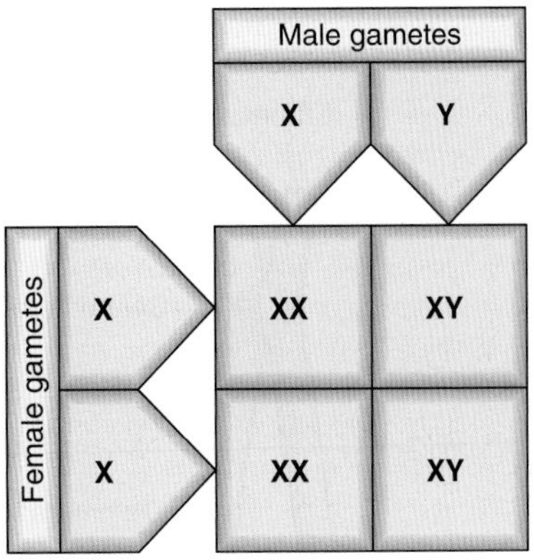

• **Fig. 3.3** Punnett square showing sex chromosome combinations for male and female gametes.

of their studies that the normal human somatic cell contains only 46 chromosomes (p. 3). The methods they used, with certain modifications, are now universally employed in cytogenetic laboratories to analyze the chromosome constitution of an individual, which is known as a **karyotype**. This term is also used to describe a photomicrograph of an individual's chromosomes, arranged in a standard manner.

Chromosome Preparation

Any tissue with living nucleated cells that undergo division can be used for studying human chromosomes. Most commonly, circulating lymphocytes from peripheral blood are used, although samples for chromosomal analysis can be prepared relatively easily using skin, bone marrow, chorionic villi or cells from amniotic fluid (amniocytes).

In the case of peripheral (venous) blood, a sample is added to a small volume of nutrient medium containing phytohemagglutinin, which stimulates T lymphocytes to divide. The cells are cultured under sterile conditions at 37° C for about 3 days, during which they divide, and colchicine is then added to each culture. This drug has the extremely useful property of preventing formation of the spindle, thereby arresting cell division during metaphase, the time when the chromosomes are maximally condensed and therefore most visible. Hypotonic saline is then added, which causes the blood cells to lyse and results in spreading of the chromosomes, which are then fixed, mounted on a slide and stained ready for analysis (Fig. 3.4).

Chromosome Banding

Several different staining methods can be used to identify individual chromosomes, but G (**Giemsa**) banding is used most commonly. The chromosomes are treated with trypsin, which

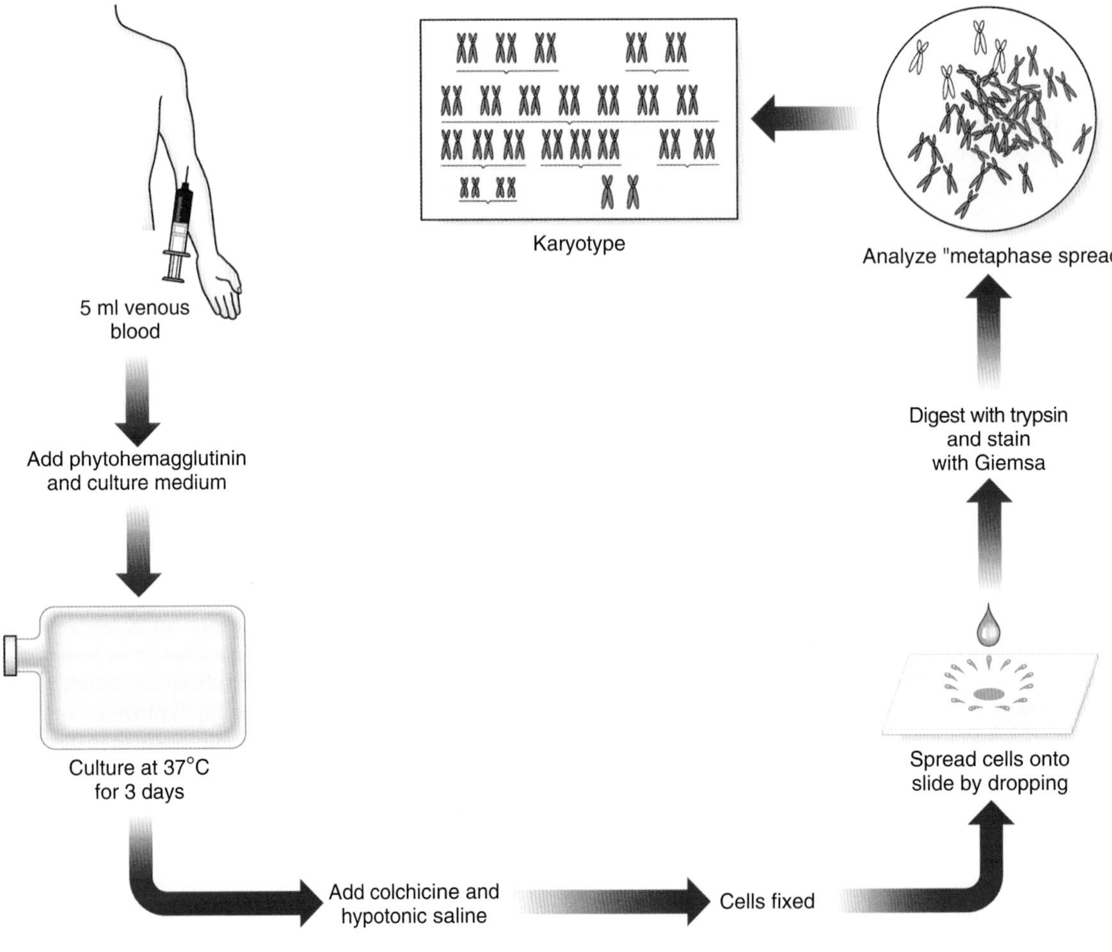

• **Fig. 3.4** Preparation of a karyotype.

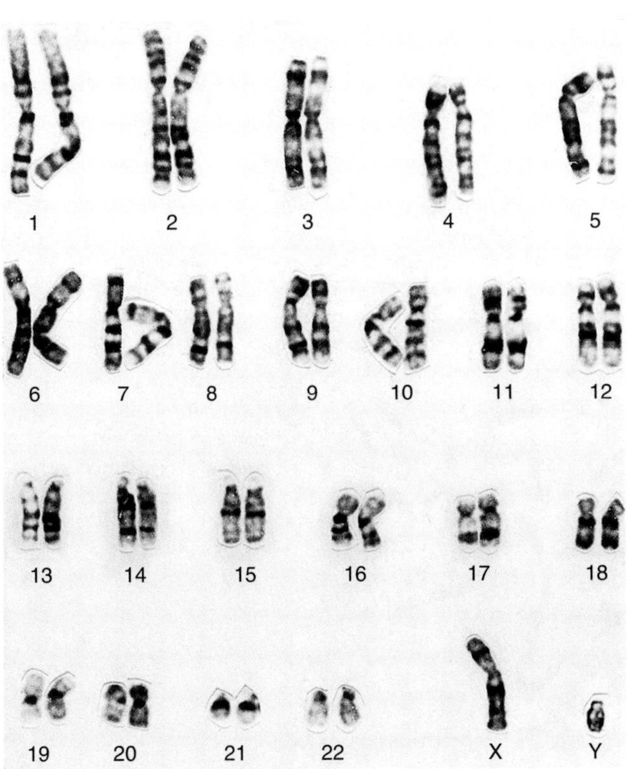

• **Fig. 3.5** A normal G-banded male karyotype.

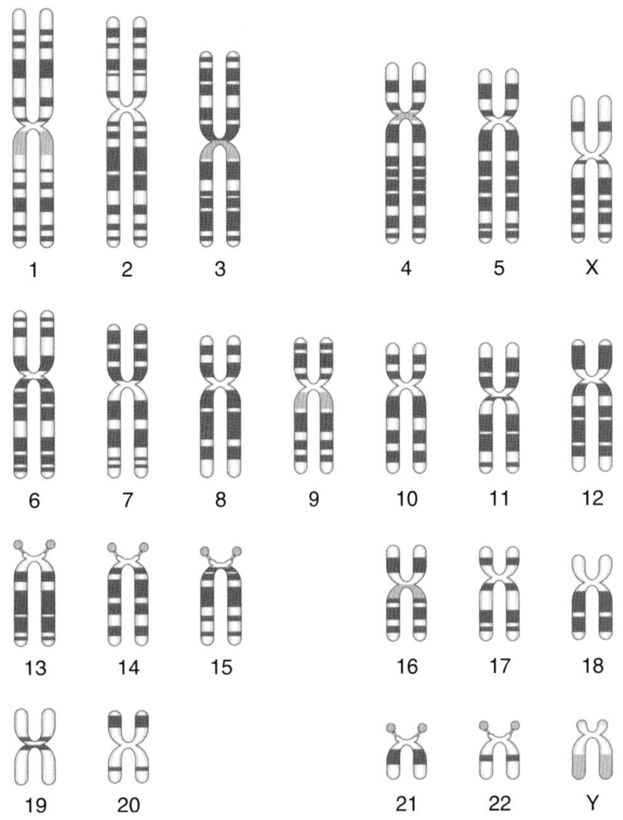

• **Fig. 3.6** An idiogram showing the banding patterns of individual chromosomes as revealed by fluorescent and Giemsa staining.

denatures their protein content, and then stained with a DNA-binding dye that gives each chromosome a characteristic and reproducible pattern of light and dark bands (Fig. 3.5).

G banding generally provides high-quality chromosome analysis with approximately 400 to 500 bands per haploid set. Each of these bands corresponds on average to approximately 6000 to 8000 kb (i.e., 6–8 megabases) of DNA.

Karyotype Analysis

The banding pattern of each chromosome is specific and can be shown in the form of a stylised ideal karyotype known as an **idiogram** (Fig. 3.6). Each pair of homologous chromosomes can be visualized either directly with a microscope, or using an image capture system to photograph the chromosomes and arrange them in the form of a karyogram (Fig. 3.7).

Molecular Cytogenetics

Fluorescence *In Situ* Hybridization

This method is based on the unique ability of a portion of single-stranded DNA (i.e., a probe) to anneal with its complementary target sequence on a metaphase chromosome, interphase nucleus or extended chromatin fiber. In **fluorescence *in situ* hybridization (FISH)**, the DNA probe is labeled with a fluorochrome which, after hybridization with the patient's sample, allows the region where hybridization has occurred to be visualized using a fluorescence microscope. FISH has been widely used for clinical diagnostic purposes during the past 30 years, and there are a number of different types of probes that may be employed.

Different Types of FISH Probes

Centromeric Probes. These consist of repetitive DNA sequences found in and around the centromere of a specific chromosome. They were the original probes used for rapid interphase FISH diagnosis of the common aneuploidy syndromes (trisomies 13, 18, 21; see pp. 250–53) from a prenatal diagnostic sample of chorionic villi until it was superseded by quantitative fluorescent polymerase chain reaction.

Chromosome-Specific Unique-Sequence Probes. These are specific for a particular single locus which can be used to identify submicroscopic deletions and duplications (Fig. 3.8) causing **microdeletion** syndromes (described in Chapter 17). Another application is the use of an interphase FISH probe to identify *HER2* overexpression in breast tumors to identify patients likely to benefit from Herceptin treatment.

Whole-Chromosome Paint Probes. These consist of a cocktail of probes obtained from different parts of a particular chromosome. When this mixture of probes is used together in a single hybridization, the entire relevant chromosome fluoresces (i.e., is "painted"). Chromosome painting is useful for characterizing complex rearrangements, such as subtle translocations (Fig. 3.9), and for identifying the origin of additional chromosomal material, such as small supernumerary markers or rings.

Chromosome Nomenclature

By convention each chromosome arm is divided into regions, and each region is subdivided into bands, numbering always from the

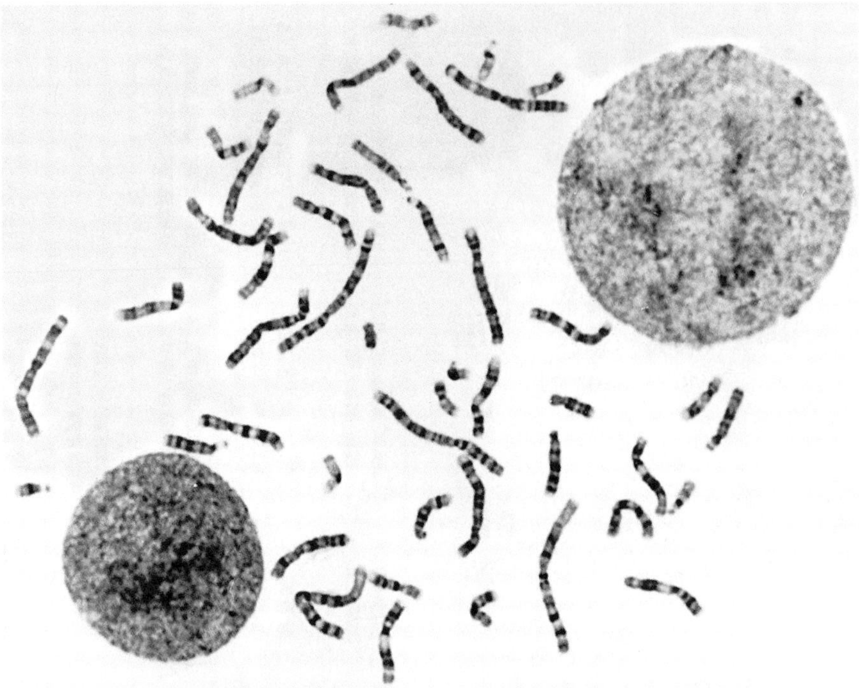

• **Fig. 3.7** A G-banded metaphase spread. (Courtesy Mr A Wilkinson, Cytogenetics Unit, City Hospital, Nottingham, UK.)

centromere outwards (Fig. 3.10). A given point on a chromosome is designated by the chromosome number, the arm (p or q), the region and the band (e.g., 15q12). Sometimes the word *region* is omitted, so that 15q12 would be referred to simply as band 12 on the long arm of chromosome 15.

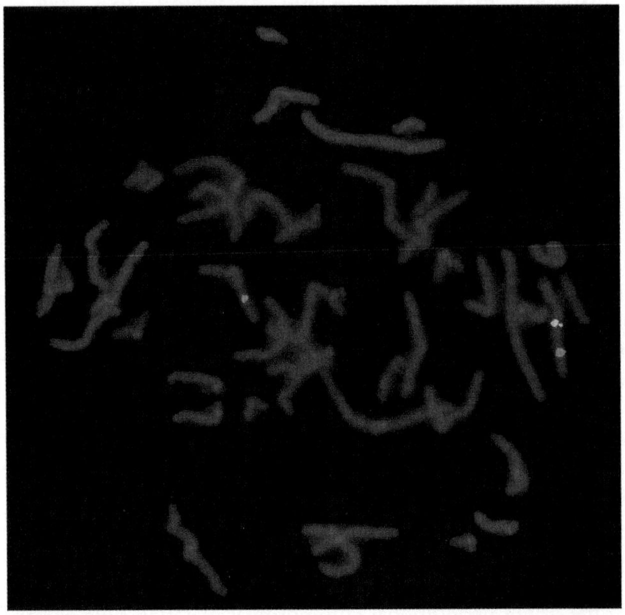

• **Fig. 3.8** Metaphase image of Williams (*ELN*) region probe (Vysis), chromosome band 7q11.23, showing the deletion associated with Williams syndrome. The normal chromosome has signals for the control probe (*green*) and the *ELN* gene probe (*orange*), but the deleted chromosome shows only the control probe signal. (Courtesy Ms C Delmege, Bristol Genetics Laboratory, Southmead Hospital, Bristol, UK.)

A shorthand notation system exists for the description of chromosome abnormalities (Table 3.2). Normal male and female karyotypes are depicted as 46,XY and 46,XX, respectively. A male with Down syndrome as a result of trisomy 21 would be represented as 47, XY, + 21, whereas a female with a deletion of the short arm of one number 5 chromosome (cri du chat syndrome; see p. 258) would be represented as 46,XX,del(5p). A chromosome report

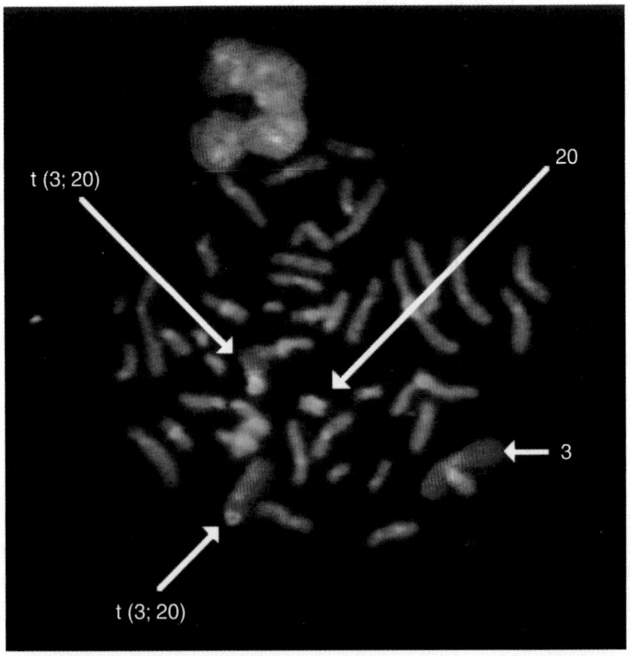

• **Fig. 3.9** Chromosome painting showing a reciprocal translocation involving chromosomes 3 (*red*) and 20 (*green*).

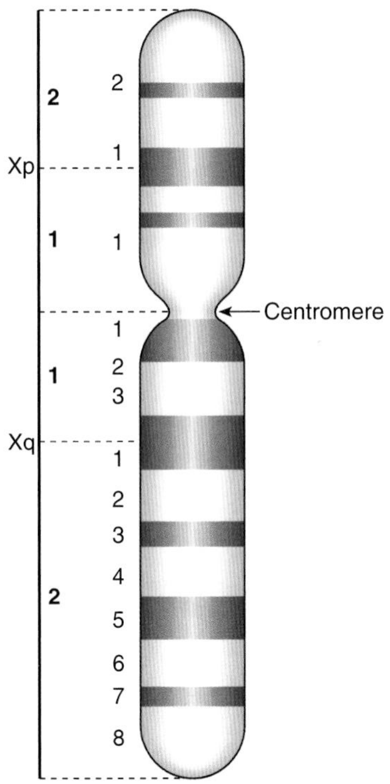

• **Fig. 3.10** X chromosome showing the short and long arms each subdivided into regions and bands.

TABLE 3.2 Symbols used in describing a karyotype

Term	Explanation	Example
p	Short arm	
q	Long arm	
cen	Centromere	
del	Deletion	46,XX,del(1)(q21)
dup	Duplication	46,XY,dup(13)(q14)
fra	Fragile site	
i	Isochromosome	46,X,i(Xq)
inv	Inversion	46,XX,inv(9)(p12q12)
ish	*In situ* hybridization	
r	Ring	46,XX,r(21)
t	Translocation	46,XY,t(2;4)(q21;q21)
ter	Terminal or end	Tip of arm; e.g., pter or qter
/	Mosaicism	46,XY/47,XXY
+ or −	Sometimes used after a chromosome arm in text to indicate gain or loss of part of that chromosome	46,XX,5p−

reading 46,XY,t(2;4)(p23;q25) would indicate a male with a reciprocal translocation involving the short arm of chromosome 2 at region 2 band 3 and the long arm of chromosome 4 at region 2 band 5.

Cell Division

Mitosis

At conception the human zygote consists of a single cell. This undergoes rapid division, leading ultimately to the mature human adult consisting of approximately 1×10^{14} cells in total. In most organs and tissues, such as bone marrow and skin, cells continue to divide throughout life. This process of somatic cell division, during which the nucleus also divides, is known as **mitosis**. During mitosis each chromosome divides into two daughter chromosomes, one of which segregates into each daughter cell. Consequently, the number of chromosomes per nucleus remains unchanged.

Before a cell enters mitosis, each chromosome consists of two identical sister chromatids as a result of DNA replication having taken place during the S phase of the cell cycle (p. 32). Mitosis is the process whereby each of these pairs of chromatids separates and disperses into separate daughter cells.

Mitosis is a continuous process that usually lasts 1 to 2 hours, but for descriptive purposes it is convenient to distinguish five distinct stages. These are prophase, prometaphase, metaphase, anaphase and telophase (Fig. 3.11).

Prophase

During the initial stage of **prophase**, the chromosomes condense and the mitotic spindle begins to form. Two **centrioles** form in each cell, from which **microtubules** radiate as the centrioles move towards opposite poles of the cell.

Prometaphase

During **prometaphase** the nuclear membrane begins to disintegrate, allowing the chromosomes to spread around the cell. Each chromosome becomes attached at its centromere to a microtubule of the mitotic spindle.

Metaphase

In **metaphase** the chromosomes become aligned along the equatorial plane or plate of the cell, where each chromosome is attached to the centriole by a microtubule forming the mature spindle. At this point the chromosomes are maximally contracted and, therefore, most easily visible. Each chromosome resembles the letter X in shape, as the chromatids of each chromosome have separated longitudinally but remain attached at the centromere, which has not yet undergone division.

Anaphase

In **anaphase** the centromere of each chromosome divides longitudinally, and the two daughter chromatids separate to opposite poles of the cell.

Telophase

By **telophase** the chromatids, which are now independent chromosomes consisting of a single double helix, have separated completely, and the two groups of daughter chromosomes each become enveloped in a new nuclear membrane. The cell cytoplasm also separates (cytokinesis), resulting in the formation of two new daughter cells, each of which contains a complete diploid chromosome complement.

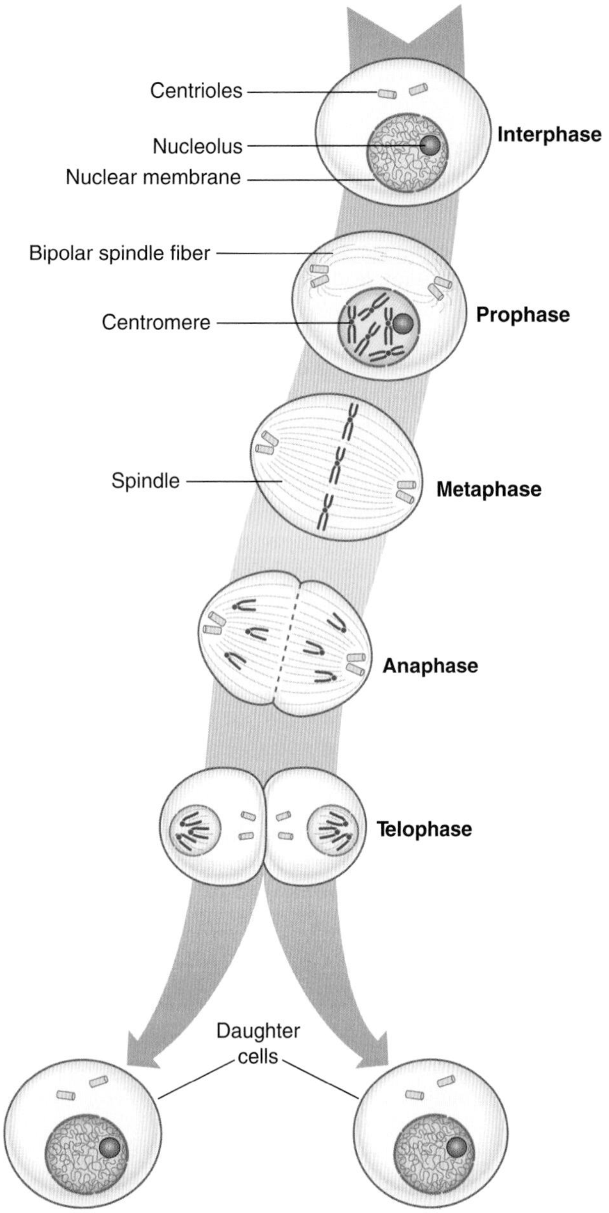

• **Fig. 3.11** Stages of mitosis.

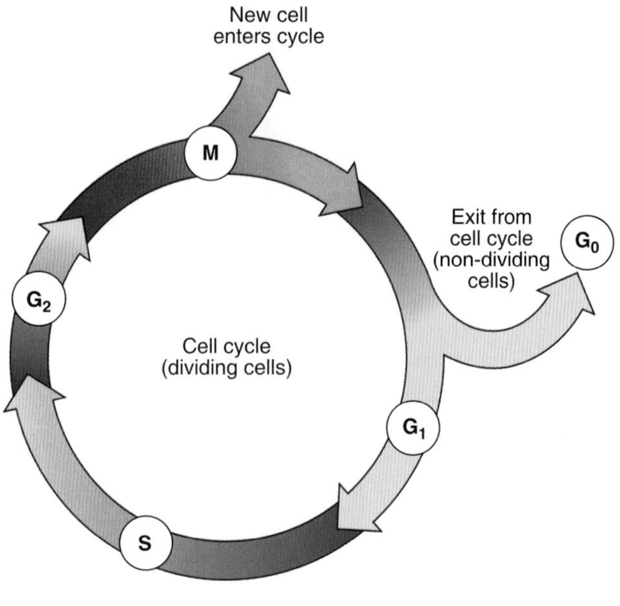

• **Fig. 3.12** Stages of the cell cycle. G1 and G2 are the first and second "resting" stages of interphase. *S* is the stage of DNA replication. *M*, mitosis.

The Cell Cycle

The period between successive mitoses is known as the **interphase** of the cell cycle (Fig. 3.12). In rapidly dividing cells this lasts for between 16 and 24 hours. Interphase commences with the G_1 (G = gap) phase during which the chromosomes become thin and extended. This phase of the cycle is very variable in length and is responsible for the variation in generation time between different cell populations. Cells that have stopped dividing, such as neurons, usually arrest in this phase and are said to have entered a non-cyclic stage known as G_0.

The G_1 phase is followed by the S phase (S = synthesis), when DNA replication occurs, and the chromatin of each chromosome is replicated. This results in the formation of two chromatids, giving each chromosome its characteristic X-shaped configuration. The process of DNA replication commences at multiple points on a chromosome (p. 11).

Homologous pairs of chromosomes usually replicate in synchrony. However, one of the X chromosomes is always late in replicating. This is the inactive X chromosome (p. 124) that forms the **sex chromatin** or so-called **Barr body**, which can be visualized during interphase in female somatic cells. This used to be the basis of a rather unsatisfactory means of sex determination based on analysis of cells obtained by scraping the buccal mucosa—a "buccal smear."

Interphase is completed by a relatively short G_2 phase during which the chromosomes begin to condense in preparation for the next mitotic division.

Meiosis

Meiosis is the process of nuclear division that occurs during the final stage of gamete formation. Meiosis differs from mitosis in three fundamental ways:

1. Mitosis results in each daughter cell having a diploid chromosome complement (46). During meiosis the diploid count is halved so that each mature gamete receives a haploid complement of 23 chromosomes.
2. Mitosis takes place in somatic cells and during the early cell divisions in gamete formation. Meiosis occurs only at the final division of gamete maturation.
3. Mitosis occurs as a one-step process. Meiosis can be considered as two cell divisions known as meiosis I and meiosis II, each of which can be considered as having prophase, metaphase, anaphase and telophase stages, as in mitosis (Fig. 3.13).

Meiosis I

This is sometimes referred to as the reduction division because it is during the first meiotic division that the chromosome number is halved.

Prophase I. Chromosomes enter this stage already split longitudinally into two chromatids joined at the centromere. Homologous chromosomes pair and, with the exception of the X and Y

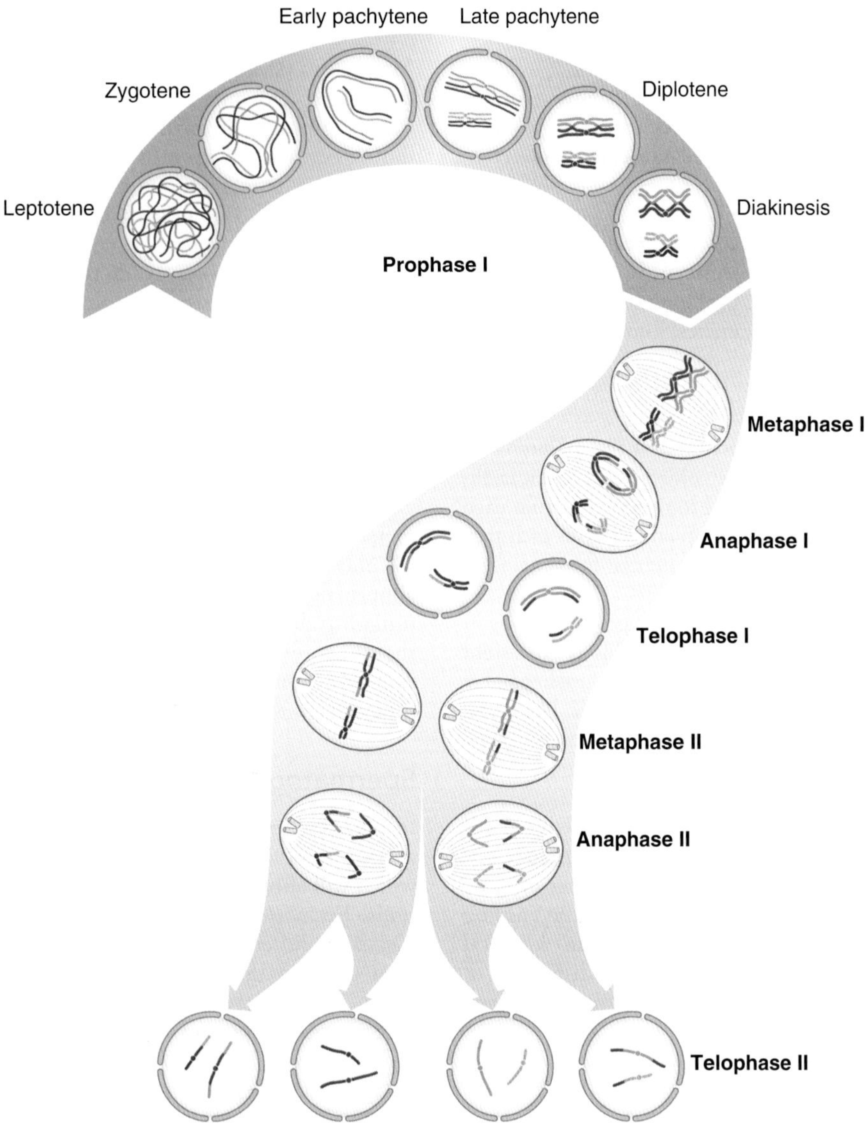

• **Fig. 3.13** Stages of meiosis.

chromosomes in male meiosis, exchange of homologous segments occurs between non-sister chromatids; that is, chromatids from each of the pair of homologous chromosomes. This exchange of homologous segments between chromatids occurs as a result of a process known as **crossing over** or **recombination**. The importance of crossing over in linkage analysis and risk calculation is considered later (pp. 45, 91).

During prophase I in the male, pairing occurs between homologous segments of the X and Y chromosomes at the tips of their short arms, with this portion of each chromosome being known as the **pseudoautosomal** region (p. 128).

The prophase stage of meiosis I is relatively lengthy and can be subdivided into five stages.

Leptotene: The chromosomes become visible as they start to condense.

Zygotene: Homologous chromosomes align directly opposite each other, a process known as synapsis, and are held together at several points along their length by filamentous structures known as synaptonemal complexes.

Pachytene: Each pair of homologous chromosomes, known as a bivalent, becomes tightly coiled. Crossing over occurs, during which homologous regions of DNA are exchanged between chromatids.

Diplotene: The homologous recombinant chromosomes now begin to separate but remain attached at the points where crossing over has occurred. These are known as chiasmata. On average, small, medium and large chromosomes have one, two and three chiasmata, respectively, giving an overall total of approximately 40 recombination events per meiosis per gamete.

Diakinesis: Separation of the homologous chromosome pairs proceeds as the chromosomes become maximally condensed.

Metaphase I. The nuclear membrane disappears, and the chromosomes become aligned on the equatorial plane of the cell where they have become attached to the spindle, as in metaphase of mitosis.

Anaphase I. The chromosomes now separate to opposite poles of the cell as the spindle contracts.

Telophase I. Each set of haploid chromosomes has now separated completely to opposite ends of the cell, which cleaves into two new daughter gametes, so-called **secondary spermatocytes** or **oocytes**.

Meiosis II

This is essentially the same as an ordinary mitotic division. Each chromosome, which exists as a pair of chromatids, becomes aligned along the equatorial plane and then splits longitudinally, leading to the formation of two new daughter gametes, known as spermatids or ova.

The Consequences of Meiosis

When considered in terms of reproduction and the maintenance of the species, meiosis achieves two major objectives. First, it facilitates halving of the diploid number of chromosomes so that each child receives half of its chromosome complement from each parent. Second, it provides an extraordinary potential for generating genetic diversity. This is achieved in two ways:

1. When the bivalents separate during prophase of meiosis I, they do so independently of one another. This is consistent with Mendel's third law (p. 3). Consequently, each gamete receives a selection of parental chromosomes. The likelihood that any two gametes from an individual will contain exactly the same chromosomes is 1 in 2^{23}, or approximately 1 in 8 million.
2. As a result of crossing over, each chromatid usually contains portions of DNA derived from both parental homologous chromosomes. A large chromosome typically consists of three or more segments of alternating parental origin. The ensuing probability that any two gametes will have an identical genome is therefore infinitesimally small. This dispersion of DNA into different gametes is sometimes referred to as **gene shuffling**.

Gametogenesis

The process of gametogenesis shows fundamental differences in males and females (Table 3.3). These have quite distinct clinical consequences if errors occur.

TABLE 3.3 Differences in gametogenesis in males and females

	Males	Females
Commences	Puberty	Early embryonic life
Duration	60–65 days	10–50 years
Numbers of mitoses in gamete formation	30–500	20–30
Gamete production per meiosis	4 spermatids	1 ovum + 3 polar bodies
Gamete production	100–200 million per ejaculate	1 ovum per menstrual cycle

Oogenesis

Mature ova develop from oogonia by a complex series of intermediate steps. Oogonia themselves originate from primordial germ cells by a process involving 20 to 30 mitotic divisions that occur during the first few months of embryonic life. By the completion of embryogenesis at 3 months of intrauterine life, the oogonia have begun to mature into primary oocytes that start to undergo meiosis. At birth, all of the primary oocytes have entered a phase of maturation arrest, known as **dictyotene**, in which they remain suspended until meiosis I is completed at the time of ovulation, when a single secondary oocyte is formed. This receives most of the cytoplasm. The other daughter cell from the first meiotic division consists largely of a nucleus and is known as a polar body. Meiosis II then commences, during which fertilization can occur. This second meiotic division results in the formation of a further polar body (Fig. 3.14).

It is probable that the very lengthy interval between the onset of meiosis and its eventual completion, up to 50 years later, accounts for the well-documented increased incidence of chromosome abnormalities in the offspring of older mothers (p. 36). The accumulating effects of "wear and tear" on the primary oocyte during the dictyotene phase probably damage the cell's spindle formation and repair mechanisms, thereby predisposing to nondisjunction (p. 35).

Spermatogenesis

In contrast, spermatogenesis is a relatively rapid process with an average duration of 60 to 65 days. At puberty, spermatogonia, which will already have undergone approximately 30 mitotic divisions, begin to mature into primary spermatocytes which enter meiosis I and emerge as haploid secondary spermatocytes. These then undergo the second meiotic division to form spermatids, which in turn develop without any subsequent cell division into mature spermatozoa, of which 100 to 200 million are present in each ejaculate.

Spermatogenesis is a continuous process involving many mitotic divisions, possibly as many as 20 to 25 per annum, so that mature spermatozoa produced by a man 50 years of age or older could well have undergone several hundred mitotic divisions. The observed paternal age effect for new dominant mutations (p. 70) is consistent with the concept that many mutations arise as a consequence of DNA copy errors occurring during mitosis.

Chromosome Abnormalities

Specific disorders caused by chromosome abnormalities are considered in Chapter 17. In this section, discussion is restricted to a review of the different types of abnormalities that may occur. These can be divided into numerical and structural, with a third category consisting of different chromosome constitutions in two or more cell lines (Box 3.1).

Numerical Abnormalities

Numerical abnormalities involve the loss or gain of one or more chromosomes, referred to as **aneuploidy**, or the addition of one or more complete haploid complements, known as **polyploidy**. Loss of a single chromosome results in **monosomy**. Gain of one or two homologous chromosomes is referred to as **trisomy** or **tetrasomy**, respectively.

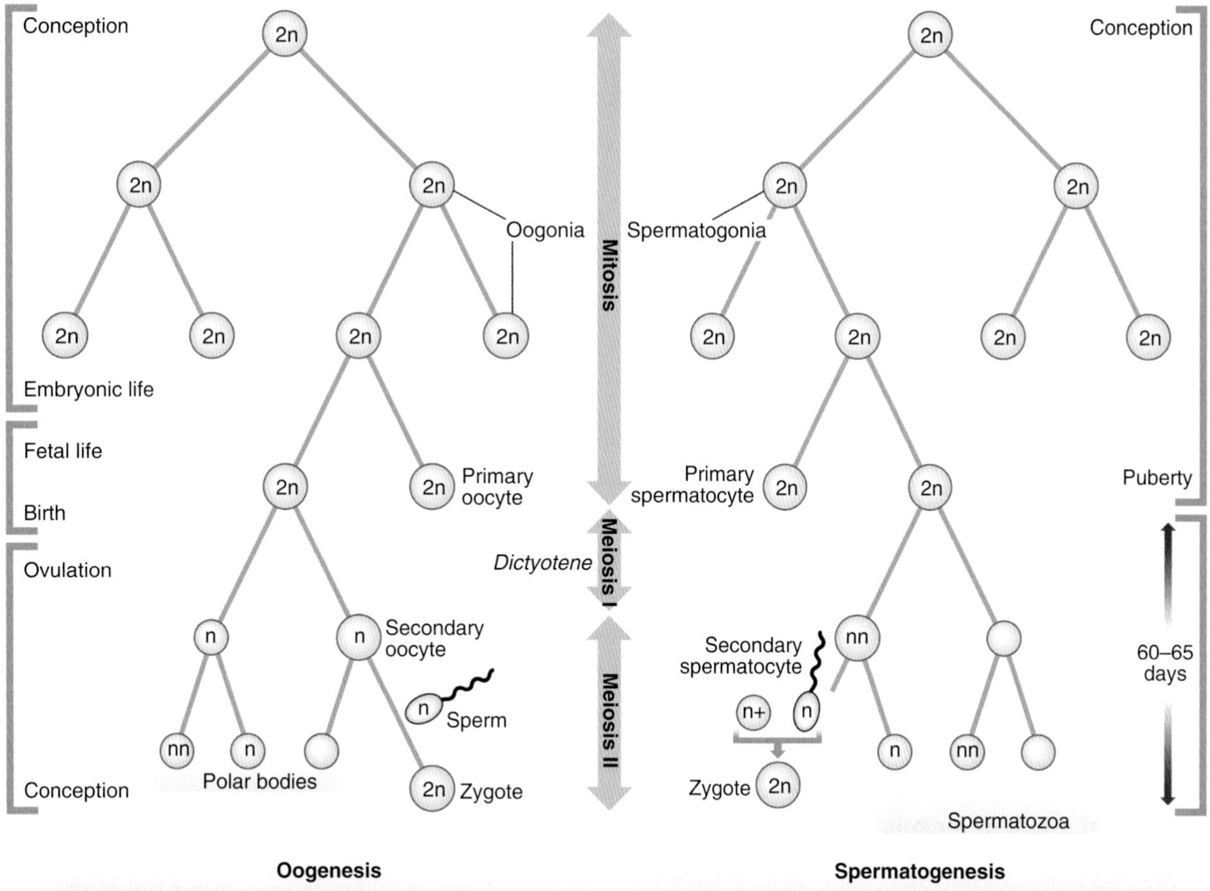

• **Fig. 3.14** Stages of oogenesis and spermatogenesis. *n*, haploid number.

• BOX 3.1 Types of Chromosome Abnormality

Numerical
Aneuploidy
Monosomy
Trisomy
Tetrasomy
Polyploidy
Triploidy
Tetraploidy

Structural
Translocations
Reciprocal
Robertsonian
Deletions
Insertions
Inversions
Paracentric
Pericentric
Rings
Isochromosomes

Different Cell Lines (Mixoploidy)
Mosaicism
Chimerism

Trisomy

The presence of an extra chromosome is referred to as **trisomy**. Most cases of Down syndrome are caused by the presence of an additional number 21 chromosome; hence, Down syndrome is often known as trisomy 21. Other autosomal trisomies compatible with survival to term are Patau syndrome (trisomy 13, p. 253) and Edwards syndrome (trisomy 18, p. 253). Most other autosomal trisomies result in early pregnancy loss, with trisomy 16 being a particularly common finding in first-trimester spontaneous miscarriages. The presence of an additional sex chromosome (X or Y) has only mild phenotypic effects (p. 254).

Trisomy 21 is usually caused by failure of separation of one of the pairs of homologous chromosomes during anaphase of maternal meiosis I. This failure of the bivalent to separate is called **nondisjunction**. Less often, trisomy can be caused by nondisjunction occurring during meiosis II when a pair of sister chromatids fails to separate. Either way the gamete receives two homologous chromosomes (**disomy**); if subsequent fertilization occurs, a trisomic conceptus results (Fig. 3.15).

The Origin of Nondisjunction. The consequences of nondisjunction in meiosis I and meiosis II differ in the chromosomes found in the gamete. An error in meiosis I leads to the gamete containing both homologs of one chromosome pair. In contrast, nondisjunction in meiosis II results in the gamete receiving two copies of one

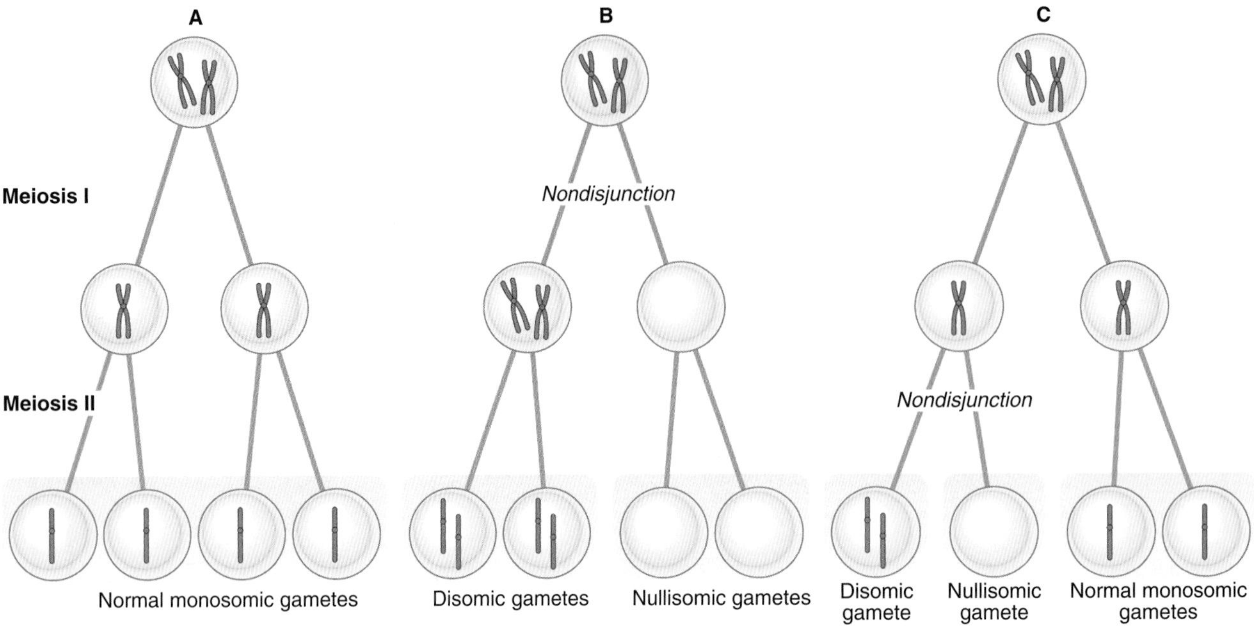

• **Fig. 3.15** Segregation at meiosis of a single pair of chromosomes in (A) normal meiosis, (B) nondisjunction in meiosis I, and (C) nondisjunction in meiosis II.

TABLE 3.4 Parental origin of meiotic error leading to aneuploidy

Chromosome Abnormality	Paternal (%)	Maternal (%)
Trisomy 13	15	85
Trisomy 18	10	90
Trisomy 21	5	95
45,X	80	20
47,XXX	5	95
47,XXY	45	55
47,XYY	100	0

of the homologs of the chromosome pair. Studies using DNA markers have shown that most children with an autosomal trisomy have inherited their additional chromosome as a result of nondisjunction occurring during one of the maternal meiotic divisions (Table 3.4).

Nondisjunction can also occur during an early mitotic division in the developing zygote. This results in the presence of two or more different cell lines, a phenomenon known as **mosaicism** (pp. 42, 77).

The Cause of Nondisjunction. The cause of nondisjunction is uncertain. The most favored explanation is that of an aging effect on the primary oocyte, which can remain in a state of suspended inactivity for up to 50 years (p. 34). This is based on the well-documented association between advancing maternal age and increased incidence of Down syndrome in offspring (see Table 17.4; see p. 251). A maternal age effect has also been noted for trisomies 13 and 18.

It is not known how or why advancing maternal age predisposes to nondisjunction, although research has shown that absence of recombination in prophase of meiosis I predisposes to subsequent nondisjunction. This is not surprising because the chiasmata that are formed after recombination are responsible for holding each pair of homologous chromosomes together until subsequent separation occurs in diakinesis. Thus failure of chiasmata formation could allow each pair of homologs to separate prematurely and then segregate randomly to daughter cells. In the female, however, recombination occurs before birth, whereas the nondisjunctional event occurs any time between 15 and 50 years later. This suggests that at least two factors can be involved in causing nondisjunction: an absence of recombination between homologous chromosomes in the fetal ovary, and an abnormality in spindle formation many years later.

Monosomy

The absence of a single chromosome is referred to as **monosomy**. Monosomy for an autosome is almost always incompatible with survival to term. Lack of contribution of an X or a Y chromosome results in a 45,X karyotype, which causes the condition known as Turner syndrome (p. 254).

As with trisomy, monosomy can result from nondisjunction in meiosis. If one gamete receives two copies of a homologous chromosome (**disomy**), the other corresponding daughter gamete will have no copy of the same chromosome (**nullisomy**). Monosomy can also be caused by loss of a chromosome as it moves to the pole of the cell during anaphase, an event known as **anaphase lag**.

Polyploidy

Polyploid cells contain multiples of the haploid number of chromosomes, such as 69, **triploidy**, or 92, **tetraploidy**. In humans, triploidy is found relatively often in material grown from

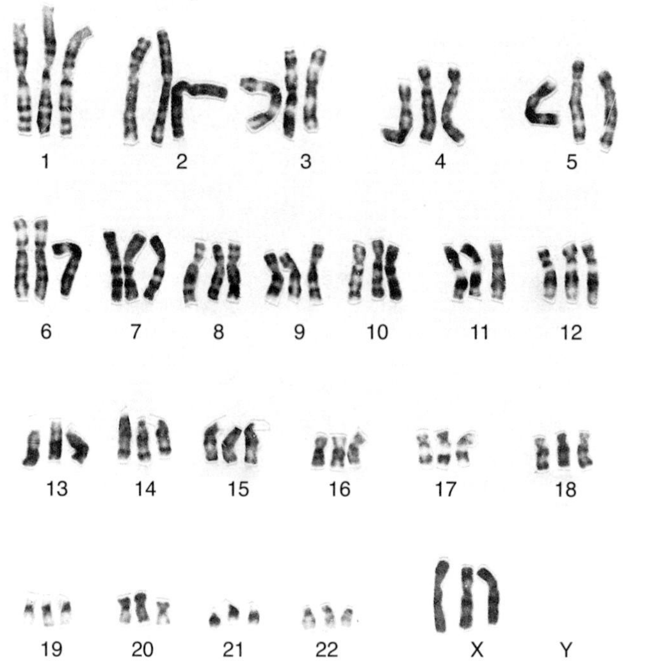

• **Fig. 3.16** Karyotype from products of conception of a spontaneous miscarriage showing triploidy.

spontaneous miscarriages, but survival beyond midpregnancy is rare. Only a few triploid live births have been described, and all died soon after birth.

Triploidy can be caused by failure of a maturation meiotic division in an ovum or sperm, leading, for example, to retention of a polar body or formation of a diploid sperm. Alternatively, it can be caused by fertilization of an ovum by two sperm: this is known as **dispermy**. When triploidy results from the presence of an additional set of paternal chromosomes, the placenta is usually swollen with what are known as hydatidiform changes (p. 122). In contrast, when triploidy results from an additional set of maternal chromosomes, the placenta is usually small. Triploidy usually results in early spontaneous miscarriage (Fig. 3.16). The differences between triploidy resulting from an additional set of **paternal** chromosomes or **maternal** chromosomes provide evidence for important "epigenetic" and "parent of origin" effects with respect to the human genome. These are discussed in more detail in Chapter 6.

Structural Abnormalities

Structural chromosome rearrangements result from chromosome breakage with subsequent reunion in a different configuration. They can be balanced or unbalanced. In balanced rearrangements the chromosome complement is complete, with no loss or gain of genetic material. Consequently, balanced rearrangements are generally harmless, with the exception of rare cases in which one of the breakpoints damages an important functional gene. However, carriers of balanced rearrangements are often at risk of producing children with an unbalanced chromosomal complement.

When a chromosome rearrangement is unbalanced, the chromosomal complement contains an incorrect amount of chromosome material, and the clinical effects are usually serious.

Translocations

A **translocation** refers to the transfer of genetic material from one chromosome to another. A reciprocal translocation is formed when a break occurs in each of two chromosomes with the segments being exchanged to form two new derivative chromosomes. A Robertsonian translocation is a particular type of reciprocal translocation in which the breakpoints are located at, or close to, the centromeres of two acrocentric chromosomes (Fig. 3.17).

Reciprocal Translocations. A reciprocal translocation involves breakage of at least two chromosomes with exchange of the fragments. Usually the chromosome number remains at 46 and, if the exchanged fragments are of roughly equal size, a reciprocal translocation can be identified only by detailed chromosomal banding studies or FISH (see Fig. 3.9). In general, reciprocal translocations are unique to a particular family, although, for reasons that are unknown, a particular balanced reciprocal translocation involving the long arms of chromosomes 11 and 22 is relatively common. The overall incidence of reciprocal translocations in the general population is approximately 1 in 500.

Segregation at Meiosis. The importance of balanced reciprocal translocations lies in their behavior at meiosis, when they can segregate to generate significant chromosome imbalance. This can lead to early pregnancy loss or to the birth of an infant with multiple abnormalities. Problems arise at meiosis because the chromosomes involved in the translocation cannot pair normally to form bivalents. Instead they form a cluster known as a pachytene quadrivalent (Fig. 3.18). The key point to note is that each chromosome aligns with homologous material in the quadrivalent.

2:2 Segregation. When the constituent chromosomes in the quadrivalent separate during the later stages of meiosis I, they can do so in several different ways (Table 3.5). If alternate chromosomes segregate to each gamete, the gamete will carry a normal or balanced haploid complement (Fig. 3.19), and with fertilization

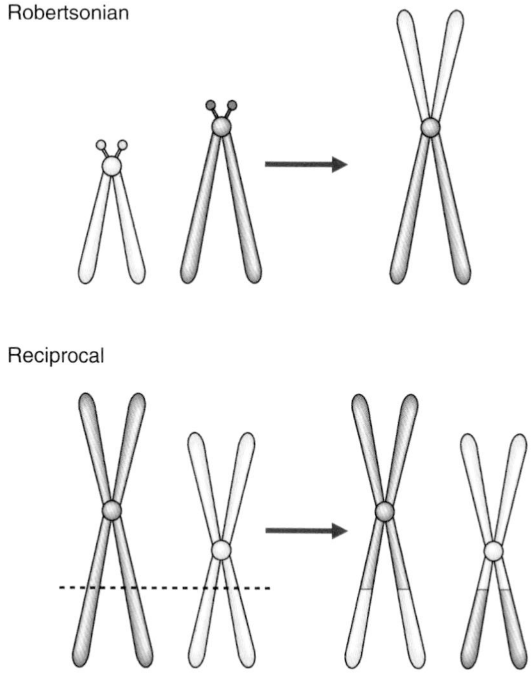

• **Fig. 3.17** Types of translocation.

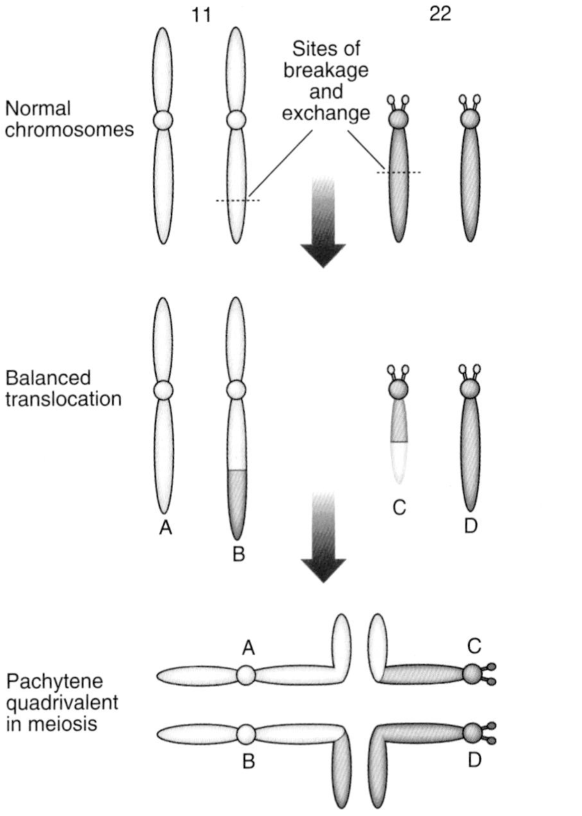

• **Fig. 3.18** How a balanced reciprocal translocation involving chromosomes 11 and 22 leads to the formation of a quadrivalent at pachytene in meiosis I. The quadrivalent is formed to maintain homologous pairing.

TABLE 3.5 Patterns of segregation of a reciprocal translocation

Pattern of Segregation	Segregating Chromosomes	Chromosome Constitution in Gamete
2:2		
Alternate	A + D	Normal
	B + C	Balanced translocation
Adjacent-1 (non-homologous centromeres segregate together)	A + C or B + D	Unbalanced, leading to a combination of partial monosomy and partial trisomy in the zygote
Adjacent-2 (homologous centromeres segregate together)	A + B or C + D	
3:1		
Three chromosomes	A + B + C A + B + D A + C + D B + C + D	Unbalanced, leading to trisomy in the zygote
One chromosome	A B C D	Unbalanced, leading to monosomy in the zygote

(See Fig. 3.18 and Fig. 3.19)

the embryo will either have normal chromosomes or carry the balanced rearrangement. If, however, adjacent chromosomes segregate together, this will invariably result in the gamete acquiring an unbalanced chromosome complement. For example, in Fig. 3.18, if the gamete inherits the normal number 11 chromosome (A) and the derivative number 22 chromosome (C), then fertilization will result in an embryo with monosomy for the distal long arm of chromosome 22 and trisomy for the distal long arm of chromosome 11.

3:1 Segregation. Another possibility is that three chromosomes segregate to one gamete with only one chromosome in the other gamete. If, for example, in Fig. 3.18 chromosomes 11 (A), 22 (D) and the derivative 22 (C) segregate together to a gamete that is subsequently fertilized, this will result in the embryo being trisomic for the material present in the derivative 22 chromosome. This is sometimes referred to as **tertiary trisomy**. Experience has shown that, with this particular reciprocal translocation, tertiary trisomy for the derivative 22 chromosome is the only viable unbalanced product. All other patterns of malsegregation lead to early pregnancy loss. Unfortunately, tertiary trisomy for the derivative 22 chromosome is a serious condition in which affected children have multiple congenital abnormalities and severe learning difficulties.

Risks in Reciprocal Translocations. When counseling a carrier of a balanced translocation, it is necessary to consider the particular rearrangement to determine whether it could result in the birth of an abnormal baby. This risk is usually somewhere between 1% and 10%. For carriers of the 11;22 translocation discussed, the risk has been shown to be 5%.

Robertsonian Translocations. A Robertsonian translocation results from the breakage of two acrocentric chromosomes (numbers 13, 14, 15, 21 and 22) at or close to their centromeres, with subsequent fusion of their long arms (see Fig. 3.17). This is also referred to as **centric fusion**. The short arms of each chromosome are lost, this being of no clinical importance as they contain genes only for ribosomal RNA, for which there are multiple copies on the various other acrocentric chromosomes. The total chromosome number is reduced to 45. Because there is no loss or gain of important genetic material, this is a functionally balanced rearrangement. The overall incidence of Robertsonian translocations in the general population is approximately 1 in 1000, with by far the most common being fusion of the long arms of chromosomes 13 and 14 (13q14q).

Segregation at Meiosis. As with reciprocal translocations, the importance of Robertsonian translocations lies in their behavior at meiosis. For example, a carrier of a 14q21q translocation can produce gametes with (Fig. 3.20):

1. A normal chromosome complement (i.e., a normal 14 and a normal 21).
2. A balanced chromosome complement (i.e., a 14q21q translocation chromosome).
3. An unbalanced chromosome complement possessing both the translocation chromosome and a normal 21. This will result in the fertilized embryo having Down syndrome.
4. An unbalanced chromosome complement with a normal 14 and a missing 21.

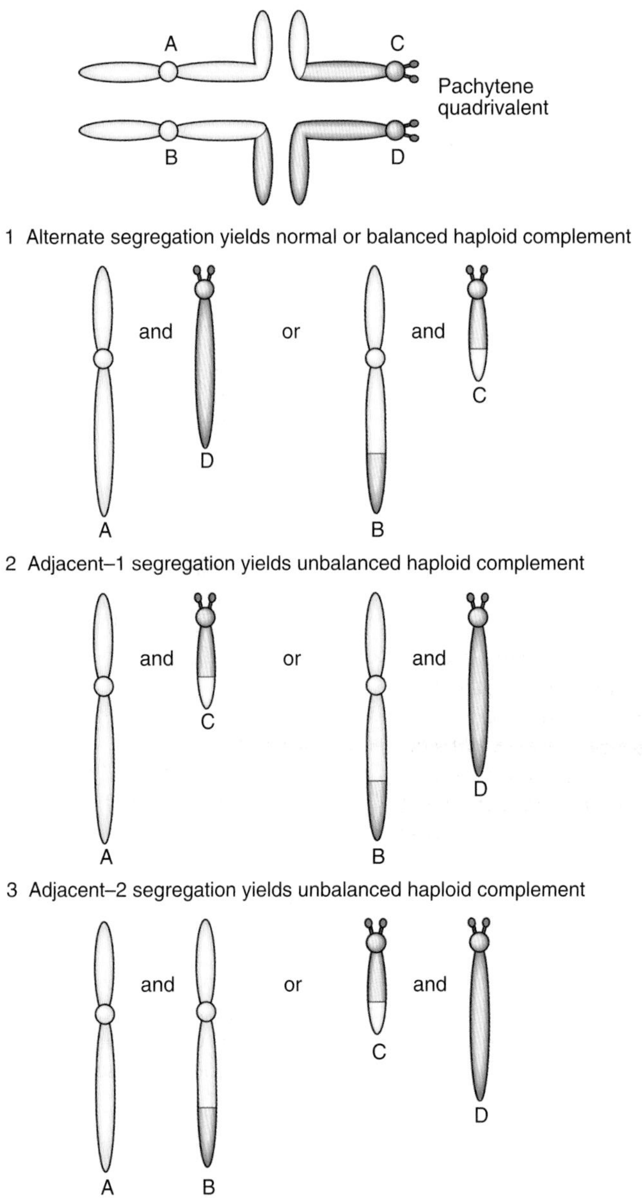

• **Fig. 3.19** The different patterns of segregation that can occur from the quadrivalent shown in Fig. 3.18. (See Table 3.5.)

5. An unbalanced chromosome complement with a normal 21 and a missing 14.
6. An unbalanced chromosome complement with the translocation chromosome and a normal 14 chromosome.

The last three combinations will result in zygotes with monosomy 21, monosomy 14, and trisomy 14, respectively. All of these combinations are incompatible with survival beyond early pregnancy.

Translocation Down Syndrome. The major practical importance of Robertsonian translocations is that they can predispose to the birth of babies with Down syndrome as a result of the embryo inheriting two normal number 21 chromosomes (one from each parent) plus a translocation chromosome involving a number 21 chromosome (Fig. 3.21). Translocation Down syndrome accounts for 2% to 3% of cases, and the clinical consequences are exactly the same as those seen in pure trisomy 21. However, unlike trisomy 21, the parents of a child with translocation Down syndrome have a relatively high risk of having further affected children if one of them carries the rearrangement in a balanced form.

Consequently, the importance of performing a chromosome analysis in a child with Down syndrome lies not only in confirmation of the diagnosis, but also in identification of those children with a translocation. In roughly two-thirds of these latter children with Down syndrome, the translocation will have occurred as a new (*de novo*) event in the child, but in the remaining one-third one of the parents will be a carrier. Other relatives might also be carriers. Therefore it is regarded as essential that efforts are made to identify all adult translocation carriers in a family so that they can be alerted to possible risks to future offspring. This is sometimes referred to as translocation **tracing**, or "chasing."

Risks in Robertsonian Translocations. Studies have shown that the female carrier of either a 13q21q or a 14q21q Robertsonian translocation runs a risk of approximately 10% for having a baby with Down syndrome, whereas for male carriers the risk is 1% to 3%. It is worth sparing a thought for the unfortunate carrier of a 21q21q Robertsonian translocation. All gametes will be either nullisomic or disomic for chromosome 21. Consequently, all pregnancies will end either in spontaneous miscarriage or in the birth of a child with Down syndrome. This is one of the very rare situations in which offspring are at a risk of greater than 50% for having an abnormality. Other examples are parents who are both heterozygous for the same autosomal dominant disorder (p. 67) and parents who are both homozygous for the same gene mutation causing an autosomal recessive disorder (p. 71), such as sensorineural deafness.

Deletions

A **deletion** involves loss of part of a chromosome and results in monosomy for that segment of the chromosome. A very large deletion is usually incompatible with survival to term, and as a general rule any deletion resulting in loss of more than 2% of the total haploid genome will have a lethal outcome.

Deletions are now recognized as existing at two levels. A "large" chromosomal deletion can be visualized under the light microscope. Such deletion syndromes include Wolf-Hirschhorn and cri du chat, which involve loss of material from the short arms of chromosomes 4 and 5, respectively (p. 258). Submicroscopic microdeletions were identified with the help of high-resolution prometaphase cytogenetics augmented by FISH studies and include Prader-Willi and Angelman syndromes (p. 78).

Insertions

An **insertion** occurs when a segment of one chromosome becomes inserted into another chromosome. If the inserted material has moved from elsewhere in another chromosome then the karyotype is balanced. Otherwise an insertion causes an unbalanced chromosome complement. Carriers of a balanced deletion–insertion rearrangement are at a 50% risk of producing unbalanced gametes, as random chromosome segregation at meiosis will result in 50% of the gametes inheriting either the deletion or the insertion, but not both.

Inversions

An inversion is a two-break rearrangement involving a single chromosome in which a segment is reversed in position (i.e., inverted). If the inversion segment involves the centromere, it is termed a **pericentric inversion** (Fig. 3.22A). If it involves only one arm of the chromosome, it is known as a **paracentric inversion** (Fig. 3.22B).

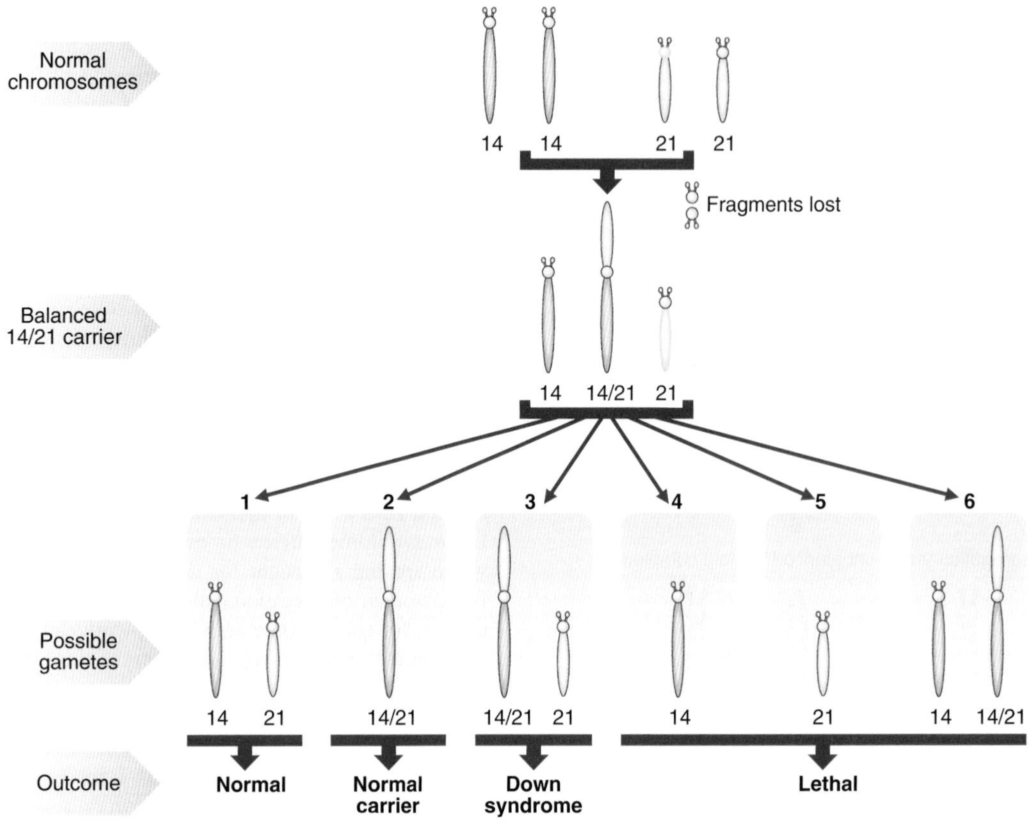

• **Fig. 3.20** Formation of a 14q21q Robertsonian translocation and the possible gamete chromosome patterns that can be produced at meiosis.

Inversions are balanced rearrangements that rarely cause problems in carriers unless one of the breakpoints has disrupted an important gene. A pericentric inversion involving chromosome number 9 occurs as a common structural variant or polymorphism, also known as a **heteromorphism**, and is not thought to be of any functional importance. However, other inversions, although not causing any clinical problems in balanced carriers, can lead to significant chromosome imbalance in offspring, with important clinical consequences.

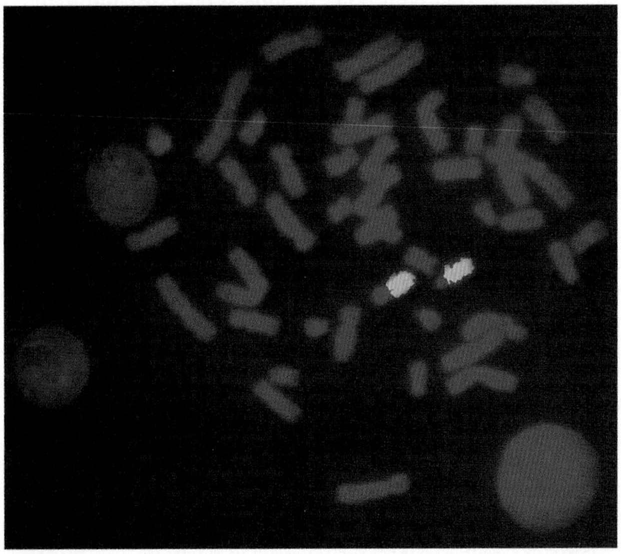

• **Fig. 3.21** Chromosome painting showing a 14q21q Robertsonian translocation in a child with Down syndrome. Chromosome 21 is shown in *blue* and chromosome 14 in *yellow*. (Courtesy Ms M Heath, City Hospital, Nottingham, UK.)

Segregation at Meiosis

Pericentric Inversions. An individual who carries a pericentric inversion can produce unbalanced gametes if a crossover occurs within the inversion segment during meiosis I, when an inversion loop forms as the chromosomes attempt to maintain homologous pairing at synapsis. For a pericentric inversion, a crossover within the loop will result in two complementary recombinant chromosomes, one with duplication of the distal non-inverted segment and deletion of the other end of the chromosome, and the other having the opposite arrangement (Fig. 3.23A).

If a pericentric inversion involves only a small proportion of the total length of a chromosome then, in the event of crossing over within the loop, the duplicated and deleted segments will be relatively large. The larger these are, the more likely it is that their effects on the embryo will be so severe that miscarriage ensues. For a large pericentric inversion, the duplicated and deleted segments will be relatively small, so that survival to term and beyond becomes more likely. Thus, in general, the larger the size of a pericentric inversion the more likely it becomes that it will result in the birth of an abnormal infant.

The pooled results of several studies have shown that a carrier of a balanced pericentric inversion runs a risk of approximately 5% to 10% for having a child with viable imbalance if that inversion has already resulted in the birth of an abnormal baby. The risk is nearer

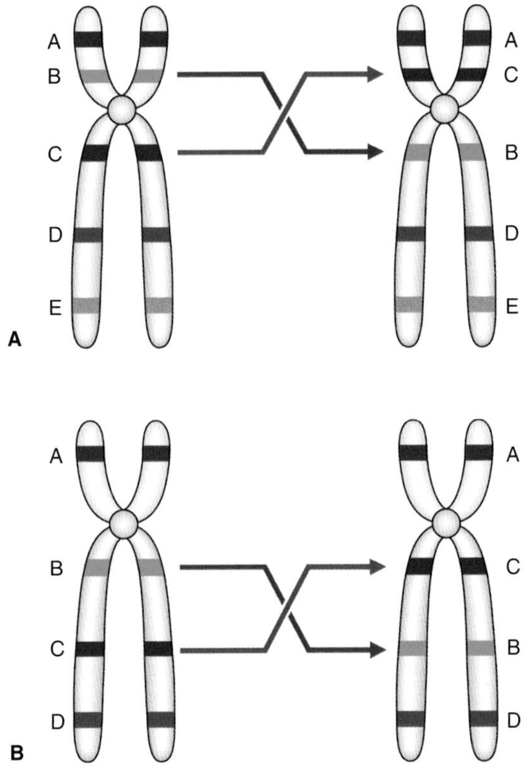

• **Fig. 3.22** (A) Pericentric and (B) paracentric inversions. (Courtesy Dr J Delhanty, Galton Laboratory, London.)

1% if the inversion has been ascertained because of a history of recurrent miscarriage.

Paracentric Inversions. If a crossover occurs in the inverted segment of a paracentric inversion, this will result in recombinant chromosomes that are either acentric or dicentric (Fig. 3.23B). Acentric chromosomes, which strictly speaking should be known as chromosomal fragments, cannot undergo mitotic division, so that survival of an embryo with such a rearrangement is extremely uncommon. Dicentric chromosomes are inherently unstable during cell division and are, therefore, also unlikely to be compatible with survival of the embryo. Thus overall, the likelihood that a balanced parental paracentric inversion will result in the birth of an abnormal baby is extremely low.

Ring Chromosomes

A **ring chromosome** is formed when a break occurs on each arm of a chromosome leaving two "sticky" ends on the central portion that reunite as a ring (Fig. 3.24). The two distal chromosomal fragments are lost, so that, if the involved chromosome is an autosome, the effects are usually serious.

Ring chromosomes are often unstable in mitosis, so that it is common to find a ring chromosome in only a proportion of cells. The other cells in the individual are usually monosomic because of the absence of the ring chromosome.

Isochromosomes. An isochromosome shows loss of one arm with duplication of the other. The most probable explanation for the formation of an isochromosome is that the centromere has divided transversely rather than longitudinally. The most commonly encountered isochromosome is that which consists of two long

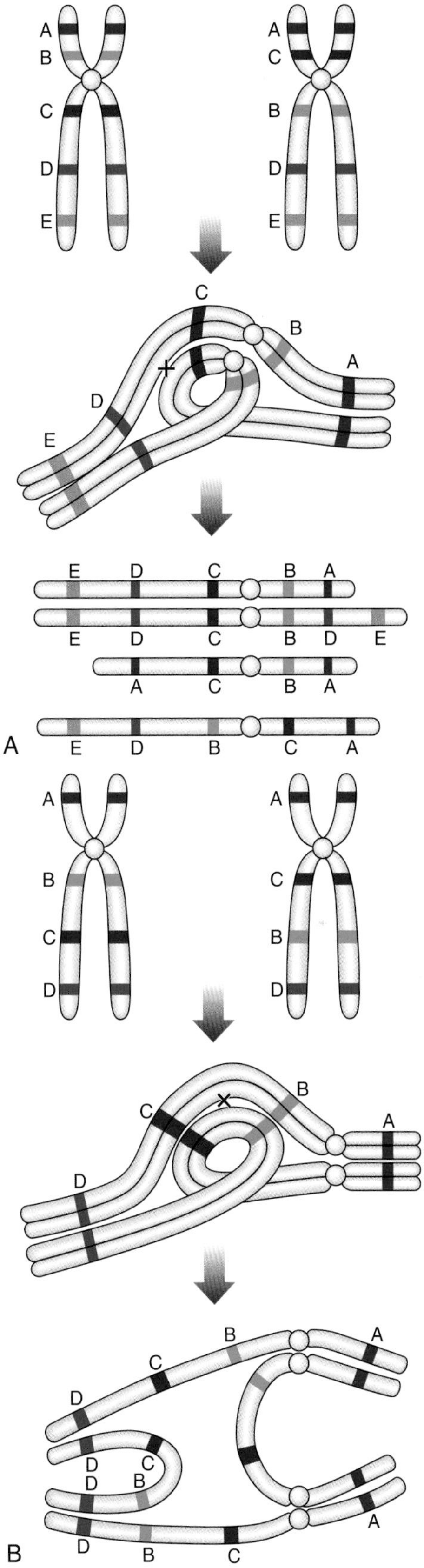

• **Fig. 3.23** Mechanism of production of recombinant unbalanced chromosomes from (A) pericentric and (B) paracentric inversions by crossing over in an inversion loop. (Courtesy Dr J Delhanty, Galton Laboratory, London.)

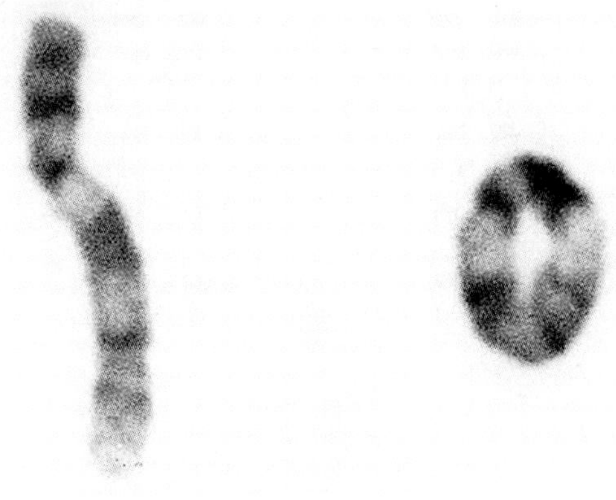

• **Fig. 3.24** Partial karyotype showing a ring chromosome 9. (Courtesy Ms M Heath, City Hospital, Nottingham.)

arms of the X chromosome. This accounts for up to 15% of all cases of Turner syndrome (p. 254).

Mosaicism and Chimerism (Mixoploidy)

Mosaicism

Mosaicism can be defined as the presence in an individual, or in a tissue, of two or more cell lines that differ in their genetic constitution but are derived from a single zygote; that is, they have the same genetic origin. Chromosome mosaicism usually results from nondisjunction in an early embryonic mitotic division with the persistence of more than one cell line. If, for example, the two chromatids of a number 21 chromosome failed to separate at the second mitotic division in a human zygote (Fig. 3.25), this would result in the four-cell zygote having two cells with 46 chromosomes, one cell with 47 chromosomes (trisomy 21) and one cell with 45 chromosomes (monosomy 21). The ensuing cell line with 45 chromosomes would probably not survive, so that the resulting embryo would be expected to show approximately 33% mosaicism for trisomy 21. Mosaicism accounts for 1% to 2% of all clinically recognized cases of Down syndrome.

Mosaicism can also exist at a molecular level if a new mutation arises in a somatic or early germline cell division (p. 77). The possibility of germline or gonadal mosaicism is a particular concern when counseling the parents of a child in whom a condition such as Duchenne muscular dystrophy (p. 299) is an isolated case.

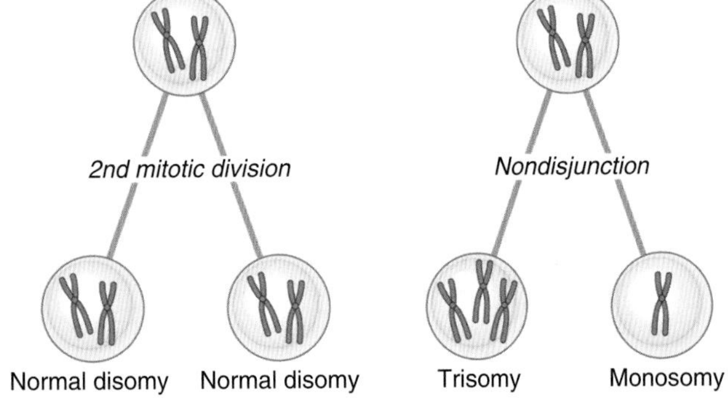

• **Fig. 3.25** Generation of somatic mosaicism caused by mitotic nondisjunction.

Chimerism

Chimerism can be defined as the presence in an individual of two or more genetically distinct cell lines derived from more than one zygote; that is, they have a different genetic origin. The word *chimera* is derived from the mythological Greek monster that had the head of a lion, the body of a goat and the tail of a dragon. Human chimeras are of two kinds: dispermic chimeras and blood chimeras.

Dispermic Chimeras. These are the result of double fertilization whereby two genetically different sperm fertilize two ova and the resulting two zygotes fuse to form one embryo. If the two zygotes are of different sex, the chimeric embryo can develop into an individual with a disorder of sex development (p. 127) and an XX/XY karyotype. Mouse chimeras of this type can now be produced experimentally in the laboratory to facilitate the study of gene transfer.

Blood Chimeras. Blood chimeras result from an exchange of cells, via the placenta, between non-identical twins *in utero*. For example, 90% of one twin's cells can have an XY karyotype with red blood cells showing predominantly blood group B, whereas 90% of the cells of the other twin can have an XX karyotype with red blood cells showing predominantly blood group A. It has long been recognized that, when twin calves of opposite sex are born, the female can have ambiguous genitalia. This is because the female calf, known as a **freemartin**, has acquired the XY component *in utero* via vascular connections between the placentas and becomes masculinised through exposure to male hormones.

ELEMENTS

1. The normal human karyotype is made up of 46 chromosomes consisting of 22 pairs of autosomes and one pair of sex chromosomes, XX in the female and XY in the male.
2. Each chromosome consists of a short (p) and long (q) arm joined at the centromere. Chromosomes are analyzed using cultured cells, and specific banding patterns can be identified by staining techniques. Fluorescence *in situ* hybridization (FISH) can be used to detect and characterize subtle chromosome abnormalities.
3. During mitosis in somatic cell division the two sister chromatids of each chromosome separate, with one chromatid passing to each daughter cell. During meiosis, which occurs during the final stage of gametogenesis, homologous chromosomes pair, exchange segments and then segregate independently to the mature daughter gametes.
4. Chromosome abnormalities can be structural or numerical. Numerical abnormalities include trisomy and polyploidy. In trisomy a single extra chromosome is present, usually as a result of nondisjunction in the first or second meiotic division. In polyploidy, three or more complete haploid sets are present instead of the usual diploid complement.
5. Structural abnormalities include translocations, inversions, insertions, rings, and deletions. Translocations can be balanced or unbalanced. Carriers of balanced translocations are at risk of having children with unbalanced rearrangements; these children are often severely affected.

Further Reading

Gardner RJM, Amor DJ. *Cytogenetic Abnormalities and Genetic Counselling*. 5th ed. Oxford: Oxford University Press; 2018.

A richly illustrated resource, combining basic concepts of chromosomal analysis with practical applications of recent advances in molecular cytogenetics.

Gersen SL, Keagle MB, eds. *The Principles of Clinical Cytogenetics*. 3rd ed. Totowa, NJ: Humana Press; 2013.

A detailed multiauthor guide to all aspects of laboratory and clinical cytogenetics.

McGowan-Jordan J, Simons A, Schmid M, eds. *An International System for Human Cytogenomic Nomenclature*. Basel, Switzerland: Karger; 2016.

An indispensable reference guide giving details of how chromosome abnormalities should be described.

Speicher MR, Carter NP. The new cytogenetics: blurring the boundaries with molecular biology. *Nat Rev Genet.* 2006;6:782–792.

A review of molecular cytogenetic techniques.

Tjio JH, Levan A. The chromosome number of man. *Hereditas.* 1956;42:1–6.

A landmark paper that described a reliable method for studying human chromosomes and gave birth to the subject of clinical cytogenetics.

4

Finding the Cause of Monogenic Disorders by Identifying Disease Genes

A disease or disorder is defined as **rare** in Europe when it affects less than 1 in 2000 people. In the United States the definition is that fewer than 200,000 Americans are affected at any given time. It is estimated that there are more than 6000 rare disorders, which means that, collectively, these rare diseases are not uncommon, and they affect up to 1 in 17 of the European population. More than 80% have a genetic basis, whereas others result from infections, allergies and environmental causes, or are degenerative and proliferative.

Identification of the gene associated with an inherited single-gene (**monogenic**) disorder, as well as having immediate clinical diagnostic application, will enable an understanding of the developmental basis of the pathology with the prospect of possible therapeutic interventions. The molecular basis for more than 5000 disease phenotypes is now known, and the rate at which single-gene disorder genes are being identified continues to increase exponentially.

The first human disease genes identified were those with a biochemical basis where it was possible to purify and sequence the gene product. The development of recombinant DNA techniques in the 1980s enabled physical mapping strategies and led to a new approach, positional cloning. This describes the identification of a gene purely on the basis of its location, without any prior knowledge of its function. Notable early successes were the identification of the gene encoding dystrophin (mutated in Duchenne muscular dystrophy) and the gene encoding the cystic fibrosis transmembrane conductance regulator (CFTR) protein. Patients with chromosome abnormalities or rearrangements have often provided important clues by highlighting the likely chromosomal region of a gene associated with disease (Table 4.1).

In the 1990s, a genome-wide set of microsatellites was constructed with approximately one marker per 10 centimorgans (cM). These 350 markers could be amplified by polymerase chain reaction and facilitated genetic mapping studies that led to the identification of thousands of genes. This approach was superseded by DNA microarrays or "single nucleotide polymorphism (SNP) chips." Although SNPs (p. 52) are less informative than microsatellites (p. 14), they can be scored automatically, and microarrays are commercially available with several million SNPs distributed throughout the genome.

The common step for all approaches to identify human disease genes is the identification of a candidate gene (Fig. 4.1). Candidate genes may be suggested from animal models of disease or by **homology**, either to a **paralogous** human gene (e.g., where multigene families exist) or to an **orthologous** gene in another species. With the sequencing of the human genome now complete, it is also possible to find new disease genes by searching through genetic databases (i.e., *in silico*).

Recent developments in sequencing technology mean that **exome** sequencing (analysis of the coding regions of all known genes) or **whole-genome** sequencing are now feasible strategies for identifying disease genes by direct identification of the causal mutation in a family (or families) with one or more affected individuals. Consequently, the timescale for identifying human disease genes has decreased dramatically from a period of years (e.g., the search for the cystic fibrosis gene in the 1980s) to sometimes just a few days.

Position-Independent Identification of Human Disease Genes

Before genetic mapping techniques were developed, the first human disease genes were identified through knowledge of the

TABLE 4.1 Historical strategies for disease gene identification

Year	Strategy	Examples of Application
1985	Patients with chromosome abnormalities	*DMD* mutations causing Duchenne muscular dystrophy
1989	Linkage mapping	*CFTR* mutations causing cystic fibrosis
1990s	Autozygosity mapping	Many recessive disease genes identified in consanguineous pedigrees
1992	Animal models	*PAX3* mutations causing Waardenburg syndrome
1999	RAPID cloning of trinucleotide repeat expansion	CTG repeat expansion causing spinocerebellar ataxia type 8
2010	Exome sequencing	*DHOD* mutations causing Miller syndrome

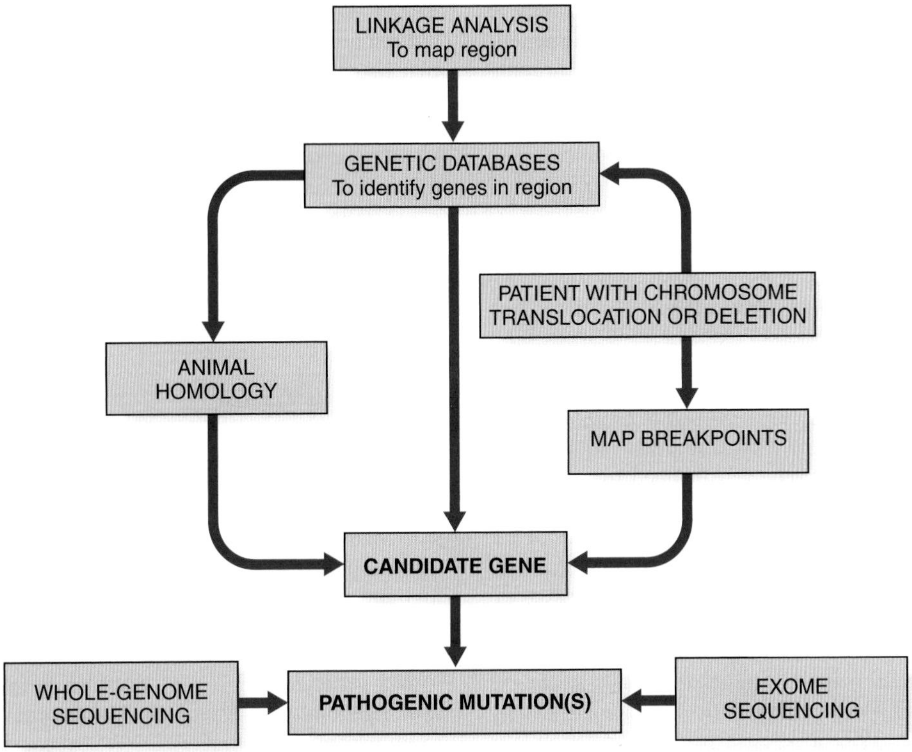

• **Fig. 4.1** Pathways towards human disease gene identification.

protein product. For disorders with a biochemical basis, this was a particularly successful strategy.

Functional Cloning

Functional cloning describes the identification of a human disease gene through knowledge of its protein product. From the amino-acid sequence of a protein, oligonucleotide probes could be synthesized to act as probes for screening complementary DNA (cDNA) libraries.

An alternative approach was to generate an antibody to the protein for screening of a cDNA expression library.

Use of Animal Models

The recognition of phenotypic features in a model organism, such as the mouse, which are similar to those seen in persons affected with an inherited disorder, allowed the possibility of cloning the gene in the model organism to lead to more rapid identification of the gene responsible in humans. An example of this approach was the mapping of the gene responsible for the inherited disorder of pigmentation and deafness known as Waardenburg syndrome (p. 113) to the long arm of human chromosome 2. This region of chromosome 2 shows extensive homology, or what is known as **synteny**, to the region of mouse chromosome 1 to which the gene for the murine pigmentary mutant known as *Splotch* had been assigned. The mapping of the murine *Pax3* gene, which codes for a transcription factor expressed in the developing nervous system, to this region suggested it as a **positional candidate gene** for the disorder. It was suggested that the pigmentary abnormalities could arise on the basis that melanocytes, in which melanin synthesis takes place, are derived from the neural crest. Identification of mutations in *PAX3*, the human homolog, confirmed it as the gene responsible for Waardenburg syndrome.

Mapping Trinucleotide Repeat Disorders

A number of human diseases are attributable to expansions of trinucleotide repeats (see Table 2.5), and in particular CAG repeat expansions which cause extended polyglutamate tracts in Huntington disease and many forms of spinocerebellar ataxia. A method developed to seek novel trinucleotide repeat expansions in genomic DNA from affected patients led to the successful identification of a CTG repeat expansion in patients with spinocerebellar ataxia type 8.

Positional Cloning

Positional cloning describes the identification of a disease gene through its location in the human genome, without prior knowledge of its function. It is also described as **reverse genetics** because it involves an approach opposite to that of functional cloning, in which the protein is the starting point.

Linkage Analysis

Genetic mapping, or linkage analysis (pp. 45, 91), is based on genetic distances that are measured in cM. A genetic distance of 1 cM is the distance between two genes that show 1% recombination; that is, in 1% of meioses the genes will not be coinherited. A distance of 1 cM is equivalent to approximately 1 megabase (Mb; 1 million bases). Linkage analysis is the first step in positional cloning that defines a genetic interval for further analysis.

Linkage analysis can be performed for a single, large family or for multiple families, although this assumes that there is no genetic heterogeneity (p. 71). The use of genetic markers located throughout the genome is described as a **genome-wide scan**. In the 1990s, genome-wide scans used microsatellite markers (a commercial set of 350 markers was popular), but were replaced with microarrays where analysis of several million SNPs provided greater statistical power.

Autozygosity mapping (also known as homozygosity mapping) is a powerful form of linkage analysis used to map autosomal recessive disorders in consanguineous pedigrees (p. 341). Autozygosity occurs when affected members of a family are homozygous at particular loci because they are identical by descent from a common ancestor.

In the mid-1980s, linkage of cystic fibrosis (CF) to chromosome 7 was found by testing nearly 50 Caucasian families with hundreds of DNA markers. The gene was mapped to a region of 500 kilobases between markers *MET* and *D7S8* at chromosome band 7q31–32, when it became evident that the majority of CF chromosomes had a particular set of alleles for these markers (shared haplotype) that was found in only 25% of towards CF chromosomes. This finding is described as **linkage disequilibrium** and suggests a common mutation from a founder effect (p. 89). Extensive physical mapping studies eventually led to the identification of four genes within the genetic interval identified by linkage analysis, and in 1989 a 3–base pair (bp) deletion was found within the cystic fibrosis transmembrane conductance regulator gene (*CFTR*). This mutation (p.Phe508del) was present in approximately 70% of CF chromosomes and 2% to 3% of towards CF chromosomes, consistent with the carrier frequency of 1 in 25 in Caucasians.

Contig Analysis

The aim of linkage analysis was to reduce the region of linkage as far as possible to identify a candidate region. Before publication of the human genome sequence, the next step was to construct a **contig**. This contig would contain a series of overlapping fragments of cloned DNA representing the entire candidate region. These cloned fragments were then used for screening cDNA libraries, searching for CpG islands (which are usually located close to genes), zoo blotting (selection based on evolutionary conservation), and exon trapping (to identify coding regions via functional splice sites). The requirement for cloning the region of interest led to the phrase "cloning the gene" for a particular disease.

Chromosome Abnormalities

Occasionally, individuals are recognize with single-gene disorders that are also found to have structural chromosomal abnormalities. The first clue that the gene responsible for Duchenne muscular dystrophy (DMD) (p. 299) was located on the short arm of the X chromosome was the identification of a number of females with DMD who were also found to have a chromosomal rearrangement between an autosome and a specific region of the short arm of one of their X chromosomes. Isolation of DNA clones spanning the region of the X chromosome involved in the rearrangement led, in one such female, to more detailed gene-mapping information, as well as to the eventual cloning of the *DMD* gene encoding dystrophin (p. 299).

At the same time as these observations, a male was reported with three X-linked disorders: DMD, chronic granulomatous disease, and retinitis pigmentosa. He also had an unusual X-linked red cell group known as the McLeod phenotype. It was suggested that he could have a deletion of a number of genes on the short arm of his X chromosome, including the *DMD* gene, or what is now termed a **contiguous gene syndrome**. Detailed prometaphase chromosome analysis revealed this to be the case. DNA from this individual was used in vast excess to hybridize in competitive reassociation, under special conditions, with DNA from persons with multiple X chromosomes to enrich for DNA sequences that he lacked, the so-called phenol-enhanced reassociation technique, which allowed isolation of DNA clones containing portions of the *DMD* gene.

Candidate Genes

Searching databases for genes with a function likely to be involved in the pathogenesis of the inherited disorder can also suggest what are known as **candidate genes**. If a disease has been mapped to a particular chromosomal region, any gene mapping to that region is a positional candidate gene. Data on the pattern of expression, timing, and distribution in tissue and cells types may suggest that a certain positional candidate gene or genes is more likely to be responsible for the phenotypic features seen in persons affected with a particular single-gene disorder. Software tools are used to search genomic DNA sequence databases for sequence homology to known genes, as well as DNA sequences specific to all genes, such as the conserved intron–exon splice junctions, promoter sequences, polyadenylation sites, and stretches of open reading frames.

Identification of a gene with homology to a known gene causing a recognized inherited disorder can suggest it as a possible candidate gene for other inherited disorders with a similar phenotype. For example, the identification of mutations in the gene encoding connexin 26, one of the proteins that constitutes the gap junctions between cells, causing sensorineural hearing impairment or deafness, has led to the identification of other connexins responsible for inherited hearing impairment or deafness.

Confirmatory Testing That a Candidate Gene is a Disease Gene

Finding loss-of-function mutations or multiple different mutations that result in the same phenotype provides supporting evidence that a potential candidate gene is associated with a disorder. For example, in the absence of functional data to demonstrate the effect of the p.Phe508del mutation on the CFTR protein, confirmation that mutations in the *CFTR* gene caused cystic fibrosis was provided by the nonsense mutation p.Gly542X.

Further evidence is sought from gene expression studies to check that the candidate gene is expressed in the appropriate tissues and at the relevant stages of development. The production of a transgenic animal model by the targeted introduction of the mutation into the homologous gene in another species that is shown to exhibit phenotypic features similar to those seen in persons affected with the disorder, or restoration of the normal phenotype by transfection of the normal gene into a cell line, provides final proof that the candidate gene and the disease gene are one and the same.

Generating transgenic animal models is a lengthy and expensive process, but a new genome-editing technology, clustered regularly

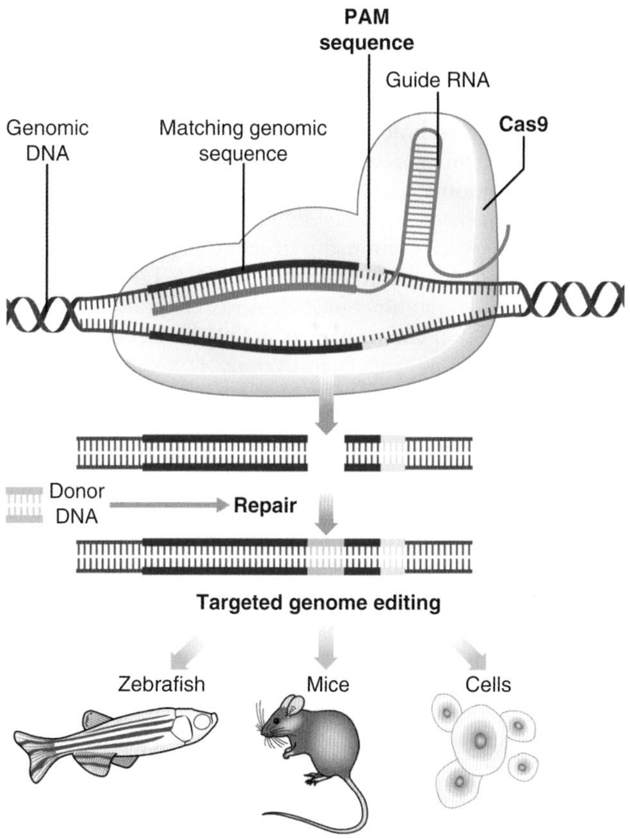

• **Fig. 4.2** Schematic illustration of genome editing using CRISPR/Cas9 technology. A guide ribose nucleic acid (gRNA) is designed to match the genomic sequence of interest. The gRNA is designed to target the genomic sequence of 19 to 23 base pairs at the 5′ side of the protospacer adjacent motif (PAM) 5'-NGG-3' sequence, where N can be any nucleotide base. The gRNA recruits Cas9 nuclease to the target locus and induces double-strand breaks (indicated by scissors). The donor DNA sequence is introduced by homology-dependent repair. CRISPR/Cas9 technology can be used to generate modified bacterial or human cells for *in vitro* studies or a range of different animal models for *in vivo* investigation.

interspaced short palindromic repeat (CRISPR)/CRISPR-associated 9 (CRISPR/Cas9), provides a powerful tool to investigate gene mutations identified in patients either in cellular systems or animal models (Fig. 4.2). This system uses a guide RNA to recruit Cas9 nuclease to the target locus by sequence complementarity and induces double-strand breaks (DSBs). These DSBs can be used to introduce specific sequence modifications through a homology-dependent repair mechanism. By microinjecting synthesized RNAs and donor DNA sequences into mouse zygotes it is possible to create a mouse model with a specific gene mutation within a few months.

The Human Genome Project

Beginning of the Human Genome Project

The concept of a map of the human genome was first proposed in 1969 by Victor McKusick (see Fig. 1.5, p. 5), one of the founding fathers of medical genetics. Human gene mapping workshops were held regularly from 1973 to collate the mapping data. The idea of a dedicated human genome project came from a meeting in 1986. The US Human Genome Project started in 1991 and is estimated to have cost approximately 2.7 billion US dollars. Other nations, notably France, the United Kingdom, and Japan, soon followed with their own major national human genome programs and were subsequently joined by a number of other countries. These individual national projects were coordinated by the Human Genome Organization, an international organization created to foster collaboration between genome scientists.

Sequencing of the Human Genome

Although sequencing of the entire human genome would have been seen to be the obvious main focus of the Human Genome Project, initially it was not the straightforward proposal it seemed. The human genome contains large sections of repetitive DNA (p. 26) that were technically difficult to clone and sequence. In addition, it would seem a waste of time to collect sequence data on the entire genome when only a small proportion is made up of expressed sequences or genes, the latter being most likely to be the regions of greatest medical and biological importance. Furthermore, the sheer magnitude of the prospect of sequencing all 3×10^9 bp of the human genome seemed overwhelming. With conventional sequencing technology, as was carried out in the early 1990s, it was estimated that a single laboratory worker could sequence up to approximately 2000 bp per day.

Projects involving sequencing of other organisms with smaller genomes showed how much work was involved, as well as how the rate of producing sequence data increased with the development of new DNA technologies. For example, with initial efforts at producing genome sequence data for yeast, it took an international collaboration involving 35 laboratories in 17 countries from 1989 until 1995 to sequence just 315,000 bp of chromosome 3, one of the 16 chromosomes that make up the 14 million bp of the yeast genome. Advances in DNA technologies meant, however, that by the middle of 1995 more than half of the yeast genome had been sequenced, with the complete genomic sequence being reported the following year.

Further advances in DNA sequencing technology led to publication of the full sequence of the nematode *Caenorhabditis elegans* in 1998 and the 50 million bp of the DNA sequence of human chromosome 22 at the end of 1999. As a consequence of these technical developments, the "working draft" sequence, covering 90% of the human genome, was published in February 2001. The finished sequence (>99% coverage) was announced more than 2 years ahead of schedule in April 2003, the 50th anniversary of the discovery of the DNA double helix. Researchers now have access to the full catalogue of approximately 20,000 genes, and the human genome sequence will underpin biomedical research for decades to come.

Ethical, Legal, and Social Issues of the Human Genome Project

The rapid advances in the science and application of developments from the Human Genome Project presented complex ethical issues for both the individual and society. These issues included ones of immediate practical relevance, such as who owns and should control genetic information with respect to privacy and confidentiality; who is entitled to have access to it and how; whether it should be used by employers, schools, and so on; the psychological impact and potential stigmatization of persons positive for genetic testing; and the use of genetic testing in reproductive decision making. Other issues include the concept of disability/differences that have a genetic basis in relation to the treatment of genetic disorders or diseases by gene therapy and the possibility of genetic enhancement (i.e., using gene therapy to supply certain characteristics, such as height). Lastly, issues needed to be resolved with regard to the appropriateness and fairness of the use of the new genetic and genomic technologies with prioritization of the use of public resources and commercial involvement and property rights, especially regarding patenting.

Development of Bioinformatics

Bioinformatics was essential to the overall success of the Human Genome Project. This is an interdisciplinary field that develops methods and software tools for understanding biological data. Bioinformaticians were responsible for the establishment of facilities for collecting, storing, organizing, interpreting, analyzing, and communicating the data from the project to the scientific community at large. It was vital for anyone involved in any aspect of the Human Genome Project to have rapid and easy access to the data/information arising from it. This dissemination of information was met by the establishment of a large number of electronic databases available on the World Wide Web on the Internet (see Appendix). These include protein and DNA sequence databases (e.g., GenBank, European Molecular Biology Laboratory), annotated genome data (Ensembl and UCSC Browser, University of California, Santa Cruz) and the catalogue of inherited diseases in humans (Online Mendelian Inheritance in Man-OMIM).

Comparative Genomics

In addition to the Human Genome Project, there were separate genome projects for a number of other species, for what are known as "model organisms." These included various prokaryotic organisms such as the bacteria *Escherichia coli* and *Haemophilus influenzae*, as well as eukaryotic organisms such as *Saccharomyces cerevisiae* (yeast), *C. elegans* (flatworm), *Drosophila melanogaster* (fruit fly), *Mus musculus* (mouse), *Rattus norvegicus* (rat), *Fugu rubripes rubripes* (puffer fish), *Anopheles gambiae* (mosquito), and *Danio rerio* (zebrafish). These **comparative genomics** projects identified many novel genes and were of vital importance in the Human Genome Project because mapping the human homologs provided new "candidate" genes for inherited diseases in humans.

Functional Genomics

The second major way in which model organisms proved to be invaluable in the Human Genome Project was by providing the means to follow the expression of genes and the function of their protein products in normal development, as well as their dysfunction in inherited disorders. This is referred to as **functional genomics**.

Beyond the Human Genome Project

The goal of functional genomics is to understand the relationship between an organism's genome and its phenotype. There are many different possible approaches. For example, the ability to introduce targeted mutations in specific genes allows the production of animal models to study the pathodevelopmental basis for inherited human disorders, as well as serve as a test system for the safety and efficacy of gene therapy and other treatment modalities (Chapter 15). Functional genomics includes a number of "-omics" such as **transcriptomics** (gene expression), **proteomics** (protein expression), and **metabolomics** (metabolites).

The activity and expression of protein-coding genes is modulated by the **regulome**, a collection of DNA elements that includes regulatory sequences (promoters, enhancers, and silencers) together with regions of chromatin structure and histone modification. The international Encyclopedia of DNA Elements project aims to identify all the functional elements of genomic DNA, in both coding and non-coding regions. In 2012 the project simultaneously published 30 papers in *Nature*, *Genome Biology*, and *Genome Research*. They reported that over 80% of the human genome is involved in the regulation of gene expression and showed enrichment of GWAS SNPs (Chapter 10) within non-coding functional elements.

Understanding the link between gene expression and DNA variation through transcriptome profiling in more than 40 different tissues from 900 postmortem donors is the focus of the Genotype-Tissue Expression Project. Early results have demonstrated that some variants affect gene expression in a single or restricted set of tissues, whereas other variants can affect gene expression of multiple tissues but to a variable degree across those different tissues.

Identifying the Genetic Etiology of Monogenic Disorders by Next-Generation Sequencing

This new sequencing technology (see Chapter 5) has revolutionized the identification of human disease genes. Since 2010, the number of disease phenotypes with a known molecular basis has increased from 2700 to over 5000. Each month more than 10 new disease genes are reported, and we anticipate that the genetic etiology of the remaining single-gene disorders will be elucidated during the next decade.

Exome Sequencing

The first successful use of next-generation sequencing technology for disease gene identification used the strategy of **exome** sequencing (Fig. 4.3). This enabled researchers to identify mutations in the *DHODH* gene as the cause of Miller syndrome. Approximately 164,000 regions encompassing exons and their conserved splice sites (a total of 27 Mb) were sequenced in a pair of affected siblings and probands from two additional families. Non-synonymous variants, splice donor/acceptor site mutations, or coding insertion/deletion mutations were identified in nearly 5000 genes in each of the two affected siblings. Filtering these variants against public databases (dbSNP and HapMap) yielded novel variants in less than 500 genes. Analysis of pooled data from the four affected patients revealed just one gene, *DHODH*, which contained two mutated alleles in each individual.

Before embarking on exome sequencing in an attempt to identify the cause of a monogenic disease, it is important to identify a suitable strategy with regard to pedigree structure, selection of cases for exome sequencing and likely mode of inheritance (Fig. 4.4). An extremely successful strategy is the "trio analysis" approach for the detection of *de novo* heterozygous mutations causing disorders with reduced biological fitness (where patients do not survive to

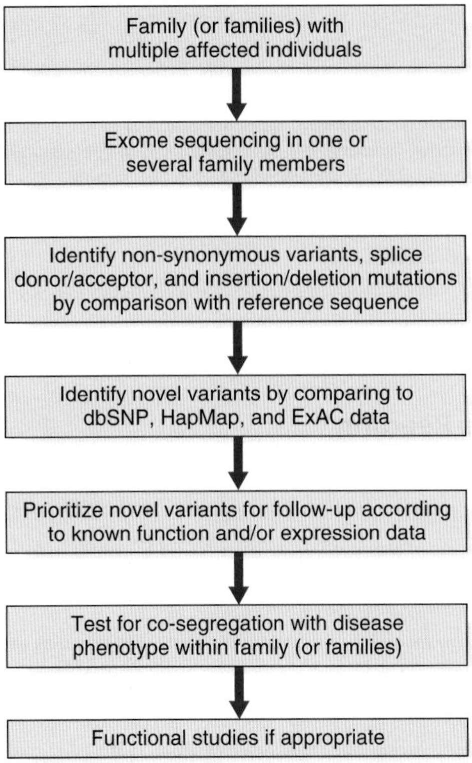

• **Fig. 4.3** A strategy for disease gene identification using exome sequencing.

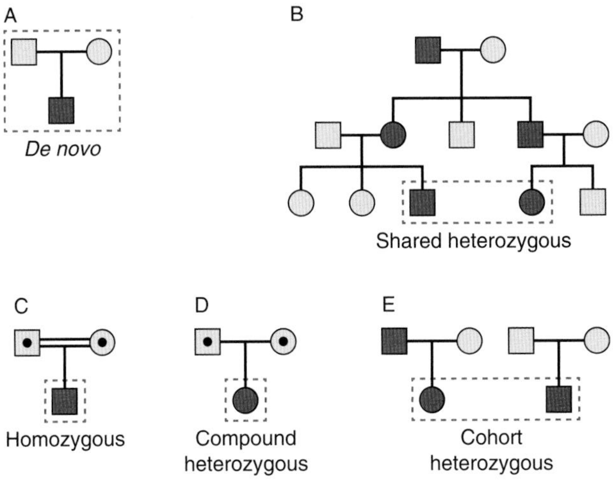

• **Fig. 4.4** Strategies for disease gene identification by exome or genome sequencing. The red dashed boxes indicate individuals within pedigrees whose samples are analyzed by exome or genome sequencing. (A) Trio analysis of an affected patient and their unrelated, unaffected parents to detect heterozygous *de novo* mutations. (B) Linkage approach of sequencing the two most distantly related, affected individuals in a dominant pedigree to identify shared heterozygous variants that include the pathogenic mutation. (C) Analysis of a proband from a consanguineous pedigree to identify homozygous variants in a gene within a homozygous region. (D) Analysis of a proband born to unaffected, unrelated parents to identify compound heterozygous mutations in a single gene. (E) Cohort analysis of unrelated, affected individuals who share a distinctive phenotype to identify heterozygous mutations in the same gene.

TABLE 4.2 Strategies for disease gene identification by exome sequencing

Strategy	Examples of Disorders With New Disease Genes Identified
Trio analysis to identify *de novo* heterozygous mutations	Intellectual disability, autism, and developmental disorders
Linkage approach of sequencing most distantly related individuals within a dominant pedigree to identify heterozygous mutations	Charcot-Marie-Tooth disease (*DYNC1H1*)
Proband sequencing in a consanguineous pedigree to identify homozygous mutations	Oculocutaneous albinism and neutropenia (in a single patient)
Proband sequencing to identify compound heterozygous mutations in an outbred family	Miller syndrome and Sensenbrenner syndrome
Cohort sequencing of affected individuals with a distinctive phenotype	Kabuki syndrome

reproductive age or do not reproduce). An affected patient and their unaffected, unrelated parents are sequenced, and the variants are filtered to identify heterozygous, potentially deleterious variants present only in the proband. If parental samples are not available, it is possible to use a cohort analysis of unrelated, affected individuals who share a distinctive phenotype to identify heterozygous mutations in the same gene. In a dominant pedigree with multiple affected patients a linkage approach can be employed where the two most distantly related affected individuals are sequenced to identify shared heterozygous variants that include the pathogenic mutation. Given that each individual has approximately 100 heterozygous potentially deleterious protein-coding variants, sequencing two family members separated by four meioses will yield a shortlist of approximately 12 gene variants. Sequencing a single affected individual to identify a recessive disorder caused by compound heterozygous mutations is also possible. For consanguineous pedigrees, sequencing of a single affected person may identify a homozygous mutation in a gene located within a homozygous region. Application of these strategies has led to the identification of hundreds of new disease genes (Table 4.2).

Having selected the most appropriate patients for exome or genome sequencing, the critical next step is to filter the identified variants to leave only a shortlist that includes the causative gene mutation or mutations. This relies upon bioinformatics selection of variants according to functional effect and exclusion of common variants using public databases. Bioinformatics as a specialty has expanded rapidly since the implementation of next-generation sequencing because of both the volume and complexity of data generated.

As the cost of next-generation sequencing has fallen, sequencing the genome instead of the exome is now feasible. Genome sequencing requires less hands-on laboratory preparation time and is able to detect nearly all types of mutations, including intronic mutations, regulatory mutations, and balanced chromosome

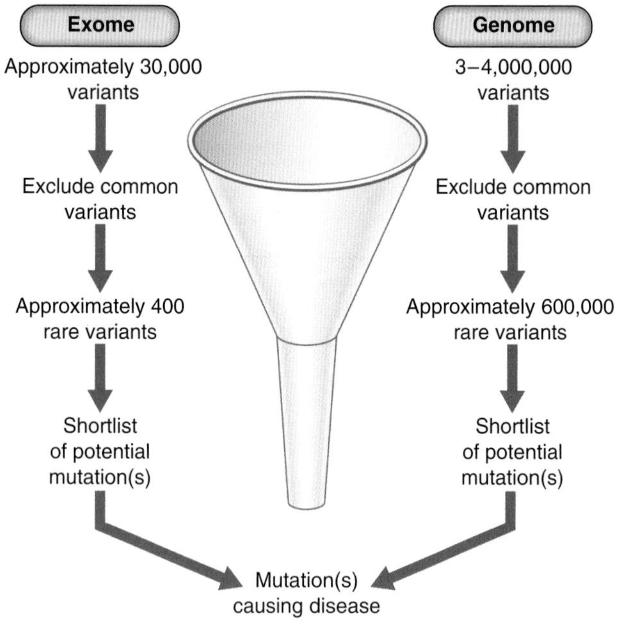

• **Fig. 4.5** Filtering variants identified by exome and genome sequencing to identify pathogenic mutations causing rare disease.

rearrangements. There is, however, an increased burden from the perspective of data storage and analysis, with 3–4 million variants per genome compared with approximately 30,000 variants per exome (Fig. 4.5). Whereas our current understanding of the clinical significance of non-coding variants is limited, much research effort is focused in this area.

ELEMENTS

1. Position-independent methods for the identification of monogenic disorders include functional cloning to identify genes from knowledge of the protein sequence and the use of animal models.
2. Positional cloning describes the identification of a gene on the basis of its location in the human genome. Chromosome abnormalities may assist this approach by highlighting particular chromosomal regions of interest. Genetic databases with human genome sequence data now make it possible to identify disease genes *in silico*.
3. Confirmation that a specific gene is responsible for a particular inherited disorder can be obtained by tissue and developmental expression studies, *in vitro* cell culture studies or the introduction and analysis of mutations in a homologous gene in another species. As a consequence, the "anatomy of the human genome" is continually being elucidated.
4. One of the goals of the Human Genome Project was to sequence the human genome. The sequencing was completed by an international consortium in 2003, and has greatly facilitated the identification of human disease genes.
5. Next-generation sequencing has hugely accelerated the pace of new disease gene discovery, and the genetic basis of approximately 80% of an estimated 6000 monogenic disorders is now known.
6. Research efforts are now focused on understanding the role of non-coding DNA in the control of gene expression and how this contributes to human disease.

Further Reading

Bernstein BE, Birney E, Dunham I, et al. An integrated encyclopedia of DNA elements in the human genome. *Nature.* 2012;489:57–74.

An overview of the results from the ENCODE project, which concluded that more than 80% of the human genome has a biochemical function in the control of gene expression.

Kerem B, Rommens JM, Buchanan JA, et al. Identification of the cystic fibrosis gene. *Genetic analysis. Science.* 1989;245:1073–1080.

Original paper describing cloning of the cystic fibrosis gene.

McKusick VA. *Mendelian Inheritance in Man*. 12th ed. London: Johns Hopkins University Press; 1998.

A computerized catalogue of the dominant, recessive, and X-linked mendelian traits and disorders in humans, with a brief clinical commentary and details of the mutational basis, if known. Also available online, updated regularly.

Ng SB, Buckingham KJ, Lee C, et al. Exome sequencing identifies the cause of a mendelian disorder. *Nat Genet.* 2010;42:30–35.

The first publication describing the use of next-generation sequencing to elucidate the genetic etiology of Miller syndrome.

Royer-Pokora B, Kunkel LM, Monaco AP, et al. Cloning the gene for an inherited human disorder—chronic granulomatous disease—on the basis of its chromosomal location. *Nature.* 1985;322:32–38.

Original paper describing the identification of a disease gene through contiguous chromosome deletions.

Strachan T, Read AP. *Human Molecular Genetics*. 5th ed. London: Garland Science; 2018.

A comprehensive textbook of all aspects of molecular and cellular biology as related to inherited disease in humans.

Sulston J. *The Common Thread: A Story of Science, Politics, Ethics and the Human Genome*. London: Joseph Henry Press; 2002.

A personal account of the human genome sequencing project by the man who led the UK team of scientists.

5 Laboratory Techniques for Diagnosis of Monogenic Disorders

In the history of medical genetics, the "chromosome breakthrough" in the mid-1950s was revolutionary. In the past 5 decades, DNA technology has had a profound effect, not only in medical genetics but also in many areas of biological science (Box 5.1).The seminal developments in the field are summarized in Table 5.1. One of the most revolutionary developments was the technique developed in the mid-1980s known as the **polymerase chain reaction**, or **PCR**, which can be used to produce vast quantities of a target DNA fragment, provided that the DNA sequence of that region is known.

Polymerase Chain Reaction

DNA sequence information is used to design two oligonucleotide primers (**amplimers**) of approximately 20 base pairs (bp) in length complementary to the DNA sequences flanking the target DNA fragment. The first step is to denature the double-stranded DNA by heating. The primers then bind to the complementary DNA sequences of the single-stranded DNA templates. DNA polymerase extends the primer DNA in the presence of the deoxynucleotide triphosphates (dATP, dCTP, dGTP and dTTP) to synthesize the complementary DNA sequence. Subsequent heat denaturation of the double-stranded DNA, followed by annealing of the same primer sequences to the resulting single-stranded DNA, will result in the synthesis of further copies of the target DNA. Some 30 to 35 successive repeated cycles result in more than 1 billion copies (**amplicons**) of the DNA target, sufficient for direct visualization by ultraviolet fluorescence after ethidium bromide staining, without the need to use indirect detection techniques (Fig. 5.1). PCR is mostly used to amplify DNA fragments up to 1 kilobase (kb), although long-range PCR allows the amplification of larger DNA fragments of up to 20 to 30 kb.

PCR allows analysis of DNA from any cellular source containing nuclei; in addition to blood, this can include less invasive samples such as saliva, buccal scrapings, or pathological archival material. It is also possible to start with quantities of DNA as small as those from a single cell, as is the case in preimplantation genetic diagnosis (p. 332). Great care has to be taken with PCR, however, because DNA from a contaminating extraneous source, such as desquamated skin from a laboratory worker, will also be amplified. This can lead to false-positive results unless the appropriate control studies are used to detect this possible source of error.

Another advantage of PCR is the rapid turnaround time of samples for analysis. Use of the heat-stable *Taq* DNA polymerase isolated from the bacterium *Thermophilus aquaticus*, which grows naturally in hot springs, generates PCR products in a matter of hours. Real-time PCR machines have reduced this time to less than 1 hour, and fluorescence technology is used to monitor the generation of PCR products during each cycle, thus eliminating the need for gel electrophoresis.

• BOX 5.1 Applications of DNA technology

- Gene structure/mapping/function
- Population genetics
- Clinical genetics
  - Preimplantation genetic diagnosis
  - Prenatal diagnosis
  - Presymptomatic diagnosis
  - Carrier detection
- Diagnosis and pathogenesis of disease
  - Genetic
  - Acquired—infective, malignant
- Biosynthesis (e.g., insulin, growth hormone, interferon, immunization)
- Treatment of genetic disease
- Gene therapy
- Agriculture (e.g., nitrogen fixation)

TABLE 5.1 Development of DNA technology

Decade	Development	Examples of Application
1980s	Recombinant DNA technology, Southern blot and Sanger sequencing	Recombinant erythropoietin (1987), DNA fingerprinting (1984) and DNA sequence of Epstein–Barr virus genome (1984)
1990s	Polymerase chain reaction	Diagnosis of genetic disorders
2000s	Capillary sequencing and microarray technology	Human genome sequence (2003)
2010s	Next-generation sequencing	First acute myeloid leukemia cancer genome sequenced (2008) Human genome sequenced at a cost of approx. $1000 (2014)

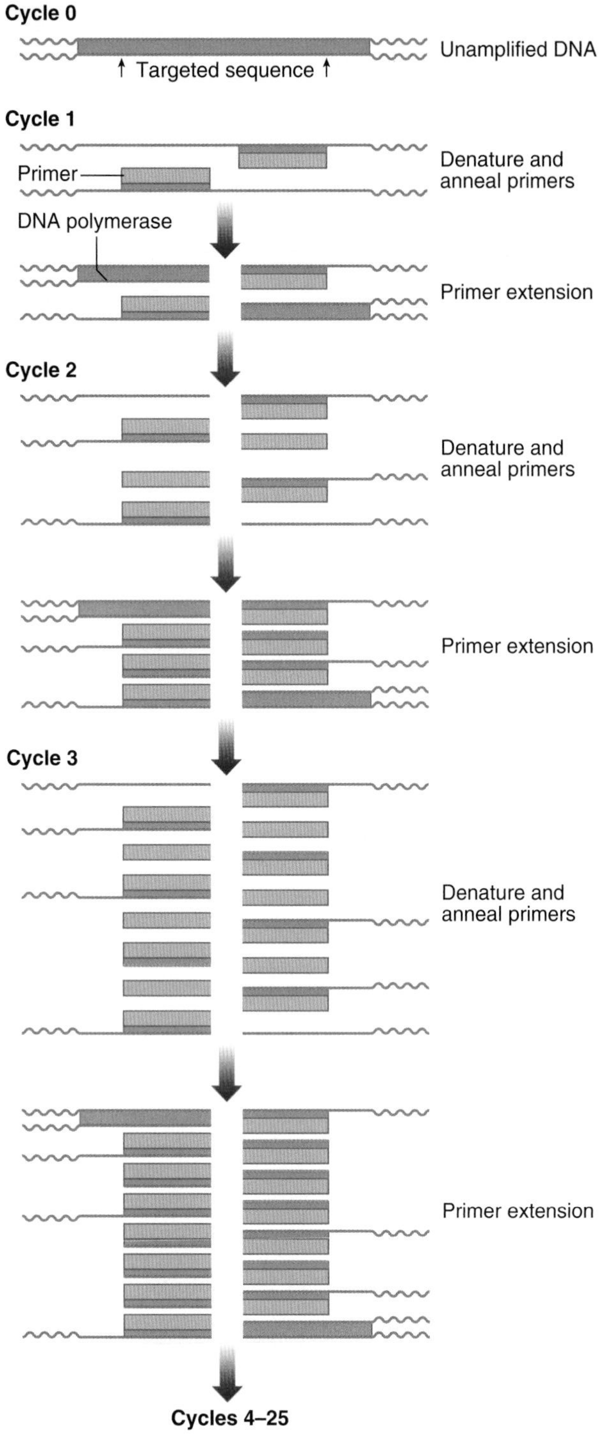

• **Fig. 5.1** Diagram of the polymerase chain reaction showing serial denaturation of DNA, primer annealing and extension, with doubling of the target DNA fragment numbers in each cycle.

Application of DNA Sequence Polymorphisms

There is an enormous amount of DNA sequence variation in the human genome. Two main types, single nucleotide polymorphisms (SNPs) and variable number tandem repeat (VNTR) DNA length polymorphisms, are predominantly used in genetic analysis.

TABLE 5.2 Some examples of restriction endonucleases with their nucleotide recognition sequence and cleavage sites

Enzyme	Organism	CLEAVAGE SITE 5′ 3′
*Bam*HI	*Bacillus amyloliquefaciens* H	G · G A T C C
*Eco*RI	*Escherichia coli* RY 13	G · A A T T C
*Hae*III	*Haemophilus aegyptius*	G G · C C
*Hind*III	*Haemophilus influenzae* Rd	A · A G C T T
*Hpa*I	*Haemophilus parainfluenzae*	G T T · A A C
*Pst*I	*Providencia stuartii*	C T G C A · G
*Sma*I	*Serratia marcescens*	C C C · G G G
*Sal*I	*Streptomyces albus* G	G · T C G A C

Single Nucleotide Polymorphisms

Approximately 1 in 1000 bases within the human genome shows variation. SNPs are most frequently biallelic and occur in coding and non-coding regions. An early way of using SNPs as genetic markers was the analysis of **restriction fragment length polymorphisms (RFLPs)**. In the 1970s, it was recognized that certain microbes contain enzymes that cleave double-stranded DNA within or near a particular sequence of nucleotides. These enzymes restrict the entry of foreign DNA into bacterial cells and were therefore called **restriction enzymes**. They recognize a palindromic nucleotide sequence of DNA of between four and eight nucleotides in length (i.e., the same sequence of nucleotides occurring on the two complementary DNA strands when read in one direction of polarity, e.g., 5′ to 3′) (Table 5.2). The longer the nucleotide recognition sequence of the restriction enzyme, the less frequently that particular nucleotide sequence will occur by chance, and therefore the larger the average size of the DNA fragments generated.

More than 3000 different restriction enzymes have been isolated from various bacterial organisms. Restriction endonucleases are named according to the organism from which they are derived (e.g., *Eco*RI is from *Escherichia coli* and was the first restriction enzyme isolated from that organism).

The complementary pairing of bases in the DNA molecule means that cleavage of double-stranded DNA by a restriction endonuclease always creates double-stranded breaks, which, depending on the cleavage points of the particular restriction enzyme used, results in either a staggered or a blunt end (Fig. 5.2). Digestion of DNA from a specific source with a particular restriction enzyme will produce the same reproducible collection of DNA fragments each time the process is carried out.

If an SNP lies within the recognition sequence of a restriction enzyme, the DNA fragments produced by that restriction enzyme will be of different lengths in different people. This can be recognized by the altered mobility of the restriction fragments on gel electrophoresis, so-called **RFLPs**. Early genetic mapping studies used Southern blotting to detect RFLPs, but current technology enables

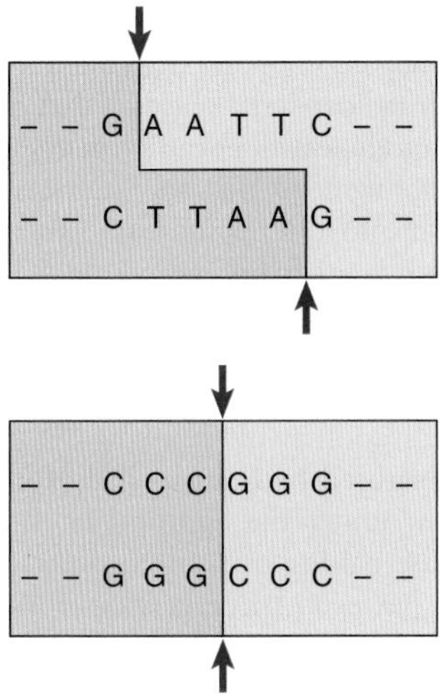

• **Fig. 5.2** The staggered and blunt ends generated by restriction digest of double-stranded DNA by *Eco*RI and *Sma*I. Sites of cleavage of the DNA strands are indicated by arrows.

the detection of any SNP. DNA microarrays have led to the creation of a dense SNP map of the human genome and assist genome searches for linkage studies in mapping single-gene disorders (see Chapter 4) and association studies in common diseases. They are also the technology of choice for generating polygenic risk scores (see Chapter 10).

Variable Number Tandem Repeats

Variable number tandem repeats (VNTRs) are highly polymorphic and are caused by the presence of variable numbers of tandem repeats of a short DNA sequence that have been shown to be inherited in a mendelian codominant fashion (p. 70). The advantage of using VNTRs over SNPs is the large number of alleles for each VNTR compared with SNPs, which are mostly biallelic.

Minisatellites

Alec Jeffreys identified a short 10-bp to 15-bp "core" sequence with homology to many highly variable loci spread throughout the human genome (p. 14). Using a probe containing tandem repeats of this core sequence, a pattern of hypervariable DNA fragments could be identified. The multiple variable-size repeat sequences identified by the core sequence are known as **minisatellites**. These minisatellites are highly polymorphic, and a profile unique to an individual (unless they have an identical twin!) is described as a **DNA fingerprint**. The technique of DNA fingerprinting is still used widely in paternity testing and for forensic purposes.

Microsatellites

The human genome contains some 50,000 to 100,000 blocks of a variable number of tandem repeats of the dinucleotide CA, so-called CA repeats or **microsatellites** (p. 14). The difference in the number of CA repeats at any one site between individuals is highly polymorphic, and these repeats have been shown to be inherited in a mendelian codominant manner. In addition, highly polymorphic trinucleotide and tetranucleotide repeats have been identified, and can be used in a similar way (Fig. 5.3). These microsatellites can be analyzed by PCR, and the use of fluorescent detection systems allows relatively high-throughput analysis. Consequently, microsatellite analysis has replaced DNA fingerprinting for paternity testing and establishing zygosity.

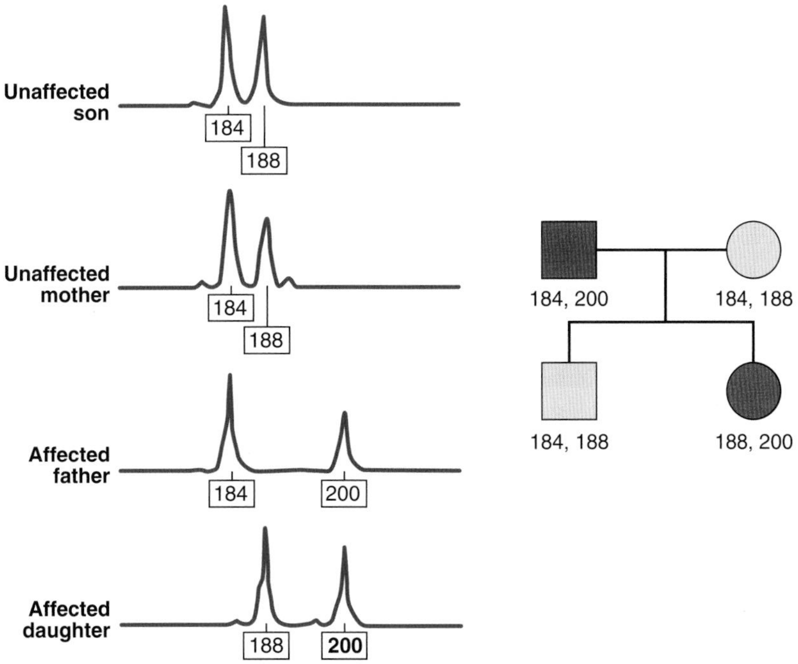

• **Fig. 5.3** Analysis of a tetranucleotide microsatellite marker in a family with a dominant disorder. *Genotyper* software was used to label the peaks with the size of the polymerase chain reaction products. The 200–base pair allele is segregating with the disorder in the affected members of the family. (Courtesy M Owens, Genomic Laboratory, Royal Devon and Exeter Hospital, Exeter, UK.)

Clinical Applications of Gene Tracking

If a gene has been mapped by linkage studies but not identified, it is possible to use the linked markers to "track" the disease-linked haplotype within a family. This approach may also be used for known genes where a causative variant has not been found. Closely flanking or intragenic microsatellites are used most commonly because of the lower likelihood of finding informative SNPs within families. Fig. 5.4 illustrates a family in which gene tracking has been used to determine carrier risk in the absence of a known pathogenic variant. There are some pitfalls associated with this method; recombination between the microsatellite and the gene may give an incorrect risk estimate, and the possibility of genetic heterogeneity (where mutations in more than one gene cause a disease) should be borne in mind.

Nucleic Acid Hybridization Techniques

Many methods of DNA analysis involve the use of nucleic acid probes and the process of nucleic acid hybridization.

Nucleic Acid Probes

Nucleic acid probes are usually single-stranded DNA sequences that have been radioactively or non-radioactively labeled and can be used to detect DNA or RNA fragments with sequence homology. DNA probes can come from a variety of sources, including random genomic DNA sequences, specific genes, cDNA sequences, or oligonucleotide DNA sequences produced synthetically based on knowledge of the protein amino-acid sequence. A DNA probe can be labeled by a variety of processes, including isotopic labeling with ^{32}P and non-isotopic methods using modified nucleotides containing fluorophores (e.g., fluorescein or rhodamine). Hybridization of a radioactively labeled DNA probe with cDNA sequences on a nitrocellulose filter can be detected by autoradiography, whereas DNA fragments that are fluorescently labeled can be detected by exposure to the appropriate wavelength of light, for example fluorescence *in situ* hybridization (pp. 55, 259).

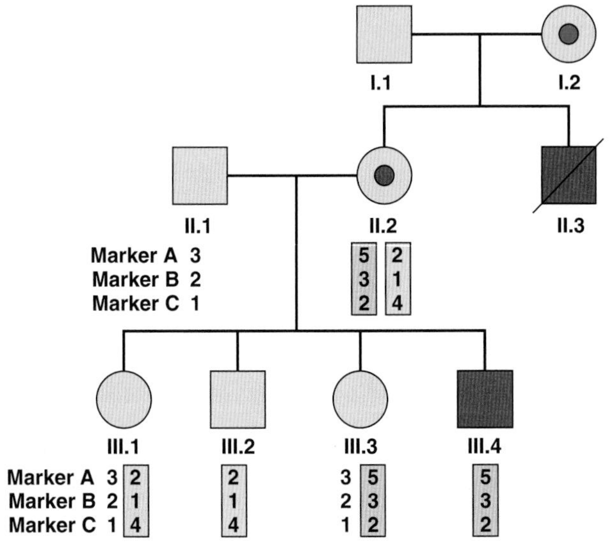

• **Fig. 5.4** Gene tracking in a family with Duchenne muscular dystrophy where no mutation has been found in the affected proband, III.4. Analysis of markers A, B and, C has enabled the construction of haplotypes; the affected haplotype is shown by an orange box. Both of the proband's sisters were at 50% prior risk of being carriers. Gene tracking shows that III.1 has inherited the low-risk haplotype and is unlikely to be a carrier, but III.3 has inherited the high-risk haplotype and is therefore likely to be a carrier of Duchenne muscular dystrophy. The risk of recombination should not be forgotten.

Nucleic Acid Hybridization

Nucleic acid hybridization involves mixing DNA from two sources that have been denatured by heat or alkali to make them single-stranded and then, under the appropriate conditions, allowing complementary base pairing of homologous sequences. If one of the DNA sources has been labeled in some way (i.e., is a DNA probe), this allows identification of specific DNA sequences in the other source.

Southern Blotting

Southern blotting, named after Edwin Southern (who developed the technique), involves digesting DNA with a restriction enzyme and then subjecting it to electrophoresis on an agarose gel. This separates the DNA or restriction fragments by size, the smaller fragments migrating faster than the larger ones. The DNA fragments in the gel are then denatured with alkali, making them single stranded. A "permanent" copy of these single-stranded fragments is made by transferring them on to a nitrocellulose filter that binds the single-stranded DNA, the so-called **Southern blot**. A particular target DNA fragment of interest from the collection on the filter can be visualized by adding a single-stranded ^{32}P radioactively labeled DNA probe that will hybridize with homologous DNA fragments in the Southern blot, which can then be detected by autoradiography (Fig. 5.5). Non-radioactive Southern blotting techniques have been developed with the DNA probe labeled with digoxigenin and detected by chemiluminescence. This approach is safer and generates results more rapidly. An example of the use of Southern blotting for clinical diagnostic fragile-X testing in patients is shown in Fig.5.6.

Northern Blotting

Northern blotting differs from Southern blotting by the use of mRNA as the target nucleic acid in the same procedure; mRNA is very unstable because of intrinsic cellular ribonucleases. Use of ribonuclease inhibitors allows isolation of mRNA that, if run on an electrophoretic gel, can be transferred to a filter. Hybridizing the blot with a DNA probe allows determination of the size and quantity of the mRNA transcript, a so-called **northern blot**. With the advent of real-time reverse transcriptase PCR, microarray technology for gene expression studies and next generation RNA sequencing, northern blotting is now rarely used.

DNA Microarrays

DNA microarrays are based on the same principle of hybridization but on a miniaturized scale, which allows simultaneous analysis of several million targets. Short, fluorescently labeled oligonucleotides attached to a glass microscope slide can be used to detect hybridization of target DNA under appropriate conditions. The color pattern of the microarray is then analyzed automatically by computer. Four classes of application have been described: (1) expression studies to look at the differential expression of thousands of genes at the mRNA level; (2) analysis of DNA variation for mutation detection and SNP typing; (3) testing for genomic

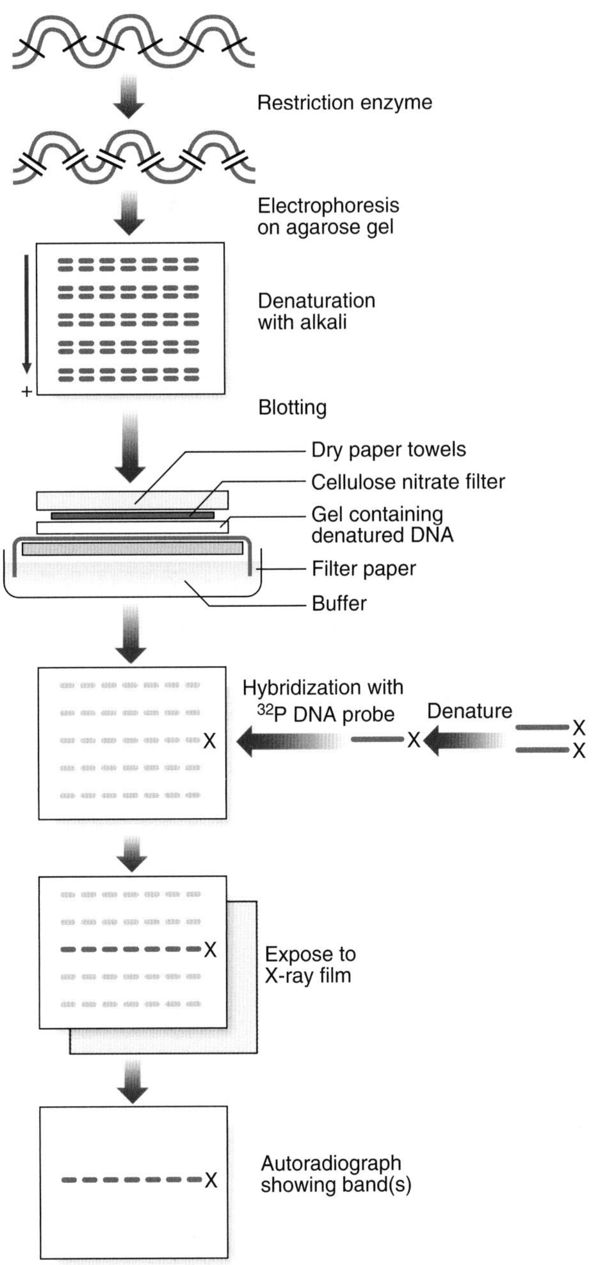

• **Fig. 5.5** Diagram of the Southern blot technique showing size fractionation of the DNA fragments by gel electrophoresis, denaturation of the double-stranded DNA to become single-stranded, and transfer to a nitrocellulose filter that is hybridized with a ^{32}P radioactively labeled DNA probe.

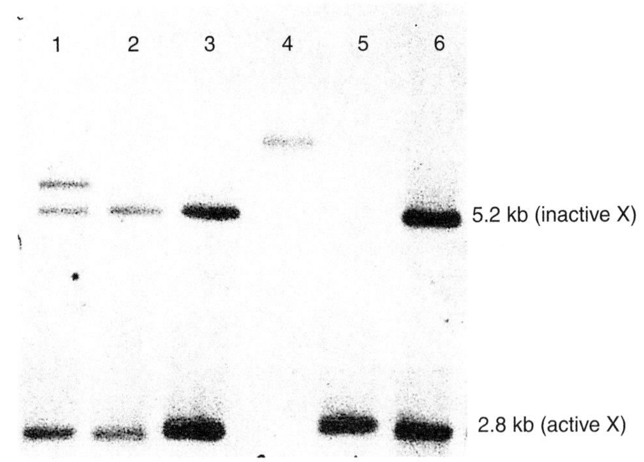

• **Fig. 5.6** Southern blot to detect methylation of the *FMR1* promoter in patients with fragile X syndrome. DNA digested with *Eco*R1 and the methylation-sensitive enzyme *Bst* Z1 was probed with Ox1.9, which hybridizes to a CpG island within the *FMR1* promoter. Lanes 1–6 show samples from Patient 1, a female with a methylated expansion; Patients 2, 3 and 6, who are unaffected females; Patient 4, who is an affected male; and Patient 5, who is an unaffected male. (Courtesy A Gardner, formerly at the Bristol Genetics Laboratory, Southmead Hospital, Bristol, UK.)

gains and losses by array comparative genomic hybridization (CGH); and (4) a combination of the latter two, SNP–CGH, which allows the detection of copy-neutral genetic anomalies such as uniparental disomy (p. 71).

Array CGH

Array CGH involves the hybridization of fluorescently labeled patient and reference DNA to large numbers of DNA sequences bound to glass slides (Fig. 5.7). The DNA target sequences are oligonucleotides (up to 1 million) spotted onto the microscope slides using robotics to create a microarray in which each DNA target has a unique location. Following hybridization and washing to remove unbound DNA, the relative levels of fluorescence are measured using computer software.

Array CGH is able to detect copy number changes at a level of 5 to 10 kb of DNA. It is faster and more sensitive than conventional metaphase analysis for the identification of constitutional rearrangements (but cannot detect balanced translocations or inversions). Array CGH is often the first-line test in the investigation of patients with severe developmental delay/learning difficulties and/or congenital abnormalities, and when abnormalities are detected by ultrasound scanning in the prenatal setting.

Mutation Detection

The choice of method depends primarily on whether the test is for a known sequence change or to identify the presence of any mutation within a particular gene. A number of techniques can be used to screen for mutations that differ in their ease of use and reliability (Table 5.3). Some of the most common techniques in current use are described in the following section.

PCR-Based Methods

Many PCR-based mutation detection methods have been developed over the past 3 decades to detect known mutations.

Size Analysis of PCR Products

Deletion or insertion mutations can sometimes be detected simply by determining the size of a PCR product. For example, the most common mutation that causes cystic fibrosis, p.Phe508del, is a 3-bp deletion that can be detected on a polyacrylamide gel. Some trinucleotide repeat expansion mutations can be amplified by PCR (Fig. 5.8).

Restriction Fragment Length Polymorphism

If a base substitution creates or abolishes the recognition site of a restriction enzyme, it is possible to test for the mutation by

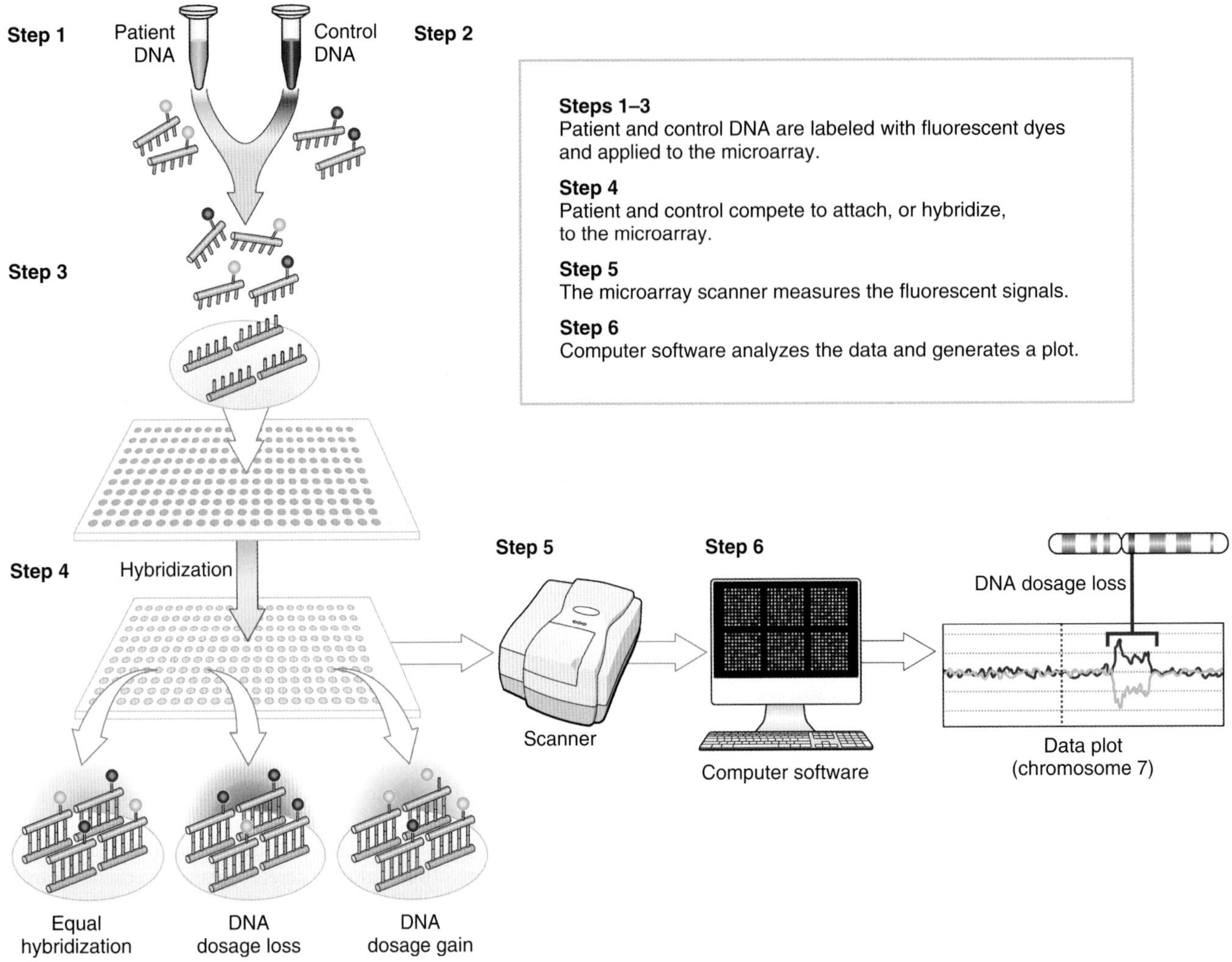

• **Fig. 5.7** Diagram of array comparative genomic hybridization to detect copy number changes across the genome to a resolution of 5 to 10 kilobases.

TABLE 5.3 Methods for detecting mutations

Method	Known/Unknown Mutations	Examples	Advantages/Disadvantages
Southern blot	Known (or unknown rearrangement)	Trinucleotide expansions in fragile X syndrome and myotonic dystrophy	Laborious
Sizing of PCR products	Known	p.Phe508del *CFTR* mutation; trinucleotide expansions in *HTT* and *SCA* genes	Simple, cheap
ARMS-PCR	Known	*CFTR* mutations	Multiplex possible
Real-time PCR	Known	Factor V Leiden	Expensive equipment
Droplet digital PCR	Known	Any gene	Expensive equipment
Sanger sequencing	Known or unknown	Any gene	Gold standard
Next-generation sequencing	Known or unknown	Any gene	Expensive equipment, enormous capacity, but vast amount of data to analyze, and interpretation of novel variants can be difficult

ARMS, Amplification-refractory mutation system; *PCR*, polymerase chain reaction.

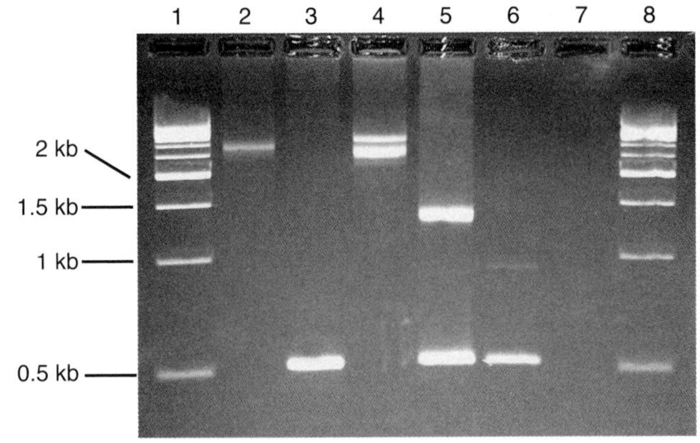

• **Fig. 5.8** Amplification of the GAA repeat expansion mutation by polymerase chain reaction to test for Friedreich ataxia. Products are stained with ethidium bromide and electrophoresed on a 1.5% agarose gel. Lanes 1 and 8 show 500–base pair ladder-size standards, Lanes 2 and 4 show patients with homozygous expansions, Lanes 3 and 6 show unaffected controls, Lane 5 shows a heterozygous expansion carrier, and Lane 7 is the negative control. (Courtesy Dr K Thomson, formerly at the Genomic Laboratory, Royal Devon and Exeter Hospital, Exeter, UK.)

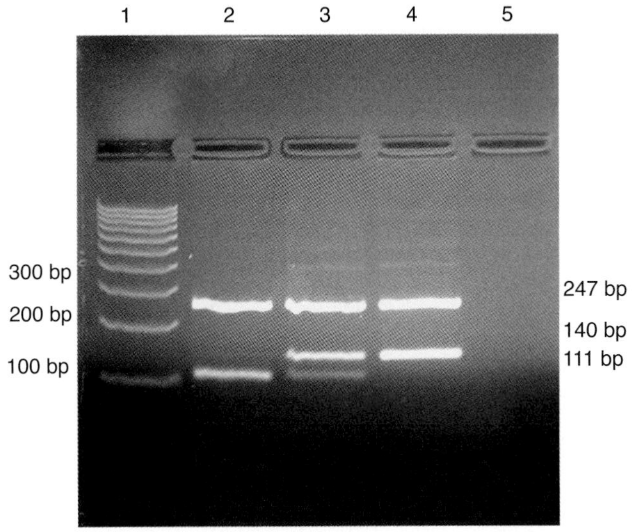

• **Fig. 5.9** Detection of the *HFE* variant C282Y (p.Cys282Tyr) by restriction fragment length polymorphism analysis. The normal 387–base pair (bp) polymerase chain reaction product is digested with *RsaI* to give products of 247 bp and 140 bp. The C282Y variant creates an additional recognition site for *RsaI*, giving products of 247 bp, 111 bp and 29 bp. Lane 1 shows a 100-bp ladder-size standard. Lanes 2 tp 4 show patients homozygous, heterozygous and normal for the C282Y (p.Cys282Tyr) variant, respectively. Lane 5 is the negative control. (Courtesy N Goodman, Genomic Laboratory, Royal Devon and Exeter Hospital, Exeter, UK.)

digesting a PCR product with the appropriate enzyme and separating the products by electrophoresis (Fig. 5.9).

Amplification-Refractory Mutation System PCR

Allele-specific PCR uses primers specific for the normal and variant sequences. The most common design is a multitube assay with normal and variant primers in separate reactions together with control primers to ensure that the PCR reaction has worked. An example of a multiplex amplification-refractory mutation system assay to detect the 50 most common *CFTR* mutations in the European population is shown in Fig. 5.10.

Real-Time PCR

There are multiple hardware platforms for real-time PCR and "fast" versions that can complete a PCR reaction in less than 30 minutes. Fluorescence technology is used to detect mutations by allelic discrimination of PCR products. Fig. 5.11 illustrates the factor V Leiden mutation detected by TaqMan methodology.

Real-time PCR platforms are very popular in clinical microbiology laboratories, where an array of commercial kits has been developed to provide rapid testing for many different viral infections. PCR can be used to detect the presence of DNA sequences specific to a particular infectious organism before conventional evidence, such as an antibody response or the results of cultures, is available. Real-time PCR techniques generate rapid results, with some test results being available within 1 hour of a sample being taken. This is particularly useful in the fight against methicillin-resistant *Staphylococcus aureus* (MRSA) because patients can be rapidly tested on admission to hospital. Anyone found to be MRSA-positive can be isolated to minimize the risk of infection to other patients.

PCR may assist in the diagnosis of lymphomas and leukemias by identifying translocations, for example t(9;22), which is characteristic of chronic myeloid leukemia. The extreme sensitivity of PCR means that minimal residual disease may be detected after treatment for these disorders, and early indication of impending relapse will inform treatment options.

Droplet Digital PCR

This technique involves PCR performed within thousands of nanolitre-sized droplets to achieve highly precise, absolute nucleic acid quantification. A genomic DNA sample is diluted to incorporate either one or zero molecules of DNA in each droplet and mixed with PCR primers, TaqMan allelic discrimination probes (as per conventional real-time PCR) and reagents. After PCR amplification the fluorescence is measured in each droplet and the droplets are counted to measure the number with a signal from either the normal or mutant allele. This provides an extremely sensitive method for identifying very low levels of mutation such as mosaic or acquired mutations, or paternally inherited mutations in cell-free fetal DNA samples.

Sequencing-Based Methods

Sequencing methods are the most frequently used technique for mutation "screening" where a patient is suspected of having a mutation within a specific gene or genes but the disease could be caused by many different mutations within that gene (or genes).

Sanger Sequencing

The "gold standard" method of mutation screening is DNA sequencing using the dideoxy chain termination method developed in the 1970s by Fred Sanger. This method originally employed radioactive labeling with manual interpretation of data. The use of fluorescent labels detected by computerized laser systems has improved ease of use and increased throughput and accuracy. Today's capillary sequencers can sequence approximately 1 megabase (Mb; 1 million bases) per day.

Dideoxy sequencing involves using a single-stranded DNA template (e.g., denatured PCR products) to synthesize new complementary strands using a DNA polymerase and an appropriate oligonucleotide primer. In addition to the four normal deoxynucleotides, a proportion of each of the four respective dideoxynucleotides is included, each labeled with a different fluorescent dye. The dideoxynucleotides lack a hydroxyl group at the 3′ carbon

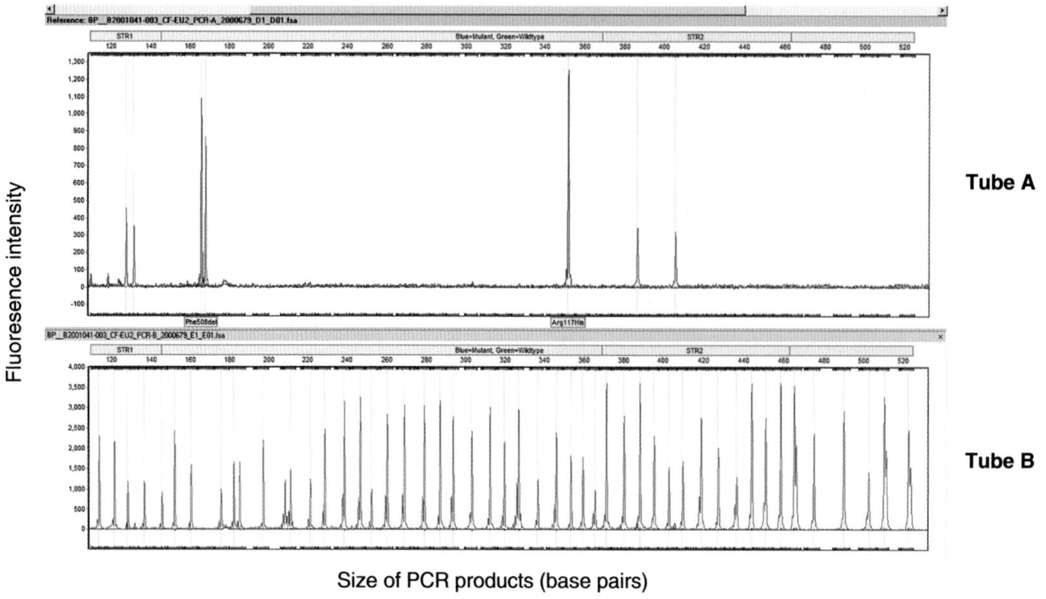

• **Fig. 5.10** Detection of *CFTR* mutations by two-tube amplification-refractory mutation system–polymerase chain reaction. The patient is a compound heterozygote for the p.Phe508del and p.Arg117His variants (see blue peaks in the upper panel—tube A). Heterozygosity is indicated by amplification of the reference sequence at Phe508 (green peak, upper panel—tube A) and at the corresponding positions for the other variants included in the assay (green peaks, lower panel—tube B). Primers for four short tandem repeats are included in both tubes for quality control and sample identification purposes (red peaks, both panels—tubes A and B). (Courtesy Dr J Evans, Bristol Genetics Laboratory, Southmead Hospital, Bristol, UK.)

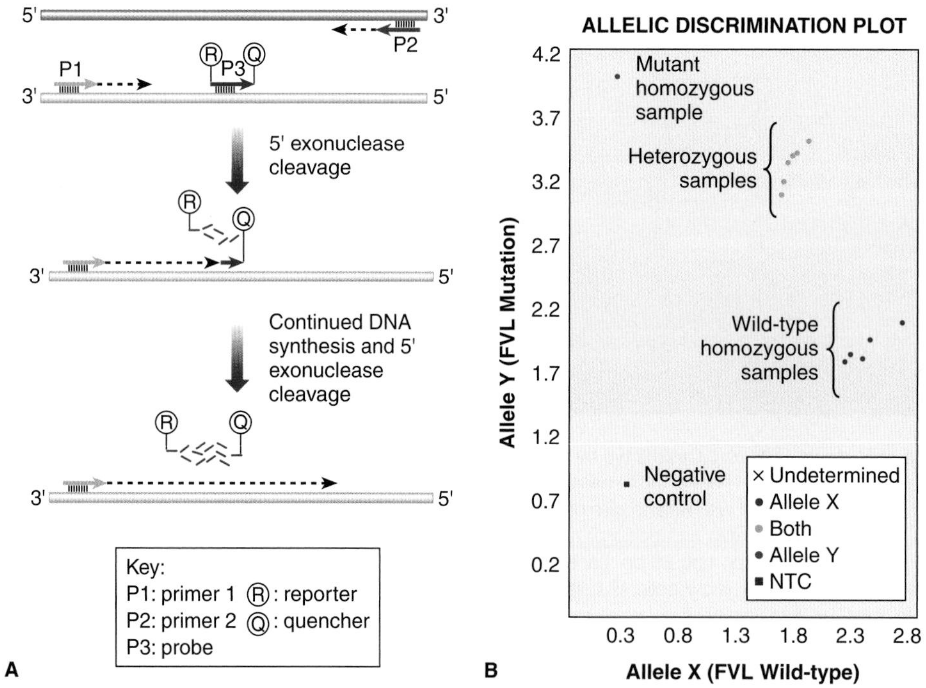

• **Fig. 5.11** Real-time polymerase chain reaction (PCR) to detect the factor V Leiden mutation. (A) TaqMan technique. The sequence encompassing the mutation is amplified by PCR primers P1 and P2. A probe, P3, specific to the mutation, is labeled with two fluorophores. A reporter fluorophore, R, is attached to the 5′ end of the probe, and a quencher fluorophore, Q, is attached to the 3′ end. During the PCR reaction, the 5′ exonuclease activity of the polymerase enzyme progressively degrades the probe, separating the reporter and quencher dyes, which results in a fluorescent signal from the reporter fluorophore. (B) TaqMan genotyping plot. Each sample is analyzed with two probes, one specific for the wild-type sequence and one for the mutation. The strength of fluorescence from each probe is plotted on a graph (wild-type on the X-axis, mutant on the Y-axis). Each sample is represented by a single point. The samples fall into three clusters representing the possible genotypes: homozygous wild-type, homozygous mutant or heterozygous. NTC – No template control. (Courtesy Dr E Young, formerly of the Genomic Laboratory, Royal Devon and Exeter Hospital, Exeter, UK.)

position; this prevents phosphodiester bonding, resulting in each reaction container consisting of a mixture of DNA fragments of different lengths that terminate in their respective dideoxynucleotide, owing to chain termination occurring at random in each reaction mixture at the respective nucleotide. When the reaction products are separated by capillary electrophoresis, a ladder of DNA sequences of differing lengths is produced. The DNA sequence complementary to the single-stranded DNA template is generated by the computer software, and the position of a mutation may be highlighted with an appropriate software package (Fig. 5.12).

Next-Generation Sequencing

The demand for low-cost sequencing has driven the development of high-throughput **sequencing** technologies that produce

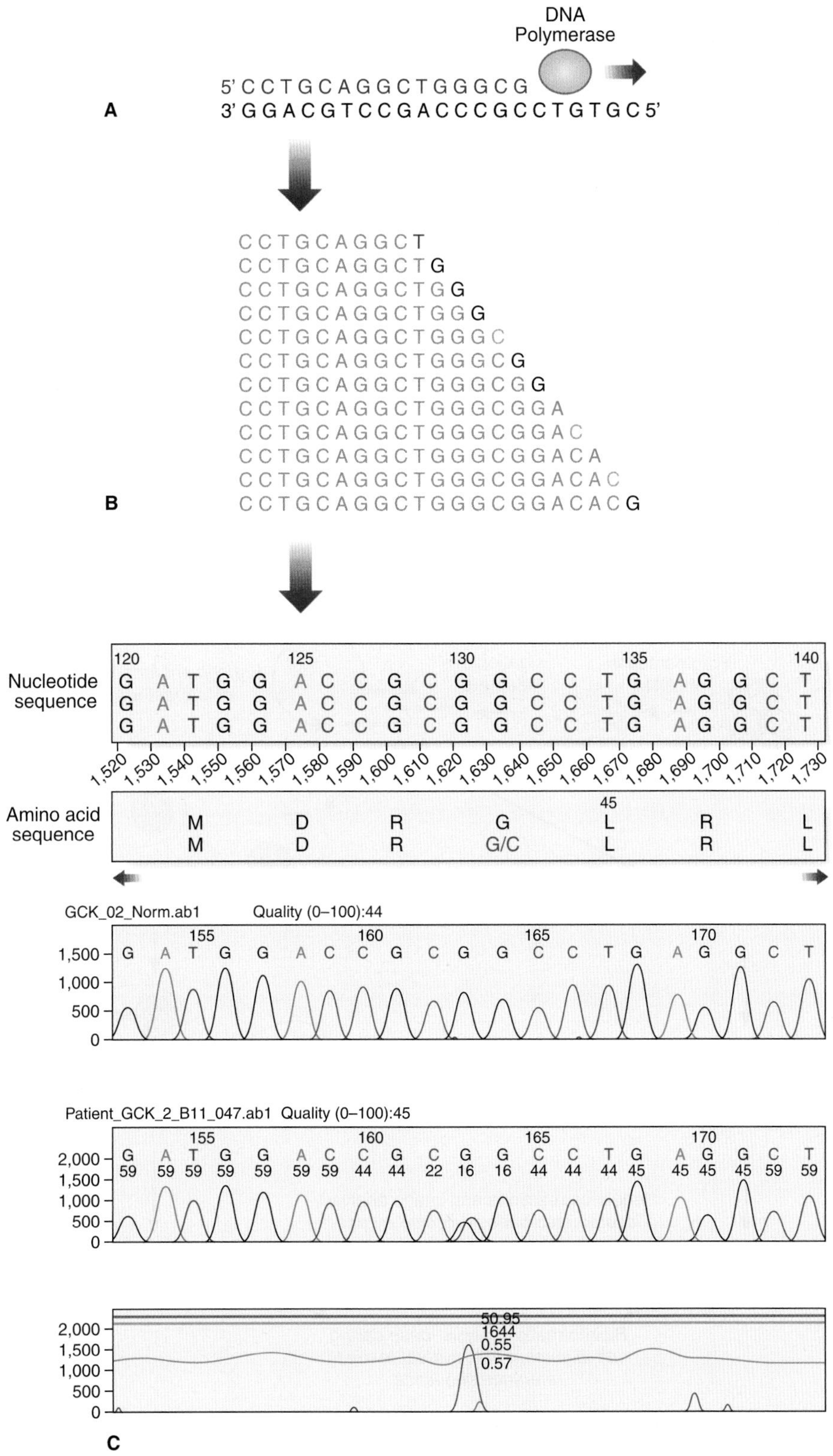

• **Fig. 5.12** Fluorescent dideoxy DNA sequencing. The sequencing primer (*shown in red*) binds to the template and primes synthesis of a complementary DNA strand in the direction indicated (A). The sequencing reaction includes four dNTPs and four ddNTPs, each labeled with a different fluorescent dye. Competition between the dNTPs and ddNTPs results in the production of a collection of fragments (B), which are then separated by electrophoresis to generate an electropherogram (C). A heterozygous mutation, p.Gly44Cys (GGC > TGC; glycine > cysteine), is identified by the software.

millions of sequences at once. Next- (or second-) generation "clonal" sequencers use an *in vitro* cloning step to amplify individual DNA molecules by emulsion or bridge PCR (Fig. 5.13). The cloned DNA molecules are then sequenced in parallel using a sequencing by synthesis where incorporated fluorescent bases are detected by laser scanning. The sequence reads are relatively short (150–250 bp) and need to be aligned to a reference sequence to identify variants that may be causative of disease (Fig. 5.14). A comparison with Sanger sequencing is shown in Table 5.4, and examples of variants identified by next-generation sequencing are shown in Fig. 5.14. So-called third-generation sequencers generate long sequence reads (kb in length) from single molecules in real time. They are better able to sequence through repetitive regions where alignment of short reads is difficult.

The **sequencing by synthesis** method was developed in the mid-1990s by Cambridge scientists Shankar Balasubramanian and David Klenerman. Their ideas of using clonal arrays and massively parallel sequencing of short reads using solid-phase sequencing by reversible terminators created the basis for the technology that enables sequencing of a human genome in just a few days at a cost of less than US$1000. By comparison, the first human genome took over a decade to sequence and was estimated to have cost US$2.7 billion!

In the clinical diagnostic setting, next-generation sequencing is particularly useful for the genetic diagnosis of rare diseases that exhibit genetic heterogeneity. Rather than sequencing single genes sequentially, all the genes in which variants have been reported to cause the disease can be analyzed simultaneously in a single test. This can be achieved either through physical targeting, where a defined set of genes is selected for capture by hybridization or PCR amplification, or through virtual gene panel analysis of exome (p. 48) or genome sequence data. These gene panel tests range from two genes (*BRCA1* and *BRCA2* for familial breast and ovarian cancer) to approximately 100 genes (for example, congenital cataract) to more than 1000 genes for intellectual disability. Exome sequencing is used routinely as a clinical diagnostic test, where variants can be filtered on the basis of a genetic strategy rather than by a gene list, for example *trio* sequencing to identify *de novo* mutations in an affected proband born to unaffected, unrelated parents.

Long-Read Next-Generation Sequencing

Second-generation sequencing generates short reads from 75 to 300 bases, as described, that need to be mapped to a human reference sequence. Long-read sequencing (third-generation) produces far longer reads of 10 to 100,000 bases in length, with 2 million bases the current maximum. Single molecules are sequenced in real time, often without the need for amplification. The two main methodologies use either protein nanopore technology, where changes to an electric current are monitored as the DNA (or RNA) molecule passes through the pore, or template-directed real-time DNA synthesis using four fluorescently distinguishable deoxyribonucleoside triphosphates.

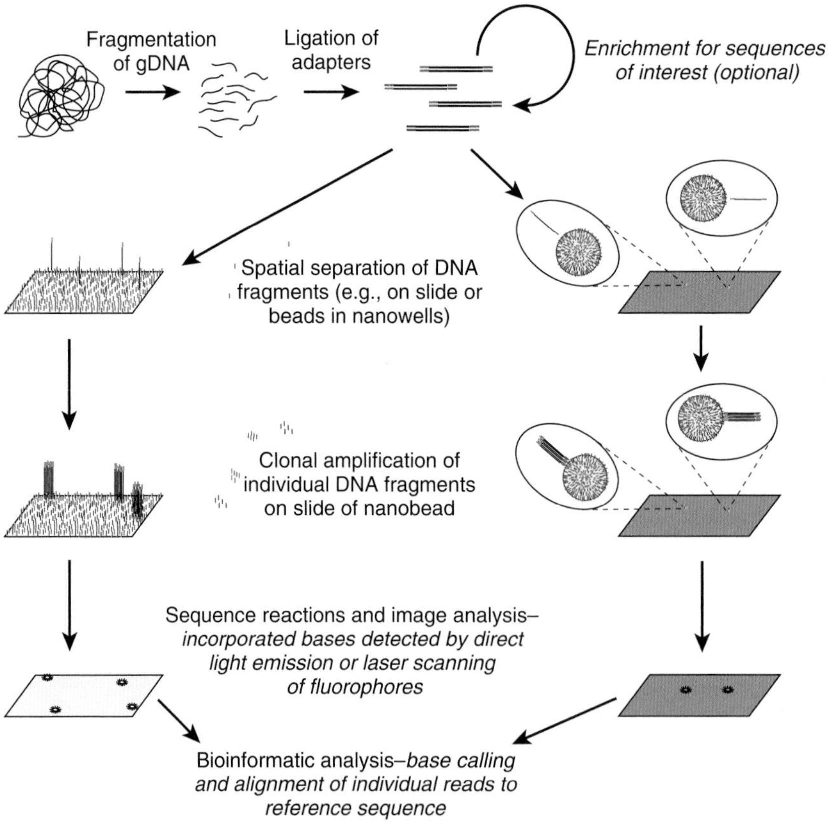

• **Fig. 5.13** Next-generation "clonal" sequencing. DNA is fragmented and adaptors ligated before clonal amplification on a bead or glass slide. Sequencing takes place *in situ*, and incorporated bases are detected by direct light emission or scanning of fluorophores. Data analysis includes base calling and alignment to a reference sequence in order to identify mutations or polymorphisms. (Courtesy Dr R Caswell, Genomic Laboratory, Royal Devon and Exeter Hospital, Exeter, UK.)

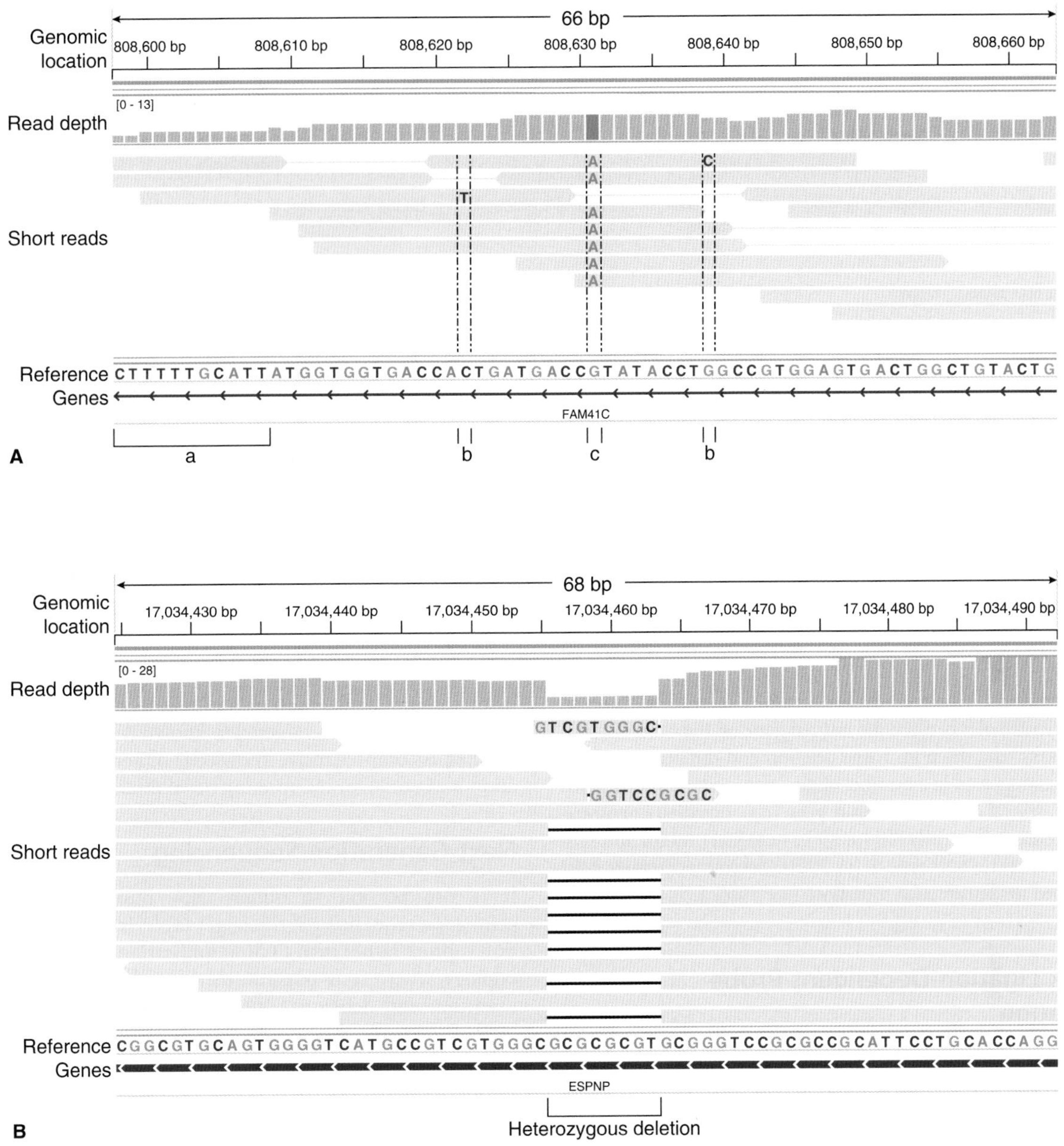

• **Fig. 5.14** (A) Aligning individual paired-end reads to the reference genome. Nucleotides in the reads that differ from the reference sequence are marked. (a) A region with poor coverage. (b) The variants at these positions are most likely sequencing errors. (c) At this position the subject is homozygous for the A alleles. A real example would have longer reads and greater read depth. (B) Aligned reads with a heterozygous deletion. Reads with an 8–base pair deletion identified are marked with a black bar. Images produced using the IGV software package. (Courtesy Dr M Wakeling, University of Exeter Medical School, UK.)

TABLE 5.4 Sanger sequencing compared with next-generation "clonal" sequencing

Sanger Sequencing	Next-Generation "Clonal" Sequencing
One sequence read per sample	Massively parallel sequencing
500–1000 bases per read	100–400 bases per read
Approx. 1 million bases per day per machine	Approx. 2 billion bases per day per machine
Approx. US$1 per 1000 bases	Approx. US$1 per 10,000,000 bases

The advantages of long-read sequencing for clinical genomic analysis include: (1) improved genome assembly, as the long reads can span repetitive regions, (2) better detection of large and/or complex rearrangements and variants within repetitive regions, and (3) the capacity to perform haplotype phasing to determine whether variants are inherited "in cis" (together).

Dosage Analysis

Most of the methods described previously will detect point mutations, small insertions and deletions. Deletions of one or more exons are common in boys with Duchenne muscular dystrophy and may be identified by a multiplex PCR that reveals the absence of one or

TABLE 5.5 Methods for detecting copy number changes

Method	Known/Unknown Copy Number Change	Example	Advantages/Disadvantages
Multiplex ligation-dependent probe amplification	Known	Gene-specific or subtelomere deletion analysis	Suited to the clinical diagnostic setting, but labor intensive and requires good quality DNA
Quantitative fluorescent PCR	Known	Prenatal aneuploidy testing	Rapid, but requires informative microsatellite markers
Droplet digital PCR	Known	Confirming deletions or duplications found by a different method	Flexible; can use standard PCR primers, but gene-centric approach
Array CGH	Known/unknown	Testing for severe developmental delay, learning difficulties, congenital abnormalities	Detects any deletion or duplication, but interpretation of novel variants can be difficult
Next-generation sequencing	Known/unknown	Analysis of all genes that are sequenced	Expensive equipment, enormous capacity, but vast amount of data to analyze, and interpretation of novel variants can be difficult

more PCR products. However, these mutations are more difficult to detect in carrier females because the normal gene on the other X chromosome "masks" the deletion. Large deletion and duplication mutations have been reported in a number of disorders and may encompass a single exon, several exons or an entire gene (e.g., hereditary neuropathy with pressure palsies [HNPP] [p. 293]; hereditary motor and sensory neuropathy [HMSN] type 1 [p. 292]). Several techniques have been developed to identify such mutations (see Table 5.5).

Multiplex Ligation-Dependent Probe Amplification

This is a high-resolution method used to detect deletions and duplications (Fig. 5.15). Each multiplex ligation-dependent probe amplification consists of two fluorescently labeled oligonucleotides that can hybridize, adjacent to each other, to a target gene sequence. When hybridized, the two oligonucleotides are joined by a ligase, and the probe is then amplified by PCR (each oligonucleotide includes a universal primer sequence at its terminus). The probes include a variable-length stuffer sequence that enables separation of the PCR products by capillary electrophoresis. Up to 40 probes can be amplified in a single reaction.

Quantitative Fluorescent PCR

Dosage analysis by quantitative fluorescent PCR (QF-PCR) is routinely used for rapid aneuploidy screening; for example, in prenatal diagnosis (p. 322). Microsatellites (see the following section) located on chromosomes 13, 18 and 21 may be amplified within a multiplex, and trisomies detected, either by the presence of three alleles or by a dosage effect where one allele is overrepresented (Fig. 5.16).

Microarray Comparative Genomic Hybridization

Array CGH provides a way to detect deletions and duplications on a genome-wide scale (Fig. 5.17). Arrays used in clinical diagnostic laboratories include both genome-wide probes to detect novel mutations and probes targeted to known deletion/duplication syndromes. A comprehensive knowledge of normal copy number variation is essential for interpreting novel mutations.

Next-Generation Sequencing

It is also possible to obtain copy number data from next-generation sequencing if the target DNA is enriched by hybridization capture rather than PCR amplification. This is the first methodology where it is possible to detect base substitutions, small insertions and deletions, as well as copy number changes at the level of an exon or entire gene.

Droplet Digital PCR

This technique is most useful for confirming deletion or duplication mutations identified by other methods. It involves PCR performed within thousands of nanolitre-sized droplets to achieve highly precise, absolute nucleic acid quantification. A genomic DNA sample is diluted to incorporate either one or zero molecules of DNA in each droplet and mixed separately with PCR primers for the gene of interest and a reference housekeeping gene. After PCR amplification the fluorescence is measured in each droplet, and the concentration of target DNA is calculated as copies per microliter from the fraction of positive reactions using Poisson statistics. The ratio of target DNA copies compared with the reference gene provides an estimate of copy number for the gene with suspected abnormal dosage.

Variant Interpretation

Sequencing a human genome will identify approximately 4 to 5 million variants compared with the reference sequence. Identifying a disease-causing variant, or variant pair (for an autosomal recessive disorder caused by compound heterozygous variants), has been likened to finding a needle in a haystack! Bioinformatic pipelines are used to filter the variants to generate a shortlist of variants for manual review (see Fig. 5.18). This last stage is usually undertaken by laboratory scientists and may involve discussion with the patient's clinical team.

In the clinical diagnostic setting, variants in genes that are associated with mendelian (single-gene) disorders are classified as pathogenic, likely pathogenic, likely benign, benign, or of uncertain significance. The variant classification is reported in the context of the disorder and the inheritance pattern. The 2015 guidelines published by the American College of Medical Genetics and Genomics and the Association for Molecular Pathology provide a framework for classifying variants into these five categories according to criteria using typical types of variant evidence (e.g., population data, computational data, functional data, segregation data). You will notice that the terms "mutation" and "polymorphism" are no longer used to describe variants identified in the clinical diagnostic setting. This change in language recognizes that each individual has millions of genetic variants, and a binary classification is overly simplistic, in addition to the negative connotation of the word 'mutation'.

Genome Sequencing as a Clinical Diagnostic Test

It is now possible to sequence a human genome in just two days at a cost of less than US$1000. Compared with exome sequencing, in the clinical setting genome sequencing offers a higher diagnostic yield through the detection of deep intronic mutations that cause aberrant splicing, mutations in regulatory elements and balanced chromosome rearrangements (Table 5.6). Although the mean read depth is generally lower than that obtained by exome sequencing, coverage is more even, and this is expected to increase the sensitivity for detecting copy number changes. The major challenge is data storage and processing of the vast volume of genome sequence data. Although much of the

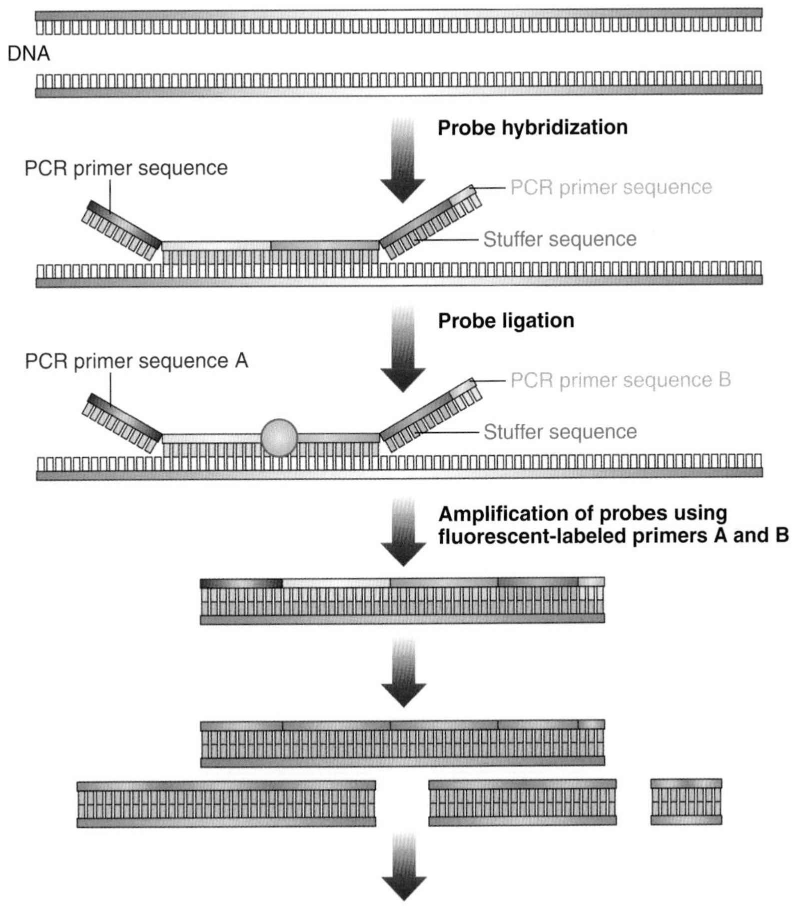

A

• **Fig. 5.15** (A) Illustration of the multiplex ligation-dependent probe amplification (MLPA) method. (B) Detection of a whole-gene deletion encompassing exons 1 to 9 of the *HNF1B* gene (*lower panel*) compared with a normal reference sample (*upper panel*). This MLPA kit also includes probes for the *GCK, HNF1A* and *HNF4A* genes. (C) Peak ratio plots showing in graphical form the ratio of normalized peak intensities between the normal reference and patient sample. Each point represents one peak: green or purple = peak within the normal range (0.75–1.25), red = peak either deleted (ratio <0.75) or duplicated (> 1.25). The data were analyzed using GeneMarker, SoftGenetics LLC. (Courtesy M Owens, Genomic Laboratory, Royal Devon and Exeter Hospital, Exeter, UK.)

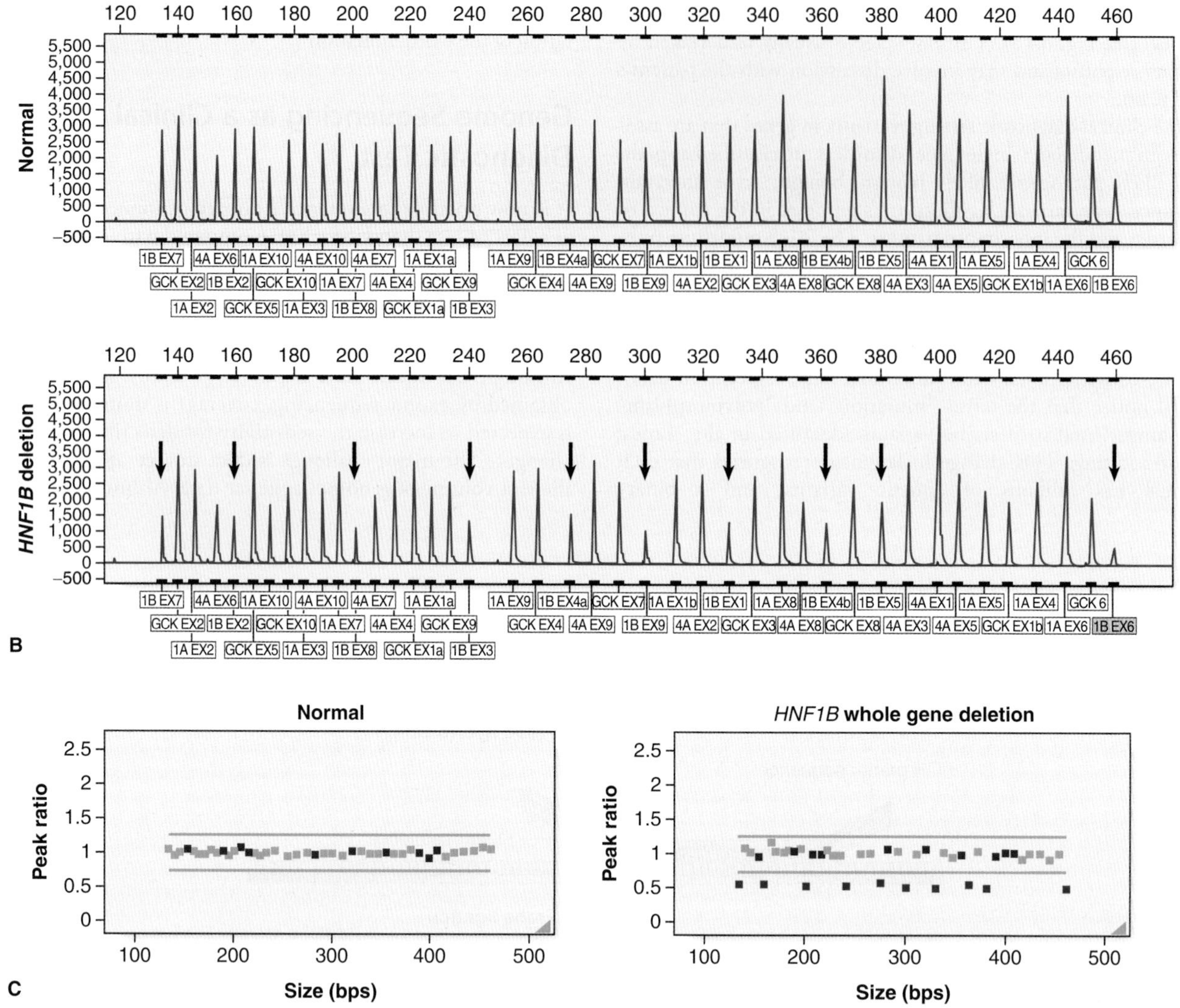

• **Fig. 5.15** (Continued)

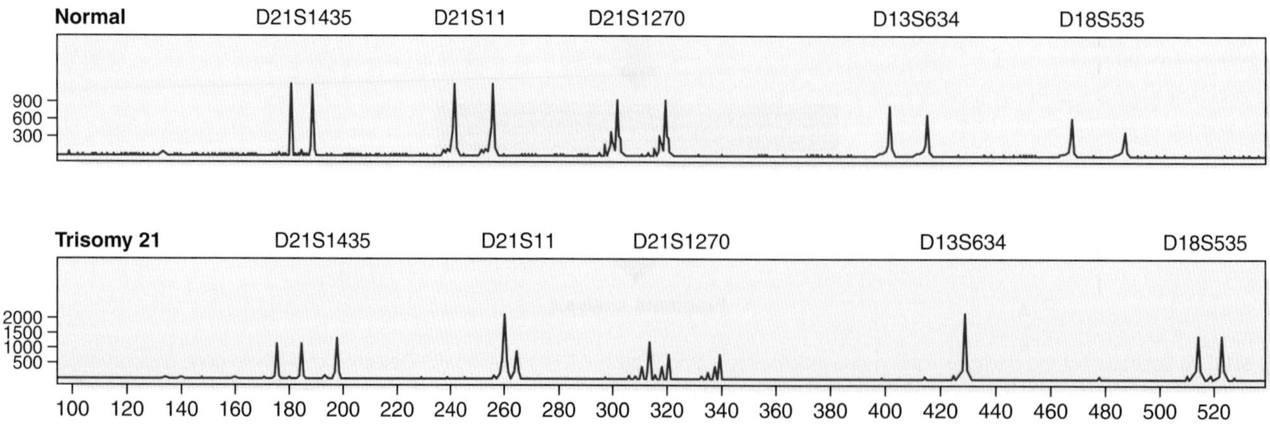

• **Fig. 5.16** Quantitative fluorescent–polymerase chain reaction for rapid prenatal aneuploidy testing. The upper panel shows a normal control, with two alleles for each microsatellite marker. The lower panel illustrates trisomy 21 with either three alleles (microsatellites D21S1435, D21S1270) or a dosage effect (D21S11). Microsatellite markers for chromosomes 13 and 18 show a normal profile. (Courtesy of C Anderson, Institute of Medical Genetics, University Hospital of Wales, Cardiff, UK.)

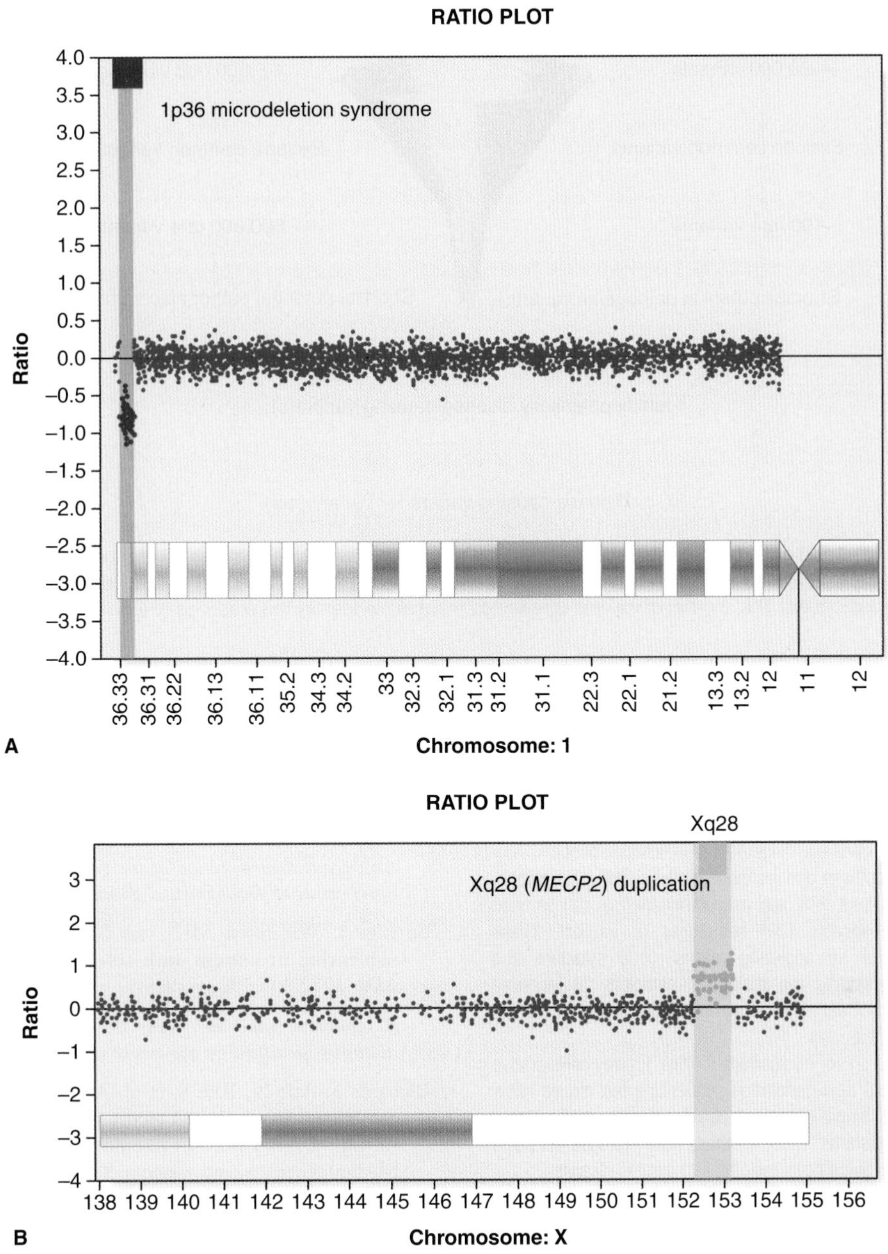

• **Fig. 5.17** Identification of copy number changes by array comparative genomic hybridization (this array includes 135,000 oligonucleotide probes). (A) A patient with the 1p36 microdeletion syndrome. (B) An *MECP2* duplication of chromosome Xq28. (Courtesy of R Palmer, North East Thames Regional Genetics Service Laboratories, Great Ormond Street Hospital for Children, London.)

non-coding sequence is currently not interpretable in the context of human disease, scientific understanding of the "regulome" is gathering pace as initiatives such as the Encyclopedia of DNA Elements project identify novel regulatory elements. In the future it may be possible to analyze the entire genome of a person and detect all known disease-associated variants, in addition to variants that determine drug response. The unanswered question is to what degree it will be possible to implement predictive medicine strategies based on this knowledge. Will genome sequencing become so routine that all babies have their genomes sequenced at birth? There are many ethical and social issues to debate around autonomy, genetic discrimination, data sharing, and privacy.

TABLE 5.6 The advantages and disadvantages of genome sequencing compared with exome sequencing

Advantages	Disadvantages
Faster library preparation	Greater cost of sequencing
Includes introns	Greater cost of data storage
Includes regulatory elements	Many more variants to analyze
Better detection of copy number variants	Difficulty in interpreting non-coding variants
Detection of structural variants	

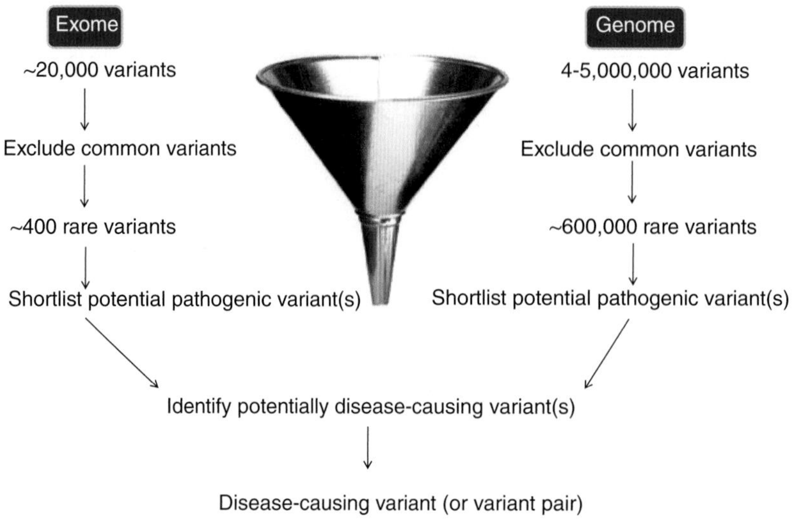

• **Fig. 5.18** Identification of a disease-causing variant (or variant pair) by exome or genome sequencing. Each human exome or genome has around 20,000 or 4 to 5 million variants compared with the reference sequence. Bioinformatic pipelines are used to filter out common variants and select those variants that are potentially pathogenic. The shortlist of variants is reviewed manually to identify the presence of a disease-causing variant (or variant pair).

ELEMENTS

1. Polymerase chain reaction (PCR) has revolutionized medical genetics. Within hours, more than a million copies of a gene can be amplified from a patient's DNA sample. The PCR product may be analyzed for the presence of a pathogenic mutation, gene rearrangement or infectious agent.
2. Techniques including Southern and northern blotting, DNA sequencing, mutation screening, real-time PCR, and microarray analysis can be used to identify or analyze specific DNA sequences of interest. These techniques can be used for analyzing normal gene structure and function, as well as revealing the molecular pathology of inherited disease. This provides a means for presymptomatic diagnosis, carrier detection, and prenatal diagnosis.
3. Single nucleotide polymorphism microarrays ("chips"), array comparative genomic hybridization and next-generation sequencing techniques allow genome-wide analysis of single nucleotide polymorphisms, copy number variants, and sequence variants. These methods have changed the scale of genetic analysis and provide novel insights into genetic disease.
4. Next-generation sequencing allows simultaneous testing for all genes in which mutations are known to cause a monogenic disorder. The gene panel may be targeted physically by hybridization capture or PCR of selected genes, or it may be a virtual panel where the entire exome is sequenced but only specific genes are analyzed. The ability to sequence a genome for less than US$1000 allows the use of genome sequencing as a clinical diagnostic test to detect base substitutions, small insertions or deletions, copy number changes, and chromosomal rearrangements in a single test.
5. Sequencing of a human genome is relatively straightforward, but interpreting genetic variants to diagnose and predict disease is a complex undertaking. With increased scientific knowledge, our ability to do this more accurately will improve. There are many ethical and social issues to consider in the context of using genomic information for prediction.

Further Reading

Deciphering Developmental Disorders Study. Large-scale discovery of novel genetic causes of developmental disorders. *Nature*. 2015;519: 223–228.

An elegant demonstration of the power of genome-wide analysis to find novel causes of developmental disorders.

de Ligt J, Willemsen MH, van Bon BW, et al. Diagnostic exome sequencing in persons with severe intellectual disability. *N Engl J Med*. 2012;367:1921–1929.

A landmark paper describing de novo *mutations causing intellectual disability identified by trio exome sequencing.*

Richards S, Aziz N, Bale S, et al. ACMG laboratory quality assurance committee. Standards and guidelines for the interpretation of sequence variants: a joint consensus recommendation of the American College of Medical Genetics and Genomics and the Association for Molecular Pathology. *Genet Med*. 2015;17:405–424.

A framework for classifying genetic variants in clinical laboratories.

Strachan T, Read AP. *Human Molecular Genetics*. 5th ed. London: Garland Science; 2019.

A comprehensive textbook of all aspects of molecular and cellular biology as related to inherited disease in humans.

6

Patterns of Inheritance

That the fundamental aspects of heredity should have turned out to be so extraordinarily simple supports us in the hope that nature may, after all, be entirely approachable.

Thomas Hunt Morgan (1919)

Family Studies

To investigate whether a particular trait or disorder in humans is genetic and hereditary, we have traditionally relied either on observation of the way in which it is transmitted within a family or on study of its frequency among relatives. This enables advice to be given to family members regarding the likelihood of their developing it or passing it on to their children (i.e., **genetic counseling**; see Chapter 21). In all clinical medicine, good history taking is vital, and a good family history can sometimes provide a diagnosis. For example, a child may see a doctor with a fracture after a minor injury. A family history of relatives with a similar tendency to fracture, together with blue sclerae, would suggest the diagnosis of osteogenesis imperfecta, but the absence of a positive family history would suggest a non-genetic diagnosis.

Pedigree Drawing and Terminology

A family tree, or pedigree, records relevant family information in a diagram. It usually begins with the person through whom the family came to medical attention: the **index case**, or **proband**. The proband in the pedigree is indicated by an arrow. Information about the health of the rest of the family is obtained by asking direct questions about brothers, sisters, parents, and maternal and paternal relatives, with the relevant information about the sex of the individual, affection status, and relationship to other individuals being carefully recorded on the chart (Fig. 6.1). Attention to detail can be crucial because patients do not always appreciate the potential importance of miscarriages, or the difference between siblings and half siblings, for example.

Mendelian Inheritance

More than 16,000 traits or disorders in humans exhibit single-gene **unifactorial** or **mendelian inheritance**. However, characteristics such as height and many common familial disorders such as diabetes or hypertension do not usually follow a simple pattern of mendelian inheritance (see Chapter 10).

A trait or disorder determined by a gene on an autosome is said to show **autosomal inheritance**, whereas a trait or disorder determined by a gene on one of the sex chromosomes is said to show **sex-linked inheritance**.

Autosomal Dominant Inheritance

An autosomal dominant trait or condition is one that manifests in the heterozygous state, that is, in a person possessing both a variant allele and a normal allele. It is often possible to trace a dominantly inherited trait or condition through many generations of a family (Fig. 6.2). In South Africa, the vast majority of cases of porphyria variegata can be traced back to one couple in the late 17th century. This is a metabolic disorder characterized by skin blistering as a result of increased sensitivity to sunlight (Fig. 6.3) and urine that becomes "port wine"–colored on standing as a result of the presence of porphyrins (p. 282). This pattern of inheritance is sometimes referred to as "vertical" transmission and is confirmed when male–male (i.e., father to son) transmission has occurred.

Genetic Risks

Each gamete from an individual with a dominant trait or condition will contain either the normal allele or the variant allele. If we represent the dominant variant allele as "D" and the normal allele as "d," then the possible combinations of the gametes is seen in Fig. 6.4. Any child born to a person affected with a dominant condition has a 1 in 2 (50%) chance of inheriting it and being similarly affected. These diagrams are often used in the genetic clinic to explain segregation to patients and are more user-friendly than a Punnett square (see Figs. 1.3 and 7.1).

Pleiotropy

Autosomal dominant traits may involve only one organ or part of the body; for example, the eye in congenital cataracts. However, it is common for them to manifest in different systems of the body in a variety of ways. This is **pleiotropy**—a single gene that may give rise to two or more apparently unrelated effects. In tuberous sclerosis, affected individuals can present with a range of problems including learning difficulties, epilepsy, a facial rash known as adenoma sebaceum (histologically composed of blood vessels and fibrous tissue known as angiokeratoma), or subungual fibromas (Fig. 6.5); some affected individuals have all features, whereas others may have almost none. Some discoveries are challenging our conceptual understanding of the term **pleiotropy** on account of the remarkably diverse syndromes that can result from different variants in the same gene—for example, the *LMNA* gene (which encodes lamin A/C) and the X-linked filamin A (*FLNA*) gene. Mutations in *LMNA* may cause Emery-Dreifuss muscular dystrophy, a form of limb girdle muscular dystrophy, a form of Charcot-Marie-Tooth disease (p. 292), dilated cardiomyopathy (p. 308) with conduction abnormality, Dunnigan-type familial partial lipodystrophy (Fig. 6.6), mandibuloacral dysplasia, and Hutchinson-Gilford progeria, a very rare condition that has always been a great curiosity. These are attributed to heterozygous variants, with the

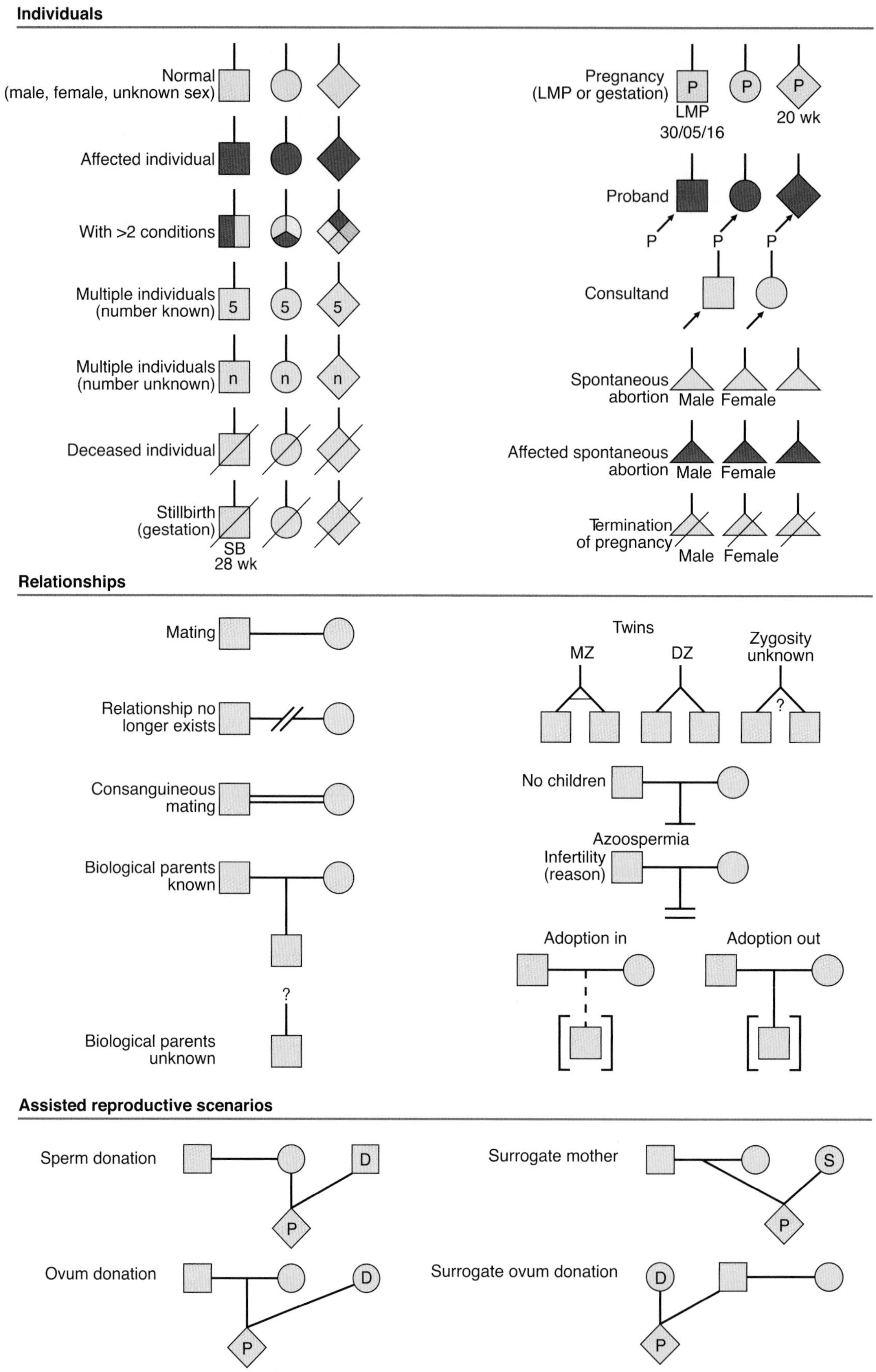

• **Fig. 6.1** Symbols used to represent individuals and relationships in family trees. DZ, *LMP, MZ.*

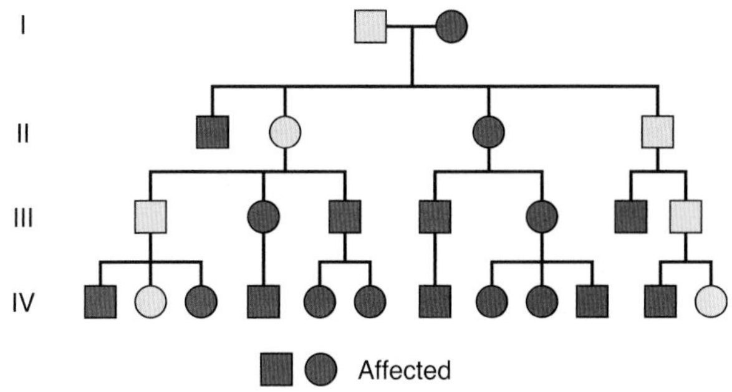

• **Fig. 6.2** Family tree of an autosomal dominant trait. Note the presence of male-to-male transmission.

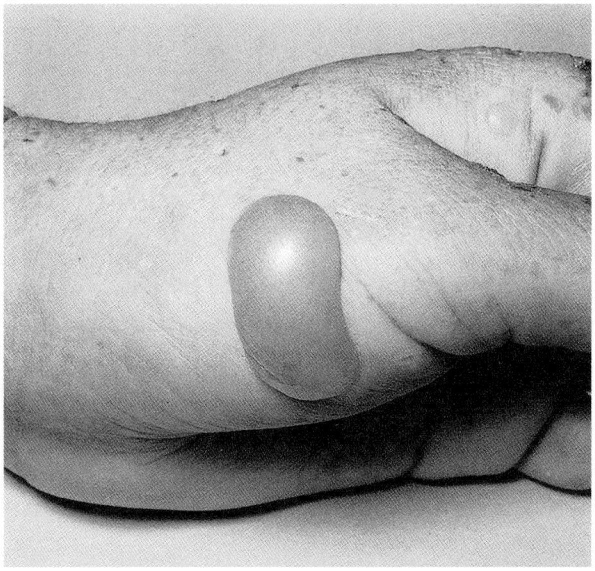

• **Fig. 6.3** Blistering skin lesions on the hand in porphyria variegata.

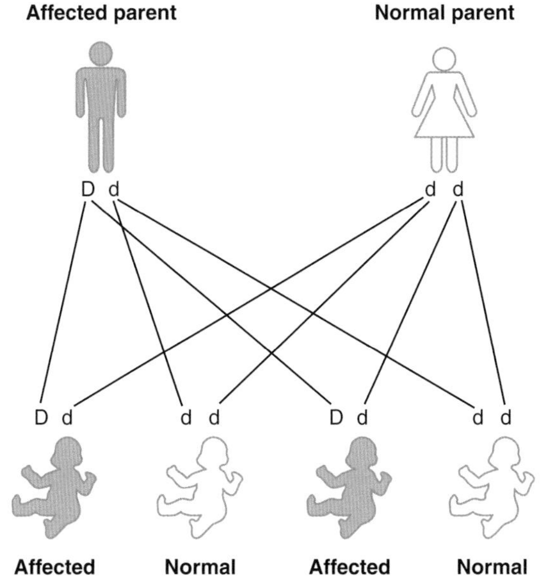

• **Fig. 6.4** Segregation of alleles in autosomal dominant inheritance. *D* represents the mutated allele, whereas *d* represents the normal allele.

exception of Charcot-Marie-Tooth disease and mandibuloacral dysplasia, which are recessive—affected individuals are therefore homozygous for *LMNA* mutations. Sometimes an individual with a variant is entirely normal. Variants in the gene encoding filamin A have been implicated in the distinct, although overlapping, X-linked dominant dysmorphic conditions oto-palato-digital syndrome, Melnick-Needles syndrome, and frontometaphyseal dysplasia. However, it was not foreseen that a form of X-linked dominant epilepsy in women, called periventricular nodular heterotopia, is also due to variants in this gene.

Variable Expressivity

The clinical features in autosomal dominant disorders can show striking variation from person to person, even in the same family. This difference between individuals is referred to as **variable expressivity**. In autosomal dominant polycystic kidney disease, for example, some affected individuals develop renal failure in early

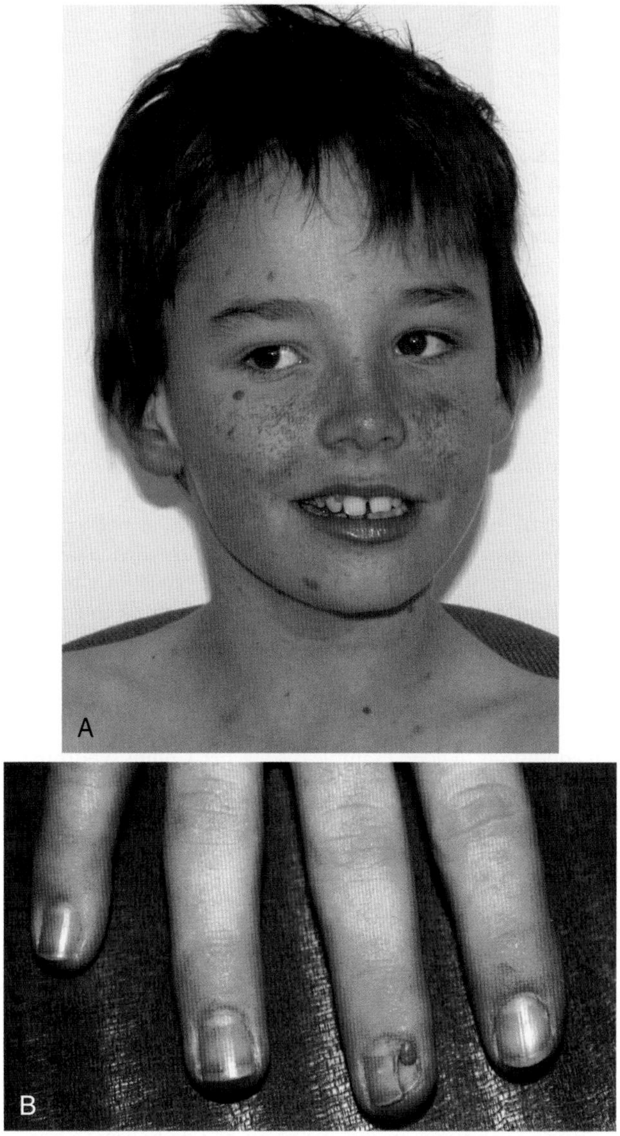

• **Fig. 6.5** The facial rash (A) of angiokeratoma (adenoma sebaceum) in a male with tuberous sclerosis, and a typical subungual fibroma of the nail bed (B).

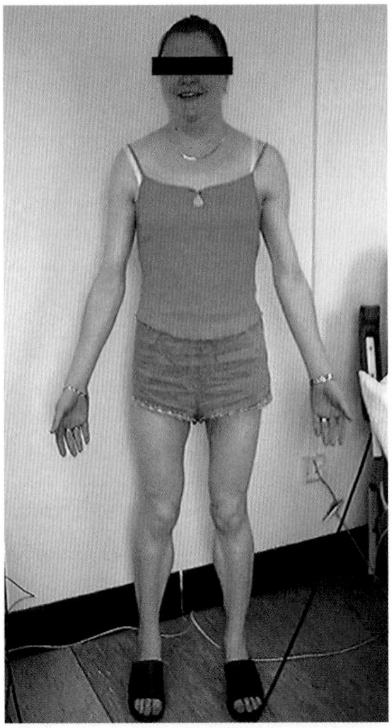

• **Fig. 6.6** Dunnigan-type familial partial lipodystrophy attributed to a variant in the gene encoding LAMIN A/C. The patient lacks adipose tissue, especially in the distal limbs. A wide variety of clinical phenotypes is associated with variants in this one gene.

adulthood whereas others have just a few renal cysts that do not affect renal function significantly.

Reduced Penetrance

In some individuals heterozygous for gene variants giving rise to certain autosomal dominant disorders, there may be minimal clinical features, and this demonstrates **reduced penetrance**. This may be the result of the modifying effects of other genes, as well as interaction of the gene with environmental factors. An individual with no features of a condition, despite being heterozygous for a particular gene variant, is said to demonstrate **non-penetrance**; in lay terms, the condition "skips a generation" (see also p. 97).

Reduced penetrance and variable expressivity, together with the pleiotropic effects of a variant allele, all need to be considered when trying to interpret family history information for autosomal dominant conditions. A good example is Treacher-Collins syndrome. In its most obvious manifestation the facial features are unmistakable (Fig. 6.7). However, the mother of the child illustrated is also known to harbor the gene (*TCOF1*) variant, and she has other close relatives who manifest the condition.

New Variants

In autosomal dominant disorders an affected person commonly has an affected parent. However, this is not always so, and it is not unusual for a condition to appear in an individual when there is no preceding family history. A striking example is achondroplasia, a form of short-limbed dwarfism (Figure 9.21), in which the parents usually have normal stature. The sudden unexpected appearance of a genetic condition arising as a result of a pathogenic heterozygous gene variant is called a ***de novo* variant**. Dominant inheritance in achondroplasia was confirmed by the observation that the offspring of an affected individual had a 50% chance of also being

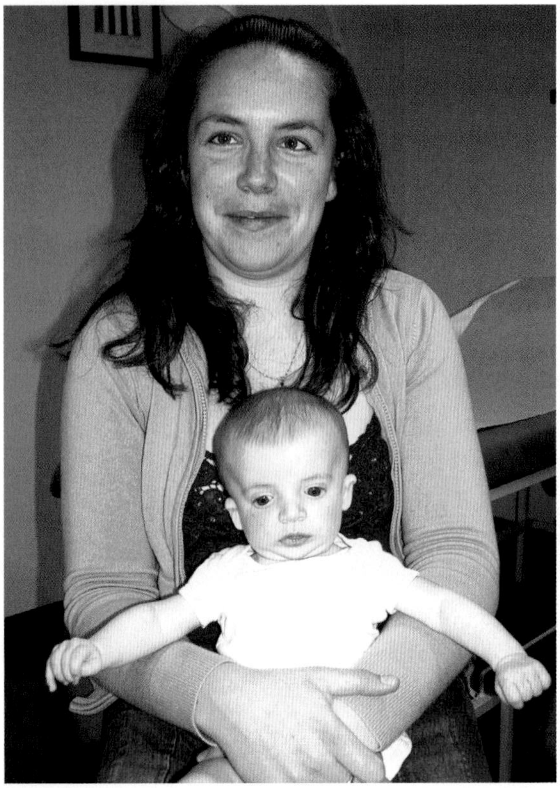

• **Fig. 6.7** The baby in this picture has Treacher-Collins syndrome, resulting from a variant in *TCOF1*. The mandible is small, the palpebral fissures slant downward, there is usually a defect (coloboma) of the lower eyelid, the ears may show microtia, and hearing impairment is common. The condition follows autosomal dominant inheritance but is very variable—the baby's mother also has the variant, but she shows no obvious signs of the condition.

affected. In less obvious conditions other explanations for their "sudden" appearance must be considered. This includes non-penetrance and variable expression, as previously mentioned. However, the astute clinician also needs to be aware that the family relationships may not be as stated; that is, there may be undisclosed **nonpaternity** (or, rarely, **non-maternity**).

New heterozygous variants, in some conditions, have been associated with older-than-average fathers. Traditionally, this is believed to be a consequence of the large number of mitotic divisions that male gamete stem cells undergo during a man's reproductive lifetime (p. 34). However, this may well be a simplistic view. In relation to variants in *FGFR2* (craniosynostosis syndromes), Wilkie's group in Oxford demonstrated that causative gain-of-function variants confer a selective advantage to spermatogonial stem cells, so that mutated cell lines accumulate in the testis.

Codominance

Codominance is the term used for two allelic traits that are both expressed in the heterozygous state. In persons with blood group AB it is possible to demonstrate both A and B blood group substances on the red blood cells, so the A and B blood groups are therefore codominant (p. 181).

Homozygosity for Autosomal Dominant Traits

The rarity of most autosomal dominant conditions means that they usually occur only in the heterozygous state. Occasionally, however, children are born to couples where both parents are heterozygous for a dominantly inherited disorder. Such offspring are at risk of being homozygous for the gene variants. In some instances, affected individuals appear either to be more severely affected, as with achondroplasia, or to have an earlier age of onset, as in familial hypercholesterolemia (p. 147). Conversely, with other dominantly inherited conditions, homozygous individuals are not more severely affected than heterozygotes—for example, Huntington disease (p. 289) and myotonic dystrophy (p. 302). These different phenotypic effects may be explained by the nature of the variant—whether they are gain-of-function (p. 22) or loss-of-function (p. 22).

Autosomal Recessive Inheritance

Recessive traits and conditions are manifest only when the variant allele is present in a double dose (i.e., homozygosity). Individuals heterozygous for such variant alleles show no features of the disorder and are perfectly healthy; they are **carriers**. The family tree for recessively inherited conditions (Fig. 6.8) differs markedly from the autosomal dominant pattern. It is not possible to trace an autosomal recessive trait or disorder through the family (except sometimes in highly inbred families), as all the affected individuals in a family are usually in a single **sibship** (i.e., brothers and sisters). This was sometimes referred to as "horizontal" transmission, but this is a misleading term.

Consanguinity

Enquiry into the family history of individuals affected with rare recessive conditions might reveal that their parents are related (i.e., **consanguineous**). The rarer a recessive trait or disorder, the greater the frequency of consanguinity among the parents of affected individuals. In cystic fibrosis, the most common "serious" autosomal recessive disease in western Europeans (p. 303), the frequency of parental consanguinity is only slightly greater than that seen in the general population. By contrast, when Bateson and Garrod originally described the very rare alkaptonuria, they observed that a quarter or more of the parents were first cousins, and rightly reasoned that rare alleles are more likely to "meet up" in the offspring of cousins than unrelated parents. In large inbred kindreds, an autosomal recessive condition may be present in more than one branch of the family.

Genetic Risks

If we represent the normal dominant allele as "R" and the recessive variant allele as "r," then each parental gamete carries either the variant or the normal allele (Fig. 6.9). At conception the various possible combinations of gametes mean that the offspring of two heterozygotes have a 1 in 4 (25%) chance of being homozygous affected, a 1 in 2 (50%) chance of being heterozygous unaffected, and a 1 in 4 (25%) chance of being homozygous unaffected.

Pseudodominance

If an individual who is homozygous for an autosomal recessive condition has children with a carrier of the same condition, their offspring have a 1 in 2 (50%) chance of being affected. Such a pedigree is said to exhibit **pseudodominance** (Fig. 6.10).

Locus Heterogeneity

Some clinical conditions occur due to variants in more than one gene, thus demonstrating **locus heterogeneity**. For example, early-onset sensorineural hearing loss/deafness most commonly follows autosomal recessive inheritance. Deaf persons, by virtue of their schooling and involvement in the deaf community, often partner with another deaf person. For two deaf persons homozygous for the same recessively inherited condition, all of their

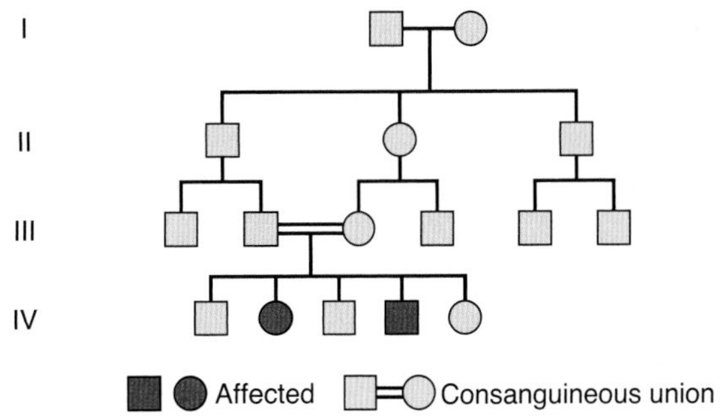

• **Fig. 6.8** Family tree of an autosomal recessive trait.

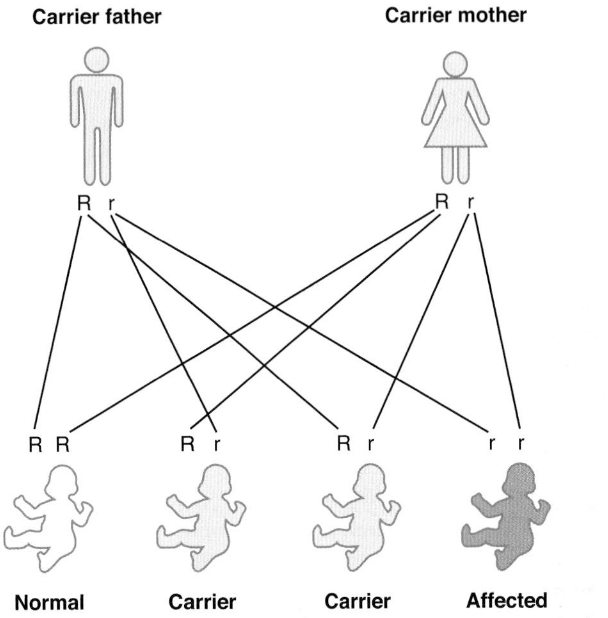

• **Fig. 6.9** Segregation of alleles in autosomal recessive inheritance. *R* represents the normal allele, *r* the mutated allele.

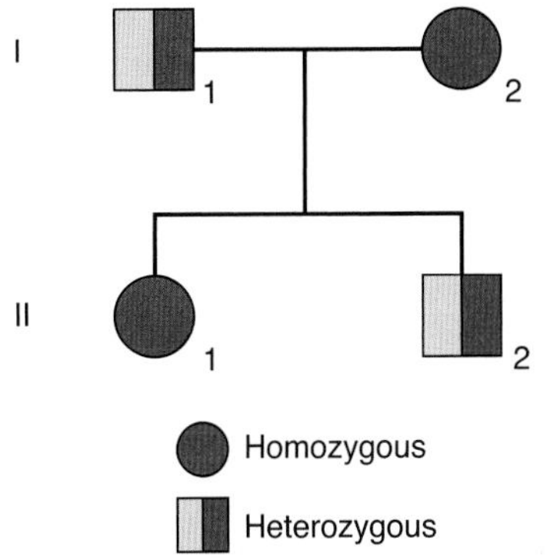

• **Fig. 6.10** A pedigree with a woman (I_2) homozygous for an autosomal recessive disorder whose husband is heterozygous for the same disorder. They have a homozygous affected daughter, so that the pedigree shows pseudodominant inheritance.

children will be affected. However, there are families in which all children born to parents with autosomal recessive deafness have normal hearing because they are **double heterozygotes** (or carriers). The parents are therefore homozygous for gene variants at different loci. In fact, there are more than 80 genes or gene loci known to be implicated in recessively inherited deafness, and a similar story applies to autosomal recessive retinitis pigmentosa.

Disorders with the same phenotype from different genetic loci are known as **genocopies**, whereas when the same phenotype results from environmental causes, it is known as a **phenocopy**.

Variant Heterogeneity

Heterogeneity can also occur at the allelic level. In the majority of single-gene disorders, for example, β-thalassemia, a large number of different variants have been identified as being responsible (p. 167). There are individuals who have two different variants at the same locus and are known as **compound heterozygotes**, constituting what is known as **allelic heterogeneity**. Most individuals affected with an autosomal recessive condition are compound heterozygotes rather than true homozygotes, unless their parents are related, in which case they are likely to be homozygous for the same variant by descent, that is, inherited from a common ancestor.

Sex-Linked Inheritance

Sex-linked inheritance refers to the pattern of inheritance shown by genes that are located on either of the sex chromosomes. Genes carried on the X chromosome are referred to as being **X-linked**, and those carried on the Y chromosome (very rare) are referred to as exhibiting **Y-linked** or **holandric inheritance**.

X-Linked Recessive Inheritance

An X-linked recessive trait is one determined by a gene carried on the X chromosome and usually manifests only in males. A male with a variant allele on his single X chromosome is said to be **hemizygous** for that allele. Conditions inherited in an X-linked recessive manner are transmitted by (usually) healthy heterozygous female carriers to affected males, as well as by affected males to their obligate carrier daughters, with a consequent risk to male grandchildren through these daughters (Fig. 6.11). This was sometimes referred to as a "diagonal" or "knight's move" pattern of transmission.

The mode of inheritance whereby only males are affected by a disease that is transmitted by normal females was appreciated by Jews 2000 years ago. They excused from circumcision the sons of all the sisters of a mother who had sons with the "bleeding disease," in other words, hemophilia (p. 316). The sons of the father's siblings were not excused. Queen Victoria was a carrier of hemophilia, and her unaffected carrier daughters introduced the gene into the Russian and Spanish royal families. Her eldest son, later Edward VII, did not inherit the gene (see Fig. 19.26).

Genetic Risks. A male transmits his X chromosome to each of his daughters and his Y chromosome to each of his sons. If a male with hemophilia has children with a normal female, then all of his daughters will be **obligate carriers**, but none of his sons will be affected (Fig. 6.12). A male cannot transmit an X-linked trait to his son, with the very rare exception of uniparental heterodisomy (p. 78).

For a carrier female of an X-linked recessive condition having children with a normal male, each son has a 1 in 2 (50%) chance of being affected, and each daughter has a 1 in 2 (50%) chance of being a carrier (Fig. 6.13).

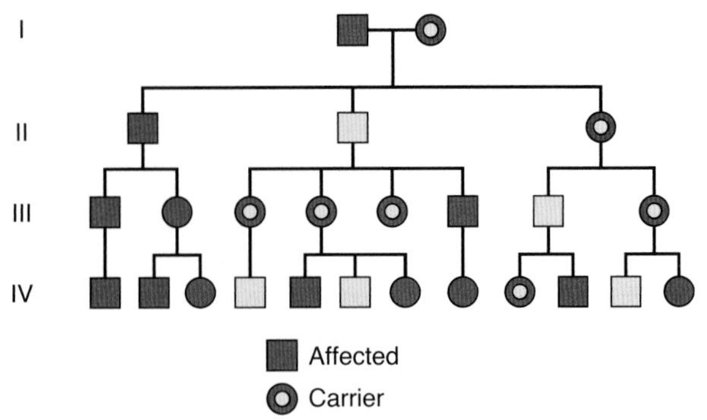

• **Fig. 6.11** Family tree of an X-linked recessive trait in which affected males reproduce.

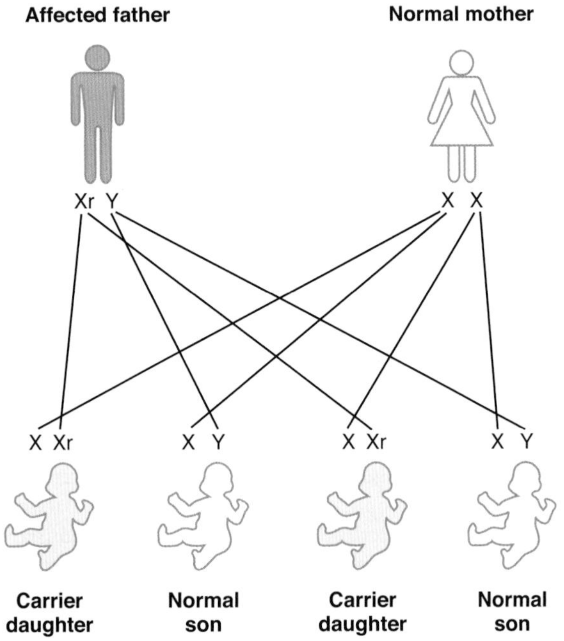

• **Fig. 6.12** Segregation of alleles in X-linked recessive inheritance, relating to the offspring of an affected male. *r* represents the mutated allele.

Some X-linked conditions are not compatible with survival to reproductive age and are not, therefore, transmitted by affected males. Duchenne muscular dystrophy is the most common severe muscle disease (p. 299). The first sign is delayed walking followed by a waddling gait, difficulty in climbing stairs unaided, and frequent falls. By approximately 10 years of age affected boys usually require a wheelchair. The muscle weakness is progressive, and affected males become bedbound and often die in their early 20s, although survival has improved significantly with steroids and respiratory support (Fig. 6.14). Because affected boys rarely survive to reproduce, the disease is transmitted by female carriers (Fig. 6.15), or may arise as a new variant.

Variable Expression in Heterozygous Females. In X-linked conditions, heterozygous females may have a mosaic phenotype with a mixture of features of the normal and variant alleles. In X-linked ocular albinism, the iris and ocular fundus of affected males lack pigment. Careful examination of the ocular fundus in

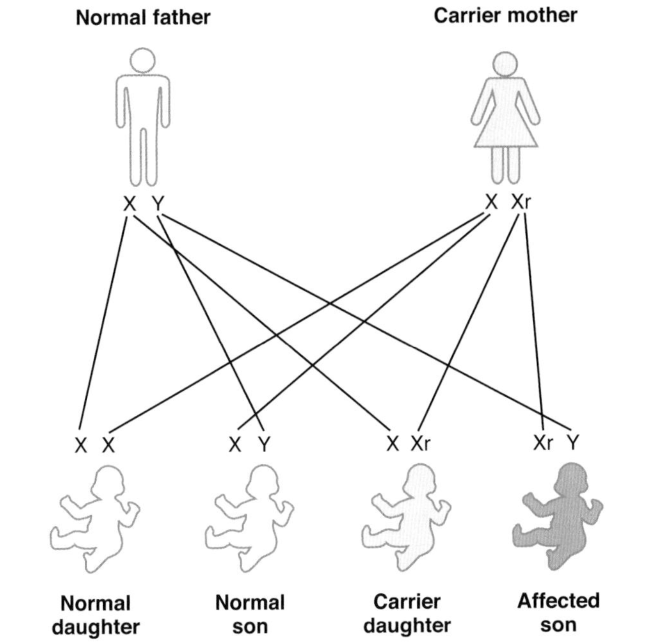

• **Fig. 6.13** Segregation of alleles in X-linked recessive inheritance, relating to the offspring of a carrier female. *r* represents the mutated allele.

females heterozygous for ocular albinism reveals a mosaic pattern of pigmentation (see Fig. 11.1, p. 152). This is explained by the random process of X-inactivation (p. 124); in the pigmented areas the normal gene is on the active X chromosome, and in depigmented areas the variant allele is on the active X chromosome.

Females Affected With X-Linked Recessive Disorders. Sometimes a woman may manifest features of an X-linked recessive trait. There are several possible explanations.

Homozygosity for X-Linked Recessive Disorders. A common X-linked recessive trait is red-green color-blindness—the inability to distinguish between the colors red and green. Approximately 8% of males are red-green color-blind, and, although it is unusual, because of the high frequency of this allele in the population, approximately 1 in 150 women are red-green color-blind by virtue of both parents having the allele on the X chromosome. Thus a female can be homozygous for an X-linked allele, although the rarity of most X-linked conditions means that the phenomenon is uncommon. A female could also be homozygous if her father was affected and her mother was normal, but a new variant occurred on the X chromosome transmitted to the daughter; vice versa, it could happen if her mother was a carrier and her father was normal, but a new variant occurred on the X chromosome he transmitted to his daughter—but these scenarios are rare.

Skewed X-Inactivation. The process of X-inactivation (p. 124) usually occurs randomly, there being an equal chance of either of the two X chromosomes in a heterozygous female being inactivated in any one cell. After X-inactivation in embryogenesis, therefore, in roughly half the cells one of the X chromosomes is active, whereas in the other half it is the other X chromosome that is active. Sometimes this process is not random, allowing for the possibility that the active X chromosome in most of the cells of a heterozygous female carrier is the one bearing the variant allele. If this happens, a carrier female would exhibit some of the symptoms and signs of the disease and be a so-called **manifesting heterozygote** or **carrier**. This occasionally

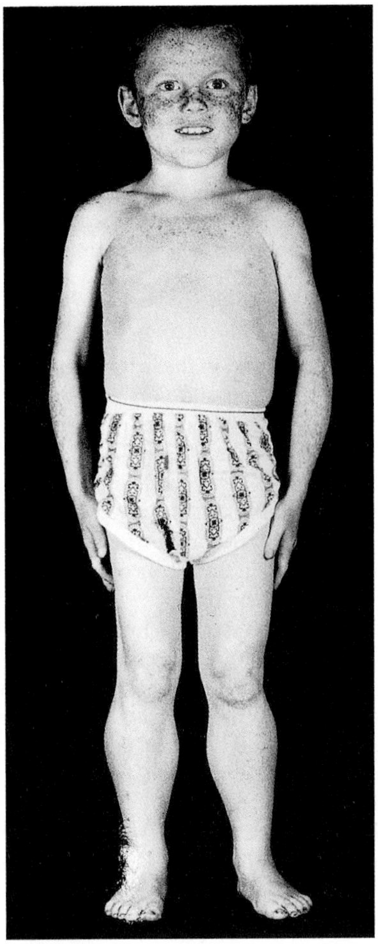

• **Fig. 6.14** Boy with Duchenne muscular dystrophy; note the enlarged calves and wasting of the thigh muscles.

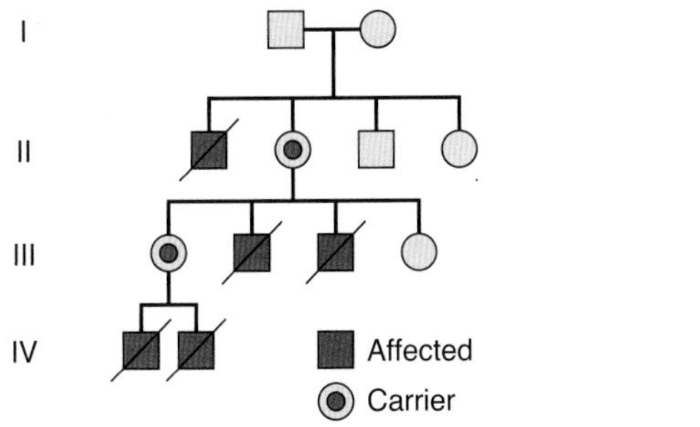

• **Fig. 6.15** Family tree of Duchenne muscular dystrophy, with the disorder being transmitted by carrier females and affecting males, who do not survive to transmit the disorder.

occurs in Duchenne muscular dystrophy and hemophilia A, for example. In addition, there are reports of X-linked disorders in which several manifesting carriers cluster in the same family, consistent with the coincidental inheritance of an abnormality of X-inactivation.

Numerical X-Chromosome Abnormalities. A female could manifest an X-linked recessive disorder if she carries an X-linked recessive variant and has a single X chromosome (i.e., Turner syndrome, see p. 254). Women with Turner syndrome and hemophilia A, or Duchenne muscular dystrophy, have been reported.

X-Autosome Translocations. Females with a translocation involving one of the X chromosomes and an autosome can be affected with an X-linked recessive disorder. If the breakpoint of the translocation disrupts an X chromosome gene, then a female can be affected. This is because the X chromosome involved in the translocation survives preferentially so as to maintain functional disomy of the autosomal genes (Fig. 6.16). The observation of females affected with Duchenne muscular dystrophy and having X-autosome translocations involving the same region of Xp helped to map the Duchenne muscular dystrophy gene (p. 299).

X-Linked Dominant Inheritance

Some conditions are manifest in the heterozygous female as well as the male who has the variant allele on his single X chromosome. This is known as X-linked dominant inheritance (Fig. 6.17). Superficially this resembles an autosomal dominant trait because both the daughters and sons of an affected female have a 1 in 2 (50%) chance of being affected. However, in X-linked dominant inheritance an affected male transmits the trait to his daughters but not to his sons, resulting in an excess of affected females and no direct male-to-male transmission.

X-linked dominant conditions include X-linked hypophosphatemia, also known as vitamin D–resistant rickets. Rickets can be caused by a dietary deficiency of vitamin D, but in vitamin D–resistant rickets the disorder occurs despite adequate dietary intake of vitamin D. In the X-linked dominant form of vitamin D–resistant rickets, both males and females have short stature because of short, and often bowed, long bones, although the females usually have less severe skeletal changes than males. The X-linked form of Charcot-Marie-Tooth disease (hereditary motor and sensory neuropathy, p. 292) is another example.

A mosaic pattern of involvement may be apparent in females heterozygous for some X-linked dominant disorders. An example is the mosaic pattern of abnormal skin pigmentation that follows developmental lines seen in females heterozygous for the X-linked dominant disorder incontinentia pigmenti (Fig. 6.18). This is also an example of a disorder that is usually lethal for male embryos that inherit the mutated allele. Others include the neurological conditions Rett syndrome (*MECP2* gene) and periventricular nodular heterotopia as a result of variants in *FLNA*.

Paradoxical X-Linked Inheritance. Recently it has been observed that patients who are hemizygous for variants in the X-linked gene *PCDH19* demonstrate the complete reversal of what is expected—males are unaffected and females are severely affected with a form of early infantile epileptic encephalopathy (EIEE–type 9). This is totally counter intuitive to our understanding of X-linked inheritance, and several possible explanations have been proposed. This includes the theory that the heterozygous state produces a harmful effect because of "metabolic interference" between the protein product of the mutated allele and that of the normal allele, whereas the mutated allele alone is benign. Another possibility is that X-inactivation is disturbed by the variant allele, giving rise in females to "functional disomy" for genes not inactivated. This parallels the situation in learning-disabled, dysmorphic females with a ring X-chromosome, which is not activated because there is no functional X-inactivation center.

Y-Linked Inheritance

Y-linked or **holandric inheritance** implies that only males are affected. An affected male transmits Y-linked traits to all of his sons but none of his daughters. In the past it has been suggested that

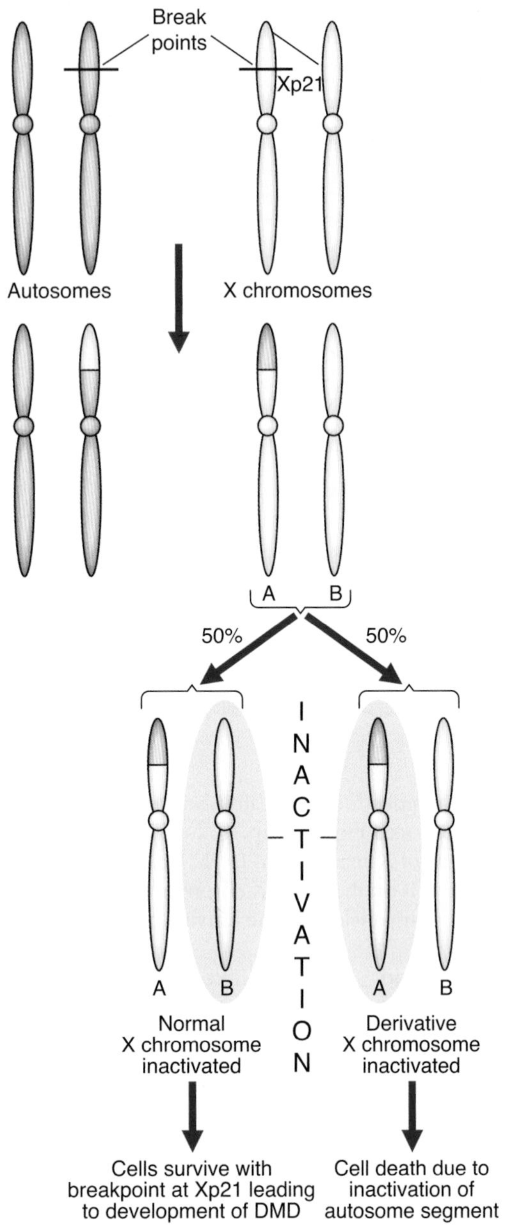

• **Fig. 6.16** Generation of an X-autosome translocation with breakpoint in a female and how this results in the development of Duchenne muscular dystrophy (*DMD*).

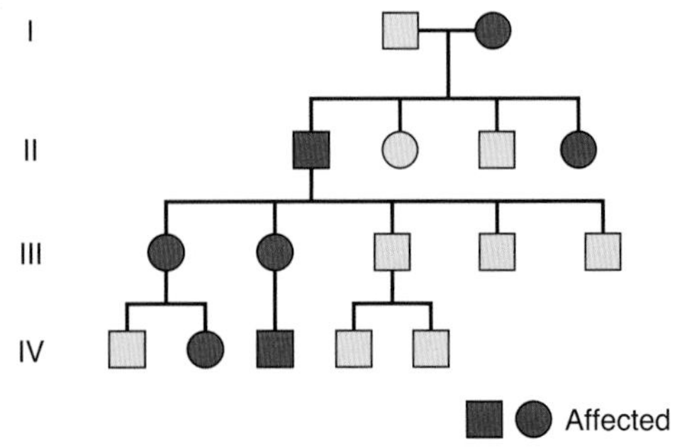

• **Fig. 6.17** Family tree of an X-linked dominant trait.

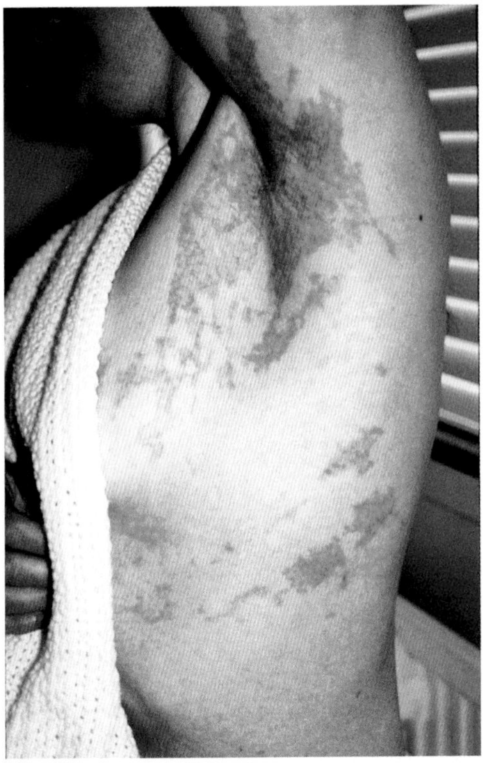

• **Fig. 6.18** Mosaic pattern of skin pigmentation in a female with the X-linked dominant disorder, incontinentia pigmenti. The patient has a variant in a gene on one of her X chromosomes; the pigmented areas indicate tissue in which the normal X chromosome has been inactivated. This developmental pattern follows Blaschko's lines (see Chapter 17, p. 253).

bizarre-sounding conditions such as porcupine skin, hairy ears, and webbed toes are Y-linked traits. With the possible exception of hairy ears, these claims of holandric inheritance can be dismissed. Evidence clearly indicates, however, that the H-Y histocompatibility antigen (p. 177) and genes involved in spermatogenesis are carried on the Y chromosome and, therefore, manifest holandric inheritance. The latter, if deleted, leads to infertility from azoospermia in males. The recent advent of techniques of assisted reproduction, particularly the technique of intracytoplasmic sperm injection, means that, if a pregnancy with a male conceptus results after the use of this technique, the child will also necessarily be infertile.

Partial Sex-Linkage

Partial sex-linkage has been used in the past to account for certain conditions that appear to exhibit autosomal dominant inheritance in some families and X-linked inheritance in others. In fact, this is because of genes present on the tip of Xp, which share homology with the Y chromosome (which escapes X-inactivation). During meiosis, pairing occurs between the homologous Xp and Yp chromosomal regions, the so-called **pseudoautosomal regions** (p. 128; Fig. 9.29). As a result of a meiotic crossover, a gene could be transferred from the X to the Y chromosome, or vice versa, allowing the possibility of male-to-male transmission. The latter instances would be consistent with autosomal dominant inheritance. A rare skeletal dysplasia, Leri-Weil dyschondrosteosis, in which affected individuals have short stature and a characteristic "Madelung" wrist deformity, shows both autosomal dominant and X-linked inheritance, and is due to deletions of, or variants in, the short stature homeobox (*SHOX*) gene, located in the pseudoautosomal region.

Sex Influence

Some autosomal traits are expressed more frequently in one sex than in another—so-called **sex influence**. In males, gout and presenile baldness are examples of sex-influenced autosomal dominant traits, probably through the effect of male hormones. Gout is very rare in women before the menopause but more frequent later; baldness does not occur in males who have been castrated. In hemochromatosis (p. 284), the most common autosomal recessive disorder in Western society, homozygous females are much less likely than homozygous males to develop iron overload and associated symptoms—the usual explanation being that women lose blood naturally through menstruation.

Sex Limitation

Sex limitation refers to the appearance of certain features only in individuals of a particular sex. Examples include virilization of female infants affected with the autosomal recessive endocrine disorder, congenital adrenal hyperplasia (p. 277).

Establishing the Mode of Inheritance of a Genetic Disorder

In clinical genetic practice, when a likely genetic condition is being assessed, the geneticist relies heavily on pedigree information, and subsequently molecular genetic testing, to try to establish the inheritance pattern. This is not necessarily straightforward with a single family and may be greatly helped by studying several families with the same condition or phenotype. For autosomal and X-linked patterns of inheritance, each is characterized by three key features, as follows (Box 6.1).

Autosomal Dominant Inheritance

Autosomal dominant inheritance (1) affects males and females in equal proportions; (2) is transmitted from one generation to the next; and (3) all forms of transmission between the sexes are observed (i.e., male to male, female to female, male to female, and female to male). Male-to-male transmission excludes the possibility of the gene being on the X chromosome.

Autosomal Recessive Inheritance

Autosomal recessive inheritance (1) affects males and females in equal proportions; (2) usually affects only individuals in one generation in a single sibship (i.e., brothers and sisters) and does not occur in previous and subsequent generations; and (3) consanguinity in the parents provides further support.

X-Linked Recessive Inheritance

X-linked recessive inheritance (1) should affect males almost exclusively; (2) transmitted through unaffected carrier females to their sons, and affected males, if able to reproduce, can have affected grandsons through their daughters who are obligate carriers; and (3) male-to-male transmission does not occur.

X-Linked Dominant Inheritance

X-linked dominant inheritance (1) is when males and females are affected, but there are more affected females than males; (2) females are usually less severely affected than males; and (3) although affected females can transmit the disorder to both male and female offspring, affected males transmit the disorder only to their daughters (except in partial sex-linkage), all of whom will be affected. In the case of X-linked dominant disorders that

• BOX 6.1 Features that support the single-gene or mendelian patterns of inheritance

Autosomal Dominant

Males and females affected in equal proportions
Affected individuals in multiple generations
Transmission by individuals of both sexes (i.e., male to male, female to female, male to female, and female to male)

Autosomal Recessive

Males and females affected in equal proportions
Affected individuals usually in only a single generation
Parents can be related (i.e., consanguineous)

X-Linked Recessive

Only males usually affected
Transmitted through unaffected females
Males cannot transmit the disorder to their sons (i.e., no male-to-male transmission)

X-Linked Dominant

Males and females affected, but often an excess of females
Females less severely affected than males
Affected males can transmit the disorder to their daughters but not to sons

Y-Linked Inheritance

Only males affected
Affected males must transmit it to their sons

are almost invariably lethal in male embryos, for example, incontinentia pigmenti (Fig. 6.18), only females will be affected, and families may show an excess of females over males, as well as a number of male-gender miscarriages. Next-generation sequencing has identified many new X-linked genes where moderate-to-severe intellectual disability is seen predominantly in females, that is, conforming to X-linked dominant inheritance.

Y-Linked Inheritance

Here, *two* features help establish Y-linked inheritance: (1) only males are affected; (2) affected males must transmit the disorder only to their sons.

Multiple Alleles and Complex Traits

So far, we have considered traits involving only two alleles—the normal and the variant. However, some traits and diseases are neither **monogenic** nor **polygenic**. Some genes have more than two allelic forms (i.e., multiple alleles). Multiple alleles are the result of a normal gene having variants that produce different alleles, some of which determine dominant inheritance and others recessive. In the ABO blood group system (p. 181) there are at least four alleles (A_1, A_2, B, and O). An individual can possess any two of these alleles, which may be the same or different (AO, A_2B, OO, etc.). Alleles are carried on homologous chromosomes, and therefore a person transmits only one allele for a certain trait to any particular offspring. For example, a person with the genotype AB will transmit either the A allele or the B allele to offspring, but never both (Table 6.1). This relates only to autosomal genes, not those on the X chromosome, where males have only one allele to transmit.

Next-generation sequencing has greatly facilitated the investigation of so-called **complex traits**—conditions that are usually much more common than mendelian disorders and likely to be because of the interaction of more than one gene. The effects may be additive, one may be rate limiting over the action of another, or one may enhance or multiply the effect of another (see Chapter 10). The possibility of a small number of gene loci being implicated in some disorders has given rise to the concept of **oligogenic** inheritance, examples of which include the following.

TABLE 6.1 Possible genotypes, phenotypes, and gametes formed from the four alleles A_1, A_2, B, and O at the ABO locus

Genotype	Phenotype	Gametes
A_1A_1	A_1	A_1
A_2A_2	A_2	A_2
BB	B	B
OO	O	O
A_1A_2	A_1	A_1 or A_2
A_1B	A_1B	A_1 or B
A_1O	A_1	A_1 or O
A_2B	A_2B	A_2 or B
A_2O	A_2	A_2 or O
BO	B	B or O

Digenic Inheritance

This refers to the situation where a disorder has been shown to be because of the additive effects of heterozygous variants at two different gene loci. This is seen in certain transgenic mice. Mice that are homozygotes for *rv* (rib-vertebrae) or *Dll1 (Delta–like-1)* manifest abnormal phenotypes, whereas their respective heterozygotes are normal. However, mice that are **double heterozygotes** for *rv* and *Dll1* show vertebral defects. In humans, a form of retinitis pigmentosa (RP), a disorder of progressive visual impairment, is caused by double heterozygosity for variants in two unlinked genes, *ROM1* and *PRPH2* (*Peripherin*), which both encode proteins present in photoreceptors. Individuals with only one of these variants are not affected. A similar example is established for recessively inherited Usher syndrome, in which RP occurs with sensorineural deafness. In the field of inherited cardiac arrhythmias and cardiomyopathies (p. 306), it is becoming clear that digenic inheritance may be essential to causing the phenotype, thus complicating genetic counseling. Inherited deafness, Bardet-Biedl syndrome, and Joubert syndrome are all further examples of a growing list of conditions sometimes demonstrating digenic inheritance.

Other patterns of inheritance that are not classically mendelian are also recognized and explain some unusual phenomena.

Anticipation

In some autosomal dominant traits or disorders, such as myotonic dystrophy, the onset of the disease occurs at an earlier age in the offspring than in the parents, or the disease occurs with increasing severity in subsequent generations. This is called **anticipation**. Before the modern era many believed this observation was because of bias of ascertainment (i.e., the way families were collected). It was argued that persons in whom the disease begins earlier, or is more severe, are more likely to reach medical attention, and only those individuals who are less severely affected tend to have children. In addition, it was thought that, because the observer is in the same generation as the affected presenting probands, many individuals who at present are unaffected will, by necessity, develop the disease later in life.

However, anticipation was shown to have a real biological basis, occurring as a result of the expansion of unstable DNA triplet repeat sequences (p. 20). An expansion of the CTG triplet repeat in the 3′ untranslated end of the myotonic dystrophy gene, occurring predominantly in **maternal** meiosis, appears to be the explanation for the severe neonatal form of myotonic dystrophy that usually only occurs when the gene is transmitted by the mother (Fig. 6.19). Fragile X syndrome (CGG repeats) (p. 255) behaves in a similar way, with major instability in the expansion occurring during **maternal** meiosis. A similar expansion—in this case CAG repeats—in the 5′ end of the Huntington disease gene (Fig. 6.20) in **paternal** meiosis accounts for the increased risk of early-onset Huntington disease, occasionally in childhood or adolescence, when the gene is transmitted by the father. The inherited spinocerebellar ataxia group of conditions (p. 291) is another example.

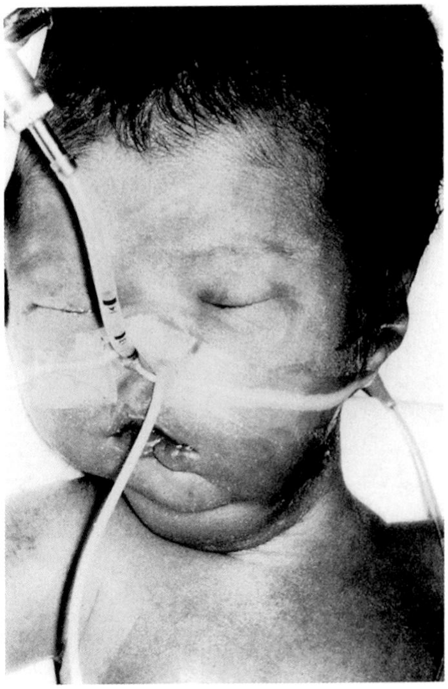

• **Fig. 6.19** Newborn baby with severe hypotonia requiring ventilation as a result of having inherited myotonic dystrophy from his mother.

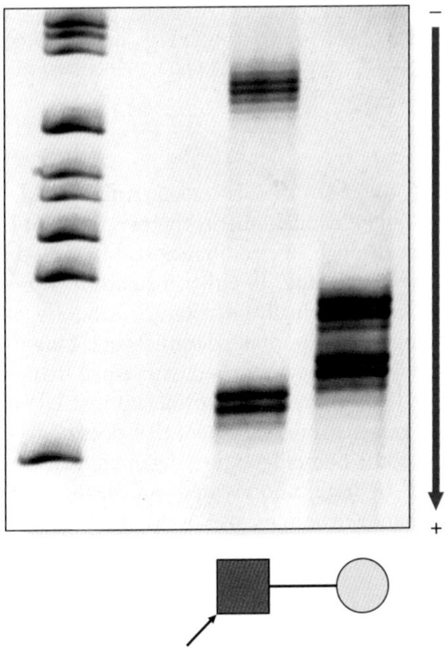

• **Fig. 6.20** Silver staining of a 5% denaturing gel of the polymerase chain reaction products of the CAG triplet in the coding sequence of the *huntingtin* gene from an affected male and his wife, showing her to have two similar-sized repeats in the normal range (20 and 24 copies) and him to have one normal-sized triplet repeat (18 copies) and an expanded triplet repeat (44 copies). The bands in the left lane are standard markers to allow sizing of the CAG repeat. (Courtesy Alan Dodge, Regional DNA Laboratory, St. Mary's Hospital, Manchester, UK.)

Mosaicism

An individual, or a particular tissue of the body, can consist of more than one cell type or line, through an error occurring during mitosis at any stage after conception. This is known as **mosaicism.** Mosaicism of either somatic tissues or germ cells can account for some instances of unusual patterns of inheritance or phenotypic features in an affected individual.

Somatic Mosaicism

The possibility of somatic mosaicism is suggested by the features of a single-gene disorder being less severe in an individual than is usual, or by being confined to a particular part of the body in a segmental distribution— for example, as occurs occasionally in neurofibromatosis type I (p. 296). The timing of the variant arising in early development may determine whether it is transmitted to the next generation with full expression—this will depend on the variant being present in gonadal tissue, and hence germline cells.

Gonadal Mosaicism

There have been many reports of families with autosomal dominant disorders, such as achondroplasia and osteogenesis imperfecta, and X-linked recessive disorders, such as Duchenne muscular dystrophy and hemophilia, in which the parents are phenotypically normal, and the results of genetic tests also normal, but in which more than one of their children has been affected. The most favored explanation for these observations is gonadal, or germline, mosaicism in one of the parents (i.e., the variant is present in a proportion of the gonadal or germline cells). An elegant example of this was provided by the demonstration of a variant in the collagen gene responsible for osteogenesis imperfecta in a proportion of individual sperm from a clinically normal father who had two affected infants with different partners. It is important to keep germline mosaicism in mind when providing recurrence risks in genetic counseling for apparently *de novo* autosomal dominant and X-linked recessive variants.

Uniparental Disomy

Individuals normally inherit one of a pair of homologous chromosomes from each parent. Occasionally, however, inheritance of both homologues of a chromosome pair from only one parent occurs, which is called **uniparental disomy (UPD)**. If an individual inherits two copies of the same homologue from one parent through an error

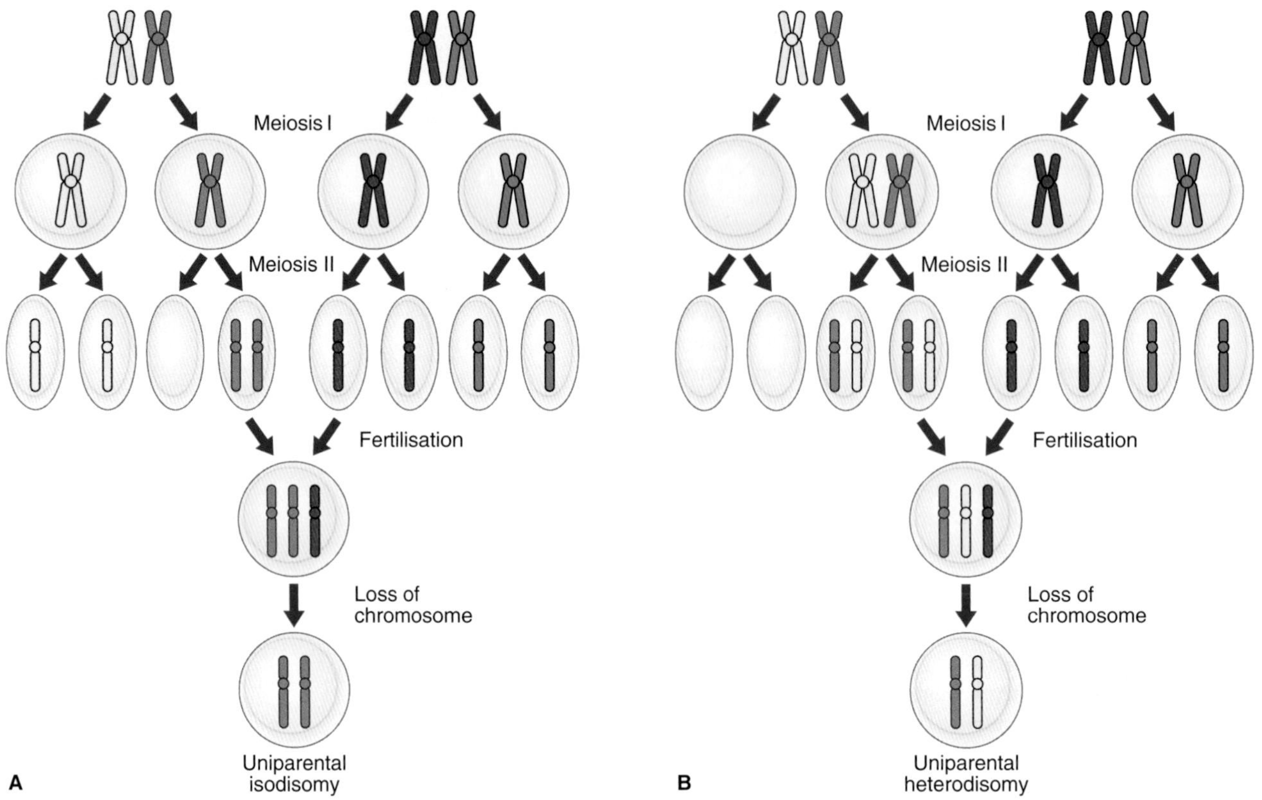

• **Fig. 6.21** Mechanism of origin of uniparental disomy. (A) Uniparental isodisomy occurring through a disomic gamete arising from nondisjunction in meiosis II fertilizing a monosomic gamete with loss of the chromosome from the parent contributing the single homolog. (B) Uniparental heterodisomy occurring through a disomic gamete arising from nondisjunction in meiosis I fertilizing a monosomic gamete with loss of the chromosome from the parent contributing the single homologue.

in meiosis II (p. 34), this is called **uniparental isodisomy** (Fig. 6.21). If the individual inherits the two different homologues from one parent through an error in meiosis I (p. 32), this is termed **uniparental heterodisomy**. In either instance it is presumed that the conceptus would originally be trisomic, with early loss of a chromosome leading to the "normal" disomic state. One-third of such chromosome losses, if they occurred with equal frequency, would result in UPD. Alternatively, it is postulated that UPD could arise as a result of a gamete from one parent that does not contain a particular chromosome homologue (i.e., a gamete that is **nullisomic**) being "rescued" by fertilization with a gamete that, through a second separate chance error in meiosis, is disomic.

UPD has been shown to be the cause of a father with hemophilia having an affected son, and of a child with cystic fibrosis being born to a couple in which only the mother was a carrier (with proven paternity). UPD for chromosome 15 gives rise to either Prader-Willi syndrome (PWS; maternal UPD) or Angelman syndrome (AS; paternal UPD), and paternal UPD for chromosome 11 is one of the causes of the overgrowth condition known as the Beckwith-Wiedemann syndrome (BWS; see the following section).

Genomic Imprinting

Genomic imprinting is an **epigenetic** phenomenon, referred to in Chapter 9 (p. 123). Epigenetics and genomic imprinting give the lie to Thomas Hunt Morgan's quotation at the start of this chapter! Although it was originally thought that genes on homologous chromosomes were expressed equally, it is now recognized that different clinical features can result depending on whether a gene is inherited from the father or from the mother. This "parent of origin" effect is referred to as **genomic imprinting**, and DNA **methylation**, occurring mostly at a CpG site, is the main mechanism by which expression is modified. Methylation is the **imprint** applied to certain DNA sequences in their passage through gametogenesis, although only a small proportion of the human genome is subject to this process. The differential allele expression (i.e., maternal or paternal) may occur in all somatic cells, or in specific tissues or stages of development. Thus far, at least 80 human genes are known to be imprinted, and the regions involved are known as differentially methylated regions (DMRs). These DMRs include imprinting control regions (ICRs) that control gene expression across imprinted domains.

Evidence of genomic imprinting has been observed in two pairs of well-known dysmorphic syndromes: PWS and AS (chromosome 15q) and BWS and Russell-Silver syndrome (RSS) (chromosome 11p). The mechanisms giving rise to these conditions, although complex, reveal much about imprinting and will therefore now be considered in more detail.

Prader-Willi Syndrome

PWS occurs in approximately 1 in 20,000 births and is characterized by short stature, obesity, hypogonadism, and learning difficulty (Fig. 6.22). Some 50% to 60% of individuals with PWS can be shown to have an approximately 2-megabase (Mb) interstitial deletion of the proximal region of chromosome 15q11-q13, visible by conventional cytogenetic means, and in a further 15% a submicroscopic deletion can be demonstrated by fluorescence *in situ* hybridization (pp. 55, 259) or molecular means. DNA analysis has revealed that the chromosome containing the deletion is almost always the paternally derived homologue. Most of the remaining 25% to 30% of individuals with PWS without a chromosome deletion have been shown to have maternal UPD. Functionally, this is equivalent to a deletion in the paternally derived chromosome 15.

It is now known that only the paternally inherited allele of this critical region of 15q11-q13 is expressed. The molecular organization of the region is shown in Fig. 6.23. PWS is a multigene disorder, and in the normal situation the gene encoding small nuclear ribonucleoprotein polypeptide N (*SNRPN*) and adjacent genes (*MKRN3*, etc.) are paternally expressed. Expression is under the control of a specific ICR. Analysis of DNA from patients with PWS and observation of various submicroscopic deletions enabled the ICR to be mapped to a segment of approximately 4 kilobases, spanning the first exon and promoter of *SNRPN* and the upstream reading frame (*SNURF*). The 3′ end of the ICR is required for expression of the paternally expressed genes and also the origin of the long *SNURF/SNRPN* transcript. The maternally expressed genes are not differentially methylated, but they are silenced on the paternal allele, probably by an antisense RNA generated from *SNURF/SNRPN*. In normal cells, the 5′ end of the ICR, needed for maternal expression and involved in AS (see later), is methylated on the maternal allele.

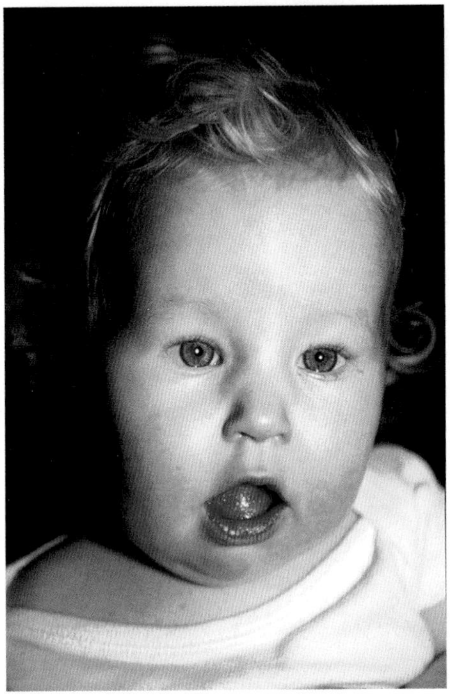

• **Fig. 6.22** Female child with Prader-Willi syndrome.

Angelman Syndrome

AS occurs in approximately 1 in 15,000 births and is characterized by epilepsy, severe learning difficulties, an unsteady or ataxic gait, and a happy demeanor (Fig. 6.24). Approximately 70% of individuals with AS have been shown to have an interstitial deletion of the same 15q11-q13 region as that involved in PWS, but in this case on the maternally derived homologue. In a further 5% of individuals with AS, the syndrome can be shown to have arisen through paternal UPD. Unlike PWS, the features of AS arise through loss of a single gene, *UBE3A*. In up to 10% of individuals with AS, variants have been identified in *UBE3A*, a ubiquitin ligase gene, which appears to be preferentially or exclusively expressed from the maternally derived chromosome 15 in the brain. How variants in *UBE3A* lead to the features seen in persons with AS is not clear, but could involve ubiquitin-mediated destruction of proteins in the central nervous system in development, particularly where *UBE3A* is expressed most strongly, namely the hippocampus and Purkinje cells of the cerebellum. *UBE3A* is under control of the AS ICR (see Fig. 6.23), which was mapped slightly upstream of *SNURF/SNRPN* through analysis of patients with AS who had various different microdeletions.

Approximately 2% of individuals with PWS and approximately 5% of those with AS have abnormalities of the ICR itself; these patients tend to show the mildest phenotypes. Patients in this last group, unlike the other three, have a risk of recurrence. In the case of AS, if the mother carries the same variant as the child, the recurrence risk is 50%, but even if she tests negative for the variant, there is an appreciable recurrence risk from gonadal mosaicism.

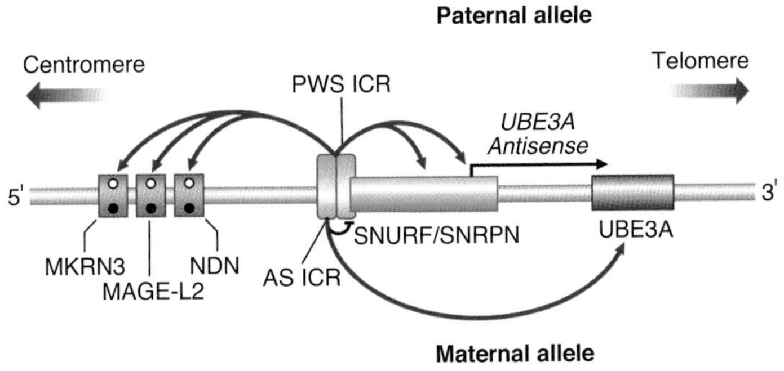

• **Fig. 6.23** Molecular organization (simplified) at 15q11-q13: Prader-Willi syndrome (*PWS*) and Angelman syndrome (*AS*). The imprinting control region (*ICR*) for this locus has two components. The more telomeric acts as the PWS ICR and contains the promoter of *SNURF/SNRPN*. *SNURF/SNRPN* produces several long and complex transcripts, one of which is believed to be an RNA antisense inhibitor of *UBE3A*. The more centromeric ICR acts as the AS ICR on *UBE3A*, which is the only gene whose maternal expression is lost in AS. The AS ICR also inhibits the PWS ICR on the maternal allele. The PWS ICR also acts on the upstream genes *MKRN3*, *MAGE-L2* and *NDN*, which are unmethylated (○) on the paternal allele but methylated (●) on the maternal allele.

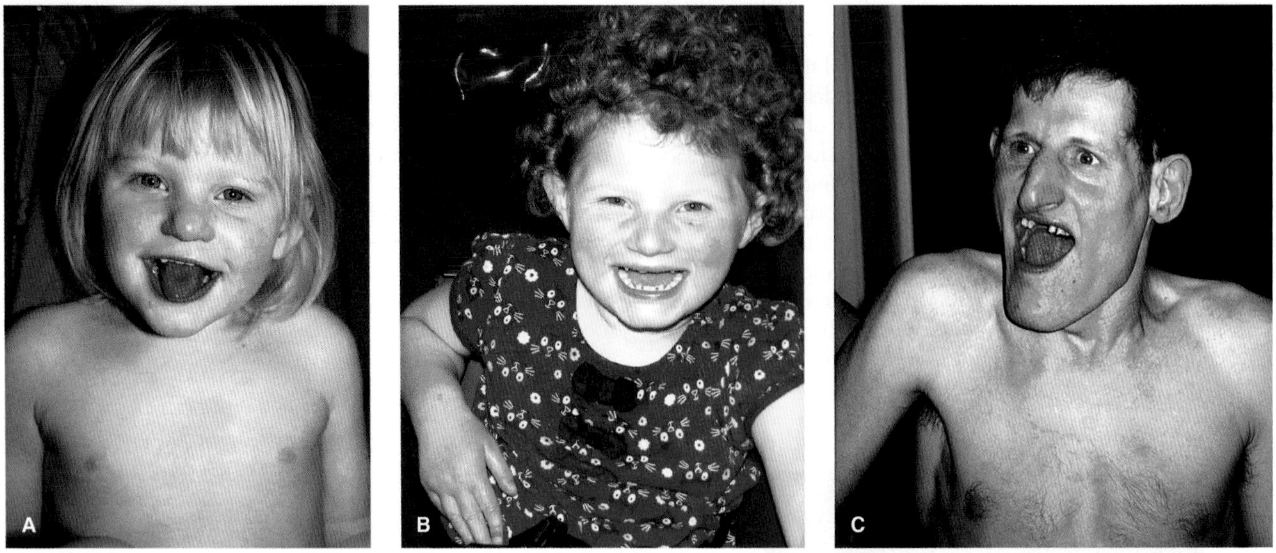

• **Fig. 6.24** (A) and (B) Two young girls with Angelman syndrome. (C) Adult male with Angelman syndrome.

Rare families have been reported in which a translocation of the proximal portion of the long arm of chromosome 15 is segregating. Depending on whether the translocation is transmitted by the father or the mother, affected offspring within the family have had either PWS or AS. In approximately 10% of AS cases the molecular defect is unknown—but it may well be that some of these alleged cases have a different, albeit phenotypically similar, diagnosis.

In most laboratories a simple DNA test is used to diagnose both PWS and AS, exploiting the differential DNA methylation characteristics at the 15q11-q13 locus, superseding southern blot analysis (Fig. 6.25).

Beckwith-Wiedemann Syndrome

BWS is a well-known "overgrowth" condition. First described in 1963 and 1964, the main features are macrosomia (prenatal and/or postnatal overgrowth), macroglossia (large tongue), abdominal wall defect (omphalocele, umbilical hernia, diastasis recti), and neonatal hypoglycemia (Fig. 6.26). Hemihyperplasia may be present, as well as visceromegaly, renal abnormalities, ear anomalies (anterior ear-lobe creases, posterior helical pits), and cleft palate, and there may be embryonal tumors (particularly Wilms tumor).

BWS is known for the multiple different (and complex) molecular mechanisms that underlie it. Genomic imprinting, somatic mosaicism, and multiple genes are involved, all within a 1-Mb region at chromosome 11p15 (Fig. 6.27). Within this region lie two independently regulated imprinted domains. The more telomeric (differentially methylated region 1 [DMR1] under control of ICR1) contains paternally expressed *IGF2* (insulin growth factor 2) and maternally expressed *H19*. The more centromeric imprinted domain (DMR2, under control of ICR2) contains the maternally expressed *KCNQ1* (previously known as *KvLQT1*) and *CDKN1C* genes, and the paternally expressed antisense transcript *KCNQ1OT1*, the promoter for which is located within the *KCNQ1* gene.

Disruption to the normal regulation of methylation can give rise to altered gene expression dosage and, consequentially, features of BWS. In DMR1, **gain of methylation** on the maternal allele leads to loss of *H19* expression and biallelic *IGF2* expression (i.e., effectively two copies of the paternal epigenotype). This occurs in up to 7% of BWS cases and is usually sporadic. In DMR2, **loss of methylation** results in two copies of the paternal epigenotype and a reduction in expression of *CDKN1C;* this mechanism is implicated in 50% to 60% of sporadic BWS cases. *CDKN1C* may be a growth inhibitory gene, and variants have been found in 5% to 10% of cases of BWS. Approximately 15% of BWS cases are familial, and *CDKN1C* variants are found in approximately half of these. In addition to imprinting errors in DMR1 and DMR2, other mechanisms may account for BWS: (1) paternally derived

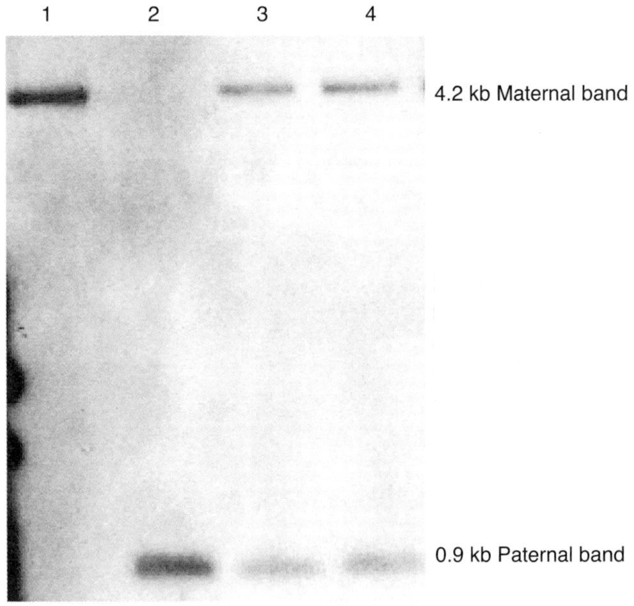

• **Fig. 6.25** Southern blot to detect methylations of *SNRPN*. DNA digested with *Xba*I and *Not*I was probed with KB17, which hybridises to a CpG island within exon 1 of *SNRPN*. Patient 1 has Prader-Willi syndrome, patient 2 has Angelman syndrome, and patients 3 and 4 are unaffected. (Courtesy A. Gardner, Department of Molecular Genetics, Southmead Hospital, Bristol.)

duplications of chromosome 11p15.5 (these cases were the first to identify the BWS locus); (2) paternal UPD for chromosome 11—invariably present in mosaic form—often associated with neonatal hypoglycemia and hemihypertrophy, and associated with the highest risk (approximately 25%) of embryonal tumors, particularly Wilms tumor; and (3) maternally inherited balanced translocations involving rearrangements of 11p15.

Russell-Silver Syndrome

This well-known condition has "opposite" characteristics to BWS by virtue of marked prenatal and postnatal growth retardation. The head circumference is relatively normal, the face rather small and triangular, giving rise to a "pseudohydrocephalic" appearance (Fig. 6.28), and there may be body asymmetry. Approximately 10% of cases appear to be as a result of maternal UPD, indicating that this chromosome is subject to imprinting. In contrast to paternally derived duplications of 11p15, which give rise to overgrowth and BWS, maternally derived duplications of this region are associated with growth retardation. Up to 50% of RSS cases are as a result of abnormalities of imprinting at the 11p15.5 locus. Whereas hypermethylation of DMR1 leads to upregulated *IGF2* and overgrowth, hypomethylation of *H19* leads to downregulated *IGF2*, the opposite molecular and biochemical consequence, and these patients have features of RSS. Interestingly, in contrast to BWS, there are no cases of RSS with altered methylation of the more centromeric DMR2 region.

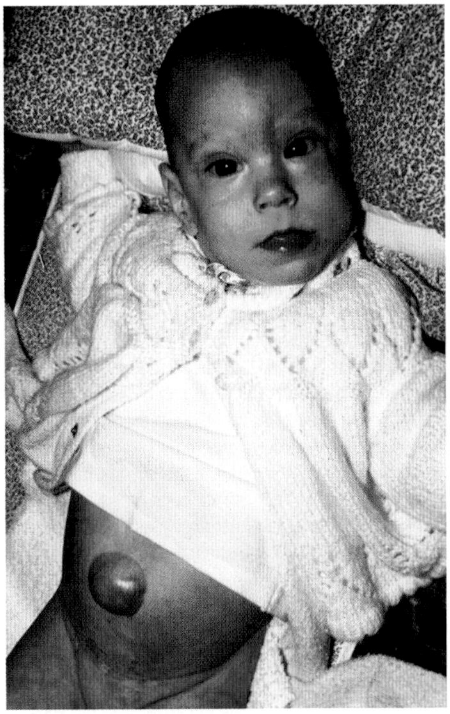

• **Fig. 6.26** Baby girl with Beckwith-Wiedemann syndrome. Note the large tongue and umbilical hernia.

Mitochondrial Inheritance

Each cell contains thousands of copies of mitochondrial DNA, with more being found in cells that have high energy requirements, such as brain and muscle. Mitochondria, and therefore their DNA, are inherited almost exclusively from the mother through the oocyte (p. 34). Mitochondrial DNA has a higher rate of spontaneous variation than nuclear DNA, and the accumulation of variants in mitochondrial DNA has been proposed as being responsible for some of the somatic effects seen with aging.

In humans, **cytoplasmic** or **mitochondrial inheritance** explains the pattern of inheritance observed in some rare disorders that affect both males and females but are transmitted only through females, so-called maternal or matrilinear inheritance (Fig. 6.29).

A number of rare disorders with unusual combinations of neurological and myopathic features, sometimes occurring in association with other conditions such as cardiomyopathy and conduction defects, diabetes, or deafness, have been characterized as being attributed to variants in mitochondrial genes (p. 286). Because mitochondria are crucial to cellular metabolism through oxidative phosphorylation, it is not surprising that the organs most susceptible to mitochondrial variants are the central nervous system, skeletal muscle, and heart.

In most persons, the mitochondrial DNA across different mitochondria is identical, or shows what is termed **homoplasmy**. If a variant occurs in the mitochondrial DNA of an

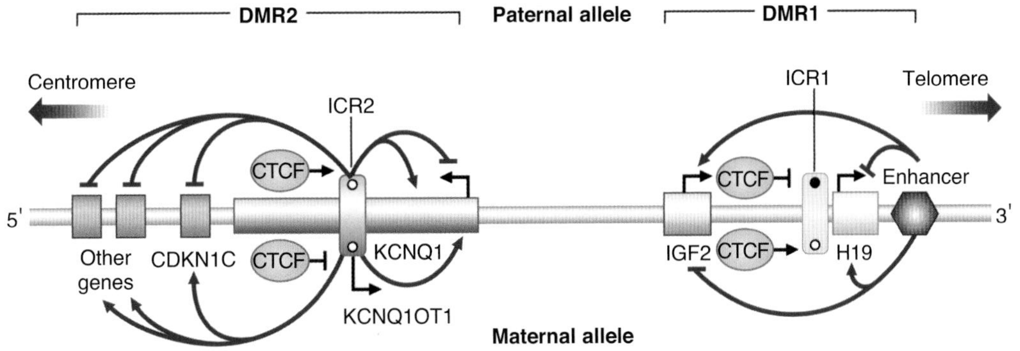

• **Fig. 6.27** Molecular organization (simplified) at 11p15.5: Beckwith-Wiedemann and Russell-Silver syndromes. The region contains two imprinted domains (*DMR1* and *DMR2*) that are regulated independently. The imprinting control regions (*ICRs*) are differentially methylated (● methylated; o unmethylated). CCCTC-binding factor (*CTCF*) binds to the unmethylated alleles of both ICRs. In DMR1, coordinated regulation leads to expression of *IGF2* only on the paternal allele and *H19* expression only on the maternal allele. In DMR2, coordinated regulation leads to *maternal* expression of *KCNQ1* and *CDKN1C* (plus other genes) and paternal expression of *KCNQ1OT1* (a non-coding RNA with antisense transcription to *KCNQ1*). Angled black arrows show the direction of the transcripts.

individual, there will initially be two populations of mitochondrial DNA, so-called **heteroplasmy**. The proportion of mitochondria with a variant in the DNA varies between cells and tissues, and this, together with variant heterogeneity, explains the range of phenotypic severity seen in persons affected with mitochondrial disorders (Fig. 6.30).

Whereas matrilinear inheritance applies to disorders that are directly attributed to variants in mitochondrial DNA, it is essential to appreciate that mitochondrial **proteins** are encoded mainly by nuclear genes. Variants in these genes can have a devastating impact on respiratory chain functions within mitochondria. Examples include genes encoding proteins within the cytochrome *c* (COX) system, for example *SURF1*, which follow autosomal recessive inheritance, and the *G4.5* (*TAZ*) gene that is X-linked and causes Barth syndrome (endocardial fibroelastosis) in males. Mitochondrial myopathy following autosomal dominant inheritance, in which multiple mitochondrial DNA deletions can be detected, may be caused by variants in *POLG* genes. Further discussion of mitochondrial disorders can be found in Chapter 18.

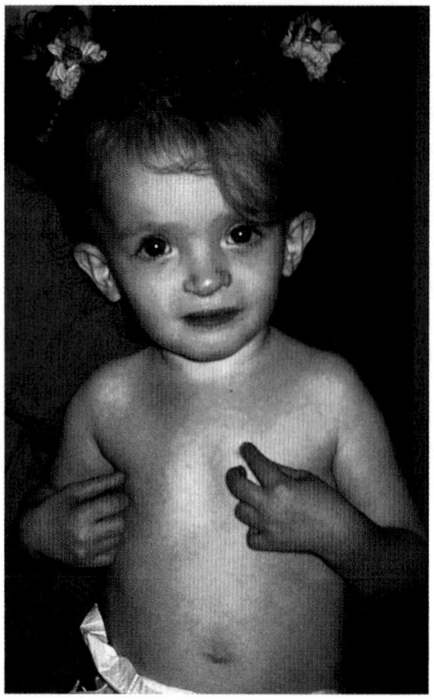

• **Fig. 6.28** Girl with Russell-Silver syndrome. Note the bossed forehead, triangular face, and "pseudohydrocephalic" appearance.

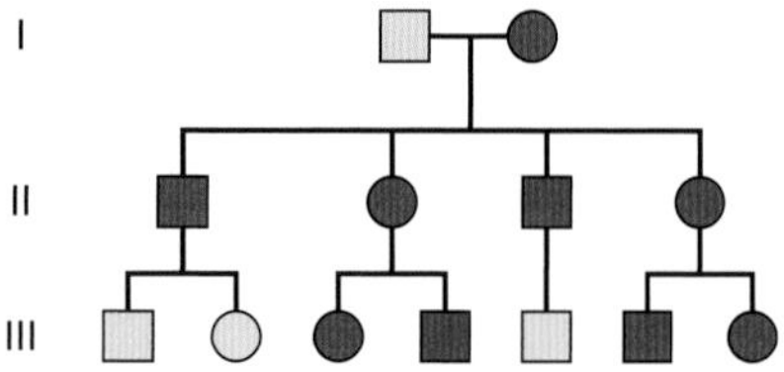

• **Fig. 6.29** Family tree consistent with mitochondrial inheritance.

ELEMENTS

1. Family studies are usually necessary to determine the mode of inheritance of a trait or disorder and to give appropriate genetic counseling. A standard shorthand convention exists for pedigree documentation of the family history.
2. Mendelian, or single-gene, disorders can be inherited in five ways: autosomal dominant, autosomal recessive, X-linked dominant, X-linked recessive, and, rarely, Y-linked inheritance.
3. Autosomal dominant alleles are manifest in the heterozygous state and are usually transmitted from one generation to the next but also arise as a new variant. They usually affect both males and females equally. Each offspring of a parent with an autosomal dominant gene has a 1 in 2 chance of inheriting it from the affected parent. Autosomal dominant alleles can exhibit reduced penetrance, variable expressivity, and sex limitation.
4. Autosomal recessive disorders are manifest only in the homozygous state and normally only affect individuals in one generation, usually in one sibship in a family. They affect both males and females equally. Offspring of parents who are heterozygous for the same autosomal recessive allele have a 1 in 4 chance of being homozygous for that allele. The less common an autosomal recessive allele, the greater the likelihood that the parents of a homozygote are consanguineous.
5. X-linked recessive alleles are normally manifest only in males. Offspring of females heterozygous for an X-linked recessive allele have a 1 in 2 chance of inheriting the allele from their mother. Daughters of males with an X-linked recessive allele are obligate heterozygotes, but sons cannot inherit

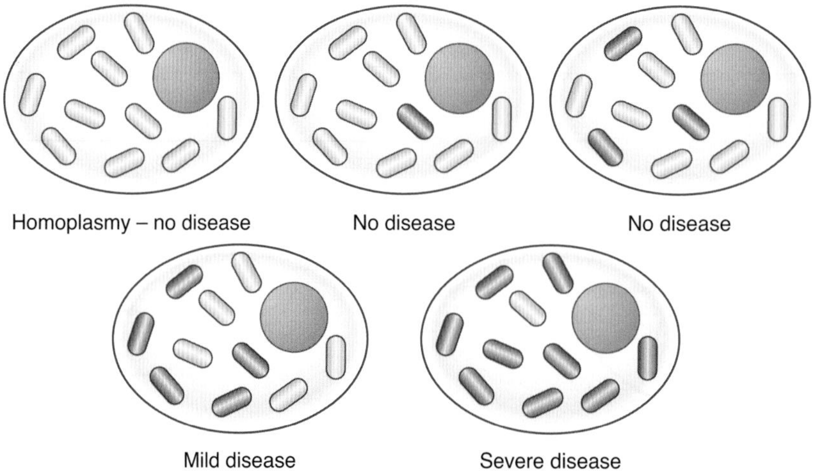

• **Fig. 6.30** Progressive effects of heteroplasmy on the clinical severity of disease from variants in the mitochondrial genome. Low proportions of variant mitochondria are tolerated well, but as the proportion increases, different thresholds for cellular, and hence tissue, dysfunction are breached (mauve circle represents the cell nucleus).

the allele. Rarely, females manifest an X-linked recessive trait because they are homozygous for the allele, have a single X chromosome, have a structural rearrangement of one of their X chromosomes, or are heterozygous but show skewed or non-random X-inactivation.

6. Some disorders are inherited in an X-linked dominant manner. In X-linked dominant disorders, hemizygous males are usually more severely affected than heterozygous females.
7. Unusual features in single-gene patterns of inheritance can be explained by phenomena such as genetic heterogeneity, mosaicism, anticipation, imprinting, uniparental disomy, and mitochondrial inheritance.

CLINICAL SCENARIO 1

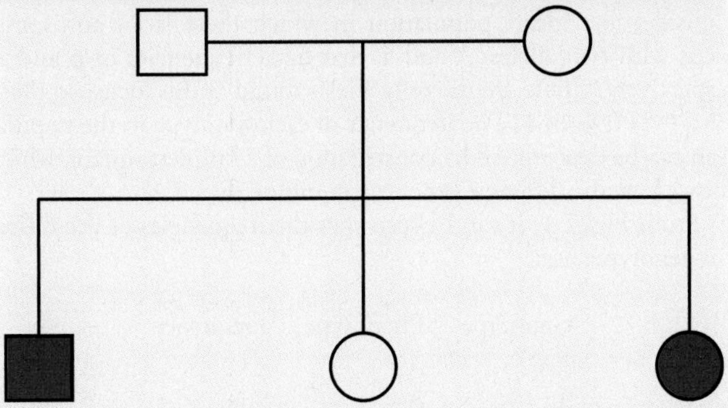

The affected children have similar problems (i.e., phenotypes), but the diagnosis is not known

This is a common scenario when assessing patients and families for learning disability, sometimes with dysmorphic features or neurological problems such as epilepsy

Exercise: List the different patterns of inheritance and mechanisms that might explain the phenotype in these siblings

CLINICAL SCENARIO 2

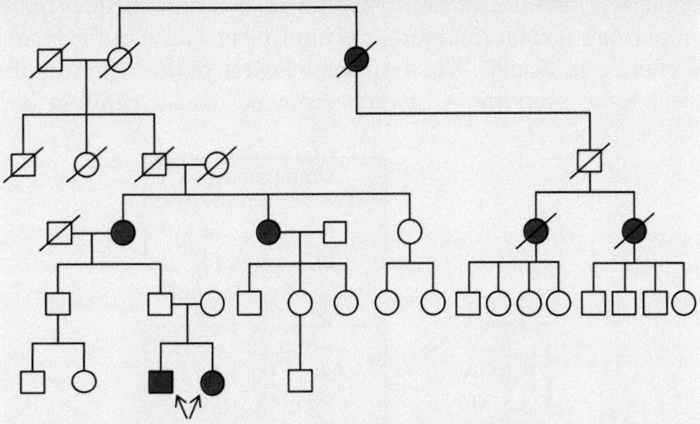

In this extensive pedigree the two arrowed siblings were diagnosed with precocious puberty by a pediatrician. Their paternal grandmother and her sister reached their menarche at 7½ and 8½ years, respectively, and had relatively short stature. At a later consultation, the wider family history of mild short stature and early menarche was ascertained.

Exercise: Which pattern(s) of inheritance might explain the family history?

Further Reading

Bateson W, Saunders ER. *Experimental Studies in the Physiology of Heredity*. London: Harrison and Sons; 1902:132–134. Royal Society Reports to the Evolution Committee, 1902.

Early observations on mendelian inheritance.

Bennet RL, Steinhaus KA, Uhrich SB, et al. Recommendations for standardized human pedigree nomenclature. *Am J Hum Genet.* 1995;56:745–752.

The main reference for modern pedigree nomenclature.

Goriely A, McVean GAT, Röjmyr M, Ingemarsson B, Wilkie AO. Evidence for selective advantage of pathogenic *FGFR2* variants in the male germ line. *Science.* 2000;301:643–646.

This paper describes the research leading to a new understanding of the increased risk of de novo mutations occurring in the male germ line.

Hall JG. Somatic mosaicism: observations related to clinical genetics. *Am J Hum Genet.* 1988;43:355–363.

Good review of findings arising from somatic mosaicism in clinical genetics.

Hall JG. Genomic imprinting: review and relevance to human diseases. *Am J Hum Genet.* 1990;46:857–873.

Extensive review of examples of imprinting in inherited diseases in humans.

Heinig RM. *The Monk in the Garden: The Lost and Found Genius of Gregor Mendel.* London: Houghton Mifflin; 2000.

The life and work of Gregor Mendel as the history of the birth of genetics.

Kingston HM. *An ABC of Clinical Genetics.* 2nd ed. London: British Medical Association; 1994.

A simple outline primer of the basic principles of clinical genetics.

Reik W, Surami A, eds. *Genomic Imprinting (frontiers in molecular biology).* London: IRL Press; 1997.

Detailed discussion of examples and mechanisms of genomic imprinting.

Schäffer AA. Digenic inheritance in medical genetics. *J Med Genet.* 2013;50:641–652.

A good early review of digenic inheritance.

7

Population and Mathematical Genetics

Do not worry about your difficulties in mathematics. I can assure you mine are still greater.

Albert Einstein

In this chapter some of the more mathematical aspects of gene inheritance are considered, together with how genes are distributed and maintained at particular frequencies in populations. This subject constitutes what is known as **population genetics**. Genetics lends itself to a numerical approach, with many of the most influential and pioneering figures in human genetics having come from a mathematical background, attracted by the challenges of trying to determine the frequencies of genes in populations and the rates at which they mutate. This still has relevance for clinical genetics, particularly genetic risk counseling, and by the end of this chapter it is hoped that the reader will have gained an understanding of the following:

1. Why a dominant trait does not increase in a population at the expense of a recessive one.
2. How the carrier frequency and mutation rate can be determined from the disease incidence.
3. Why a particular genetic disorder can be more common in one population or community than another.
4. How it can be confirmed that a genetic disorder shows a particular pattern of inheritance.
5. The concept of genetic linkage and how this differs from linkage disequilibrium.
6. The potential effects of medical intervention on gene frequencies.

Allele Frequencies in Populations

On first reflection, it would be reasonable to predict that dominant genes and traits in a population would tend to increase at the expense of recessive ones. On average, three-quarters of the offspring of two heterozygotes will manifest the dominant trait, and only one-quarter will have the recessive trait. It might be thought, therefore, that eventually almost everyone in the population would have the dominant trait. However, it can be shown that, in a large randomly mating population in which there is no disturbance by outside influences, dominant traits do not increase at the expense of recessive ones. In fact, in such a population, the relative proportions of the different genotypes (and phenotypes) remain constant from one generation to another. This is known as the Hardy-Weinberg principle, proposed independently by the English mathematician G H Hardy and a German physician, W Weinberg, in 1908, and it remains important.

The Hardy-Weinberg Principle

Consider an "ideal" population in which there is an autosomal locus with two alleles, A and a, that have frequencies of p and q, respectively. These are the only alleles found at this locus, so that $p + q = 100\%$, or 1. The frequency of each genotype in the population can be determined by construction of a Punnett square, which shows how the different genes can combine (Fig. 7.1).

From Fig. 7.1, it can be seen that the frequencies of the different genotypes are:

Genotype	Phenotype	Frequency
AA	A	p^2
Aa	A	$2pq$
aa	a	q^2

If there is random mating of sperm and ova, the frequencies of the different genotypes in the first generation will be as shown. If these individuals mate with one another to produce a second generation, a Punnett square can again be used to show the different matings and their frequencies (Fig. 7.2).

From Fig. 7.2 the total frequency for each genotype in the second generation can be derived (Table 7.1). This shows that the relative frequency or proportion of each genotype is the same in the second generation as in the first. In fact, no matter how many generations are studied, the relative frequencies will remain constant. The actual numbers of individuals with each genotype will change as the population size increases or decreases, but their relative frequencies or proportions remain constant—the fundamental tenet of the Hardy-Weinberg principle. When epidemiological studies confirm that the relative proportions of each genotype remain constant with

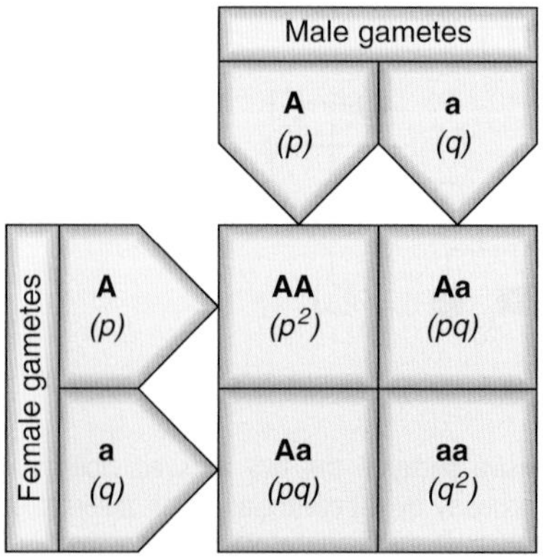

• **Fig. 7.1** Punnett square showing allele frequencies and resulting genotype frequencies for a two-allele system in the first generation.

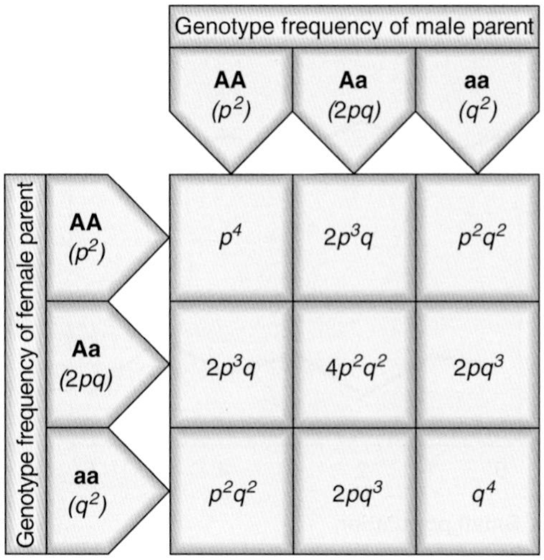

• **Fig. 7.2** Punnett square showing frequencies of the different matings in the second generation.

frequencies of p^2, 2pq and q^2, then that population is said to be in Hardy-Weinberg equilibrium for that particular genotype.

Factors That Can Disturb Hardy-Weinberg Equilibrium

So far, this relates to an "ideal" population. By definition such a population is large and shows random mating with no new mutations and no selection for or against any particular genotype. For some human characteristics, such as neutral genes for blood groups or enzyme variants, these criteria can be fulfilled. However, several factors can disturb Hardy-Weinberg equilibrium, either by influencing the distribution of genes in the population or by altering the gene frequencies. These factors include:

1. Non-random mating
2. Mutation
3. Selection
4. Small population size
5. Gene flow (migration).

Non-random Mating

Random mating, or panmixis, refers to the selection of a partner regardless of that partner's genotype. Non-random mating can lead to an increase in the frequency of affected homozygotes by two mechanisms, either assortative mating or consanguinity.

Assortative Mating. This is the tendency for human beings to choose partners who share characteristics such as height, intelligence and racial origin. If assortative mating extends to conditions such as autosomal recessive (AR) deafness, which accounts for a large proportion of all congenital hearing loss, this will lead to a small increase in the relative frequency of affected homozygotes.

Consanguinity. Consanguinity is the term used to describe childbearing between blood relatives who have at least one common ancestor no more remote than a great-great-grandparent. Widespread consanguinity in a community will lead to a relative increase in the frequency of affected homozygotes but a relative decrease in the frequency of heterozygotes.

Mutation

The validity of the Hardy-Weinberg principle is based on the assumption that no new mutations occur. If a particular locus shows a high mutation rate, then there will be a steady increase in the proportion of mutant alleles in a population. In practice, mutations do occur at almost all loci, albeit at different rates, but the effect of their introduction is usually balanced by the loss of mutant alleles because of reduced fitness of affected individuals. If a population is found to be in Hardy-Weinberg equilibrium, it is generally assumed that these two opposing factors have roughly equal effects—discussed further in the section that follows on the estimation of mutation rates.

Selection

In the "ideal" population there is no selection for or against any particular genotype. In reality, for deleterious characteristics there is likely to be negative selection, with affected individuals having reduced reproductive (= biological = "genetic") fitness. This implies that they do not have as many offspring as unaffected members of the population. In the absence of new mutations, this reduction in fitness will lead to a gradual reduction in the

TABLE 7.1 Frequency of the various types of offspring from the matings shown in Fig. 7.2

		FREQUENCY OF OFFSPRING		
Mating Type	Frequency	AA	Aa	aa
AA × AA	p^4	p^4	—	—
AA × Aa	$4p^3q$	$2p^3q$	$2p^3q$	—
Aa × Aa	$4p^2q^2$	p^2q^2	$2p^2q^2$	p^2q^2
AA × aa	$2p^2q^2$	—	$2p^2q^2$	—
Aa × aa	$4pq^3$	—	$2pq^3$	$2pq^3$
aa × aa	q^4	—	—	q^4
Total		$p^2(p^2 + 2pq + q^2)$	$2pq(p^2 + 2pq + q^2)$	$q^2(p^2 + 2pq + q^2)$
Relative frequency		p^2	$2pq$	q^2

frequency of the mutant gene, and hence disturbance of Hardy-Weinberg equilibrium.

Selection can act in the opposite direction by increasing fitness. For some AR disorders there is evidence that heterozygotes show a slight increase in biological fitness compared with unaffected homozygotes—referred to as heterozygote advantage. The best understood example is sickle-cell disease, in which affected homozygotes have severe anemia and often show persistent ill health (p. 158). However, heterozygotes are relatively immune to infection with *Plasmodium falciparum* malaria because their red blood cells undergo sickling and are rapidly destroyed when invaded by the parasite. In areas where this form of malaria is endemic, carriers of sickle-cell (SC) anemia (SC trait) have a biological advantage compared with unaffected homozygotes. Therefore in these regions the proportion of heterozygotes tends to increase relative to the proportions of normal and affected homozygotes, and Hardy-Weinberg equilibrium is disturbed.

Small Population Size

In a large population, the numbers of children produced by individuals with different genotypes, assuming no alteration in fitness for any particular genotype, will tend to balance out, so that gene frequencies remain stable. However, in a small population it is possible that, by random statistical fluctuation, one allele could be transmitted to a high proportion of offspring by chance, resulting in changes in allele frequency from one generation to the next, resulting in Hardy-Weinberg *dis*equilibrium. This is known as random genetic drift. In extreme cases one allele may be lost altogether, and the other "fixed" (Fig. 7.3).

Gene Flow (Migration)

If new alleles are introduced into a population through migration and intermarriage, a change will occur in the relevant allele frequencies. This slow diffusion of alleles across racial or geographical boundaries is known as gene flow. The most widely quoted example is the gradient shown by the incidence of the B blood group allele throughout the world (Fig. 7.4), which is thought to have originated in Asia and spread slowly westward from admixture through invasion.

Validity of Hardy-Weinberg Equilibrium

It is relatively simple to establish whether a population is in Hardy-Weinberg equilibrium for a particular trait if all possible genotypes can be identified. Consider a system with two alleles, A and a, with three resulting genotypes, AA, Aa/aA and aa. Among 1000 individuals selected at random, the following genotype distributions are observed:

AA	800
Aa/aA	185
aa	15

From these figures, the incidence of the "A" allele (p) equals $[(2 \times 800) + 185]/2000 = 0.8925$, and the incidence of the "a" allele (q) equals $[185 + (2 \times 15)]/2000 = 0.1075$.

However, if the population were in Hardy-Weinberg equilibrium, the expected gene frequencies would be:

Genotype	Observed	Expected
AA	800	796.5 ($p^2 \times 1000$)
Aa/aA	185	192 ($2pq \times 1000$)
aa	15	11.5 ($q^2 \times 1000$)

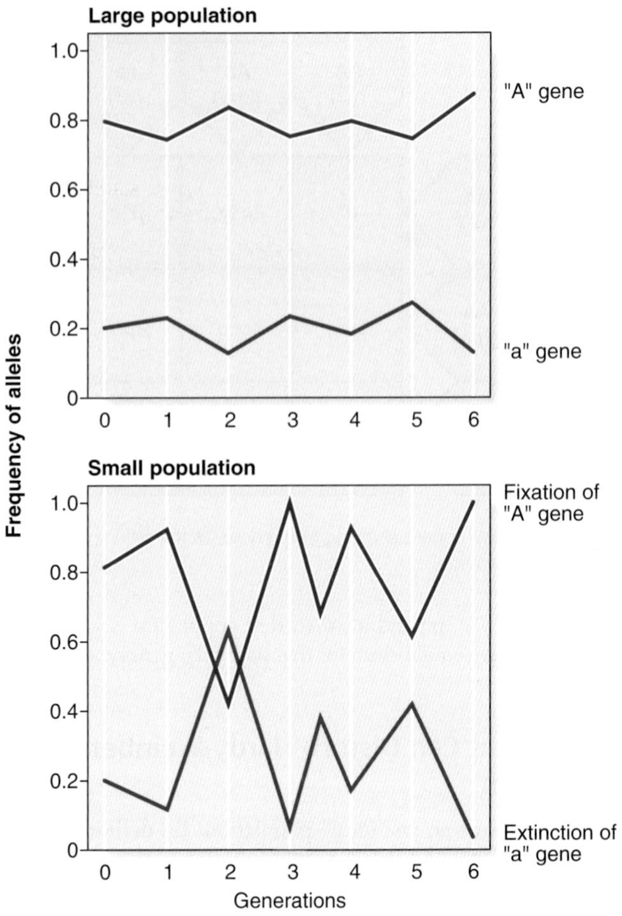

• **Fig. 7.3** Possible effects of random genetic drift in large and small populations.

The observed and expected allele frequencies can be statistically compared by a χ^2 test, which confirms that they do not differ significantly.

Next, consider a different system with two alleles, B and b. Among 1000 randomly selected individuals the observed genotype distributions are:

BB	430
Bb/bB	540
bb	30

From these values, the incidence of the "B" allele (p) equals $[(2 \times 430) + 540]/2000 = 0.7$, and the incidence of the "b" allele (q) equals $[540 + (2 \times 30)]/2000 = 0.3$.

Using these values for p and q, the observed and expected genotype distributions can be compared:

Genotype	Observed	Expected
BB	430	490 ($p^2 \times 1000$)
Bb/bB	540	420 ($2pq \times 1000$)
bb	30	90 ($q^2 \times 1000$)

These values differ significantly, with an increased number of heterozygotes at the expense of homozygotes. Such deviation from Hardy-Weinberg equilibrium should prompt a search for factors that could result in increased numbers of heterozygotes, such as heterozygote advantage or negative assortative mating—that is, the attraction of opposites!

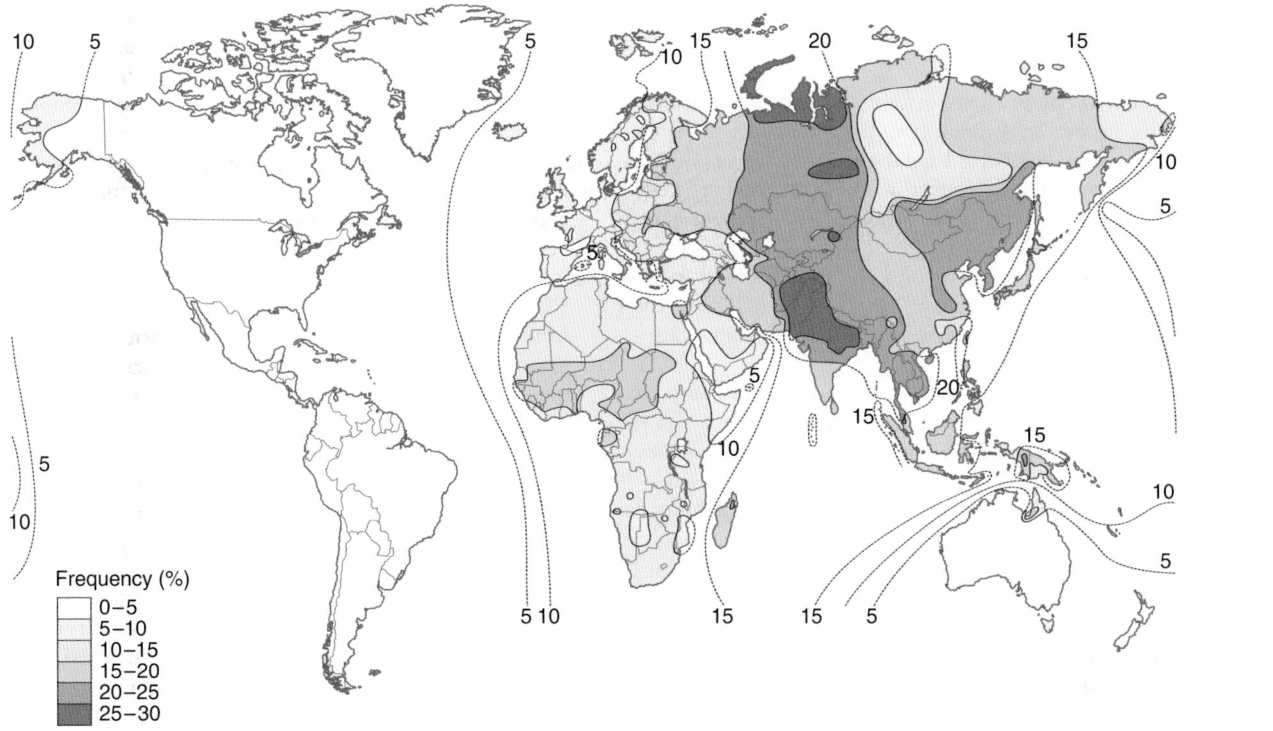

• **Fig. 7.4** Distribution of blood group B throughout the world. (From Mourant AE, Kopéc AC, Domaniewska-Sobczak K. *The Distribution of the Human Blood Groups and other Polymorphisms*. 2nd ed. London: Oxford University Press; 1976. With permission.)

Despite the number of factors that can disturb Hardy-Weinberg equilibrium, most populations are in equilibrium for most genetic traits, and significant deviations from expected genotype frequencies are unusual.

Applications of Hardy-Weinberg Equilibrium

Estimation of Carrier Frequencies

If the incidence of an AR disorder is known, it is possible to calculate the carrier frequency using some relatively simple algebra. For example, if the disease incidence is 1 in 10,000, then $q^2 = {}^1/_{10,000}$ and $q = {}^1/_{100}$. Because $p + q = 1$, therefore $p = {}^{99}/_{100}$. The carrier frequency can then be calculated as $2 \times {}^{99}/_{100} \times {}^1/_{100}$ (i.e., 2pq), which approximates to 1 in 50. Thus a rough approximation of the carrier frequency can be obtained by doubling the square root of the disease incidence. Approximate values for gene frequency and carrier frequency derived from the disease incidence can be extremely useful in genetic risk counseling (see Chapter 21) (Table 7.2). However, if the disease incidence includes cases resulting from a high proportion of consanguineous relationships, then it is not valid to use the Hardy-Weinberg principle to calculate heterozygote frequencies because consanguinity disturbs the equilibrium, leading to a relative increase in the proportion of affected homozygotes.

For an X-linked recessive (XLR) disorder, the frequency of affected males equals the frequency of the mutant allele, q. Thus, for a trait such as red-green color blindness, which affects approximately 1 in 12 male western European Caucasians, $q = {}^1/_{12}$ and $p = {}^{11}/_{12}$. This means that the frequency of affected females (q^2) and carrier females (2pq) is ${}^1/_{144}$ and ${}^{22}/_{144}$, respectively.

TABLE 7.2 **Approximate values for gene frequency and carrier frequency calculated from the disease incidence assuming Hardy-Weinberg equilibrium**

Disease Incidence (q^2)	Gene Frequency (q)	Carrier Frequency (2pq)
1/1000	1/32	1/16
1/2000	1/45	1/23
1/5000	1/71	1/36
1/10,000	1/100	1/50
1/50,000	1/224	1/112
1/100,000	1/316	1/158

Estimation of Mutation Rates

Direct Method. If an autosomal dominant (AD) disorder shows full penetrance, and is therefore always expressed in heterozygotes, an estimate of its mutation rate can be made relatively easily by counting the number of new cases in a defined number of births. Consider a sample of 100,000 children, 12 of whom have the AD disorder achondroplasia (p. 117). Only two of these children have an affected parent, so the remaining 10 must have acquired their disorder as a result of new mutations. Therefore 10 new mutations have occurred among the 200,000 genes inherited by these children (because each child inherits two copies of each gene), giving a mutation rate of 1 per 20,000 gametes per generation. In fact, this example is unusual because all new mutations in achondroplasia occur on the paternally derived chromosome 4; therefore, the mutation rate is 1 per 10,000 in spermatogenesis and, as far as we know, zero in oogenesis.

Indirect Method. For an AD disorder with reproductive fitness (f) equal to zero, all cases must result from new mutations. If the incidence of a disorder is denoted as I and the mutation rate as μ, then as each child inherits two alleles, either of which can mutate to cause the disorder, the incidence equals twice the mutation rate (i.e., $I = 2\mu$).

If fitness is greater than zero, and the disorder is in Hardy-Weinberg equilibrium, then genes lost through reduced fitness must be counterbalanced by new mutations. Therefore $2\mu = I(1 - f)$ or $\mu = [I(1 - f)]/2$.

Thus if an estimate of genetic fitness can be made by comparing the average number of offspring born to affected parents with the average number of offspring born to controls such as their unaffected siblings, it will be possible to calculate the mutation rate.

A similar approach can be used to estimate mutation rates for AR and XLR disorders. With an AR condition, two genes will be lost for each homozygote that fails to reproduce. These will be balanced by new mutations. Therefore $2\mu = I(1 - f) \times 2$ or $\mu = I(1-f)$.

For an XLR condition with an incidence in males equal to I^M, three X chromosomes are transmitted per couple per generation. Therefore, $3\mu = I^M(1 - f)$ or $\mu = [I^M(1 - f)]/3$.

Why Is It Helpful to Know Mutation Rates?

There is a tendency to either love or hate mathematical formulae, but the link among mutation rates, disease incidence, and fitness does hold practical value.

Estimation of Gene Size. If a disorder has a high mutation rate, the gene may be large. Alternatively, it may contain a high proportion of GC residues and be prone to copy error, or contain a high proportion of repeat sequences (p. 17), which could predispose to misalignment in meiosis, resulting in deletion and duplication.

Determination of Mutagenic Potential. Accurate methods for determining mutation rates may be useful in relation to predicted and observed differences in disease incidence in the aftermath of events such as nuclear accidents, for example Chernobyl in 1986 (p. 23).

Consequences of Treatment of Genetic Disease. As discussed later, improved treatment for serious genetic disorders may increase biological fitness, which may result in an increase in disease incidence.

Why Are Some Genetic Disorders More Common Than Others?

It follows that, if a gene has a high mutation rate, the disease incidence may be relatively high. However, factors other than the mutation rate and biological fitness may be involved, as mentioned previously. These are now considered in the context of population size.

Small Populations

Several rare AR disorders show a relatively high incidence in certain population groups (Table 7.3). High allele frequencies are usually

TABLE 7.3 Rare autosomal recessive disorders that are relatively common in certain groups of people

Group	Disorder	Clinical Features
Finns	Congenital nephrotic syndrome	Edema, proteinuria, susceptibility to infection
	Aspartylglycosaminuria	Progressive mental and motor deterioration, coarse features
	Mulibrey nanism	Muscle, liver, brain and eye involvement
	Congenital chloride diarrhoea	Reduced Cl^- absorption, diarrhea
	Diastrophic dysplasia	Progressive epiphyseal dysplasia with dwarfism and scoliosis
Amish	Cartilage–hair hypoplasia	Dwarfism, fine, light-colored and sparse hair
	Ellis–van Creveld syndrome	Dwarfism, polydactyly, congenital heart disease
	Glutaric aciduria type 1	Episodic encephalopathy and cerebral palsy–like dystonia
Hopi and San Blas Indians	Albinism	Lack of pigmentation
Ashkenazi Jews	Tay-Sachs disease	Progressive mental and motor deterioration, blindness
	Gaucher disease	Hepatosplenomegaly, bone lesions, skin pigmentation
	Dysautonomia	Indifference to pain, emotional lability, lack of tears, hyperhidrosis
Karaite Jews	Werdnig-Hoffmann disease	Infantile spinal muscular atrophy
Afrikaners	Sclerosteosis	Tall stature, overgrowth of craniofacial bones with cranial nerve palsies, syndactyly
	Lipoid proteinosis	Thickening of skin and mucous membranes
Ryukyan Islands (off Japan)	"Ryukyan" spinal muscular atrophy	Muscle weakness, club foot, scoliosis

explained by the combination of a founder effect together with social, religious, or geographical isolation—hence the term genetic isolates. In some situations, genetic drift may have played a role.

For example, several very rare AR disorders occur at relatively high frequency in the Old Order Amish living in Pennsylvania—Christians originating from the Anabaptist movement who fled Europe during religious persecution in the 18th century. Original founders of the group must have carried abnormal alleles that became established at relatively high frequency because of the restricted number of partners available to members of the community.

Founder effects can also be observed in AD disorders. Variegate porphyria, which is characterized by photosensitivity and drug-induced neurovisceral disturbance, has a high incidence in the Afrikaner population of South Africa, traceable to one of two early Dutch settlers having transmitted the condition to many descendants (p. 282).

Interestingly, the Hopi Indians of Arizona show a high incidence of albinism. Affected males were excused from outdoor farming activities because of the health and visual problems of bright sunlight, thus providing more opportunity to reproduce relative to unaffected group members.

Large Populations

When a serious AR disorder resulting in reduced fitness in affected homozygotes has a high incidence in a large population, the explanation is presumed to lie in either a very high mutation rate and/or a heterozygote advantage. The latter explanation is the more probable for most AR disorders (Table 7.4).

Heterozygote Advantage. For SC anemia (p. 164) and thalassemia (p. 166) there is very good evidence that heterozygote advantage results from reduced susceptibility to *P. falciparum* malaria, as explained in Chapter 12. Americans of Afro-Caribbean origin are no longer exposed to malaria, so it would be expected that the frequency of the SC allele in this group would gradually decline. However, the predicted rate of decline is so slow that it will be many generations before it is detectable.

For several AR disorders the mechanisms proposed for heterozygote advantage are largely speculative (see Table 7.4). The discovery of the cystic fibrosis (CF) gene, with the subsequent elucidation of the role of its protein product in membrane permeability (p. 303), supports the hypothesis of selective advantage through increased resistance to the effects of gastrointestinal infections, such as cholera and dysentery, in the heterozygote. This relative resistance could result from reduced loss of fluid and electrolytes. It is likely that this selective advantage was of greatest value several hundred years ago when these infections were endemic in Western Europe. If so, a gradual decline in the incidence of CF would be expected. However, if this theory is correct, one has to ask why CF has not become relatively common in other parts of the world where gastrointestinal infections are endemic, particularly the tropics; in fact, the opposite is the case, for CF is rarer in these regions.

An alternative, but speculative, mechanism for the high incidence of a condition such as CF is that the mutant allele is preferentially transmitted at meiosis. This type of segregation distortion, whereby an allele at a particular locus is transmitted more often than would be expected by chance (i.e., in more than 50% of gametes), is referred to as meiotic drive. Firm evidence for this phenomenon in CF is lacking, although it has been demonstrated in the AD disorder myotonic dystrophy (p. 302).

A major practical problem when studying heterozygote advantage is that even a tiny increase in heterozygote fitness compared with the fitness of unaffected homozygotes can be sufficient to sustain a high allele frequency. For example, in CF, with an allele frequency of approximately 1 in 50, a heterozygote advantage of 2% to 3% would be sufficient to account for the high allele frequency.

Genetic Polymorphism

Polymorphism is the occurrence in a population of two or more genetically determined forms (alleles, sequence variants) in such frequencies that the rarest of them could not be maintained by mutation alone. By convention, a polymorphic locus is one at which there are at least two alleles, each with a frequency greater than 1%. Alleles with frequencies of less than 1% are referred to as rare variants.

In humans, at least 30% of structural gene loci are polymorphic, with each individual being heterozygous at between 10%

TABLE 7.4 Presumed increased resistance in heterozygotes that could account for the maintenance of various genetic disorders in certain populations

Disorder	Genetics	Region/Population	Resistance or Advantage
Sickle-cell disease	AR	Tropical Africa	Falciparum malaria
α- and β-thalassemia	AR	Southeast Asia and the Mediterranean	Falciparum malaria
G6PD deficiency	XLR	Mediterranean	Falciparum malaria
Cystic fibrosis	AR	Western Europe	Tuberculosis? The plague? Cholera?
Tay-Sachs disease	AR	Eastern European Jews	Tuberculosis?
Congenital adrenal hyperplasia	AR	Yupik Eskimos	Influenza B
Type 2 diabetes	AD	Pima Indians and others	Periodic starvation
Phenylketonuria	AR	Western Europe	Spontaneous abortion rate lower?

AD, autosomal dominant; *AR*, Autosomal recessive; *G6PD*, glucose 6-phosphate dehydrogenase; *XLR*, X-linked recessive.

and 20% of all loci. Known polymorphic protein systems include the ABO blood groups (p. 181) and many serum proteins, which may exhibit polymorphic electrophoretic differences—or isozymes.

DNA polymorphisms, including single nucleotide polymorphisms (SNPs), have been crucial to positional cloning, gene mapping, the isolation of many disease genes (p. 52), studying population migrations and forensic science. They are also used in gene tracking in the clinical context of preimplantation genetic diagnosis (p. 332) and exclusion testing. The value of a particular polymorphic system is assessed by determining its polymorphic information content (PIC). The higher the PIC value, the more likely it is that a polymorphic marker will be of value in various applications.

Segregation Analysis

Segregation analysis refers to the study of the way in which a disorder is transmitted in families so as to establish the underlying mode of inheritance. The mathematical aspects of complex segregation analysis are far beyond the scope of this book—as well as many clinical geneticists! However, it is an important part of human genetics, and some understanding of the principles involved, and the pitfalls, is relevant for the clinician meeting families.

Autosomal Dominant Inheritance

For an AD disorder, the simplest approach is to compare the observed numbers of affected offspring born to affected parents with what would be expected based on the disease penetrance (i.e., 50% if penetrance is complete). A χ^2 test can be used to see whether the observed and expected numbers differ significantly. Care must be taken to ensure that a bias is not introduced by excluding parents who were ascertained through an affected child.

Autosomal Recessive Inheritance

For disorders thought to follow AR inheritance, formal segregation analysis is much more difficult. This is because some couples who are both carriers will by chance not have affected children, and therefore not feature in ascertainment. To illustrate this, consider 64 possible sibships of size 3 in which both parents are carriers, drawn from a large hypothetical population (Table 7.5). The sibship structure shown in Table 7.5 is that which would be expected, on average.

In this population, on average, 27 of the 64 sibships will not contain any affected individuals. This can be calculated simply by cubing $^{3}/_{4}$—that is, $^{3}/_{4} \times {}^{3}/_{4} \times {}^{3}/_{4} = {}^{27}/_{64}$. Therefore, when the families are analyzed these 27 sibships containing only healthy individuals will not be ascertained—referred to as incomplete ascertainment. If this is not taken into account, a falsely high segregation ratio of 0.43 will be obtained instead of the correct value of 0.25.

Mathematical methods have been devised to cater for incomplete ascertainment, but analysis is usually further complicated by problems associated with achieving full or complete ascertainment. In practice, "proof" of AR inheritance requires accurate molecular or biochemical markers for carrier detection. Affected siblings (especially when at least one is female) born to unaffected parents usually suggest AR inheritance, but somatic and germline parental mosaicism (p. 77), nonpaternity and other possibilities need to be considered. There are some good examples of conditions originally reported to follow AR inheritance but subsequently shown to be dominant with germline or somatic mosaicism; for example, osteogenesis imperfecta and pseudoachondroplasia. However, a high incidence of parental consanguinity undoubtedly provides strong supportive evidence for AR inheritance, as first noted by Bateson and Garrod in 1902 (pp. 4, 71).

Genetic Linkage

Mendel's third law—the principle of independent assortment—states that members of different gene pairs assort to gametes independently of one another (p. 3). Stated more simply, the alleles of genes at different loci segregate independently. Although this is true for genes on different chromosomes, it is not always true for genes that are located on the same chromosome (i.e., close together, or syntenic).

Two loci positioned adjacent, or close, to each other on the same chromosome will tend to be inherited together, and are said to be linked. The closer they are, the less likely they will be separated by a crossover, or recombination, during meiosis I (Fig. 7.5).

TABLE 7.5 Expected sibship structure in a hypothetical population that contains 64 sibships, each of size 3, in which both parents are carriers of an autosomal recessive disorder

Number of Affected in Sibship	Structure of Sibship	Number of Sibships	Number of Affected	Total Number of Sibs
3	■■■	1	3	3
2	■■□	3	6	9
	□■■	3	6	9
	■□■	3	6	9
1	■□□	9	9	27
	□■□	9	9	27
	□□■	9	9	27
0	□□□	27	0	81
Total		64	48	192

If no allowance is made for truncate ascertainment, in that the 27 sibships with no affected cases will not be ascertained, then a falsely high segregation ratio of 48/111 (= 0.43) will be obtained.

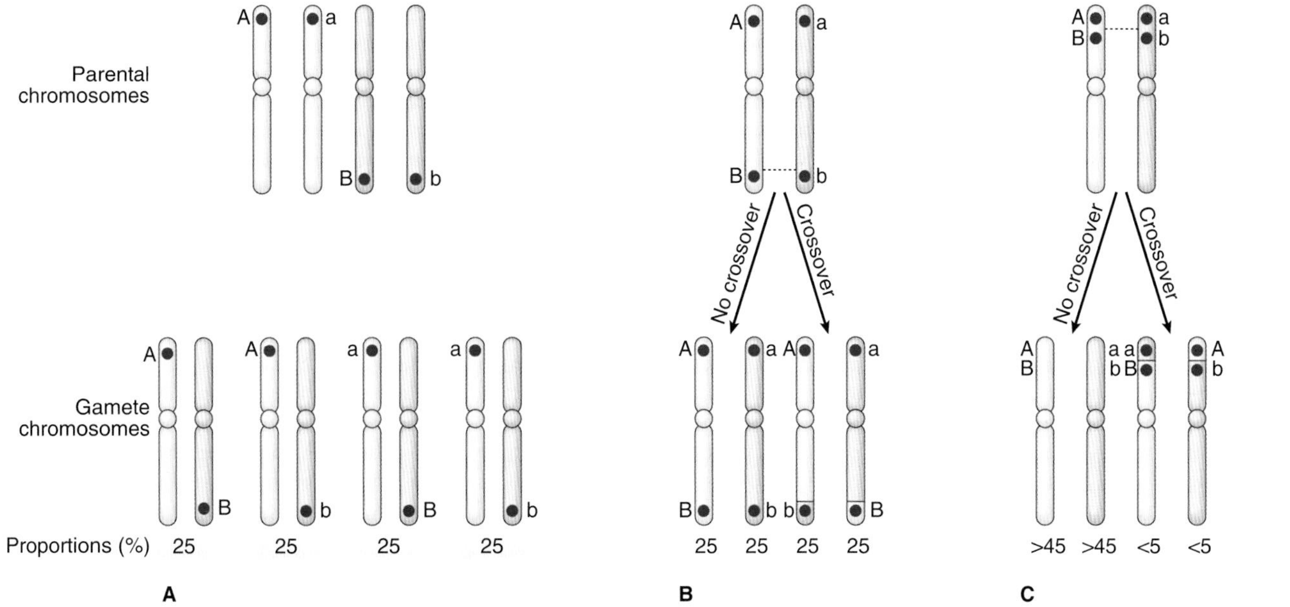

• **Fig. 7.5** Segregation at meiosis of alleles at two loci. In (A) the loci are on different chromosomes, and in (B) they are on the same chromosome but widely separated. Hence these loci are not linked, and there is independent assortment. In (C) the loci are closely adjacent so that separation by a crossover is unlikely (i.e., the loci are linked).

Linked alleles on the same chromosome, and a pattern of associated markers, are known as the **linkage phase**. Thus in the parental chromosomes in Fig. 7.5, C, A and B, as well as a and b, are in phase, whereas A and b, as well as a and B, are unlinked, in trans.

Recombination Fraction

The recombination fraction, usually designated as θ (Greek theta), is a measure of the distance separating two loci, or more precisely an indication of the likelihood that a crossover will occur between them. If two loci are not linked, then θ equals 0.5 because, on average, genes at unlinked loci will segregate together during 50% of all meioses. If θ equals 0.05, this means that on average the syntenic alleles will segregate together 19 times out of 20 (i.e., a crossover will occur between them during, on average, only 1 in 20 meioses).

Centimorgans

The unit of measurement for genetic linkage is known as a map unit or centimorgan (cM). If two loci are 1 cM apart, a crossover occurs between them, on average, only once in every 100 meioses (i.e., $\theta = 0.01$). The cM is a measure of the genetic, or linkage, distance between two loci. This is not the same as physical distance, which is measured in base pairs (bp) (kb – kilobases: 1000 base pairs; Mb – megabases: 1,000,000 base pairs).

The human genome has been estimated by recombination studies to be approximately 3000 cM in length in males. Because the physical length of the haploid human genome is approximately 3×10^9 bp, 1 cM corresponds to approximately 10^6 bp (1 Mb or 1000 kb). However, the relationship between linkage map units and physical length is not linear. Some chromosome regions appear to be particularly prone to recombination—so-called "hotspots"—and recombination occurs less often during meiosis in males than in females, in whom the genome "linkage" length has been estimated to be 4200 cM. Generally, in humans one or two recombination events take place between each pair of homologous chromosomes in meiosis I, with a total of ~40 across the entire genome. Recombination events are rare close to the centromeres but relatively common in telomeric regions.

Linkage Analysis

Linkage analysis proved invaluable for mapping genes in the past (see Chapter 4) but is now largely redundant following complete sequencing of the human genome and next-generation methodologies, although the principles still apply in genome-wide association studies. It is based on studying the segregation of the disease with polymorphic markers from each chromosome—preferably in large families. Eventually a marker will be identified that cosegregates with the disease more often than would be expected by chance (i.e., the marker and disease locus are linked). The mathematical analysis tends to be very complex, particularly if many closely adjacent markers are being used, as in multipoint linkage analysis. However, the underlying principle is relatively straightforward and involves the use of likelihood ratios, the logarithms of which are known as LOD scores (logarithm of the odds).

Logarithm of the Odds Scores

When studying the segregation of alleles at two loci that could be linked, a series of likelihood ratios is calculated for different values of the recombination fraction (θ), ranging from $\theta = 0$ to $\theta = 0.5$. The likelihood ratio at a given value of θ equals the likelihood of the observed data, if the loci are linked at recombination value of θ, divided by the likelihood of the observed data if the loci are not linked ($\theta = 0.5$). The logarithm to the base 10 of this ratio is known as the LOD score (Z)—that is, LOD (θ) = $\log_{10}$ [Lθ/L (0.5)]. Logarithms are used because they allow results from different families to be added together.

For example, a LOD score of 4 at recombination fraction (θ) 0.05 means that the results, in the families studied, indicate that it is 10,000 (10^4) times more likely that the disease and marker loci are closely linked (i.e., 5 cM apart) than that they are not linked. A LOD score of +3 or more would be confirmation of linkage, yielding a ratio of 1000 to 1 in favor of linkage; however, because there is a prior probability of only 1 in 50 that any two given loci are linked, a LOD score of +3 means that the overall probability that the loci are linked is approximately 20 to 1—that is, [1000 × 1/50]:1. The importance of taking prior probabilities into account in probability theory is discussed in the section on Bayes' theorem (p. 96).

A "Simple" Example

Consider a three-generation family in which several members have an AD disorder (Fig. 7.6). A and B are alleles at a locus that is being tested for linkage to the disease locus.

To establish whether it is likely that these two loci are linked, the LOD score is calculated for various values of θ. The value of θ that gives the highest LOD score is taken as the best estimate of the recombination fraction. This is known as a **maximum likelihood method.**

To demonstrate the underlying principle, the LOD score is calculated for a value of θ equal to 0.05. If θ equals 0.05, then the loci are linked, in which case the disease gene and the B marker must be on the same chromosome in II2, as both of these characteristics have been inherited from the mother. Thus in II2 the linkage phase is known: the disease allele and the B allele are linked. Therefore the probability that III1 will be affected and will also inherit the B marker equals 0.95 (i.e., 1 − θ). A similar result is obtained for the remaining three members of the sibship in generation III, giving a value for the numerator of $(0.95)^4$. If the loci are not linked, the likelihood of observing both the disease and marker B in III1 equals 0.5. A similar result is obtained for his three siblings, giving a value for the denominator of $(0.5)^4$.

Therefore the LOD score for this family, given a value of $\theta = 0.05$, equals $\log\ 0.95^4/0.5^4 = \log_{10}\ 13.032 = 1.12$. For a value of $\theta = 0$, the LOD score equals $\log_{10}\ 14/0.54 = \log_{10}\ 16 = 1.20$. For a value of $\theta = 0.1$, the LOD score equals $\log_{10}\ 0.94/0.54 = \log_{10}\ 10.498 = 1.02$. The highest LOD score is obtained for a value of θ equals 0, consistent with close linkage of the disease and marker loci, such that no recombination has occurred between the two loci in members of generation III.

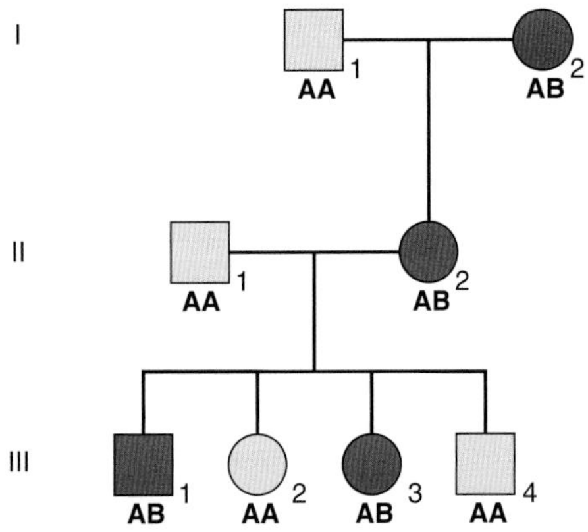

• **Fig. 7.6** Three-generation pedigree showing segregation of an autosomal dominant disorder and alleles (A and B) at a locus that may or may not be linked to the disease locus.

To confirm linkage other families would have to be studied by pooling all the results until a LOD score of +3 or greater was obtained. A LOD score of −2 or less is taken as proof that the loci are not linked. This less stringent requirement for proof of non-linkage (i.e., a LOD score of −2 compared with +3 for proof of linkage) is attributed to the high prior probability that any two loci are not linked.

Multipoint Linkage Analysis

Initial linkage results using a limited number of markers would be followed up by a multipoint linkage analysis using a series of polymorphic markers known to map to the disease region, allowing fine tuning of the likely position of the disease locus within the interval previously defined. A computer program would then calculate the overall likelihood of the position of the disease locus in relation to the marker loci, and a graph constructed of the "location score" against map distance (Fig. 7.7). On this graph the peaks represent possible positions of the disease locus, with the tallest peak being the most probable location. The troughs represent the positions of the polymorphic marker loci.

Once the smallest interval for the disease locus was located, physical mapping methods were applied to identify the disease gene (see Chapter 4), although sophisticated sequencing methods are now used.

Autozygosity Mapping

This form of linkage analysis has been used to map and identify many rare AR disorders. Autozygosity occurs when individuals are homozygous at particular loci by descent from a common ancestor. In an inbred pedigree containing two or more children with a rare AR disorder, it is very likely that the children will be homozygous not only at the disease locus but also at closely linked loci. Thus all affected relatives in an inbred family will be homozygous for markers close to the disease locus (Fig.7.8). By searching the genome

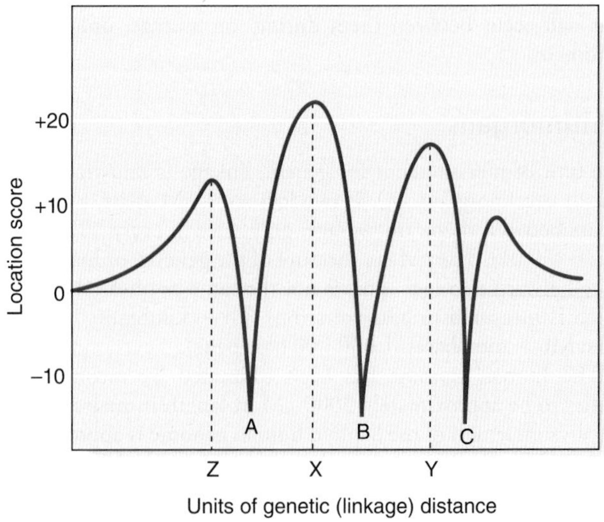

• **Fig. 7.7** Multipoint linkage analysis. (A), (B), and (C) represent the known linkage relationships of three polymorphic marker loci. X, Y, and Z represent in descending order of likelihood the probable position of the disease locus.

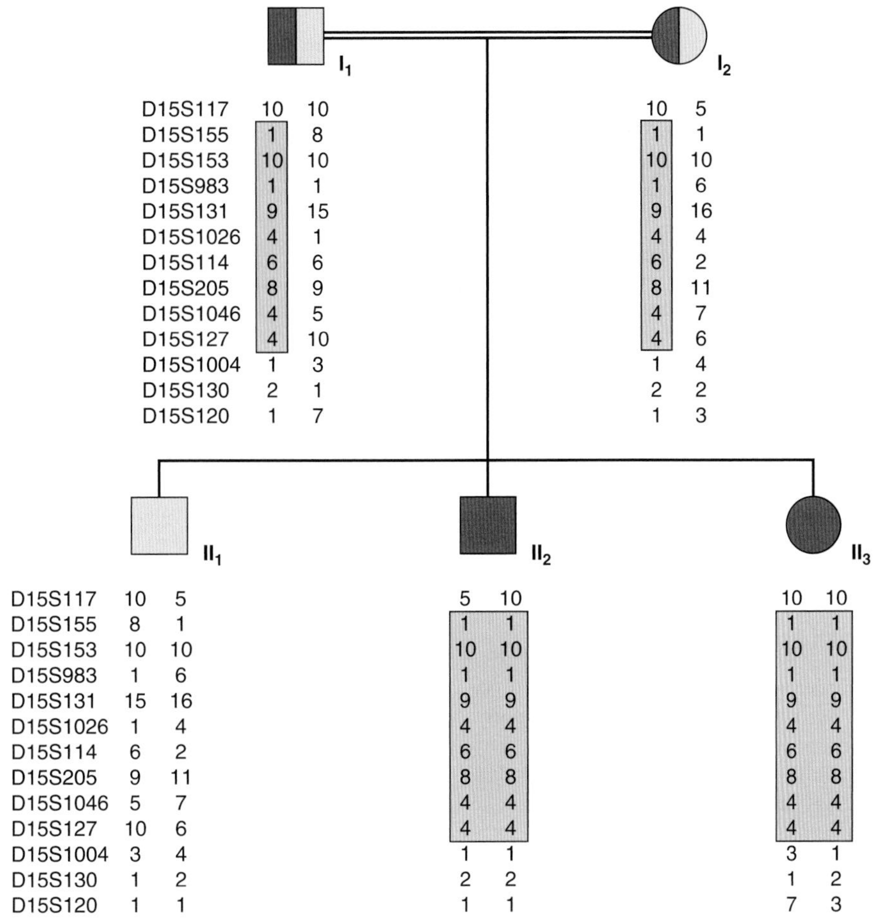

• **Fig. 7.8** Autozygosity mapping in a family with spondylocostal dysostosis. The father of individual I1 is the brother of I2's grandfather. The region of homozygosity is defined by markers D15S155 and D15S127. A mutation in the *MESP2* gene was subsequently shown to be the cause of spondylocostal dysostosis in this pedigree.

for regions of homozygosity in the affected members of a sibship, and perhaps other affected relatives, only a small number of such regions will be identified. One of these can be expected to harbor the disease locus, and sequencing of candidate genes can go ahead.

Where more than one branch of a large inbred family can be studied, autozygosity is very powerful, and many rare disease genes have been found in this way, for example, the genes for AR sensorineural hearing loss, various skeletal dysplasias, and primary microcephalies.

Linkage Disequilibrium

Linkage disequilibrium is defined formally as the association of two alleles at linked loci more frequently than would be expected by chance and is also referred to as allelic association. The concept and the term relate to the study of diseases in populations rather than families. In the latter, an association between specific alleles and the disease in question holds true only within an individual family; in a separate affected family a different pattern of alleles, or markers, at the same locus may show association with the disease—because the alleles themselves are polymorphic.

The rationale for studying allelic association in populations assumes that a mutation occurred in a founder case some generations previously and is still causative of the disease. If this is true, the pattern of markers in a small region close to the mutation will have been maintained, and thus constitutes what is termed the founder haplotype. The underlying principles used in mapping are the same as those for linkage analysis in families, the difference being the degree of relatedness of the individuals under study. In the pedigree shown in Fig. 7.6, support was obtained for linkage of the disease gene with the B marker allele. If we assume that further studies confirm linkage of these loci and that the A and B alleles have an equal frequency of 0.5, it would be reasonable to expect that the disease gene is linked with allele A in approximately 50% of families and with allele B in the remaining 50%. If, however, the disease allele was found to be linked exclusively with one particular marker allele, this would be an example of linkage disequilibrium.

The demonstration of linkage disequilibrium in a particular disease suggests that the mutation causing the disease has occurred relatively recently and that the marker locus studied is very closely linked to the disease locus. There may be pitfalls, however, in interpreting haplotype data that suggest linkage disequilibrium. Other possible reasons for linkage disequilibrium include: (1) the rapid growth of genetically isolated populations leading to large regions of allelic association throughout the genome; (2) selection, whereby particular alleles enhance or diminish reproductive fitness; and (3) population admixture, where population subgroups with different patterns of allele frequencies are combined into a single study. Allowance for the latter problem can be made by using family-based controls and analysing the transmission of alleles using a method called the transmission/disequilibrium test. This uses the fact that transmitted and non-transmitted alleles from a given parent are paired observations, and examines the preferential transmission of one allele over the other in all heterozygous parents. The method has been applied, for example, to studies of genetic conditions based on discordant sibling pairs.

Medical and Societal Intervention

The ability of modern medicine to enable patients with serious disease to live much longer raises the prospect that biological fitness may be increased, leading to increased numbers of "bad genes" in society, potentially adding adversely to humanity's future genetic load. Such long-term consequences generally carry no weight, however, and may in any case be offset by greater use of prenatal genetic testing, which for many is a focus of ethical concern (see Chapter 22). The ethical debate is very important, but it is worth considering the possible long-term effects of artificial selection for or against genetic disorders, according to pattern of inheritance.

Autosomal Dominant Disorders

If everyone with an AD disorder were successfully encouraged not to reproduce, the incidence of that disorder would decline rapidly, with all future cases being the result only of new mutations. This would have a particularly striking effect on the incidence of relatively mild conditions such as familial hypercholesterolemia, in which genetic fitness is close to 1.

Alternatively, if successful treatment became available for all patients with a serious AD disorder that at present is associated with a marked reduction in genetic fitness, there would be an immediate increase in the frequency of the disease gene followed by a more gradual leveling off at a new equilibrium level. If, at one time, all those with a serious AD disorder died in childhood ($f = 0$), then the incidence of affected individuals would be $2\ \mu$. If treatment raised the fitness from 0 to 0.9, the incidence of affected children in the next generation would rise to $2\ \mu$ because of new mutations plus $1.8\ \mu$ inherited, which equals $3.8\ \mu$. Eventually a new equilibrium would be reached, by which time the disease incidence would have risen tenfold to $20\ \mu$. This can be calculated relatively easily with the formula $\mu = [I(1 - f)]/2$ (p. 88), which can also be expressed as $I = 2\ \mu/(1 - f)$. The net result would be that the proportion of affected children who died would be lower (from 100% down to 10%), but the total number affected would be much greater, although the actual number who died from the disease would remain unchanged at $2\ \mu$.

Autosomal Recessive Disorders

In contrast to an AD disorder, artificial selection against an AR condition will have only a very slow effect. The reason for this difference is that in AR conditions most of the genes in a population are present in healthy heterozygotes who would not be affected by selection measures. It can be shown that if there is complete selection against an AR disorder, so that no homozygotes reproduce, the number of generations (n) required for the allele frequency to change from q^0 to q^n equals $1/q^n - 1/q^0$. Therefore, for a condition with an incidence of approximately 1 in 2000 and an allele frequency of roughly 1 in 45, if all affected patients refrained from reproduction then it would take more than 500 years (18 generations) to reduce the disease incidence by half, and more than 1200 years (45 generations) to reduce the gene frequency by half, assuming an average generation time of 27 years.

Now consider the opposite situation, where selection operating against a serious AR disorder is relaxed because of improvement in medical treatment. More affected individuals will reach adult life and transmit the mutant allele to their offspring. The result will be that the frequency of the mutant allele will increase until a new equilibrium is reached. Using the formula $\mu = I(1 - f)$, it can be shown that, when the new equilibrium is eventually reached, an increase in fitness from 0 to 0.9 will have resulted in a tenfold increase in the disease incidence.

X-Linked Recessive Disorders

Here it is necessary to take into account the fact that a large proportion of the relevant genes are present in entirely healthy female carriers, who are often unaware of their carrier status. For a very serious condition, such as Duchenne muscular dystrophy (p. 99), with fitness equal to 0 in affected males, selection will have no effect unless female carriers choose to limit their families. If all female carriers opted not to have any children, the incidence would be reduced by two-thirds (i.e., from $3\ \mu$ to μ).

More plausibly, effective treatment for these disorders may result in a steady increase in the disease incidence. For example, an increase in fitness from 0 to 0.5 will lead to a doubling of the disease incidence by the time a new equilibrium has been established. This can be calculated using the formula $\mu = [I^M(1 - f)]/3$ (p. 88).

Conclusion

In reality, it is extremely difficult to predict the long-term impact of medical intervention on the incidence and burden of genetic disease. Although it is true that improvements in medical treatment could result in an increased genetic load in future generations, it is also possible that successful therapies will ease the overall burden of these disorders in terms of human suffering. Some of these arguments applied to other major medical developments, such as immunization and the discovery of insulin and antibiotics, which have had immeasurable financial implications in terms of the pharmaceutical industry, as well as contributing to an aging population. Ultimately, how society copes with these advances and challenges provides a measure of civilization.

ELEMENTS

According to the Hardy-Weinberg principle, the relative proportions of the possible genotypes at a particular locus remain constant from one generation to the next.

Factors that may disturb Hardy-Weinberg equilibrium are non-random mating, mutation, selection for or against a particular genotype, small population size and migration.

If an autosomal recessive disorder is in Hardy-Weinberg equilibrium, the carrier frequency can be estimated by doubling the square root of the disease incidence.

The mutation rate for an autosomal dominant disorder can be measured directly by estimating the proportion of new mutations among all members of one generation. Indirect estimates of mutation rates can be made using the formula:

a. $= [I(1 - f)]/2$ for autosomal dominant inheritance
b. $= I(1 - f)$ for autosomal recessive inheritance
c. $= [I^M(1 - f)]/3$ for X-linked recessive inheritance.

Otherwise rare single-gene disorders can show a high incidence in a small population because of a founder effect coupled with genetic isolation.

When a serious autosomal recessive disorder has a relatively high incidence in a large population, it is likely because of heterozygote advantage.

Closely adjacent loci on the same chromosome are regarded as linked if genes at these loci segregate together during more than 50% of meioses. The recombination fraction (θ) indicates how often two such genes will be separated (recombine) at meiosis.

The logarithm of the odds (LOD) score is a mathematical indication of the relative likelihood that two loci are linked. A LOD score of +3 or greater is taken as confirmation of linkage.

The principle of autozygosity (or homozygosity) mapping has facilitated the discovery of many genes for autosomal recessive disorders.

Further Reading

Allison AC. Protection afforded by sickle-cell trait against subtertian malarial infection. *BMJ.* 1954;1:290–294.

A landmark paper providing clear evidence that the sickle-cell trait provides protection against parasitemia by falciparum malaria.

Emery AEH. *Methodology in Medical Genetics.* 2nd ed. Edinburgh: Churchill Livingstone; 1986.

A useful handbook of basic population genetics and mathematical methods for analysing the results of genetic studies.

Francomano CA, McKusick VA, Biesecker LG, eds. Medical genetic studies in the Amish: historical perspective. *Am J Med Genet C Semin Med Genet.* 2003;121:1–4.

A short letter discussing the events which led to the study of medical genetics in the Pennsylvania Amish community in the early 1960s.

Hardy GH. Mendelian proportions in a mixed population. *Science.* 1908;28:49–50.

A short letter in which Hardy pointed out that in a large randomly mating population dominant "characters" would not increase at the expense of recessives.

Khoury MJ, Beaty TH, Cohen BH. *Fundamentals of Genetic Epidemiology.* New York: Oxford University Press; 1993.

A comprehensive textbook of population genetics and its areas of overlap with epidemiology.

Ott J. *Analysis of Human Genetic Linkage.* Baltimore: Johns Hopkins University Press; 1991.

A detailed mathematical explanation of linkage analysis.

Vogel F, Motulsky AG. *Human Genetics, Problems and Approaches.* 3rd ed. Berlin: Springer; 1997.

The definitive textbook of human genetics with extensive coverage of mathematical aspects.

8 Risk Calculation

As far as the laws of mathematics refer to reality, they are not certain; and as far as they are certain, they do not refer to reality.

Albert Einstein

One of the most important aspects of genetic counseling (Chapter 21) is the provision of risk information, often referred to as **recurrence** risk with respect to a couple who have had at least one affected child. Estimation of the recurrence risk usually requires careful consideration and takes into account:

1. The diagnosis, its mode of inheritance, and epidemiological data relating to the natural history (e.g., age of onset)
2. Analysis of the family pedigree
3. The results of different forms of both positive and negative genetic analysis, and clinical data from conventional investigations

Sometimes the provision of a risk figure can be quite easy, but a surprisingly large number of complicating factors arise that make the calculation very difficult. For example, the mother of a boy who is an isolated case of a sex-linked recessive disorder could very reasonably wish to know the recurrence risk for her next child. This is a very simple question, but the solution may be far from straightforward, as discussed later.

It is helpful to clarify what we mean by **probability** and review the different ways in which it can be expressed. The probability of an outcome can be defined as the number or, more correctly, the **proportion** of times it occurs in a large series of events. Conventionally, probability is indicated as a proportion of 1, so that a probability of 0 implies that an outcome will never be observed, whereas a probability of 1 implies that it will always be observed. Therefore, a probability of 0.25 indicates that, on average, a particular outcome or event will be observed on 1 in 4 occasions, or 25%. The probability that the outcome will not occur is 0.75, which can also be expressed as 3 chances out of 4, or 75%. Alternatively, this probability could be expressed as **odds** of 3 to 1 against, or 1 to 3 in favor of the particular outcome being observed. Here we use **fractions** where possible as these tend to be more easily understood than proportions of 1 expressed as decimals.

Probability Theory

To calculate genetic risk it is necessary to have a basic understanding of probability theory. This will be discussed insofar as it is relevant to genetic counseling.

Laws of Addition and Multiplication

When considering the probability of two different events or outcomes, it is essential to clarify whether they are mutually exclusive or independent. If the events are mutually exclusive, then the probability that either one or the other will occur equals the **sum** of their individual probabilities. This is known as the **law of addition**.

If, however, two or more events or outcomes are independent, then the probability that both the first and the second will occur equals the **product** of their individual probabilities. This is known as the **law of multiplication**.

As a simple illustration of these laws, consider parents who have embarked upon their first pregnancy. The probability that the baby will be either a boy or a girl equals 1 (i.e., $1/2 + 1/2$). If the mother is found on ultrasonography to be carrying twins who are non-identical, then the probability that *both* the first *and* the second twin will be boys equals 1/4 (i.e., $1/2 \times 1/2$).

Bayes' Theorem

Bayes' theorem, first devised by Reverend Thomas Bayes (1702–1761) and published after his death in 1763, is widely used in genetic counseling. Essentially it provides a very valuable method for determining the overall probability of an event or outcome, such as carrier status, by considering all initial possibilities (e.g., carrier or non-carrier) and then modifying or "conditioning" these by incorporating information, such as test results or pedigree information, that indicates which is the more likely. Thus the theorem combines the probability that an event will occur with the probability that it will not occur. The theorem lay fairly dormant for a long time but has been enthusiastically employed by geneticists. In recent years, its simplicity and usefulness have been recognized in many other fields—for example, legal work, computing, and statistical analysis—such that it has truly come of age.

The initial probability of each event is known as its **prior probability**, and is based on ancestral or **anterior information**. The observations that modify these prior probabilities allow **conditional probabilities** to be determined. In genetic counseling these are usually based on numbers of offspring and/or the results of tests. This is **posterior information**. The resulting probability for each event or outcome is known as its **joint probability**. The final probability for each event is known as its **posterior** or **relative probability** and is obtained by dividing the joint probability for that event by the sum of all the joint probabilities.

This is not an easy concept to grasp! To make it easier, consider a pedigree with two males, I_3 and II_1, who have a sex-linked recessive disorder (Fig. 8.1). The sister, II_2, of one of these men wishes to know the probability that she is a carrier. Her mother, I_2, must be a carrier because she has both an affected brother and an affected son (i.e., she is an **obligate** carrier). Therefore the prior probability that II_2 is a carrier equals 1/2. Similarly, the prior probability that II_2 is not a carrier equals 1/2.

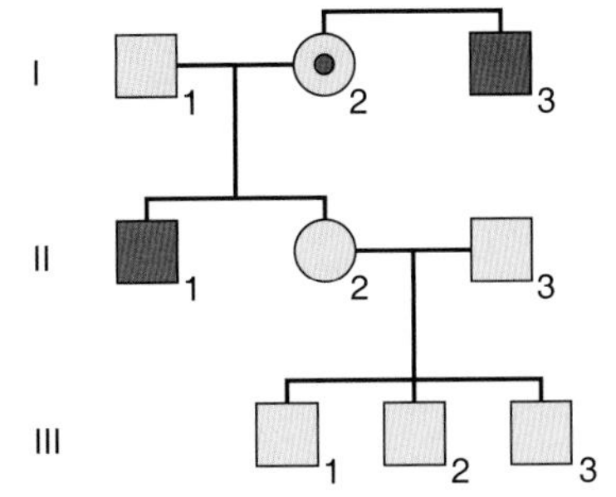

• **Fig. 8.1** Pedigree showing sex-linked recessive inheritance. When calculating the probability that II_2 is a carrier, it is necessary to take into account her three unaffected sons.

The fact that II_2 already has three healthy sons must be taken into consideration because intuitively this makes it less likely that she is a carrier. Bayes' theorem provides a way to quantify this intuition. These three healthy sons provide posterior information. The conditional probability that II_2 will have three healthy sons if she is a carrier is $1/2 \times 1/2 \times 1/2$, which equals 1/8. These values are multiplied, as they are independent events, in that the health of one son is not influenced by the health of his brother(s). The conditional probability that II_2 will have three healthy sons if she is not a carrier equals 1.

This information is now incorporated into a bayesian calculation (Table 8.1). From this table, the posterior probability that II_2 is a carrier equals $1/16/(1/16+1/2)$, which reduces to 1/9. Similarly, the posterior probability that II_2 is not a carrier equals $1/2/(1/16+1/2)$, which reduces to 8/9. Another way to obtain these results is to consider that the odds for II_2 being a carrier versus not being a carrier are 1/16 to 1/2 (i.e., 1 to 8, which equals 1 in 9). Thus by taking into account the fact that II_2 has three healthy sons, we have been able to reduce her risk of being a carrier from 1 in 2 to 1 in 9.

By now the use of Bayes' theorem should be a little clearer. Remember that the basic approach is to draw up a table showing all of the possibilities (e.g., carrier, not a carrier), then establish the background (prior) risk for each possibility, next determine the chance (conditional possibility) that certain observed events (e.g., healthy children) would have happened if each possibility were true, then work out the combined (joint) likelihood for each possibility, and finally weigh up each of the joint probabilities to calculate the exact (posterior) probability for each of the original possibilities. Here are more examples.

TABLE 8.1 **Bayesian calculation for II_2 in Fig. 8.1**

Probability	II_2 is a Carrier	II_2 is not a Carrier
Prior	1/2	1/2
Conditional		
Three healthy sons	$(1/2)^3 = 1/8$	$(1)^3 = 1$
Joint	1/16	1/2 (= 8/16)
Expressed as odds	1 to	8
Posterior	1/9	8/9

Autosomal Dominant Inheritance

For someone with an autosomal dominant disorder, the risk that each of his or her children will inherit the mutant gene equals 1 in 2. This will apply whether the affected individual inherited the disorder from a parent or developed the condition as the result of a *de novo* mutation. Therefore the provision of risks for disorders showing autosomal dominant inheritance is usually straightforward as long as: (1) there is a clear family history; (2) the condition is characterized by being fully penetrant; and (3) there is a reliable means of diagnosing heterozygotes. However, if penetrance is incomplete or there is a delay in the age of onset so that heterozygotes cannot always be diagnosed, the risk calculation becomes more complicated. Two examples illustrate the problems that can arise.

Reduced Penetrance

A disorder is said to show **reduced penetrance** when it has clearly been demonstrated that individuals who must possess the abnormal gene, who by pedigree analysis must be obligate heterozygotes, show no manifestations of the condition. For example, if someone who was completely unaffected had both a parent and a child with the same autosomal dominant disorder, this would be an example of **non-penetrance**. Penetrance is usually quoted as a percentage (e.g., 80%) or as a proportion of 1 (e.g., 0.8). This would imply that 80% of all heterozygotes express the condition in some way.

For a condition showing reduced penetrance, the risk that the child of an affected individual will be affected equals 1/2; that is, the probability that the child will inherit the mutant allele, $\times P$, the proportion of heterozygotes who are affected. Therefore, for a disorder such as hereditary retinoblastoma, an embryonic eye tumor (p. 189), which shows dominant inheritance in some families with a penetrance of $P = 0.8$, the risk that the child of an affected parent will develop a tumor equals $1/2 \times 0.8$, which equals 0.4. A more difficult calculation arises when a risk is sought for the future child of someone who is healthy but whose parent has, or had, an autosomal dominant disorder showing reduced penetrance (Fig. 8.2).

Let us assume the penetrance, P, equals 0.8. Calculation of the risk that III_1 will be affected can be approached in two ways. The first simply involves a little logic. The second uses Bayes' theorem.

1. Imagine that I_2 has 10 children. On average, five children will inherit the gene, but because $P = 0.8$, only four will be affected (Fig. 8.3). Therefore 6 of the 10 children will be

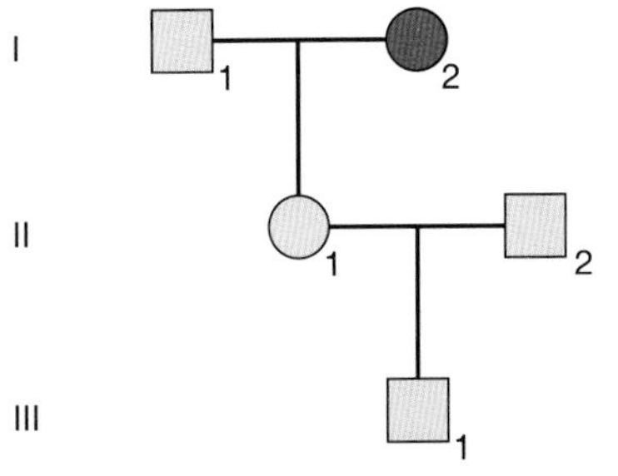

• **Fig. 8.2** I_2 has an autosomal dominant disorder that shows reduced penetrance. The probability that III_1 will be affected has to take into account the possibility that his mother (II_1) is a non-penetrant heterozygote.

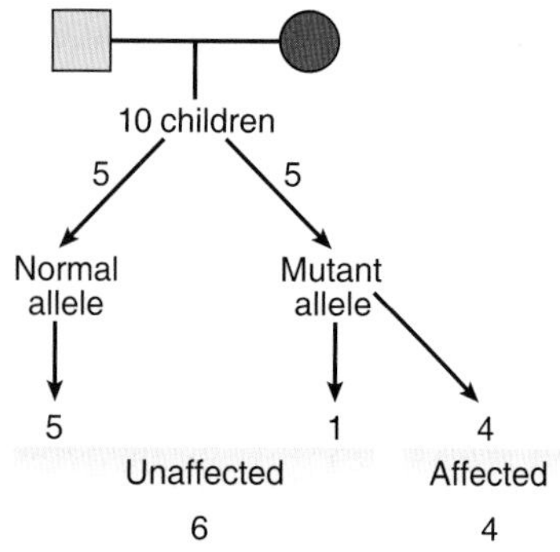

• **Fig. 8.3** Expected genotypes and phenotypes in 10 children born to an individual with an autosomal dominant disorder with penetrance equal to 0.8.

TABLE 8.2 **Bayesian calculation for II_1 in Fig. 8.2**

Probability	II_1 is Heterozygous	II_1 is not Heterozygous
Prior	1/2	1/2
Conditional		
Not affected	1 − P	1
Joint	1/2 (1 − P)	1/2

unaffected, one of whom has the mutant allele, with the remaining 5 having the normal allele. II_1 is unaffected, so there is a probability of 1 in 6 that she is, in fact, a heterozygote. Consequently, the probability that III_1 will both inherit the mutant gene and be affected equals $1/6 \times 1/2 \times P$, which equals 1/15 if P is 0.8.

2. Now consider II_1 in Fig. 8.2. The prior probability that she is a heterozygote equals 1/2. Similarly, the prior probability that she is not a heterozygote equals 1/2. Now a bayesian table can be constructed to determine how these prior probabilities are modified by the fact that II_1 is not affected (Table 8.2).

The posterior probability that II_1 is a heterozygote equals $1/2(1-P)/[1/2(1-P)+1/2]$, which reduces to $[1-P/2-P]$. Therefore, the risk that III_1 will both inherit the mutant allele and be affected equals $(1-P/2-P) \times 1/2 \times P$, which reduces to $[(P-P^2)/(4-2P)]$. If P equals 0.8, this expression equals 1/15 or 0.067.

By substituting different values of P in the above expression, it can be shown that the maximum risk for III_1 being affected equals 0.086, approximately 1/12, which is obtained when P equals 0.6. This maximum risk figure can be used when counseling people at risk for late-onset autosomal disorders with reduced penetrance and who have an affected grandparent and unaffected parents.

Delayed Age of Onset

Many autosomal dominant disorders do not present until well into adult life. Healthy members of families in which these disorders are segregating often wish to know whether they themselves will develop the condition and/or pass it on to their children. Risks for these individuals can be calculated in the following way.

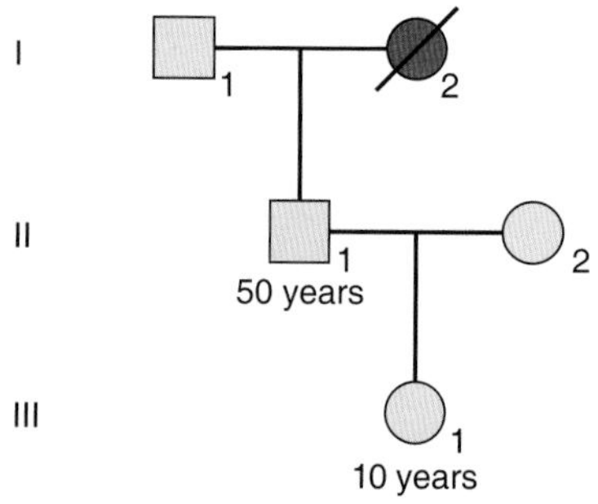

• **Fig. 8.4** I_2 had an autosomal dominant disorder showing delayed age of onset. When calculating the probability that III_1 will develop the disorder, it is necessary to determine the probability that II_1 is a heterozygote who is not yet clinically affected.

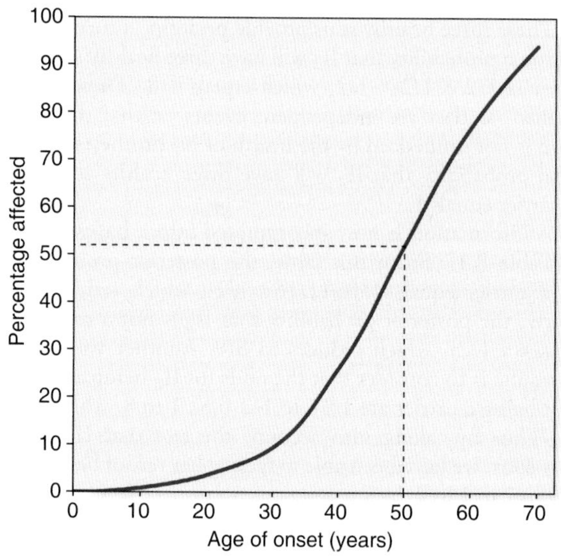

• **Fig. 8.5** Graph showing age of onset in years of clinical expression in Huntington disease heterozygotes. Approximately 50% show clinical signs or symptoms by age 50 years. (Data from Newcombe RG. A life table for onset of Huntington's chorea. *Ann Hum Genet*. 1981;45:375–385.)

Consider someone who has died with a confirmed diagnosis of Huntington disease (Fig. 8.4). This is a late-onset autosomal dominant disorder. The son of I_2 is entirely healthy at age 50 years and wishes to know the probability that his 10-year-old daughter, III_1, will develop Huntington disease in later life. In this condition, the first signs usually appear between the ages of 30 and 60 years, and approximately 50% of all heterozygotes show signs by the age of 50 years (Fig. 8.5).

To answer the question about the risk to III_1, it is first necessary to calculate the risk for II_1 (if III_1 was asking about her own risk, her father might be referred to as the **dummy consultand**). The probability that II_1 has inherited the gene, given that he shows no signs of the condition, can be determined by a simple bayesian calculation (Table 8.3).

The posterior probability that II_1 is heterozygous equals $1/4/(1/4+1/2)$, which equals 1/3. Therefore, the prior probability that his daughter III_1 will have inherited the disorder equals $1/3 \times 1/2$, or 1/6.

TABLE 8.3 Bayesian calculation for II_1 in Fig.8.4

Probability	II_1 is Heterozygous	II_1 is not Heterozygous
Prior	1/2	1/2
Conditional		
Unaffected at age 50 years	1/2	1
Joint	1/4	1/2

There is a temptation when doing calculations such as these to conclude that the overall risk for II_1 being a heterozygote simply equals $1/2 \times 1/2$; that is, the prior probability that he will have inherited the mutant gene times the probability that a heterozygote will be unaffected at age 50 years, giving a risk of 1/4. This is correct inasmuch as it gives the joint probability for this possible outcome, but it does not consider the possibility that II_1 is not a heterozygote. Consider the possibility that I_2 has four children. On average, two will inherit the mutant allele, one of whom will be affected by the age of 50 years. The remaining two children will not inherit the mutant allele. By the time these children have grown up and reached the age of 50 years, on average one will be affected and three will not. Therefore, on average, one-third of the healthy 50-year-old offspring of I_2 will be heterozygotes. Hence the correct risk for II_1 is 1/3 and not 1/4.

Autosomal Recessive Inheritance

With an autosomal recessive condition, the **biological** parents of an affected child are both heterozygotes. Apart from undisclosed nonpaternity and donor insemination, there are two possible exceptions, both of which are very rare. These arise when only one parent is a heterozygote, in which case a child can be affected if either a *de novo* mutation occurs on the gamete inherited from the other parent, or uniparental disomy occurs resulting in the child inheriting two copies of the heterozygous parent's mutant allele (p. 77). For practical purposes, it is usually assumed that both parents of an affected child are carriers.

Carrier Risks for the Extended Family

When both parents are heterozygotes, the risk that each of their children will be affected is 1 in 4. On average, three of their four children will be unaffected, of whom, on average, two will be carriers (Fig. 8.6). Therefore the probability that the healthy sibling of someone with an autosomal recessive disorder will be a carrier equals 2/3. Carrier risks can be derived for other family members, starting with the assumption that both parents of an affected child are carriers (Fig. 8.7).

When calculating risks in autosomal recessive inheritance, the underlying principle is to establish the probability that each prospective parent is a carrier and then multiply the product of these probabilities by 1/4, this being the risk that any child born to two carriers will be affected. Therefore, in Fig. 8.7, if the sister, III_3, of the affected boy was to marry her first cousin, III_4, the probability that their first baby would be affected would equal $2/3 \times 1/4 \times 1/4$; that is, the probability that III_3 is a carrier times the probability that III_4 is a carrier times the probability that a child of two carriers will be affected. This gives a final risk of 1/24.

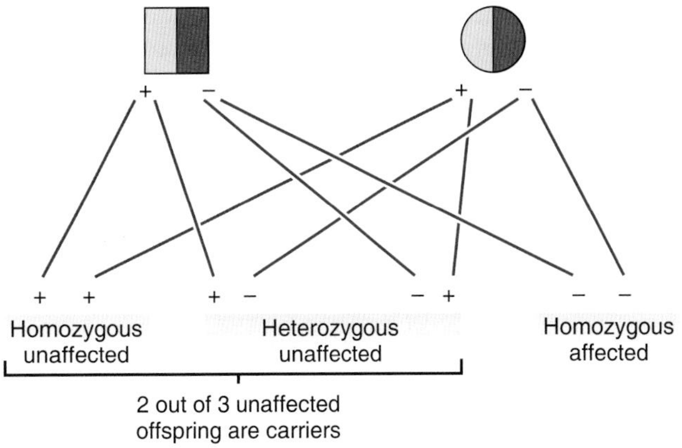

• **Fig. 8.6** Possible genotypes and phenotypes in the offspring of parents who are both carriers of an autosomal recessive disorder. On average, two of three healthy offspring are carriers.

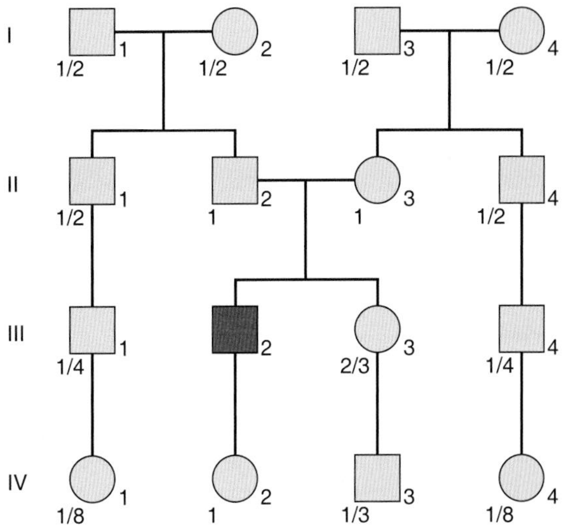

• **Fig. 8.7** Autosomal recessive inheritance. The probabilities that various family members are carriers are indicated as fractions.

If this same sister, III_3, was to marry a healthy unrelated individual, the probability that their first child would be affected would equal $2/3 \times 2pq \times 1/4$; that is, the probability that III_3 is a carrier times the carrier frequency in the general population times the probability that a child of two carriers will be affected. For a condition such as cystic fibrosis (CF), with a disease incidence of approximately 1 in 2500 (in the United Kingdom), $q^2 = 1/2500$ and therefore $q = 1/50$ and thus $2pq = 1/25$. Therefore the final risk would be $2/3 \times 1/25 \times 1/4$, or 1 in 150.

Modifying a Carrier Risk by Mutation Analysis

Newborn screening for CF has been introduced in the United Kingdom after pilot studies (p. 159). More than 2000 different pathogenic variants have been identified in the *CFTR* gene, so that carrier detection by DNA analysis is not straightforward. However, a relatively simple test has been developed for the most common variants, which enables about 90% of all carriers of Western European origin to be detected. What is the probability that a healthy individual who has no family history of CF, and who tests negative on the common variant screen, is a carrier?

The answer is obtained, once again, by drawing up a simple bayesian table (Table 8.4). The prior probability that this healthy member of the general population is a carrier equals 1/25; therefore the prior probability that he or she is not a carrier equals 24/25. If this individual is a carrier, then the probability that the common variant test will be normal is 0.10, as only 10% of carriers do not have one of the common pathogenic variants. The probability that someone who is not a carrier will have a normal test result is 1.

This gives a joint probability for being a carrier of 1/250 and for not being a carrier of 24/25. Therefore the posterior probability that this individual is a carrier equals 1/250 / (1/250+24/25), which equals 1/241. Thus, the normal result on common variant testing has reduced the carrier risk from 1/25 to 1/241.

X-Linked Recessive Inheritance

Among mendelian disorders this pattern of inheritance can generate the most complicated risk calculations. In severe sex-linked conditions, affected males are often unable to have their own children. Consequently, these conditions are usually transmitted only by healthy female carriers. The carrier of a sex-linked recessive disorder transmits the gene on average to half of her daughters, who are therefore carriers, and to half of her sons, who will thus be affected. If an affected male does have children, he will transmit his Y chromosome to all of his sons, who will be unaffected, and his X chromosome to all of his daughters, who will be carriers (Fig. 8.8).

An example of how the birth of unaffected sons to a possible carrier of an X-linked disorder results in a reduction of her carrier risk has already been discussed in the introduction to Bayes' theorem (p. 96). Here we consider two further factors that can complicate risk calculation in sex-linked recessive disorders.

TABLE 8.4 Bayesian table for cystic fibrosis carrier risk if common mutation screen is negative

Probability	Carrier	Not a Carrier
Prior	1/25	24/25
Conditional		
Normal result on common mutation screening	0.10	1
Joint	1/250	24/25

The Isolated Case

If a woman has only one affected son, then, in the absence of a positive family history, there are three possible ways in which this can have occurred.

1. The woman is a carrier of the pathogenic variant, in which case there is a risk of 1/2 that any future son will be affected.
2. The disorder in the son arose because of a *de novo* pathogenic variant that occurred during meiosis in the gamete that led to his conception. The recurrence risk in this situation is negligible.
3. The woman is a **gonadal mosaic** (p. 77) for the pathogenic variant that occurred in an early mitotic division during her own embryonic development. The recurrence risk will be equal to the proportion of ova that carry the variant (i.e., between 0% and 50%).

It may be very difficult to distinguish between these three possibilities without reliable molecular genetic sequencing. If a woman is found to be a carrier, then risk calculation is straightforward. If the tests indicate that she is not a carrier, the recurrence risk is probably low but not negligible because of the possibility of **gonadal mosaicism.**

For example, in Duchenne muscular dystrophy (DMD; p. 299) it has been estimated that, among the mothers of isolated cases, approximately two-thirds are carriers, 5% to 10% are

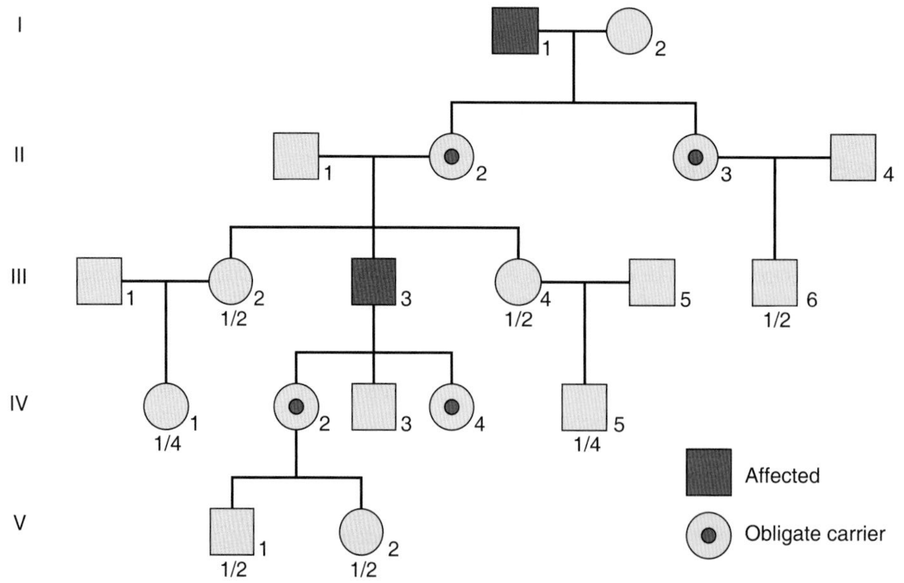

• **Fig. 8.8** Probabilities of male relatives being affected and female relatives being carriers of an X-linked recessive disorder. All the daughters of an affected male are obligate carriers.

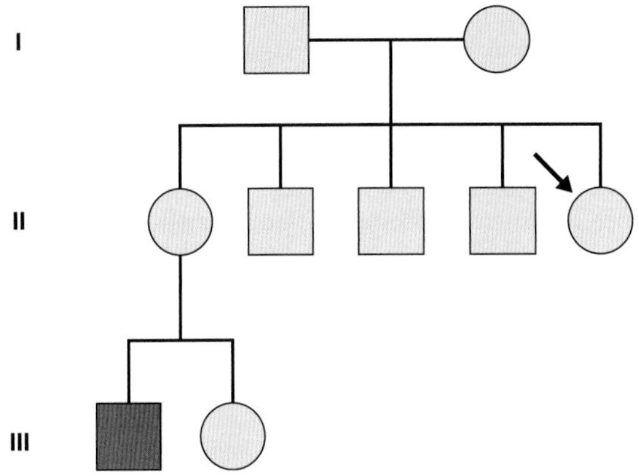

• **Fig. 8.9** In this pedigree, III_1 is affected by Duchenne muscular dystrophy and is an isolated case (i.e., there is no history of the condition in the wider family). The consultand, II_5 (*arrow*), wishes to know whether she is at risk of having affected sons. To calculate her risk, the risk that her mother, I_2, is a carrier is first calculated; this requires consideration of the mutation rate, μ. I_2 is the *dummy consultand* in this scenario.

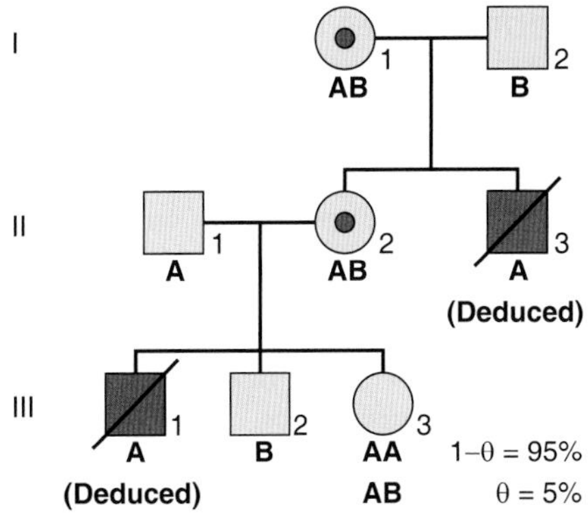

• **Fig. 8.10** Pedigree showing a Duchenne muscular dystrophy family where the affected individuals are deceased and no DNA is available. (A) and (B) represent alleles closely linked to the gene encoding dystrophin.

TABLE 8.5 **Bayesian calculation for II_2 in Fig. 8.1**

Probability	II_2 is a Carrier	II_2 is not a Carrier
Prior	1/2	1/2
Conditional		
Three healthy sons	1/8	1
Normal creatine kinase	1/3	1
Joint	1/48	1/2

gonadal mosaics, and in the remaining 25% to 30% the disorder has arisen as a *de novo* mutation in meiosis.

Leaving aside the complicating factor of gonadal mosaicism, risk calculation in the context of an isolated case (Fig. 8.9) is possible, but may require calculation of the risk for a **dummy consultand** within the pedigree, as well as taking account of the **mutation rate**, or **μ**. For a fuller understanding of μ, the student is referred to one of the more detailed texts listed at the end of the chapter.

Incorporating Carrier Test Results

Where sequencing analysis is not available, biochemical tests may help in detecting carriers of sex-linked recessive disorders. Unfortunately, there is often overlap in the values obtained for controls and women known to be obligate carriers. Although an abnormal result in a potential carrier would suggest that she is likely to be a carrier, a normal test result does not exclude a woman from being a carrier. Consider the example of DMD.

In DMD the serum creatine kinase (CK) level is raised in approximately two out of three obligate carriers (see Fig. 11.2; p. 152). Therefore, if a possible carrier such as II_2 in Fig. 8.1 is found to have a normal level of CK, this would provide further support for her not being a carrier. The test result therefore provides a conditional probability, which is included in a new bayesian calculation (Table 8.5).

The posterior probability that II_2 is a carrier equals 1/48 / (1/48 + 1/2), or 1/25. Consequently, by first taking into account this woman's three healthy sons, and second her normal CK test result, it has been possible to reduce her carrier risk from 1 in 2 to 1 in 9 and then to 1 in 25.

The Use of Linked Markers

Today, for most single-gene disorders, sequence analysis is possible if not always routine. Linked DNA markers are therefore rarely used but still sometimes have a role in clarifying the genetic status of an individual in a pedigree, for example where the affected individual died and no DNA was stored. There must be certainty that the genetic condition in question is caused by a variant at just one gene locus rather than being **genetically** heterogeneous.

To illustrate, consider the sister of a boy affected with DMD, now deceased, whose mother is an obligate carrier because she herself had an affected brother (Fig. 8.10). A DNA marker with alleles A and B is available and is known to be closely linked to the DMD disease locus with a recombination fraction (θ) equal to 0.05. The disease allele must, by deduction, be linked with the A marker allele in II_2, because II_2 must have inherited the B allele from her normal father, which she has passed to her unaffected son III_2. If II_1 also has the A allele (not in this case linked to DMD because he is not a relative and is unaffected), the combination of alleles in III_3 is either AA or AB. If AA, III_3 has inherited the high-risk allele from her mother but if AB, she has inherited the low-risk B allele. The final probability is a function of the chance of a crossover (the recombination fraction, θ) having occurred between the actual pathogenic variant and marker locus at meiosis in the ovum from which she was conceived. Therefore, with markers AA the carrier risk is 0.95 or 95%, and with AB the carrier risk for III_3 0.05 or 5%.

It follows that, the smaller the value of θ, the smaller the likelihood of a predictive error. If DNA markers "bridge" or "flank" the disease locus, this greatly reduces the risk of a predictive error, as only a double crossover will go undetected, which is extremely unlikely.

Bayes' Theorem and Prenatal Screening

To further illustrate the potential of Bayes' theorem in genetic risk calculation counseling, an example from prenatal screening follows. A woman age 20 presents at 13 weeks' gestation with a fetus that has been shown on ultrasound to have significant nuchal translucency (NT) (see Fig. 20.6). NT may be present in about 75% of fetuses with Down syndrome (p. 322). In contrast, the incidence in babies not affected with Down syndrome is approximately 5%. Therefore, NT is 15 times more common in Down syndrome than in unaffected fetuses.

Does this mean that the odds are 15 to 1 that this unborn baby has Down syndrome? No! This risk, or more precisely **odds ratio**, would be correct only if the prior probabilities that the baby would be affected or unaffected were equal. In reality the prior probability that the baby will be unaffected is much greater than the prior probability that it will have Down syndrome.

Actual values for these prior probabilities can be obtained by reference to a table showing maternal age-specific risks for Down syndrome (see Table 17.4; p. 251). For a woman age 20, the incidence of Down syndrome is approximately 1 in 1500; hence, the prior probability that the baby will be unaffected equals 1499/1500. If these prior probability values are used in a bayesian calculation, it can be shown that the posterior probability risk that the unborn baby will have Down syndrome is approximately 1 in 100 (Table 8.6)—thus far removed from the conditional odds of 15 to 1 in favor of the baby being affected.

In practice, the demonstration of NT on ultrasonography in a fetus would usually prompt an offer of definitive chromosome analysis by chorionic villous biopsy, amniocentesis, or non-invasive prenatal testing (see Chapter 20). This example emphasizes that an observed conditional probability ratio should always be combined with prior probability information to calculate the actual risk.

TABLE 8.6 Bayesian calculation to show the posterior probability that a fetus with nuchal translucency conceived by a 20-year-old mother will have Down syndrome

Probability	Fetus Unaffected	Fetus Affected
Prior	1499/1500	1/1500
Conditional		
Nuchal translucency	1	15
Joint	1499/1500 = 1	1/100
Expressed as odds	100 to	1
Posterior	100/101	1/101

Empiric Risks

Up to this point, risks have been calculated for single-gene disorders using knowledge of basic mendelian genetics and applied probability theory. In many counseling situations it is not possible to arrive at an accurate risk figure in this way, either because the disorder in question does not show single-gene inheritance or because the clinical diagnosis in the family shows causal heterogeneity (see later). In these situations, it is usually necessary to resort to the use of observed or **empiric risks**. These are based on observations derived from family and population studies rather than theoretical calculations.

TABLE 8.7 Empiric recurrence risks for common multifactorial disorders

Disorder	Incidence (Per 1000)	Sex Ratio (M:F)	Unaffected Parents Having a Second Affected Child (%)	Affected Parents Having an Affected Child (%)
Cleft lip ± cleft palate	1–2	3:2	4	4
Clubfoot (talipes)	1–2	2:1	3	3
Congenital heart defect	8	1:1	1–4	2 (father affected) 6 (mother affected)
Congenital dislocation of the hip	1	1:6	6	12
Hypospadias (in males)	2	—	10	10
Manic depression	4	2:3	10–15	10–15
Neural Tube Defect				
Anencephaly	1.5	1:2	4–5	—
Spina bifida	2.5	2:3	4–5	4
Pyloric Stenosis				
Male index	2.5	—	2	4
Female index	0.5	—	10	17
Schizophrenia	10	1:1	10	14

TABLE 8.8 **Empiric recurrence risks for conditions showing causal heterogeneity**

Disorder	Incidence (Per 1000)	Sex Ratio (M:F)	Unaffected Parents Having a Second Affected Child (%)	Affected Parents Having an Affected Child (%)
Autism	1–2	4:1	2–3	—
Epilepsy (idiopathic)	5	1:1	5	5
Hydrocephalus	0.5	1:1	3	—
Learning disability (idiopathic)	3	1:1	3–5	10
Profound childhood sensorineural hearing loss	1	1:1	10–15	5–10

Multifactorial Disorders

One of the basic principles of multifactorial inheritance is that the risk of recurrence in first-degree relatives, siblings, and offspring equals the square root of the incidence of the disease in the general population (p. 140)—that is, $P^{1/2}$, where P equals the general population incidence. For example, if the general population incidence equals 1/1000, then the theoretical risk to a first-degree relative equals the square root of 1/1000, which approximates to 1 in 32 or 3%. The theoretical risks for second- and third-degree relatives can be shown to approximate to $P^{3/4}$ and $P^{7/8}$, respectively—that is, much lower values. Therefore, if there is strong support for multifactorial inheritance, it is reasonable to use these theoretical risks when counseling close family relatives.

However, when using this approach it is important to remember that the confirmation of multifactorial inheritance will often have been based on the study of observed recurrence risks. Consequently, it is generally more appropriate to refer back to the original family studies and counsel on the basis of the derived risks (Table 8.7).

Ideally, reference should be made to local studies, as recurrence risks may differ in specific communities, ethnic groups, and geographical locations. For example, in the United Kingdom, the recurrence risk for neural tube defects in siblings used to be quoted as 4% (before the promotion of periconceptional maternal folate intake). This, essentially, was an average risk. The actual risk varied from 2% to 3% in southeast England up to 8% in Northern Ireland, and also showed an inverse relationship with the family's socioeconomic status, being greatest for mothers in poorest circumstances.

Unfortunately, empiric risks are rarely available for families in which there are several affected family members, or for disorders with variable severity or different sex incidences. For example, in a family where several members have been affected by cleft lip/palate, the empiric risks based on population data may not apply—the condition may appear to be segregating as an autosomal dominant trait with a high penetrance. In the absence of a syndrome diagnosis being made and positive results from whole exome sequencing (WES) being obtained, the clinical geneticist has to make the best judgment about recurrence risk.

Conditions Showing Causal Heterogeneity

Many referrals to genetic clinics relate to a clinical phenotype rather than to a precise underlying diagnosis (Table 8.8). In these situations, great care must be taken to ensure that all appropriate diagnostic investigations have been undertaken, including WES if available, before resorting to the use of empiric risk data.

It is worth emphasizing that the use of empiric risks for conditions such as sensorineural hearing loss in childhood is at best a compromise because the figure quoted to an individual family will rarely be the correct one for their particular diagnosis. Severe sensorineural hearing loss in a young child is usually caused either by single-gene inheritance, most commonly autosomal recessive, but occasionally autosomal dominant or X-linked recessive, or by an environmental condition such as rubella embryopathy. Therefore for most families the correct risk of recurrence will be either 25% or 0%. In practice, it is often not possible to establish the precise cause, so that the only option available is to offer the family an empiric or "average" risk.

ELEMENTS

1. Risk calculation in genetic counseling requires a knowledge and understanding of basic probability theory. Bayes' theorem enables initial background "prior" risks to be modified by "conditional" information to give an overall probability or risk for a particular event such as carrier status.
2. For disorders showing autosomal dominant inheritance, it is often necessary to consider factors such as reduced penetrance and age of onset. For disorders showing autosomal recessive inheritance, risks to offspring are determined by calculating the probability that each parent is a carrier and then multiplying the product of these probabilities by 1/4.
3. In X-linked recessive inheritance, a particular problem arises when only one male in a family is affected. The results of biochemical carrier tests that show overlap between carriers and non-carriers can be incorporated in a bayesian calculation in some circumstances.
4. When interpreting odds ratios, it is crucial to use this in the context of prior probabilities to avoid giving spurious and widely inaccurate genetic risk information.
5. Empiric (observed) risks are available for multifactorial disorders and for etiologically heterogeneous conditions such as cleft lip/palate and non-syndromic sensorineural hearing loss.

CLINICAL SCENARIO 1

A couple attend clinic, and they are expecting their first baby. The young woman is 8 weeks pregnant. She never met her maternal aunt who died from spinal muscular atrophy type 1 (SMA1) aged 7 months. The incidence of the condition in the general population is approximately 1:10,000.

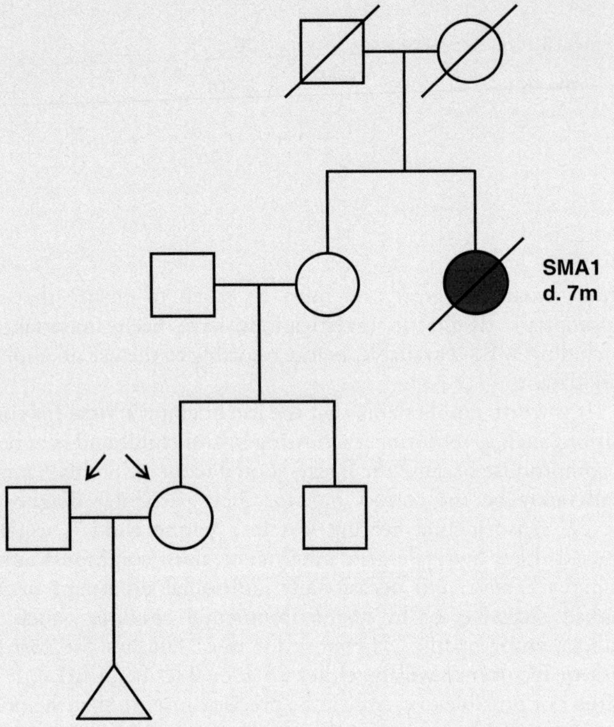

Before any genetic carrier testing is undertaken, what is the risk of their unborn baby being affected by SMA1?

CLINICAL SCENARIO 2

A 26-year-old man, John, is referred to your genetic clinic to discuss predictive testing for Huntington disease (HD). He attends with his partner, and they would like to start a family. His paternal grandfather had confirmed HD by genetic testing and died aged 83. His father, who was not tested, had no signs or symptoms of HD and died from lung cancer at the age of 60. John's two older sisters have had predictive testing, both yielding normal results.

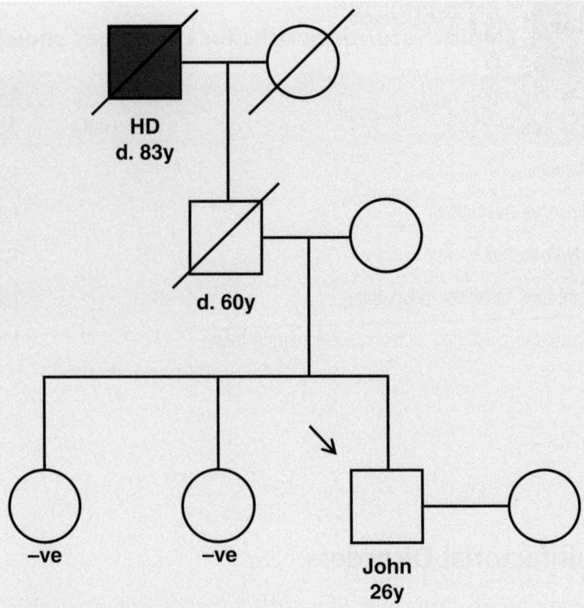

Data suggest that the risk of being unaffected and heterozygous for the HD pathogenic triplet repeat at the age of 60 years is 20%.

What is the risk of John having the pathogenic HD triplet repeat and therefore developing the disease in later life, which would also mean his offspring will be at risk?

Further Reading

Bayes T. An essay towards solving a problem in the doctrine of chances. *Biometrika*. 1958;45:296–315.

A reproduction of the Reverend Bayes' original essay on probability theory that was first published, posthumously, in 1763.

Emery AEH. *Methodology in Medical Genetics*. 2nd ed. Edinburgh, UK: Churchill Livingstone; 1986.

An introduction to statistical methods of analysis in human and medical genetics.

Murphy EA, Chase GA. *Principles of Genetic Counseling*. Chicago: Year Book Medical; 1975.

A very thorough explanation of the use of Bayes' theorem in genetic counseling.

Young ID. *Introduction to Risk Calculation in Genetic Counselling*. 2nd ed. Oxford, UK: Oxford University Press; 1999.

A short introductory guide to all aspects of risk calculation in genetic counselling. Highly recommended.

9

Developmental Genetics

The history of man for the nine months preceding his birth would, probably, be far more interesting and contain events of greater moment than all the three score and ten years that follow it.

Samuel Taylor Coleridge

At fertilization the nucleus from a spermatozoon penetrates the cell membrane of an oocyte to form a zygote. This single cell divides to become two, then four, and when the number has doubled some 50 times, the resulting organism comprises more than 200 distinct cell types and a total cell number of approximately 10,000 trillion. This is a fully formed human being with complex biochemistry and physiology, having consciousness, and is capable of exploring both the cosmos and subatomic particles. Not surprisingly, biologists and geneticists are intrigued by the mechanisms of early development and, whereas many mysteries remain, the rate of progress in understanding key events and signaling pathways is rapid. Nongenetic influences on the developing fetus and young child are legion, but more difficult to analyze with precision.

A fetus is recognizably human after approximately 12 weeks of pregnancy—the first trimester. Normal development requires an optimum maternal environment, but genetic integrity is fundamental, which has given rise to the field of developmental genetics. Most of what we know about the molecular processes inevitably comes from the study of animal models, with great emphasis on the mouse, whose genome closely resembles our own.

Prenatal life can be divided into three main stages: **preembryonic**, **embryonic**, and **fetal** (Table 9.1). During the preembryonic stage, a small collection of cells becomes distinguishable, first as a double-layered or **bilaminar disc**, and then as a triple-layered or **trilaminar disc** (Fig. 9.1), which is destined to develop into the human infant. During the embryonic stage, craniocaudal, dorsoventral, and proximodistal axes are established as cellular aggregation and differentiation lead to tissue and organ formation. The final fetal stage is characterized by rapid growth and development as the embryo, now a fetus, matures into a viable human infant.

On average, this extraordinary process takes approximately 38 weeks. By convention pregnancy is usually dated from the first day of the last menstrual period, which usually precedes conception by around 2 weeks, so that the normal period of gestation is often stated (incorrectly) as 40 weeks.

Fertilization and Gastrulation

Fertilization, the process by which the male and female gametes fuse, occurs in the Fallopian tube. Of the 100 to 200 million spermatozoa deposited in the female genital tract, only a few hundred reach the site of fertilization. Of these, usually only a single spermatozoon succeeds in penetrating first the corona radiata, then the zona pellucida and finally the oocyte cell membrane, whereupon the oocyte completes its second meiotic division (p. 32; and see Fig. 3.15, p. 34). After the sperm has penetrated the oocyte and the meiotic process has been completed, the two nuclei, known as

TABLE 9.1 Main events in the development of a human infant

Stage	Time From Conception	Length of Embryo/Fetus
Preembryonic Stage		
First cell division	30 h	
Zygote reaches uterine cavity	4 d	
Implantation	5–6 d	
Formation of bilaminar disc	12 d	0.2 mm
Lyonization in female	16 d	
Formation of trilaminar disc and primitive streak	19 d	1 mm
Embryonic Stage		
Organogenesis	4–8 wk	
Brain and spinal cord are forming, and first signs of heart and limb buds	4 wk	4 mm
Brain, eyes, heart and limbs developing rapidly, and bowel and lungs beginning to develop	6 wk	17 mm
Digits have appeared. Ears, kidneys, liver, and muscle are developing	8 wk	4 cm
Palate closes, and joints form	10 wk	6 cm
Sexual differentiation almost complete	12 wk	9 cm
Fetal Stage		
Fetal movements felt	16–18 wk	20 cm
Eyelids open. Fetus is now viable with specialized care	24–26 wk	35 cm
Rapid weight gain as a result of growth and accumulation of fat as lungs mature	28–38 wk	40–50 cm

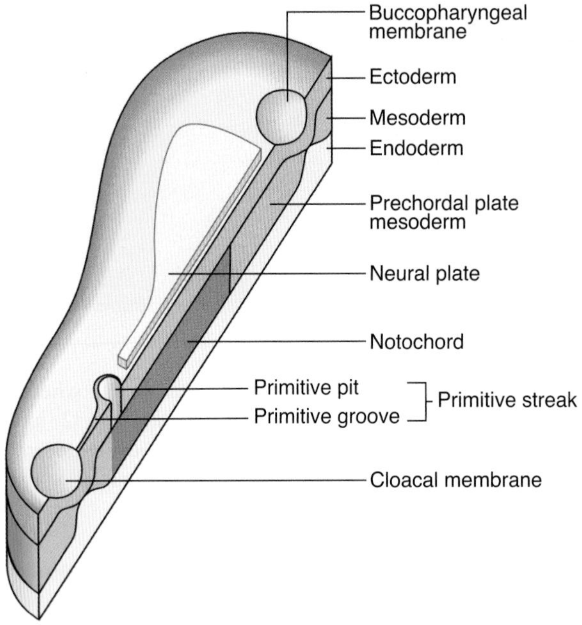

• **Fig. 9.1** A schematic trilaminar disc sectioned along the rostrocaudal axis. Cells from the future ectoderm (*top layer*) migrate through the primitive streak to form the endoderm (*bottom layer*) and mesoderm (*blue*). Formation of the neural plate in the overlying ectoderm, destined to be the central nervous system, involves Sonic hedgehog signaling (p. 107) from the notochord and prechordal plate mesoderm. (Modified from Larsen WJ. *Essentials of human embryology*. New York: Churchill Livingstone; 1998. With permission.)

pronuclei, and then fuse, thereby restoring the diploid number of 46 chromosomes. This is a potentially chaotic molecular encounter with a high chance of failure, as we know from observations of the early human embryo from *in vitro* fertilization programs. It may be likened, somewhat flippantly, to "speed dating," whereby couples test whether they might be compatible on the basis of only a brief encounter.

Germ cell and very early embryonic development are two periods characterized by widespread changes in DNA methylation patterns—epigenetic reprogramming (see p. 123). Primordial germ cells are globally *de*methylated as they mature and are subsequently methylated *de novo* during gametogenesis, the time when most DNA methylation **imprints** are established. After fertilization a second wave of change occurs. The oocyte rapidly removes methyl imprints from sperm DNA, which has the effect of resetting the developmental stopwatch to zero. By contrast, the maternal genome is more passively demethylated because the imprinting is more resistant to the process. A third wave of methylation, *de novo*, establishes the somatic cell pattern of DNA methylation after implantation. These alternating methylation states help to control which genes are active, or expressed, at a time when two genomes, initially alien to each other, collide.

The fertilized ovum, or zygote, undergoes a series of mitotic divisions to consist of two cells by 30 hours, four cells by 40 hours and 12 to 16 cells by 3 days, when it is known as a **morula**. A key concept in development at all stages is the emergence of **polarity** within groups of cells—part of the process of differentiation that generates multiple cell types with unique identities. Although precise mechanisms remain elusive, observations suggest that this begins at the very outset; in the fertilized egg of the mouse, the point of entry of the sperm determines the plane through which the first cell cleavage division occurs. This seminal event is the first step in the development of the so-called dorso-ventral, or primary body, axis in the embryo.

Further cell division leads to formation of a **blastocyst**, which consists of an inner cell mass or **embryoblast**, destined to form the embryo, and an outer cell mass or **trophoblast**, which gives rise to the placenta. The process of converting the inner cell mass into first a bilaminar, and then a trilaminar, disc (see Fig. 9.1) is known as **gastrulation** and takes place between the beginning of the second and the end of the third weeks.

Between 4 and 8 weeks, the body form is established, beginning with the formation of the primitive streak at the caudal end of the embryo. The germinal layers of the trilaminar disc give rise to **ectodermal**, **mesodermal**, and **endodermal** structures (Box 9.1). The neural tube is formed, and neural crest cells migrate to form sensory ganglia, the sympathetic nervous system, pigment cells and both bone and cartilage in parts of the face and branchial arches.

Disorders involving cells of neural crest origin, such as neurofibromatosis (p. 296), are sometimes referred to as **neurocristopathies**. This period between 4 and 8 weeks is described as the period of organogenesis, because during this interval all of the major organs are formed as regional specialization proceeds in a craniocaudal direction along the axis of the embryo.

Developmental Gene Families

Information about the genetic factors that initiate, maintain, and direct embryogenesis is incomplete. However, extensive genetic studies of the fruit fly, *Drosophila melanogaster*, and vertebrates such as mouse, chick, and zebrafish have identified several genes and gene families that play important roles in early developmental processes. It has also been possible through painstaking gene expression studies to identify several key developmental pathways, or cascades, to which more detail and complexity is continually being added. The gene families identified in vertebrates usually show strong sequence homology with developmental regulatory genes in *Drosophila*. Studies in humans have revealed that mutations in various members of these gene families can result in either isolated malformations or multiple congenital anomaly syndromes (see Table 16.5, p. 236). Many developmental genes produce

• BOX 9.1 Organ and Tissue Origins

Ectodermal

Central nervous system
Peripheral nervous system
Epidermis, including hair and nails
Subcutaneous glands
Dental enamel

Mesodermal

Connective tissue
Cartilage and bone
Smooth and striated muscle
Cardiovascular system
Urogenital system

Endodermal

Thymus and thyroid
Gastrointestinal system
Liver and pancreas

proteins called **transcription factors** (p. 17), which control RNA transcription from the DNA template by binding to specific regulatory DNA sequences to form complexes that initiate transcription by RNA polymerase.

There are a number of different regulatory elements and mechanisms for developmental genes besides transcription factors, namely promoters, enhancers and repressors. It is becoming clear that the relationships between these elements and their target genes in the molecular space of the nucleus may be crucial to gene expression and easily disrupted by a small intervening deletion, duplication, or inversion in the region. This helps to explain why the search for gene mutations in families with some monogenic disorders, particularly limb abnormalities, is sometimes fruitless, which is well illustrated by the molecular complexities that explain ectrodactyly, or split-hand-foot malformation (SHFM). For example, the locus for SHFM type 1 is chromosome 7q21.3, and several cases were reported in association with a reciprocal translocation or chromosome rearrangement at this locus. It is now apparent that the key gene is *DLX5*, but its enhancer must be intact, as well as the spatial relationship with the enhancer. Curiously, the enhancer in this case is found within the terminal exons of an upstream gene called *DYNC1I1* (Fig. 9.2), which has its own role in neuronal development. It is frequently the case that SHFM shows reduced or non-penetrance, which is not easily explained.

Besides these regulatory elements switching genes on and off by activating or repressing gene expression, in normal development this occurs as a highly coordinated and complex series of sequential cascades and feedback loops involving the regulation of fundamental embryological processes such as **induction** (the process in which extracellular signals give rise to a change from one cell fate to another in a particular group of cells), **segmentation**, **migration**, **differentiation**, and **programmed cell death** (known as **apoptosis**). It is believed that these processes are mediated by growth factors, cell receptors, and chemicals known as **morphogens**. Across species, the signaling molecules involved are very similar. The protein signals identified over and over again tend to be members of the transforming growth factor-β (TGF-β) family, the wingless (Wnt) family and the hedgehog (HH) family (see the following section). In addition, it is clear within any given organism that the same molecular pathways are reused in different developmental domains. In addition, it has become clear that these pathways are closely interlinked with each other and, in molecular terms, multidimensional. The known interactions of these networks are sometimes represented in schematic form, as illustrated in relatively simple form in Fig. 9.3.

Early Patterning

The emergence of the mesoderm heralds the transition from the stage of **bilaminar** to **trilaminar** disc, or **gastrulation**. Induction of the mesoderm—the initiation, maintenance, and subsequent patterning of this layer—involves several key families of signaling factors. The Nodal family is involved in initiation, fibroblast growth factors (FGFs), and WNTs are involved in maintenance, and bone morphogenetic proteins (BMPs) are involved in patterning the mesoderm. Signaling pathways are activated when a key ligand binds specific membrane-bound protein receptors. This usually leads to the phosphorylation of a cytoplasmic factor, and this in turn leads to binding with other factor(s). These factors translocate to the nucleus where transcriptional activation of specific targets occurs.

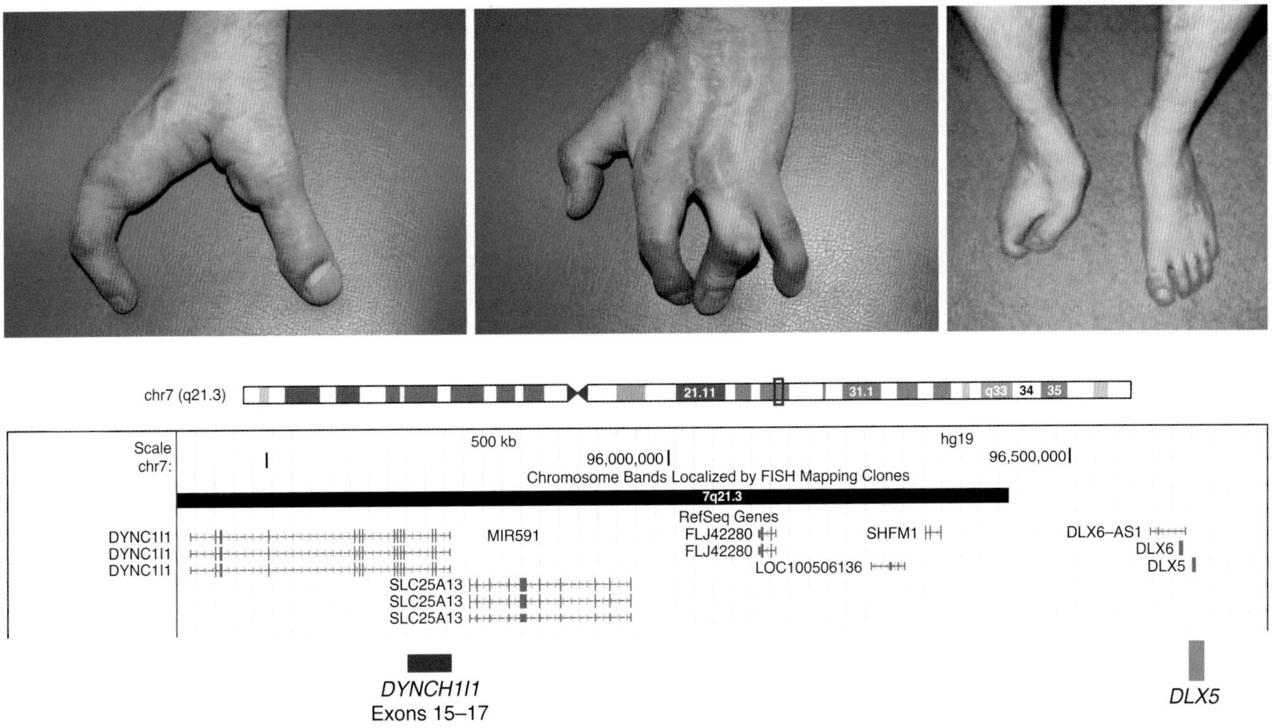

• **Fig. 9.2** Split-hand-foot malformation (*SHFM*), also known as ectrodactyly, and chromosome 7q21.3. In this individual with SHFM (and other family members) a deletion of approximately 100 kilobases has occurred, removing exons 15–17 of the *DYNCH1I1* gene which incorporates an enhancer of the downstream *DLX5* gene. Any disruption of the relationship between *DLX5* and its enhancer causes SHFM.

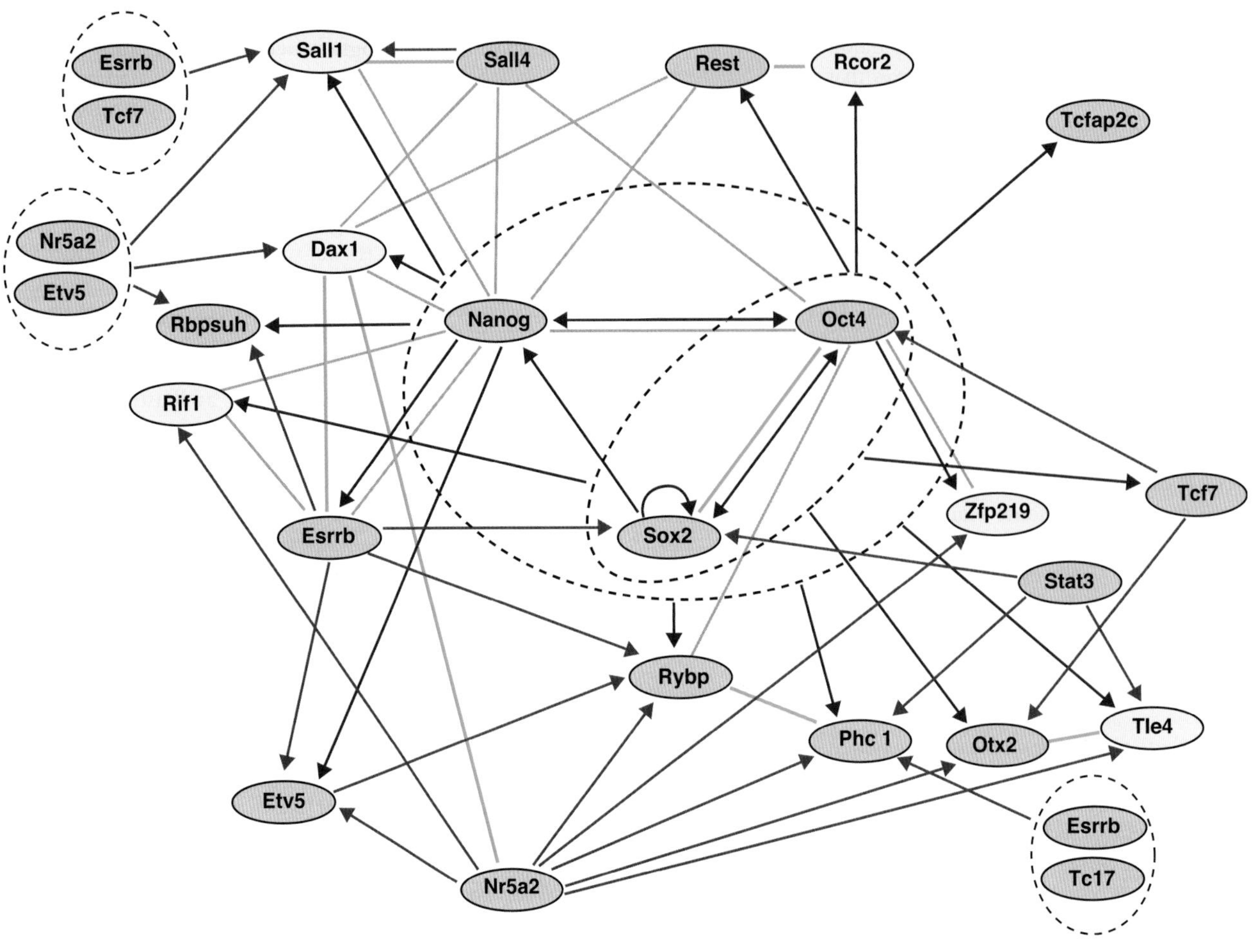

• **Fig. 9.3** Example of a complex gene/protein network in development. Proposed regulatory network in mouse embryonic stem cells centred on the master regulators OCT4, SOX2, and NANOG. Core regulators (pink) and their protein-interaction partners (yellow). Blue and pink arrows indicate inferred regulatory interactions. Orange and green lines represent reported protein interactions. Some regulators appear multiple times to reduce the number of intersecting arrows. Arrows from a dashed ellipse show that targets are regulated by all regulators within the ellipse. (From Qing Zhou, Hiram Chipperfield, Douglas A. Melton, Wing Hung Wong: A gene regulatory network in mouse embryonic stem cells. *Proceedings of the National Academy of Sciences*, October 2007, 104 (42) 16438–16443. Copyright (2007) National Academy of Sciences, U.S.A.)

In the case of the Nodal and BMP pathways, ligand binding of a specific heterotetramer membrane-bound protein initiates the signaling, which is common to all members of the TGF-β family, the cytoplasmic mediators being SMAD factors (see the following section). The embryo appears to have gradients of Nodal activity along the dorsal-ventral axis, although the significance and role of these gradients in mesoderm induction are uncertain.

The WNT pathway has two main branches: one that is β-catenin–dependent (canonical) and the other independent of β-catenin. In the canonical pathway, WNT ligand binds to a Frizzled/low density lipoprotein receptor–related protein membrane-bound heterodimeric protein complex, and the downstream intracellular signaling involves a G protein. The effect of this is to disrupt a large cytoplasmic protein complex that includes APC, the adenomatous polyposis coli protein (see p. 189) and the glycogen synthase kinase-3β protein. This prevents the phosphorylation of β-catenin, but when β-catenin is not degraded, it accumulates and translocates to the nucleus where it activates the transcription of dorsal-specific regulatory genes. Binding of the ligand to the FGF receptor results in dimerization of the receptor and transphosphorylation of the receptor's cytoplasmic domain, with activation of RAS and other kinases, one of which enters the nucleus and activates target transcription factors. Mutated *WNT10A* in humans results in a form of ectodermal dysplasia (odonto-onycho-dermal dysplasia), and *WNT4* is one of the genes implicated in the rare Mayer-Rokitansky-Kuster syndrome, featuring Müllerian (female genital) tract malformations.

The TGF-β Superfamily in Development and Disease

Thus far it is recognized that there are some 33 members of this family of secreted growth factors and **cytokines** in mammalian cells. Cytokines are a category of signaling molecules—polypeptide regulators—that enable cells to communicate. They differ from hormones in that they are not produced by discrete glands. These extracellular signaling polypeptides are transduced through a cascade to regulate gene expression within the cell nucleus. This is achieved through binding with cell surface receptors, which, through a series of reactions, induces phosphorylation and activation of specific receptor kinases. This leads to the translocation of

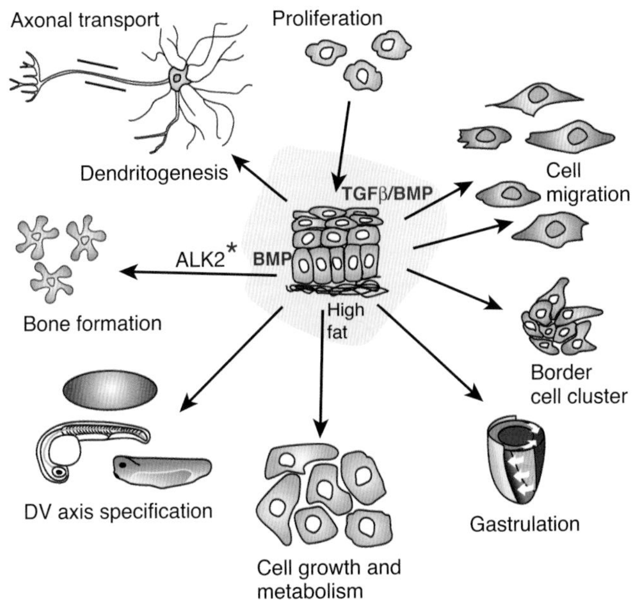

• **Fig. 9.4** A summary of biological responses to transforming growth factor family signaling. The range of processes that come under the influence of this superfamily is very broad. (Modified from Wharton K, Derynck R. TGFβ family signaling: novel insights in development and disease. *Development*. 2009;136:3693.)

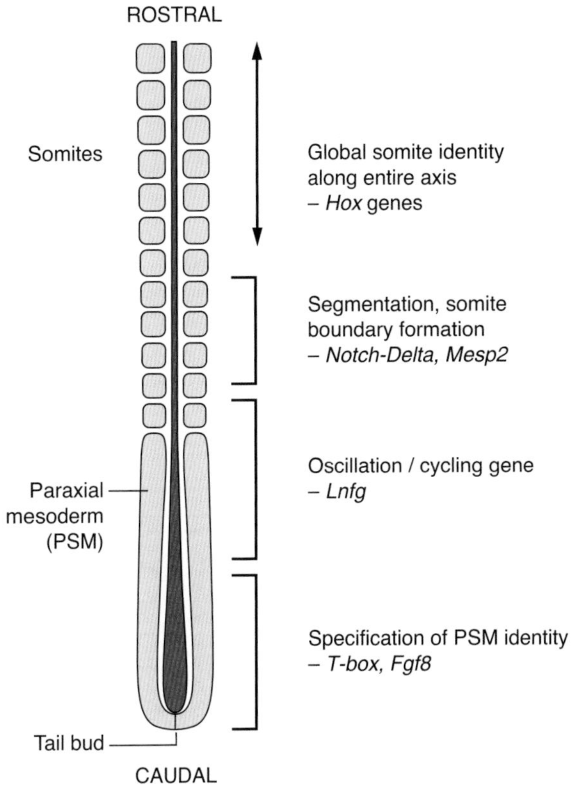

• **Fig. 9.5** Somatogenesis and Notch-Delta pathway. *T-box* genes have a role in presomitic mesoderm specification, whereas the segmentation clock depends on oscillation, or cycling, genes that are important in somite boundary formation where genes of the Notch-Delta pathway establish rostrocaudal polarity. *HOX* genes have a global function in establishing somite identity along the entire rostrocaudal axis. (Modified from Tickle C. Patterning in vertebrate development. Oxford: Oxford University Press; 2003.)

complexes into the nucleus, where they execute transcriptional activation or repression of responsive target genes. The TGF-β family can be divided into two groups: (1) the BMPs and (2) the TGF-βs, Activins, Nodal, and Myostatin, acting through various SMAD proteins. Ultimately, this superfamily is actively involved in a very broad range of cellular and developmental processes (Fig. 9.4), most prominent being the control on differentiation of all cell lineages at multiple stages in development. This includes regulation of the cell cycle, cell migration, cell size, gastrulation, and axis specification and metabolic processes. In relation to health and disease, there are consequences for immunity, cancer, heart disease, diabetes and Marfan and Loeys-Dietz syndromes (p. 309). Generally, deregulation of TGF-β–family signaling leads to developmental anomalies and disease, whereas activation of TGF-β–signaling contributes to cancer and fibrosis. Overexpression of *BMP4* has been found in the rare bony condition fibrodysplasia ossificans progressiva, where disabling heterotopic bone deposition occurs, which is as a result of variants in *ACVR1*, which encodes a BMP type 1 receptor. A mutated BMP receptor 2 has been shown to be a cause of familial primary pulmonary hypertension (p. 288). BMP signaling is also involved in both dendritogenesis and axonal transport.

Somatogenesis, Notch Signaling, and the Axial Skeleton

The vertebrate axis is closely linked to the development of the primary body axis during gastrulation, and during this process the presomitic mesoderm (PSM), where somites arise, is laid down in higher vertebrates. WNT and FGF signals play vital roles in the specification of the PSM. The somites form as blocks of tissue from the PSM in a rostrocaudal direction (Fig. 9.5), each being laid down with a precise periodicity that, in the 1970s, gave rise to the concept of the "clock and wavefront" model. Since then, molecular techniques have given substance to this concept, and the key pathway here is **Notch-delta signaling** and the "oscillation clock"—a precise, temporally defined wave of **cycling gene** expression (*c-hairy* in the chick, *lunatic fringe* and *hes* genes in the mouse) that sweeps from the tail-bud region in a rostral direction and has a key role in the process leading to the defining of somite boundaries. It has become clear that the integrity of the segmentation oscillation clock is dependent on complex interactions and cross-talk between the Notch, WNT, and FGF signaling pathways (Fig. 9.6).

Not all of the components of Notch signaling are fully understood, but the Notch receptor and its ligands, Delta-like-1 and Delta-like-3, together with Presenilin-1 and Mesoderm posterior-2, work in concert to establish rostrocaudal polarity within the PSM such that somite blocks are formed. Human phenotypes from mutated genes in this pathway are now well-known, and include presenile dementia (*presenilin-1*), which is dominantly inherited, and spondylocostal dysostosis (Delta-like-3, Mesoderm posterior-2, lunatic fringe, and hairy enhancer of split-7), which is recessively inherited (Fig. 9.7). *T-box6* is implicated in some cases of dominantly inherited as well as recessive spondylocostal dysostosis. Variants in *NOTCH1* are a rare cause of some forms of congenital heart disease, whereas pathogenic variants in *JAGGED1* result in the dominantly inherited and very variable condition Alagille

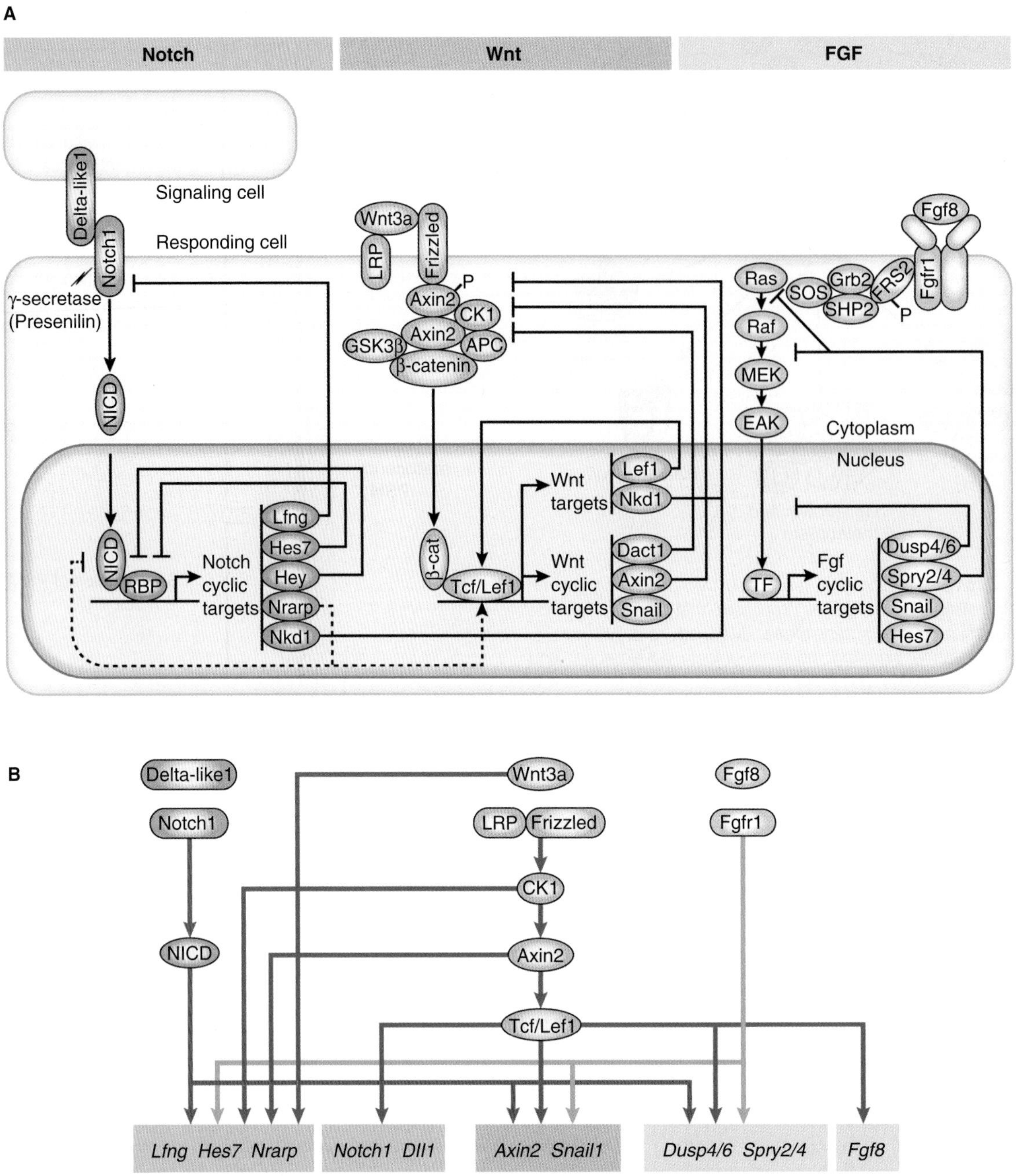

• **Fig. 9.6** The Notch, Wnt, and Fgf signaling pathways, and their interactions. This diagram highlights the basic but complex circuitry of the three distinct "oscillator" developmental pathways in the mouse presomitic mesoderm (PSM). (A) The Notch and Fgf-regulated genes oscillate asynchronously to those of the Wnt pathway, and many are involved in negative feedback loops. Mutations in the human orthologues of some of these genes give rise to distinct malformations or syndromes. The hashed line represents interactions in tissues outside the PSM; and (B) this shows the interactions between the three pathways that have been demonstrated in the mouse PSM through the study of mouse mutants, relying on analysis of mRNA expression. (Modified from Gibb S, Maroto M, Dale JK. The segmentation clock mechanism moves up a notch. *Trends Cell Biol*. 2010;20:593–600. With permission.)

syndrome (arteriohepatic dysplasia) (Fig. 9.8), which also includes congenital heart disease. Pathogenic variants in *NOTCH2* are a rare cause of Alagille syndrome, as well as Hajdu-Cheney syndrome.

The Sonic Hedgehog–Patched Gli Pathway

The Sonic hedgehog (SHH) gene is as well known for its quirky name as it is for its function. *SHH* induces cell proliferation in a tissue-specific distribution and is expressed in the notochord, the brain and the zone of polarizing activity of developing limbs. After cleavage and modification by the addition of a cholesterol moiety, the SHH protein binds with its receptor, Patched (PTCH), a transmembrane protein. The normal action of PTCH is to inhibit another transmembrane protein called Smoothened (SMO), but when bound by SHH this inhibition is released, and a signaling cascade within the cell is activated. The key intracellular targets are the GLI (glioma-associated oncogene) family of transcription factors (Fig. 9.9).

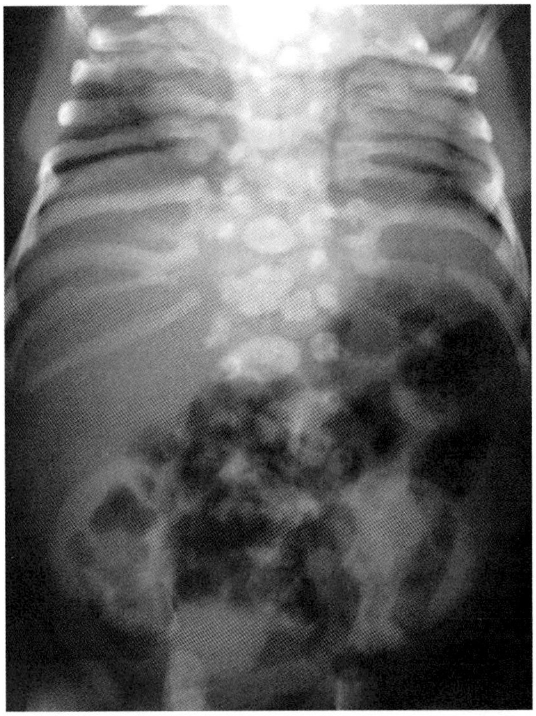

• **Fig. 9.7** Disrupted development of the vertebrae in a patient with spondylocostal dysostosis type 1 resulting from mutations in the *delta-like-3* gene, part of the notch signaling pathway. (Courtesy Dr Meriel McEntagart, Kennedy-Galton Centre, London.)

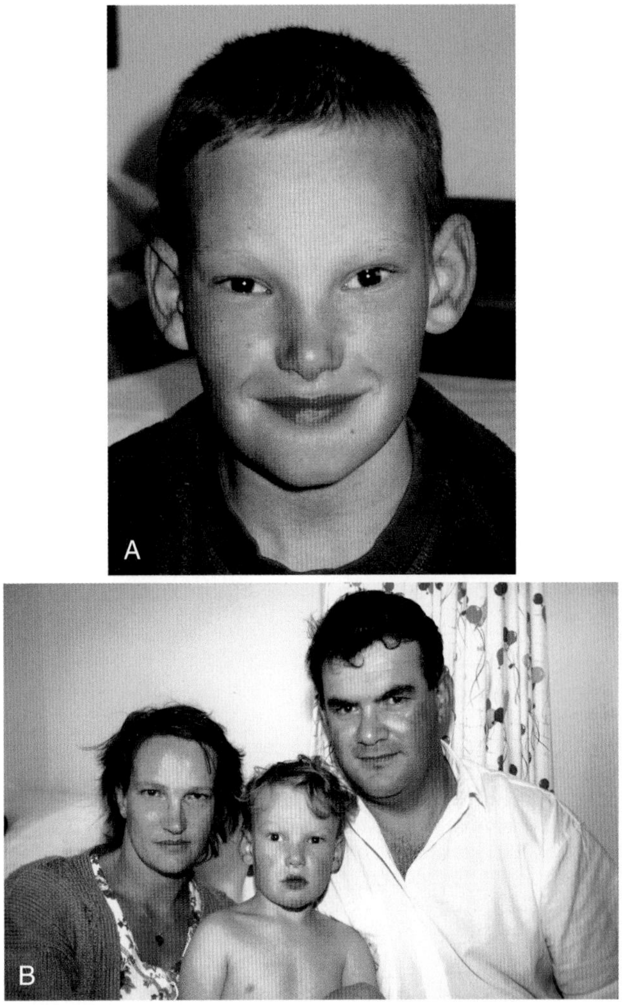

• **Fig. 9.8** (A) Boy with Alagille syndrome and confirmed mutation in *JAGGED1* who presented with congenital heart disease. (B) The same boy a few years earlier with his parents. His mother has a pigmentary retinopathy and was positive for the same gene mutation.

Molecular defects in any part of this pathway lead to a number of apparently diverse malformation syndromes (Fig. 9.9). Mutations in, or deletions of, *SHH* (chromosome 7q36) cause holoprosencephaly (Fig. 9.10), in which the primary defect is incomplete cleavage of the developing brain into separate hemispheres and ventricles. The most severe form of this malformation is cyclopia—the presence of a single central eye. The complexity of early development can be appreciated by the fact that at least a dozen chromosomal regions have so far been implicated in the pathogenesis of holoprosencephaly (p. 235). Mutations in *PTCH* (9q22) result in Gorlin syndrome (nevoid basal cell carcinoma syndrome; Fig. 9.11), which comprises multiple basal cell carcinomas, odontogenic keratocysts, bifid ribs, calcification of the falx cerebri, and ovarian fibromata. Mutations in *SMO* (7q31) are found in some basal cell carcinomas and medulloblastomas. Mutations in *GLI3* (7p13) cause Pallister-Hall and Grieg syndromes, which are distinct entities with more or less the same body systems affected. However, there are also links to other conditions, in particular the very variable Smith-Lemli-Opitz syndrome (SLOS), which may include holoprosencephaly as well as some characteristic facial features, pulmonary segmentation defects, genital anomalies, postaxial polydactyly, and syndactyly. This condition is because of a defect in the final step of cholesterol biosynthesis, which in turn may disrupt the binding of SHH with its receptor, PTCH. Some, or all, of the features of SLOS may therefore be as a result of loss of integrity in this pathway. Furthermore, a cofactor for the GLI proteins, cAMP response element–binding protein (CREBBP) (16p13), is mutated in Rubenstein-Taybi syndrome (Fig. 9.12). Disturbance of different components of the SHH is also clearly implicated in many types of tumor formation.

Homeobox (*HOX*) Genes

In *Drosophila* a class of genes known as the homeotic genes has been shown to determine segment identity. Incorrect expression of these genes results in major structural abnormalities; the *Antp* gene, for example, which is normally expressed in the second thoracic segment, will transform the adult fly's antennae into legs if incorrectly expressed in the head. Homeotic genes contain a conserved 180–base pair sequence known as the homeobox, which is believed to be characteristic of genes involved in spatial pattern control and development. This encodes a 60–amino acid domain that binds to DNA in Hox-response enhancers. Proteins from homeobox-containing (or *HOX*) genes are therefore important transcription factors that activate and repress batteries of downstream genes. At least 35 downstream targets are known. The HOX proteins regulate other "executive" genes that encode transcription factors or morphogen signals, as well as operating at many other levels, on genes that mediate cell adhesion, cell division rates, cell death, and cell movement. They specify cell fate and help to establish the embryonic pattern along the primary (rostrocaudal) axis as well as the secondary (genital and limb bud) axis.

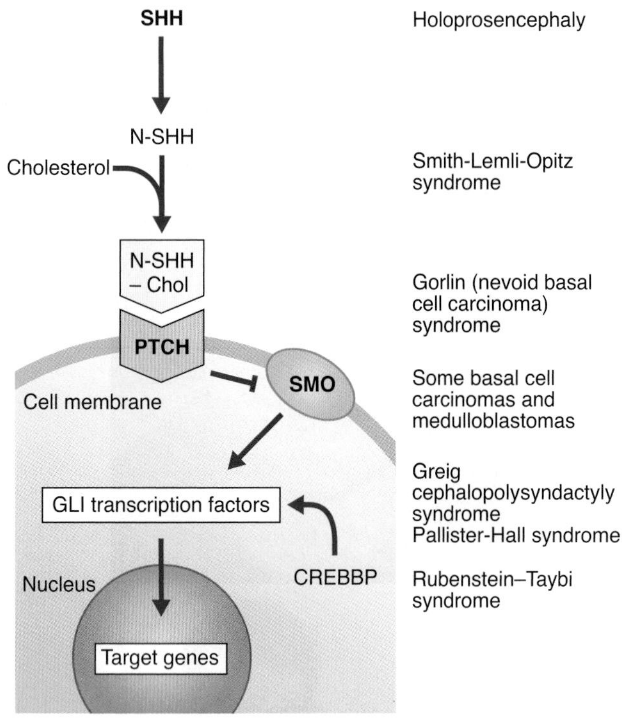

• **Fig. 9.9** The Sonic hedgehog (*SHH*)-patched (*PTCH*)-Gli pathway and connection with disease. Different elements in the pathway act as activators (*arrows*) or inhibitors (*bars*). The SHH protein is initially cleaved to an active N-terminal form, which is then modified by the addition of cholesterol. The normal action of PTCH is to inhibit SMO, but when PTCH is bound by SHH this inhibition is removed, and the downstream signaling proceeds. *CREBBP*, cAMP response element–binding protein.

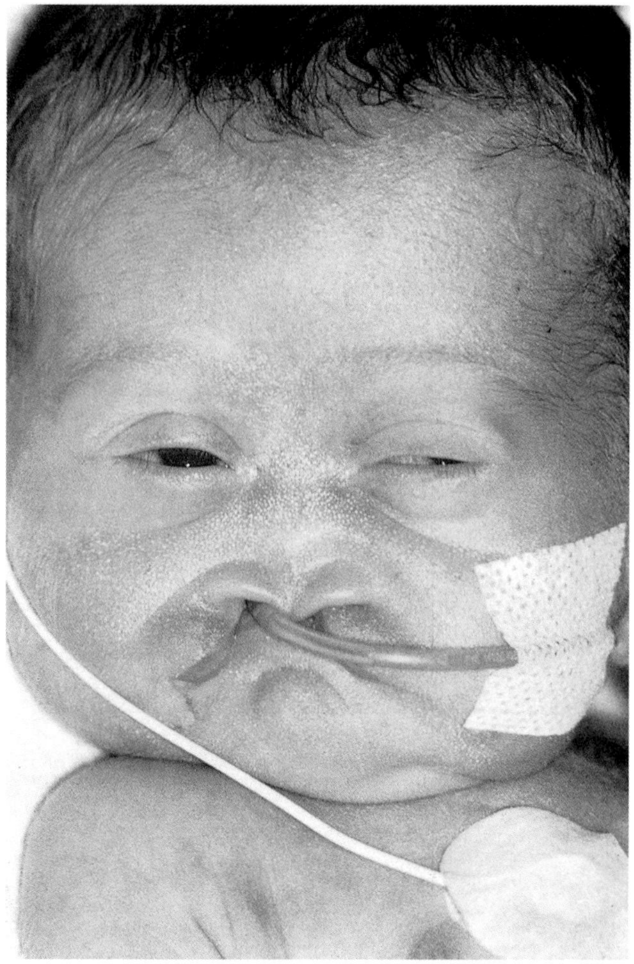

• **Fig. 9.10** Facial features in holoprosencephaly. The eyes are close together and there is a midline cleft lip because of a failure of normal prolabia development.

They therefore play a major part in the development of the central nervous system, the axial skeleton and limbs, the gastrointestinal and urogenital tracts, and the external genitalia.

Drosophila has eight *HOX* genes arranged in a single cluster, but in humans, as in most vertebrates, there are four homeobox gene clusters containing a total of 39 *HOX* genes (Fig. 9.13). Each cluster contains a series of closely linked genes. In vertebrates such as mice, it has been shown that these genes are expressed in segmental units in the hindbrain and in global patterning of the somites formed from axial presomitic mesoderm. In each *HOX* cluster, there is a direct linear correlation between the position of the gene and its temporal and spatial expression. These observations indicate that these genes play a crucial role in early morphogenesis. Thus, in the developing limb bud (Fig. 9.26) *HOXA9* is expressed both anterior to, and before, *HOX10*, and so on.

Mutations in *HOXA13* cause a rare condition known as the hand-foot-genital syndrome. This shows autosomal dominant inheritance and is characterized by shortening of the first and fifth digits, with hypospadias in males and bicornuate uterus in females. Experiments with mouse *HOXA13* mutants have shown that expression of another gene, *EphA7*, is severely reduced. Therefore, if this gene is not activated by *HOXA13*, there is failure to form the normal chondrogenic condensations in the primordial distal limb. Mutations in *HOXD13* result in an equally rare limb developmental abnormality known as synpolydactyly. This also shows autosomal dominant inheritance and is characterized by insertion of an additional digit between the third and fourth fingers and the fourth and fifth toes, which are webbed (Fig. 9.14). The phenotype in homozygotes is more severe, and reported mutations take the form of an increase in the number of residues in a polyalanine tract. This triplet-repeat expansion probably alters the structure and function of the protein, thereby constituting a gain-of-function mutation (p. 22). Mutated *HOXA1* has been found in the rare, recessively inherited, Bosley-Saleh-Alorainy syndrome, consisting of central nervous system abnormalities, deafness and cardiac and laryngotracheal anomalies. A mutation in *HOXD10* was found in isolated congenital vertical talus in a large family demonstrating autosomal dominant inheritance, and duplications of *HOXD* have been found in mesomelic limb abnormality syndromes.

Given that there are 39 *HOX* genes in mammals, it is surprising that so few syndromes or malformations have been attributed to *HOX* gene mutations. One possible explanation is that most *HOX* mutations are so devastating that the embryo cannot survive. Alternatively, the high degree of homology between *HOX* genes in the different clusters could lead to functional redundancy so that one *HOX* gene compensates for a loss-of-function mutation in another. In this context *HOX* genes are said to be paralogous because family members from different clusters, such as *HOXA13* and *HOXD13*, are more similar than adjacent genes in the same cluster.

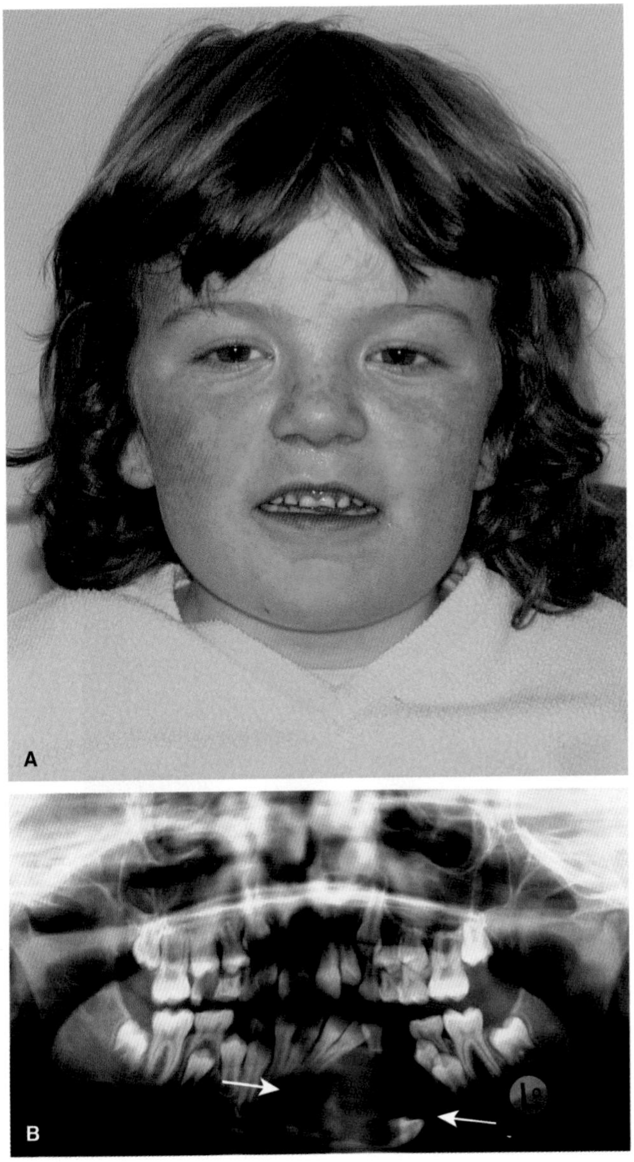

• **Fig. 9.11** Gorlin (nevoid basal cell carcinoma) syndrome. (A) This 6-year-old girl from a large family with Gorlin syndrome has macrocephaly and a cherubic appearance. (B) Her affected sister developed a rapidly enlarging odontogenic keratocyst (*arrows*) in the mandible at the age of 9 years, displacing the roots of her teeth.

Several other developmental genes also contain a homeobox-like domain. These include *MSX2*, mutations in which can cause craniosynostosis—premature fusion of the cranial sutures.

Paired-Box (*PAX*) Genes

The paired-box is a highly conserved DNA sequence that encodes a 130–amino acid DNA-binding transcription regulator domain. Nine *PAX* genes have been identified in mice and humans. In mice these have been shown to play important roles in the developing nervous system and vertebral column. In humans, loss-of-function mutations in five *PAX* genes have been identified in association with developmental abnormalities (Table 9.2). Waardenburg syndrome type 1 is caused by mutations in *PAX3*. It shows autosomal dominant inheritance and is characterized by sensorineural hearing loss, areas of depigmentation in hair and skin, abnormal patterns of pigmentation in the iris, and widely spaced inner canthi (Fig. 9.15). Waardenburg syndrome shows clinical and genetic heterogeneity; the more common type 2 form, in which the inner canthi are not widely separated, may be caused by mutations in *MITF* or *SOX10*, with other cases as yet unexplained.

The importance of expression of the *PAX* gene family in eye development is illustrated by the effects of mutations in *PAX2* and *PAX6*. Mutations in *PAX2* cause the renal-coloboma syndrome, in which renal malformations occur in association with structural defects in various parts of the eye, including the retina and optic nerve. Mutations in *PAX6* lead to absence of the iris, which is known as aniridia (Fig. 9.16). This is a key feature of the WAGR syndrome (p. 258), which results from a contiguous gene deletion involving the *PAX6* locus on chromosome 11.

SRY-Type HMG Box (*SOX*) Genes

SRY is the Y-linked gene that plays a major role in male sex determination (p. 128). A family of genes known as the *SOX* genes show homology with *SRY* by sharing a 79–amino acid domain known as the high-mobility group (HMG) box. This HMG domain activates transcription by bending DNA in such a way that other regulatory factors can bind with the promoter regions of genes that encode for important structural proteins. These *SOX* genes are thus transcription regulators which are expressed in specific tissues during embryogenesis. For example, *SOX1*, *SOX2*, and *SOX3* are expressed in the developing mouse nervous system.

In humans it has been shown that loss-of-function mutations in *SOX9* on chromosome 17 cause campomelic dysplasia (Fig. 9.17). This rare disorder is characterized by bowing of the long bones, sex reversal in chromosomal males, and very poor long-term survival. *In situ* hybridization studies in mice have shown that *SOX9* is expressed in the developing embryo in skeletal primordial tissue, where it regulates type II collagen expression, as well as in the genital ridges and early gonads. *SOX9* is now thought to be one of several genes that are expressed downstream of *SRY* in the process of male sex determination. Mutations in *SOX10* are one cause of Waardenburg syndrome type 2 and may include a peripheral neuropathy as well as Hirschsprung disease. Mutations in *SOX2* (3q26) have been shown to cause anophthalmia or microphthalmia, but also a wider syndrome of esophageal atresia and genital hypoplasia in males—the anophthalmia-esophageal-genital syndrome.

T-Box (*TBX*) Genes

The *T* gene in mice plays an important role in specification of the paraxial mesoderm and notochord differentiation. Heterozygotes for loss-of-function mutations have a short tail and malformed sacral vertebrae. This gene, which is also known as *Brachyury*, encodes a transcription factor that contains both activator and repressor domains. It shows homology with a series of genes through the shared possession of the T domain, which is also referred to as the T-box. These T-box or *TBX* genes are dispersed throughout the human genome, with some family members existing in small clusters. One of these clusters on chromosome 12 contains *TBX3* and *TBX5*. Loss-of-function mutations in *TBX3* cause the ulnar-mammary syndrome in which ulnar ray developmental abnormalities in the upper limbs are associated with hypoplasia of the mammary glands. Loss-of-function mutations in *TBX5* cause Holt-Oram syndrome. This autosomal dominant disorder is

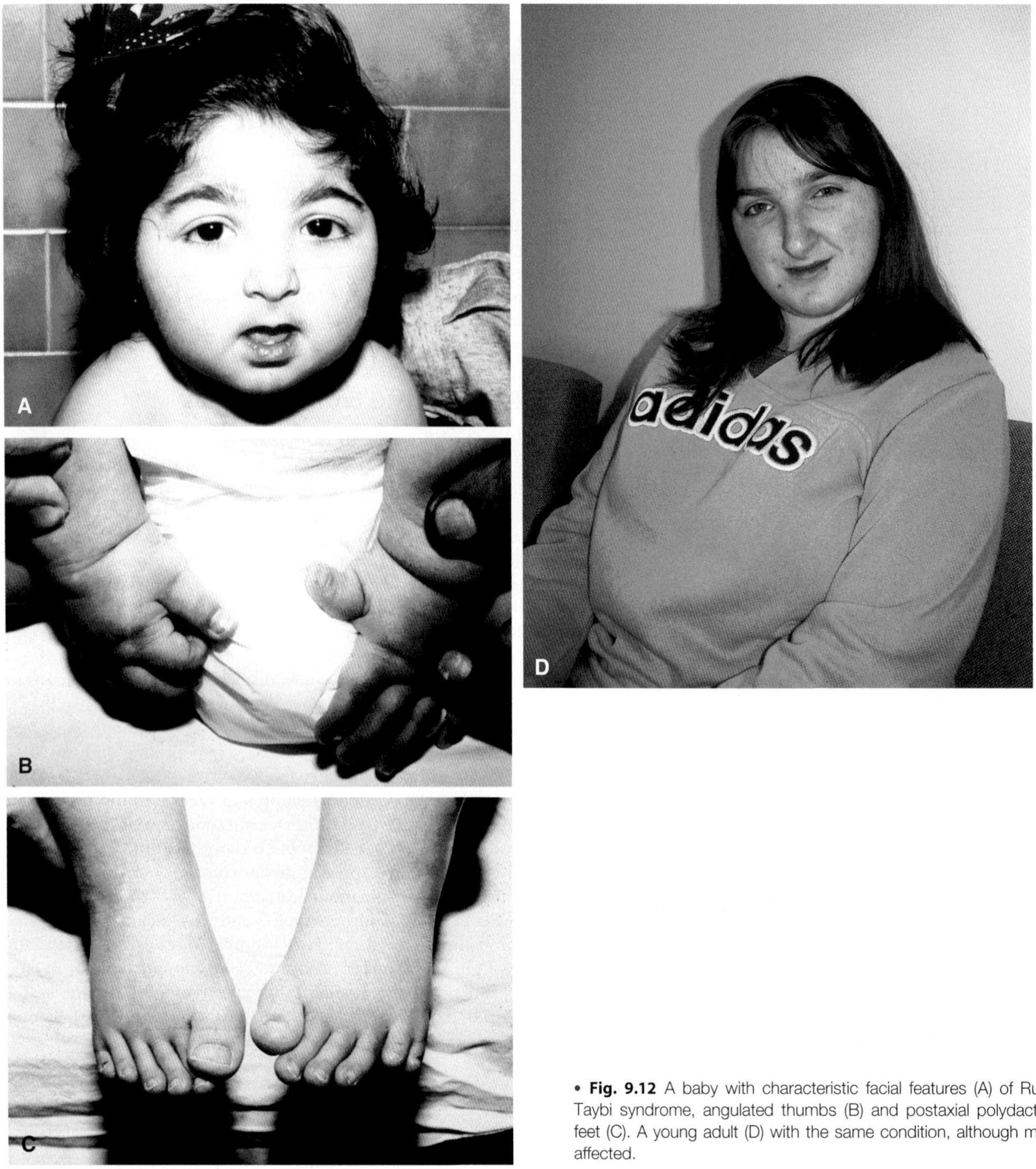

• **Fig. 9.12** A baby with characteristic facial features (A) of Rubenstein-Taybi syndrome, angulated thumbs (B) and postaxial polydactyly of the feet (C). A young adult (D) with the same condition, although more mildly affected.

characterized by congenital heart abnormalities, most notably atrial septal defects, and upper limb radial ray reduction defects that can vary from mild hypoplasia (sometimes duplication) of the thumbs to almost complete absence of the forearms. *TBX6* is implicated in congenital scoliosis, autosomal dominant and recessive forms of spondylocostal dysostosis, and Müllerian aplasia (abnormalities of the female genital tract).

Zinc Finger Genes

The term **zinc finger** refers to a finger-like loop projection consisting of a series of four amino acids that form a complex with a zinc ion. Genes that contain a zinc finger motif act as transcription factors through binding of the zinc finger to DNA. Consequently they are good candidates for single-gene developmental disorders (Table 9.3).

For example, a zinc finger motif–containing (zfm-c) gene known as *GLI3* on chromosome 7 (as mentioned, a component of the SHH pathway) has been implicated as the cause of two developmental disorders. Large deletions or translocations involving *GLI3* cause Greig cephalopolysyndactyly, which is characterized by head, hand, and foot abnormalities such as polydactyly and syndactyly (Fig. 9.18A). In contrast, frameshift mutations in *GLI3* have been reported in the Pallister-Hall syndrome (Fig. 9.18B), in

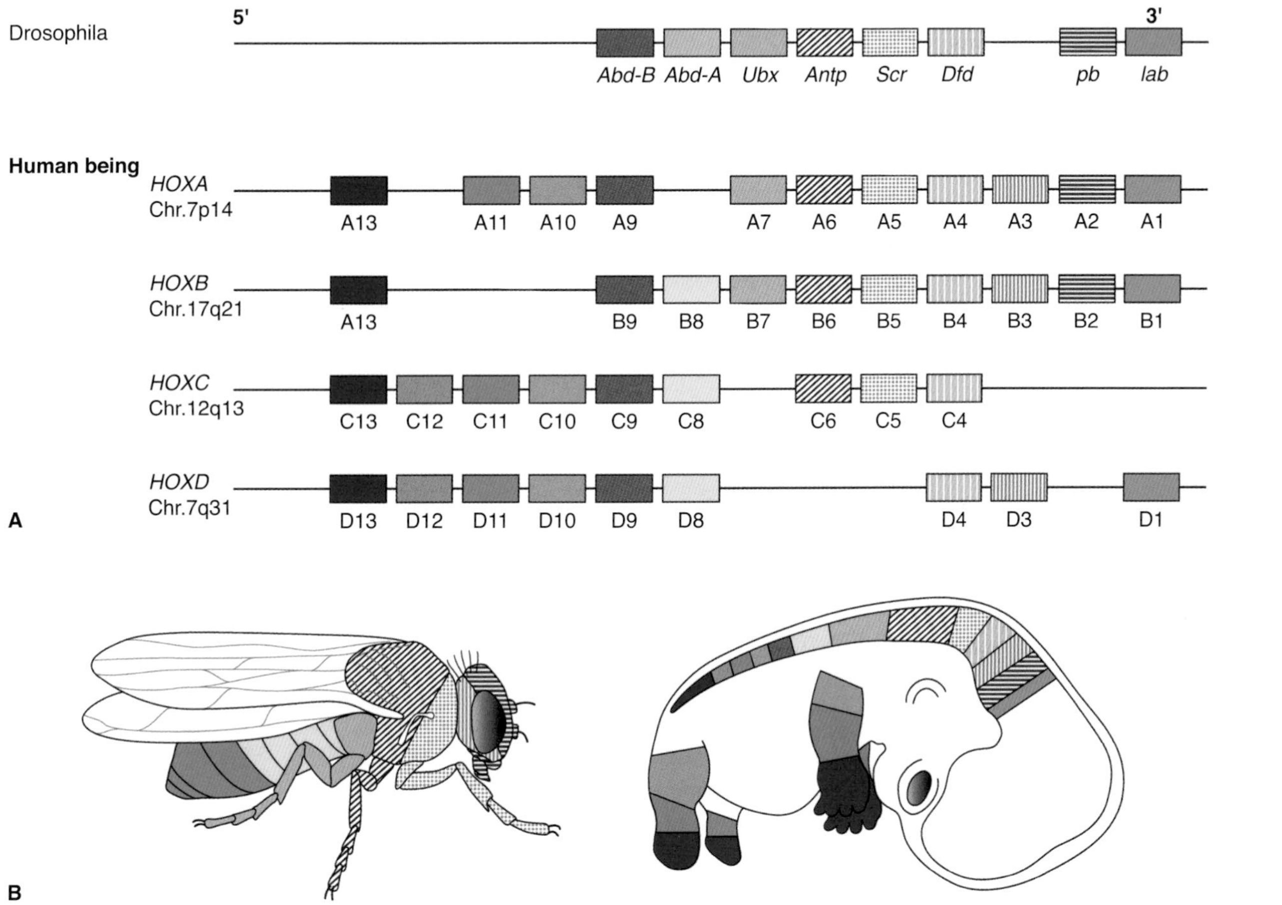

• **Fig. 9.13** (A) *Drosophila* has eight *Hox* genes in a single cluster, whereas there are 39 *HOX* genes in humans, arranged in four clusters located on chromosomes 7p, 17q, 12q, and 2q for the A, B, C, and D clusters, respectively. (B) Expression patterns of *Hox* and *HOX* genes along the rostrocaudal axis in invertebrates and vertebrates, respectively. In vertebrates the clusters are *paralogous* and appear to compensate for one another. (Modified from Veraksa A, Del Campo M, McGinnis W. Developmental patterning genes and their conserved functions: from model organisms to humans. *Mol Genet Metab*. 2000;69:85–100. With permission.)

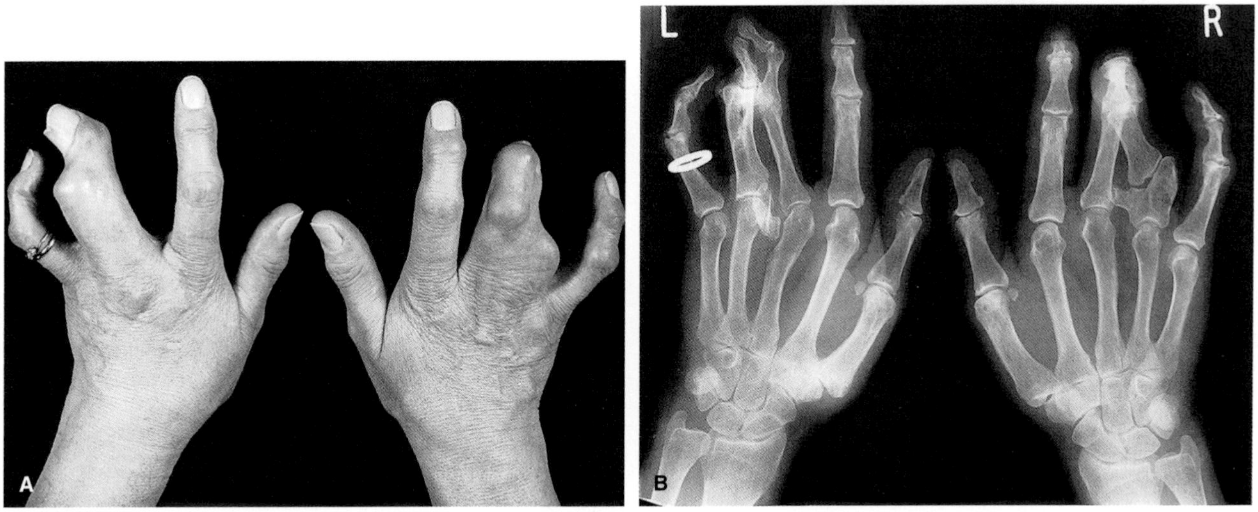

• **Fig. 9.14** Clinical (A) and radiographic (B) views of the hands in synpolydactyly as a result of mutated *HOXD13*.

which the key features are polydactyly, hypothalamic hamartomata, and imperforate anus.

Mutations in another zfm-c gene known as *WT1* on chromosome 11 can cause both Wilms' tumor and a rare developmental disorder, the Denys-Drash syndrome, in which the external genitalia are ambiguous and there is progressive renal failure as a result of nephritis. Mutations in two other zfm-c genes, *ZIC2* and *ZIC3*, have been shown to cause holoprosencephaly and laterality defects, respectively.

TABLE 9.2 Developmental abnormalities associated with *PAX* gene mutations

Gene	Chromosome Location	Developmental Abnormality
PAX2	10q24	Renal-coloboma syndrome
PAX3	2q35	Waardenburg syndrome type 1
PAX6	11p13	Aniridia
PAX8	2q12	Absent or ectopic thyroid gland
PAX9	14q12	Oligodontia

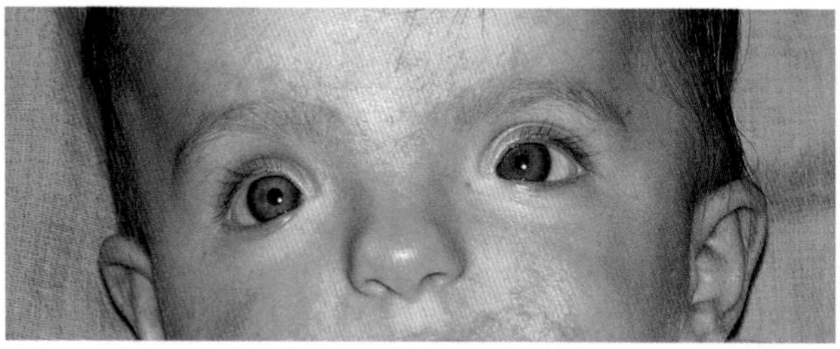

• **Fig. 9.15** Iris heterochromia and marked dystopia canthorum in an infant with Waardenburg syndrome type 1, caused by a mutation in *PAX3*.

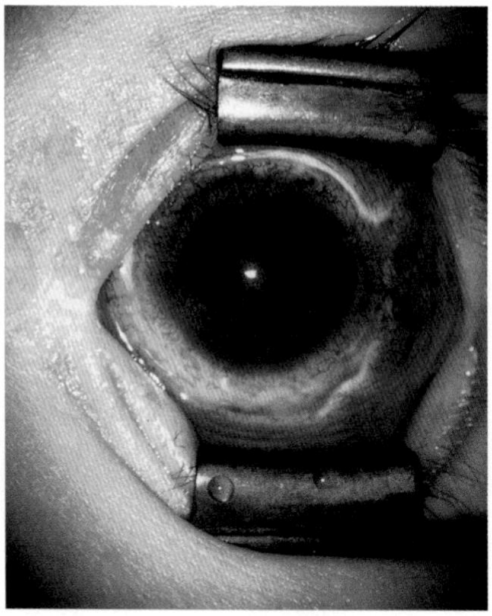

• **Fig. 9.16** An eye showing absence of the iris (aniridia). The cornea shows abnormal vascularization. (Courtesy Mr R. Gregson, Queen's Medical Centre, Nottingham, UK.)

Just as **polarity** is a key concept in development, so too is **laterality**, with implications for the establishment of a normal left-right body axis. In very early development, integrity of many of the same gene families previously mentioned—Nodal, SHH, and Notch—is essential to the establishment of this axis. Clinically, **situs solitus** is the term given to normal left-right asymmetry and **situs inversus** to reversal of the normal arrangement. Up to 25% of individuals with situs inversus have an autosomal recessive condition—Kartagener syndrome, or primary ciliary dyskinesia. Other terms used are **isomerism sequence**, **heterotaxy**, **asplenia/polyasplenia**, and **Ivemark syndrome**. Laterality defects are characterized by abnormal positioning of unpaired organs such as the heart, liver, and spleen, and more than 20 genes are now implicated from studies in vertebrates, with a number identified in humans by the study of affected families, with all of the main patterns of inheritance represented.

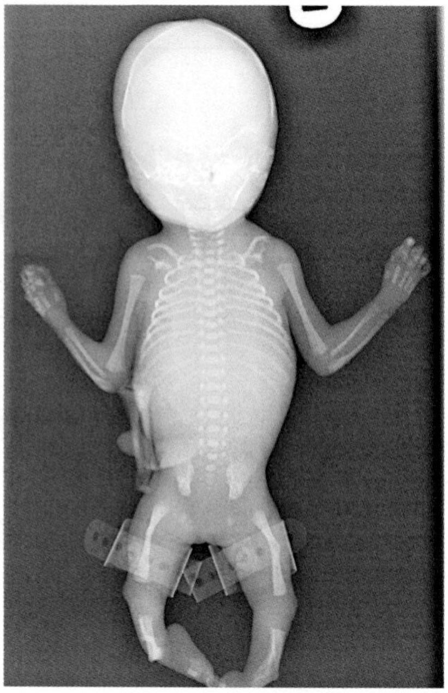

• **Fig. 9.17** Campomelic dysplasia. This skeletal dysplasia is characterised by angulation of the long bones, especially in the legs, very small scapulae, and sex reversal in males. Severe and life-threatening respiratory distress in the neonatal period is usual. It is caused by mutations in the *SOX9* gene.

TABLE 9.3 Developmental abnormalities associated with genes containing a zinc finger motif

Gene	Chromosome Location	Developmental Abnormality
GLI3	7p13	Greig syndrome and Pallister-Hall syndrome
WT1	11p13	Denys-Drash syndrome
ZIC2	13q32	Holoprosencephaly
ZIC3	Xq26	Laterality defects

Signal Transduction ("Signaling") Genes

Signal transduction is the process whereby extracellular growth factors regulate cell division and differentiation by a complex pathway of genetically determined intermediate steps. Mutations in many of the genes involved in signal transduction play a role in causing cancer (p. 188). In some cases they can also cause developmental abnormalities. The RAS-MAPK pathway and associated syndromes are discussed in Chapter 16 (p. 234; Fig. 16.12), and

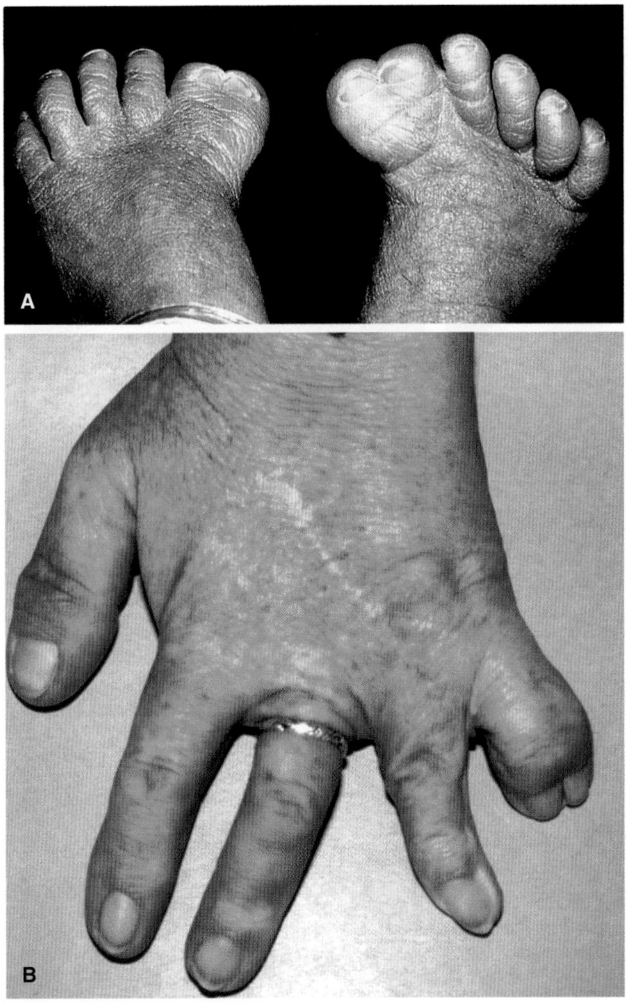

• **Fig. 9.18** (A) The feet of a child with Greig cephalopolysyndactyly. Note that they show both preaxial polydactyly (extra digits) and syndactyly (fused digits). (B) The left hand of a woman with Pallister-Hall syndrome and a proven mutation in *GLI3*. Note the postaxial polydactyly and the surgical scar, where an extra digit arising from between the normal metacarpal rays (mesoaxial polydactyly) was removed.

the mTOR pathway and syndromes in Chapter 19 (p. 298; Fig. 19.11).

The RET *Proto-oncogene*

The proto-oncogene *RET* on chromosome 10q11.2 encodes a cell-surface tyrosine kinase (Fig. 9.27). Gain-of-function mutations, whether inherited or acquired, are found in a high proportion of medullary thyroid cancers. Loss-of-function mutations in *RET* have been identified in approximately 50% of familial cases of Hirschsprung disease, in which there is failure of migration of ganglionic cells to the submucosal and myenteric plexuses of the large bowel. The clinical consequences are usually apparent shortly after birth when the child presents with abdominal distension and intestinal obstruction.

Fibroblast Growth Factor Receptors

FGFs play key roles in embryogenesis, including cell division, migration, and differentiation. The transduction of extracellular FGF signals is mediated by a family of four transmembrane

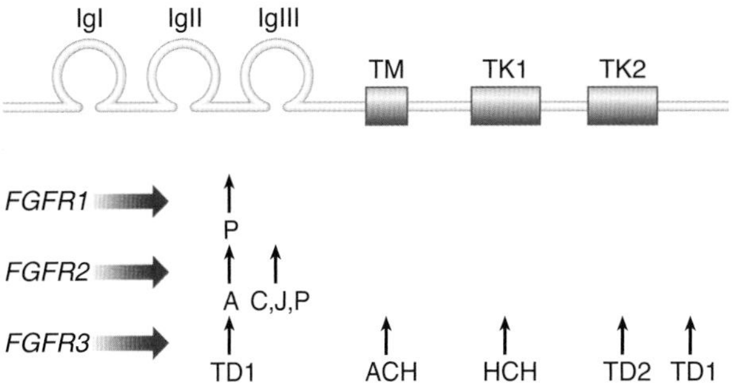

• **Fig. 9.19** Structure of the fibroblast growth factor receptor (FGFR). Arrows indicate the location of mutations in the craniosynostosis syndromes and achondroplasia group of skeletal dysplasias. *A*, Apert syndrome; *ACH*, achondroplasia; *C*, Crouzon syndrome; *HCH*, hypochondroplasia. *Ig*, Immunoglobulin-like domain; *J*, Jackson-Weiss syndrome; *P*, Pfeiffer syndrome; *TD*, thanatophoric dysplasia; *TK*, tyrosine kinase domain; *TM*, transmembrane domain.

tyrosine kinase receptors. These are the fibroblast growth factor receptors (FGFRs), each of which contains three main components—an extracellular region with three immunoglobulin-like domains, a transmembrane segment and two intracellular tyrosine kinase domains (Fig. 9.19).

Pathogenic variants in the genes that encode FGFRs have been identified in two groups of developmental disorders (Table 9.4), and they are activating or gain-of-function mutations (p. 22). These are the craniosynostosis syndromes and the achondroplasia family of skeletal dysplasias. The craniosynostosis syndromes, of which Apert syndrome (Fig. 9.20) is the best known, are characterized by premature fusion of the cranial sutures, often in association with hand and foot abnormalities such as syndactyly (fusion of the digits). Apert syndrome is caused by a mutation in one of the adjacent FGFR2 residues in the peptides that link the second and third immunoglobulin loops (see Fig. 9.19). In contrast, mutations in the third immunoglobulin loop can cause either Crouzon syndrome, in which the limbs are normal, or Pfeiffer syndrome, in which the thumbs and big toes are broad. Achondroplasia is the most commonly encountered genetic form of extreme short stature (Fig. 9.21). The limbs show proximal ("rhizomelic") shortening, and the head is enlarged with frontal

TABLE 9.4 Developmental disorders caused by mutations in fibroblast growth factor receptors

Gene	Chromosome	Syndrome
Craniosynostosis Syndromes		
FGFR1	8p11	Pfeiffer
FGFR2	10q25	Apert Crouzon Jackson-Weiss Pfeiffer
FGFR3	4p16	Crouzon (with acanthosis nigricans)
Skeletal Dysplasias		
FGFR3	4p16	Achondroplasia Hypochondroplasia Thanatophoric dysplasia

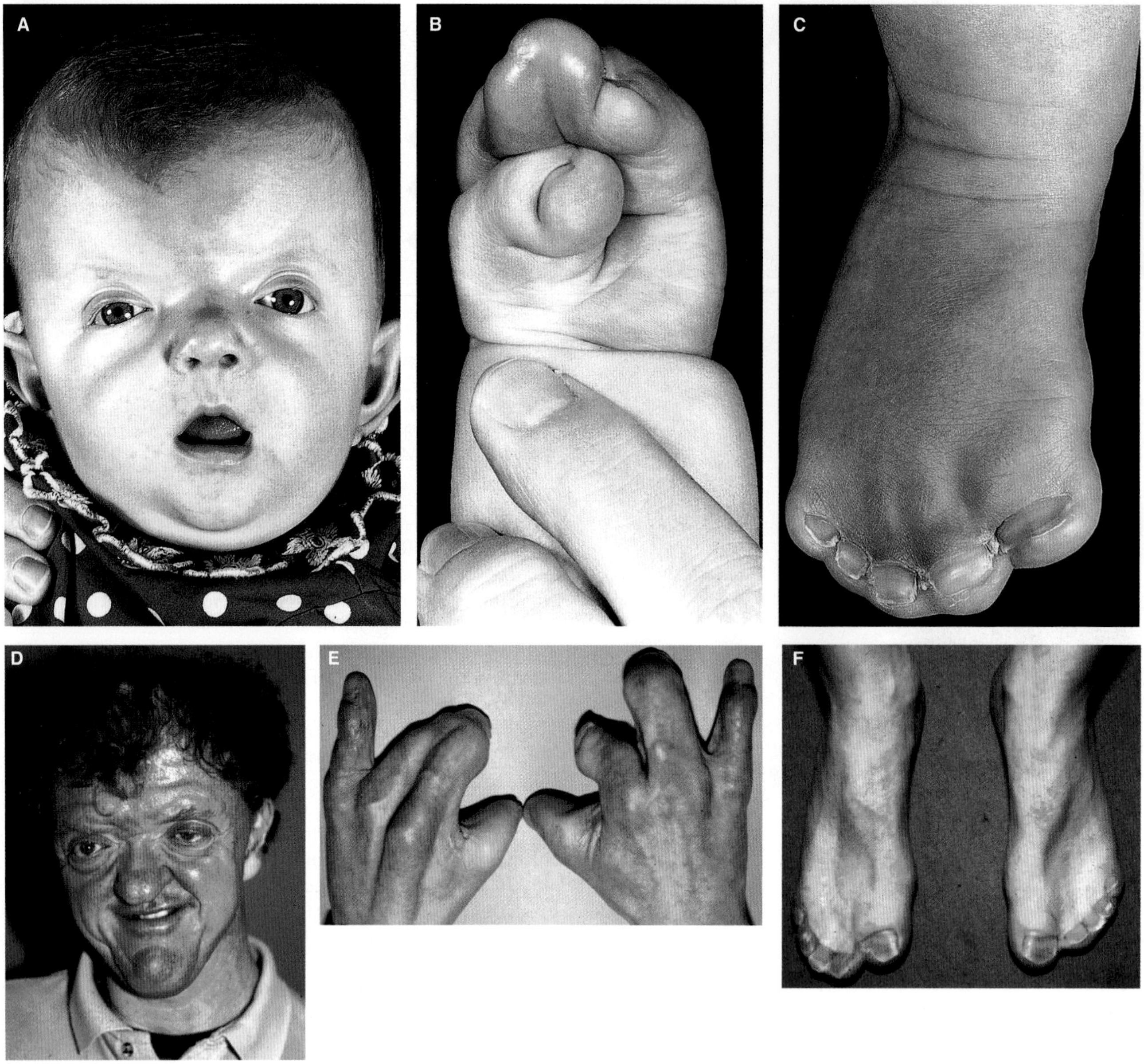

• **Fig. 9.20** Apert syndrome, as a result of mutated *FGFR2*. Views of the face (A), hand (B), and foot (C) of a child. An affected adult is shown in (D), (E), and (F).

bossing. Intelligence and life expectancy are near normal, but there is an increased risk of death in infancy attributed to craniocervical junction compression, and surveillance is important. Other complications include obstructive sleep apnea, middle ear dysfunction, kyphosis, and spinal stenosis. Achondroplasia is almost always caused by a variant in, or close to, the transmembrane domain of *FGFR3*. The common (~98% of cases) transmembrane domain variant, G380R or c.1138 G>A, results in the replacement of a glycine residue by arginine—an amino acid never normally found in cell membranes. This in turn appears to enhance dimerization of the protein that catalyzes downstream signaling. Approximately 1% of cases are caused by a different substitution, c.1138 G>C (also resulting in G380R).

Hypochondroplasia, a milder form of skeletal dysplasia with similar trunk and limb changes but normal head shape and size, is caused by mutations in the proximal tyrosine kinase domain (intracellular) of *FGFR3*. Finally, thanatophoric dysplasia, a much more severe and invariably lethal form of skeletal dysplasia, is caused by mutations in either the peptides linking the second and third immunoglobulin domains (extracellular) of *FGFR3*, or the distal *FGFR3* tyrosine kinase domain. Loss-of-function effects in *FGFR3* do not give rise to a skeletal dysplasia, as children with Wolf-Hirschhorn syndrome (p. 243), attributed to chromosome 4p microdeletions that include *FGFR3*, do not show skeletal anomalies.

The Pharyngeal Arches

The pharyngeal (or branchial) arches correspond to the gill system of lower vertebrates and appear in the fourth and fifth weeks of development. Five (segmented) pharyngeal arches in humans arise lateral to the structures of the head (Fig. 9.22), and each comprises

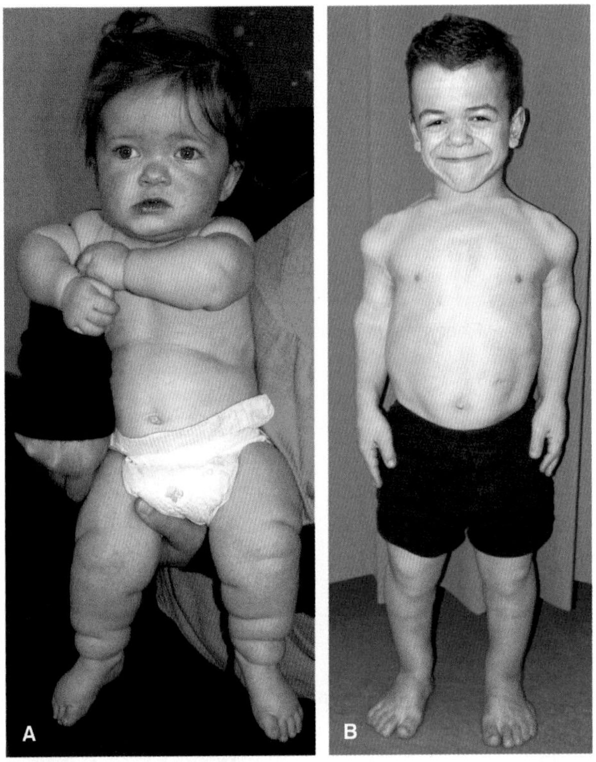

• **Fig. 9.21** Two young patients with achondroplasia. (A) An infant showing typical frontal bossing and excess skin folds as a result of short long bones. (B) An older child who is part of a family with achondroplasia.

cells from the three germ layers and the neural crest. The lining of the pharynx, thyroid, and parathyroids arises from the **endoderm**, and the outer epidermal layer arises from the **ectoderm**. The musculature arises from the **mesoderm**, and bony structures from **neural crest** cells. Separating the arches are the pharyngeal clefts externally and the pharyngeal pouches internally—these have important destinies. Numbered from the rostral end, the first arch forms the jaw and muscles of mastication; the first cleft is destined to be the external auditory meatus, and the first pouch the middle ear apparatus. The second arch forms the hyoid apparatus and muscles of facial expression, whereas the third pouch develops into the thymus, and the third and fourth pouches become the parathyroids. The arteries within the arches have important destinies too and, after remodeling, give rise to the aortic and pulmonary arterial systems. Some of the syndromes, malformations, inheritance patterns and genetic mechanisms associated with the first and second pharyngeal arches are listed in Table 9.5. One of these, branchio-oculo-facial syndrome, is illustrated in Fig. 9.23. However, the most well-known condition attributed to disturbed development of pharyngeal structures—the third and fourth pouches—is DiGeorge syndrome, also known as velocardiofacial syndrome, and well described earlier by Sedláčková of Prague in 1955. This is covered in more detail in Chapter 17 (p. 259) and results from a 3-megabase submicroscopic chromosome deletion at band 22q11.2 with the loss of some 30 genes. Studies in mice (the equivalent, or **syntenic**, region is on mouse chromosome 16) suggest that the most significant gene loss is that of *Tbx1*, strongly expressed throughout the pharyngeal apparatus. Heterozygous *Tbx1* knock-out mice show hypoplastic or absent fourth pharyngeal arch arteries, suggesting that *TBX1* in humans is the key. Indeed, mutations in this gene have been found in some congenital heart abnormalities and other features of deletion 22q11.2, except cognitive impairment.

The Role of Cilia in Developmental Abnormalities

The vital role of the humble cilium in driving movement or particle flow across epithelial surfaces has become increasingly apparent. As with other areas of cell and molecular biology, we learn most about motile cilia when they are dysfunctional—the result may be major developmental abnormalities.

Cilia are the equivalent of flagella in wider biology, and they share structural identity. They are hair-like protrusions from the cell surface (Fig. 9.24), up to 20 μm long, are present in large numbers on the apical cell surface and beat in coordinated waves. In cross-section they consist of a scaffold of nine microtubule doublets surrounding a central pair. The central and outer doublets are connected by radial spokes, which produce the force necessary to bend the cilium; dynein arms facilitate this movement. Among other functions they clear mucus from the respiratory epithelium, drive sperm along the Fallopian tube and move cerebrospinal fluid in the cavities of the central nervous system. In development, the cilia at the organizational node of the vertebrate embryo conduct a circular motion, wafting molecules unidirectionally and helping to establish left-right asymmetry.

Apart from their obvious mechanical function, which conceptually is straightforward, it appears increasingly likely that cilia behave like molecular antennae that sense extracellular signaling molecules. The SHH and Wnt signaling pathways depend to an extent on cilial functional integrity for optimal signaling. Defective cilial function can therefore impact on a broad range of developmental processes and pathways. Defects in the cilial proteins themselves lead to wide-ranging phenotypic effects that include retinal degeneration, anosmia, renal, hepatic, and pancreatic cyst formation, postaxial polydactyly, and situs inversus. The associated syndromes are referred to as "ciliopathies" (Table 9.6). One of these, short-rib polydactyly syndrome (also known as short-rib thoracic dysplasia), which follows autosomal recessive inheritance and in type 3 is as a result of mutated *DYNC2H1*, is shown in Fig. 9.25. The features of the listed syndromes in Table 9.6 overlap with many other multiple congenital abnormality syndromes, and the role of functioning cilia in development cannot be underestimated.

The Limb as a Developmental Model

Four main phases are recognized in limb development: (1) initiation, (2) specification, (3) tissue differentiation, and (4) growth. Understanding of these stages and their molecular mechanisms continues to grow, and insights have been gleaned from the study of limb development in chicks and mice in particular, as well as elucidation of the causes of various limb abnormalities in humans.

Initiation and Specification

Limb bud formation is thought to be initiated at approximately 28 days by a member of the *FGF* family as illustrated by the development of an extra limb if *FGF1*, *FGF2*, or *FGF4* is applied to the side of a developing chick embryo. During normal limb initiation *FGF8* transcripts have been identified in mesenchyme near the

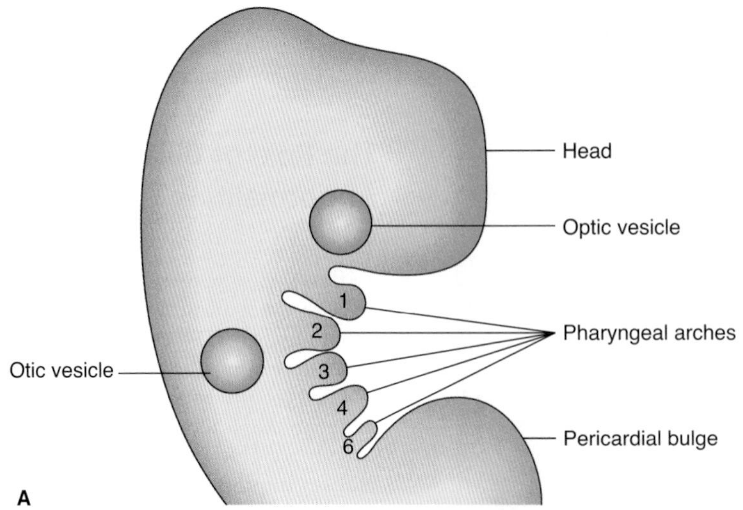

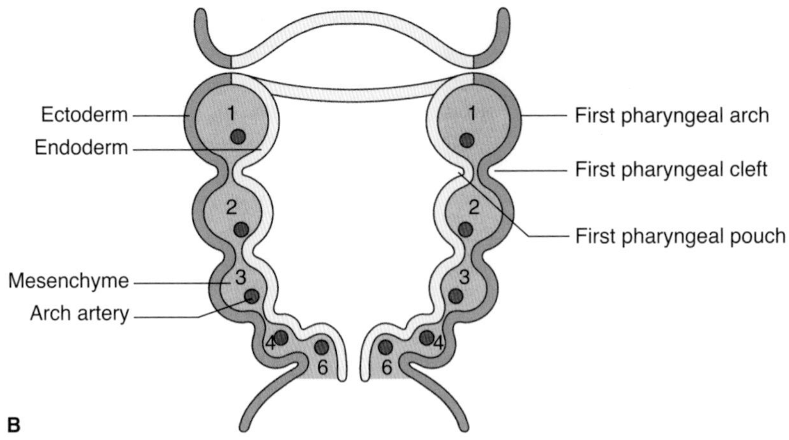

• **Fig. 9.22** The pharyngeal (or branchial) apparatus. The lateral view (A) shows the five pharyngeal arches close to the embryonic head, and the cross-section (B) shows the basic arrangement from which many head and neck structures, as well as the heart, develop. Humans and mice do not have arch number 5. (Modified from Graham A, Smith A. Patterning the pharyngeal arches. *Bioessays*. 2001;23:54–61. With permission of Wiley-Liss Inc., a subsidiary of John Wiley & Sons, Inc.)

initiation site. FGF8 expression is probably controlled by *HOX* genes, which determine limb type (forelimb or hindlimb) and number.

Tissue Differentiation and Growth

Once limb formation has been initiated, a localized area of thickened ectoderm at the limb tip, known as the **apical ectodermal ridge** (**AER**), produces growth signals such as FGF4 and FGF8, which maintain further growth and establish the proximo-distal axis (Fig. 9.26). Expression of the gene *TP63* is crucial for sustaining the AER, and when this gene is mutated split hand-foot malformations result, often together with oral clefting and other anomalies—ectrodactyly-ectodermal dysplasia-clefting syndrome. Signals from another localized area on the posterior (ulnar) margin of the developing bud, known as the **zone of polarizing activity (ZPA)**, determine the anteroposterior axis. Downregulation of ZPA results in loss of digits on the ulnar side, whereas upregulation results in postaxial polydactyly. One of the key ZPA signals is *SHH* (p. 107), which acts in concert with other *FGF* genes, *GLI3* and another gene family that encodes BMPs. Another morphogen, retinoic acid, is believed to play a major role at this stage in determining development at the anterior margin of the limb bud.

Subsequent development involves the activation of genes from the *HOXA* and *HOXD* clusters in the undifferentiated proliferating mesenchymal cells beneath the AER. This area is known as the **progress zone**. Cells in different regions express different combinations of *HOX* genes that determine local cell proliferation, adhesion, and differentiation. Downstream targets of the *HOX* gene clusters remain to be identified. Other genes that clearly have a key role are those of the *T-box* family, previously discussed, and *SALL4*, which is mutated in Okihiro syndrome (radial ray defects with abnormal eye movements resulting from congenital palsy affecting the sixth cranial nerve).

FGFs continue to be important during the later stages of limb development. In this context it becomes easy to understand why limb abnormalities are a feature of disorders such as Apert syndrome (see Fig. 9.20), in which mutations have been identified in the extracellular domains of *FGFR2*. Wnt signaling is also integral to limb development with expression in the posterior aspect of the

TABLE 9.5 Some syndromes and malformations associated with the first and second pharyngeal arches

Syndrome	Malformations	Inheritance	Mechanisms
Oculo-auriculo-vertebral spectrum (Goldenhar syndrome)	Hemifacial microsomia, ear malformations; epibulbar dermoids; occasional clefts; (cervical vertebral anomalies)	Usually sporadic. Occasional AD and AR families reported	Probable non-genetic factors Possible locus at 14q32.1
Treacher-Collins syndrome	Hypoplasia of the maxilla and mandible; downslanting palpebral fissures with coloboma of the lower lid; cleft palate; hearing impairment	AD	Mutation in *TCOF1*
Branchio-oculo-facial syndrome	Branchial cleft sinus defects; a cleft or pseudocleft lip/palate; ocular anomalies including microphthalmia and lacrimal duct obstruction	AD	Mutation in *TFAP2A*
Branchio-oto-renal syndrome	Long, narrow face; aplasia or stenosis of lacrimal duct; ear anomalies—external and inner—and preauricular pits	AD	Mutation in *EYA1*, *SIX5*
Pierre-Robin sequence	Micrognathia, cleft palate, glossoptosis (posteriorly placed tongue); if syndromic, may be associated with limb anomalies and/or congenital heart disease	Various: sporadic if occurring as an isolated malformation complex; syndromic forms—both AD and AR families reported	Sporadic cases may be a deformation sequence secondary to oligohydramnios. Mendelian forms rare
Townes-Brock syndrome	Malformed ("satyr") ears, sensorineural hearing loss, preauricular skin tags; (imperforate anus, triphalangeal thumbs, cardiac/renal defects)	AD	Mutation in *SALL1*
Auriculo-condylar syndrome	Prominent, malformed ears; abnormal temporomandibular joint; microstomia	AD/AR	*GNA13*, *PLCB4*, *EDN1*
Oro-facial-digital (OFD) syndromes (types I–X)	Cleft or lobulated tongue; cleft palate; oral frenulae; (digital anomalies—brachydactyly, polydactyly, syndactyly, clinodactyly)	XLD (OFD1, OFD7) XLR (OFD8, OFD9) AR (OFD2, OFD3, OFD4, OFD5), OFD6, OFD9) AD (OFD7)	OFD1 as a result of mutation in *CXORF5* (Xp22)
Oto-palato-digital syndrome	Prominent supraorbital ridge, wide nasal bridge, downslanting palpebral fissures, low-set ears, microstomia, micrognathia; skeletal abnormalities (restricted growth, narrow thorax, platyspondyly, bowed long bones)	XL semidominant	Mutation in *FLNA* (Xq28)

AD, Autosomal dominant; *AR*, autosomal recessive; *XLD*, X-linked dominant; *XLR*, X-linked recessive.

progress zone, and homozygous (or compound heterozygous) mutations of *LRP4*, whose gene product forms a complex with Frizzled in the Wnt canonical pathway (see Fig. 9.6), give rise to Cenani-Lenz syndrome, a condition characterized by digital fusion/syndactyly, oligodactyly, renal anomalies, and facial dysmorphism.

Developmental Genes and Cancer

Several genes that play important roles in embryogenesis have also been shown to play a role in causing cancer (Table 9.7). This is not surprising, given that many developmental genes are expressed throughout life in processes such as signal transduction and signal transcription (see Fig. 14.5, p. 188). It has been shown that several different mechanisms can account for the phenotypic diversity demonstrated by this group of genes.

Gain-of-Function Versus Loss-of-Function Mutations

Mention has already been made of the causal role of the *RET* proto-oncogene in familial Hirschsprung disease, as well as in both inherited and sporadic medullary thyroid cancer (p. 117). The protein encoded by *RET* consists of three main domains: an extracellular domain that binds to a glial cell line–derived neurotrophil factor, a transmembrane domain, and an intracellular tyrosine kinase domain that activates signal transduction (Fig. 9.27). Mutations causing loss-of-function result in Hirschsprung disease. These include whole gene deletions, small intragenic deletions, nonsense mutations, and splicing mutations leading to synthesis of a truncated protein.

In contrast, mutations causing a gain-of-function effect result in either type 2A or type 2B multiple endocrine neoplasia (MEN).

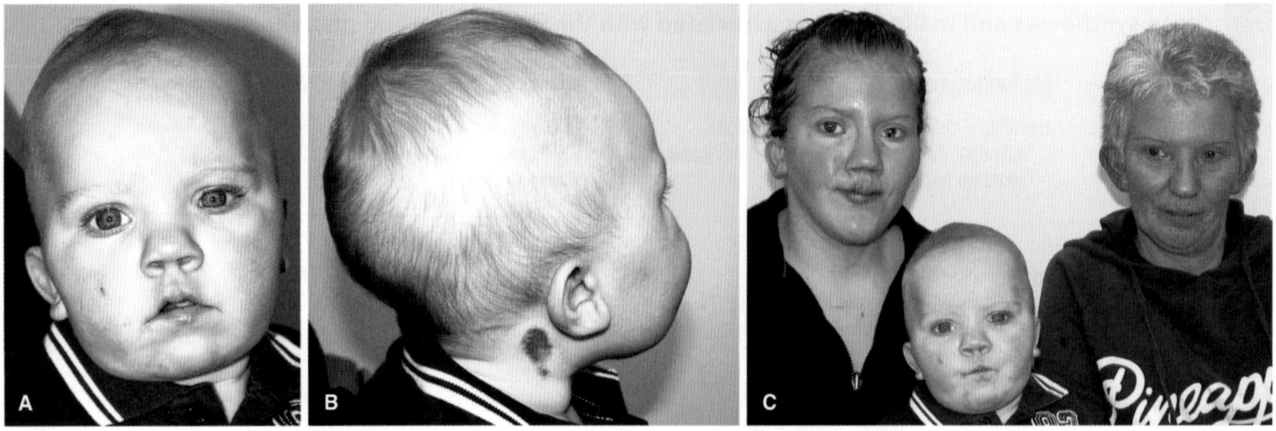

• **Fig. 9.23** Branchio-oculo-facial syndrome, a condition affecting the first and second pharyngeal arches. (A) A young child with a pseudocleft of the upper lip, flattened nasal tip, and anteverted nares; (B) the same child showing a typical cutaneous branchial sinus lesion; (C) the child with his mother (who also has small ears) and grandmother—all clearly affected with pseudoclefts.

These disorders are characterized by a high incidence of medullary thyroid carcinoma and pheochromocytoma. The activating mutations that cause MEN-2A are clustered in five cysteine residues in the extracellular domain. MEN-2B, which differs from MEN-2A in that affected individuals are tall and thin, is usually caused by a unique mutation in a methionine residue in the tyrosine kinase domain.

Somatic Rearrangements

Activation of the *RET* proto-oncogene can occur by a different mechanism whereby the genomic region encoding the intracellular domain is juxtaposed to one of several activating genes that are normally preferentially expressed in the thyroid gland. The newly formed hybrid *RET* gene produces a novel protein whose activity is not ligand-dependent. These somatic rearrangements are found in a high proportion of papillary thyroid carcinomas, which show a particularly high incidence in children who were exposed to radiation following the Chernobyl nuclear accident in 1986.

PAX3 provides another example of a developmental gene that can cause cancer if it is fused to new DNA sequences. A specific translocation between chromosomes 2 and 13 that results in a new chimeric transcript leads to the development in children of a rare lung tumor called alveolar rhabdomyosarcoma.

Positional Effects and Developmental Genes

The discovery of a chromosomal abnormality such as a translocation or inversion in a person with a single-gene developmental syndrome provides a strong indication of the probable position of the disease locus, because it is likely that one of the breakpoints involved in the rearrangement will have disrupted the relevant gene. However, in a few instances, it has emerged that the chromosome breakpoint actually lies approximately 10 to 1000 kilobases upstream or downstream of the gene that is subsequently shown to be mutated in other affected individuals (Table 9.8). The probable explanation is that the breakpoint has separated the coding part of the gene from contiguous regulatory elements, similar to the scenario discussed in relation to SHFM type 1 (see Fig. 9.2).

Hydatidiform Moles

Occasionally conception results in an abnormal pregnancy in which the placenta consists of a proliferating disorganized mass known as a hydatidiform mole. These changes can be either partial or complete (Table 9.9).

Partial Hydatidiform Mole

Chromosome analysis of tissue from partial moles reveals the presence of 69 chromosomes—that is, triploidy (p. 253). Using DNA polymorphisms, it has been shown that 46 of these chromosomes are always derived from the father, with the remaining 23 being maternal in origin. This doubling of the normal haploid paternal contribution of 23 chromosomes can be caused by either fertilization by two sperm, which is known as **dispermy**, or to duplication of a haploid sperm chromosome set by a process known as **endoreduplication**.

In these pregnancies the fetus rarely, if ever, survives to term. Triploid conceptions survive to term only when the additional chromosome complement is maternally derived, in which case partial hydatidiform changes do not occur. Even in these situations, it is extremely uncommon for a triploid infant to survive for more than a few hours or days after birth.

Complete Hydatidiform Mole

Complete moles have only 46 chromosomes, but these are exclusively paternal in origin. A complete mole is caused by fertilization of an empty ovum either by two sperm or by a single sperm that undergoes endoreduplication. The opposite situation of an egg undergoing development without being fertilized by a sperm, a process known as parthenogenesis, occurs in lower animals such as arthropods but has been reported in a human, this being in the form of chimeric fusion with another cell line that had a normal male-derived complement.

The main importance of complete moles lies in their potential to undergo malignant change into invasive choriocarcinoma. This can usually be treated successfully by chemotherapy, but if untreated the outcome can be fatal. Malignant change is seen only very rarely with partial moles.

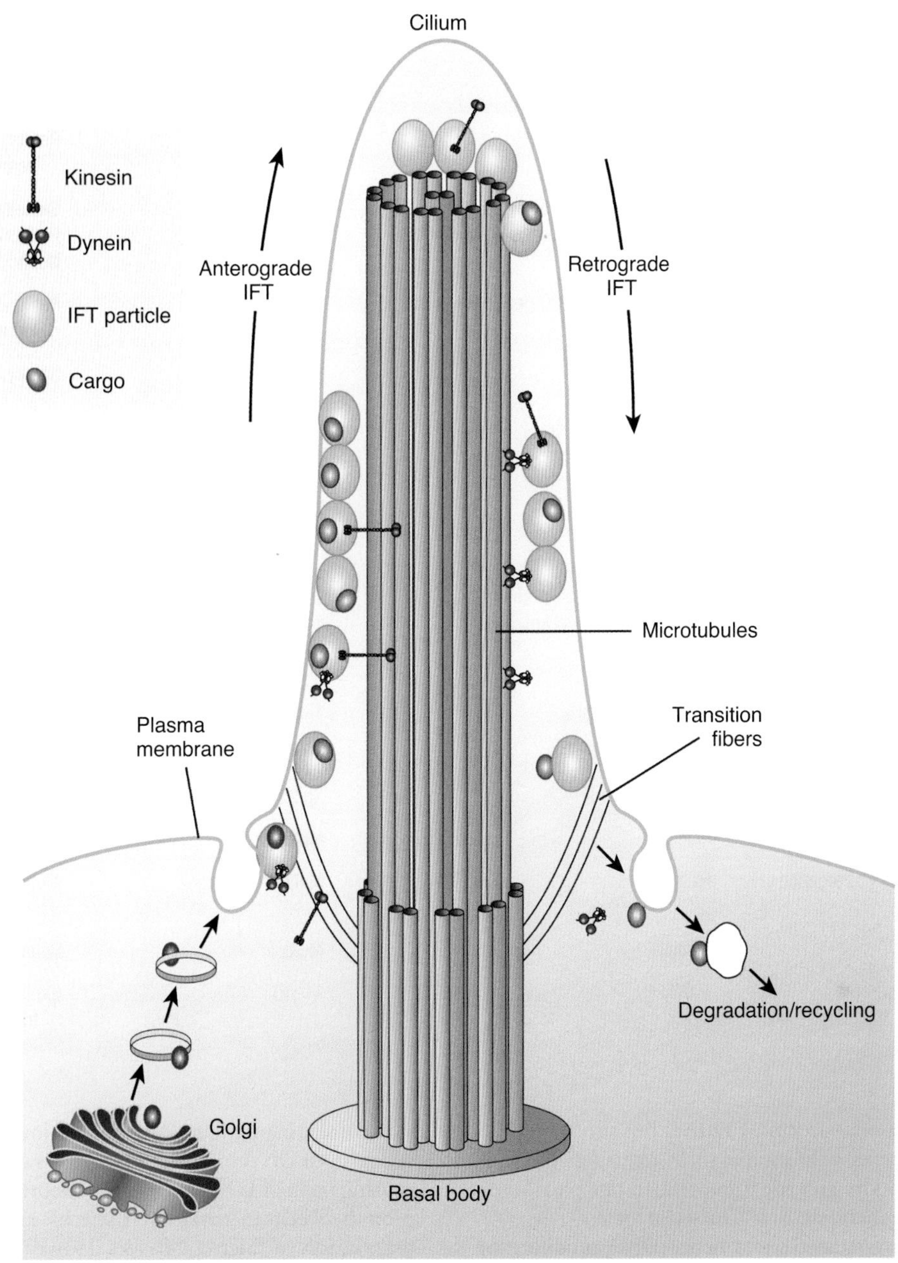

• **Fig. 9.24** The structure of a cilium. Nine microtubule doublets provide the main scaffold and surround one microtubule doublet in the centre. *IFT*, Intraflagellar transport.

Different Parental Expression in Trophoblasts and Embryoblasts

Studies in mice have shown that, when all nuclear genes in a zygote are derived from the father, the embryo fails to develop, whereas trophoblast development proceeds relatively unimpaired. In contrast, if all of the nuclear genes are maternal in origin, the embryo develops normally, but extraembryonic development is poor. The observations outlined previously on partial and complete moles indicate that a comparable situation exists in humans, with paternally derived genes being essential for trophoblast development and maternally derived genes being necessary for early embryonic development. These phenomena are relevant to the concept of epigenetics.

Epigenetics and Development

The concept of "epigenetics" is not recent. Epigenesis was first mooted as a theme by Conrad Waddington in 1942 and referred, in essence, to the unfolding of developmental programs and processes from an undifferentiated zygote—the very heart of embryonic development. This roughly equates with our modern understanding of the control of developmental gene expression and signaling pathways. It incorporated the concept of molecular mechanisms being "wiped clean" and "reset" at some point in the life cycle, as mentioned earlier. Although this is still valid, the term in current usage is extended to include heritable changes to gene expression that are not caused by sequence variation in the genetic code. Such gene expression states may be transmitted

TABLE 9.6 **The human ciliopathies: diseases of development known to be caused by defective cilia**

Disease/Syndrome	Gene	Chromosome Locus	Body System(s) Affected
Alstrom syndrome	*ALMS1*	2p13	Retina, adipose, endocrine, heart
Jeune asphyxiating thoracic dystrophy (or short-rib thoracic dystrophy, SRTD)	SRTD1 mapped to 15q31, *IFT80* (SRTD2), and another 18 genes up to SRTD20	Multiple	Skeleton Periportal fibrosis Nephritis
Bardet-Biedl syndrome	*BBS1* and another 20 genes up to BBS type 21	Multiple	Multisystem, including retina, kidney, skeleton
Cranioectodermal dysplasia (Sensenbrenner syndrome)	*IFT122*	3q21.3	Kidney, liver
	WDR35	2p24.1	
	IFT43	14q24.3	
	WDR19	4p14	
Ellis–van Crefeld syndrome	*EVC1, EVC2*	4p16	Skeleton, heart
Joubert syndrome	*JBTS1* (+ others)	9q34.3	Brain
Leber congenital amaurosis	*GUCY2D, RPE65* (+ others)	17p13, 11p31 (+ others)	Retina
McKusick-Kaufman syndrome	*BBS6*	20p12	Limb, heart, urogenital tract
Meckel-Gruber syndrome	*MKS1* (+ others)	17q23 (+ others)	Brain, kidney, liver
Nephronophthisis (types 1–4)	*NPHP1* (+ others)	Multiple	Kidney
Oro-facio-digital syndrome type 1	*OFD1* (+ others)	Xp.22 (+ others)	Skeleton (limb, face)
Polycystic kidney disease	Multiple	Multiple	Kidney
Primary ciliary dyskinesia (Kartegener syndrome)	Multiple	Multiple	Multisystem
Senior-Loken syndrome	Multiple	Multiple	Retina, kidney
Short-rib polydactyly syndrome	*DYNC2H1*	11q13	Skeleton, kidney, urogenital tract

stably through cell divisions—certainly mitosis but also sometimes meiosis (thereby not necessarily subject to a "resetting" process). One genotype can therefore give rise to more than one phenotype, depending on the "epigenetic state" of a locus, or loci.

The mechanism for epigenesis, and hence DNA modification with the consequence of downstream influences on gene regulation, is usually the biochemical, covalent **methylation** of CpG nucleotides. This appears to lead to a series of steps that alters local chromatin structure. In human genetics the best recognized epigenetic phenomena are X-chromosome inactivation (initiated by the *XIST* gene), described later, and parent-of-origin specific gene expression (parental imprinting), which is realized when errors occur to give rise to Prader-Willi and Angelman syndromes (pp. 78–79) and Beckwith-Wiedemann and Russell-Silver syndromes (pp. 80–81).

There is much interest, however, in the possibility that epigenetic states can be influenced by environmental factors *in utero*, such as maternal obesity and type 2 diabetes mellitus, as well as ingested toxins. In animal studies there is evidence that the nutritional and behavioral environment may lead to different "epialleles," and in human populations epidemiological studies have shown convincing correlations of maternal (and in some cases grandparental) nutritional status with late-onset cardiovascular and metabolic-endocrine disease. Some of this evidence has come from correlating periconceptional famine exposure, where reliable data exist, to DNA methylation patterns 60 years later. Other studies using banked DNA from birth cohorts have found some correlation between methylation patterns and subsequent body fat composition in later childhood. However, there is still much to learn about the causal mechanisms.

X-Chromosome Inactivation

As techniques were developed for studying chromosomes, it was noted that in female mice one of the X chromosomes often differed from all other chromosomes in the extent to which it was condensed. In 1961 Dr Mary Lyon proposed that this heteropyknotic X chromosome was inactivated, citing as evidence her observations on the mosaic pattern of skin coloration seen in mice known to be heterozygous for X-linked genes that influence coat color. Subsequent events have confirmed the validity of Lyon's hypothesis, and in recognition of her foresight the process of X-chromosome inactivation (XCI) is often referred to as **lyonization.**

The process of XCI probably begins at the earliest stages of embryogenesis, as it has been shown that *XIST* RNA progressively accumulates on one of the two X chromosomes in female preimplantation embryos, starting around the 8-cell stage. Either of the

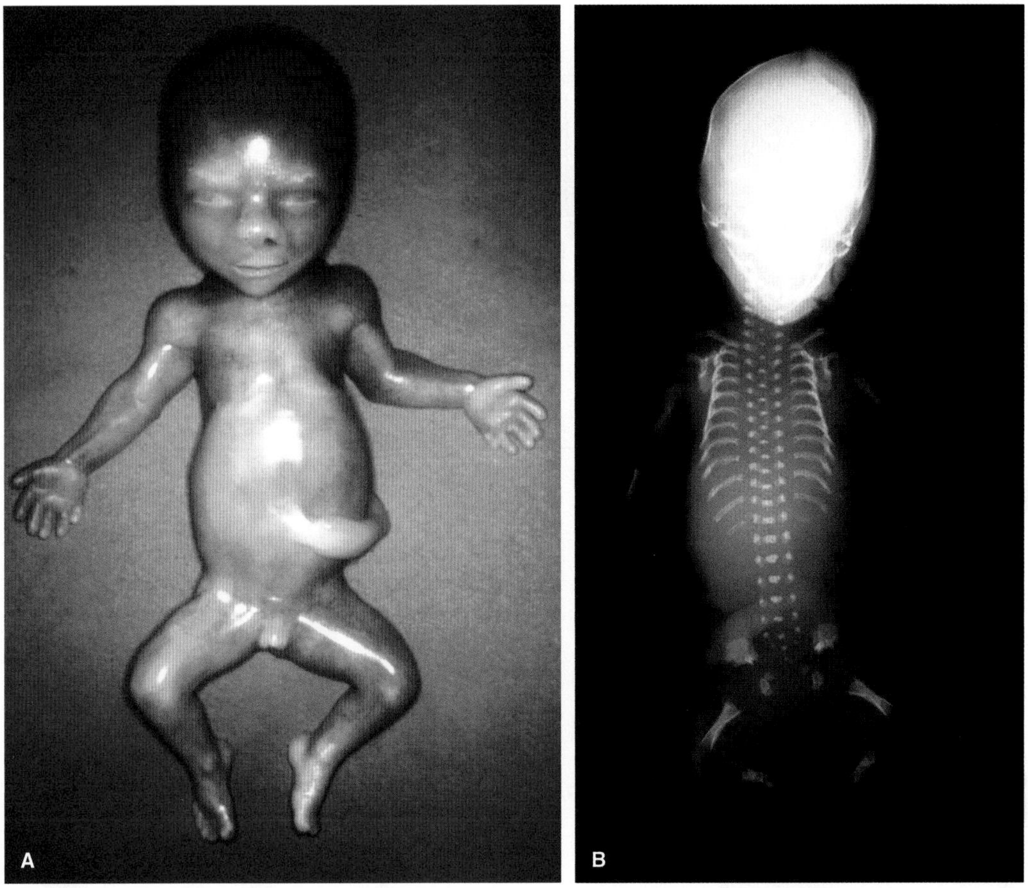

• **Fig. 9.25** Short-rib polydactyly syndrome (also known as short-rib thoracic dysplasia). (A) The chest of the fetus is narrow, and postaxial polydactyly affects all four limbs. (B) As seen in this x-ray, the ribs of the fetus are very short.

two X chromosomes can be inactivated in any particular cell, and thereafter the same X chromosome is inactivated in all daughter cells (Fig. 9.28). This differs from marsupials, where the paternally derived X chromosome is consistently inactivated.

The inactive X chromosome exists in a condensed form during interphase when it appears as a darkly staining mass of "sex chromatin," or Barr body (p. 32). In men and women with more than one X chromosome, the number of Barr bodies visible at interphase is always one less than the total number of X chromosomes. Thus, men with Klinefelter syndrome (p. 254) (47,XXY) have a single Barr body, whereas women with a 47,XXX karyotype (p. 255) have two.

During mitosis the inactive X chromosome is late replicating. Laboratory techniques can distinguish which X is late replicating in each cell. This may be useful for identifying structurally abnormal X chromosomes because they are usually preferentially inactivated—or, more correctly, only those hematopoietic stem cells in which the normal X chromosome is active will have survived. Such apparent non-random XCI is usual when one X is involved in a translocation with an autosome (p. 74).

The epigenetic process of XCI is achieved by differential methylation, initiated by the gene *XIST* at Xq13.3. *XIST* is expressed only from the inactive X chromosome and produces RNA that spreads an inactivation methylation signal in both directions along the X chromosome. This differential methylation of the X chromosomes has been used in carrier detection studies for X-linked immunodeficiency diseases (e.g., Wiskott-Aldrich syndrome) using methylation-sensitive probes (p. 181). But not all of the X chromosome is inactivated. Genes in the pseudoautosomal region (PAR) at the tip of the short arm (Fig. 9.29) remain active, as do other loci elsewhere on both long and short arms, including *XIST* itself. More genes escape XCI in Xp (PAR1) compared with Xq (PAR2), which probably explains why more severe phenotypic effects are seen in women with small Xp deletions compared with women with small deletions in Xq. If all loci on the X chromosome were inactivated, then all women would have Turner syndrome, and more than one X in a male (e.g., 47,XXY), or two in a female (e.g., 47,XXX), would have no phenotypic effects. In fact, these disorders have characteristic clinical features (see Chapter 17).

Dosage Compensation and X-Linked Disorders Involving the PAR

For most X-chromosome genes the levels of their protein products are equivalent between the sexes by virtue of XCI in women, for example the blood clotting Factor VIII which is implicated in hemophilia A. However, the level of steroid sulfatase in blood, encoded by the *STS* gene, is increased in women compared with men, and this is attributed to the fact that it escapes XCI, and two copies are therefore expressed. Deficiency of steroid sulfatase caused either by a mutation in *STS* or a microdeletion causes the skin disorder X-linked ichthyosis.

Within the PAR1 itself, the only known gene with a clear role in human development, giving rise to a recognizable phenotype when mutated, is *SHOX* (short stature homeobox; see Fig. 9.29).

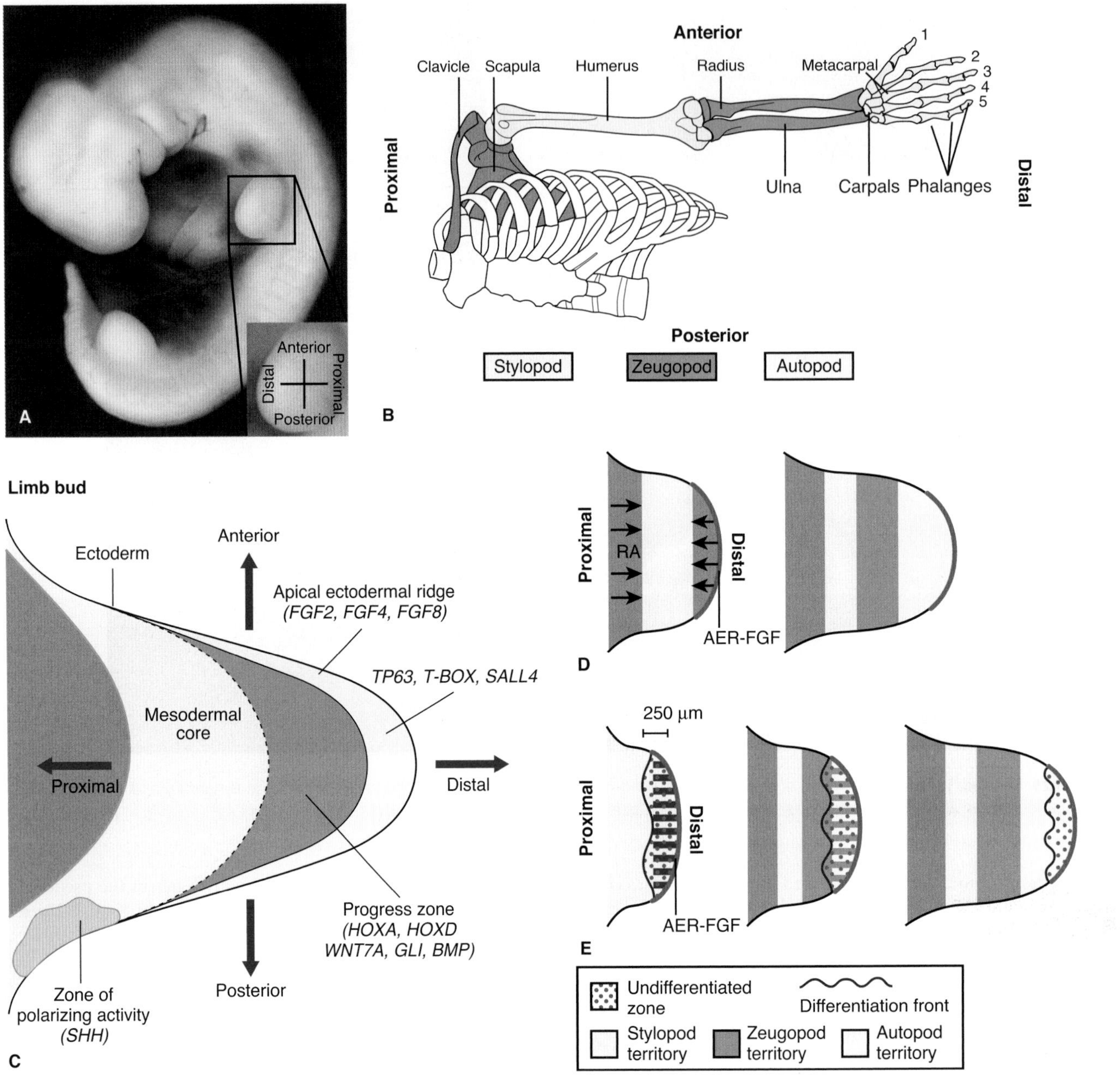

• **Fig. 9.26** Simplified representation of vertebrate limb development. (A) The emerging limb bud in a vertebrate embryo, with axes defined. (B) Diagram of the human upper limb skeleton; the colors of the component parts corresponding to the regions depicted in (C), (D), and (E). (C) The various developmental regions of the limb bud, with the expression regions of key genes highlighted. (D), (E) The role of retinoic acid and FGF in determining segmental regions within the limb bud.

Mutations in, or deletions of, the gene cause either Leri-Weill dyschondrosteosis with mesomelic limb shortening and Madelung deformity, or non-syndromic short stature. Deletions may also occur outside the gene itself, affecting the *SHOX* gene regulatory elements. Importantly in genetic counseling, the inheritance pattern behaves like autosomal dominant rather than X-linked.

X-Chromosome Mosaicism

Mice that are heterozygous for X-linked genes affecting coat color show mosaicism with alternating patches of different color rather than a homogeneous pattern. This is consistent with patches of skin being clonal in origin, in that they are derived from a single stem cell in which one or other of the X chromosomes is expressed, but not both. Thus, each skin patch reflects which of the X chromosomes was active in the original stem cell. Similar effects are seen in tissues of clonal origin in women who are heterozygous for X-linked mutations, such as ocular albinism (see Fig. 11.1, p. 152) and incontinentia pigmenti (see Fig. 6.18, p. 75).

Carrier detection for X-linked recessive disorders based only on examination of clinical features, or on biochemical assay of the gene product in Fabry disease or X-linked adrenoleukodystrophy, for example, is unreliable (see Chapter 18). Today, DNA sequencing methods usually resolve carrier status, but previously molecular methods using PCR primers that distinguish the products of methylated and unmethylated DNA were used, assuming there had been selection against the cell line in which the mutant-bearing

TABLE 9.7 Genes that can cause both developmental anomalies and cancer

Gene	Chromosome	Developmental Anomaly	Cancer
PAX3	2q35	Waardenburg syndrome type 1	Alveolar rhabdomyosarcoma
KIT	4q12	Piebaldism	Mast cell leukemia
PTCH	9q22	Gorlin syndrome	Basal cell carcinoma
RET	10p11	Hirschsprung disease	MEN2A, MEN2B, medullary thyroid carcinoma
WT1	11p13	Denys-Drash syndrome	Wilms' tumor

MEN, Multiple endocrine neoplasia.

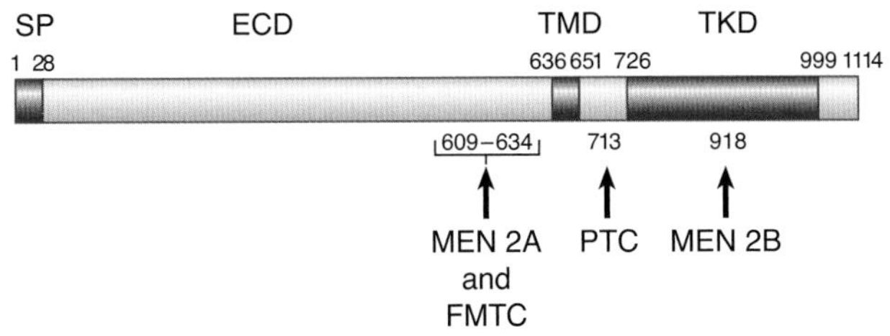

• **Fig. 9.27** The *RET* proto-oncogene. The most common mutation sites in the different clinical entities associated with *RET* are indicated. Numbers refer to amino-acid residues. *SP*, Signal peptide; *ECD*, extracellular domain; *TMD*, transmembrane domain; *TKD*, tyrosine kinase domain; *MEN*, multiple endocrine adenomatosis; *FMTC*, familial medullary thyroid carcinoma. The arrow above *PTC* (papillary thyroid carcinoma) indicates the somatic rearrangement site for the formation of new hybrid forms of *RET*. (Modified from Pasini B, Ceccherini I, Romeo G. RET mutations in human disease. *Trends Genet*. 1996;12:138–144.)

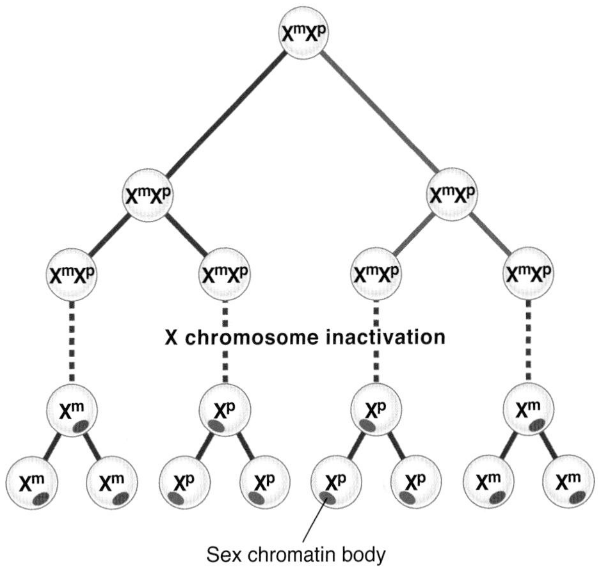

• **Fig. 9.28** X-chromosome inactivation during development. The maternally and paternally derived X chromosomes are represented as X^m and X^p, respectively.

TABLE 9.8 Developmental genes that show a position effect

Gene	Chromosome	Developmental Anomaly
GLI3	7p13	Greig cephalopolysyndactyly
SHH	7q36	Holoprosencephaly
PAX6	11p13	Aniridia
SOX9	17q24	Campomelic dysplasia

TABLE 9.9 Characteristics of partial and complete hydatidiform moles

	Partial Mole	Complete Mole
No. of chromosomes	69	46
Parental origin of chromosomes	23 maternal 46 paternal	All 46 paternal
Fetus present	Yes, but not viable	No
Malignant potential	Very low	High

X chromosome was active (Fig. 9.30). Some female carriers of X-linked recessive conditions manifest clear features of the disorder, and this is most likely to be caused by skewed X-inactivation (p. 73).

It also appears that XCI is not necessarily an all-or-none phenomenon for every gene. In a study of skin fibroblasts, which express more than 600 of the 1098 genes identified on the X chromosome, approximately 20% were found to be inactivated in some but not all samples. Approximately 15% escaped XCI completely, whereas only 65% were fully silenced, and thus expressed in one dose. In addition to non-random, or skewed, XCI, the variable dosage of genes that escape XCI may account for variation among normal females as well as those who are heterozygous for X-linked recessive disease genes.

Sex Determination and Disorders of Sex Development

The determination of gender is a crucial aspect of physical development, as well as procreation and the survival of our species, but

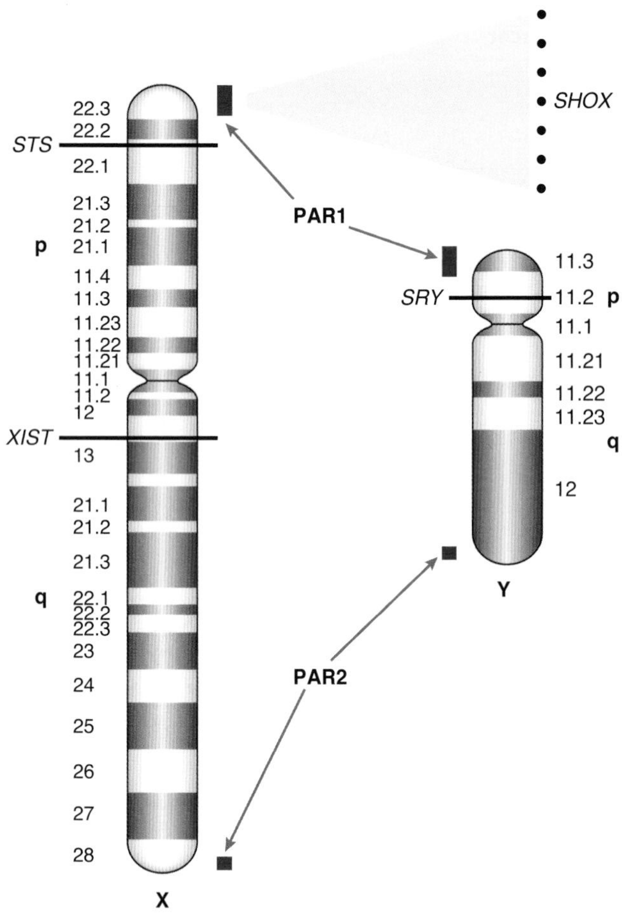

• **Fig. 9.29** The X and Y chromosomes showing the pseudoautosomal regions, PAR1 and PAR2, at the tips of Xp-Yp and Xq-Yq, respectively, and the relative positions of the *XIST*, *SRY*, *STS*, and *SHOX* genes, referred to in the text.

when it goes wrong, the impact may be extremely challenging for the parents and family as well as the affected child, with lifelong emotional and psychological consequences. In many societies serious cultural taboos are associated with the birth of a child whose gender is indeterminate. The term Disorders of Sex Development (DSD) is now preferred to cover congenital conditions in which chromosomal, gonadal, or anatomical sex is atypical, and terms such as "intersex" and "pseudohermaphrodite" are considered anachronistic and derogatory, and are therefore strongly discouraged. In a clinical setting, good management of each case requires expert input from the disciplines of endocrinology, genetics, surgery and psychology, as well as radiology and laboratory science.

Normal Development

In man the default developmental pathway is, in fact, woman! The presence of an intact Y chromosome is essential for male development regardless of the number of X chromosomes present, and absence of a functioning Y chromosome results in female development.

Although the sex chromosomes are present from conception, differentiation into a phenotypic male or female does not commence until approximately 6 weeks. Up to this point both the Müllerian and Wolffian duct systems are present, and the embryonic gonads, although consisting of cortex and medulla, are still undifferentiated (Fig. 9.31). From 6 weeks onwards, the embryo develops into a female unless the "testis-determining factor"—encoded by the *SRY* gene—initiates a sequence of events that prompt the undifferentiated gonads to develop into testes (Fig. 9.32).

The SRY *Gene*

In 1990 it was shown that the *SRY* gene is located on chromosome Yp close to the pseudoautosomal region (see Fig. 9.29) and derives its name from being in the "**s**ex-determining **r**egion" of the **Y** chromosome. It consists of a single exon that encodes a protein of 204 amino acids, including a 79–amino acid DNA-binding HMG motif (p. 113), indicating its role as a transcription factor. Evidence that the *SRY* gene determines *gonadal* and *anatomic* (but not necessarily chromosomal) maleness is given in Box 9.2.

From a biological fitness viewpoint (i.e., maintenance of the species), it would clearly be impossible for the *SRY* gene to be involved in crossing over with the X chromosome during meiosis I. Hence *SRY* has to lie outside the pseudoautosomal region. However, there has to be pairing of X and Y chromosomes because otherwise they would segregate together into the same gamete during, on average, 50% of meioses. Nature's compromise has been to ensure that only small regions of the X and Y are homologous, and therefore pair during meiosis I. Unfortunately, the close proximity of *SRY* to the pseudoautosomal region means that occasionally it is caught up in a recombination event (see Fig. 9.29). This appears to account for approximately 80% of XX males, in whom molecular and fluorescence *in situ* hybridization studies have shown evidence of Y-chromosome sequences at the distal end of one X-chromosome short arm (Fig. 9.33).

Expression of *SRY* triggers a series of events that involves inhibition of an upstream repressor of *SOX9* (17q24), allowing the latter to be upregulated to stimulate the medulla of the undifferentiated gonad to develop into a testis and for pre-Sertoli cells to become Sertoli cells. Concomitantly, and by the end of week 9, interstitial cells derived from mesenchyme give rise to steroid-secreting Leydig cells and the production of testosterone (Fig. 9.34). This leads to stimulation of the Wolffian ducts and formation of male internal genitalia, as well as masculinization of the external genitalia. This latter step is mediated by dihydrotestosterone, produced from testosterone by the action of 5α-reductase (Fig. 18.6, p. 278). The Sertoli cells produce anti-Müllerian hormone, also known as Müllerian inhibitory factor, which causes the Müllerian duct system to regress. In campomelic dysplasia (see Fig. 9.17), resulting from mutated *SOX9*, sex reversal occurs in cases with a 46,XY karyotype, (i.e., the child appears to be female). Sex reversal is also frequent in cases of deletion 9p24.3 syndrome, probably caused by haploinsufficiency for the *DMRT1* gene, which encodes a transcriptional regulator expressed in Sertoli cells, spermatogonia and spermatocytes.

In the absence of normal *SRY* expression, the cortex of the undifferentiated gonad develops into an ovary. The Müllerian duct forms the internal female genitalia. The external genitalia fail to fuse and instead evolve into normal female external genitalia. Without the stimulating effects of testosterone, the Wolffian duct system regresses.

Members of the Wnt family of developmental signaling molecules are also important in gonadal differentiation. WNT4 is expressed in the developing mesonephros and activates *DAX1*. It is downregulated in the testis by SRY but persists in the ovary, and is expressed in the Müllerian ducts but is absent from Wolffian ducts.

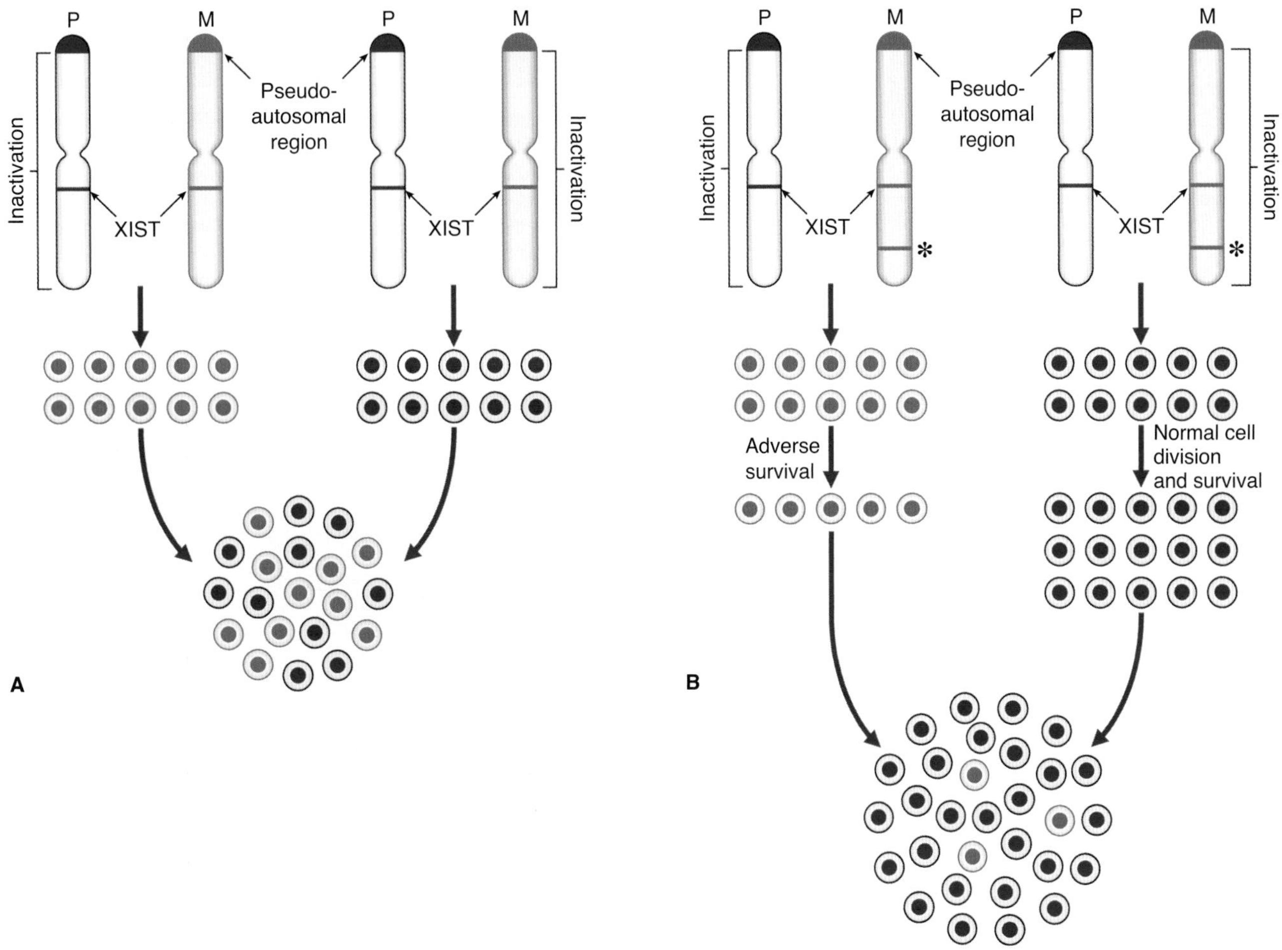

• **Fig. 9.30** (A) Normal X-chromosome inactivation resulting in survival of roughly equal numbers of cells with the paternally (*P*) and maternally (*M*) derived X chromosome active. (B) In this situation the maternally derived X chromosome has a mutation (*) that results in selection against the cells in which it is active. Thus surviving cells show preferential expression of the paternally derived X chromosome.

Disruption of WNT4 in females results in masculinized ovaries, production of androgens from Leydig-like cells, and is a rare cause of Müllerian aplasia. Another member of the family, *WNT7A*, is needed to complete development of Müllerian ducts into the internal female genital tract.

Normally, sexual differentiation is complete by 12 to 14 weeks' gestation, although the testes do not migrate into the scrotum until late pregnancy (see Fig. 9.32).

Abnormalities of sexual differentiation are uncommon, but they are important causes of infertility and sexual ambiguity, and their management involves multidisciplinary teams. We now turn our attention to an overview of the various DSDs, although sex chromosome aneuploidy conditions are described in Chapter 17, and congenital adrenal hyperplasia is covered in Chapter 18.

Classification of Disorders of Sex Development

This is a complex area and dissatisfaction with existing classifications led to a major multidisciplinary and far-ranging international review of DSDs, with the establishment of a new system known as the Chicago Consensus in 2006. However, this remains a "work in progress," as a definitive diagnosis is not always reached, and there is more to be discovered in the molecular pathways of sexual differentiation. Around 80 genes, for example, are now known to have a role in male infertility, so there is much to be unraveled. The main proposals for changes in nomenclature are shown in Table 9.10. Apart from the sex chromosome aneuploidies the starting point for the classification is the chromosomal sex, and an outline diagnostic tree or algorithm is shown in Fig. 9.35.

46,XY Disorders of Sex Development

In the current classification the causes of XY DSDs are shown in Box 9.3. This is the largest group of DSDs, but the likelihood of reaching a definitive genetic diagnosis is lower than in the XX DSD group. No more than 15% of cases of complete gonadal dysgenesis are caused by *SRY* gene defects, so other genes are implicated, including *SF1*, also known as *NR5A1*, which encodes the protein steroidogenic factor 1. Some are implicated in various syndromes, such as *SOX9* in campomelic dysplasia (see Fig. 9.17).

Androgen Insensitivity Syndrome. Overall, resistance to the action of androgens is the most common cause of XY DSD, with complete androgen insensitivity syndrome (CAIS) being the classic condition. This usually results from mutations in the androgen receptor (*AR*) gene on the X-chromosome but can be secondary to

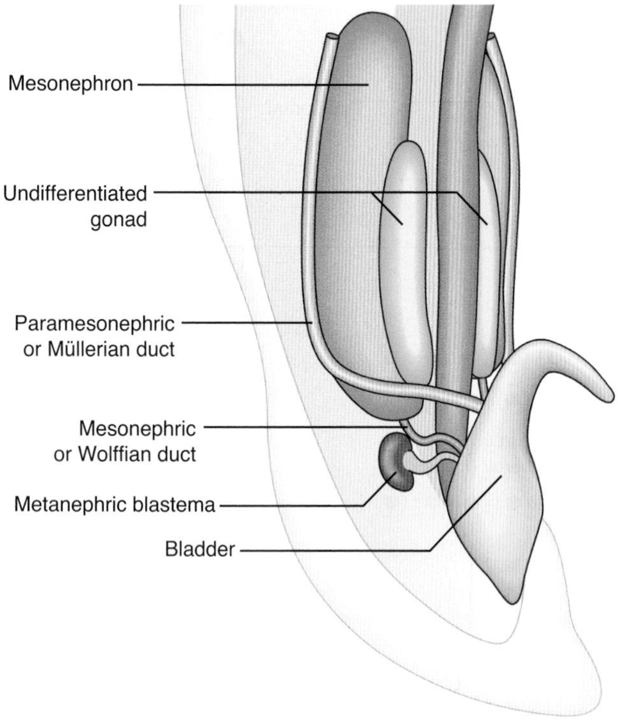

• **Fig. 9.31** Both male and female genital ducts are present in the embryo at the end of 6 weeks' gestation, derived from the mesonephrons. Anatomical sex has the potential to differentiate either way.

abnormalities of AR intracellular transport, which is dependent on a number of coregulator proteins. Partial AIS, where incomplete undermasculinization occurs, is only occasionally caused by variants in the *AR* gene, and in many cases the cause currently remains undetermined. Individuals with CAIS have female external genitalia and develop breasts at puberty, but the uterus and Fallopian tubes are absent. They often present with primary amenorrhea, although in girls with inguinal hernia, especially if bilateral, the diagnosis should be considered. Androgen production by the testes is normal, but it is ineffective because the receptor is nonfunctional. Testicular tissue must be removed because of the risk of malignancy.

• BOX 9.2 Evidence That the *SRY* Gene Determines Gonadal and Anatomic Maleness

- *SRY* sequences are present in approximately 80% of 46,XX individuals, who are infertile phenotypic males.
- Up to 20% of infertile phenotypic females with a 46,XY karyotype have mutations or deletions in *SRY*.
- In mice, the *Sry* gene is expressed only in the male gonadal ridge as testes are developing in the embryo.
- Transgenic XX mice with tiny portions of Y chromosome containing the *Sry* region develop into males with testes.

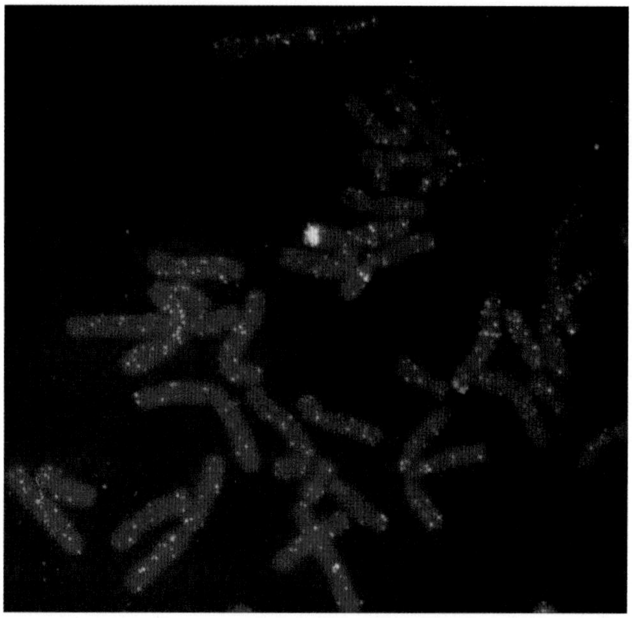

• **Fig. 9.33** Fluorescence *in situ* hybridization showing hybridization of a Y chromosome paint to the short arm of an X chromosome in a 46,XX male. (Courtesy Nigel Smith, City Hospital, Nottingham, UK.)

46,XX Disorders of Sex Development

The causes of XX DSDs are shown in Box 9.4. Congenital adrenal hyperplasia is the most common form of XX DSD, caused by

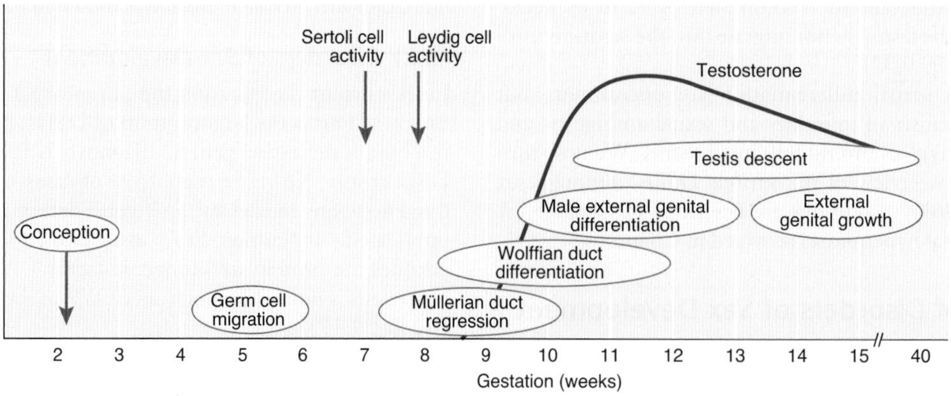

• **Fig. 9.32** The timing of embryological events in male sex differentiation. At approximately 6–7 weeks' gestation the first sign of testis determination is seen with the aggregation of pre-Sertoli cells to form primary sex cords. Steroid-secreting Leydig cells emerge from differentiation of interstitial cells by the end of week 9, which secrete anti-Müllerian hormone to cause Müllerian duct regression. Testosterone levels rise in fetal serum to approach concentrations close to the lower end of the adult male range.

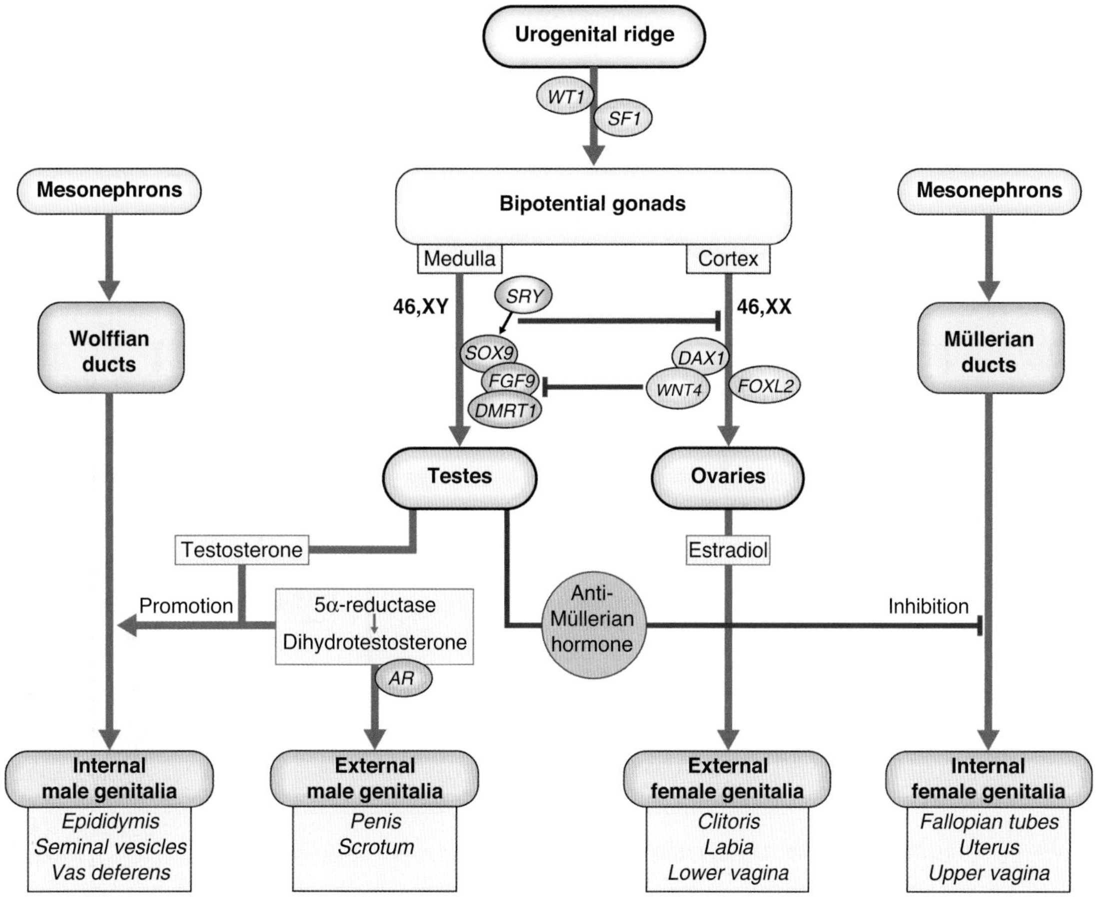

• **Fig. 9.34** A simplified scheme of the main genetic and hormonal events of sex determination. *SRY* is crucial to driving testis development, whereas *WNT4* and *FOXL2* are important for ovarian development. The promotion of either male or female gonads is accompanied by inhibition of the pathways in the alternative gonad. *DAX1* has a positive role in testis development, but overexpression inhibits testis formation, and WNT4 upregulates *DAX1* to assist this inhibition.

TABLE 9.10 Nomenclature relating to disorders of sex development

Previous	Proposed
Intersex	Disorders of sex development (DSDs)
Male pseudohermaphrodite	46,XY DSD
Undervirilization of an XY male	
Female pseudohermaphrodite	46,XX DSD
Overvirilization of an XX female	
Masculinization of an XX female	
True hermaphrodite	Ovotesticular DSD
XX male or XX sex reversal	46,XX testicular DSD
XY sex reversal	46,XY complete gonadal dysgenesis

defects in steroidogenesis leading to excess androgens in the developing female fetus. This is covered in detail in Chapter 18 (p. 277). Also within this group are those cases caused by mutations in the cytochrome P450 oxidoreductase (*POR*) gene (also implicated in some cases of the rare Antley-Bixler syndrome) and aromatase deficiency.

A normal male phenotype occurs in 46,XX DSD where Wolffian structures (testes) are present and Müllerian structures absent, and these patients are often diagnosed when a karyotype analysis is undertaken for infertility. Approximately 80% to 90% of these patients have Y chromosomal material, including a translocated *SRY* gene, which is only rarely detected in 46,XX DSD where testicular structures alone (and sometimes ovarian structures—"ovotestis") are present. Such "dysgenetic" gonads are often at risk of later gonadoblastoma, and in many DSDs prophylactic gonadectomy is recommended when this tissue has been located.

Twinning

Twinning occurs frequently in humans, although the incidence in early pregnancy as diagnosed by ultrasonography is greater than at delivery, presumably as a result of death and subsequent resorption of one of the twins in a proportion of twin pregnancies. The overall incidence of twinning in the United Kingdom is approximately 1 in 80 of all pregnancies, so that approximately 1 in 40 (i.e., 2 of 80) of all individuals is a twin. However, the spontaneous twinning rate varies enormously, from approximately 1 in 125 pregnancies in Japan to 1 in 22 in Nigeria.

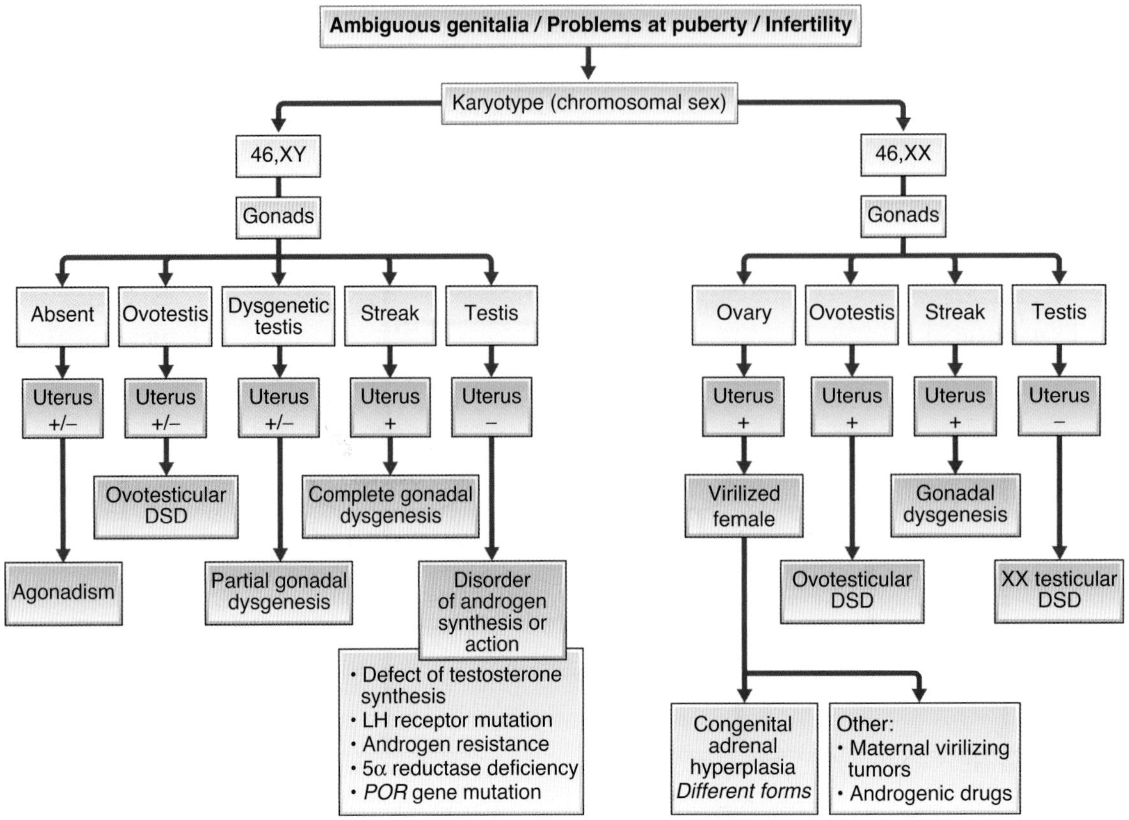

• **Fig. 9.35** A disorders of sex development (*DSD*) diagnostic tree or algorithm.

• BOX 9.3 Causes of 46,XY Disorders of Sex Development

A: Disorders of gonadal (testicular) development

1. Complete or partial gonadal dysgenesis (e.g., *SRY, SOX9, SF1, WT1, DHH*, etc.)
2. Ovotesticular disorder of sex development
3. Testis regression

B: Disorders in androgen synthesis or action

1. **Disorders of androgen synthesis**
   LH receptor mutations
   Smith-Lemli-Opitz syndrome
   Steroidogenic acute regulatory protein mutations
   Cholesterol side-chain cleavage (*CYP11A1*)
   3β-hydroxysteroid dehydrogenase 2 (*HSD3B2*)
   17α-hydroxylase/17,20-lyase (*CYP17*)
   P450 oxidoreductase (*POR*)
   17β-hydroxysteroid dehydrogenase (*HSD17B3*)
   5α-reductase 2 (*SRD5A2*)
2. **Disorders of androgen action**
   Androgen insensitivity syndrome (*AR* gene)
   Drugs and environmental modulators

C: Other

1. Syndromic associations of male genital development, e.g., cloacal anomalies
2. Persistent Müllerian duct syndrome
3. Vanishing testis syndrome
4. Isolated hypospadias (*CXorf6*)
5. Congenital hypogonadotropic hypogonadism
6. Cryptorchidism (*INSL3, LGR8*)
7. Environmental influences

Twins can be identical or non-identical—that is, **monozygotic** (MZ) (uniovular) or **dizygotic** (DZ) (biovular)—depending on whether they originate from a single conception or from two separate conceptions (Table 9.11). Comparison of the incidence of disease in MZ and DZ twins reared apart and together can provide information about the relative contributions of genetics and the environment to the cause of many of the common diseases of adult life (p. 137), including cancer, diabetes, mental health, and behavior.

Monozygotic Twins

MZ twinning occurs, fairly consistently, in approximately 1 in 300 births in all populations that have been studied. MZ twins originate from a single egg that has been fertilized by a single sperm. A very early division, occurring in the zygote before separation of the cells that make the chorion, results in dichorionic twins. Division during the blastocyst stage from days 3 to 7 results in monochorionic diamniotic twins. Division after the first week leads to monoamniotic twins. However, the reason(s) why MZ twinning occurs at all in humans is not clear. As an event, the incidence is increased two- to fivefold in babies born by *in vitro* fertilization. There are rare cases of familial MZ twinning that can be transmitted by the father or mother, suggesting a single-gene defect that predisposes to the phenomenon.

There is a tendency to think of MZ twins as being genetically identical, and basically this is of course true. However, they can be discordant for structural birth defects that may be linked to the twinning process itself—especially those anomalies affecting midline structures. There is probably a two- to threefold increased

• BOX 9.4 Causes of 46,XX Disorders of Sex Development

A: Disorders of gonadal (ovarian) development

1. Gonadal dysgenesis
2. Ovotesticular disorder of sex development (DSD)
3. Testicular DSD (e.g., *SRY*, dup *SOX9*, *RSPO1*)

B: Androgen excess

1. **Fetal (different forms of congenital adrenal hyperplasia)**
   3β-hydroxysteroid dehydrogenase 2 (*HSD3B2*)
   21-hydroxylase (*CYP21A2*)
   P450 oxidoreductase (*POR*)
   11β-hydroxylase (*CYP11B1*)
   Glucocorticoid receptor mutations
2. **Fetoplacental**
   Aromatase (*CYP19*) deficiency
   Oxidoreductase (*POR*) deficiency
3. **Maternal**
   Maternal virilising tumors (e.g., luteomas)
   Androgenic drugs

C: Other

1. Syndromic associations (e.g., cloacal anomalies)
2. Müllerian agenesis/hypoplasia, (e.g., MURCS)
3. Uterine abnormalities (e.g., MODY5—*HNF1B*)
4. Vaginal atresias (e.g., McKusick-Kaufman)
5. Labial adhesions

TABLE 9.11 Summary of differences between monozygotic and dizygotic twins

	Monozygotic	Dizygotic
Origin	Single egg fertilized	Two eggs, each fertilized by a single sperm
Incidence	1 in 300 pregnancies	Varies from 1 in 100 to 1 in 500 pregnancies
Proportion of genes in common	100%	50% (on average)
Fetal membranes	70% monochorionic and diamniotic; 30% dichorionic and diamniotic; rarely monochorionic and monoamniotic	Always dichorionic and diamniotic

risk of congenital anomalies in MZ twins (i.e., 5%–10% of MZ twins overall). Discordance for single-gene traits or chromosome abnormalities may occur because of a postzygotic somatic mutation or nondisjunction, respectively. One example of the latter is the very rare occurrence of MZ twins of different sex: one 46,XY and the other 45,X. Curiously, MZ female twins can show quite striking discrepancy in X-chromosome inactivation. There are several reports of female MZ twin pairs of which only one is affected by an X-linked recessive condition such as DMD or hemophilia A. In these rare examples, both twins have the mutation and both show non-random X-inactivation, but in opposite directions.

MZ twins have traditionally provided ideal research material for the study of genetic versus environmental influences. In a study of 40 pairs of MZ twins, geneticists measured levels of two epigenetic modifications, DNA methylation and histone acetylation. Two-thirds of the twin pairs had essentially identical profiles, but significant differences were observed in the remaining third. These differences were broadly correlated with the age of the twins, the amount of time spent apart and the differences in their medical histories, suggesting a cumulative effect on DNA modification over time. It also suggests a possible causal link between epigenetic modification and susceptibility to disease for which MZ twins may be discordant.

Very late division occurring more than 14 days after conception can result in conjoined twins. This occurs in about 1 in 100,000 pregnancies, or approximately 1 in 400 MZ twin births. Conjoined twins are sometimes referred to as Siamese, in memory of Chang and Eng, who were born in 1811 in Thailand (then known as Siam). They were joined at the upper abdomen and made a successful living as celebrities at traveling shows in the United States, where they settled and married. They both managed to have large numbers of children and died within a few hours of each other at age 61.

The sex ratio for conjoined twins is markedly distorted, with approximately 75% being female. The later the twinning event, the more distorted the sex ratio in favor of females, and it is possible that the process of X-inactivation in female zygotes predisposes to division of the embryo.

Dizygotic Twins

DZ twins result from the fertilization of two ova by two sperm and are no more closely related genetically than brothers and sisters, as they share, on average, 50% of the same genes from each parent; hence, they are sometimes referred to as **fraternal twins**. DZ twins are dichorionic and diamniotic, although they can have a single fused placenta if implantation occurs at closely adjacent sites. Unlike MZ twinning, the incidence of DZ twinning varies significantly from approximately 1 in 100 deliveries in Afro-Caribbean populations to 1 in 500 deliveries in Asia and Japan. In Europeans, the incidence is approximately 1 in 120 deliveries and has been observed to fall with both urbanization and starvation, but increase in relation to the amount of seasonal light (e.g., in northern Scandinavia during the summer). Factors that convey an increased likelihood of DZ twinning are increased maternal age, a positive family history (from a familial increase in follicle-stimulating hormone levels) and the use of ovulation-inducing drugs such as clomiphene.

Determination of Zygosity

Zygosity used to be established by study of the placenta and membranes and also by analysis of polymorphic systems such as the blood groups, the human leukocyte antigens and other biochemical markers. Now it is determined most reliably by the use of highly polymorphic molecular (DNA) markers (pp. 50–52) and single nucleotide polymorphisms.

ELEMENTS

1. The earliest stages of successful development are characterized by extensive sequential epigenetic reprogramming in the embryo, (i.e., the modification of both the paternal and maternal genomes through methylation status to control and facilitate gene expression).
2. Overall, development from zygote to fully formed human being is subject to a vast array of influences, both genetic and non-genetic, many remaining to be elucidated.
3. Developmental gene families first identified in *Drosophila* and mice also play equivalent roles in human morphogenesis. These include segment polarity genes, homeobox-containing (*HOX*) genes and paired-box containing (*PAX*) genes. Many of these genes encode transcription factors that regulate sequential developmental processes, but there is also extensive and complex interaction, giving rise to gene/protein networks. Many genes and their proteins are important in cell signaling. Many human malformations and multiple malformation syndromes are caused by mutations in these genes.
4. Many well-recognized syndromes are now known to be linked through their relationships to developmental signaling pathways (e.g., Sonic hedgehog, Notch-Delta, TGF-β, HOX, and PAX).
5. The conformational alignment and spatial relationship of a developmental gene with its promoter, enhancer, or repressor is key to normal developmental processes, particularly in the limb bud.
6. For normal development a haploid chromosome set must be inherited from each parent. A paternal diploid complement results in a complete hydatidiform mole if there is no maternal contribution, and in triploidy with a partial hydatidiform mole if there is a haploid maternal contribution.
7. The gene encoding testis-determining factor on the Y chromosome, known as *SRY*, is crucial in stimulating the undifferentiated gonads to develop into testes. This, in turn, sets off a series of events leading to male development and suppression of female gonadal development. Without *SRY* expression the anatomic gender development of the human embryo defaults to female.
8. In females one of the X chromosomes is inactivated in each cell in early embryogenesis. This can be either the maternally derived or the paternally derived X chromosome. Thereafter, in all daughter cells the same X chromosome is inactivated. This process of X-inactivation, also known as lyonization, explains the presence of the Barr body in female nuclei and achieves dosage compensation of most X-chromosome gene products in males and females.
9. Twins can be monozygotic (identical) or dizygotic (fraternal). Monozygotic twins originate from a single zygote that divides into two during the first 2 weeks after conception. Monozygotic twins are genetically identical. Dizygotic twins originate from two separate zygotes and are no more genetically alike than brothers and sisters.

CLINICAL SCENARIO 1

A 3-year-old girl is referred to you with "polydactyly in the extremities" and very little other information. The parents, reported to be unaffected, are planning to extend their family and would like genetic risk information.

Exercise: To give accurate genetic risk information, you require a precise diagnosis. What other clinical information are you going to explore to help you reach a diagnosis?

CLINICAL SCENARIO 2

A baby is born with ambiguous genitalia. A small phallus is present with features of hypospadias and no testes are palpable in either the rudimentary scrotum or inguinal canals. The baby has a good birthweight and appears normal in all other respects.

Exercise:

Describe a plan of investigation and consider the diagnostic possibilities.

Further Reading

Baker K, Beales PL. Making sense of cilia in disease: the human ciliopathies. *Am J Med Genet C Semin Med Genet.* 2009;151C: 281–295.

An overview of ciliopathy conditions.

Dequéant ML, Pourquié O. Segmental patterning of the vertebrate embryonic axis. *Nat Rev Genet.* 2008;9:370–382.

A review of the process of vertebral segmentation.

Gibb S, Maroto M, Dale JK. The segmentation clock mechanism moves up a notch. *Trends Cell Biol.* 2010;20:593–600.

An overview of Notch signaling.

Hall JG. Twinning. *Lancet.* 2003;362:735–743.

Describes the mechanism of twinning.

Hughes IA. Disorders of sex development: a new definition and classification. *Best Pract Res Clin Endocrinol Metab.* 2008;22: 119–134.

Describes the most recent international classification of DSDs.

Krumlauf R. Hox genes in vertebrate development. *Cell.* 1994; 78:191–201.

An early overview of HOX genes.

Lyon MF. Gene action in the X chromosome of the mouse (Mus musculus L). *Nature.* 1961;190:372–373.

The original proposal of X-inactivation—very short and easily understood.

Muragaki Y, Mundlos S, Upton J, Olsen BR. Altered growth and branching patterns in synpolydactyly caused by mutations in HOXD13. *Science.* 1996;272:548–551.

The long-awaited first report of a human malformation caused by a mutation in a HOX gene.

Passos-Bueno MR, Ornelas CC, Fanganiello RD. Syndromes of the first and second pharyngeal arches: a review. *Am J Med Genet A.* 2009;149A:1853–1859.

A review of syndromes associated with embryonic processes in pharyngeal arches.

Robson MI, Ringel AR, Mundlos S. Regulatory Landscaping: How Enhancer-Promoter Communication Is Sculpted in 3D. *Mol Cell.* 2019;74(6):1110–1122.

A review of gene transcription in space and time as it relates to embryogenesis and development.

An excellent short overview of pharyngeal arches and associated syndromes.

Saga Y. The mechanism of somite formation in mice. *Curr Opin Genet Dev*. 2012;22:331–338.

An excellent review of somite development.

Tickle C. *Patterning in Vertebrate Development*. Oxford: Oxford University Press; 2003.

A detailed, multiauthor collection handling very early development from mainly molecular perspectives.

Villavicencio EH, Walterhouse DO, Iannaccone PM. The Sonic hedgehog-patched-Gli pathway in human development and disease. *Am J Hum Genet*. 2000;67:1047–1054.

An excellent short overview of the Sonic hedgehog pathway.

10 Common Disease, Polygenic, and Multifactorial Genetics

Many disorders demonstrate familial clustering that does not conform to any recognized pattern of mendelian inheritance. Examples include several of the most common congenital malformations and many common acquired diseases (Box 10.1). These conditions show a definite familial tendency, but the incidence in close relatives of affected individuals is much lower than would be seen if these conditions were caused by mutations in single genes. Medical genetics usually concentrates on the study of rare unifactorial chromosomal and single-gene disorders. Diseases such as diabetes, cancer, cardiovascular and coronary artery disease, mental health, and neurodegenerative disorders are responsible, however, for the majority of the morbidity and mortality in developed countries.

Because it is likely that many factors, both genetic and environmental, are involved in causing these disorders, they are generally referred to as showing **multifactorial** inheritance, although sometimes one can appear more important than the other (Fig. 10.1).

• BOX 10.1 Disorders that show multifactorial inheritance

Congenital Malformations

Cleft lip/palate
Congenital dislocation of the hip
Congenital heart defects
Neural tube defects
Pyloric stenosis
Talipes

Acquired Diseases of Childhood and Adult Life

Asthma
Autism
Diabetes mellitus
Epilepsy
Glaucoma
Hypertension
Inflammatory bowel disease (Crohn disease and ulcerative colitis)
Ischemic heart disease
Ischemic stroke
Bipolar disorder
Multiple sclerosis
Parkinson disease
Psoriasis
Rheumatoid arthritis
Schizophrenia

At one extreme are diseases such as Duchenne muscular dystrophy; these are exclusively genetic in origin, and the environment plays little or no direct part in the etiology. At the other extreme are infectious diseases that are almost entirely the result of environmental factors. Between these two extremes are the common diseases and disorders such as diabetes mellitus (DM), hypertension, cerebrovascular and coronary artery disease, schizophrenia, the common cancers, and certain congenital abnormalities in which both genetic and environmental factors are involved.

Types and Mechanisms of Genetic Susceptibility

Genetic susceptibility for a particular disease can occur through single-gene inheritance of an abnormal gene product involved in a particular metabolic pathway, such as occurs in early coronary artery disease arising from familial hypercholesterolemia (FH) (p. 147). In an individual with a mutation in the *LDLR* gene, the genetic susceptibility is the main determinant of the development of coronary artery disease, but this can be modified by environmental alteration like reduction in dietary cholesterol and avoidance of other risk factors such as obesity, lack of exercise, and smoking.

Inheritance of single-gene susceptibility does not, however, necessarily lead to development of a disease. For some diseases, exposure to specific environmental factors will be the main determinant in the development of the disease (e.g., smoking or occupational dust exposure in the development of pulmonary emphysema in persons with α_1-antitrypsin deficiency [p. 305]).

In other instances, the mechanism of the genetic susceptibility is less clear-cut. This can involve inheritance of a single nucleotide polymorphism (p. 52) that leads to differences in susceptibility to a disease (e.g., acetaldehyde dehydrogenase activity and alcoholism). In addition, inherited single-gene polymorphisms appear to determine the response to as yet undefined environmental factors—for example, the antigens of the major histocompatibility (HLA) complex and specific disease associations (p. 176) such as type 1 diabetes and rheumatoid arthritis. Lastly, genetic susceptibility can determine differences in responses to medical treatment; isoniazid inactivation status in the treatment of tuberculosis (p. 211) is a good example.

Many common diseases however are **polygenic**, being determined by variation in many genes at different loci, with each variant exerting a small, generally **additive** effect. Additive means that the

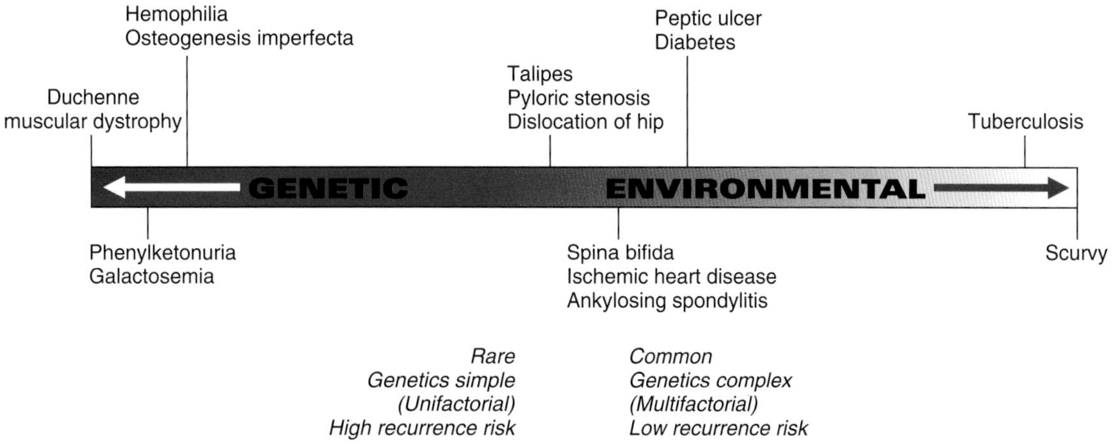

• **Fig. 10.1** Human diseases represented as being on a spectrum ranging from those that are entirely genetic in causation to those that are largely environmental.

influence of each genetic variant on the phenotype is cumulative, not dominant or recessive. For instance if a variant doubles the risk for coronary heart disease compared with homozygous carriers of the low-risk allele, heterozygotes will have a twofold increased risk and alternative homozygotes a fourfold increased risk of heart disease.

Approaches to Demonstrating Genetic Susceptibility to Common Diseases

In attempting to understand the genetics of a particular condition, the investigator can approach the problem in a number of ways. These can include comparing the prevalence and incidence in various different population groups and the effects of migration. Studies of migrant groups moving from a population group with a low incidence of a disease to one with a high incidence, in which the incidence of the disease in the migrant group rises to that of its new population group, would suggest that environmental factors are more important. Conversely, maintenance of a low incidence of the disease in the migrant group would suggest that genetic factors are more important.

Family and Twin Studies

Genetic susceptibility to a disease can be suggested by the finding of a higher frequency of the disease in relatives than in the general population. Familial aggregation does not, however, prove a genetic susceptibility because families share a common environment. This problem can be partly resolved by comparing differences in the frequency of a disease or disorder between non-identical or dizygotic (DZ) and identical or monozygotic (MZ) twin pairs. Both members of a pair of twins are said to be **concordant** when either both are affected or neither is affected. The term **discordant** is used when only one member of a pair of twins is affected. Both types of twins will have a tendency to share the same environment but, whereas identical twins basically have identical genotypes, non-identical twins are no more similar genetically than brothers and sisters. If a disease is entirely genetically determined, then apart from rare events such as chromosome nondisjunction or a new mutation occurring in one of a twin pair, both members of a pair of identical twins will be similarly affected, but non-identical twins will be more likely to differ. If a disease is entirely caused by environmental factors, then identical and non-identical twins will have similar concordance rates.

Although all twins tend to share the same environment, it is probably more likely in identical twins than in non-identical twins. Similarities between identical twins can therefore reflect their shared environment as much as their identical genotypes. In one study of identical twins reared separately, the data clearly showed that each pair of twins differed little in height but differed considerably in body weight. These observations suggest that heredity plays a bigger part in determining stature than it does in determining body weight.

Heritability

The similarity between individuals in a family for a particular phenotype can be used to calculate the heritability of the disease or trait. The heritability gives a mathematical estimate of the relative contributions of genetic variation and environmental factors to the trait variability. Heritability (often denoted H^2 or h^2) is the proportion of a trait that is attributed to genetic variation divided by the total variation in the trait in a given population. The total variation is a combination of genetic and environmental variation. Genetic variability is best calculated by measuring the difference in disease concordance in identical twins compared with non-identical twins, who only share 50% of their genes on average, but like identical twins have a shared environment. The calculation assumes that environmental variation for twin pairs is identical, which may not be true, and may differ for MZ versus DZ twins. A more accurate estimate can be achieved by comparing twin pairs separated at birth, but these studies are not feasible for most diseases because there are not enough individuals that meet these criteria. Where such studies have been carried out they give estimates comparable to the MZ versus DZ comparisons. Heritability estimates for some common multifactorial diseases are given in Table 10.1.

The degree of familial clustering shown by a multifactorial disorder can be estimated by measuring the ratio of the risk to siblings of affected individuals compared with the general population incidence. This ratio of sib risk to population incidence is known as λ_s. For example, in type 1 diabetes, where the UK population incidence is 0.4% and the risk to siblings is 6%, λ_s is 15. For type 2 diabetes in Europe, λ_s is estimated at a more modest 3.5 (35% sibling risk; 10% population risk).

Polymorphism Association Studies

Sequencing of the human genome has shown that the around 3 billion base pairs (bp) are 99.9% identical in every person. This also

TABLE 10.1 Examples of complex diseases with heritability estimates based on twin/family studies and calculated from genome-wide association studies

Trait or Disease	Twin/Family Study Heritability	Top GWAS SNPs (a)	All common SNPs (b)
Type 1 diabetes	0.9	0.6	0.3
Type 2 diabetes	0.3–0.6	0.05–0.1	
Obesity (BMI)	0.4–0.6	0.01–0.02	0.2
Crohn disease	0.6–0.8	0.1	0.4
Ulcerative colitis	0.5	0.05	
Multiple sclerosis	0.3–0.8	0.1	
Ankylosing spondylitis	>0.90	0.21	
Rheumatoid arthritis	0.6		
Schizophrenia	0.7–0.8	0.01	0.3
Bipolar disorder	0.6–0.7	0.02	0.4
Breast cancer	0.3	0.08	
Von Willebrand factor	0.66–0.75	0.13	0.2
Height	0.8	0.1	0.5
Bone mineral density	0.6–0.8	0.05	
QT interval	0.37–0.60	0.07	0.2
HDL cholesterol	0.5	0.1	
Platelet count	0.8	0.05–0.1	

(From Visscher PM, Brown MA, McCarthy MI, Yang J. Five years of GWAS discovery. *Am J Hum Genet.* 2012;90:7–24.)
GWAS estimates are either based on the known top signals associated with the trait (a) or by using all common variants without invoking a p value threshold (b). *BMI,* Body mass index; *GWAS,* genome-wide association studies; *HDL,* high-density lipoprotein; *SNP,* single nucleotide polymorphism.

means that individuals are, on average, 0.1% different genetically from every other person on the planet. And within that 0.1% lies the mystery of why some people are more susceptible to a particular illness, or more likely to be healthy, than another member of the population. The human genome contains more than 10 million single nucleotide polymorphisms (SNPs) that occur in more than 1% of individuals, and our increased knowledge of genetic variation, together with high throughput SNP genotyping platforms, has revolutionized our ability to identify disease susceptibility loci for many common diseases and traits.

It is possible to determine whether particular variants occur more commonly in individuals affected with a particular disease than in the population in general, or what is known as **association.** Although demonstration of a polymorphic association can suggest that the inherited variation is involved in the etiology of the disorder, such as the demonstration of HLA associations in the immune response in the causation of the autoimmune disorders (p. 178), it may only reflect that a gene nearby in linkage disequilibrium (p. 93) is involved in causation of the disorder.

Polygenic Inheritance and the Normal Distribution

The concept of **polygenic** inheritance, the cornerstone of **quantitative** genetics, was first proposed by Ronald Fisher in 1918, and is exemplified by variation in human height, the classic polygenic trait. The result is a normal distribution of the trait generated by many genes, known as **polygenes**, each acting in an additive fashion. Individuals who lie at the extreme ends of the distribution curve may be of clinical interest, (e.g., those with idiopathic short or tall stature).

• BOX 10.2 Human characteristics that show a continuous normal distribution

Blood pressure
Dermatoglyphics (ridge count)
Head circumference
Height
Intelligence
Body mass index

Several human characteristics (Box 10.2) show a continuous distribution in the general population, which closely resembles a normal distribution. This takes the form of a symmetrical bell-shaped curve distributed evenly about a mean (Fig. 10.2). The spread of the distribution about the mean is determined by the standard deviation (SD). Approximately 68%, 95% and 99.7% of observations fall within the mean plus or minus one, two or three SDs, respectively.

It is possible to show that a phenotype with a normal distribution in the general population can be generated by polygenic inheritance involving the action of many genes at different loci, each of which exerts an equal additive effect. This can be illustrated by considering a trait such as height. If height were to be determined by two equally frequent alleles, "a" (tall) and "b" (short), at a single locus, then this would result in a discontinuous phenotype with three groups in a ratio of 1 (tall-aa) to 2 (average-ab/ba) to 1 (short-bb). If the same trait were to be determined by two alleles at each of two loci interacting in a simple additive way, this would lead to a phenotypic distribution of five groups in a ratio of 1 (4 tall genes) to 4 (3 tall + 1 short) to 6 (2 tall + 2 short) to 4 (1 tall + 3 short)

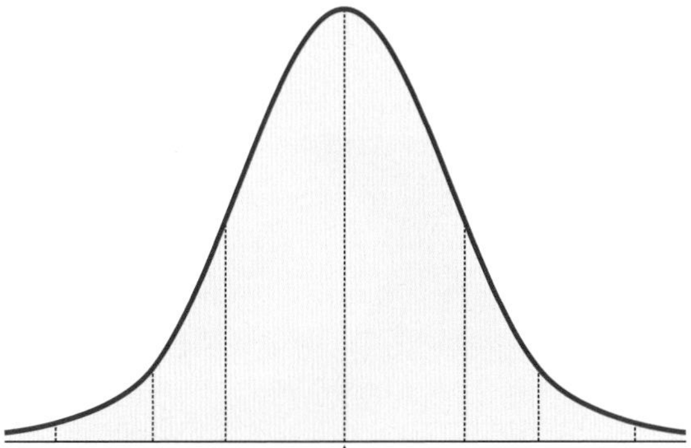

• **Fig. 10.2** The normal (Gaussian) distribution.

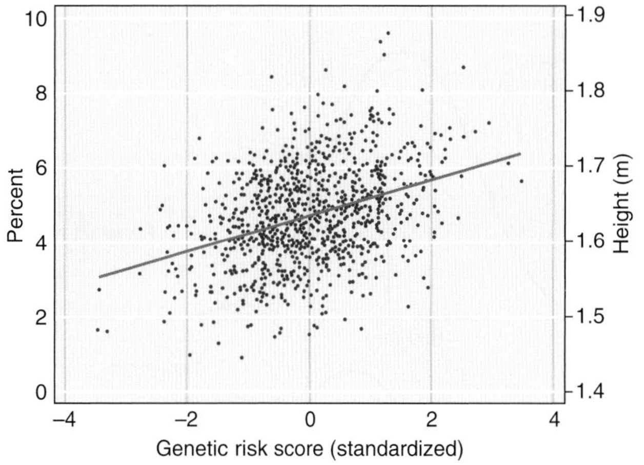

• **Fig. 10.4** The combined effect of 697 common variants, which explain 20% of the heritability of height, on the variation of height in a population of 1000 adult women. The scatter plot indicates the mean height for individuals carrying each risk score for height genes and the histogram illustrates the percentage of individuals carrying that risk score. The risk score has been standardized so that it has a mean of 0 and standard deviation of 1. There is a difference in mean height of about 1.5 cm between those individuals with the fewest compared with the greatest number of height-increasing variants.

to 1 (4 short). For a system with three loci each with two alleles the phenotypic ratio would be 1-6-15-20-15-6-1 (Fig. 10.3).

It can be seen that, as the number of loci increases, the distribution increasingly comes to resemble a normal curve, thereby supporting the concept that characteristics such as height are determined by the additive effects of many genes at different loci. The prediction from this model has now been demonstrated with empirical data (Fig. 10.4). Correlation is a statistical measure of the degree of resemblance or relationship between two parameters. First-degree relatives share, on average, 50% of their genes (see Table 10.1). Therefore, if height is polygenic, the correlation between first-degree relatives should be 0.5. Several studies have shown that the sib–sib correlation for height is indeed close to 0.5.

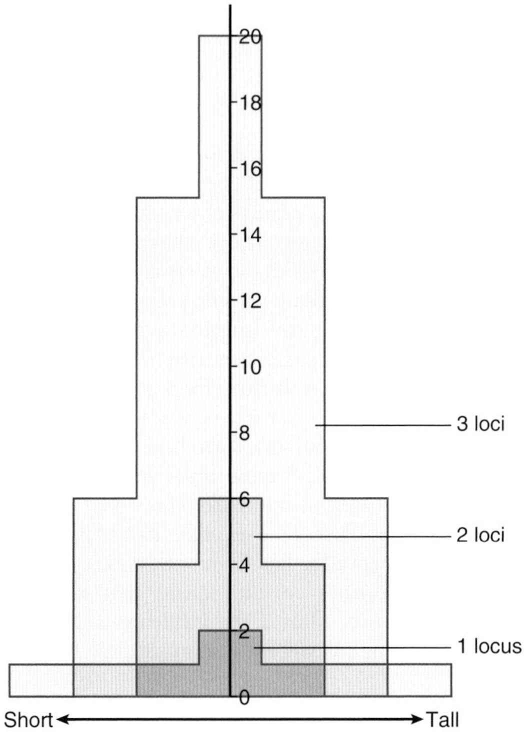

• **Fig. 10.3** Distribution of genotypes for a characteristic such as height with one, two, and three loci each with two alleles of equal frequency. The values for each genotype can be obtained from the binomial expansion $(p + q)^{(2n)}$, where $p = q = 1/2$ and n equals the number of loci.

In reality, human characteristics such as height and intelligence are also influenced by environment, and possibly also by genes that are not additive in that they exert a dominant effect. These factors probably account for the observed tendency of offspring to show what is known as **regression to the mean**. This is demonstrated by tall or intelligent parents (the two are not mutually exclusive) having children whose average height or intelligence is slightly lower than the average or midparental value. Similarly, parents who are very short or of low intelligence tend to have children whose average height or intelligence is lower than the general population average, but higher than the average value of the parents. If a trait were to show true polygenic inheritance with no external influences, then the measurements in offspring would be distributed evenly around the mean of their parents' values.

Multifactorial Inheritance—the Liability/Threshold Model

For disease states such as type 1 DM (T1DM), the genetic contribution involves many loci, but the phenotype does not have a continuous distribution, it is either present or absent. The polygenic theory for the inheritance of quantitative or continuous traits accounts for **discontinuous** multifactorial disorders, such as T1DM or cleft lip, with the **liability/threshold** model, proposed by Sewall Wright in 1934. All of the factors that influence the development of a multifactorial disorder, whether genetic or environmental, can be considered as a single entity known as liability. The liabilities of all individuals in a population form a continuous variable, which has a normal distribution in both the general population and in relatives of affected individuals. However, the curves

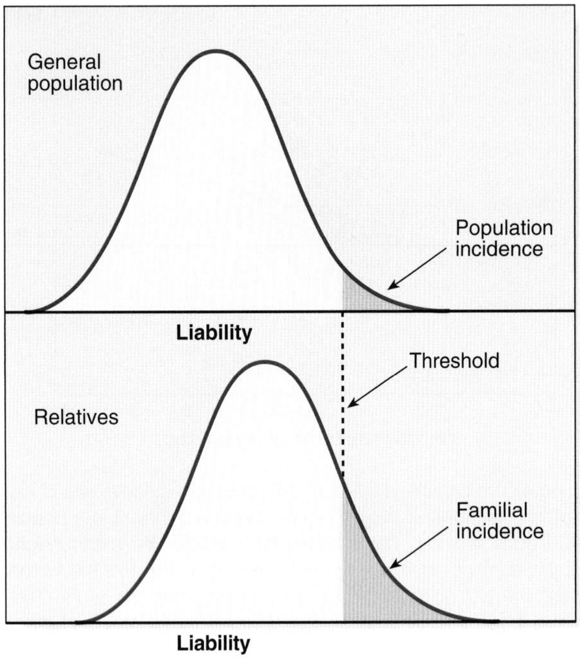

• **Fig. 10.5** Hypothetical liability curves in the general population and in relatives for a hereditary disorder in which the genetic predisposition is multifactorial.

for these relatives will be shifted to the right, with the extent to which they are shifted being directly related to the closeness of their relationship to the affected index case, indicating an increased shared genetic burden (Fig. 10.5).

It is important to emphasize again that liability includes all factors that contribute to the cause of the condition. Looked at very simply, a deleterious liability can be viewed as consisting of a combination of several "bad" genes and adverse environmental factors. This model of inheritance has been supported by numerous multifactorial discontinuous traits through **genome-wide association studies (GWAS)** (p. 142), including schizophrenia, type 2 DM (T2DM), rheumatoid arthritis, Crohn disease, and various cancers.

Consequences of the Liability/Threshold Model

Part of the attraction of this model is that it provides a simple explanation for the observed patterns of familial risks in conditions such as cleft lip/palate, pyloric stenosis, and spina bifida.

1. The incidence of the condition is greatest among relatives of the most severely affected patients, presumably because they are the most extreme deviants along the liability curve. For example, in cleft lip/palate the proportion of affected first-degree relatives (parents, siblings, and offspring) is 6% if the index patient has bilateral cleft lip and palate, but only 2% if the index patient has a unilateral cleft lip (Fig. 10.6).
2. The risk is greatest among close relatives of the index case and decreases rapidly in more distant relatives. For example, in spina bifida the risks to first-, second-, and third-degree relatives of the index case are approximately 4%, 1%, and less than 0.5%, respectively.
3. If there is more than one affected close relative, then the risks for other relatives are increased. In spina bifida, if one sibling is affected, the risk to the next sibling (if folic acid is not taken by the mother periconceptionally) is approximately 4%; if two siblings are affected, the risk to a subsequent sibling is approximately 10%.
4. If the condition is more common in individuals of one sex, then relatives of an affected individual of the less frequently affected sex will be at higher risk than relatives of an affected individual of the more frequently affected sex. This is illustrated by the condition pyloric stenosis. Pyloric stenosis shows a male to female ratio of 5 to 1. The proportions of affected offspring of male index patients are 5.5% for sons and 2.4% for daughters, whereas the risks to the offspring of female index patients are 19.4% for sons and 7.3% for daughters. The probable explanation for these different risks is that, for a female to be affected, she has to lie at the extreme of the liability curve, so that her close relatives will also have a very high liability for developing the condition. Because males are more susceptible to developing the disorder, risks in male offspring are higher than in female offspring regardless of the sex of the affected parent.
5. The risk of recurrence for first-degree relatives (i.e., siblings and offspring) approximates to the square root of the general population incidence. Thus if the incidence is 1 in 1000, the sibling and offspring risk will equal approximately 1 in 32, or 3%.

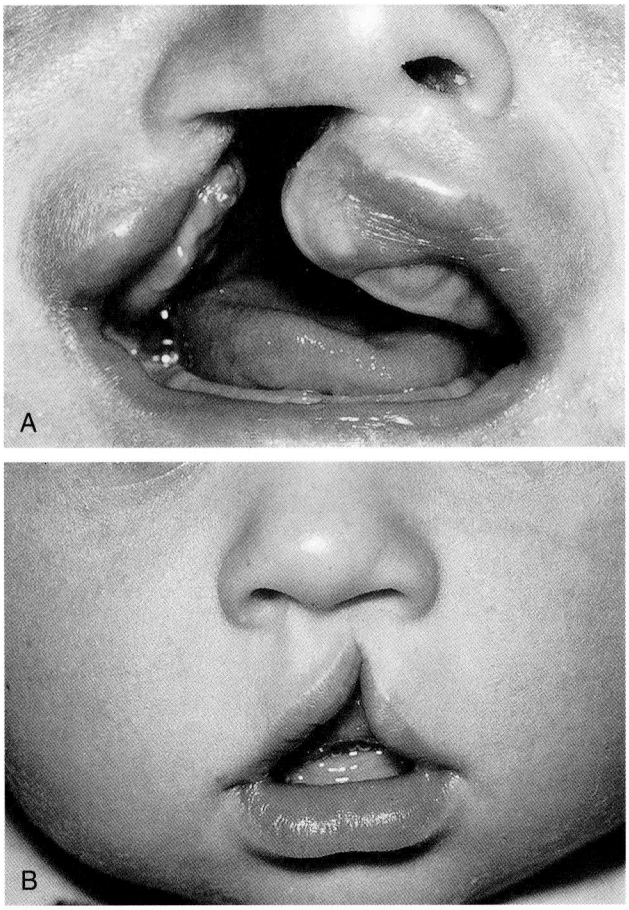

• **Fig. 10.6** Severe (A) and mild (B) forms of cleft lip/palate.

Identifying Genes That Cause Multifactorial Disorders

Multifactorial disorders are common and make a major contribution to human morbidity and mortality (p. 103). Vigorous efforts

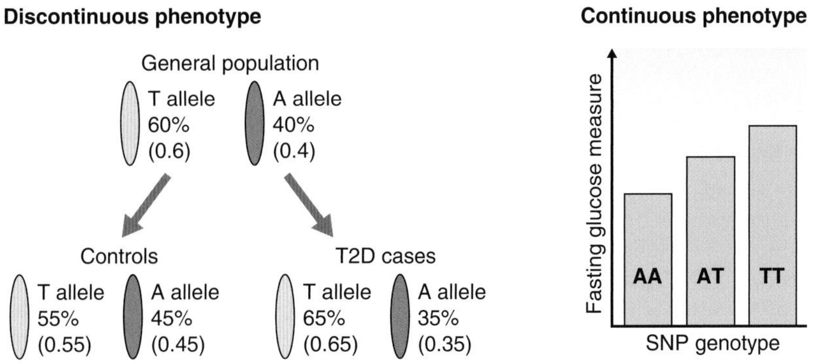

• **Fig. 10.7** Illustration of the principle of association testing, using diabetes as an example, with a single nucleotide polymorphism (*SNP*). Studies may either test allele frequency differences between cases and controls for a disease phenotype, or compare mean trait values for each genotype group (e.g., for fasting glucose).

have been made over recent years to identify genes that contribute to their etiology. Early studies focused on methods used in monogenic disease, such as linkage analysis (p. 91), but these were largely unsuccessful. In 2007 the results from the first large-scale GWAS were published, and this has revolutionized the field of complex trait genetics.

Association Studies

Association studies are undertaken by comparing the frequency of a particular variant in affected patients with its frequency in a control group. This approach is often described as a **case-control** study. If the frequencies in the two groups differ significantly, this provides evidence for an association. For quantitative traits the mean trait value for each genotype group is compared, and significant differences provide evidence for an association (Fig. 10.7).

The polymorphic HLA histocompatibility complex on chromosome 6 (p. 176) has been frequently studied. One of the strongest known HLA associations is that between ankylosing spondylitis and the B27 allele. This is present in approximately 90% of all patients and in only 5% of controls. The strength of an association is indicated by the ratio of the odds of developing the disease in those with the antigen to the odds of developing the disease in those without the antigen (Table 10.2). This is known as the **odds ratio (OR)**, and it gives an indication of how much more frequently the disease occurs in individuals with a specific marker than in those without that marker. For the HLA-ankylosing spondylitis association, the OR is 171. However, for most markers associated with multifactorial disease, the frequency difference between cases and controls is small, giving rise to modest ORs (usually between 1.1 and 1.5).

If evidence for association is forthcoming, this suggests that the allele encoded by the marker is either directly involved in causing the disease (i.e., a susceptibility variant) or that the marker is in linkage disequilibrium with a closely linked susceptibility variant. When considering disease associations, remember that the identification of a susceptibility locus does not mean that the definitive disease gene has been identified. For example, although it is one of the strongest disease associations known, only 1% of all HLA B27 individuals develop ankylosing spondylitis, so that many other factors, genetic and/or environmental, must be involved in causing this condition.

Before 2006, association studies were carried out by first selecting a candidate gene or genomic region, which would either have plausible biological links to the disease of interest or be situated in a region of linkage. One or more genetic variants were selected from the gene or gene region and genotyped in cases and controls to test for association with the disease. Many studies showing evidence of association with candidate genes were published for a variety of diseases and traits. However, in numerous cases, these associations did not replicate in independent studies, leaving the validity of many of the initially reported associations unclear. The reasons for this inconsistency included (1) small sample sizes, (2) weak statistical support, and (3) the low prior probability of any of the few selected variants being genuinely associated with the disease. All of these features increased the chances of false-positive associations. In addition, false-positive associations were found to be caused by population stratification, where the population contains subgroups of different ancestries in which both the disease and the allele happen to be common. A famous example was reported in a study by Lander and Schork which showed, in a San Francisco population, that HLA-A1 is associated with the ability to eat with chopsticks. This association is simply explained by the fact that HLA-A1 is more common among Chinese than Europeans.

The candidate gene approach led to only a handful of widely replicated associations. Two important developments made it possible to move away from this approach, toward a genome-wide approach to association studies: the first was the development of microarray technology to genotype hundreds of thousands of SNPs in thousands of individuals quickly and at little cost; the second was the creation of a reference catalogue of SNPs and linkage disequilibrium, the International Haplotype Map (HapMap).

TABLE 10.2 Calculation of odds ratio for a disease association

	Allele 1	Allele 2
Patients	a	b
Controls	c	d
Odds ratio	= a/c ÷ b/d = ad/bc	

HapMap Project

Although it is estimated that there are over 10 million SNPs in the human genome, many SNPs are in linkage disequilibrium (p. 93) and therefore coinherited. Regions of linked SNPs are known as haplotypes. The International HapMap project (www.1000genomes.org or ftp://ftp.ncbi.nlm.nih.gov/hapmap/)

was set up to identify SNP frequencies and haplotypes in different populations and make that data freely and publically available. The project genotyped more than 3 million SNPs in 270 samples from Europe, East Asia, and West Africa.

Genome-Wide Association Studies

In GWAS, researchers compare variants across the entire genome, rather than looking at just one variant at a time. Since 2006 this powerful new method has produced an explosion in the number of widely replicated associations between SNPs and common diseases, which are catalogued at http://www.ebi.ac.uk/gwas/. To date, GWAS have identified thousands of reproducible associations with over 600 common diseases or traits from over 3500 studies. The results of a GWAS of autism are shown in Fig. 10.8. In a typical GWAS, 500,000 to 1,000,000 SNPs are genotyped in each subject using a single microarray ("SNP chip").

A clear advantage of GWAS over the candidate gene approach is that they are "hypothesis-free." No prior assumption is made about the genes likely to be involved in the disease, and as a result associations have been uncovered which provide new insights into biological pathways, opening up new avenues for research.

It has been important to develop new statistical criteria for GWAS. If we were to perform a statistical test of association comparing the frequency of one SNP between cases and controls, we might interpret a P value of less than .05 as being unlikely to have occurred by chance. However, when testing associations with increasing numbers of SNPs, the P value threshold needs to

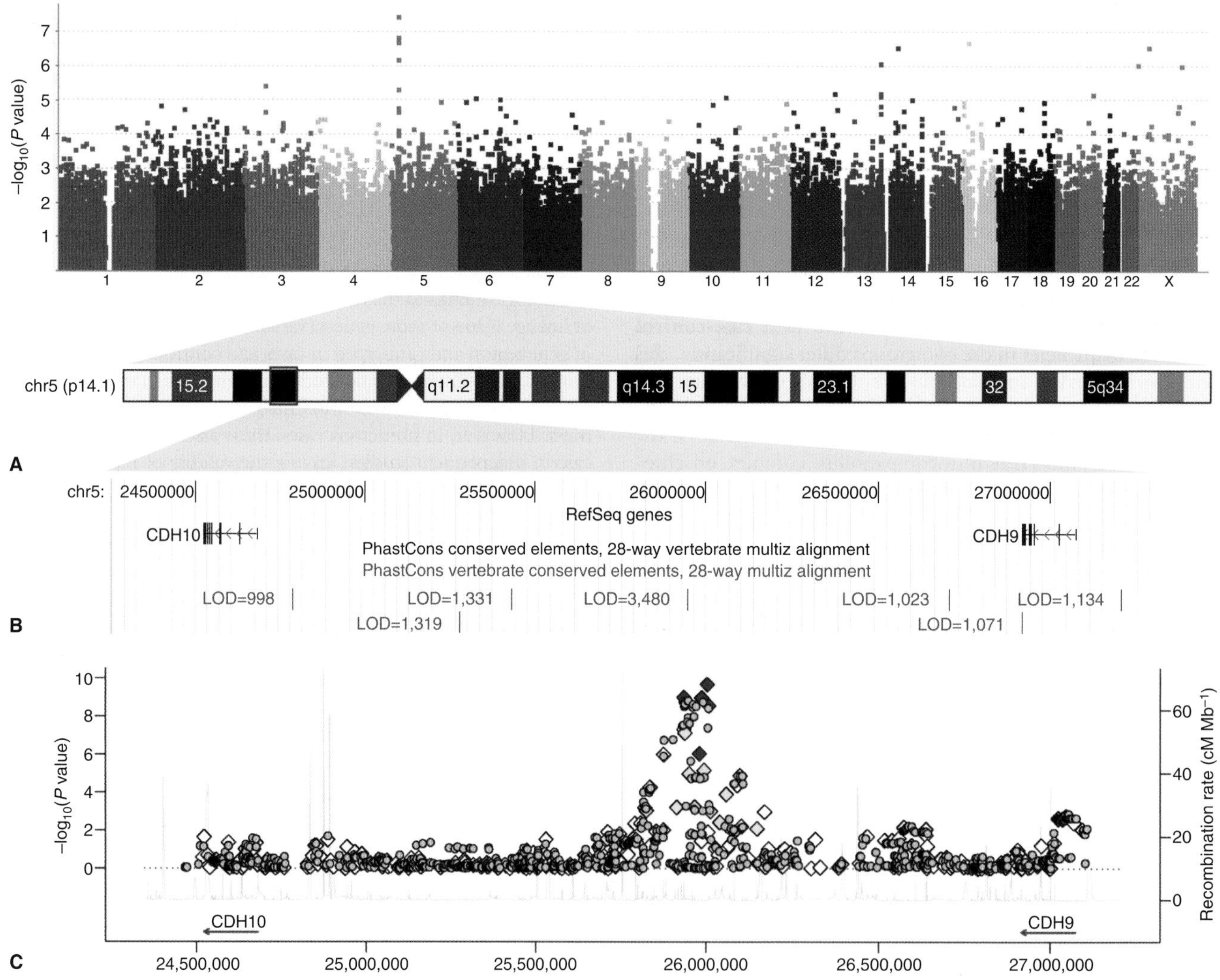

• **Fig. 10.8** Results of a genome-wide association study of autism spectrum disorders. (A) "Manhattan plot" of $-\log_{10}$ (P value) against genomic position. Each data point represents the association between an individual single nucleotide polymorphism (SNP) and autism. SNPs are ordered according to their position in the genome, and each chromosome is colored differently. The higher the position on the y-axis, the stronger the evidence for association. SNPs on chromosome 5p14.1 show the strongest associations. (B) The 5p14.1 genomic region as displayed in the University of California Santa Cruz genome browser (http://genome.ucsc.edu/). (C) Zooming in on the 5p14.1 region: both genotyped SNPs (*diamonds*) and imputed SNPs (inferred from linkage disequilibrium with genotyped SNPs; *grey circles*) are plotted with $-\log_{10}$ (P value) (y-axis) against genomic position (x-axis). Genotyped SNPs are colored on the basis of their correlation with the most strongly associated SNP (*red* = high, *yellow* = medium, *white* = low). Estimated recombination rates from HapMap data are plotted to reflect the local linkage disequilibrium structure. *LOD*, Logarithm of odds; *RefSeq*, reference sequence. (From Wang K, Zhang H, Ma D, et al. Common genetic variants on 5p14.1 associated with autism spectrum disorders. *Nature*. 2009;459:528–533. With permission.)

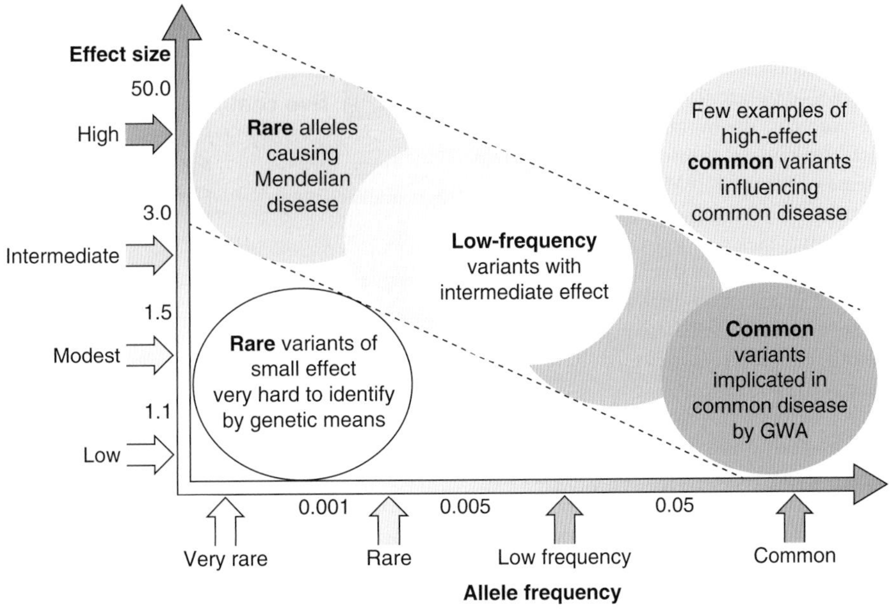

• **Fig. 10.9** Feasibility of identifying genetic variants by risk allele frequency and strength of genetic effect (odds ratio). *GWA*, genome-wide association. (From Manolio TA, Collins FS, Cox NJ, et al. Finding the missing heritability of complex diseases. *Nature*. 2009;461[7265]:747–753. With permission.)

change: 1 in 20 tests will have a *P* value less than .05 just by chance. Based on HapMap European data, there are approximately 1 million common SNPs in the genome that are independent (i.e., in very low linkage disequilibrium with all others). Therefore, a comprehensive GWAS of common variants is equivalent to testing approximately 1 million hypotheses. Consequently, in GWAS, $P = 5 \times 10^{-8}$ is the accepted threshold below which an association is unlikely to be a false positive. Large sample sizes are needed to achieve such low *P* values, and metaanalysis of multiple studies is a common approach to enlarge the sample size. Dense SNP data can be used to identify population stratification in GWAS. For example, if an individual shows allele frequency differences from the rest of the study sample at thousands of SNPs, this may indicate that they are of different ancestry, and may lead to their exclusion from the study.

Initially, GWAS focused on common variation, (i.e., SNPs with a minor allele frequency >5%). However, despite identifying multiple loci, for most traits initial studies were only able to explain a relatively small proportion of the trait variability, typically less than 10%. Rarer variants not captured by the GWAS approach may explain some of this **missing heritability**. Common variants found to date have relatively modest effect sizes. For example, a SNP identified as being associated with human height through a GWAS will typically alter adult height by less than 1 mm per allele. This has led to the hypothesis that much of the missing heritability lies in rarer variation that has a larger effect size per allele, that is, intermediate between classic monogenic disease-causing alleles and the typical, common GWAS SNPs (Fig. 10.9). Some of this rarer variation is captured with specialized SNP arrays, or **exome chips**, that are enriched for SNPs in coding sequences. Rarer variation in noncoding regions can also be evaluated by using **imputation**.

Imputation

Most SNPs are strongly correlated to one or more others nearby, and by genotyping only a proportion of SNPs we can infer genotypes for others based on these linkage disequilibrium patterns. This means that, by genotyping approximately 500,000 SNPs in most populations, we can capture information on the majority of common SNPs in the human genome (with minor allele frequency >5%). The added advantage of imputation is that studies that have used different genotyping arrays can impute missing SNPs, and thus studies can be metaanalyzed easily. Imputation relies on using a **reference panel** of genomic data. Larger and more detailed reference panels allow for more and rarer untyped SNPs to be imputed.

Reference Panels

The first commonly used reference panel was provided by the HapMap consortium, but since 2013, additional reference panels have become available based on whole-genome sequence data rather than SNP genotypes derived from microarrays. The **1000 Genomes Project** (www.1000genomes.org) provides an accurate map of common and lower frequency alleles found in multiple ancestral groups for SNPs and other types of variation, including copy number polymorphisms (duplications, deletions, and other structural variation). The **Haplotype Reference Consortium** (http://www.haplotype-reference-consortium.org/) also provides a comprehensive map of the human genome, and is currently derived nearly entirely from individuals of European ancestry, allowing for more detailed analysis of rarer variation in European-based studies.

Despite the success of GWAS, many challenges remain. To date, the associations identified only explain a small fraction of the susceptibility to most diseases studied (e.g., <20% in T2DM). Over 10,000 SNPs have been reported from GWAS, associated with hundreds of traits and diseases, but 90% of those SNPs fall in noncoding regions of the genome. In addition, the loci identified generally range from 10 to 100 kilobases (kb) in length and include numerous associated SNPs. This means that it has not been possible in most cases to identify the causal variants or even the causal genes. Further techniques, including resequencing of the associated regions, testing in different ethnic groups, examining expression data, and performing functional studies will be necessary to understand the associations fully.

Polygenic Risk Scores

Effect estimates of multiple genetic variants from a GWAS can be combined into a single variable—a polygenic risk score (PRS). For a given individual, this score represents the overall genetic susceptibility for a disease or for raised or lowered measures of a continuous trait. For multifactorial diseases, such as T2DM and coronary artery disease, a genetic score is calculated based on summing over the number of disease risk–increasing alleles an individual carries for a variant, weighted by the respective effect on disease risk. It is more informative to weight counts of disease risk–increasing alleles than to simply count alleles because not all effects are equal, and there may be a relatively small number of genetic variants that have disproportionate effect on disease risk over others.

Weightings for disease-risk alleles are usually based on ORs. For continuous outcomes, such as body mass index (BMI) and low-density lipoproteins (LDL)-cholesterol levels, a genetic score is calculated in a similar way but weighted using linear-regression coefficients. Weights should be derived from effect estimates obtained from studies that are independent of the study in which the PRS is being created to avoid "overfitting." Overfitting can lead to upwardly biased estimates of the amount of variation in disease risk the PRS explains.

Polygenic Risk Score Feature Selection

There are a number of approaches in determining which genetic variants should be incorporated into polygenic risk scores. An intuitive approach is to take all variants that pass the genome-wide significance level threshold for GWAS ($P < 5 \times 10^{-8}$). Using this method, only genetic variants that have been robustly associated with the disease or continuous outcome are included in the genetic predictor.

However, researchers may be interested in incorporating additional data from the rest of the genome that may have not been associated through GWAS to date owing to several factors, including limited statistical power—that is, the probability of identifying an association that exists at genome-wide significance may be reduced if the sample size is not large enough to detect associations of relatively small effects. By incorporating more genetic variation from the genome, it may be possible to increase disease-risk prediction or the variation in a continuous outcome. One method to construct a PRS that incorporates more genetic variation combines linkage disequilibrium (LD)-pruning and *P*-value thresholding. In summary, association statistics from a GWAS are linked to LD-pruned (uncorrelated) variants before a number of *P*-value inclusion thresholds are applied (e.g., $P < 5 \times 10^{-8}$, $P < 5 \times 10^{-7}$, $P < 5 \times 10^{-6}$, $P < 0.05$) to create several polygenic risk scores that incorporate different genetic variants. Once several PRSs have been created, they are compared across the set to find the optimal genetic predictor that either maximizes disease prediction or variation explained for a continuous outcome. Although commonly used, this is a relatively naïve approach, and more complex statistical methods exist to optimize PRSs that consider distributions of effect sizes and LD without the need for several to be generated through subjective *P*-value thresholding.

Polygenic Risk Score Utility in Disease Discrimination

Polygenic risk scores have potential utility in stratifying individuals into disease subgroups. For example, previous studies have shown that combining genetics associated with T1DM risk results in a strong discriminatory power to separate T1DM cases from other forms of diabetes. This is mainly attributed to large effects on T1DM disease risk that have been observed in the HLA region on chromosome 6p21 (see section later). Additional regions of the genome have been associated with T1DM risk through GWAS, but the observed effects are modest. Recent studies have shown that combining all genetic factors robustly associated with T1DM results in greater than 90% discriminatory power to classify someone correctly as having T1DM over other disease groups, such as T2DM. However, this is one of few examples where such high discriminatory power exists for disease classification. For many other traits, predictive accuracy is currently less than 80% owing to a variety of reasons—including the modest effect sizes and the absence of disproportionately large-effect associations.

TABLE 10.3 Proportion (%) of individuals from the UK Biobank with the highest polygenic risk scores at three-, four-, and fivefold increased risk of five common diseases

Odds Ratio	Coronary Artery Disease	Atrial Fibrillation	Type 2 Diabetes	Inflammatory Bowel Syndrome	Breast Cancer
≥3	8	6.1	3.5	3.2	1.5
≥4	2.3	1.5	0.2	0.8	0.3
≥5	0.5	0.7	0.05	0.2	0.1

(From Khera AV, Chaffin M, Aragam KG, et al. Genome-wide polygenic scores for common diseases identify individuals with risk equivalent to monogenic mutations. *Nat Genet.* 2018;50:1219–1224.)

Polygenic Risk Score Utility in Stratifying Individuals for Prioritized Health Screening

Screening individuals who are more likely to develop a disease is important for disease prevention strategies and clinical trials where disease events are more likely to occur. Recently, researchers used data from the UK Biobank to examine the risk of five common diseases among groups of individuals who had the highest PRSs for the respective disease. The researchers found that individuals had a threefold increased risk of coronary artery disease, atrial fibrillation, T2DM, inflammatory bowel disease, and breast cancer if they were within the top 8%, 6.1%, 3.5%, 3.2%, and 1.5% of the respective PRS distribution (Table 10.3). For some diseases, these risks are equivalent to those that have monogenic disease-causing variants, but the number of people affected is many-fold higher. For example, an exome-sequencing study identified 35 pathogenic variants in the *LDLR*, *APOB*, and *PCSK9* genes associated with familial hypercholesterolemia—a condition that increases the risk of coronary artery disease. When combining all heterozygous individuals for at least one of the variants, the OR among this group was 2.6 for coronary heart disease. Furthermore, the OR for premature coronary heart disease, defined as coronary heart disease among males younger than 55 years and females younger than 65 years, was 3.7. In the future, identifying groups of individuals with a several-fold increase in disease risk based on a PRS may facilitate the design and implementation of targeted intervention strategies in larger groups of individuals, but will require genome-wide genetic data collection.

Disease Models for Multifactorial Inheritance

The search for susceptibility loci in human multifactorial disorders has met with increasing success in recent years, largely as a result of the success of GWAS. Examples of recent research in some common conditions will be considered to illustrate the progress to date and the extent of the challenges that lie ahead.

Diabetes Mellitus

There are two main forms of DM that are clinically distinct. T1DM is the rarer juvenile-onset, insulin-dependent form (previous abbreviation IDDM) which affects 0.4% of the population and shows a high incidence of potentially serious renal, retinal, and vascular complications. T1DM has a peak age of onset in adolescence and can only be controlled by regular injection of insulin. T2DM is the more common later-onset, non-insulin-dependent form that affects up to 10% of the population and is strongly associated with overweight and obesity. It usually affects older persons and may respond to simple weight loss, although many people with T2DM require oral hypoglycaemic medication, and some require insulin. An additional 1% to 2% of persons with diabetes have **monogenic** (single gene) forms of diabetes.

Up to 10% of women develop glucose intolerance during pregnancy. This is known as **gestational** diabetes. Their abnormal glucose tolerance usually reverts to normal after the pregnancy; although these women have an increased risk of developing T2DM later in life.

Diabetes can also occur secondary to a variety of other rare genetic syndromes and non-genetic disorders. Examples include Prader-Willi syndrome (p. 78), Bardet-Biedl syndrome, Wolfram syndrome, and Friedreich ataxia (p. 292). DM is therefore etiologically heterogeneous.

Type 1 Diabetes Mellitus

Initial research into the genetics of diabetes tended to focus on T1DM, where there is greater evidence for familial clustering (λ_s is 15 for T1DM versus 3.5 for T2DM [p. 139]). The concordance rates in MZ and DZ twins are approximately 50% and 12%, respectively. These observations point to a multifactorial etiology with both environmental and genetic contributions. Known environmental factors include diet, viral exposure in early childhood, and certain drugs. The disease process involves irreversible destruction of insulin-producing islet β cells in the pancreas by the body's own immune system, perhaps as a result of an interaction between infection and an abnormal genetically programmed immune response.

The first major breakthrough came with the recognition of strong associations with the HLA region on chromosome 6p21. The original associations were with the HLA B8 and B15 antigens that are in linkage disequilibrium with the DR3 and DR4 alleles. It is with these that the T1DM association is strongest, with 95% of affected individuals having DR3 and/or DR4 compared with 50% of the general population. Following the development of PCR analysis for the HLA region, it was shown that the HLA contribution to T1DM susceptibility is determined by the 57th amino acid residue at the DQ locus, where aspartic acid conveys protection, in contrast to other alleles that increase susceptibility. The HLA region contributes approximately 50% of the genetic susceptibility to T1DM.

The next locus to be identified was the insulin gene on chromosome 11p15, where it was shown that variation in the number of tandem repeats of a 14-bp sequence upstream of the gene (known as the *INS* variable number tandem repeat [**VNTR**]) influences disease susceptibility. It is hypothesized that long repeats convey protection by increasing expression of the insulin gene in the fetal thymus gland, thereby reducing the likelihood that insulin-producing β cells will be viewed as foreign by the mature immune system.

These two loci contribute λ_s values of approximately 3 and 1.3, respectively. However, the total risk ratio for T1DM is approximately 15. Numerous GWAS of increasing size have led to an explosion in the number of T1DM susceptibility loci supported by robust statistical evidence, bringing the total to over 50 distinct genomic locations. It is likely that many more remain to be identified through future, even larger, efforts. Most of the identified loci confer a modest increase in the risk of T1DM, with ORs (Table 10.2) ranging from 1.1 to 1.3 for each inherited allele, in contrast with the much larger role of the HLA locus. In most cases, the causal genes and variants underlying the associations have yet to be identified. However, the regions of association often encompass strong biological candidates—for example, the interleukin genes *IL10*, *IL19*, *IL20*, and *IL27*. In two notable cases, follow-up studies have already enabled the causal gene to be confirmed, deepening our understanding of the biological pathways behind the associations.

The first example was a study of the *IL2RA* (*CD25*) locus by Dendrou et al (2009). It used the United Kingdom–based Cambridge BioResource, a collection of approximately 5000 volunteers who can be recalled to participate in research on the basis of their genotype. Using fewer than 200 of these individuals, and by means of flow cytometry to assay the levels of CD25 protein expressed on the surface of T-regulatory cells, the study showed that people with the T1DM-protective haplotype expressed higher CD25 levels. This confirmed that *IL2RA* is indeed the causal gene, and that the genotype-phenotype association is mediated via differences in expression of the gene product.

In the second study by Nejentsev et al (2009), the exons and splice sites of 10 candidate genes situated in regions of genomewide association were resequenced in 480 T1DM patients and 480 controls. Variants identified were then tested for association with the disease in 30,000 further subjects. Four rare variants (minor allele frequency ≈ 1%–2%) in the *IFIH1* gene were identified, each of which independently reduced the odds of T1DM by about 50%. This finding demonstrated that the *IFIH1* gene is important in the etiology of T1DM. Because its function is to mediate the induction of an interferon response to viral RNA, this adds to the evidence implicating viral infection in the development of the disease. These results also demonstrate that there may be both high- and low-frequency susceptibility variants at the same locus, with varying effect sizes. Future follow-up by resequencing of other loci, both in T1DM and in other diseases, should lead to the identification of even more of these variants and a better understanding of the loci.

Type 2 Diabetes

The prevalence of T2DM is increasing and is predicted to reach 300 million affected worldwide by 2025. Although commonly believed to be more benign than the earlier-onset, insulin-dependent T1DM, patients with T2DM are also prone to both macrovascular and microvascular diabetic complications, with corresponding excess morbidity and mortality.

GWAS have identified over 240 susceptibility loci for T2DM. There is no overlap with the T1DM loci, illustrating that these two diseases have very different etiologies. Unlike the HLA and *INS* VNTR loci in T1DM, there are no major predisposing loci commonly associated with T2DM. Most ORs for common variants are modest (between 1.03 and 1.37 per allele), with higher ORs for lower-frequency or rare variants (1.08–8.05 per allele). The latest GWAS of T2DM has shown that the prevalence of T2DM among the 18% of individuals carrying the highest polygenic risk scores is ninefold higher compared with individuals with a lower burden of risk alleles. Analysis of the susceptibility loci for T2DM suggests several mechanisms are involved in disease etiology, including cAMP response element–binding protein (CREB)-related transcription, adipocytokine signaling, and cell cycle regulation.

The *TCF7L2* locus has the largest OR of all T2DM loci found in multiple populations. Individuals who inherit two risk alleles (approximately 9% of Europeans) are at nearly twice the risk of developing T2DM as those who inherit none. The locus was discovered in large-scale association studies of a region on chromosome 10, which was originally identified in linkage studies. However, the *TCF7L2* variant does not account for the linkage in this region, suggesting that other rarer but more penetrant variants may be close by. As with many of the other loci, the *TCF7L2* risk allele is associated with impaired β-cell function, highlighting the importance of the β-cell and insulin secretion in T2DM etiology. As more loci for T2DM have been discovered, the role of insulin sensitivity in the etiology has also been highlighted. Thus a more complex picture is emerging.

Obesity is a well-known risk factor for T2DM, and there are examples of obesity-related genes associated with T2DM, for example, the *FTO* gene, which was previously of unknown function. Recent research has shown, using mouse models and CRISPR/Cas9 genome editing techniques, that the obesity-predisposing allele of FTO represses mitochondrial thermogenesis, preventing adipocytes from converting from fat storage to fat burning functions. However, most T2DM susceptibility loci are not associated with obesity (Fig. 10.10), suggesting that there are BMI-independent mechanisms involved in the etiology of T2DM.

It is likely that many more loci will be identified through future metaanalyzes of GWAS, and that detailed follow-up of the associated regions will lead to identification of the causal variants. The large number of predisposing loci highlights multiple targets for intervention, but there is more work to be done to translate these findings into clinical applications.

Crohn Disease

Inflammatory bowel disease (IBD) includes two clinical subtypes: Crohn disease and ulcerative colitis. The prevalence of IBD in Western countries is 0.15% to 0.5%, and the estimated λ_s is between 23 and 25. Crohn disease is characterized by perturbed control of inflammation in the gut and its interaction with bacteria.

In 2001, two groups working independently and using different approaches identified disease-predisposing variants in the *CARD15* gene (previously known as *NOD2*). One of the groups, Ogura et al,

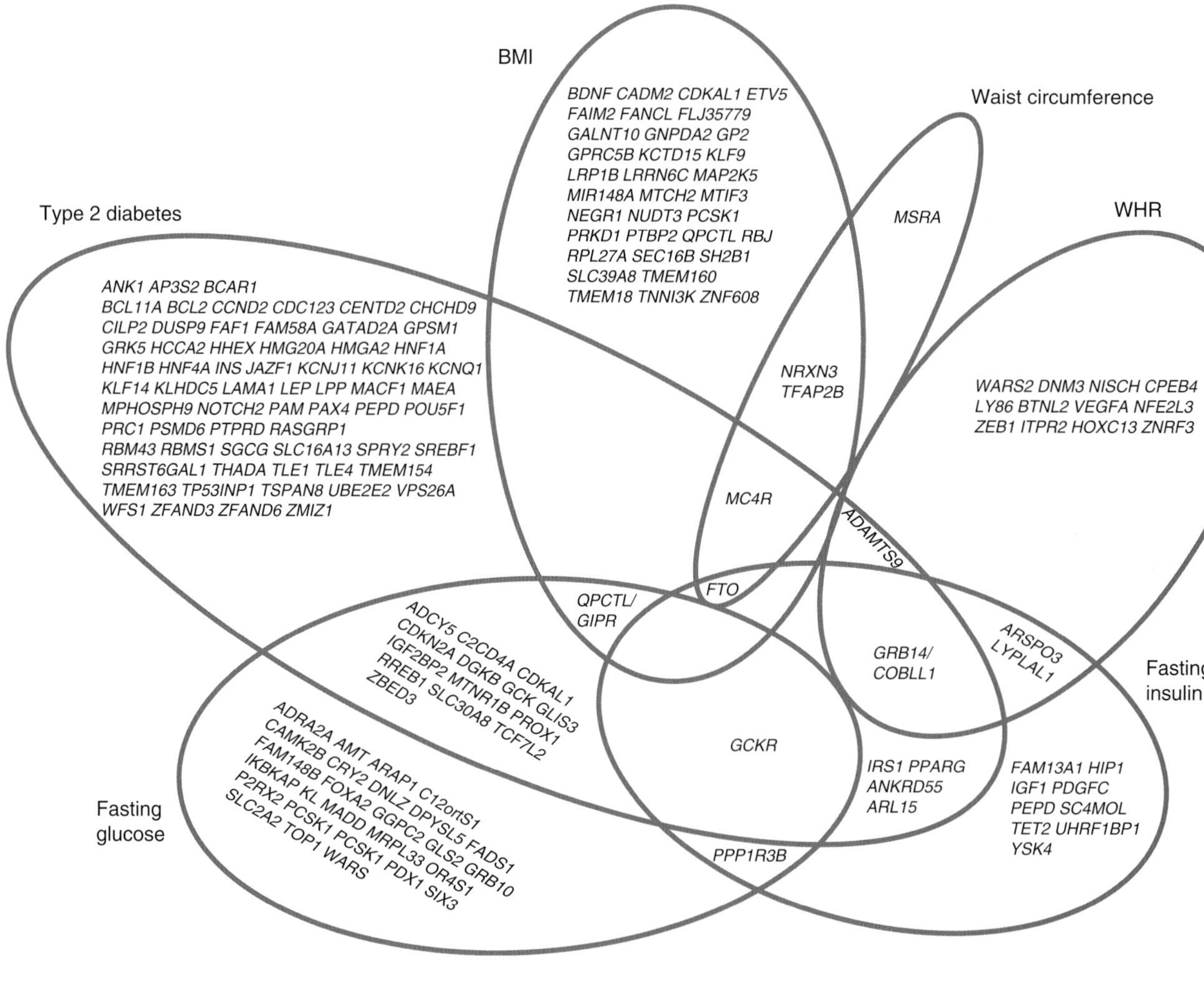

• **Fig. 10.10** Venn diagram of intersection between loci associated at genome-wide significance with type 2 diabetes, measures of adiposity and glucose homeostasis. Genome-wide significant associations for six metabolic traits are shown. Gene symbols shown in the plot are by convention the closest gene and not necessarily the functional gene. (From Grarup N, Sandholt CH, Hansen T, Pedersen O. Genetic susceptibility to type 2 diabetes and obesity: from genome-wide association studies to rare variants and beyond. *Diabetologia* 2014;57:1528–1541.)

had previously identified a Toll-like receptor (p. 171), NOD2, which activates nuclear factor Kappa-B (NFκB) (p. 178), making it responsive to bacterial lipopolysaccharides. Sequence analysis revealed three variants (p.(Arg702Trp), p.(Gly908Arg), and c.3020insC) that were shown by case-control and transmission disequilibrium tests to be associated with Crohn disease. The second group, Hugot et al, fine-mapped the 16p12 region by genotyping SNPs within the 20-megabase interval and also arrived at the same variants within the *CARD15* gene. These variants are found in up to 15% of patients with Crohn disease but only 5% of controls. The relative risk conferred by heterozygous and homozygous genotypes was approximately 2.5 and 40, respectively. For therapy, drugs which target the NFκB complex are already the most effective drugs currently available.

Since 2006, GWAS have identified over 200 susceptibility loci for IBD, all of which confer more modest risks of disease than the *CARD15* variants (ORs per allele between 1.1 and 2.5). The genes identified implicate innate immunity, T-cell signaling and epithelial barrier function as the predominant etiological mechanisms in IBD. Discoveries of loci containing the *IRGM* and *ATG16L1* genes were particularly exciting findings because these genes are essential for autophagy, a biological pathway whose relevance to the disease was previously unsuspected. Further studies of the *IRGM* locus by McCarroll et al (2008) identified that the causal variant is a 20-kb deletion immediately upstream of *IRGM*, which is in linkage disequilibrium (p. 93) with the associated SNPs. The deletion results in altered patterns of gene expression, which in turn were shown to modulate the autophagy of bacteria inside cells.

Coronary Artery Disease

Coronary artery disease is the most common cause of death in industrialized countries and is rapidly increasing in prevalence in developing countries. It results from atherosclerosis, a process taking place over many years which involves the deposition of fibrous plaques in the subendothelial space (intima) of arteries, with a consequent narrowing of their lumina. Narrowing of the coronary arteries compromises the metabolic needs of the heart muscle, leading to myocardial ischemia, which if severe, results in myocardial infarction.

For the majority of persons, their risk of coronary artery disease is multifactorial or polygenic in origin. A variety of different genetic and environmental risk factors have been identified that predispose to early onset of the atherosclerotic process, including lack of exercise, dietary saturated fat, and smoking.

Lipid Metabolism

The metabolic pathways by which the body absorbs, synthesizes, transports and catabolizes dietary and endogenous lipids are complex. Lipids are packaged in intestinal cells as a complex with various proteins known as **apolipoproteins** to form triglyceride-rich chylomicrons. These are secreted into the lymph and transported to the liver, where, in association with endogenous synthesis of triglyceride and cholesterol, they are packaged and secreted into the circulation as triglyceride-rich very low-density lipoproteins (VLDLs). VLDL is degraded to intermediate-density lipoprotein (IDL), which is further broken down into cholesterol-rich LDLs. High-density lipoproteins (HDLs) are formed from lipoproteins secreted by the liver, chylomicrons, and VLDL remnants.

High levels of LDLs are associated with an increased risk of coronary artery disease. Conversely, high levels of HDLs are inversely correlated with a risk of coronary artery disease. Consequently, the LDL:HDL ratio has been used as a risk predictor for coronary artery disease and as an indicator for therapeutic intervention. Statins are effective drugs for lowering LDL cholesterol levels.

Family and Twin Studies

The risk to a first-degree relative of a person with premature coronary artery disease, defined as occurring before age 55 years in males and age 65 years in females, varies between two and seven times that for the general population (Table 10.4). Twin studies of concordance for coronary artery disease vary from 15% to 25% for DZ twins and from 39% to 48% for MZ twins. Although these figures support the involvement of genetic factors, the low concordance rate for MZ twins clearly supports the importance of environmental factors.

Single-Gene Disorders of Lipid Metabolism Leading to Coronary Artery Disease

Although there are a number of individually rare inherited disorders of specific lipoproteins, levels of the various lipoproteins and the hyperlipidemias are determined by a complex interaction of genetic and environmental factors. Family studies of some of the hyperlipidemias are, however, consistent with a single gene being a major factor determining genetic susceptibility.

Familial Hypercholesterolemia

The best-known disorder of lipid metabolism is FH (p. 277). FH is associated with a significantly increased risk of early coronary artery disease and is inherited as an autosomal dominant disorder. It has been estimated that about 1 person in 500 in the general population, and about 1 in 20 persons presenting with early coronary artery disease, are heterozygous for a mutation in the low-density lipoprotein receptor (*LDLR*) gene. Molecular studies in FH have revealed that it is because of a variety of defects in the number, function or processing of the LDL receptors on the cell surface (Fig. 18.9, p.280).

Susceptibility Genes

Since 2007, numerous large-scale GWAS and follow-up replication studies have identified over 160 susceptibility loci for coronary artery disease and myocardial infarction. Of these loci many are also associated with lipid levels and blood pressure, and the key pathways implicated in the pathogenesis of coronary artery disease from GWAS are lipid metabolism, inflammation, and artery vessel wall structure. One of the strongest associations identified is on chromosome 9p21 (OR per allele $\approx$ 1.3). The nearest genes, *CDKN2A* and *CDKN2B*, are over 100 kb away. Interestingly, the SNPs most strongly associated with coronary artery disease are only 10 kb

TABLE 10.4 Recurrence risks for premature coronary artery disease

Proband	Relative Risk
Male (< 55 years old)	
Brother	5
Sister	2.5
Female (< 65 years old)	
Siblings	7

(From Slack J, Evans KA. The increased risk of death from ischemic heart disease in first degree relatives of 121 men and 96 women with ischemic heart disease. *J Med Genet.* 1966;3:239–257.)

away from those associated with T2DM. However, the two disease associations are independent and not in linkage disequilibrium with one another. Much work is already being done to investigate the role of *ANRIL*, a large non-coding RNA which overlaps with the coronary artery disease-associated haplotype. It is expressed in tissues associated with atherosclerosis, and studies have shown correlations between expression of *ANRIL* transcripts and severity of atherosclerosis. However, additional evidence from large-scale association studies has shown that the same haplotype on 9p21 is associated with abdominal aortic aneurysm and intracranial aneurysm, suggesting that its role is not limited to atherosclerotic disease. Together with other loci, the locus at 9p21 only explains a small fraction (approximately 9%) of the heritability of coronary artery disease, and it is likely that many more loci will be identified.

Progress in uncovering susceptibility loci has also come from large GWAS of lipid levels. Over 380 loci have been robustly associated with circulating levels of lipids through large-scale GWAS metaanalysis. In addition to common variants, low frequency variants have also been associated with lipid levels, and together these variants explain up to 11.7%, 13.7%, 14.6% and 15.0% of the variance in triglycerides, HDL cholesterol, LDL cholesterol and total cholesterol concentrations, respectively. The frequency of LDL-raising alleles is higher in patients with coronary artery disease than in controls, indicating that they predispose to the disease via their primary effect on LDL levels. In many cases, the genes implicated by the loci are already associated with single-gene disorders. For example, *PCSK9* harbors a full spectrum of LDL-altering alleles, from rare mutations which cause large differences in LDL (> 100 mg/dL), through low-frequency variants with more modest effects (e.g., *PCSK9* p.(Arg46Leu) has a 1% minor allele frequency and a 16 mg/dL effect size), to common variants at 20% minor allele frequency which change LDL levels by less than 5 mg/dL. Monoclonal antibody PCSK9 inhibitors have now been approved for use as cholesterol-lowering agents and could provide an alternative to statin treatment. The resequencing of further loci is likely to uncover rarer variants and mutations at lipid trait loci, which may further explain genetic susceptibility to coronary artery disease.

Schizophrenia

Schizophrenia is a serious psychotic illness with an onset usually in late adolescence or early adult life. It is characterized by grossly disorganized thought processes and behavior, together with a marked deterioration of social and occupational functioning, and can be accompanied by hallucinations and delusions.

Epidemiology

Schizophrenia is a principal cause of chronic mental illness. There is a 1% lifetime risk for a person to develop schizophrenia, and at any one time approximately 0.2% of the population is affected. Schizophrenia occurs more commonly in individuals of poorer socioeconomic status and has an earlier age of onset and worse prognosis in males. There is an excess of winter births in schizophrenic individuals, which has suggested that environmental factors such as certain viral infections or nutritional factors could be contributory.

Evidence for Genetic Factors

The nature and extent of the genetic contribution to schizophrenia is unclear. This is partly because of past and continuing controversy concerning the definition of schizophrenia and the term schizoid. The latter term refers to the schizophrenia-like traits often seen in relatives of schizophrenics. The problem arises because clinical criteria to distinguish schizoid personality from normal personality are lacking. For the sake of simplicity, we can regard the term schizoid as referring to a person with the fundamental symptoms of schizophrenia but in a milder form. It has been estimated that roughly 4% of the general population have schizophrenia or a schizoid personality disorder.

Family and Twin Studies

The results of several studies of the prevalence of schizophrenia and schizoid disorder among the relatives of schizophrenics are summarized in Table 10.5. If only schizophrenia is considered, the concordance rate for identical twins is only 46%, suggesting the importance of environmental factors. If, however, schizophrenia and schizoid personality disorder are considered together, then almost 90% of identical twins are concordant.

Susceptibility Genes

GWAS of copy number variations have identified large (> 500 kb) deletions associated with the condition—for example on chromosomes 1q21.1, 15q13.3, and 22q11.2 (p. 259). These deletions are rare but penetrant: the OR for the 15q13.3 deletion

TABLE 10.5 Proportions (%) of first-degree relatives of individuals with schizophrenia who are similarly affected or have a schizoid disorder[a]

	PROPORTION (%) OF RELATIVES		
Relatives	**Schizophrenia[b]**	**Schizoid**	**Total Schizophrenia + Schizoid**
Identical twins	46	41	87
Offspring (of one schizophrenic)	16	33	49
Siblings	14	32	46
Parents	9	35	44
Offspring (of two schizophrenics)	34	32	66
General population	1	3	4

[a]From Heston LL. The genetics of schizophrenia and schizoid disease. *Science.* 1970;167:249–256.

[b]Age corrected.

has been estimated at between 16 and 18 in two independent studies. A key observation is that these deletions are not only associated with schizophrenia. The 1q21.1 deletion (p. 262) has also been associated with autism, learning disability, and epilepsy. Thus, current clinically defined disease boundaries are not mirrored by the underlying genetics. Although these deletions explain some of the genetic susceptibility to schizophrenia, they also explain susceptibility to other conditions. It is likely that a better understanding of the genetics will lead to better definition of clinical phenotypes.

Common genetic variants are also implicated in the etiology of schizophrenia. Recent metaanalyzes of GWAS have identified over 100 associated loci, including the HLA region on chromosome 6p21.3–6p22.1, suggesting an immune system component to the risk of disease. Robust associations have also been observed with variants near the *NRGN* gene and in the *TCF4* gene, which implicate biological pathways involved in brain development, cognition and memory. To date, researchers have shown that polygenic risk scores have low predictive power for schizophrenia presently, explaining 7% of variation in risk as measured on the liability scale. There are likely to be many more common and rare variants that collectively contribute to the heritability of schizophrenia.

Alzheimer Disease

Dementia is characterized by an irreversible and progressive global impairment of intellect, memory, social skills and control of emotional reactions, in the presence of normal consciousness. Dementia is etiologically heterogeneous, occurring secondarily to both a variety of non-genetic causes such as vascular disease and infections such as acquired immunodeficiency syndrome, as well as genetic causes. Alzheimer disease (AD) is the most common cause of dementia in persons with either early-onset (<60 years, or presenile) or late-onset (> 60 years, or senile) dementia. The classic neuropathological finding in persons with AD is the presence at postmortem examination of amyloid deposits in neurofibrillary tangles and neuronal or senile plaques. In addition, individuals with Down syndrome have an increased risk of developing dementia (p. 250), which at postmortem has identical central nervous system findings to those seen in persons with typical AD.

Epidemiology

Limited numbers of studies of the incidence and prevalence of AD are available, owing to problems of ascertainment. However, the risk of developing AD clearly increases dramatically with age (Table 10.6).

TABLE 10.6 Estimates of age-specific cumulative prevalence of dementia

Age Interval (Years)	Prevalence (%)
<70	1.3
70–74	2.3
75–79	6.4
80–84	15.3
85–89	23.7
90–94	42.9
>95	50.9

(From Heston LL. Alzheimer's disease, in King RA, Rotter JI, Motulsky AG, eds. *The genetic basis of common diseases.* New York: Oxford University Press; 1992.)

Twin and Family Studies

Differences in the age of onset of AD in identical twins are consistent with the importance of environmental factors, but there are difficulties with family studies in AD. Many studies are based on a clinical diagnosis. However, a significant proportion of persons with a clinical diagnosis of AD are found to have other causes at postmortem, such as cerebrovascular atherosclerotic disease. Attempts to confirm diagnoses in relatives who have died previously are often unsuccessful. Obviously, given the age of onset, it is generally neither practical nor possible to obtain funding for prospective studies of the risk to offspring. Therefore family studies of the risk to siblings are the only practical type of family study to provide reliable data. Although there are numerous retrospective reports of families with AD that are consistent with autosomal dominant inheritance, recurrence risks in a number of studies for first-degree relatives are less than 10%. The risks are age-related and are greater the younger the age at diagnosis in the affected individual.

Biochemical Studies

The amyloid deposits in the neurofibrillary tangles and neuronal plaques have been shown to consist of the amyloid-β A4 precursor protein (APP). The major protein component of the neurofibrillary tangles has been shown to be derived from a microtubule-associated protein (MAP) called *tau* (τ). Along with other MAPs, it interacts with β-tubulin to stabilize microtubules.

Single-Gene Disorders

The identification of APP in the amyloid deposits of the neuronal plaques, its mapping in or near the critical region of the distal part of chromosome 21q associated with the phenotypic features of Down syndrome (p. 250) and the increased risk of AD in persons with Down syndrome led to the suggestion that duplication of the *APP* gene could be a cause of AD. Evidence of linkage to the *APP* locus was found in studies of families with early-onset AD, and it is now known that mutations in the *APP* gene account for a small proportion of cases.

Evidence of linkage to early-onset AD was found for another locus on chromosome 14q. Mutations were identified in a proportion of affected individuals in one of a novel class of genes known as *presenilin-1* (*PSEN1*), now known to be a component of the Notch signaling pathway (p. 109). A large number of mutations in *PSEN1* have now been identified and account for up to 70% of familial early-onset AD. A second gene, *presenilin-2* (*PSEN2*), with homology to *PSEN1*, was mapped to chromosome 1q and has been shown to have mutations in a limited number of families with AD. *PSEN1* and *PSEN2* encode integral membrane proteins containing multiple transmembrane domains that localize to the endoplasmic reticulum and the Golgi complex. All of the presenile dementias following autosomal dominant inheritance demonstrate high penetrance.

Susceptibility Genes

Polymorphisms in the apolipoprotein E (*APOE*) gene are the most important genetic risk factor identified for late-onset AD. The locus was initially identified in the early 1990s through linkage studies. The *APOE* gene has three major protein isoforms, ε2, ε3, and ε4. Numerous studies in various populations and ethnic groups have shown an increased frequency of the ε4 allele in persons with both sporadic and late-onset familial AD. In addition, the ε2 allele is associated with a decreased risk of the disease. The finding of apolipoprotein E in senile plaques and neurofibrillary tangles, along with its role in lipid transport, possibly in relation to the nerve injury and regeneration seen in AD, provides further evidence for a possible role in the acceleration of the neurodegenerative process in AD.

Although the *APOE* ε4 allele, found in up to 40% of cases, is a clearly an important risk factor, the strongest association is with the age of onset rather than the absolute risk of developing AD. The *APOE* ε4 allele is therefore neither necessary nor sufficient for the development of AD, emphasising the importance of other genetic and environmental etiological factors.

GWAS of AD have found over 20 loci associated with disease risk, but none has an effect comparable with *APOE*, the ORs ranging from 1.1 to 2.0. In fact, even in combination, the attributable risk of all common variants is less than that for *APOE*. Polygenic risk scores that include all associated loci do not presently have sufficient discriminatory power for clinical use. The loci do however shed light on the pathogenesis of AD, and there appear to be three predominant pathways involved: cholesterol and lipid metabolism; immune system and inflammatory response; and endosomal vesicle cycling. Further work will be needed to uncover the mechanisms underlying these associations, and it is likely that many more loci with more modest effects remain to be discovered.

ELEMENTS

1. The concept of multifactorial inheritance has been proposed to account for the common congenital malformations and acquired disorders that show non-Mendelian familial aggregation. These disorders are thought to result from the interaction of genetic and environmental factors.
2. Human characteristics such as height and intelligence, which show a normally distributed continuous distribution in the general population, are probably caused by the additive effects of many genes (i.e., polygenic inheritance).
3. According to the liability/threshold model for multifactorial inheritance, the population's genetic and environmental susceptibility, which is known as liability, is normally distributed. Individuals are affected if their liability exceeds a threshold superimposed on the liability curve.
4. Recurrence risks to relatives for multifactorial disorders are influenced by the disease severity, the degree of relationship to the index case, the number of affected close relatives and, if there is a higher incidence in one particular sex, the sex of the index case.
5. Heritability is a measure of the proportion of the total variance of a character or disease that is because of the genetic variance. Heritability is best calculated in twin and family studies.
6. Thousands of genetic susceptibility loci for multiple common diseases have been identified. Major progress has been enabled in recent years by genome-wide association studies revealing new biological pathways involved in disease pathogenesis and leading to future therapeutic advances.
7. Polygenic risk scores constructed from genome-wide association study data have the potential to stratify sub–disease groups and target groups of individuals with the highest genetic risk for preventative strategies.

Further Reading

Albert FW, Kruglyak L. The role of regulatory variation in complex traits and disease. *Nat Rev Genet.* 2015;16:197–212.

This article highlights the challenges and approaches that can be used to take a region of association identified by genome-wide association studies through to understanding how that locus causes disease or variation in a trait.

Falconer DS. The inheritance of liability to certain diseases estimated from the incidence among relatives. *Ann Hum Genet.* 1965;29: 51–76.

The original exposition of the liability/threshold model and how correlations between relatives can be used to calculate heritability.

Fraser FC. Evolution of a palatable multifactorial threshold model. *Am J Hum Genet.* 1980;32:796–813.

An amusing and "reader-friendly" account of models proposed to explain multifactorial inheritance.

Khera AV, Chaffin M, Aragam KG, et al. Genome-wide polygenic scores for common diseases identify individuals with risk equivalent to monogenic mutations. *Nat Genet.* 2018;50:1219–1224.

An example of constructing and using polygenic risk scores to determine groups at high risk of common disease.

Lloyd-Jones LR, Zeng J, Sidorenko J, et al. Improved polygenic prediction by Bayesian multiple regression on summary statistics. *Nat Commun.* 2019;10:5086.

Provides examples of computer programs that implement statistical modeling to generate polygenic risk scores, and also compares predictive accuracy for continuous traits of different scores.

McCarthy MI, Abecasis GR, Cardon LR, et al. Genome-wide association studies for complex traits: consensus, uncertainty and challenges. *Nat Rev Genet.* 2008;9:356–369.

Detailed review article on genome-wide association studies, which gives a comprehensive overview of the methods and highlights the various challenges which still need to be addressed in the search for complex disease genes.

Visscher PM, Brown MA, McCarthy MI, Yang J. Five years of GWAS discovery. *Am J Hum Genet.* 2012;90:7–24.

Summarizes the progress made as a result of the first five years of GWAS. It focuses on autoimmune and metabolic disease, but gives an excellent general overview of the field.

Witte JS, Visscher PM, Wray NR. The contribution of genetic variants to disease depends on the ruler. *Nat Rev Genet.* 2014;15:765–776.

Assesses the different methods that can be used to determine the genetic contribution or heritability of a trait or disease.

11

Screening for Genetic Disease

A lot of politicians are beginning to be aware that it actually does save money to prevent nonlethal, lifelong handicapping conditions, because they require so damn much money.

Robert Guthrie (1916–1995), writing in the* Buffalo Courier-Express Sunday Magazine *in 1980.

Genetic disease may affect individuals and their families dramatically, but every couple having children is at some risk of seeing a disorder with a genetic component suddenly appear. Our concepts and approaches to screening reflect the different burdens that these two realities impose. First, there is screening of individuals and couples known to be at significant or high risk because of a positive family history—sometimes referred to as **targeted** or **family screening**. This includes **carrier**, or **heterozygote**, **screening**, as well as **presymptomatic testing**. Second, there is the screening offered to the general population, who are at low risk—sometimes referred to as **community genetics**—and very much within the remit of public health. Population screening involves the offer of genetic testing on an equitable basis to all relevant individuals in a defined group. The objectives are to prevent morbidity and suffering resulting from genetic disease and to enhance individual autonomy through better information about genetic risks and reproductive options.

Screening Those at High Risk

Here we focus on the wide range of general genetic disease rather than screening in the field of cancer genetics, which is addressed in Chapter 14. Prenatal screening is also covered in more detail in Chapter 20. If it were easy to recognize carriers of autosomal and X-linked recessive disorders and persons who are heterozygous for autosomal dominant disorders that show reduced penetrance or a late age of onset, much doubt and uncertainty would be removed when providing information in genetic counseling. Increasingly, analysis of DNA variants in causative genes is making the task easier. Where this is not possible, either because no gene test is available or because sequencing is negative or yields variants of uncertain significance, a number of strategies are available to detect carriers of autosomal recessive and X-linked recessive disorders, and for presymptomatic diagnosis of heterozygotes for autosomal dominant disorders.

Carrier Testing for Autosomal Recessive and X-Linked Disorders

In a number of autosomal recessive disorders, such as some inborn errors of metabolism (e.g., Tay-Sachs disease; p. 281) and the hemoglobinopathies (e.g., sickle-cell disease; p. 164), carriers can be recognized with a high degree of certainty using biochemical or hematological techniques, and DNA analysis is not essential. In other single-gene disorders it is possible to detect or confirm carrier status by biochemical means in only a proportion of carriers; for example, mildly abnormal coagulation study results in a woman at risk of being a carrier for hemophilia (p. 316). A significant proportion of obligate carriers of hemophilia will have normal coagulation, however, so a normal result does not exclude carrier status.

There are several ways to recognize carriers of genetic disease.

Clinical Manifestations in Carriers

Occasionally, carriers for certain disorders have mild clinical manifestations of the disease (Table 11.1), particularly with some of the X-linked disorders. These manifestations are usually so slight that they are apparent only on careful clinical examination; for instance, the mosaic pattern of retinal pigmentation seen in female carriers of X-linked ocular albinism (Fig. 11.1), or the characteristic lens opacities seen in Fabry disease. Such manifestations, although minimal, are often reliable, but they are the exception rather than the rule. In most autosomal recessive and X-linked recessive disorders there are either no reliable manifestations in carriers or the manifestations overlap with the variation seen in the general population. Female carriers of hemophilia, for example, may have a tendency to bruise easily, but this is far too common in the general population to determine carrier status definitively. In X-linked adrenoleukodystrophy, a proportion of female carriers manifest mild neurological problems relatively late in life, but these might easily be confused with the aging process.

Biochemical Abnormalities in Carriers

Historically, the demonstration of detectable biochemical abnormalities in carriers of certain conditions has been important. The biochemical abnormality may be a direct product of the gene, and carrier status can be investigated with confidence. For example, in carriers of Tay-Sachs disease the range of enzyme (**hexosaminidase**) activity is intermediate between levels found in normal and affected people. Carrier testing for Tay-Sachs disease in many orthodox Jewish communities, where the carrier frequency is relatively high, is highly developed. Because of faith-based objections to termination of pregnancy, carrier testing may be crucial in the selection of life partners. A couple considering betrothal will first see their rabbi, who will counsel them and arrange carrier testing for Tay-Sachs disease. If both prove to be carriers, the proposed engagement will be called off, leaving them free to look for a new partner. If only one proves to be a carrier the engagement can

TABLE 11.1 Clinical and biochemical abnormalities in carriers of X-linked disorders

Disorder	Abnormality
Clinical	
Anhidrotic ectodermal dysplasia	Sweat pore counts reduced, dental anomalies
Alport syndrome	hematuria
Fabry disease	Corneal and lens opacities
Lowe syndrome	Lens opacities
Ocular albinism	Mosaic retinal pigmentary pattern
Retinitis pigmentosa	Mosaic retinal pigmentation, abnormal electroretinographic findings
Biochemical	
Becker muscular dystrophy	Raised serum creatine kinase level
Duchenne muscular dystrophy	Raised serum creatine kinase level
Glucose 6-phosphate dehydrogenase (G6PD) deficiency	Erythrocyte G6PD activity reduced
Hemophilia A	Reduced factor VIII activity:antigen ratio
Hemophilia B	Reduced levels of factor IX
Hunter syndrome	Reduced sulfoiduronate sulfatase activity in skin fibroblasts
Lesch-Nyhan syndrome fibroblasts	Reduced hypoxanthine-guanine phosphoribosyl transferase activity in skin
Vitamin D–resistant rickets	Serum phosphate level reduced

In many cases these methods have been superseded by direct gene tests.

proceed, although the rabbi does not disclose which one is the carrier. Although such a strategy to prevent genetic disease would theoretically be possible in many communities where inbreeding is the norm, and their "private" diseases have been well characterized, in practice this is very rare.

In many single-gene disorders, the biochemical abnormality used to diagnose the affected individual is not a direct result of action of the gene product but a secondary or downstream consequence. However, because these may be removed from the primary action of the gene they may be only partially useful in identifying carriers. For example, in Duchenne muscular dystrophy (DMD) there is an increased permeability of the muscle membrane, resulting in escape of the muscle enzyme creatine kinase (CK) into the blood. A grossly raised serum CK level often confirms the diagnosis of DMD in a boy presenting with features of the disorder (p. 299). Obligate female carriers of DMD have, on average, serum CK levels that are increased compared with those of the general female population (Fig. 11.2), but there is substantial overlap of CK values between normal and obligate carrier females. Where DNA is not available from an affected male for dystrophin gene sequencing, and sequencing in the at-risk female carrier has been inconclusive, this information can be used in conjunction with pedigree risk information and perhaps linked DNA markers (p. 101) to help calculate the likelihood of a woman

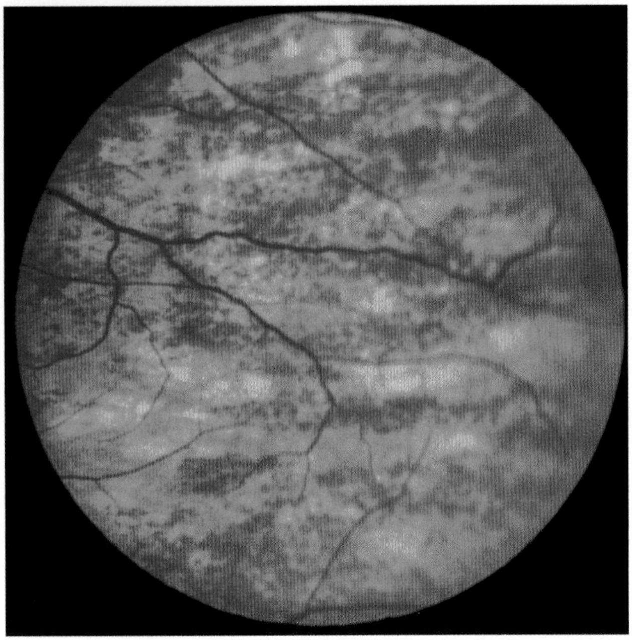

• **Fig. 11.1** The fundus of a carrier of X-linked ocular albinism showing a mosaic pattern of retinal pigmentation. (Courtesy Mr S.J. Charles, The Royal Eye Hospital, Manchester, UK.)

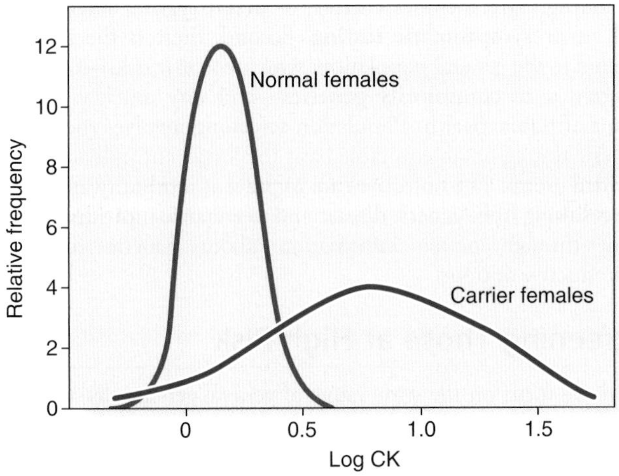

• **Fig. 11.2** Creatine kinase levels in obligate carrier females of Duchenne muscular dystrophy and women from the general population. (Modified from Tippett PA, Dennis NR, Machin D, et al. Creatine kinase activity in the detection of carriers of Duchenne muscular dystrophy: comparison of two methods. *Clin Chim Acta*. 1982;121:345–359.)

being a carrier. The use of linked markers requires DNA samples to be available from key family members, particularly unaffected males. The markers used need to be sufficiently polymorphic to be **informative**, and must tightly flank the locus if possible, and genetic heterogeneity for the condition (where the disease phenotype may be associated with mutations in more than one gene) should not be an issue.

Difficulty with biochemical carrier testing in X-linked recessive disorders is often as a result of random inactivation of the X chromosome in females (p. 73). In some situations "X-inactivation studies" are possible, whereby the analysis of individual clones to look for evidence of two populations of cells is performed, for example, with peripheral blood lymphocytes in carriers of some of the X-linked immunodeficiency syndromes (p. 181).

Presymptomatic Diagnosis of Autosomal Dominant Disorders

Many autosomal dominant single-gene disorders either have a delayed age of onset or exhibit reduced penetrance. **Presymptomatic** or **predictive genetic testing** is often possible, but clinical examination, specialist investigations and biochemical studies may also have a place in determining the at-risk individual's genetic status.

Direct Genetic Testing

As our knowledge of the human genome has grown, direct DNA variant analysis has become the investigation of choice to clarify the genetic status of individuals at risk of inherited conditions. In the majority of clinical situations it is both desirable and necessary to first identify a pathogenic variant in an affected individual within a family. Where this is achieved with confidence, presymptomatic testing can be offered to family members at risk, subject to age-appropriateness and consent/autonomy issues relating to children and minors. A common problem in the outcome of testing, however, is determining the pathogenicity of many DNA findings such as missense variants and intronic changes, especially where they are novel and not previously listed in DNA databases. In these circumstances the help of bioinformatics tools can be crucial. Box 11.1 lists some of the more common conditions in which direct testing is regularly used to offer presymptomatic diagnosis, but there are of course many more.

Clinical Examination

In some dominantly inherited disorders, simple clinical means can be used for presymptomatic diagnosis, taking into account possible pleiotropic effects of a gene (p. 67). For example, individuals with neurofibromatosis type I (NF1) can have a variety of clinical features (p. 296). It is not unusual to examine an apparently unaffected relative of someone with NF1, who has had no medical problems, only to discover that they have sufficient numbers of café-au-lait spots or cutaneous **neurofibromas** to confirm that they are affected. NF1 is a relatively rare example of a dominantly inherited disorder that is virtually 100% penetrant by the age of 5 or 6 years, with visible external features. With many other disorders, clinical examination is less reliable.

In tuberous sclerosis (TSC) a number of body systems may be involved, and the external manifestations, such as the facial rash of angiokeratoma (Fig. 6.5A, p. 69) may not be present. Similarly, seizures and learning difficulties are not inevitable. In autosomal dominant polycystic kidney disease, which is extremely variable and may have a delayed age of onset, there may be no suspicion of the condition from routine examination, and hypertension may be borderline without raising suspicions of an underlying problem. Reaching a diagnosis in Marfan syndrome (p. 308) can be difficult because of variable features and overlap with other joint hypermobility disorders, even though very detailed diagnostic criteria have been established. However, other inherited cardiac conditions, such as the cardiomyopathies or familial arrhythmias (e.g., long QT and Brugada syndromes) present very significant challenges (p. 306). These conditions are clinically variable with reduced penetrance, are genetically very heterogeneous, and in a proportion of cases are the result of digenic inheritance (p. 76).

Specialist Investigation

In conditions where clinical assessment leaves diagnostic doubt or ambiguity, special investigations of relevant body systems can serve to clarify status and deliver presymptomatic diagnosis. In TSC, imaging studies of the brain by computed tomography to look for intracranial calcification (Fig. 11.3) are more or less routine, as

• BOX 11.1 Autosomal Disorders that Show a Delayed Age of Onset, or exhibit Reduced Penetrance, for Which Mutational Analysis (Occasionally Linked Markers) can be used to Offer Presymptomatic Testing

Breast cancer
Familial adenomatous polyposis
Hereditary motor and sensory neuropathy type I
Hereditary non-polyposis colonic cancer
Huntington disease
Inherited cardiac arrhythmias
Marfan syndrome
Myotonic dystrophy
Neurofibromatosis type I
Neurofibromatosis type II
Tuberous sclerosis
Von Hippel–Lindau disease

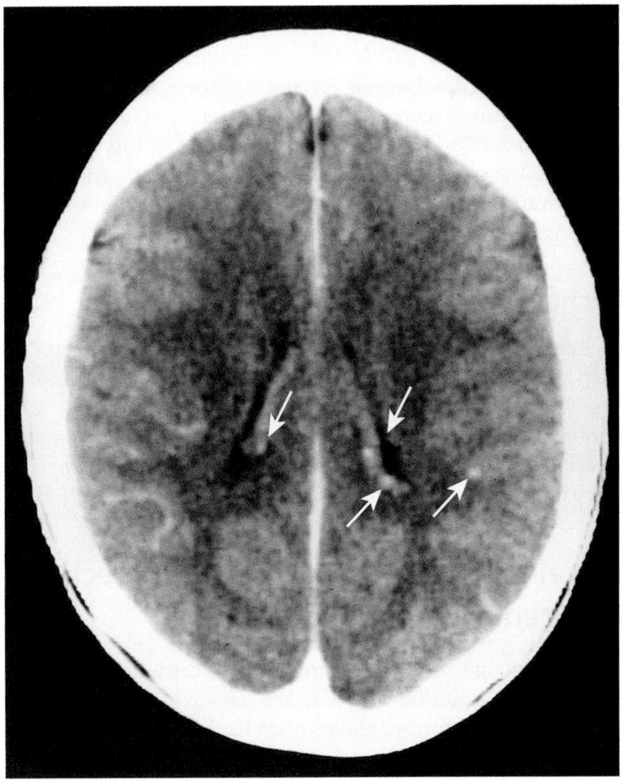

• **Fig. 11.3** Intracranial calcification (*arrows*) in an asymptomatic person with tuberous sclerosis.

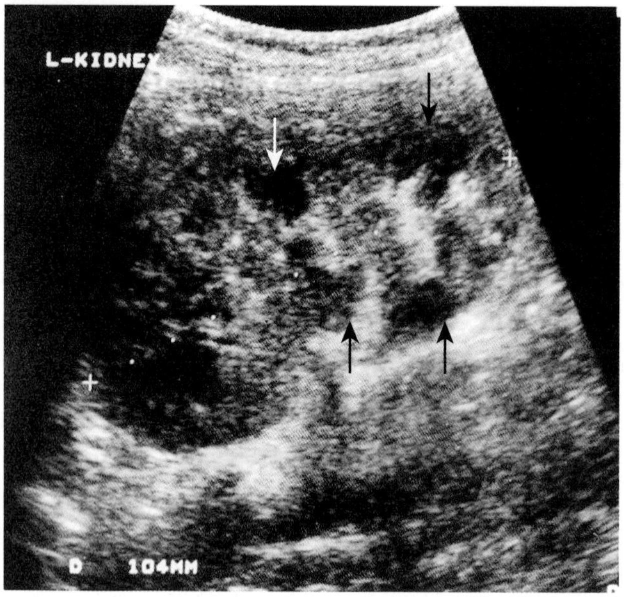

• **Fig. 11.4** Renal ultrasonogram of an asymptomatic person with tuberous sclerosis showing abnormal echogenicity attributed to presumed angiomyolipomata (*arrows*).

well as renal ultrasonography to identify the cysts known as angiomyolipoma(ta) (Fig. 11.4). Use of these relatively non-invasive tests in relatives of persons with TSC can often detect evidence of the condition in asymptomatic persons, especially as sequencing of the *TSC1* and *TSC2* genes is not guaranteed to identify a pathogenic variant.

Similarly, assessment for Marfan syndrome involves ophthalmic examination for evidence of ectopia lentis, echocardiography for measurement of the aortic root diameter, and sometimes magnetic resonance imaging of the lumbar spine to look for evidence of dural ectasia—all of which are important criteria. Their absence does not exclude the diagnosis, and further assessments are necessary if sequencing of the Marfan gene, *FBN1*, reveals a variant of uncertain significance, which is not uncommon for this gene.

Biochemical Tests

Biochemical tests are very useful in some autosomal dominant disorders. Examples include the use of serum cholesterol levels in those at risk of familial hypercholesterolemia (pp. 147, 277), although genetic testing is increasingly available, as well as assay of the appropriate urinary porphyrins or the specific enzyme deficiency in the various dominantly inherited porphyrias (p. 282).

Ethical Considerations in Carrier Detection and Predictive Testing

One of the main reasons for determining the carrier status of a person at risk of an autosomal or X-linked recessive disorder is to help couples make an informed choice when having children. For some, however, the knowledge that there is a significant risk of having an affected child may present options and choices that they would rather avoid. Knowledge of the risk and the awareness that prenatal diagnosis is available may create a sense of guilt whichever decision is taken—either to have a child knowing it could be affected, or to have prenatal testing that may lead to termination of pregnancy. The latter option is especially difficult when the prognosis of the disease cannot be stated with certainty because of its variability or reduced penetrance, or if treatment may be developed in time to help the child.

Experience with these potential dilemmas has resulted in normal practice promoting the flow of information within families, rather than from professionals. In general this approach works well, but professional dilemmas can arise if family members refuse to communicate with one another even when the condition carries significant morbidity and the risk is high, particularly with X-linked conditions.

Presymptomatic diagnosis for some late-onset autosomal dominant disorders has clear medical advantages in relation to early intervention and prevention. In familial adenomatous polyposis, for example (p. 197), colonoscopy looking for the presence of colonic polyps can be offered as a regular screening procedure to those who have been shown to be at high risk of developing colonic cancer by molecular studies. Conversely, individuals who have not inherited a pathogenic variant in the *APC* gene do not need to be screened.

In contrast, for persons at risk for Huntington disease (HD), a disorder for which there is currently no effective treatment to delay onset or progression, the benefit of predictive testing is not immediately obvious. The same is true for familial forms of Alzheimer disease, motor neurone disease, cerebral autosomal dominant arteriopathy with subcortical infarcts and leukoencephalopathy, and the spinocerebellar ataxias. Although choice is often considered to be of paramount importance in genetic counseling for those at risk of inherited disorders, remember that those considering presymptomatic or predictive testing should proceed only if they can give truly informed consent and are free from coercion from others. It is possible that employers, life insurance companies, and society in general will put indirect, and on occasion direct, pressure on those at high risk to be tested (p. 350). Indeed, there are examples in which individuals at risk of HD have received prejudicial treatment in relation to employment, and higher than average insurance premiums can be expected on the basis of the family history alone.

Predictive testing for late-onset disorders can, in theory, be used for children and minors, but this can be a contentious issue. Parents sometimes argue that it is their right to know the status of their child(ren). However, this conflicts with upholding the principle of individual autonomy wherever possible. Presymptomatic testing of children is therefore usually discouraged unless an early medical intervention or screening is beneficial for the disorder, which is certainly true for a number of the familial cancer conditions. The issue of genetic testing of children is addressed more fully in Chapter 22 (p. 348).

Population Screening

One definition of population screening is: "The systematic application of a test or inquiry, to identify individuals at sufficient risk of a specific disorder to warrant further investigation or treatment, amongst persons who have not sought medical attention on account of symptoms of that disorder." Neonatal screening for phenylketonuria is the paradigm of a good screening program and has been available since 1969 in the United Kingdom, with screening for congenital hypothyroidism from 1981. In the United Kingdom, since 1996, population screening has been overseen by the UK National

• BOX 11.2 Current Nationally-Managed Screening Programs in the United Kingdom (for Conditions With Genetic or Potentially Genetic Causes)

Antenatal

Down syndrome
Sickle-cell disease
Thalassemia
Structural abnormalities (fetal anomaly scanning at 18–20 weeks' gestation)

Newborn Bloodspot

Phenylketonuria
Congenital hypothyroidism
Sickle-cell disease
Cystic fibrosis
Medium-chain acyl-CoA dehydrogenase deficiency
Maple syrup urine disease
Isovaleric acidemia
Glutaric aciduria type 1
Homocystinuria

Newborn and Infant Physical Examination

Newborn hearing

Adult

Breast cancer (women >50 years old)
Bowel cancer (>60 years old, fecal occult blood)
Sight-threatening diabetic retinopathy
Abdominal aortic aneurysm (men >65 years old)

Screening Committee (NSC) and Public Health England (PHE). The current, nationally managed, screening programs are listed in Box 11.2. The implementation of a screening program is a huge logistical exercise requiring financial and statistical expertise and technology resources, as well as practical mechanisms to introduce the program and monitor outcomes and quality assurance.

Criteria for a Screening Program

Criteria for a screening program can be considered under the headings of the disease, the test and the practical aspects of the program (Box 11.3). These criteria apply equally to prenatal screening, also addressed in Chapter 20.

• BOX 11.3 Criteria for a Screening Program

Disease

High incidence in target population
Serious effect on health
Treatable or preventable

Test

Non-invasive and easily carried out
Accurate and reliable (high sensitivity and specificity)
Inexpensive

Program

Widespread and equitable availability
Voluntary participation
Acceptable to the target population
Full information and counseling provided

The Disease

To justify the applied effort and resources allocated to screening, the disease should be sufficiently common and have potentially serious effects that are amenable to prevention or amelioration. This may involve early treatment, as for phenylketonuria diagnosed in the neonatal period (p. 271), or the offer of termination of pregnancy for disorders that cannot be treated effectively and are associated with serious morbidity and/or mortality.

The Test

The test should be accurate and reliable with high **sensitivity** and **specificity**. Sensitivity refers to the proportion of cases that are detected. A measure of sensitivity can be made by determining the proportion of false-negative results (i.e., how many cases are missed). Thus, if a test detects only 70 of 100 cases, it shows a sensitivity of 70%. Specificity refers to the extent to which the test detects only affected individuals. If unaffected people test positive, these are referred to as false positives. Thus, if 10 of 100 unaffected individuals have a false-positive test result, the test shows a **specificity** of 90%. Table 11.2 explains this further. This feeds into the **positive predictive value** of a screening test, which is the proportion of positive tests that are true positives; this is illustrated in Table 11.3.

The Program

The program should be offered in a fair and equitable manner and should be widely available. It must also be morally acceptable to a substantial proportion of the population to which it is offered.

TABLE 11.2 Sensitivity and specificity

	DISEASE STATUS	
	Affected	**Unaffected**
Screening Test Result		
Positive	a (true positive)	b (false positive)
Negative	c (false negative)	d (true negative)

Sensitivity: a/(a + c) – proportion of true positives

Specificity: d/(d + b) – proportion of true negatives

TABLE 11.3 In this hypothetical scenario a screening test for congenital adrenal hyperplasia has been implemented, with the following results

CONGENITAL ADRENAL HYPERPLASIA PRESENT		CONGENITAL ADRENAL HYPERPLASIA ABSENT	
Positive	**Negative**	**Positive**	**Negative**
96	4	4980	510,100

Positive predictive value: 96/(96 + 4980) = 2%

Sensitivity: 96/(96 + 4) = 96%

Specificity: 510,100/(510,100 + 4980) = 99%

TABLE 11.4 Incidence of conditions in the United Kingdom detected by newborn bloodspot screening, based on 6 million births 2005–2011

Phenylketonuria	1:10,000
Congenital hypothyroidism	1:3000
Medium-chain acyl-CoA dehydrogenase deficiency	1:10,000
Cystic fibrosis	1:2500
Sickle-cell disease	1:2400

Participation must be entirely voluntary in the case of prenatal programs, but the ethical principles are more complex in neonatal screening for conditions where early treatment is essential and effective in preventing morbidity. In these situations, the principles of **beneficence** (doing good) and **non-maleficence** (not doing harm) are relevant. Easily understood information and well-informed counseling should both be readily available.

It is often stated that the cost of a screening program should be reasonable and affordable. This does not mean that the potential savings gained through a reduction in the number of affected cases requiring treatment should exceed or even balance the cost of screening. The incidence of several conditions screened for in the United Kingdom, based on data from 2005 to 2011, is shown in Table 11.4. Financial considerations can never be ignored, but cost-benefit analysis must also take into account non-tangible factors such as the emotional costs of human suffering born by both the affected individuals and those who care for them.

Prenatal and Postnatal Screening

In the United Kingdom the NSC and PHE have overseen comprehensive programs of screening through pregnancy and the neonatal period (Fig. 11.5), and to a greater or lesser extent similar programs are in place worldwide where public healthcare systems exist. This comprises fetal anomaly screening, newborn bloodspot screening (NBS), the newborn and infant physical examination, and newborn hearing screening. In addition, the National Health Service Sickle Cell and Thalassemia (SCT—see later) screening program is available both prenatally, aimed at identifying mothers and parents who are carriers for sickle-cell, thalassemia and other hemoglobin disorders, and as part of the NBS for sickle-cell disease and β-thalassemia major. Screening is constantly evolving, with one-off adult screening in males older than 65 years for abdominal aortic aneurysm having been introduced. Early detection of "critical" congenital heart disease by newborn pulse oximetry, for cases not detected through fetal ultrasound, has been recommended.

Fetal Anomaly Screening

Aspects of prenatal screening and testing are covered in more detail in Chapter 20. Fetal anomaly screening essentially consists of the combined test, optimally performed between 11^{+2} to 14^{+1} weeks of pregnancy, aimed mainly at the detection of Down syndrome but also trisomies 13 and 18. It has four components: maternal age, the nuchal translucency measurement, free beta human chorionic gonadotropin, and pregnancy-associated plasma protein A. Subsequently, the program consists of ultrasound scanning of the fetus sometime between 18^{+0} and 20^{+6} weeks' gestation.

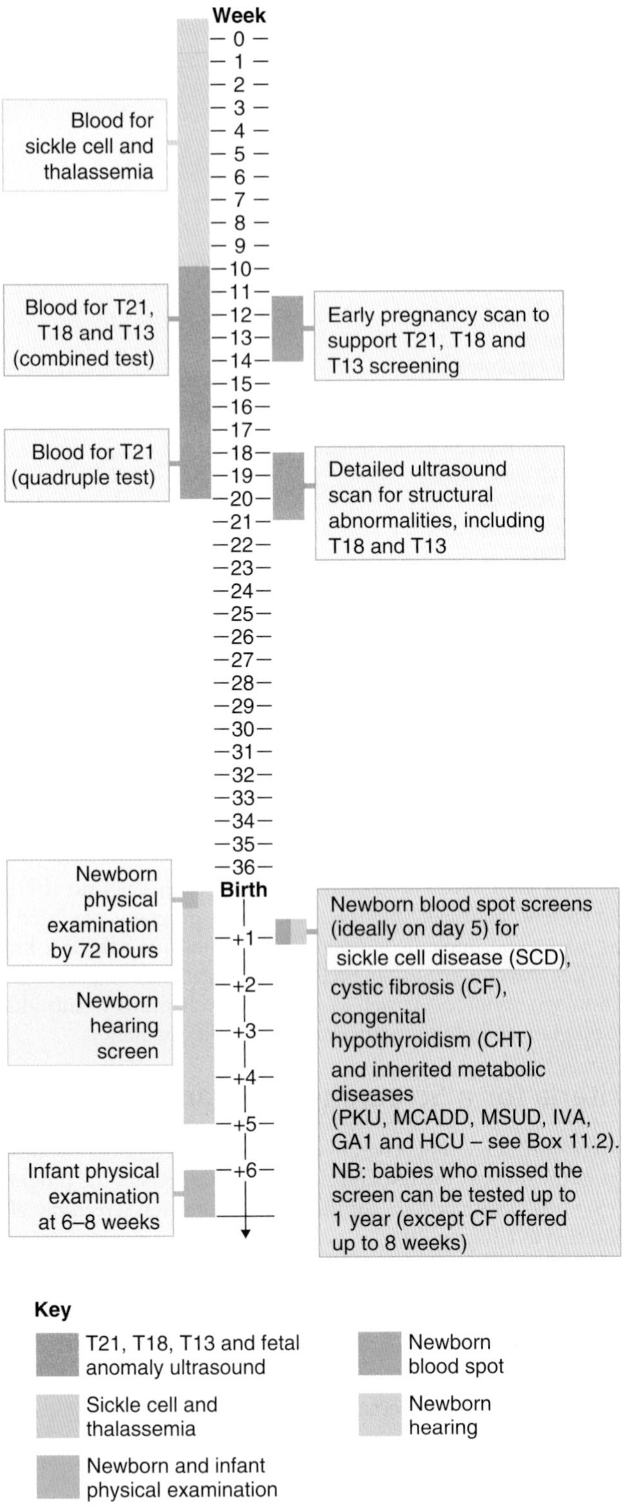

• **Fig. 11.5** Prenatal and postnatal screening timeline indicating the key routine events.

Newborn Screening

Clinical Examination

A competent and thorough clinical examination of the newborn infant within 2 to 3 days of birth is a fundamental screening episode and should be performed by a trained clinician or health visitor who is familiar with the normal range. It is part of the Newborn and Infant Physical Examination screening program in the United Kingdom. To miss developmental dysplasia of the hip at these early stages and not embark on treatment, for example, may have lifelong disabling consequences. Follow-up examinations are usually performed by health visitors who refer to a pediatrician if they have concerns about developmental progress or hearing, vision and vocalization/speech.

Newborn Bloodspot Screening

For this methodology we are indebted to Robert Guthrie, an American microbiologist, whose niece was diagnosed with phenylketonuria (PKU) in 1958. Using a bacterial inhibition assay, he developed a method that could detect high levels of phenylalanine in blood shortly after a baby was born, which he pioneered from 1961. For this he introduced the filter paper on which blood spots could be easily collected and transported—still used today—and overcame commercial pressures to see his methods introduced at low cost. NBS programs have been extended significantly after being limited to PKU, galactosemia, and congenital hypothyroidism for many years, and the analytical methods vary, with tandem mass spectrometry greatly extending the range (Tables 11.4 and 11.5).

In the United Kingdom nine conditions are now screened for, the most recent of which was introduced in 2014 (see Box 11.2).

TABLE 11.5 Some conditions for which neonatal screening is undertaken, and the methods of testing

Disorder	Test/Method
Phenylketonuria	Guthrie test[a] or tandem mass spectrometry
Congenital hypothyroidism	Thyroid-stimulating hormone (fluoroimmunoassay)
Biotinidase deficiency	Enzymatic assay (fluorescence measurement)
Galactosemia	Enzymatic assay (fluorescence measurement)
Maple syrup urine disease	Tandem mass spectrometry
Glutaric aciduria, type 1	Tandem mass spectrometry
Isovaleric academia	Tandem mass spectrometry
Medium-chain acyl-CoA dehydrogenase deficiency	Tandem mass spectrometry
Very long–chain acyl-CoA dehydrogenase deficiency	Tandem mass spectrometry
Long-chain 3-hydroxyacyl-CoA-dehydrogenase deficiency	Tandem mass spectrometry
Congenital adrenal hyperplasia	17-Hydroxyprogesterone assay (fluoroimmunoassay)
Cystic fibrosis	Immunoreactive trypsin and DNA analysis
Duchenne muscular dystrophy	Creatine kinase
Sickle-cell disease	Hemoglobin electrophoresis

[a]The Guthrie test is based on reversal of bacterial growth inhibition by a high level of phenylalanine.

For all these disorders early diagnosis leads either to treatment that essentially prevents the development of learning disability, or to other interventions that prevent or ameliorate medical problems. Worldwide, there is significant variation in NBS programs, with the United States leading the way. Here the Newborn Screening Saves Lives Act was signed into law in 2007 with the intention of unifying and expanding the program nationwide. This is overseen by the Centers for Disease Control and Prevention, and at least 29 conditions are screened for in all states, and more than 50 in some. The list includes severe combined immunodeficiency, as well as a wide range of metabolic disorders. Germany screens for 15 conditions, and across the Middle East and North Africa, where rates of consanguinity are high, there is wide variation. In Saudi Arabia, for example, NBS covers more than 10 disorders, but this does not reach the whole population. In the Netherlands, newborn screening is voluntary with informed parental consent, although strongly recommended. Generally speaking, screening is mandatory, or consent is implied.

The importance of adhering to the principle of screening for a disorder that needs to be treated early is illustrated by the Swedish experience of neonatal screening for α_1-antitrypsin deficiency. In this condition neonatal complications occur in up to 10% of cases, but for most cases the morbidity is seen in adult life, and the main message on diagnosing the disorder is avoidance of smoking. Between 1972 and 1974, 200,000 newborns were screened, and follow-up studies showed that considerable anxiety was generated when the information was conveyed to parents, who perceived their children to be at risk of a serious, life-threatening disorder. The case of newborn screening for DMD also deviates from the screening paradigm because, thus far, no early intervention is helpful. Here, the parents (or mother) can be counseled before having more children and, in the wider family, identification of female carriers (of reproductive age) may be possible. However, parental reaction has not been uniformly favorable. The rationale of screening for the following conditions is well established.

Phenylketonuria

This was introduced in the United Kingdom in 1969 after it had been shown (some 10 years earlier) that a low-phenylalanine diet could prevent the severe learning disabilities that previously had been a hallmark of this condition (p. 271). The bloodspot is obtained by heel-prick at approximately 6 to 7 days of age, and an abnormal test result is followed by repeat analysis of phenylalanine levels in a venous blood sample. A low-phenylalanine diet is not particularly palatable, but affected children can be persuaded to adhere to it until early adult life, when it can be relaxed. However, because high phenylalanine levels are toxic to the developing brain, a woman with phenylketonuria who is contemplating pregnancy should adhere to a strict low-phenylalanine diet both before and during pregnancy (p. 240).

Galactosemia

Classic galactosemia affects approximately 1 in 50,000 newborn infants and usually presents with vomiting, lethargy, and severe metabolic collapse within the first 2 or 3 weeks of life. Early introduction of appropriate dietary restriction can prevent the development of serious complications such as cataracts, liver failure, and learning disability. Newborn screening was based on a modification of Guthrie's early methods with subsequent confirmation by specific enzyme assay, but was discontinued in the United

Kingdom around 2000 on the recommendation of the NSC, the rationale being that, if present, it will manifest within the first few days of life and should be clinically recognizable. However, it is included in the extended screening programs of some countries.

Congenital Hypothyroidism

Screening was introduced in the United States in 1974 and the United Kingdom in 1981, and is now widespread. The test is usually based on assay of **thyroid-stimulating hormone**. This disorder is particularly suitable for screening as it is relatively common, with an incidence of approximately 1 in 4000, and treatment with lifelong thyroxine replacement is extremely effective in preventing the severe developmental problems associated with the classic picture of "cretinism." The most common cause of congenital hypothyroidism is absence of the thyroid gland rather than an inborn error of metabolism (see Chapter 18). Congenital absence of the thyroid gland is usually not caused by genetic factors but on rare occasion is part of a wider syndrome.

Cystic Fibrosis

Newborn screening for cystic fibrosis ([CF], p. 303) is particularly relevant for northern European countries with a high population carrier frequency and was introduced in England in 2006. It is based on the detection of a raised blood level of **immunoreactive trypsin**, which is a consequence of blockage of pancreatic ducts *in utero*, supplemented by DNA analysis. Early treatment with physiotherapy and antibiotics improves the long-term prognosis.

Sickle-Cell Disease and Thalassemia

Newborn screening for sickle-cell disease and thalassemia (SCT) based on **hemoglobin electrophoresis** is undertaken in many countries with a significant Afro-Caribbean community. As with CF, early prophylaxis reduces morbidity and mortality and the long-term outlook. In the case of sickle-cell disease, treatment involves the use of oral penicillin to reduce the risk of pneumococcal infection resulting from immune deficiency secondary to splenic infarction (p. 165). Even in Western countries with good medical facilities, a significant proportion of sickle-cell homozygotes, possibly as many as 15%, die as a result of infection in early childhood. In the case of thalassemia, early diagnosis makes it possible to optimize transfusion regimens and iron-chelation therapy from an early stage. Newborn screening programs for SCT were implemented in the United Kingdom in 2005, with antenatal screening (of the mother, followed by the father if necessary) also in place. In some low-risk areas there is a preference for antenatal screening to be targeted to high-risk couples after completion of an ethnicity questionnaire.

Newborn Hearing Screening

The acquisition of language skills is an early developmental process in postnatal life and is crucially dependent on adequate hearing. Although individuals with hearing impairment, and their community, make the best of life opportunities, and should not be subject to discrimination, most would concur that good communication skills are very important through life. If hearing impairment is identified early, then aids can be fitted. The assessment should be performed in the first month of life and consists of the automated otoacoustic emission (AOAE) test for well babies followed by the automated auditory brainstem response test where there is no clear AOAE response.

Population Carrier Screening

Widespread screening for carriers of autosomal recessive disorders in high-incidence populations was first introduced for the hemoglobinopathies (see Chapter 12) and has been extended to other disorders (Table 11.6). The rationale behind these programs is that carrier detection can be supported by genetic counseling so that carrier couples can be forewarned of the 1 in 4 risk that each of their children could be affected. The example of Tay-Sachs disease in orthodox Jewish communities has been discussed (p. 151), but this does not amount to "population" screening.

Experience with SCT illustrates the extremes of success and failure that can result from well or poorly planned screening programs.

Thalassemia

α-Thalassemia and β-thalassemia are caused by abnormal globin chain synthesis because of variants involving the α- and β-globin genes or their promoter regions (p. 166) and follow autosomal recessive inheritance. They are very common in South-East Asia (α-thalassemia), Cyprus and the Mediterranean region, Italy and the Indian subcontinent (β-thalassemia).

In Cyprus in 1974 the birth incidence of β-thalassemia was 1 in 250 (carrier frequency 1 in 8). After the introduction of a comprehensive screening program to determine the carrier status of young adults, which had the support of the Greek Orthodox Church, the incidence of affected babies declined by more than 95% within 10 years. Similar programs in Greece and Italy have seen a drop in the incidence of affected homozygotes of more than 50%.

Sickle-Cell Disease

In contrast to the Cypriot response to β-thalassemia screening, early attempts to introduce sickle-cell carrier detection in African-Americans were disastrous. Information pamphlets tended to

TABLE 11.6 Autosomal recessive disorders suitable for population carrier screening

Disorder	Ethnic Group or Community	Test
α-Thalassemia	China and eastern Asia	Mean corpuscular hemoglobin and hemoglobin electrophoresis
β-Thalassemia	Indian subcontinent and Mediterranean countries	Mean corpuscular hemoglobin and hemoglobin electrophoresis
Sickle-cell disease	Afro-Caribbean	Sickle-cell test and hemoglobin electrophoresis
Cystic fibrosis	Europeans	Common mutation analysis
Tay-Sachs disease	Ashkenazi Jews	Hexosaminidase A

confuse the sickle-cell carrier state, or trait, which is usually harmless, with the homozygous disease, which conveys significant morbidity (p. 164). Several US states passed legislation making sickle-cell screening in people of Afro-Carribean origin mandatory, and carriers suffered discrimination by employers and insurance companies, resulting in screening programs being abandoned. This experience emphasizes the importance of ensuring voluntary participation and providing adequate and appropriate information and counseling. Later pilot studies in the United States and in Cuba have shown that individuals of Afro-Caribbean origin are perfectly receptive to well-planned, nondirective sickle-cell screening programs.

Cystic Fibrosis

In Europeans within the United Kingdom population of the United Kingdom, the CF carrier frequency is approximately 1 in 25, and the Phe508del variant accounts for 75% to 80% of all heterozygotes. Initial studies of attitudes to CF carrier detection yielded quite divergent results. A casual, written invitation generates a poor take-up response of approximately 10%, whereas personal contact during early pregnancy, whether mediated through general practice or an antenatal clinic, results in uptake rates of more than 80%. Studies have been undertaken to explore attitudes to CF screening among specific groups, such as school leavers and women in early pregnancy.

Two approaches for screening pregnant women were researched. One was a **two-step** process starting with pregnant mothers at the antenatal clinic. Those who tested positive for a common pathogenic variant (approximately 85% of all cystic fibrosis carriers) were informed of the result and invited to bring their partners for testing—the second step. If both partners were carriers, an offer of prenatal diagnosis was made. This approach had the advantage that all carriers detected were informed of their result, and further family studies—**cascade screening**—can be initiated.

The second approach was **couple screening**, whereby both partners were tested together and positive results disclosed only if both were found to be carriers. In this way less anxiety was generated, but the opportunity for offering cascade screening was lost. The results suggested that both screening approaches were equally acceptable to pregnant women, with take-up rates of approximately 70%. However, there is no publicly available CF screening for adults in the United Kingdom, and newborn screening is now established.

Positive and Negative Aspects of Population Screening

High-quality population screening enhances informed choice and offers the prospect of a significant reduction in the incidence of disabling genetic disorders. This has to be weighed against the potential disadvantages that may arise from the overenthusiastic pursuit of a poorly planned or ill-judged screening program (Box 11.4). Experience to date indicates that in relatively small, well-informed groups, such as the Greek Cypriots and American Ashkenazi Jews, community screening is welcomed. When screening is offered to larger populations the outcome is less certain.

A 3-year follow-up of almost 750 individuals screened for CF carrier status in the United Kingdom revealed that a positive test result did not cause undue anxiety, although some carriers had a relatively poor perception of their own general health. A more worrying outcome was that almost 50% of the individuals tested could not accurately recall or interpret their results. This emphasizes the importance of good pretest counseling and the provision of accurate information that is easily processed and understood.

• BOX 11.4 Potential Advantages and Disadvantages of Population Genetic Screening

Advantages

Informed choice
Improved understanding
Early treatment when available
Reduction in births of affected homozygotes

Disadvantages and hazards

Pressure to participate causing mistrust and suspicion
Stigmatization of carriers (social, insurance, and employment)
Irrational anxiety in carriers
Inappropriate reassurance if test is not 100% sensitive

Genetic Registers

Regional genetic centers maintain confidential patient information systems and **registers** of families and individuals according to specific disease groups. The main difference compared with conventional medical records is the linking of biological relatives—whether affected or unaffected. They greatly assist patient and family management, and calls for their destruction at a given time after death will be vigorously resisted. Confidentiality and data security are of course paramount.

One important function of registers is the facility to rapidly identify patients eligible for new or modified screening programs and modalities when introduced, for example, in cancer genetics (Chapter 14). Similarly, patients with specific diagnoses or phenotypes can be readily found for new research projects. The uses of genetic registers are listed in Box 11.5. In addition, many international databases facilitate variant and phenotype registry, for example, the Human Genome Mutation Database (http://www.hgmd.cf.ac.uk/ac/index.php) and Decipher (https://decipher.sanger.ac.uk/). GeneMatcher (https://www.genematcher.org/) is proving invaluable in linking patients with rare disease, which in turn enables verification of variant pathogenicity.

• BOX 11.5 Roles and Benefits of Genetic Registers

- To maintain a communication process between the family and the genetics center when necessary, thus providing information and long-term support
- To link biological relatives to understand the genetic risks that may apply to individuals, and help coordinate predictive testing and prenatal testing when requested
- To offer carrier detection to relevant family members when age-appropriate (e.g., young women for X-linked disorders)
- To schedule the start (and continuation) of conventional screening investigations and multidisciplinary management when age-appropriate (e.g., inherited cardiac conditions)
- To rapidly identify individuals eligible for new or modified screening programs (e.g., in cancer genetics) and, increasingly, treatment
- To readily identify suitable patients for new research projects
- To contribute to national and international efforts to assemble information in the genomic era and thus determine the significance of DNA sequence data through good phenotyping

ELEMENTS

1. Targeted or family screening in genetics concerns those who are at relatively high risk because of their family history. Direct gene testing is often possible, but there remains a vital role for detailed clinical examination and specialist clinical investigations, such as biochemical tests and imaging.
2. Consideration should be given to the advantages and disadvantages of presymptomatic or predictive testing from both a practical and an ethical point of view.
3. Population screening involves the offer of genetic testing to all members of a particular population, with the objectives of preventing later ill health and providing informed personal choice. A good screening test has a high sensitivity and specificity.
4. Participation should be voluntary, and each program should be widely available, equitably distributed, acceptable to the target population, and supported by full information and counseling.
5. Prenatal screening based on ultrasound examination at approximately 12 and 20 weeks' gestation is routinely available, as well as combined testing to refine the risk for aneuploidies such as Down syndrome, which may lead to the offer of amniocentesis for genetic testing of the fetus.
6. Newborn screening for phenylketonuria was introduced in the 1960s but has now expanded to incorporate a wide range of metabolic conditions, as well as hearing testing.
7. Population screening programs for carriers of β-thalassemia have resulted in a major fall in the incidence of births of affected homozygotes. This has provided the paradigm for the introduction of screening for other disorders with serious long-term morbidity.
8. Well-organized genetic registers provide an effective means of identifying individuals eligible for testing and screening when new programs or modalities are introduced.

CLINICAL SCENARIO 1

Consideration is being given to the introduction of a newborn screening program for a metabolic disease not yet covered by the current program. The criteria for early screening, in terms of the medical need, are satisfied.

The data for the new test are as follows:

Affected	Unaffected
Screening Test Result	
True positives: 115	False positives: 1312
False negatives: 22	True negatives: 460,364

Regarding this test, what is the:

a. Sensitivity?
b. Specificity?
c. Positive predictive value?

CLINICAL SCENARIO 2

With reference to **Clinical Scenario 1**, a technical modification of the screening test has been made, and it has been reevaluated.

The data for this modified new test are as follows:

Affected	Unaffected
Screening Test Result	
True positives: 83	False positives: 9529
False negatives: 2	True negatives: 348,109

Regarding this modified test, what is the:

a. Sensitivity?
b. Specificity?
c. Positive predictive value?

Which is the better test, this one or the earlier test (Clinical Scenario 1), and why?

Further Reading

Axworthy D, Brock DJH, Bobrow M, Marteau TM. Psychological impact of population-based carrier testing for cystic fibrosis: 3-year follow-up. *Lancet.* 1996;347:1443–1446.

A review of the impact of carrier testing for cystic fibrosis on over 700 individuals.

Baily MA, Murray TH, eds. *Ethics and Newborn Genetic Screening: New Technologies, New Challenges.* Baltimore, MD: Johns Hopkins University Press; 2009.

A multiauthor volume with a focus on the health economics of newborn screening and distributive justice.

Harper PS. *Practical Genetic Counselling.* 7th ed. London: Hodder Arnold; 2010.

A very good starting point in almost every aspect of genetic counseling, including carrier testing.

Marteau T, Richards M, eds. *The Troubled Helix.* Cambridge: Cambridge University Press; 1996.

Perspectives on the social and psychological implications of genetic testing and screening.

Nuffield Council on Bioethics. Genetic Screening: Ethical Issues. London: Nuffield Council on Bioethics; 1993.

This report remains a very helpful read even though technologies have progressed.

Websites

Centers for Disease Control and Prevention. Newborn Screening. (http://www.cdc.gov/newbornscreening/).

A source of information on newborn screening in the United States.

Burton H, Moorthie S. *Expanded Newborn Screening. A Review of the Evidence.* Cambridge: PHG Foundation; 2010 (https://www.phgfoundation.org/documents/229_1275040921.pdf).

National Health Service websites offering information on screening programs. (https://www.nhs.uk/conditions/nhs-screening/; https://phescreening.blog.gov.uk/about/)

UK National Screening Committee (https://www.gov.uk/government/groups/uk-national-screening-committee-uk-nsc).

A source of up-to-date information on screening in the United Kingdom.

12 Hemoglobin and the Hemoglobinopathies

Blood is a very special juice.

Johann Wolfgang von Goethe, in Faust I (1808)

Over a quarter of a million people are born in the world each year with one of the disorders of the structure or synthesis of hemoglobin (Hb)—the hemoglobinopathies. Originally conditions of the tropics and subtropics, migration has seen these conditions have worldwide impact. In fact, the impact on morbidity and mortality is the greatest of any single group of disorders following mendelian inheritance and, as such, has served as a paradigm for our understanding of the pathology of inherited disease at the clinical, protein and DNA levels. The mobility of modern society means that new communities with a high frequency of Hemoglobinopathies have become established in countries whose indigenous populations have a low frequency. Because they are a major public health concern, many countries have introduced screening programs. In England and Wales, there are an estimated 600,000 healthy carriers of Hb variants.

To understand the various Hemoglobinopathies and their clinical consequences, it is first necessary to consider the structure, function, and synthesis of Hb.

Structure of Hemoglobin

Hb is the protein present in red blood cells that is responsible for oxygen transport. There are approximately 15 g of Hb in every 100 mL of blood, making it amenable to analysis.

Protein Analysis

In 1956, by fractionating the peptide products of digestion of human Hb with the proteolytic enzyme trypsin, Ingram found 30 discrete peptide fragments. Trypsin cuts polypeptide chains at the amino acids arginine and lysine. Analysis of the 580 amino acids of human Hb had previously revealed a total of 60 arginine and lysine residues, suggesting that Hb was made up of two identical peptide chains with 30 arginine and lysine residues on each chain.

At about the same time, a family was reported in which two Hb variants, HbS and Hb Hopkins II, were both present in some family members. Several members of the family who possessed both variants had children with normal Hb—offspring who were heterozygous for only one Hb variant, as well as offspring who, like their parents, were doubly heterozygous for the two Hb variants. These observations provided further evidence that at least two different genes were involved in the production of human Hb.

Soon after, the amino-terminal amino acid sequence of human Hb was determined and showed valine–leucine and valine–histidine sequences in equimolar proportions, with two moles of each of these sequences per mole of Hb. This was consistent with human Hb being made up of a tetramer consisting of two pairs of different polypeptides, referred to as the α- and β-globin chains.

Analysis of the iron content of human Hb revealed that iron constituted 0.35% of its weight, from which it was calculated that human Hb should have a minimum molecular weight of 16,000 Daltons (Da). In contrast, determination of the molecular weight of human Hb by physical methods gave values of the order of 64,000 Da, consistent with the suggested tetrameric structure, $\alpha_2\beta_2$, with each of the globin chains having its own iron-containing group—heme (Fig. 12.1).

Subsequent investigators demonstrated that Hb from normal adults also contained a minor fraction, constituting 2% to 3% of the total Hb, with an electrophoretic mobility different from the majority of human Hb. The main component was called HbA, whereas the minority component was called HbA_2. Subsequent

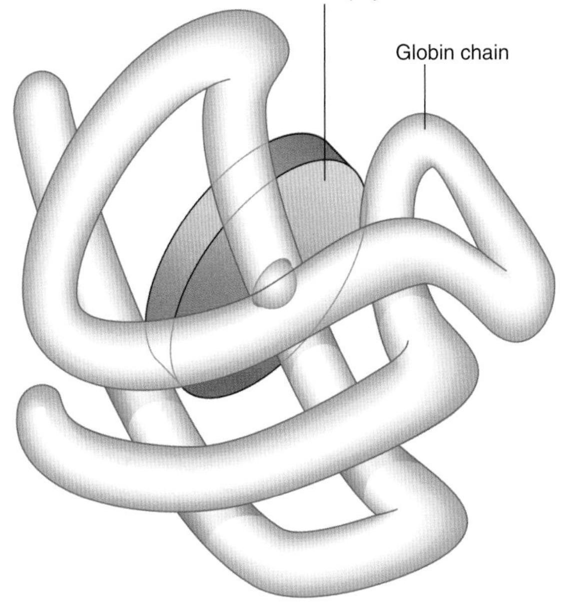

• **Fig. 12.1** Diagrammatic representation of one of the globin chains and associated porphyrin molecule of human hemoglobin.

studies revealed HbA_2 to be a tetramer of two normal α chains and two other polypeptide chains whose amino-acid sequence resembled most closely the β chain and were designated delta (δ).

Developmental Expression of Hemoglobin

Analysis of Hb from a human fetus revealed it to consist primarily of an Hb with a different electrophoretic mobility from normal HbA, and it was designated fetal Hb or HbF. Subsequent analysis showed HbF to be a tetramer of two α chains and two polypeptide chains whose sequence resembled the β chain and which were designated gamma (γ). HbF makes up somewhere in the region of 0.5% of Hb in the blood of normal adults.

Analysis of Hb from embryos earlier in gestation revealed a developmental, or ontological, succession of different embryonic Hbs: Hb Gower I and II, and Hb Portland, which are produced transiently in varying amounts at different gestational ages. These occur in tetramers of various combinations of α, or α-like, zeta (ζ) chains with β, or β-like, γ-, and epsilon (ε) chains (Table 12.1). Although both the ζ chain and ε chain are expressed transiently in early embryonic life, the α and γ chains are expressed throughout development, with increasing levels of expression of the β chain toward the end of fetal life (Fig. 12.2).

TABLE 12.1 Human hemoglobins

Stage in Development	Hemoglobin	Structure	Proportion in Normal Adult (%)
Embryonic	Gower I	$\zeta_2\varepsilon_2$	—
	Gower II	$\alpha_2\varepsilon_2$	—
	Portland I	$\zeta_2\gamma_2$	—
Fetal	F	$\alpha_2\gamma_2$	<1
Adult	A	$\alpha_2\beta_2$	97–98
	A_2	$\alpha_2\delta_2$	2–3

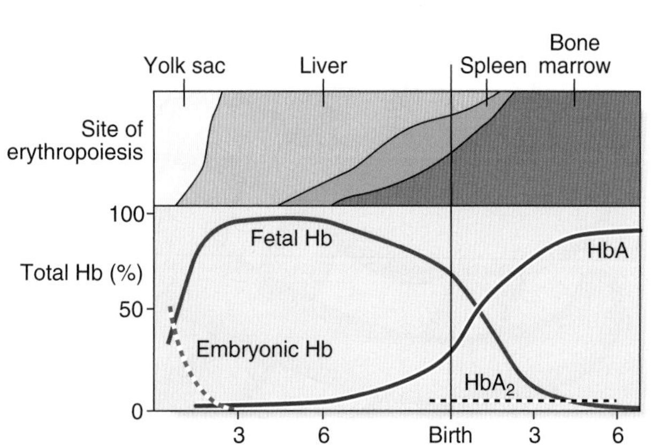

• **Fig. 12.2** Hemoglobin synthesis during prenatal and postnatal development. There are several embryonic hemoglobins. (From Huehns ER, Shooter EM. Human hemoglobins. *J Med Genet.* 1965;2:48-90. With permission.)

Globin Chain Structure

Analysis of the structure of the individual globin chains was initially carried out at the protein level.

Protein Studies

Amino acid sequencing in the 1960s showed that the α chain was 141 amino acids long, compared with the β chain's 146 amino acids. Their sequences were similar but not identical. The δ chain differs from the β chain by 10 amino acids, and analysis of the γ chain showed that it also most closely resembles the β chain, differing by 39 amino acids. In addition, two types of HbF were identified, in which the γ chain contains either the amino acid glycine or alanine at position 136, designated (G)γ and (A)γ, respectively. Partial sequence analyzes of the ζ and ε chains of embryonic Hb suggest that ζ is similar in amino acid sequence to the α chain, whereas ε resembles the β chain.

Thus, there are two groups of globin chains, the α-like and β-like, possibly derived from an ancestral Hb gene that has changed over time.

Globin Gene Mapping

Analysis of the Hb electrophoretic variant Hb Lepore helped our understanding of how globin genes are assembled on human chromosomes. Comparison of trypsin digests of Hb Lepore with normal Hb revealed normal α chains, whereas the non-α chains consisted of an amino-terminal δ-like sequence and a carboxy-terminal β-like sequence. This suggested Hb Lepore could represent a "fusion" globin chain resulting from a crossover coincidental with mispairing of the δ- and β-globin genes during meiosis because of sequence similarity of the two genes and their close proximity on the same chromosome (Fig. 12.3). If correct, it was argued that there should also be an "anti-Lepore" Hb—that is, a β−δ-globin fusion product in which the non−α-globin chains contained β-chain residues at the amino-terminal end and δ-chain residues at the carboxy-terminal end. In the late 1960s Hb Miyada was identified in Japan, and was shown to contain β-globin sequence at the amino-terminal end and δ-globin sequence at the carboxy-terminal end, as predicted.

Further evidence at the protein level for the physical mapping of globin genes came from another electrophoretic variant, Hb Kenya. Amino acid analysis suggested it was a γ−β fusion product with a crossover having occurred somewhere between amino acids 81 and 86 in the two globin chains, which in turn suggested the γ-globin structural gene must also be in close physical proximity to the β-globin gene.

Little evidence was forthcoming from protein studies about the mapping of the α-globin genes. The presence of normal HbA in individuals who, from family studies, should have been homozygous for a particular α chain variant, or obligate compound (double) heterozygotes (p. 72), suggested there could be more than one α-globin gene. In addition, the proportion of the total Hb made up by the α chain variant in subjects heterozygous for those variants was consistently lower (<20%) than that seen with the β chain variants (usually >30%), suggesting there could be more than one α-globin structural gene.

Globin Gene Structure

The detailed structure of globin genes has been made possible by DNA analysis. Immature red blood cells (reticulocytes) provide a rich source of globin mRNA for the synthesis of cDNA—

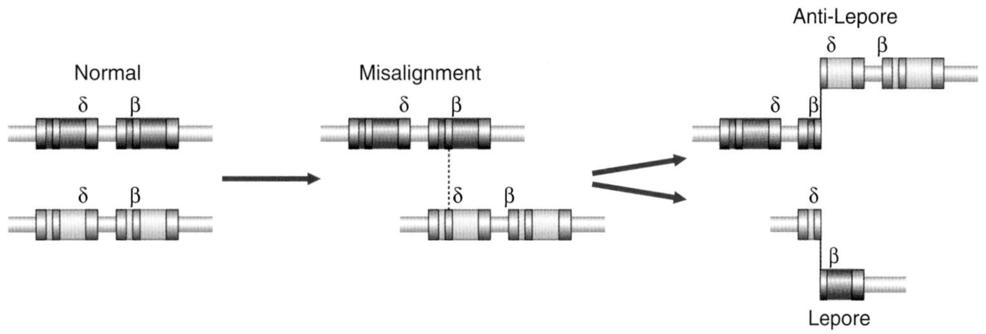

• **Fig. 12.3** Mechanism of unequal crossing over which generates Hb Lepore and Hb anti-Lepore. (Modified from Weatherall DJ, Clegg JB. *The Thalassaemia Syndromes*. Blackwell, Oxford; 1981.)

reticulocytes synthesize little else! Use of β-globin cDNA for restriction mapping studies of DNA from normal individuals revealed that the non-α, or β-like, globin genes are located in a 50-kilobase (kb) stretch on the short arm of chromosome 11 (Fig. 12.4). The entire sequence of this 50-kb stretch containing the various globin structural genes is known. Of interest are non-functional regions with sequences similar to those of the globin structural genes, (i.e., they produce no identifiable message or protein product and are pseudogenes).

Studies of the α-globin structural genes have shown that there are two α-globin structural genes—α_1 and α_2—located on chromosome 16p (see Fig. 12.4). Sequencing has revealed nucleotide differences between these two genes even though the transcribed α-globin chains have an identical amino acid sequence, considered as evidence for "degeneracy" of the genetic code. In addition, there are pseudo-α, pseudo-ζ, and ζ genes to the 5′ side of the α-globin genes, as well as an additional theta (θ)-globin gene to the 3′ side of the α_1-globin gene. The θ-globin gene, whose function is unknown, is interesting because, unlike the globin pseudogenes, which are not expressed, its structure is compatible with expression. It has been suggested that it could be expressed in very early erythroid tissue such as the fetal liver and yolk sac.

Synthesis and Control of Hemoglobin Expression

Translation studies with reticulocyte mRNA has shown that α- and β-globin chains are synthesized in roughly equal proportions. *In vitro* studies have shown, however, that β-globin mRNA is slightly more efficient in protein synthesis than α-globin mRNA, and this difference is compensated for in red blood cell precursors by a relative excess of α-globin mRNA. The most important level of regulation of expression of the globin genes, as with other eukaryotic genes, appears to occur at the level of transcription (p. 15).

The timing and tissue-specific pattern of expression of globin genes in development is attributed to the **locus control region (lcr)**. In addition to promoter sequences in the 5′ flanking regions of the various globin genes, there are sequences 6 to 20 kb 5′ to the ε-globin gene necessary for the expression of the various β-like globin genes, which constitute the lcr. This region regulates the **switching** of β-like globin genes. There is a similar region 5′ to the α-globin genes involved in the control of their expression, in both cases involved in the binding of proteins and transcription factors.

Disorders of Hemoglobin

The disorders of human Hb can be divided into two main groups: (1) structural globin chain variants, such as sickle-cell disease, and (2) disorders of synthesis of the globin chains, the thalassemias.

Structural Variants/Disorders

In 1975, Ingram demonstrated that the difference between HbA and HbS lay in the substitution of valine for glutamic acid in the β chain. In 2001 the HbVar database was established at the Globin Gene Server (http://globin.bx.psu.edu), and more than 1300 Hb electrophoretic variants have been described according to the type of variant (Table 12.2). The majority are single amino acid substitutions and are not associated with clinical disease. A number are, of course, associated with disease and are often relatively population-specific.

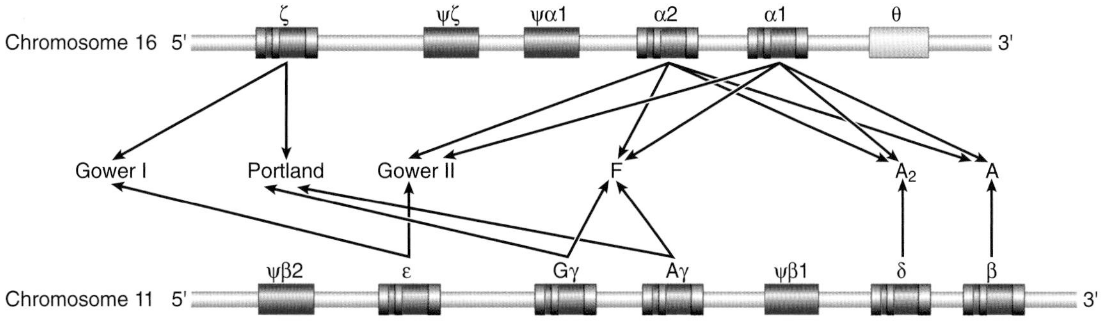

• **Fig. 12.4** The α- and β-globin regions on chromosomes 16 and 11 showing the structural genes and pseudogenes (ψ) and the various hemoglobins produced. (Modified from Carrell RW, Lehman H. The hemoglobinopathies. In: Dawson AM, Besser G, Compston N, eds. *Recent Advances in Medicine* 19, pp. 223–225. Churchill Livingstone, Edinburgh, UK; 1985.)

TABLE 12.2 Structural variants of hemoglobin

Type of Variant	Examples	Chain/Residue(s)/Alteration
Point (> 200 variants)	HbS	β, 6 Glu to Val
	HbC	β, 6 Glu to Lys
	HbE	β, 26 Glu to Lys
Deletion (shortened chain)	Hb Freiburg	β, 23 to 0
	Hb Lyon	β, 17–18 to 0
	Hb Leiden	β, 6 or 7 to 0
	Hb Gun Hill	β, 92–96 or 93–97 to 0
Insertion (elongated chain)	Hb Grady	α, 116–118 (Glu, Phe, Thr) duplicated
Frameshift (insertion or deletion of multiples other than three base pairs)	Hb Tak, Hb Cranston	β[a], +11 residues, loss of termination codon, insertion of two base pairs in codon 146/147
	Hb Wayne	α[a], +5 residues, because of loss of termination codon by single base-pair deletion in codon 138/139
	Hb McKees Rock	β[a], −2 residues, point mutation in 145, generating premature termination codon
Chain termination	Hb Constant Spring	α[a], +31 residues, point mutation in termination codon
Fusion chain (unequal crossing over)	Hb Lepore/anti-Lepore	Non-α, δ-like residues at N-terminal end and β-like residues at C-terminal end, and vice versa, respectively
	Hb Kenya/anti-Kenya	Non-α, γ-like residues at N-terminal end and β-like residues at C-terminal end, and vice versa, respectively

[a]Residues are either added (+) or lost (−).

Types of Variant

Point Mutation. A point mutation that results in substitution of one amino acid for another can lead to altered Hb, such as HbS, HbC, or HbE. These are missense variants (p. 19).

Deletion. There are a number of Hb variants in which one or more amino acids of one of the globin chains are missing or deleted (p. 20) (e.g., Hb Freiburg).

Insertion. Conversely, there are variants in which the globin chains are longer than normal because of insertions (p. 20), such as Hb Grady.

Frameshift Variant. Frameshift variants involve disruption of the normal triplet reading frame—that is, the addition or removal of a number of bases that are not a multiple of three (p. 22). In this instance, translation of the mRNA continues until a termination codon is read "in frame." These variants can result in either an elongated or a shortened globin chain.

Chain Termination. A variant in the termination codon itself can lead to an elongated globin chain (e.g., Hb Constant Spring).

Fusion Polypeptides. Unequal crossover events in meiosis can lead to structural variants called **fusion polypeptides**, of which Hbs Lepore and Kenya are examples (p. 162).

Clinical Aspects

Some Hb variants are associated with disease (the more common are shown in Table 12.3) but most are harmless, having been identified coincidentally in the course of population surveys.

If the variant is on the inside of the globin subunits, in close proximity to the heme pockets, or at the interchain contact areas, this can produce an unstable Hb molecule that precipitates in the red blood cell, damaging the membrane and resulting in hemolysis of the cell. Alternatively, variants can interfere with the normal oxygen transport function of Hb, leading to either enhanced or reduced oxygen affinity or an Hb that is more stable in its reduced form, so-called **methemoglobin**.

The structural variants of Hb identified by electrophoretic techniques represent a minority of the total number of variants that exist because it is predicted that only one-third of possible Hb variants will produce an altered charge in the Hb molecule, and thereby be detectable by electrophoresis (Fig. 12.5).

Sickle-Cell Disease

This severe hereditary hemolytic anemia was first recognized clinically early in the twentieth century, but in 1940 red blood cells from affected individuals with sickle-cell disease were noted to appear birefringent when viewed in polarized light under the microscope, reflecting polymerization of the sickle Hb. This distorts the shape of red blood corpuscles under deoxygenated conditions—so-called **sickling** (Fig. 12.6). Linus Pauling, using electrophoresis in 1949, showed that it had different mobility to HbA and called it HbS, for sickle.

Clinical Aspects of Sickle-Cell Disease

Sickle-cell disease, following autosomal recessive inheritance, is the most common hemoglobinopathy with over 11,000 affected individuals recorded by the National Hemoglobinopathy Register in England. Registration is voluntary, so it is quite possible that the actual prevalence is higher. In England, approximately 250,000

TABLE 12.3 Functional abnormalities of structural variants of hemoglobin

Clinical Features	Examples
Hemolytic Anemia	
Sickling disorders	HbS/S, HbS/C disease, or HbS/O (Arab), HbS/D (Punjab), HbS/β-thalassemia, HbS/Lepore
	Other rare homozygous sickling variants—HbS-Antilles, HbS-Oman
Unstable hemoglobin	Hb Köln
	Hb Gun Hill
	Hb Bristol
Cyanosis	
Hemoglobin M (methemoglobinemia)	HbM (Boston)
	HbM (Hyde Park)
Low oxygen affinity	Hb Kansas
Polycythemia	
High oxygen affinity	Hb Chesapeake
	Hb Heathrow

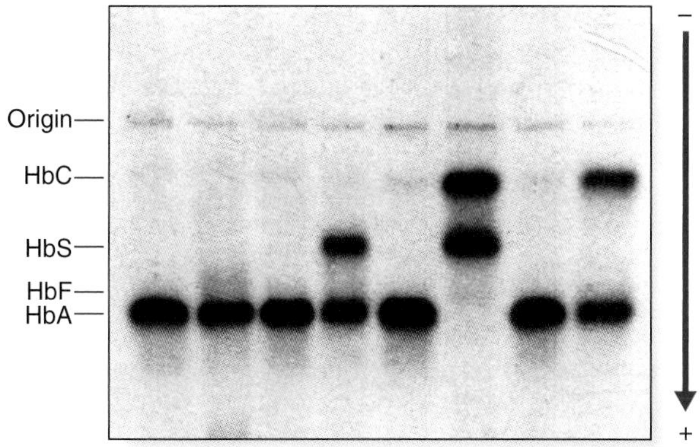

• **Fig. 12.5** Hemoglobin electrophoresis showing hemoglobins A, C and S. (Courtesy Dr D. Norfolk, General Infirmary, Leeds, UK.)

people are thought to be carriers (of the sickle-cell trait), dominated by those of African-Caribbean origin. The disease is especially prevalent in those areas of the world where malaria is endemic. The parasite *Plasmodium falciparum* is disadvantaged because the red cells of SC heterozygotes are believed to express malarial or altered self-antigens more effectively, resulting in more rapid removal of parasitized cells from the circulation. Sickle-cell heterozygotes are therefore relatively protected from malarial attacks and biologically fitter, meaning the sickle-cell gene can be passed to the next generation. Over time this has resulted in relatively high gene frequency in malaria-infested regions (see Chapter 7).

Clinical manifestations include painful **sickle-cell crisis**, chest crisis, aplastic crisis, splenic sequestration crisis, priapism, retinal disease, and cerebrovascular accident. Pulmonary hypertension may occur, and heart failure can accompany severe anemia during aplastic or splenic sequestration crises. All these result from deformed, sickle-shaped red cells, which are less able to change shape and tend to obstruct small arteries, thus reducing oxygen

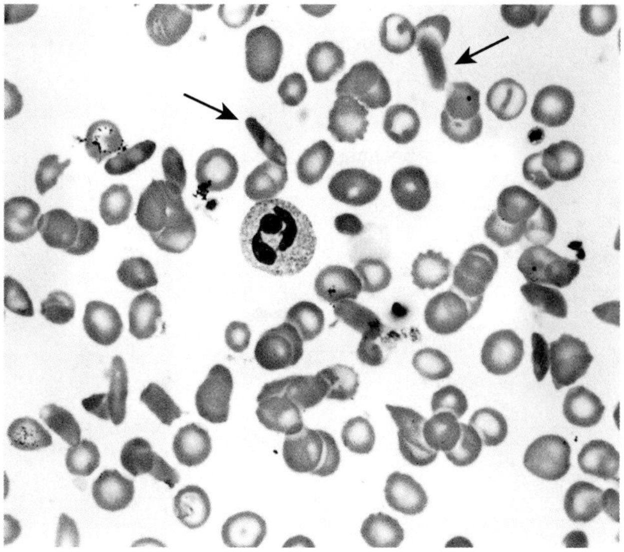

• **Fig. 12.6** Blood film showing sickling of red cells in sickle-cell disease. Sickled cells are indicated with arrows. (Courtesy Dr D. Norfolk, General Infirmary, Leeds, UK.)

supply to the tissues (Fig. 12.7). Sickled cells, with damaged cell membranes, are taken up by the reticuloendothelial system. Shorter red cell survival time leads to a more rapid red cell turnover and, consequently, anemia.

Sickling crises reduce life expectancy, so early recognition and treatment of the complications are vital. Prophylactic penicillin V should be given to reduce the risk of sepsis, especially from pneumococcus, and is recommended from the age of 3 months because this is when the levels of fetal Hb begin to decline and splenic hypofunction increases. Lifelong prophylaxis is recommended, although the evidence of benefit in adults is equivocal. Affected individuals should also follow the appropriate immunization schedule. Although there is currently little evidence of benefit, the use of folic acid is encouraged. Because chronic hemolysis increases folate turnover, replacing folate should reduce the risk of bone marrow aplasia. The other beneficial approach is the use of **hydroxyurea (hydroxycarbamide)**, a simple chemical compound that can be taken orally. Once-daily administration has been shown to increase levels of HbF through pharmacological induction, reduce the number of painful crises and reduce transfusion requirements. The HbF percentage has been shown to predict the clinical severity of SC disease, preventing intracellular sickling, which decreases vasoocclusion and hemolysis. It has been suggested that a potential threshold of 20% HbF is required to prevent recurrent vasoocclusive events. Hydroxyurea is recommended in patients with recurrent painful crises that impact on daily living, those admitted with more than three episodes of acute pain over a 12-month period and those with two or more episodes of acute chest syndrome. Patients need careful monitoring because of the risk of myelosuppression, and those of childbearing age need to be aware of the teratogenic effects of the drug, with provision of an appropriate method of contraception.

Stem cell transplant is the only cure for sickle-cell disease and may be considered in some patients, but requires a matched sibling donor. In the United Kingdom, if a donor is available, this would be considered in those under 17 years of age with sickle brain disease, or severe sickle-cell disease–related complications which have not responded to hydroxyurea. Published evidence suggests a disease-free survival of 75% to 84% following transplant.

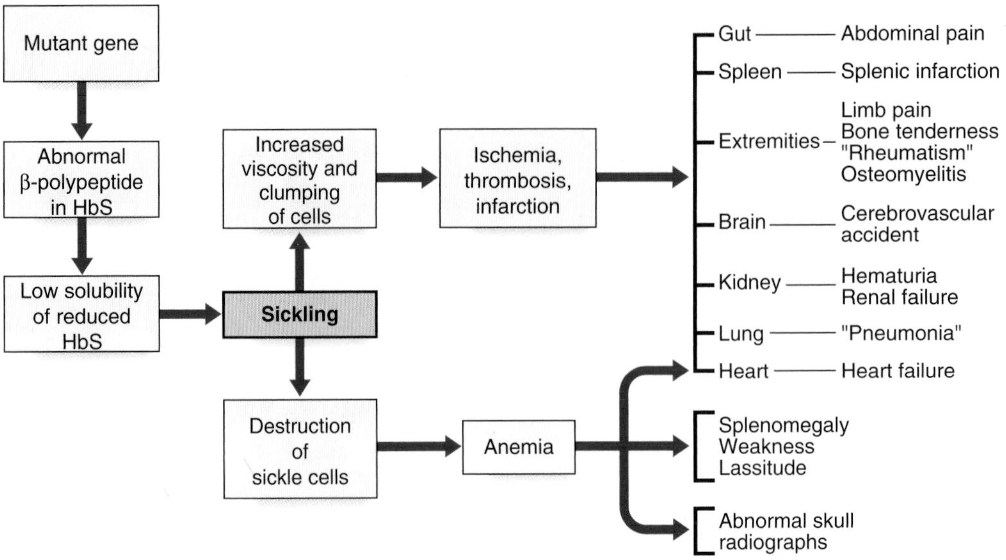

• **Fig. 12.7** The pleiotropic effects of the gene for sickle-cell disease.

Sickle-Cell Trait

The heterozygous, or carrier, state for the sickle-cell allele is known as **sickle-cell trait** and in general is not associated with any significant health risk. However, they are at risk of vasoocclusive episodes if oxygen deprived. They should avoid high altitudes/traveling in unpressurized aircraft, inform medical teams of their carrier status if having an anesthetic, and avoid extreme exhaustion if involved in intensive athletic activity.

Mutational Basis of Sickle-Cell Disease

The amino acid valine, at the sixth position of the β-globin chain, is substituted by glutamic acid, the result of a missense change from GAG to GTG, which is readily detected by PCR. In the United Kingdom, as elsewhere, both antenatal and newborn screening programs are established to identify carriers (see Chapter 11).

Disorders of Hemoglobin Synthesis

The **thalassemias** are the most common single group of inherited disorders in humans, occurring in persons from the Mediterranean region, Middle East, Indian subcontinent, and Southeast Asia. They are heterogeneous and classified according to the particular globin chain or chains synthesized in reduced amounts (e.g., α-, β-, δβ-thalassemia). There are similarities in the pathophysiology of all forms of thalassemia, although excessive α chains are more hemolytic than excessive β chains. An imbalance of globin-chain production results in the accumulation of free globin chains in the red blood cell precursors, which, being insoluble, precipitate, resulting in hemolysis of red blood cells (i.e., a hemolytic anemia). The consequence is compensatory hyperplasia of the bone marrow.

α-Thalassemia

This results from underproduction of the α-globin chains and occurs most commonly in Southeast Asia, but is also prevalent in the Mediterranean, Middle East, India, and sub-Saharan Africa, with carrier frequencies ranging from 15% to 30%. There are two main types of α-thalassemia. The severe form, α-thalassemia major, in which no α chains are produced, is associated with fetal death as a consequence of severe anemia leading to heart failure and massive edema, a condition known as *hydrops fetalis* (Fig. 12.8). Analysis of Hb from such fetuses reveals a tetramer of γ chains, originally called Hb Barts. The milder form of α-thalassemia is compatible with survival, and although one α chain is produced there is still a relative excess of β chains, resulting in production of the β-globin tetramer HbH—known as **HbH disease**. Both Hb Barts and HbH globin tetramers have an oxygen affinity similar to that of myoglobin and do not release oxygen as normal to peripheral tissues. Also, HbH is unstable and precipitates, resulting in hemolysis of red blood cells. HbH is mild to moderate in severity and does not usually require treatment except for in periods of extreme stress, for example, in pregnancy or with serious infections. Carriers of α-thalassemia are known as

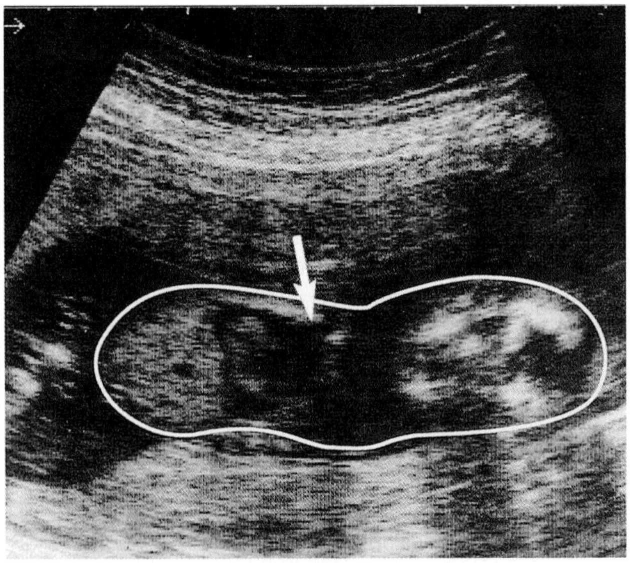

• **Fig. 12.8** Longitudinal ultrasonographic scan of a coronal section of the head (*to the right*) and thorax of a fetus with hydrops fetalis from the severe form of α-thalassemia, Hb Barts, showing a large pleural effusion (*arrow*). (Courtesy Mr J. Campbell, St. James's Hospital, Leeds, UK.)

α-thalassemia trait, which can either be termed α^+ [(-α/ α α) or (-α/- α)], or α^0 (--/α α) (Fig. 12.9).

Mutational Basis of α-Thalassemia. The absence of α chain synthesis in hydropic fetuses, and partial absence in HbH disease, was confirmed using quantitative mRNA studies from reticulocytes. Studies comparing the quantitative hybridization of radioactively labeled α-globin cDNA to DNA from hydropic fetuses, and in HbH disease, were consistent with the α-globin genes being deleted, which by restriction mapping studies were localized to chromosome 16p. The various forms of α-thalassemia are mostly the result of deletions of one or more of these structural genes (Fig. 12.9), and deletions are thought to have arisen as a result of unequal crossover events in meiosis—more likely to occur where genes with homologous sequences are in close proximity. Support for this hypothesis comes from the finding of the other product of such an event (i.e., individuals with *three* α-globin structural genes located on one chromosome).

These observations resulted in the recognition of two other milder forms of α-thalassemia that are not associated with anemia and can be detected only by the transient presence of Hb Barts in newborns. Mapping studies of the α-globin region showed that these milder forms of α-thalassemia are attributed to the deletion of one or two of the α-globin genes. Occasionally, point mutations in the α-globin genes, as well as the 5′ transcriptional region, have been found to cause α-thalassemia.

An exception to this classification of α-thalassemias is the Hb variant Constant Spring, named after the town in the United States from which the original patient came. This was detected as an electrophoretic variant in a person with HbH disease. Hb Constant Spring is attributed to an abnormally long α chain resulting from a variant in the normal termination codon at position 142 in the α-globin gene. Translation of α-globin mRNA therefore continues until another termination codon is reached, resulting in an abnormally long α-globin chain. The abnormal α-globin mRNA molecule is also unstable, leading to a relative deficiency of α chains and the presence of the β-globin tetramer, HbH.

β-Thalassemia

By now the reader will deduce that this is caused by underproduction of the β-globin chain of Hb. Production of β-globin chains may be either reduced (β^+) or absent (β^0). Individuals homozygous for β^0-thalassemia variants have severe, transfusion-dependent anemia—β-thalassemia major. Approximately 1:1000 Northern Europeans are β-thalassemia carriers, and in the United Kingdom some 20 to 30 babies with β^0 thalassemia are born annually, and approximately 1000 people live with the condition. There are an estimated 300,000 carriers in England, mainly of Cypriot, Indian, Pakistani, Bangladeshi, or Chinese ancestry.

Mutational Basis of β-Thalassemia. β-Thalassemia is rarely the result of gene deletion, and DNA sequencing is often necessary to determine the molecular pathology. Almost 300 different variants have been shown to cause β-thalassemia, including point mutations, insertions, and base-pair deletions. These occur within both the coding and non-coding portions of the β-globin genes, as well as the 5′ flanking promoter region, the 5′ capping sequences (p. 15), and the 3′ polyadenylation sequences (p. 15) (Fig. 12.10). The various variants are often unique to certain population groups and can be considered to fall into six main functional types.

Transcription Variants. Variants in the 5′ flanking TATA box or the promoter region of the β-globin gene can result in reduced transcription levels of the β-globin mRNA.

Messenger RNA Splicing Variants. Variants involving the invariant 5′ GT or 3′ AG dinucleotides of the introns in the β-globin gene or the consensus donor or acceptor sequences (p. 15) result in abnormal splicing with consequent reduced levels of β-globin mRNA. The most common Mediterranean β-thalassemia variant leads to the creation of a new acceptor AG dinucleotide splice site sequence in the first intron of the β-globin gene, creating a "cryptic" splice site (p. 22). The cryptic splice site competes with the normal splice site, leading to reduced levels of the normal β-globin mRNA. Variants in the coding regions of the β-globin region can also lead to cryptic splice sites.

Polyadenylation Signal Variants. Variants in the 3′ end of the untranslated region of the β-globin gene can lead to loss of the signal for cleavage and polyadenylation of the β-globin gene transcript.

RNA Modification Variants. Variants in the 5′ and 3′ DNA sequences, involved respectively in the capping and polyadenylation (p. 15) of the mRNA, can result in abnormal processing and transportation of the β-globin mRNA to the cytoplasm, and therefore reduced levels of translation.

Chain Termination Variants. Insertions, deletions and point mutations can all generate a nonsense or chain termination codon, leading to premature termination of translation of the β-globin mRNA. Usually this results in a shortened β-globin mRNA that is unstable and more rapidly degraded, leading to reduced levels of translation of an abnormal β-globin.

Missense Variants. Rarely, missense variants lead to a highly unstable β-globin (e.g., Hb Indianapolis).

Clinical Aspects of β-Thalassemia. Children with β-thalassemia major, or "Cooley's anemia" as it was originally known, usually present in infancy with a severe transfusion-dependent anemia. Unless adequately transfused, compensatory expansion of the bone marrow results in an unusually shaped face and skull (Fig. 12.11). Affected individuals previously died in their teens or early adulthood from organ damage resulting from iron overload caused by repeated transfusions. However, daily use of iron-chelating drugs, such as desferrioxamine, has greatly improved long-term survival. Other complications seen in β-thalassemia include delayed

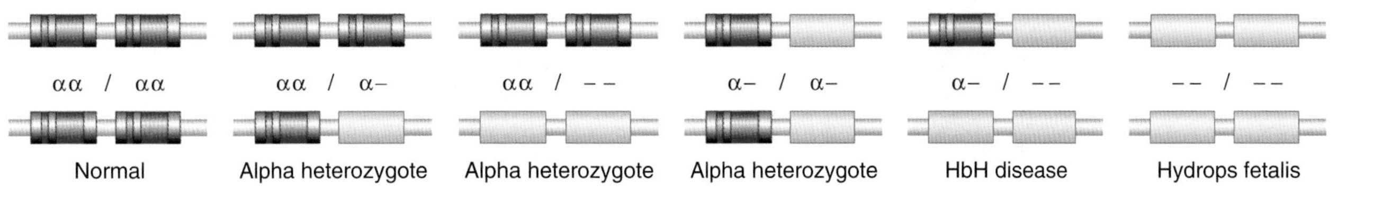

• **Fig. 12.9** Structure of the normal and deleted α-globin structural genes in the various forms of α-thalassemia. (Modified from Emery AEH. *An Introduction to Recombinant DNA*. John Wiley, Chichester; 1984.)

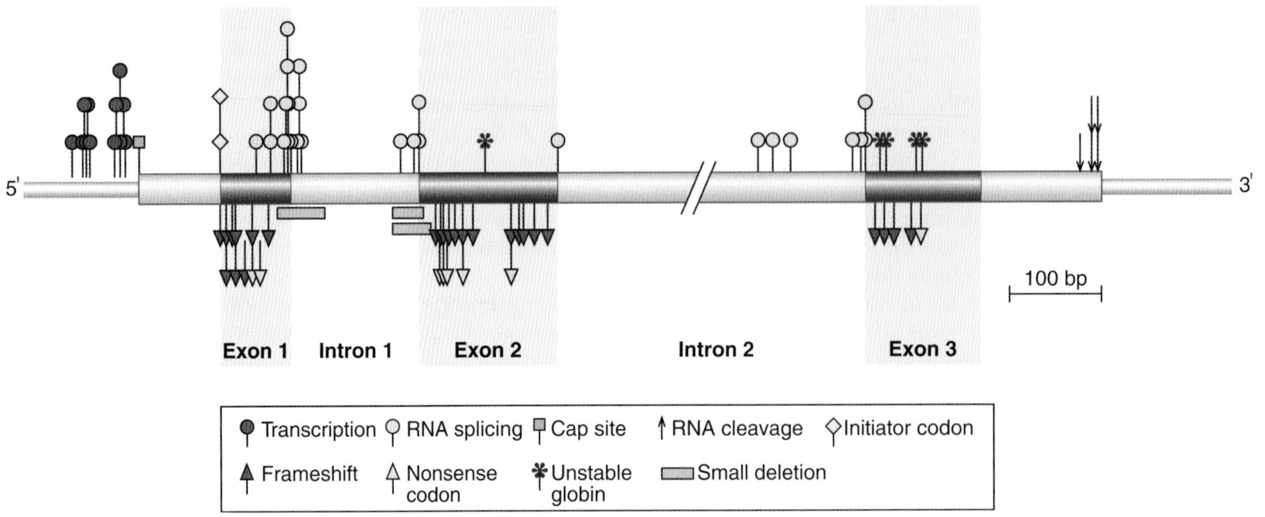

• **Fig. 12.10** Location and some of the types of variant in the β-globin gene and flanking region that result in β-thalassaemia. (Modified from Orkin SH, Kazazian HH. The mutation and polymorphism of the human β-globin gene and its surrounding DNA. *Annu Rev Genet*. 1984;18:131-171.)

puberty, hypothyroidism, osteoporosis, splenomegaly, and cardiac arrhythmia.

The only current cure for β-thalassemia is stem cell transplant from a human leukocyte antigen-matched donor, usually a sibling, which is often not possible. However, gene therapy for β-thalassemia is a very real prospect for the future. Although this is a more costly approach than stem cell transplant, it appears to have fewer complications, and better outcomes, with many patients involved in trials becoming transfusion-independent. A US biotech company, Bluebird Bio, was given conditional EU authorisation for their gene therapy, Zynteglo, in 2019 for patients over the age of 12 with transfusion-dependent β-thalassemia. Clinical trials are ongoing, but certainly promising. This is not the only hope for the future, with others looking at gene editing using the CRISPR/Cas9 stem cell modification.

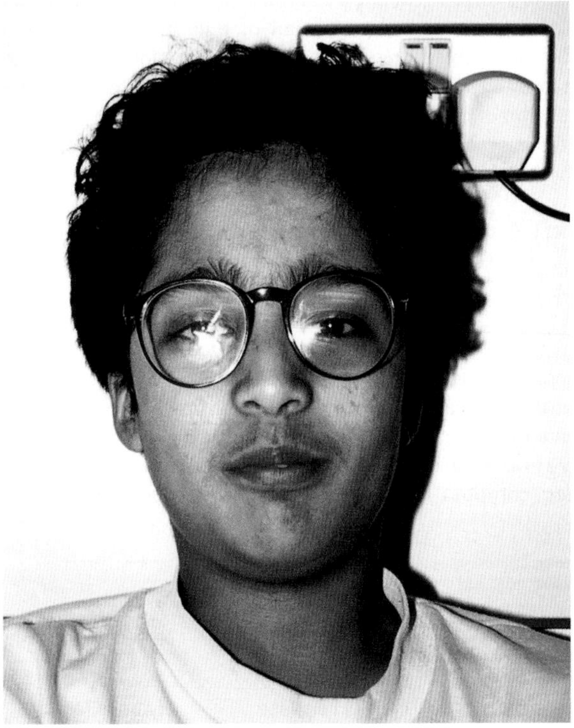

• **Fig. 12.11** Face of a child with β-thalassemia showing prominence of the forehead through changes in skull shape as a result of bone marrow hypertrophy. (Courtesy Dr D. Norfolk, General Infirmary, Leeds, UK.)

Individuals heterozygous for β-thalassemia—**thalassemia trait** or **thalassemia minor**—usually have no symptoms or signs, but do have a mild hypochromic, microcytic anemia. This can easily be confused with simple iron deficiency anemia.

δβ-Thalassemia

In this hemoglobinopathy, there is underproduction of both the δ and β chains. Homozygous individuals produce no δ- or β-globin chains, which one might expect to cause a profound illness. However, they have only mild anemia because of increased production of γ chains, such that HbF levels are much higher compared with the mild compensatory increase seen in β^0-thalassemia.

Mutational Basis of δβ-Thalassemia. The cause is extensive deletions in the β-globin region involving the δ- and β-globin structural genes (Fig. 12.12). Some large deletions include the Aγ-globin gene so that only the Gγ-globin chain is synthesized.

Hereditary Persistence of Fetal Hemoglobin

Hereditary persistence of fetal Hb (HPFH), in which HbF production persists into childhood and beyond, is included in the thalassemias. It is usually a form of δβ-thalassemia in which continued γ-chain synthesis compensates for the lack of δ and β chains. HbF may account for 20% to 30% of total Hb in heterozygotes and 100% in homozygotes. Individuals are usually symptom-free.

Mutational Basis of Fetal Hemoglobin. Some forms of HPFH are caused by deletions of the δ- and β-globin genes, whereas non-deletion forms may have point mutations in the 5′ flanking promoter region of either the Gγ or Aγ globin genes near the CAAT box sequences (p. 17), which are involved in the control of Hb gene expression.

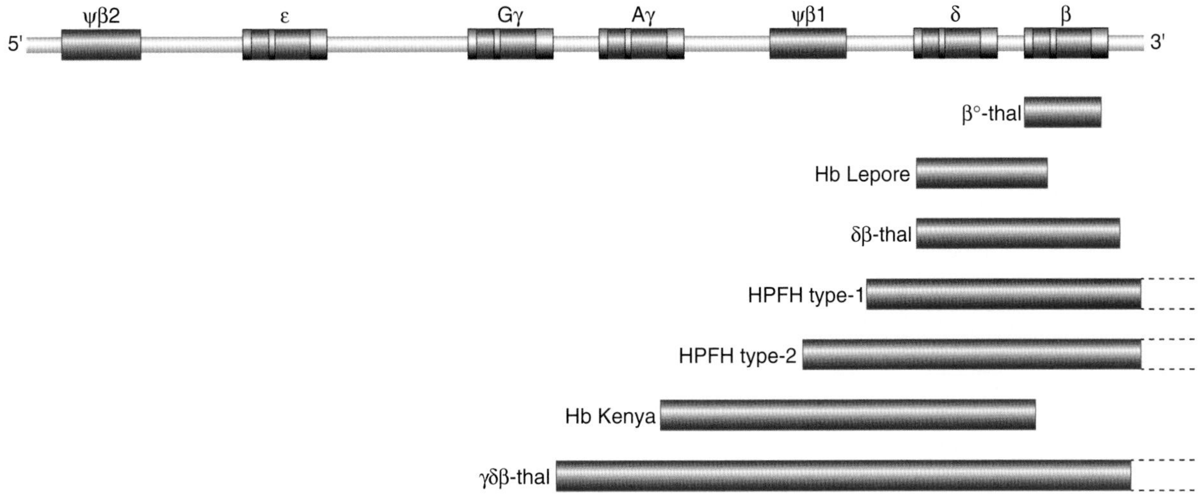

• **Fig. 12.12** Some of the deletions in the β-globin region that result in some forms of thalassemia and hereditary persistence of fetal hemoglobin.

Clinical Variation of the Hemoglobinopathies

The marked mutational heterogeneity of β-thalassemia means that affected individuals are often compound heterozygotes (p. 72), that is, they have different variants in their β-globin genes, leading to a broad spectrum of severity, including intermediate forms—**thalassemia intermedia**—which require less frequent transfusions.

Certain areas of the world show a high prevalence of all the hemoglobinopathies, and, not unexpectedly, individuals may have two different disorders of Hb. In the past, precise diagnoses were difficult, but DNA sequencing has greatly helped to solve conundrums—for example, individuals heterozygous for both HbS and β-thalassemia (i.e., compound heterozygotes). Certain combinations can result in a previously unexplained mild form of what might otherwise be anticipated to be a severe hemoglobinopathy. For example, deletion of one or two of the α-globin genes in a person homozygous for β-thalassemia results in a milder illness because there is less of an imbalance in globin chain production. Similarly, the presence of one form of HPFH in a person homozygous for β-thalassemia or sickle-cell disease can contribute to amelioration of the disease, as the increased production of γ-globin chains compensates for the deficient β-globin chain production. The relative severity of different homozygous or compound heterozygous hemoglobinopathies is helpfully summarized in a risk assessment tool produced by the National Health Service Sickle Cell and Thalassaemia Screening Programme (Fig. 12.13).

Antenatal and Newborn Hemoglobinopathy Screening

Sickle-cell and thalassemia screening were introduced in newborns in the United Kingdom in 2005 and are offered as part of antenatal

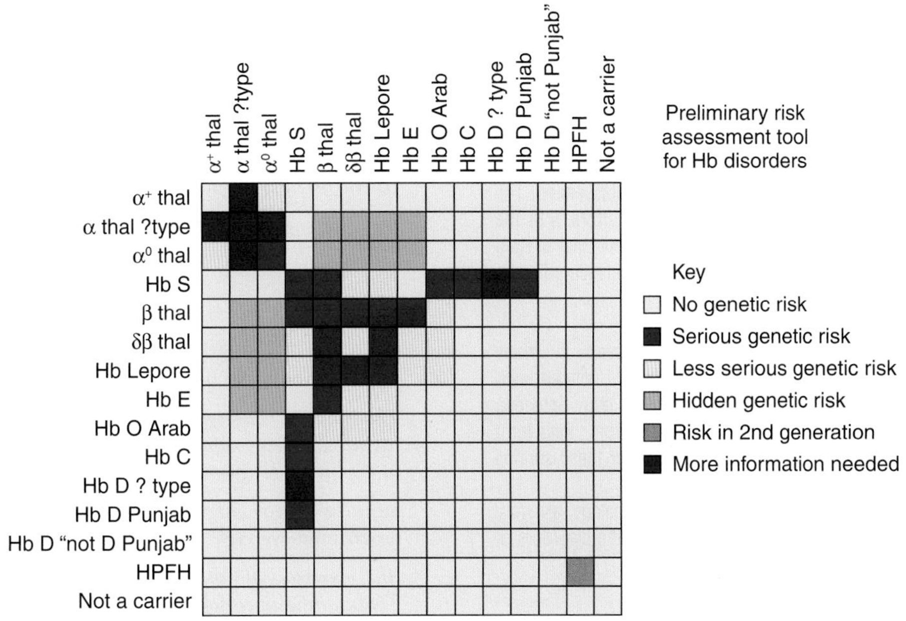

• **Fig. 12.13** A hemoglobinopathy tool depicting the anticipated clinical severity associated with the occurrence of different homozygous or compound heterozygous states.

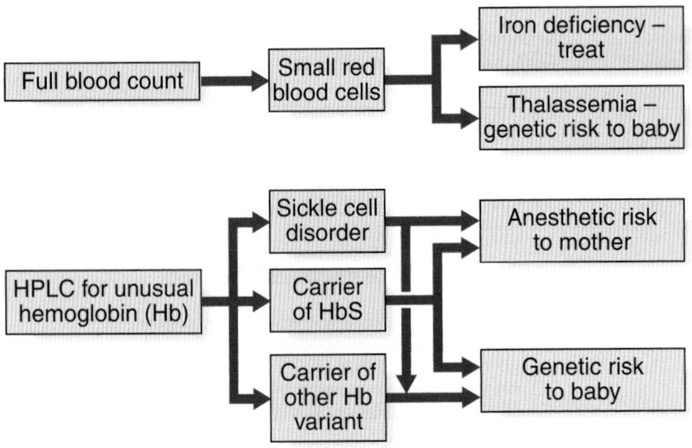

• **Fig. 12.14** Antenatal screening for hemoglobinopathies.

screening. The purpose of newborn screening is the presymptomatic diagnosis of serious hemoglobinopathies so that early treatment can be instituted, and long-term complications minimized. In the antenatal setting, in the United Kingdom, pregnant women are offered sickle-cell screening if they live in a high prevalence area, and a family origin questionnaire is used to identify those at high risk who live in lower prevalence areas. Thalassemia screening is offered to all pregnant women in the United Kingdom. Initial screening is undertaken on a full blood count, looking for anemia (Hb <11 g/dL) and microcytosis (mean corpuscular Hb <27 pg). These findings prompt electrophoresis by high performance liquid chromatography, summarized in Fig. 12.14. The antenatal screening program enables access to prenatal testing for those fetuses at risk of serious disease, where couples may choose to end an affected pregnancy.

Both programs mean that cascade screening through the wider family, and genetic counseling, can be offered.

As with all screening, these programs aim to reduce the burden of health care in the long term and improve quality of life.

ELEMENTS

1. Hemoglobin (Hb), the protein present in red blood cells responsible for oxygen transport, is a tetramer made up of two dissimilar pairs of polypeptide chains and the iron-containing molecule heme.
2. Human Hb is heterogeneous. During development, it comprises a succession of different globin chains that are expressed differentially during embryonic, fetal and adult life (e.g., $\alpha_2\varepsilon_2$, $\alpha_2\gamma_2$, $\alpha_2\delta_2$, $\alpha_2\beta_2$).
3. The disorders of Hb—the hemoglobinopathies—can be divided into two main groups: the structural disorders of Hb, such as sickle-cell anemia (HbS), and disorders of production or synthesis—the thalassemias. The former can be subdivided by the way in which they interfere with the normal function of Hb and/or the red blood cell (e.g., abnormal oxygen affinity, hemolytic anemia). The latter can be subdivided according to which globin chain is produced abnormally (i.e., α-, β-, or $\delta\beta$-thalassemia).
4. Screening for hemoglobinopathies has been introduced in many countries, not only in those areas with a high prevalence. Without such measures the burden of disease would be much higher; early detection facilitates early treatment and reduced morbidity from long-term consequences and, in many places, prenatal diagnosis for these serious disorders is accepted.
5. Gene therapy, and gene editing using CRISPR/Cas9 technology, are very likely to play a significant role in the future treatment of the disorders of hemoglobin.

CLINICAL SCENARIO 1

A female from Southeast Asia is seen in the antenatal booking clinic at 8 weeks' gestation. Routine screening shows a microcytic, hypochromic picture with normal HbA2 level on hemoglobin electrophoresis. The lab reports this as suggestive of thalassemia carrier status and recommends DNA analysis for confirmation.

Further testing confirms alpha zero thalassemia trait (- -/α α). The patients' partner is offered testing which confirms the same genotype (- -/ α α).

What are the possible outcomes of the pregnancy?

What complications would occur in a pregnancy affected with alpha-thalassemia major? What are the risks to the mother?

CLINICAL SCENARIO 2

A 5-day-old baby undergoes newborn (heel prick) screening which shows he is affected with sickle-cell disease. His parents are from West Africa and recently moved to the United Kingdom.

What are the key factors in the management of sickle-cell disease?

How will you counsel the family about their future pregnancy risks?

Further Reading

Cooley TB, Lee P. A series of cases of splenomegaly in children with anemia and peculiar bone changes. *Trans Am Pediatr Soc.* 1925;37:29–40.

The original description of β-thalassemia.

Giardine B, Borg J, Viennas E, et al. Updates of the HbVar database of human hemoglobin variants and thalassemia mutations. *Nucleic Acids Res.* 2014;42:D1063–D1069.

A helpful introduction to the HbVar database.

Pauling L, Itano HA, Singer SJ, Wells IC. Sickle-cell anaemia, a molecular disease. *Science.* 1949;110:543–548.

The first genetic disease for which a molecular basis was described, leading to a Nobel Prize.

Serjeant GR, Serjeant BE. *Sickle Cell Disease.* 3rd ed. Oxford: Oxford University Press; 2001.

Excellent, comprehensive text covering all aspects of this important disorder.

Weatherall DJ, Clegg JB. *The Thalassaemia Syndromes.* 4th ed. Blackwell Science Ltd; 2001. Available at: https://onlinelibrary.wiley.com/book/10.1002/9780470696705.

An authoritative and comprehensive text, available online.

Websites

http://www.nhr.nhs.uk/

The National Haemoglobinopathy Registry is a database of patients with red cell disorders (mainly sickle-cell disease and thalassemia major) living in the United Kingdom. Various useful reports are available online.

https://www.gov.uk/guidance/sickle-cell-and-thalassemia-screening-programme-overview

An overview of the National Health Service Sickle-Cell and Thalassaemia Screening Programme.

13 Immunogenetics

Medicinal discovery,
It moves in mighty leaps,
It leapt straight past the common cold
And gave it us for keeps.

Pam Ayers

Immunity

The immune system defends us against armies of microorganisms that numerically dwarf the human population. Without it we would not survive, and to understand the inherited disorders of immunity we must look at the fundamentals of the genetic basis of immunity.

Immune defense mechanisms can be divided into two main types: **innate immunity**, which includes a number of nonspecific systems that do not require or involve prior contact with the infectious agent, and **specific acquired** or **adaptive immunity**, which involves a tailor-made immune response that occurs after exposure to an infectious agent. Both types can involve either **humoral immunity**, which combats extracellular infections, or **cell-mediated immunity**, which fights intracellular infections.

Innate Immunity

The first simple defense against infection is the mechanical barrier of the skin, which functions most of the time as an impermeable barrier, but in addition the acidic pH of sweat is inhibitory to bacterial growth. Mucus membranes line the respiratory and gastrointestinal tracts, and the respiratory tract is further protected by ciliary movement. Other body fluids contain a variety of bactericidal agents, such as lysozymes in tears. If an organism succeeds in invading the body, a healthy immune system reacts immediately by recognizing the alien intruder, and a chain response is triggered.

Cell-Mediated Innate Immunity

Phagocytosis

Two major cell types go on the offensive when a foreign microorganism invades—**macrophages** and **neutrophils**. Macrophages are the mature form of circulating monocytes that migrate into tissues and occur primarily around the basement membrane of blood vessels in connective tissue, lung, liver, the lining of the sinusoids of the spleen and the medullary sinuses of the lymph nodes. They are believed to play a key role in the orchestration of both the innate and adaptive responses and can recognize invading microorganisms through surface receptors able to distinguish between self and pathogen. Recognition of the foreign material leads to phagocytosis by the macrophage, followed rapidly by neutrophils recruited from the circulation during the inflammatory process. The activation of the macrophage triggers the inflammatory process through the release of inflammatory mediators. The invading organism is destroyed by fusion with intracellular granules of the phagocyte and exposure to the action of hydrogen peroxide, hydroxyl radicals, and nitrous oxide (Fig. 13.1).

The Toll-Like Receptor Pathway

A key component of cell-mediated immunity is the **Toll-like receptor (TLR)** pathway. TLRs are conserved transmembrane receptors which are expressed on the membranes of leucocytes, including dendritic cells, macrophages, **natural killer** (NK) cells, and cells of the adaptive immune system—**T cells** and **B cells**. They are also present in non-immune cells—epithelial and endothelial cells and fibroblasts. In fruit fly embryos they play a critical role in dorsal-ventral development, but their mammalian homologues function in innate immune responses and microbial recognition, and belong to the interleukin-1/TLR superfamily. The superfamily has two subgroups based on the extracellular characteristics of the receptor—that is, whether they possess an

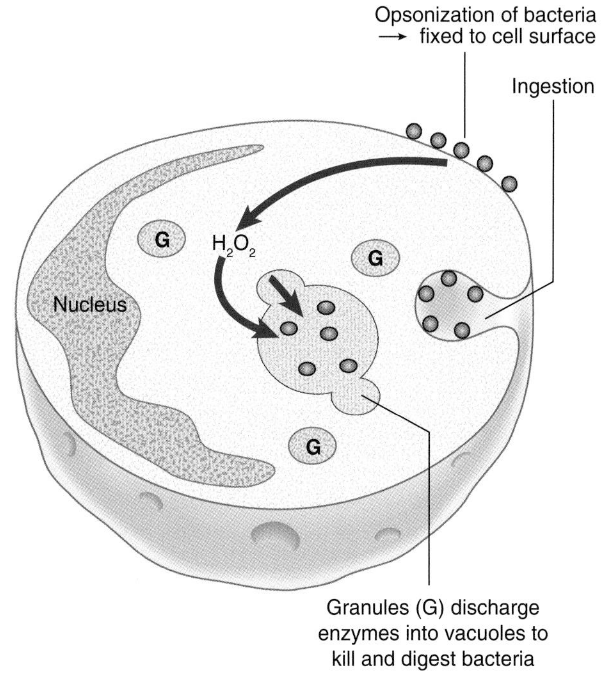

• **Fig. 13.1** Phagocytosis and the pathways involved in intracellular killing of microorganisms.

immunoglobulin (Ig)-like domain or leucine-rich repeats. TLRs typically have extracellular leucine-rich repeats.

There are 10 TLRs in humans, each receptor being responsible for recognition of a specific set of pathogen-associated molecular patterns. TLR2 has been well characterized and has an essential role in the detection of invading pathogens, recognizing peptidoglycans and lipoproteins associated with gram-positive bacteria, as well as a host of other microbial and endogenous ligands. The primary function of TLR2 is therefore lipoprotein-mediated signaling, and activation of the pathway by recognition of its ligand results in activation of the transcription factor NF-κB, which in turn results in the increased expression of co-stimulatory molecules and inflammatory cytokines (Fig. 13.2). These cytokines help mediate migration of dendritic cells from infected tissue to lymph nodes, where they may encounter and activate leucocytes involved in the adaptive immune response. The signaling pathways used by TLRs share many of the same proteins as the interleukin-1 receptor (IL-1R) pathway (Fig. 13.2). Activation of TLR leads to recruitment of the MyD88 (this is sometimes known as the MyD88-dependent pathway) which mediates the interaction between IL-1R associated kinases 1 and 4 (IRAK1 and IRAK4).

The activation of the Toll pathway has several important effects in inducing innate immunity. These effects include the production of cytokines and chemokines, including IL-1, IL-6 and tumor necrosis factor-alpha (TNF-α), which have local effects in containing infection and systemic effects with the generation of fever and induction of acute phase responses, including production of C-reactive protein. One important medical condition related to the Toll pathway is **septic shock** because activation of the Toll pathway by certain ligands induces systemic release of TNF-α. There are also important health-related consequences that result from mutated or deficient *TLR2*. *TLR2*-deficient mice are susceptible to infection by Gram-positive bacteria as well as meningitis from *Streptococcus pneumoniae*.

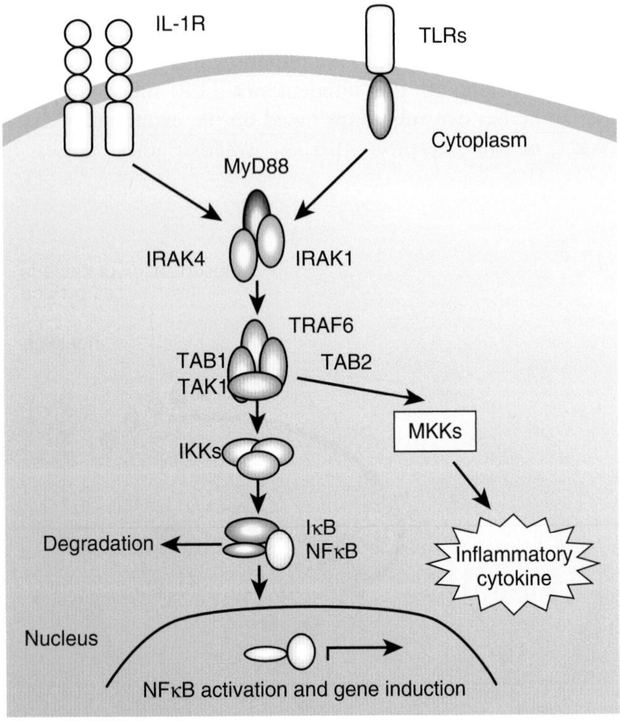

• **Fig. 13.2** The Toll-like receptor (TLR) and interleukin-1 receptor (IL-1R) pathways, which share many of the same proteins. Activation of TLR2 and other TLRs, via NFκB activation and gene induction, leads to dendritic cell maturation, upregulation of expression of the major histocompatibility complex and co-stimulatory molecules and production of immuno-stimulatory cytokines. *IKK*, I kappa kinase; *IκB*, NFκB inhibitor; *IRAK*, IL-1R–associated protein kinases; *MKK*, MAP kinases; *MyD88*, adapter molecule; *TAB1*, TAK1-binding protein 1; *TAB2*, TAK1-binding protein 2; *TAK1*, transforming growth factor-β–activated kinase; *TRAF6*, tumor necrosis factor receptor-associated factor 6.

Extracellular Killing

Virally infected cells can be killed by large granular lymphocytes, known as NK cells. These have carbohydrate-binding receptors on their cell surface that recognize high molecular weight glycoproteins expressed on the surface of the infected cell as a result of the virus taking over the cellular replicative functions. NK cells play an early role in viral infections and are activated by cytokines from macrophages. They recognize virally infected cells through changes either in glycoproteins or in the expression of major histocompatibility complex (MHC) class 1 on virally infected host cells. Binding to the infected cells results in the release of a number of agents which results in damage to the membrane of the infected cell, leading to cell death.

Humoral Innate Immunity

Several soluble factors are involved in innate immunity; they help to minimize tissue injury by limiting the spread of infectious microorganisms. These are called the **acute-phase proteins** and include C-reactive protein, mannose-binding protein, and serum amyloid P component. The first two act by facilitating the attachment of one of the components of complement, C3b, to the surface of the microorganism, which becomes opsonized (made ready) for adherence to phagocytes. The third binds lysosomal enzymes to connective tissues. In addition, cells infected by virus synthesize and secrete interferon-α and interferon-β, which have a role in promoting the cellular response to viral infection by NK cell activation and upregulation of MHC class I. Also, **interferon** interferes with viral replication by reducing messenger RNA (mRNA) stability and interfering with translation.

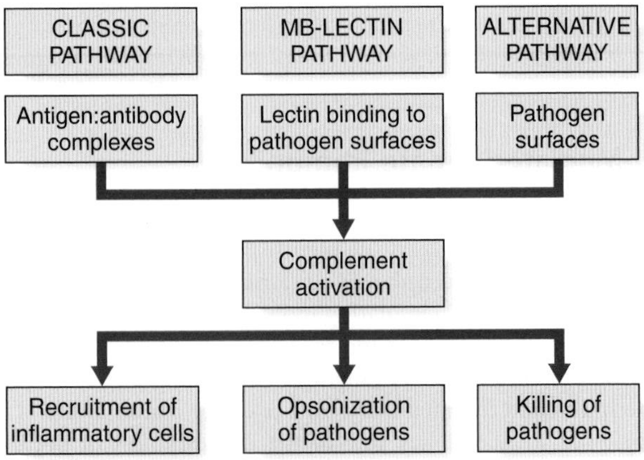

• **Fig. 13.3** The classic and alternative pathways of complement activation. The main functions of complement are recruitment of inflammatory cells, opsonization of pathogens and killing of pathogens.

Complement

The complement system is a complex of 20 or so plasma proteins that cooperate to attack extracellular pathogens. Although the critical role of the system is to opsonize pathogens, it also recruits inflammatory cells and kills pathogens directly through membrane attack complexes. This system can be activated through three pathways: (1) the classical pathway; (2) the alternative pathway; and (3) the **mannose-binding lectin** (MBL) pathway (see Fig. 13.3).

Complement nomenclature, like much else in immunology, can be confusing. Each component is designated by the letter C, followed by a number—but each component were numbered in order of their discovery rather than the sequence of reactions. The reaction sequence is C1, C4, C3, C5, C6, C7, C8 and C9. The product of each cleavage reaction is designated by letters, the larger fragment being "b" (b = big), and the smaller fragment "a." In the lectin pathway, MBL in the blood binds another protein, a serine protease called MBL-associated serine protease (MASP). When MBL binds to its target (e.g., mannose on the surface of a bacterium), the MASP protein functions like a convertase to clip C3 into C3a and C3b. C3 is abundant in the blood, so this happens very efficiently. The other two complement pathways also converge toward C3 convertase, which cleaves C3. C3a mediates inflammation, whereas C3b binds to the pathogen surface, coating it and acting as an opsonin. The effector roles of the major complement proteins can be summarized according to function as follows (Fig. 13.4):

1. Opsonization: C3b and C4b are opsonins that coat foreign organisms, greatly enhancing their phagocytosis—phagocytes have receptors that recognize complement proteins bound to a pathogen.
2. Inflammation: C5a, as well as C4a and C3a, are inflammatory activators that induce vascular permeability and recruit and activate phagocytes.
3. Lysis: C5b binds and recruits C6 and C7, eventually forming the **membrane attack complex** (MAC), C5b678, which catalyzes the polymerization of the final component C9, forming a transmembrane pore of approximately 10 nm diameter, ultimately resulting in cell lysis.
4. Immune complex clearance: Complement has a critical role in removing immune complexes from the circulation. The immune complex binds C4b and C3b, which then bind to receptors on red blood cells. The complexes are transported to the liver and spleen, where they are given up to phagocytes for destruction.

There are clinical consequences relating to variants in the genes of these pathways. The frequency of variants of the *MBL2* gene in the general population may be 5% to 10%. Although most individuals with MBL deficiency from variants and promoter polymorphisms in *MBL2* are healthy, there is an increased risk, severity and frequency of infections and autoimmunity, as reported in infants with recurrent respiratory tract infection, otitis media, and chronic diarrhea.

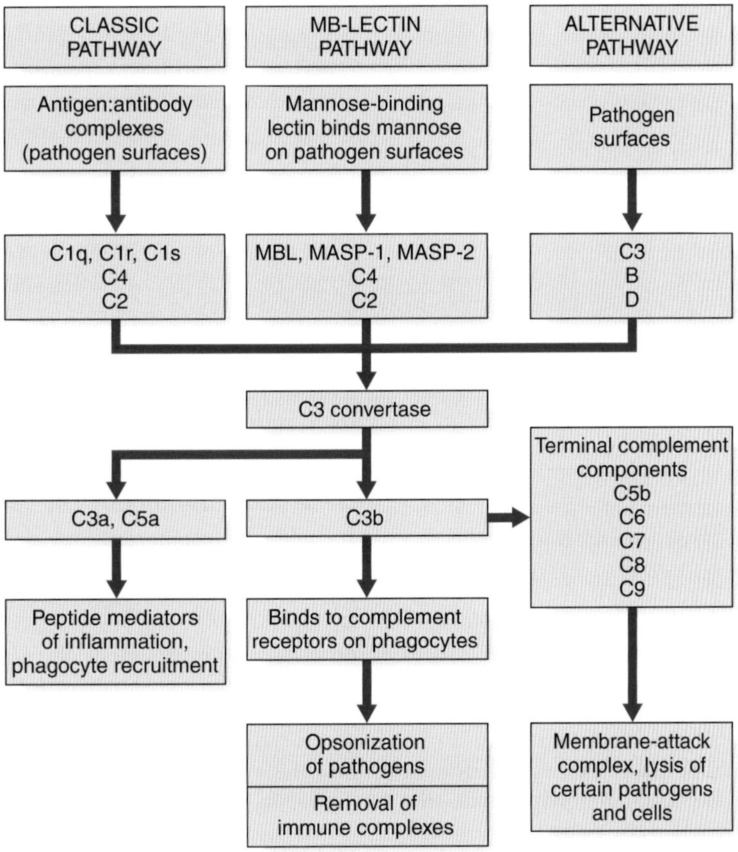

• **Fig. 13.4** Overview of the main components and effector actions of complement. Note that the Mannose-binding lectin (*MBL*) pathway involves the MBL protein, MBL-associated serine protease (MASP)-1, MASP-2, C4, and C2. MASP acts as a C3 convertase, creating a C3b fragment from C3. C3b attaches to the pathogen surface and binds to receptors on phagocytes, leading to opsonization C3b can also combine with other proteins on the pathogen surface and form a membrane attack complex.

Specific Acquired Immunity

Many infective microorganisms have, through mutation and selective pressures, developed strategies to overcome or evade the mechanisms associated with innate immunity. There is a need, therefore, to be able to generate specific acquired, or adaptive, immunity. This can, as with innate immunity, be separated into both humoral and cell-mediated processes.

Humoral Specific Acquired Immunity

The main mediators of humoral specific acquired immunity are Igs, or antibodies. Antibodies are able to recognize and bind to surface antigens of infecting microorganisms, leading to the activation of phagocytes and the initiation of the **classic pathway** of complement, resulting in the generation of the MAC (see Fig. 13.4) and other complement effector functions. Exposure to a specific antigen results in the clonal proliferation of a small ('B') lymphocyte derived from the bone marrow, resulting in mature antibody-producing cells, or **plasma cells.**

Lymphocytes that produce antibodies express copies of the Ig for which they code on their surface, then act as a surface receptor for antigen. Binding of the antigen, in conjunction with other MASPs, results in signal transduction leading to the clonal expansion and production of antibody. The **primary response** is the production of IgM, followed by IgG. Reexposure to the same antigen results in a swifter response and enhanced antibody levels, which is the **secondary response**, amounting to the antigen-specific **immunological memory**.

Immunoglobulins

The Igs, or antibodies, are one of the major classes of serum protein. Their function, both in the recognition of antigenic variability and in effector activities, was first revealed by study of their structure, and later by DNA analysis.

Immunoglobulin Structure. Papain, a proteolytic enzyme, splits the Ig molecule into three fragments. Two of the fragments are similar, each containing an antibody site capable of combining with a specific antigen and therefore referred to as the **antigen-binding fragment** or **Fab**. The third fragment can be crystalized and was called **Fc**, and this component determines the secondary biological functions of antibodies, binding complement and Fc receptors on different cell types involved in the immune response.

The Ig molecule is made up of four polypeptide chains—two 'light' (L) and two 'heavy' (H)—that are approximately 220 and 440 amino acids in length, respectively. They are held together in a Y-shape by disulfide bonds and non-covalent interactions. Each Fab fragment is composed of L chains linked to the amino-terminal portion of the H chains, whereas each Fc fragment is composed only of the carboxy-terminal portion of the H chains (Fig. 13.5).

Immunoglobulin Isotypes, Subclasses and Idiotypes. There are five different types of heavy chain, designated respectively as γ, μ, α, δ, and ε, one each for the five major antibody classes—the **isotypes**—IgG, IgM, IgA, IgD, and IgE, respectively. The L chains are of two types—kappa (κ) or lambda (λ)—and these occur in all five classes of antibody, but only one type occurs in each individual antibody. Thus the molecular formula for IgG is $\lambda_2\gamma_2$ or $\kappa_2\gamma_2$. The characteristics of the various classes of antibody are outlined in Table 13.1. In addition, there are four IgG **subclasses**—IgG1, IgG2, IgG3, and IgG4—and two IgA subclasses—IgA1 and IgA2—that differ in their amino acid sequence and interchain disulfide bonds. Individual antibody molecules that recognize specific antigens are known as **idiotypes**.

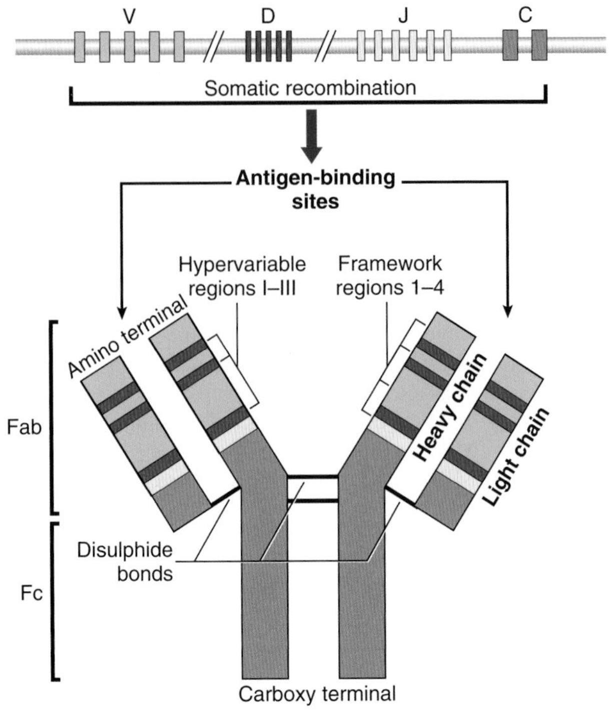

• **Fig. 13.5** Model of antibody molecule structure.

Immunoglobulin Allotypes. The five Ig classes occur in all normal individuals, but allelic variants, or what are known as antibody **allotypes** of these classes, have also been identified. These are the *Gm* system associated with the heavy chain of IgG, the *Am* system associated with the IgA heavy chain, the *Km* and *Inv* systems associated with the κ light chain, the *Oz* system for the λ light chain and the *Em* allotype for the IgE heavy chain. The Gm and Km systems are independent of each other and are polymorphic (p. 89), the frequencies of the different alleles varying in different ethnic groups.

Generation of Antibody Diversity

It could seem paradoxical for a single protein molecule to exhibit sufficient structural heterogeneity to have specificity for a large number of different antigens. Different combinations of H and L chains could, to some extent, account for this diversity. It would, however, require thousands of structural genes for each chain type to provide sufficient variability for the large number of antibodies produced in response to the equally large number of antigens to which individuals can be exposed. Our initial understanding of how this works came from persons with a malignancy of antibody-producing cells—**multiple myeloma.**

Multiple Myeloma. People with multiple myeloma make a single or monoclonal antibody species in large abundance, which in a proportion of patients is detected in their urine. This is known as **Bence Jones protein** and consists of antibody L chains. The amino-terminal ends of this protein molecule in different patients

TABLE 13.1 Classes of human immunoglobulin

Class	Mol. Wt (Da)	Serum Concentration (mg/mL)	Antibody Activity	Complement Fixation	Placental Transfer
IgG	150,000	8–16	Binds to microorganisms and neutralizes bacterial toxins	+	+
IgM	900,000	0.5–2	Produced in early immune response, especially in bacteremia	+	–
IgA	160,000	1.4–4	Guards mucosal surfaces	+	–
IgD	185,000	0–0.4	On lymphocyte cell surface, involved in control of activation and suppression	–	–
IgE	200,000	Trace	In parasitic and allergic reactions	–	–

Ig, Immunoglobin.

are quite variable in sequence, whereas the carboxy-terminal ends are relatively constant. These are called the **variable (V)** and **constant (C)** regions, respectively. However, the V regions of different myeloma proteins show four regions that vary little from one antibody to another, known as **framework regions** (FR 1–4), and three markedly variable regions interspersed between these, known as **hypervariable regions** (HV I–III) (see Fig. 13.5).

DNA Studies of Antibody Diversity. In 1965 Dreyer and Bennett proposed that an antibody could be encoded by separate 'genes' in germline cells that undergo rearrangement or, as they termed it, 'scrambling', in lymphocyte development. Comparison of the restriction maps of the DNA segments coding for the C and V regions of the Ig λ light chains in embryonic and antibody-producing cells revealed that they were far apart in the former but close together in the latter. Detailed analysis revealed that the DNA segments coding for the V and C regions of the light chain are separated by some 1500 base pairs (bp) in antibody-producing cells. The intervening DNA segment was found to code for a **joining (J)** region immediately adjacent to the V region of the light chain. The κ L-chain was shown to have the same structure. Cloning and DNA sequencing of H-chain genes in germline cells revealed that they have a fourth region, called **diversity (D)**, between the V and J regions.

There are estimated to be some 60 different DNA segments coding for the V region of the H-chain, 40 for the V region of the κ L-chain, and 30 for the λ L-chain V region. Six functional DNA segments code for the J region of the H-chain, five for the J region of the κ L-chain and four for the J region of the λ L-chain. A single DNA segment codes for the C region of the κ L-chain, seven code for the C region of the λ L-chain, and 11 functional DNA segments code for the C region of the different classes of H-chain. There are also 27 functional DNA segments that code for the D region of the H-chain (Fig. 13.6).The genomic regions in question also contain a large number of unexpressed DNA sequences or pseudogenes (p. 14).

Antibody Gene Rearrangement. The genes for the κ and λ L-chains and the H-chains are located on chromosomes 2, 22 and 14, respectively. Only one of each of the relevant types of DNA segment is expressed in any single antibody molecule. The DNA coding segments for the various portions of the antibody chains on these chromosomes are separated by DNA that is non-coding. Somatic recombination events involved in antibody production involve short conserved recombination signal sequences that flank

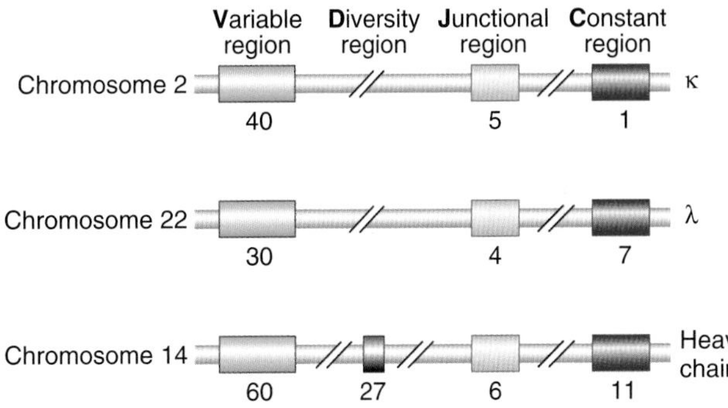

• **Fig. 13.6** Estimated number of the various DNA segments coding for the κ, λ, and various heavy chains.

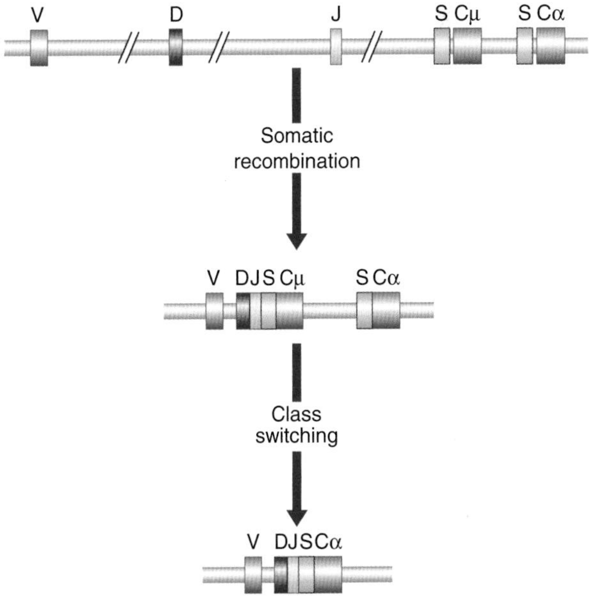

• **Fig. 13.7** Immunoglobulin heavy-chain gene rearrangement and class switching.

each germline DNA segment (Fig. 13.7). Further diversity occurs by variable mRNA splicing at the V–J junction in RNA processing and by somatic variants of the antibody genes. These mechanisms readily account for the antibody diversity seen in nature, although how particular DNA segments are selected to produce an antibody to a specific antigen is not fully resolved.

Class Switching of Antibodies

There is a normal switch of antibody class produced by B cells on continued, or further, exposure to antigen—from IgM, the initial class of antibody produced in response to exposure to an antigen, to IgA or IgG. This **class switching** retains specificity of the antibody to the same antigen. Analysis of class switching in a population of cells derived from a single B cell has shown that both classes of antibody have the same antigen-binding sites, having the same V region but differing only in their C region. Class switching occurs by a somatic recombination event that involves DNA segments, designated S (for switching), that lead to looping out and deletion of the intervening DNA. The result is to eliminate the DNA segment coding for the C region of the H-chain of the IgM molecule, and to bring the gene segment encoding the C region of the new class of H-chain adjacent to the segment encoding the V region (see Fig. 13.7).

The Immunoglobulin Gene Superfamily

Several other molecules involved in the immune response have been shown to have structural and DNA sequence homology to the Igs. This involves a 110–amino acid sequence characterized by a centrally placed disulfide bridge that stabilizes a series of antiparallel β strands into an "antibody fold." This group of structurally similar molecules has been called the **Ig superfamily** (p. 13). It consists of eight multigene families that, in addition to the κ and λ L-chains and different classes of H-chain, include the chains of the T-cell receptor (p. 13), the class I and II MHC or human leucocyte antigens (HLA) (p. 177). Other molecules in this group include the T-cell CD4 and CD8 cell surface receptors, which cooperate with T-cell receptors in antigen recognition, and the intercellular adhesion molecules-1, -2, and -3, which are involved in leucocyte-endothelial adhesion and extravasation, T-cell activation, and T-cell homing.

Antibody Engineering

At the beginning of the 20th century, Paul Ehrlich proposed the idea of the "magic bullet"—the hope that one day there might be a compound that would selectively target a disease-causing organism. Today we have **monoclonal antibodies** (mAbs), and, for almost any substance, it is possible to create a specific antibody that binds that substance. mAbs are the same because they are made by a homogenous population of immune cells which are all clones of a unique parent cell.

In the 1970s it was found that the B-cell cancer, multiple myeloma, produced a single type of antibody—a **paraprotein**. This facilitated the study of the structure of antibodies, but it was not possible to produce identical antibodies specific to a given antigen. Myeloma cells cannot grow because they lack hypoxanthine-guanine-phosphoribosyl transferase, which is necessary for DNA replication. Typically, mAbs are made by fusing myeloma cells with spleen cells from a mouse (or rabbit) that has been immunized with the desired antigen. They are then grown in medium which is selective for these hybrids—the spleen cell partner supplies hypoxanthine-guanine-phosphoribosyl transferase, and the myeloma has immortal properties because it is a cancer cell. The cell mixture is diluted, and clones are grown from single parent cells. The antibodies secreted by different clones are assayed for their ability to bind the antigen, and the healthiest clone is selected for future use. The hybrids can also be injected into the peritoneal cavity of mice to produce tumors containing antibody-rich ascitic fluid, and the mAb then has to be extracted and purified.

To overcome the problem of purification, recombinant DNA technologies have been used since the 1980s. DNA that encodes the binding portion of mouse mAb is merged with human DNA that encodes antibodies. Mammalian cell culture is then used to express this DNA, producing chimeric antibodies. The goal, of course, is to create "fully human" mAb, which has met with success in "phage display–generated" antibodies and mice that have been genetically modified to produce more human-like antibodies.

Specific mAbs have now been developed and approved for the treatment of cancer, cardiovascular disease, inflammatory diseases, macular degeneration, and transplant rejection, among others. An mAb that inhibits TNF-α has applications in rheumatoid arthritis, Crohn disease and ulcerative colitis; one that inhibits IL-2 on activated T cells is used in preventing rejection of transplanted kidneys, and another inhibits vascular endothelial growth factor with a role in antiangiogenic cancer therapy.

Cell-Mediated Specific Acquired Immunity

Certain microorganisms, viruses and parasites live inside host cells. As a result, a separate form of specific acquired immunity has developed to combat intracellular infections involving lymphocytes differentiated and matured in the thymus—hence T cells. T lymphocytes have specialized receptors on the cell surface, known as **T-cell surface antigen receptors**, which in conjunction with the MHC on the cell surface of the infected cell result in the involvement of different subsets of T cells, each with a distinct function—**T helper cells** and **cytotoxic T cells**. The battle against intracellular infections is a cooperative, coordinated response from these separate components of the immune system, leading to death of the infected cell (Fig. 13.8).

T-Cell Surface Antigen Receptor

T cells express on their surface an antigen receptor, which distinguishes them from other lymphocyte types, such as B cells and NK cells. The antigen consists of two different polypeptide chains, linked by a disulfide bridge, both of which contain two Ig-like domains, one that is relatively invariant in structure, the other highly variable like the Fab portion of an Ig. The diversity in T-cell receptors required for recognition of the range of antigenic variation that can occur is generated by a process similar to that seen with Igs. Rearrangement of variable (V), diversity (D), junctional (J), and constant (C) DNA segments during T-cell maturation, through a similar recombination mechanism as occurs in B cells, results in a contiguous VDJ sequence. Binding of antigen to the T-cell receptor, in conjunction with an associated complex of transmembrane peptides, results in signaling the cell to differentiate and divide.

The Major Histocompatibility Complex

The MHC plays a central role in the immune system. Its role is to bind antigen peptides processed intracellularly and present this material on the cell surface, with co-stimulatory molecules, where it can be recognized by T cells. MHC molecules occur in three classes: class I occur on virtually all cells and are responsible for presenting cytotoxic T cells; class II occur on B cells and macrophages and are involved in signaling T-helper cells to present further B cells and macrophages; and the non-classic class III molecules include a number of other proteins with a variety of other immunological functions. The latter include inflammatory mediators

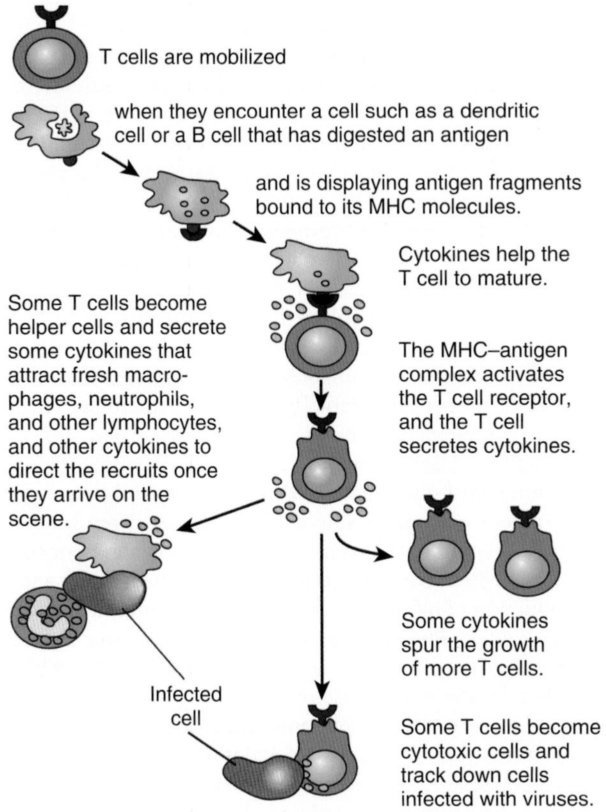

• **Fig. 13.8** T cells and the cooperative response resulting in death of an infected cell. *MHC*, Major histocompatibility complex.

such as TNF, heat-shock proteins and the various components of complement.

Structural analysis of class I and II MHC molecules reveal them to be heterodimers with homology to Ig. The genes coding for the class I (A, B, C, E, F and G), class II (DR, DQ and DP) and class III MHC molecules, or what is also known as the HLA system, are located on chromosome 6.

Transplantation Genetics

Organ transplantation has become routine in clinical medicine, and, with the exception of corneal and bone grafts, success depends on the degree of antigenic similarity between donor and recipient. The closer the similarity, the greater the likelihood that the transplanted organ or tissue (the **homograft**) will be accepted rather than rejected. Homograft rejection does not occur between identical twins or between non-identical twins where there has been mixing of the placental circulations before birth. In all other instances, the antigenic similarity of donor and recipient has to be assessed by testing them with suitable antisera or mAbs for antigens on donor and recipient tissues. These were originally known as transplantation antigens but are now known to be a result of the MHC. As a general rule, a recipient will reject a graft from any person who has antigens that the recipient lacks. HLA typing of an individual is carried out using PCR-based techniques.

The HLA system is highly polymorphic (Table 13.2). A virtually infinite number of phenotypes resulting from different combinations of the various alleles at these loci are theoretically possible.

TABLE 13.2 Alleles at the human leucocyte antigens loci

HLA Locus	Number of Alleles
A	57
B	111
C	34
D	228

HLA, Human leucocyte antigen.

Two unrelated individuals are therefore very unlikely to have identical HLA phenotypes. The close linkage of the HLA loci means that they tend to be inherited *en bloc*, the term **haplotype** being used to indicate the particular HLA alleles that an individual carries on each of the two copies of chromosome 6. Thus, any individual will have a 25% chance of having identical HLA antigens with a sibling because there are only four possible combinations of the two paternal (say, P and Q) and the two maternal (say, R and S) haplotypes, (i.e., PR, PS, QR, and QS). The siblings of a particular recipient are more likely to be antigenically similar than either of his or her parents, and the latter more than a non-relative. Therefore a sibling is frequently selected as a potential donor.

Although recombination occurs within the HLA region, certain alleles tend to occur together more frequently than would be expected by chance, that is, they tend to exhibit linkage disequilibrium (p. 93). An example is the association of the HLA antigens A1 and B8 in populations of western European origin.

H-Y Antigen (Also Known as Müllerian Inhibiting Factor). In a number of different animal species, it was noted that tissue grafts from males were rejected by females of the same inbred strain. These incompatibilities were found to be as a result of a histocompatibility antigen known as H-Y. However, H-Y seems to play little part in transplantation in humans. The H-Y antigen, also known as Müllerian inhibiting factor—which is not the *SRY* gene —is important for testicular differentiation (p. 128) and function, but its expression does not correlate with the presence or absence of testicular tissue.

Human Leucocyte Antigens Polymorphisms and Disease Associations

The association of certain diseases with certain HLA types (Table 13.3) should shed light on the pathogenesis of the disease, but in reality this is not well understood. The best documented association is between ankylosing spondylitis and HLA-B27. Narcolepsy, a condition of unknown etiology characterized by a periodic uncontrollable tendency to fall asleep, is almost invariably associated with HLA-DR2. The possession of a particular HLA antigen does not mean that an individual will necessarily develop the associated disease, only that the relative risk of being affected is greater than that in the general population. In a family, the risks to first-degree relatives of those affected are low, usually no more than 5%.

Explanations for the various HLA-associated disease susceptibilities include: (1) close linkage to a susceptibility gene near the HLA complex; (2) cross-reactivity of antibodies to environmental antigens or pathogens with specific HLA antigens; and (3) abnormal recognition of "self" antigens through defects in T-cell

TABLE 13.3 Some human leucocyte antigen-associated diseases

Disease	HLA
Ankylosing spondylitis	B27
Celiac disease	DR4
21-Hydroxylase deficiency	A3/Bw47/DR7
Hemochromatosis	A3
Insulin-dependent diabetes (type 1)	DR3/4
Myasthenia gravis	B8
Narcolepsy	DR2
Rheumatoid arthritis	DR4
Systemic lupus erythematosus	DR2/DR3
Thyrotoxicosis (Graves disease)	DR3

HLA, Human leucocyte antigen.

receptors or antigen processing. These conditions are known as **autoimmune diseases**. An example of close linkage is congenital adrenal hyperplasia from a 21-hydroxylase deficiency (p. 277) from mutated *CYP21*, which lies within the HLA MHC locus. This form of congenital adrenal hyperplasia is strongly associated with HLA-A3/Bw47/DR7 in northern European populations. Non-classical 21-hydroxylase deficiency is associated with HLA-B14/DR1, and HLA-A1/B8/DR3 is negatively associated with 21-hydroxylase deficiency.

Inherited Immunodeficiency Disorders

Inherited immunodeficiency disorders are uncommon and sometimes severe, but, with early diagnosis and optimum management, many patients with primary immune deficiency (PID) can remain healthy. Prompt diagnosis is very important in order that treatment, for example antimicrobials, Ig or bone marrow transplant, be instituted before significant irreversible end-organ damage takes place. Presentation is variable but often in childhood for more severe immune defects, especially after the benefits of maternal transplacental immunity have declined from 3 to 4 months of age. New diagnoses of PID are sometimes made in adults. Investigation of immune function should be considered in all patients with recurrent infections and in children with failure to thrive. Failure to thrive, diarrhea, and hepatosplenomegaly may also be features.

Primary Inherited Disorders of Immunity

The manifestations of at least some of the PID diseases in humans can be understood by considering whether they are disorders of either innate or specific acquired immunity. Abnormalities of *humoral* immunity are associated with reduced resistance to bacterial infections and may be lethal in infancy. Abnormalities of *cell-mediated* specific acquired immunity are associated with increased susceptibility to viral infections and are manifested experimentally in animals by prolonged survival of skin homografts.

Disorders of Innate Immunity

Primary disorders of innate immunity are considered under humoral and cell-mediated immunity categories.

Disorders of Innate Humoral Immunity. A variety of defects of complement can lead to disordered innate immunity.

Disorders of complement. If a complement defect is suspected, investigation of the integrity of the classic and alternative pathways should begin with functional assays looking at the entire pathway. If functional abnormalities are found, measurement of the individual components of that pathway can be undertaken.

The clinical effects of MBL deficiency have been described previously. Defects of the third component of complement, C3, lead to abnormalities of opsonization of bacteria, resulting in difficulties in combating pyogenic infections. Defects in the later components of complement—those involved in the formation of the MAC (p. 173)—also result in susceptibility to bacterial infection, particularly *Neisseria* (meningococcal infections). This includes deficiency of properdin (factor P), a plasma protein active in the alternative complement pathway.

C1 inhibitor (also known as C1 esterase inhibitor) deficiency follows autosomal dominant (AD) inheritance, and there are two forms—type 1 because of low levels, and type 2 resulting from nonfunctioning protein. Inappropriate activation and poor control of the complement pathway occur with breakdown of C2 and C4, and production of inflammatory mediators. C1 inhibitor also controls the kinin-bradykinin pathway, and C1 inhibitor deficiency leads to accumulation of bradykinin in the tissues, which is believed to be the main cause of edema triggered by episodes of surgery, dental work, trauma, and some drugs. Attacks vary in severity from mild cutaneous to abdominal pain and swelling, which can be severe, and laryngeal edema is potentially fatal. This is known as **hereditary angioedema**. Acute attacks were traditionally treated with C1 inhibitor concentrate, a blood product, which superseded fresh frozen plasma when available. In 2014 the US Food and Drug Administration approved a plasma-free recombinant C1 inhibitor which appears to be effective and safe. The drug Danazol, an androgen, has also been a mainstay of long-term prevention.

Other associations with disease include homozygous C2 deficiency. There are various case reports of individuals who developed cutaneous vasculitis, Henoch-Schönlein purpura, seropositive rheumatoid arthritis, polyarteritis, membranoproliferative glomerulonephritis, and an association with systemic lupus erythematosus (SLE). Similarly, C4 is associated with SLE. The copy number of C4 genes in a diploid human genome varies from 2 to 6 in Europeans. Each of these genes encodes either a C4A or C4B protein. Individuals with only two copies of total C4 are at significantly increased risk of SLE, whereas those with five copies or more are at decreased risk.

Defects in NFκB Signaling

Inappropriate **activation** of nuclear factor kappa-B (NFκB) has been linked to inflammation associated with autoimmune arthritis, asthma, septic shock, lung fibrosis, glomerulonephritis, atherosclerosis, and acquired immunodeficiency syndrome. Conversely, persistent **inhibition** of NFκB has been linked directly to apoptosis, abnormal immune cell development and delayed cell growth.

Since 2000, pathogenic variants have occasionally been found in the XL *IKK-gamma* (or *IKBKG*, or *NEMO*) gene, part of the TLR pathway (p. 171), in children demonstrating failure to thrive, recurrent digestive tract infections, often with intractable diarrhea and recurrent ulcerations, respiratory tract infections with bronchiectasis, and recurrent skin infections. Presentation is in infancy, suggesting susceptibility to various gram-positive and gram-negative bacteria. Sparse scalp hair is sometimes a feature, and in older children oligodontia and conical-shaped maxillary lateral incisors have been noted. Survival ranged from 9 months to 17 years in one study. IgG is low and IgM usually high. Interestingly, *IKKg* is the same as *NEMO*, the gene that causes X-linked dominant incontinentia pigmenti (p. 75). However, in this condition of the immune system variants occur in exon 10 of the gene.

IRAK4 is another component of the TLR pathway, and deficiency leads to recurrent infections, mainly from gram-positive microorganisms, although also from fungi. There is a reduced inflammatory response. Infections begin early in life but become less frequent with age, with some patients requiring no treatment by late childhood. It follows autosomal recessive (AR) inheritance.

Disorders of Innate Cell-Mediated Immunity. An important mechanism in innate cell-mediated immunity is phagocytosis, as previously discussed, which results in subsequent cell-mediated killing of microorganisms.

Chronic granulomatous disease (CGD). This is the best-known example of a disorder of phagocytic function and follows either an XL (*CYBB* gene) or AR (*CYBA, NCF1, NCF2, NCF4* genes) pattern of inheritance. It results from an inability of phagocytes to kill ingested microbes, because of defects in the nicotinamide adenine dinucleotide phosphate oxidase enzyme complex which generates the so-called microbicidal "respiratory burst" (see Fig. 13.1). Hypergammaglobulinemia may be present. CGD is therefore associated with recurrent bacterial or fungal infections and may present at any time between infancy and late adulthood with suppurative lymphadenitis, hepatosplenomegaly, pulmonary infiltrates, and/or eczematoid dermatitis. Childhood mortality was high until the advent of supportive treatment and prophylactic antibiotics. Bone marrow transplant has been successful, as well as transplantation of peripheral blood stem cells from an HLA-identical sibling.

The neutropenias. The neutropenias are a heterogeneous group of disorders of varying severity, following different patterns of inheritance, and characterized by very low neutrophil counts. AD or sporadic congenital neutropenia (SCN type 1) is caused by variants in the neutrophil elastase gene (*ELA2*), whereas variants in the proto-oncogene *GFI1*, which targets *ELA2*, also cause dominantly inherited neutropenia (SCN2). Pathogenic variants in the *HAX1* gene causes AR SCN3 ("classical" SCN—Kostmann disease), although AR SCN4 is caused by variants in the *G6PC3* gene. SCN patients with **acquired** variants in the granulocyte colony-stimulating factor receptor *(CSF3R)* gene in hematopoietic cells are at high risk for developing acute myeloid leukemia.

In SCN, hematopoiesis is characterized by a maturation arrest of granulopoiesis at the promyelocyte level; peripheral absolute neutrophil counts are below 0.5×10^9/L, and there is early onset of severe bacterial infections. As well as dominantly inherited SCN1, there is an XL form caused by a constitutively activating variant in the *WAS* gene, mutated in Wiskott-Aldrich syndrome (WAS).

Cyclic neutropenia is rare, characterized by regular 21-day fluctuations in the numbers of blood neutrophils, monocytes, eosinophils, lymphocytes, platelets, and reticulocytes. This results in patients experiencing periodic symptoms of fever, malaise, mucosal ulcers, and occasionally life-threatening infections. As with SCN1, it is because of mutated *ELA2*.

Leucocyte adhesion deficiency (LAD). Individuals with LAD present with life-threatening bacterial infections of the skin and mucous membranes and impaired pus formation. The increased susceptibility to infections occurs because of defective migration of phagocytes from abnormal adhesion-related functions of chemotaxis and phagocytosis. This disorder is fatal unless antibiotics are given, both for infection and prophylactically, until bone marrow transplantation can be offered. Three different forms of LAD are recognized, each with unique clinical features, although leucocytosis is a constant feature. LAD I and LAD II, and usually LAD III, follow AR inheritance; LAD II and LAD III are very rare.

LAD I is characterized by delayed separation of the umbilical cord, omphalitis, and severe recurrent infections with no pus formation. It is because of mutated *ITGB2* (21q22) and encodes the β_2 subunit of the integrin molecule.

LAD II patients have the rare Bombay blood group and suffer from psychomotor retardation and growth delay; it is also known as congenital disorder of glycosylation type IIc (CDG2C). It is caused by variants in *SLC35C1* (11p11), the gene encoding the Golgi-specific GDP-fucose transporter.

LAD III is similar to LAD I but includes severe neonatal bleeding tendency. Various defects in leucocyte chemotaxis and adhesion to endothelial cells have been found, and the diagnosis is reached by showing defects in the integrin activation process; the CD18 molecule is structurally intact. It is due to variants in *FERMT3* (11p13).

Autoimmune Polyendocrinopathy-Candidosis-Ectodermal Dysplasia Syndrome

Also known as autoimmune polyendocrinopathy syndrome, autoimmune polyendocrinopathy-candidosis-ectodermal dysplasia (APECED) syndrome type I is characterized by the presence of two of three major clinical symptoms: Addison disease, hypoparathyroidism and chronic mucocutaneous candidiasis, and is caused by pathogenic variants in the autoimmune regulator (*AIRE*) gene. Both AD and AR forms exist. Malabsorption and diarrhea can be striking and dominate the clinical picture, and immune disorders may be present, although diabetes mellitus and thyroid disease are infrequent. The onset of Addison disease is mostly in childhood or early adulthood, and frequently accompanied by chronic active hepatitis, malabsorption, juvenile-onset pernicious anemia, alopecia, and primary hypogonadism.

Disorders of Specific Acquired Immunity

Again, these can be considered under the categories of disorders of humoral and cell-mediated specific acquired immunity.

Disorders of Humoral Acquired Immunity. Abnormalities of Ig function lead to an increased tendency to develop bacterial infections.

Bruton-type agammaglobulinemia. Boys with this XL immunodeficiency usually develop multiple recurrent bacterial infections of the respiratory tract and skin after the first few months of life, having been protected initially by placentally transferred maternal IgG. Features similar to rheumatoid arthritis develop in many, and they are not prone to viral infection. Treatment of life-threatening infections with antibiotics and the use of prophylactic intravenous Igs have improved survival prospects, but children with this disorder can still die from respiratory failure through complications of repeated lung infections. The diagnosis of this type of immunodeficiency is confirmed by demonstration of Ig deficiency and absence of B lymphocytes. The disorder has been shown to result from variants in a tyrosine kinase (*BTK*) gene specific to B cells that result in loss of the signal for B cells to differentiate to mature antibody-producing plasma cells. A rarer, AR form of agammaglobulinemia shows marked depression of the circulating lymphocytes, and lymphocytes are absent from the lymphoid tissue—caused by variants in the mu heavy-chain (IGHM) gene (14q32).

Hyper-IgM syndrome (HIGM). HIGM is another genetically heterogeneous condition that includes increased levels of IgM, and also usually of IgD, with levels of the other Igs being decreased or virtually absent. Patients are susceptible to recurrent pyogenic infections, as well as opportunistic infections such as *Pneumocystis* and *Cryptosporidium*, because of primary T-cell abnormality. In the XL form (HIGM1) the mutated gene encodes a cell surface molecule on activated T cells called CD40 ligand (renamed *TNFSF5*). When the gene is not functioning, Ig class switches are inefficient, so that IgM production cannot be readily switched to IgA or IgG. IgM levels are therefore high, and IgG levels reduced. At least four other types are recognized including AR forms HIGM2 (CD40 deficiency) and HIGM3 (activation-induced cytidine deaminase) deficiency.

Hyper-IgE syndrome (HIES). Again heterogeneous, this condition is sometimes known as Job syndrome and is a PID characterized by chronic eczema, recurrent staphylococcal infections, increased serum IgE and eosinophilia. Abscesses may be "cold." that is, they lack associated warmth, erythema, or tenderness. Patients have a distinctive coarse facial appearance, abnormal dentition, hyperextensibility of the joints and bone fractures. AD HIES is caused by variants in the *STAT3* gene and AR HIES by variants in *DOCK8*.

Common variable immunodeficiency (CVID). CVID has tended to be a "wastebasket" category but constitutes the most common group of B-cell deficiencies characterized by normal numbers of Ig-bearing B-cell precursors and a broad deficiency of Ig isotypes. It is very heterogeneous, with at least 12 genetic varieties identified. The presentation is similar to other forms of immune deficiency, at any age, including nodular lymphoid hyperplasia, and males and females are equally affected. Affecting approximately 1:800 Caucasians, selective IgA deficiency is the most frequently recognized PID. Many affected people have no obvious health problems, but others may have recurrent infections, gastrointestinal disorders, autoimmune diseases, allergies, or malignancies. The pathogenesis is arrest of B-cell differentiation, giving rise to a normal number of IgA-bearing B-cell precursors but a profound deficit in IgA-producing plasma cells. The response to immunization with protein and polysaccharide antigens is abnormal.

Disorders of Cell-Mediated Specific Acquired Immunity. The most common inherited disorder of cell-mediated specific acquired immunity is severe combined immunodeficiency (SCID).

Severe combined immunodeficiency. SCID, as the name indicates, is associated with an increased susceptibility to both viral and bacterial infections because of profoundly abnormal humoral and cell-mediated immunity. Common to all forms of SCID is the absence of T cell–mediated cellular immunity because of defective T-cell development. Presentation is in infancy with recurrent, persistent, opportunistic infections by many organisms, including *Candida albicans*, *Pneumocystis carinii*, and cytomegalovirus. The incidence of all types of SCID is approximately 1:75,000. Death usually occurs in infancy because of overwhelming infection, unless a bone marrow transplant is performed. SCID is genetically heterogeneous and can be inherited as either an XL or AR disorder. The XL form (SCIDX1) is the most common form of SCID in males, accounting for 50% to 60% overall, and has been shown to be caused by variants in the γ chain of the cytokine receptor for IL-2 *(IL2RG)*. In approximately one-third to one-half of children with SCID that is not attributed to XL inheritance, the disease is AR (SCID1,) and the different forms are classified according to whether they are T- and B-cell negative (T-B-) or B-cell positive (T-B +). The presence or absence of NK cells is variable. T-B + SCID, apart from SCIDX1, includes deficiencies of the protein tyrosine phosphatase receptor type C (or CD45) deficiency. CD45 suppresses Janus kinases (JAK), and there is a specific B-cell–positive SCID caused by JAK3 deficiency, which can be very variable—from subclinical to life-threatening in early childhood. Other rare AR forms of SCID include variants in the *IL7R* gene—IL2RG is dependent on a functional interleukin-7 receptor.

T-B- SCID includes **adenosine deaminase deficiency**, which accounts for approximately 15% of all cases of SCID and one-third of all cases of AR SCID. The phenotypic spectrum is variable, the most severe being SCID presenting in infancy and usually resulting in early death. Some 10% to 15% of patients have a "delayed" clinical onset by age 6 to 24 months, and a smaller percentage of patients have "later" onset, diagnosed from 4 years to adulthood, showing less severe infections and gradual immunologic deterioration. The immune system is affected through the accumulation of purine degradation products that are selectively toxic to T cells. Rare forms of B-cell negative SCID include mutated *RAG1/RAG2* (recombination activating genes), which are normally responsible for VDJ recombinations (p. 176) that lead to mature Ig chains and T-cell receptors. In addition, cases occur because of variants in the Artemis gene (DNA cross-link repair protein 1c—*DCLRE1C*). The latter forms are sensitive to ionizing radiation. Lastly, reticular dysgenesis is a rare and very severe form of SCID characterized by congenital agranulocytosis, lymphopenia, and lymphoid and thymic hypoplasia with absent cellular and humoral immunity functions. It is due to variants in the mitochondrial *Adenylate kinase-2* gene *(AK2)*.

Secondary or Associated Immunodeficiency

There are a number of hereditary disorders in which immunological abnormalities occur as one of a number of associated features as part of a syndrome.

DiGeorge/Sedláčková Syndrome (Deletion 22q11.2)

Children with **DiGeorge/del22q11.2 syndrome** (see p. 259), well described by Eva Sedláčková in 1955, 10 years earlier than Angelo DiGeorge, present with recurrent viral illnesses and are found to have abnormal cellular immunity as characterized by reduced numbers of T lymphocytes, as well as abnormal antibody production. This is caused by partial absence of the thymus gland, leading to defects in cell-mediated immunity and T cell–dependent antibody production. Usually these defects are relatively mild and improve with age as the immune system matures, but occasionally the immune deficiency is very severe because no T cells are produced, and bone marrow transplantation is indicated. It is important for all patients diagnosed to be investigated by taking a full blood count with differential CD3, CD4, and CD8 counts made, and Ig levels assessed. The levels of diphtheria and tetanus antibodies can indicate the ability of the immune system to respond. These patients usually have a characteristic face (see Fig. 17.17, p. 261) and frequently have congenital heart disease and hypoplastic parathyroid glands. The latter can result in presentation in the newborn period with hypocalcaemic tetany secondary to low parathyroid hormone levels. The diagnosis is usually apparent from chromosome microarray.

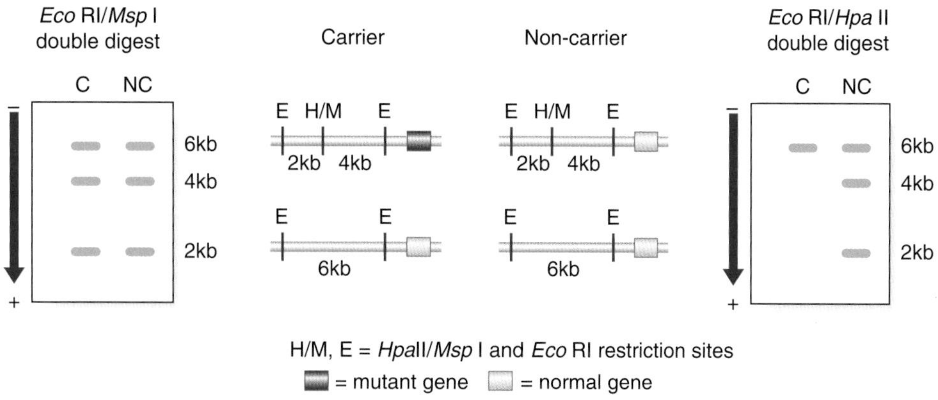

• **Fig. 13.9** Non-random inactivation in T lymphocytes for carrier testing in X-linked severe combined immunodeficiency.

Ataxia Telangiectasia

Ataxia telangiectasia is an AR disorder in which children present in early childhood with signs of cerebellar ataxia, dilated blood vessels on the sclera of the eyes, ears, and face (oculocutaneous telangiectasia) and a susceptibility to sinus and pulmonary infections. This is due to thymic hypoplasia, and low serum IgA levels as a result of a defect in the cellular response to DNA damage. The diagnosis is made by the demonstration of low or absent serum IgA and IgG, as well as characteristic chromosome abnormalities on culture of peripheral blood lymphocytes—a form of chromosome instability (p. 268) and/or DNA testing. Patients have an increased risk of developing leukemia or lymphoid malignancies.

Wiskott-Aldrich Syndrome

This XL recessive disorder affects boys who present with eczema, diarrhea, recurrent infections (chest, ears), thrombocytopenia and, usually, low serum IgM levels, and impaired T-cell function and numbers. Variants in the *WAS* gene (Xp11) result in loss of cytotoxic T-cell responses and T-cell help for B-cell response, leading to an impaired response to bacterial infections. Until the advent of bone marrow transplantation, the majority of affected boys died by midadolescence from hemorrhage or B-cell malignancy.

Carrier Tests for X-Linked Immunodeficiencies

Before it was possible to sequence the genes responsible for WAS, Bruton-type hypogammaglobulinemia and XL SCID, the availability of closely linked DNA markers allowed female carrier testing by studies of the pattern of X-inactivation (p. 124) in the lymphocytes of females at risk. A female relative of a sporadically affected male with an XL immunodeficiency would be confirmed as a carrier by the demonstration of a non-random pattern of X-inactivation—"skewed" X-inactivation (p. 73)—in the T-lymphocyte population, indicating that all her peripheral blood T lymphocytes had the same chromosome inactivated (Fig. 13.9).

The carrier (C) and non-carrier (NC) are both heterozygous for an *Hpa*II/*Msp*I restriction site polymorphism. *Hpa*II and *Msp*I recognize the same nucleotide recognition sequence, but *Msp*I cuts double-stranded DNA whether it is methylated or not, whereas *Hpa*II cuts only unmethylated DNA (i.e., only the active X chromosome). In the carrier female, the SCID gene variant is on the X chromosome on which the *Hpa*II/*Msp*I restriction site is present. *Eco*RI/*Msp*I double digests of T lymphocytes result in 6-, 4-, and 2-kilobase (kb) DNA fragments on gel analysis of the restriction fragments for both the carrier and non-carrier females. However, *Eco*RI/*Hpa*II double digests of T-lymphocyte DNA result in a single 6-kb fragment in the carrier female because in a carrier the only T cells to survive will be those in which the normal gene is on the active, unmethylated X chromosome. Thus although X-inactivation appears to be non-random, it is actually cell population survival that is non-random.

TABLE 13.4 ABO blood group phenotypes and genotypes

RED BLOOD CELLS		REACT WITH ANTISERUM		
Phenotype	Genotype	Antibodies	Anti-A	Anti-B
0	00	Anti-A, anti-B	–	–
A	AA, A0	Anti-B	+	–
B	BB, B0	Anti-A	–	+
AB	AB	–	+	+

Blood Groups

Blood groups reflect the antigenic determinants on red cells and were one of the first areas in which an understanding of basic biology led to significant advances in clinical medicine. Our knowledge of the ABO and Rhesus (Rh) blood groups has resulted in safe blood transfusion and the prevention of Rh hemolytic disease of the newborn.

The ABO Blood Groups

The ABO blood groups were discovered by Landsteiner early in the 20th century. In some cases blood transfusion resulted in rapid hemolysis because of incompatibility. Four major ABO blood groups were discovered: A, B, AB, and O. Those with blood group A possess the antigen A on the surface of their red blood cells, those with blood group B have antigen B, those with AB have both antigens, and those with blood group O have neither. People of blood group A have naturally occurring anti-B antibodies, and blood group B have anti-A, whereas blood group O have both. The alleles at the ABO blood group locus are inherited in a codominant manner but are both dominant to the gene for the O antigen. Therefore, six possible genotypes exist (Table 13.4).

Blood group AB individuals do not produce anti-A or anti-B antibodies, so they can receive a blood transfusion from people of all other ABO blood groups, and are therefore referred to as **universal recipients**. On the other hand, because individuals of group O do not express either A or B antigens on their red cells, they are referred to as **universal donors**. Antisera can differentiate two subgroups of blood group A, A1 and A2, but this is of little practical importance as far as blood transfusions are concerned.

Individuals with blood groups A, B, and AB possess enzymes with glycosyltransferase activity that convert the basic blood group, known as the "H" antigen, into the oligosaccharide antigens "A" or "B." The alleles for blood groups A and B differ in seven single-base substitutions that result in different A and B transferase activities, the A allele being associated with the addition of *N*-acetylgalactosaminyl groups, and the B allele with the addition of D-galactosyl groups. The O allele results from a critical single base-pair deletion that results in an inactive protein incapable of modifying the H antigen.

Rhesus Blood Group

The Rh blood group system involves three sets of closely linked antigens, Cc, Dd, and Ee. D is very strongly antigenic, and persons are, for practical purposes, either Rh-positive (possessing the D antigen) or Rh-negative (lacking the D antigen).

Rhesus Hemolytic Disease of the Newborn

A proportion of women who are Rh-negative have an increased chance of having a child who will either die *in utero* or be born severely anaemic because of hemolysis, unless transfused *in utero*. This occurs because, if Rh-positive blood is given to persons who are Rh-negative, the majority will develop anti-Rh antibodies. Such sensitization occurs with exposure to very small quantities of blood and once a person is sensitized, further exposure results in the production of very high antibody titres.

In the case of an Rh-negative mother carrying an Rh-positive fetus, fetal red cells that cross to the mother's circulation can induce the formation of maternal anti-Rh antibodies. In a subsequent pregnancy these antibodies can cross the placenta from the mother to the fetus, leading to hemolysis and severe anemia. In its most severe form, this is known as **erythroblastosis fetalis**, or **hemolytic disease of the newborn**. After a woman has been sensitized there is a significantly greater risk that a child in a subsequent pregnancy, if Rh-positive, will be more severely affected.

To avoid sensitizing an Rh-negative woman, Rh-compatible blood must always be used in any blood transfusion. Furthermore, the development of sensitization, and therefore Rh incompatibility after delivery, can be prevented by giving the mother an injection of anti-Rh antibodies—**anti-D**—so that fetal cells in the maternal circulation are destroyed before the mother can become sensitized.

It is routine to screen all Rh-negative women during pregnancy for the development of anti-Rh antibodies. Despite these measures, a small proportion of women do become sensitized. If anti-Rh antibodies appear, tests are carried out to see whether the fetus is affected. If so, there is a delicate balance between the choice of early delivery, with the risks of prematurity and exchange transfusion, and treating the fetus *in utero* with blood transfusions.

Molecular Basis of the Rh Blood Group

There are two types of Rh red cell membrane polypeptide. One corresponds to the D antigen and the other to the C and E series of antigens. Two genes code for the Rh system: one for *D* and *d*, and a second for both *C* and *c* and *E* and *e*. The D locus is present in most persons and codes for the major D antigen present in those who are Rh-positive. Rh-negative individuals are homozygous for a deletion of the *D* gene. Therefore an antibody has never been raised to "d."

Analysis of complementary DNA from reticulocytes in Rh-negative persons who were homozygous for dCe, dcE, and dce allowed identification of the genomic DNA sequences responsible for the different antigenic variants at the second locus, revealing that they are produced by alternative splicing of the mRNA transcript. The Ee polypeptide is a full-length product of the *CcEe* gene, very similar in sequence to the D polypeptide. The E and e antigens differ by a point mutation in exon 5. The Cc polypeptides are, in contrast, products of a shorter transcript of the same gene that occurs through alternative splicing. The difference between C and c is four amino-acid substitutions in exons 1 and 2.

Other Blood Groups

There are approximately 12 additional "common" blood group systems of clinical importance in humans, including Duffy, Lewis, MN, and S. These are usually of concern only when crossmatching blood for persons who, because of repeated transfusions, have developed antibodies to one of these other blood group antigens. Until the advent of DNA fingerprinting (p. 53), they were used in linkage studies (p. 91) and paternity testing (p. 53).

ELEMENTS

1. The immune response can be divided into two main types, innate and specific acquired, or adaptive, immunity. Both can be further subdivided into humoral and cell-mediated immunity.
2. Innate humoral immunity involves acute-phase proteins that act to minimize tissue injury by limiting the spread of infective organisms that, through the alternative pathway of complement activation, results in a localized inflammatory response and the attraction of phagocytes and opsonization of microorganisms. Complement, which consists of a series of inactive blood proteins that are activated sequentially in a cascade, can also be activated through the classic pathway by antibody binding to antigen.
3. Innate cell-mediated immunity involves phagocytosis of microorganisms by macrophages and their intracellular destruction.
4. Specific acquired humoral immunity involves production of antibodies by mature B cells or plasma cells in response to an antigen. Antibodies are Y-shaped molecules composed of two identical heavy (H) chains and two identical light (L) chains. The antibody molecule has two parts that differ in their function: two identical antigen-binding sites (Fab) and a single binding site for complement (Fc). There are five classes of antibody, IgA, IgD, IgE, IgG, and IgM, each with a specific H chain. The L chain of any class of antibody can be made up of either kappa (κ) or lambda (λ) chains.
5. Each Ig L or H chain has a variable (V) region of approximately 110 amino acids at the amino-terminal end. The carboxy-terminal end consists of a constant (C) region of approximately 110 amino acids in the κ and λ L chains and 3 to 4 times that length in the H chain. Most of the amino-acid sequence variation in both the L and H chains occurs within several small hypervariable regions, which are thought to be the sites of antigen binding. The immunoglobulin chains are produced from combinations of separate groups of DNA segments. The κ and λ L chains and the various types of H chains consist of constant (C) and joining (J) regions separated by a variable number of V regions. The H chains also contain a diversity (D) region located between the V and J regions. The total number of possible antibodies that can be produced by various combinations of these DNA segments accounts for the antibody diversity seen in humans.

6. Cell-mediated specific acquired immunity primarily involves T cells that, through the T-cell surface antigen receptor, in conjunction with the major histocompatibility complex (MHC) molecules on the surface of infected cells, engage T helper cells and cytotoxic T cells to combat intracellular infections.
7. The MHC or human leucocyte antigen (HLA) system consists of a series of closely linked loci on chromosome 6. The many different alleles that can occur at each locus mean that a very large number of different combinations can result. The HLA loci are inherited *en bloc* as a haplotype. The closer the match of HLA antigens between the donor and recipient in organ transplantation, the greater the likelihood of long-term survival of the homograft. Possession of certain HLA antigens is associated with an increased relative risk of developing specific diseases.
8. An understanding of the ABO and Rhesus blood groups has resulted in safe blood transfusions and the prevention of Rhesus hemolytic disease of the newborn.

CLINICAL SCENARIO 1

A 9-month-old infant with quite severe eczema is investigated for an episode of mucosal bleeding, and has already been an inpatient on three occasions to treat moderately severe chest and ear infections. In the family history a maternal uncle with eczema died in the second year of life from pneumonia, but no further details are available.

Investigations show thrombocytopenia.

What diagnoses should be considered?

CLINICAL SCENARIO 2

A 6-year-old girl has suffered very frequent upper respiratory infections throughout her life, sometimes resulting in chest infections, and the recovery period is prolonged compared with her peer group. She is struggling to keep up at school, quite apart from the time she is missing because of recurrent infections.

She has an indistinct nasal quality to her speech and some soft dysmorphic features with small, simple ears. She also has slightly long fingers. She had a low calcium level recorded in the neonatal period.

What is the most likely diagnosis, and how would it be confirmed? What further clinical surveillance is indicated?

Further Reading

Chapel H, Haeney M, Misbah S, Snowden N. *Essentials of Clinical Immunology*. 6th ed. Wiley-Blackwell; 2014.

Excellent basic immunology textbook.

Delves PJ, Martin SJ, Burton DR, Roitt IM. *Roitt's Essential Immunology*. 12th ed. Wiley-Blackwell; 2011.

Excellent basic immunology textbook.

Murphy K, Weaver C. *Janeway's Immunobiology*. 9th ed. Oxford: Garland Science; 2016.

Good, well-illustrated textbook of the biology of immunology.

14 The Genetics of Cancer. . .and Cancer Genetics

All cancer is genetic, but some cancers are more genetic than others.

Paraphrased from* Animal Farm, *by George Orwell

Cell biology and molecular genetics have revolutionized our understanding of cancer, especially in recent years as next-generation sequencing has been applied to analyzing the genetic architecture of tumors. This is an exciting and rapidly moving field with projects such as the 100,000 Genomes Project adding vast amounts of information through paired germline and tumor sequencing in cancer patients. This opens the door to "precision medicine," allowing clinicians to alter cancer management on the basis of the specific somatic variants and pathways driving tumorigenesis. Although there are currently few somatic findings that specifically alter treatment (which will be discussed later in the chapter), many clinical trials are in progress, and the impact they will have on cancer management in the future is certainly great.

All cancer is a genetic disease of **somatic** cells because of aberrant cell division or loss of normal programmed cell death, and the processes from the start of life as a fertilized egg through to advanced cancer are summarized schematically in Fig. 14.1. However, a small proportion of the population is strongly predisposed by inherited **germline** pathogenic variants behaving as mendelian traits, but this does not contradict our traditional understanding that, for many cancers, environmental factors are etiologically important, whereas heredity plays a lesser role. This certainly applies to the "industrial cancers," which result from prolonged exposure to carcinogenic chemicals, for example, cancer of the skin in tar workers, cancer of the bladder in aniline dye workers, angiosarcoma of the liver in process workers making polyvinyl chloride and cancer of the lung (mesothelioma) in asbestos workers. Even so, for those who have suffered cancer as a consequence of such exposures, it is possible, if not likely, that a proportion may have a genetic predisposition to the action of the carcinogen. The link between cigarette smoking and lung cancer (among others) has been recognized for half a century, but not all smokers develop a tobacco-related malignancy. Studies have shown that smokers with short chromosome telomeres (p. 26) appear to be at substantially greater risk for tobacco-related cancers than people with short telomeres who have never smoked, or smokers who have long telomeres. Lung cancer can also cluster in families, and a range of germline pathogenic variants, polymorphisms, and susceptibility loci have been identified as risk factors.

The recognition that a number of rare cancer-predisposing syndromes, as well as a small but significant proportion of common cancers having a hereditary basis, has led to an explosion in our understanding of the genetic basis and cellular biology of cancer in humans. As a general principle, it is now clear that cancers arise as the end result of an accumulation of both inherited and somatic variants, occurring throughout life, in **proto-oncogenes** and **tumor suppressor** genes. A third class of genes—the DNA **mismatch repair** genes—are also important because their inactivation is thought to contribute to the genesis of variants in other genes directly affecting DNA repair, cell-cycle control, and cell-death pathways. Pathogenic germline variants in at least 100 genes and somatic variants in hundreds of others are known to contribute to the total burden of human cancer. The relationship between cancer risk and the presence of variants with variable penetrance can be expressed graphically (Fig. 14.2). Clinical geneticists have typically been involved in the management of rare, highly penetrant gene variants, for example in *BRCA1* and *BRCA2*. Our increased understanding of, and ability to test, genes associated with a moderate increase in cancer risk, for example *RAD51C* in ovarian cancer, has expanded this role and the complexities of genetic counseling in cancer genetics.

Differentiation Between Genetic and Environmental Factors in Cancer

For many cancers, distinguishing between genetic and environmental causative factors is not obvious. There is usually neither a clear-cut mode of inheritance nor a clearly identified environmental cause. Historically, evidence to help distinguish environmental and genetic factors came from a combination of epidemiology, family and twin studies, disease associations and viral factors, all of which are considered briefly here. Increasingly, in the modern era, molecular analysis and/or DNA tumor profiling provide further evidence, and these are considered later.

Epidemiology

Breast cancer is the most common cancer in women and the second most common cancer overall, accounting for 11.6% of new cancer diagnoses worldwide in 2018. It has long been established that reproductive and menstrual histories are risk factors. Parous women, especially multiparous, are at lower risk of developing breast cancer than nulliparous women. Furthermore, the younger the age at first pregnancy and the later the age at menarche, the lower the risk of breast cancer. Breastfeeding, regular exercise, and reduced alcohol intake also appear to have a role in decreasing breast cancer risk.

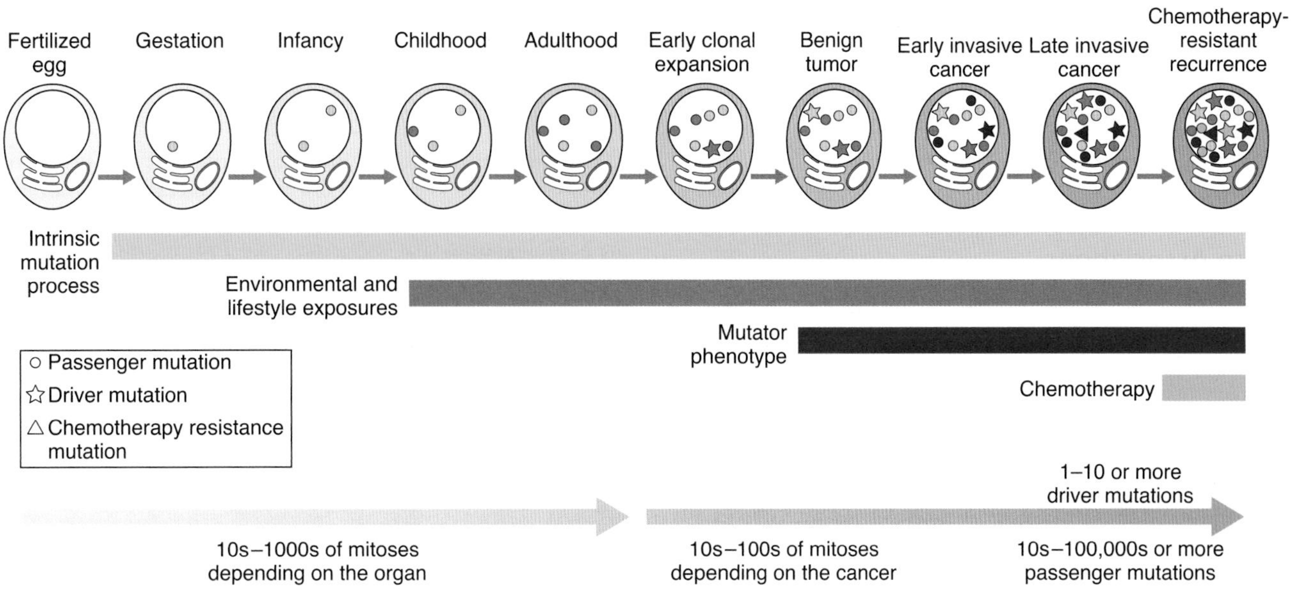

• **Fig. 14.1** The lineage of mitotic cell divisions from the fertilized egg to a single cell within a cancer showing the timing of the somatic variants acquired by the cancer cell and the processes that contribute to them. Variants may be acquired through both intrinsic cell division processes and as a result of mutagens. DNA repair defects may contribute, but driver mutations will cause clonal expansion, with passenger mutations having little overall effect. Relapse following chemotherapy may be caused by resistant variants predating treatment. (From Stratton MR, Campbell PJ, Futreal PA. The cancer genome. *Nature*. 2009;458:719–724. With permission.)

The incidence of breast cancer varies greatly between different populations, with age-standardized incidence rates highest in women in Australia and New Zealand (94.2 per 100,000) and Western Europe (92.6 per 100,000). Incidence rates up to 3.6 times lower are seen in women from the Middle Africa (27.9 per 100,000) and South-Central Asia (25.9 per 100,000). Although these differences could be attributed to genetic differences between these population groups, study of immigrant populations moving from an area with a low incidence to one with a high incidence has shown that the risk of developing breast cancer rises with time to that of the native population, supporting the view that non-genetic factors are highly significant. Some of this changing risk may be accounted for by **epigenetic** factors.

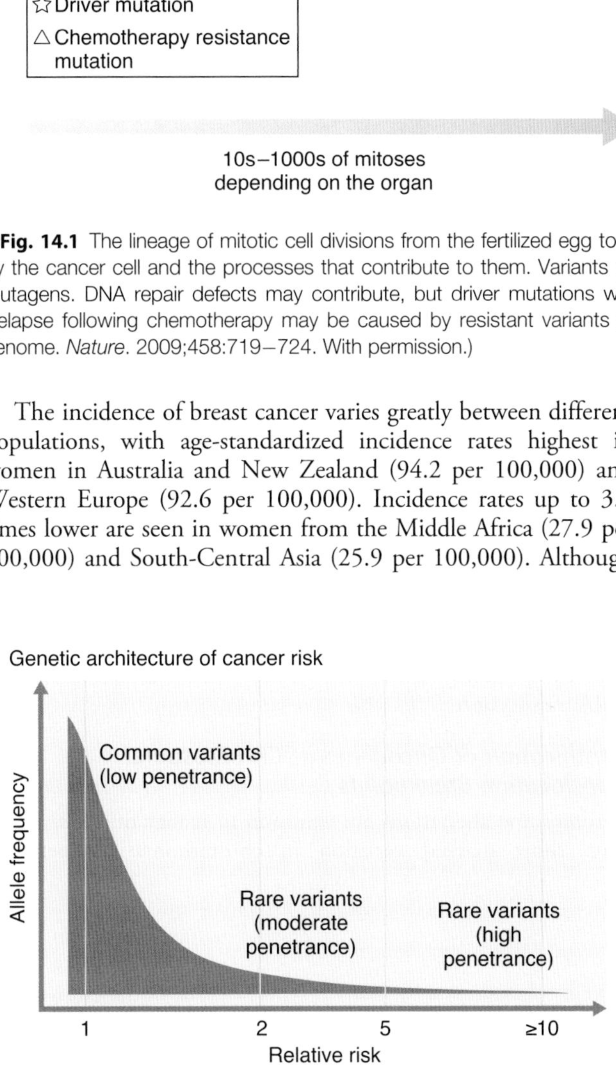

• **Fig. 14.2** Genetic architecture of cancer risk. In the majority of cancers there is a low risk to relatives because genetic associations tend to be with common, low-penetrance alleles identified in genome-wide association studies. The risk to relatives increases markedly when the cancer is associated with rare, high-penetrant genetic variants, such as variants in the *BRCA1*/*BRCA2* genes, e.g., hereditary breast and ovarian cancer, and in the mismatch repair genes associated with Lynch syndrome. (From National Cancer Institute: PDQ Cancer Genetics Overview. Bethesda, MD: National Cancer Institute. Date last modified January 15, 2016. Available at: http://www.cancer.gov/about-cancer/causes-prevention/genetics/overview-pdq. Accessed August 2020. With permission.)

It has long been recognizes that people from lower socioeconomic groups have an increased risk of developing gastric cancer. Specific dietary irritants, such as salts and preservatives, or potential environmental agents, such as nitrates, have been suggested as possible carcinogens. Gastric cancer also shows variations in incidence in different populations, with age-standardized incidence rates almost four times higher in Eastern Asia compared with Western Europe. Migration studies have shown that the risk of gastric cancer for immigrants from high-risk populations does not fall to that of the native low-risk population until two to three generations later. It has been suggested that this could be attributed to exposure to environmental factors at an early critical age, for example, early infection with *Helicobacter pylori*, causing chronic gastric inflammation and associated with a fivefold to sixfold increased gastric cancer risk.

Family and Twin Studies

The clustering of cancer cases within families can provide significant evidence supporting a genetic contribution. The lifetime risk of developing breast cancer for a woman who lives until 80 in Western Europe is now approximately 1 in 8. For a woman who has a first-degree relative with breast cancer, the risk that she will also develop breast cancer is between 1.5 and 3 times the risk for the general population. The risk varies according to the age of onset in the affected family member—the earlier the age at diagnosis, the greater the risk to close relatives (Table 14.7).

Concordance rates for breast cancer in both monozygotic (MZ) and dizygotic (DZ) twins are low, being only slightly greater in MZ female twins, at 17% compared with 13% in DZ female twins. This suggests that, overall, environmental factors are more important than genetic factors. Twin studies in gastric cancer have not shown an increased concordance rate in either MZ or DZ twins.

Disease Associations

Blood groups are genetically determined, and therefore the association of a particular blood group with a disease suggests a possible genetic contribution to the etiology. A large number of studies have shown an association between blood group A and gastric cancer. It is estimated that those with blood group A have a 20% increased risk of developing gastric cancer. Blood group A is associated with an increased risk of developing pernicious anemia, which is also closely associated with chronic gastritis. However, pernicious anemia appears to have a separate association with gastric cancer because affected individuals have a threefold to sixfold increased risk.

Viral Factors

The first indication that transmissible factors can cause cancer came from animal studies performed by Peyton Rous (among others) early in the 20th century. In due course these agents were shown to be viruses. Subsequently it was shown that certain viruses are tumor-forming or **oncogenic** in humans. A limited number of DNA viruses are associated with certain types of human tumors (Table 14.1), whereas a variety of RNA viruses, or **retroviruses**, cause neoplasia in animals.

The genetic information of retroviruses is encoded in RNA and they replicate through DNA by coding for an enzyme known as reverse transcriptase (p. 14), which makes a double-stranded DNA copy of the viral RNA. This DNA intermediate integrates into the host cell genome, facilitating appropriate protein manufacture, which results in the repackaging of new progeny virions.

Naturally occurring retroviruses have only three genes necessary to ensure replication (Fig. 14.3). Study of the virus responsible for a transmissible tumor in chickens, the so-called Rous sarcoma virus, identified a fourth gene that *transforms* host cells both *in vitro* and *in vivo*, causing malignancy. This viral gene is known as an **oncogene**.

Oncogenes

Oncogenes are the altered forms of normal genes—**protooncogenes**—that have key roles in cell growth and differentiation pathways. Normal mammalian cells contain sequences of DNA that are homologous to viral oncogenes, called **proto-oncogenes** or **cellular oncogenes**. Although the terms proto-oncogene and cellular oncogene are often used interchangeably, strictly speaking proto-oncogene is reserved for the normal gene, and cellular oncogene, or c-*onc*, refers to a mutated proto-oncogene, which has oncogenic properties such as the viral oncogenes, or v-*onc*. Approximately 100 oncogenes have been identified.

Relationship Between c-*onc* and v-*onc*

Cellular oncogenes are highly conserved in evolution, suggesting that they have important roles as regulators of cell growth, maintaining the ordered progression through the cell cycle, cell division and differentiation. Retroviral oncogenes are thought to acquire their dominant transforming activity during viral transduction through errors in the replication of the retrovirus genome following their random integration into the host DNA. The end result is a viral gene that is structurally similar to its cellular counterpart but is persistently different in its function.

Identification of Oncogenes

Oncogenes have been identified by two types of cytogenetic finding in association with certain types of leukemia and tumor in humans. These include the location of oncogenes at chromosomal translocation breakpoints, or their amplification in double-minute chromosomes or homogeneously staining regions of chromosomes (p. 188). In addition, a number of oncogenes have also been identified by the ability of tumor DNA to induce tumors *in vitro* by DNA transfection.

Identification of Oncogenes at Chromosomal Translocation Breakpoints

Chromosome aberrations are common in malignant cells, which often show marked variation in chromosome number and

TABLE 14.1 Human DNA viruses implicated in carcinogenesis

Virus Family	Type	Tumor
Papova	Papilloma	Warts (plantar and genital), urogenital cancers (cervical, vulval, vaginal and penile), skin cancer, oral (mouth/tongue/oropharynx)
Herpes	Epstein-Barr	Burkitt lymphoma[a], nasopharyngeal carcinoma, lymphomas in immunocompromised hosts
Hepadna	Hepatitis B	Hepatocellular carcinoma[b]
Hepacivirus	Hepatitis C	Hepatocellular carcinoma, non-Hodgkin lymphoma
Human gamma herpesvirus 8 (HHV-8)	KSHV[c]	Kaposi sarcoma, lymphoma (particularly in the context of HIV infection)

[a]For full oncogenicity, "cocarcinogens" are necessary

[b]E.g., aflatoxin B_1 in hepatitis B–associated hepatocellular carcinoma

[c]Kaposi sarcoma–associated herpesvirus

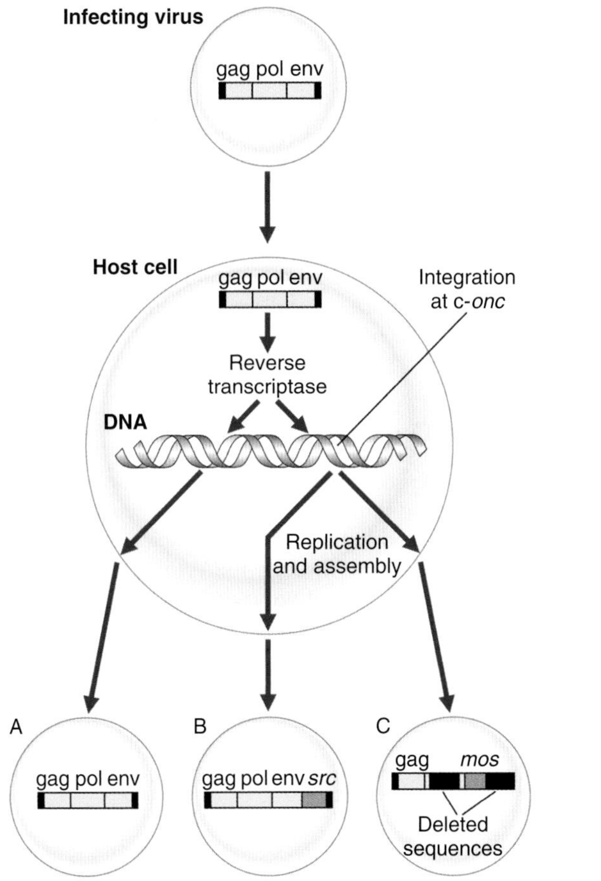

• **Fig. 14.3** Model for acquisition of transforming ability in retroviruses. (A) Normal retroviral replication. (B) The Rous sarcoma virus has integrated near a cellular oncogene. The transforming ability of this virus is attributed to the acquired homolog of the cellular oncogene, v-*src*. (C) A defective transforming virus carries an oncogene similar to *src* but is defective in the structural genes (e.g., Moloney murine sarcoma virus, which carries *mos*).

structure. Certain chromosomes seemed to be more commonly involved, and it was initially thought that these changes were secondary to the transformed state rather than causal. This understanding changed when evidence suggested that chromosomal structural changes, often translocations (p. 37), resulted in rearrangements within or adjacent to proto-oncogenes. It has been found that chromosomal translocations can lead to novel **chimeric genes** with altered biochemical function or altered proto-oncogene activity level. There are numerous examples of both types; chronic myeloid leukemia (CML) is an example of the former and Burkitt lymphoma of the latter.

Chronic Myeloid Leukemia. In 1960, investigators in Philadelphia were the first to describe an abnormal chromosome in white blood cells from patients with CML. The abnormal chromosome, referred to as the **Philadelphia**, or **Ph^1**, **chromosome**, is an acquired abnormality found in blood or bone marrow cells but not in other tissues from these patients. The Ph^1 is a tiny chromosome that is now known to be a chromosome 22 from which long arm material has been reciprocally translocated with the long arm of chromosome 9 (Fig. 14.4), that is, t(9;22)(q34;q11). This chromosomal rearrangement is seen in 90% of those with CML. This translocation has been found to transfer the cellular *Abelson (ABL)* oncogene from chromosome 9 into a region of chromosome 22 known as the **breakpoint cluster**, or *BCR*, region, resulting in a chimeric transcript derived from both the c-*ABL* (70%) and the *BCR* genes. This results in a chimeric gene expressing a **fusion protein** consisting of the BCR protein at the amino end and the ABL protein at the carboxy end, which transforms activity.

Burkitt Lymphoma. An unusual form of neoplasia seen in children in Africa is a lymphoma that involves the jaw, known as Burkitt lymphoma, named after Dennis Burkitt, a medical missionary who first described the condition in 1958. Chromosomal analysis has revealed the majority (90%) of affected children to have a translocation of the c-*MYC* oncogene from the long arm of chromosome 8 onto heavy (H) chain immunoglobulin locus on chromosome 14. Less commonly the *MYC* oncogene is translocated to regions of chromosome 2 or 22, which encode genes for the kappa (κ) and lambda (λ) light chains, respectively (p. 174). As a consequence of these translocations, *MYC* comes under the influence of the regulatory sequences of the respective immunoglobulin gene and is overexpressed tenfold or more.

Oncogene Amplification

Proto-oncogenes can also be activated by the production of multiple copies of the gene (known as **gene amplification**), a mechanism known to have survival value when cells encounter environmental stress. For example, leukemic cells exposed to the chemotherapeutic agent methotrexate acquire resistance to the drug by making multiple copies of the gene for dihydrofolate reductase, the target enzyme for methotrexate. The number of copies of the oncogene per cell can increase several hundred times,

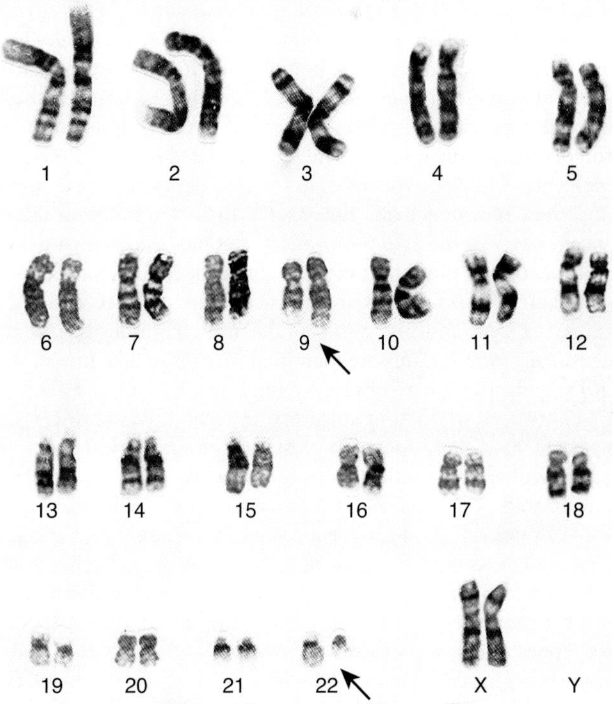

• **Fig. 14.4** Karyotype from a patient with chronic myeloid leukemia showing the chromosome 22 (*arrow*) or Philadelphia chromosome, material from which has translocated to the long arm of one of the number 9 chromosomes (*arrow*).

with greater amounts of oncoprotein as a consequence. The amplified sequence of DNA in tumor cells gives rise to small extra chromosomes (**double-minute chromosomes**) seen in approximately 10% of tumors, especially in the later stages of the malignant process.

Amplification of specific proto-oncogenes is a feature of certain tumors and is frequently seen with the *MYC* family of genes. For example, N-*MYC* is amplified in approximately 30% of neuroblastomas, but in advanced cases the proportion rises to 50%, where gene amplification can be up to 1000-fold. Human small cell carcinomas of the lung show amplification of *MYC*, N-*MYC*, and L-*MYC*. Also, in lung cancer, multiple downstream components of the EGFR-family-signaling pathway, including *CDK5*, *AKT1*, and *SHC1*, are overexpressed. Amplification of *ERBB2* (*HER2*), *MYC*, and *cyclin D1* is a feature in 20% of breast carcinomas, where it correlates with a number of well-established prognostic factors such as lymph node status, estrogen and progestogen receptor status, tumor size, and histological grade. Currently available tests of oncogene activity in breast cancer cover more than 20 genes and assign a recurrence score which, in combination with the patient's age and tumor type, can be used to prognosticate in terms of recurrence risk, but can also be used to predict the benefit of chemotherapy in early breast cancer, or radiotherapy in ductal carcinoma *in situ*.

Detection of Oncogenes by DNA Transfection Studies

The ability of DNA from a human bladder carcinoma cell line, transferred by a process known as DNA **transfection**, to transform a well-established mouse fibroblast cell line called NIH3T3, as demonstrated by the loss of contact inhibition of the cells in culture, led to the discovery of the human sequence homologous to the *ras* gene of the Harvey murine sarcoma virus more than four decades ago. The human *RAS* gene family consists of three closely related members, *HRAS (Harvey rat sarcoma virus)*, *KRAS (Kristen rat sarcoma virus)* and *NRAS (neuroblastoma ras viral oncogene)*. The RAS proteins are closely homologous to their viral counterparts and differ from one another near the carboxy termini (the C-terminal hypervariable region). The *RAS* genes code for four isoproteins whose role is to mediate signals related to cell survival and senescence. Despite similarities in the *RAS* genes and their isoproteins, there is evidence that their role is distinct in different tissues. Oncogenicity of the *RAS* proto-oncogenes has been shown to arise by acquisition of point mutations in the nucleotide sequence.

Variants in *RAS* genes were among the first to be recognized in human cancers and are some of the most commonly mutated genes. *RAS* gene variants are identified in 25% of all cancers, with *KRAS* being the most commonly mutated. Variants in *KRAS* or *NRAS* are seen in 52% of colorectal cancers (CRCs), where they appear to play a key role in both tumor progression and maintenance, with animal models showing that a loss of *KRAS* expression is associated with increased rates of apoptosis. *RAS* variants in CRC can not only add prognostic value, as certain variants appear to be associated with different outcomes, but their absence is also an indication for the addition of antiepidermal growth factor receptor monoclonal antibodies, for example cetuximab, to standard chemotherapy protocols. Wild-type RAS status is linked to improve treatment outcomes in patients with metastatic CRC, perhaps demonstrating one of the first steps towards precision medicine.

Similarly, variants in *BRAF*, which encodes a serine/threonine protein kinase, are associated with various cancers, including non-Hodgkin lymphoma, CRC, malignant melanoma, thyroid carcinoma, non-small cell lung carcinoma, and adenocarcinoma of lung. Both *RAS* and *BRAF* are key constituents of the RAS-MAPK signaling pathway, which affects cell division, differentiation, and secretion. Pathogenic germline variants in these genes are associated with neurofibromatosis type 1 (p. 296–297) and the Noonan/cardio-facio-cutaneous/Costello group of syndromes (p. 233–234), which are variably associated with an increased tumor risk.

DNA transfection studies have also led to identification of other oncogenes that have not been demonstrated through retroviral studies. These include *MET* (hereditary papillary renal cell carcinoma), *TRK* (familial medullary thyroid cancer), and *RET* (multiple endocrine neoplasia [MEN] type 2, see p. 121–122, Figure 9.27; Tables 14.4, 14.9).

Function of Oncogenes

Oncogene products consistently have a role in the control of cellular proliferation and differentiation in the process known as **intracellular signal transduction**. This is a complex multistep pathway from the cell membrane through the cytoplasm to the nucleus, involving a variety of types of proto-oncogene product involved in positive and negative feedback loops necessary for accurate cell proliferation and differentiation (Fig. 14.5).

Proto-oncogenes are highly conserved, being present in a variety of different species, indicating they are likely to have essential biological functions. They act in three main ways in the process of signal transduction: (1) through phosphorylation of serine, threonine

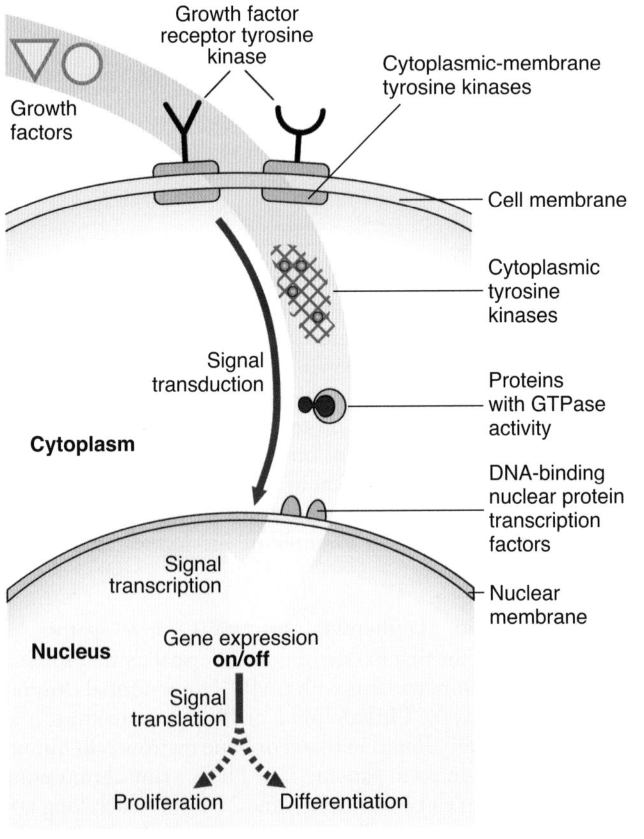

• **Fig. 14.5** Simplified schema of the steps in signal transduction and transcription from cell surface to nucleus. The intracellular pathway amplifies the signal by a cascade that involves one or more of the steps.

and tyrosine residues of proteins by the transfer of phosphate groups from adenosine triphosphate; this leads to alteration of the configuration activating the kinase activity of proteins and generating docking sites for target proteins, resulting in signal transduction; (2) through the guanosine diphosphate–guanosine triphosphate cycle as intermediates relaying the transduction signal from membrane-associated tyrosine kinases to serine threonine kinases (includes the *RAS* family); or (3) through proteins located in the nucleus that control progress through the cell cycle, DNA replication, and gene expression.

Types of Oncogene

Growth Factors

Growth factors stimulate cells to grow by binding to growth factor receptors and govern the transition of a cell from G_0 to the start of the cell cycle (p. 32). The v-*SIS* oncogene, which encodes part of the biologically active platelet-derived growth factor B subunit, acts as a growth factor. When v-SIS oncoprotein is added to cell cultures they are transformed, behaving like neoplastic cells—their growth rate increases, and they lose contact inhibition. *In vivo* they form tumors when injected into nude mice. Oncogenes showing homology to fibroblast growth factor–encoding genes include *HST* and *INT*-2, which are amplified in stomach cancers and in malignant melanomas, respectively.

Growth Factor Receptors

Many oncogenes encode proteins that form growth factor receptors, possessing tyrosine kinase domains that allow cells to bypass normal control mechanisms. More than 40 different tyrosine kinases are known, and there are two main types: those that span the cell membrane (growth factor receptor tyrosine kinases) and those located in the cytoplasm (non-receptor tyrosine kinases). Examples of genes encoding tyrosine kinases include *ERBB*, which encodes the epidermal growth factor receptor, and the related *ERBB2* (*HER2*) oncogene. Variants, rearrangements, and amplification of *ERBB2* result in ligand-independent activation, associated with cancer of the stomach, pancreas, and ovary. Variants in *KIT* and *PDGFRA* occur in sporadic and hereditary gastrointestinal stromal tumor syndrome as a result of **point mutations**. Germline variants alone do not cause carcinogenesis.

Intracellular Signal Transduction Factors

As mentioned in the previous section, there are two forms of intracellular signal transduction—proteins with GTPase activity, and cytoplasmic serine threonine kinases (see Fig. 14.5). Examples of both are found in the RAS-MAPK pathway, with variants in *RAS* genes leading to increased or sustained GTPase activity, and variants in *BRAF* resulting in sustained or increased transmission of a growth-promoting signal to the nucleus.

DNA-Binding Nuclear Proteins

These proteins bind to single- or double-stranded DNA, usually in the major groove if the binding is sequence-specific. Therefore they are specific transcription factors that activate or suppress neigboring DNA sequences. Variants in *c-MYC* are found in many cancers, and the c-MYC oncoprotein activates expression of many genes by binding enhancer box sequences and recruiting histone acetyltransferases. It also has a direct role in the control of DNA replication, and overproduction results in persistent cellular proliferation.

Cell-Cycle Factors and Apoptosis

Abnormal regulation of the cell cycle, for example, at G_1 when a cell becomes committed to DNA synthesis in the S phase, or G_2 for cell division in the mitosis (M) phase, can result in uncontrolled cell growth. This may be through growth factors, growth factor receptors, GTPases or nuclear proteins, or loss of inhibitory factors lead to activation of the cyclin-dependent kinases, such as cyclin D1. Alternatively, loss of factors that lead to normal programmed cell death, **apoptosis** (p. 107), can result in the prolonged cell survival as a mechanism of development of some tumors. Activation of the *BCL2* oncogene through chromosomal rearrangements is associated with inhibition of apoptosis, leading to certain types of lymphoma.

Signal Transduction and the Phakomatoses

Phakomatosis derives from the Greek *phakos*, meaning "lentil" (i.e., "lentil-shaped object"), originally referring to three conditions with benign lesions—neurofibromatosis, tuberous sclerosis, and von Hippel–Lindau disease. We now include nevoid basal cell carcinoma (Gorlin) syndrome, Cowden disease, familial adenomatous polyposis (FAP), Peutz-Jegher syndrome, and juvenile polyposis in this group. The genes for these conditions are known and are normally active within intracellular signal transduction, and their protein products are **tumor suppressors**.

Tumor Suppressor Genes

The study of human hereditary cancer has identified the existence of **tumor suppressor genes**, which constitute the largest group of hereditary cancer genes.

Studies in the 1960s showed that fusion of malignant cells with normal cells in culture resulted in the suppression of the malignant phenotype in the hybrids. Malignancy recurred with the loss of certain chromosomes from the hybrids, suggesting that normal cells contain one or more genes with tumor suppressor activity which, if lost or inactive, resulted in malignancy and behaved like a recessive trait. The paradigm for our understanding of the biology of tumor suppressor genes is the eye tumor retinoblastoma (Rb). It is important to appreciate, however, that a germline pathogenic variant in a tumor suppressor gene (as with an oncogene) does not by itself provoke carcinogenesis; further somatic variation at one or more loci is necessary, and environmental factors, such as ionizing radiation, may be significant in the process. More than 20 tumor suppressor genes have been identified.

Retinoblastoma

This is a rare but highly malignant childhood cancer of the developing retinal cells of the eye, usually occurring before 5 years of age (Fig. 14.6). Early diagnosis and treatment are associated with a good long-term outcome. Rb can occur either sporadically, the so-called non-hereditary form, or be familial, the so-called hereditary form, which is inherited in an autosomal dominant manner. Non-hereditary cases usually involve only one eye, whereas hereditary cases can be unilateral but are more commonly bilateral or multifocal in one eye. The familial form also tends to present at an earlier age than the sporadic form.

"Two-Hit" Hypothesis

In 1971 Knudson studied the epidemiology of both types of Rb and advanced a "two-hit" hypothesis to explain the occurrence of this rare tumor in patients with and without a positive family history. He

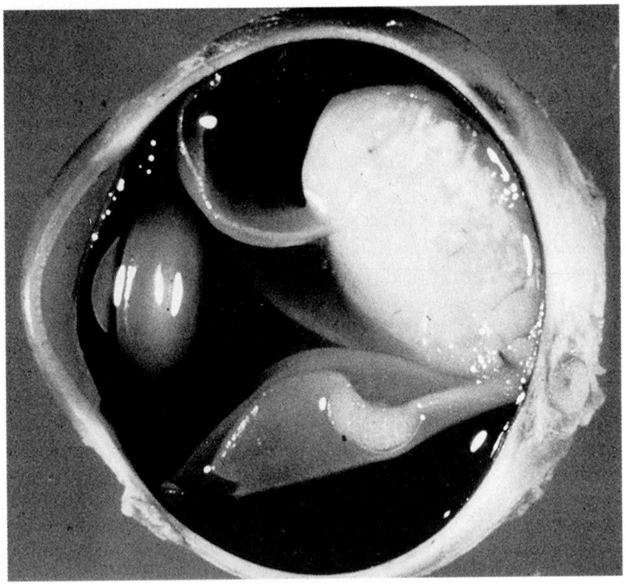

• **Fig. 14.6** Section of an eye showing a retinoblastoma *in situ*.

proposed that affected individuals with a positive family history had inherited one nonfunctional gene that was present in all cells of the individual, known as a **germline pathogenic variant**, with the second gene at the same locus becoming inactivated somatically in a developing retinal cell (Fig. 14.7A). The occurrence of a second pathogenic variant was likely, given the large number of retinal cells, explaining the autosomal dominant pattern of inheritance. This would also explain the observation that in hereditary Rb the tumors were often (but not always) bilateral and multifocal. In contrast, in the non-heritable or sporadic form, two inactivating **somatic variants** would need to occur independently in the same retinoblast cell (Fig. 14.7B), which was much less likely to occur, explaining the fact that tumors in these patients were often unilateral and unifocal and occurred at a later age than in the hereditary form. Hence, although the hereditary form of Rb follows an autosomal dominant pattern of inheritance, at the molecular level it is recessive because a tumor occurs only after the loss of both alleles.

Approximately 5% of children presenting with Rb had other physical abnormalities and developmental concerns. Some of these children had a cytogenetically visible interstitial deletion of chromosome 13q, and in due course the common critical region was determined to lie at 13q14 (Fig. 14.8). This suggested it could also be the locus for the autosomal dominant familial form of Rb, which was subsequently confirmed by linkage studies.

Loss of Heterozygosity

By comparing DNA sequences from both peripheral blood and the Rb tumor in children with inherited Rb it was shown that there was loss of an allele at the Rb locus in the tumor material. This is known as **loss of heterozygosity** (LOH). In Fig. 14.9A the mother transmits the Rb gene along with allele 2 at a closely linked marker locus. The father is homozygous for allele 1 at this locus, so the child shows heterozygosity at this locus. However, tumor tissue analysis reveals apparent homozygosity for allele 2, which is because of loss of the paternally derived allele 1—LOH in the tumor material—consistent with Knudson's "two-hit" hypothesis.

LOH may occur through several somatic mechanisms, illustrated in Fig. 14.9B—loss of a chromosome through mitotic nondisjunction (p. 35–36), nondisjunction and reduplication, mitotic recombination (leading to homozygosity for the mutant allele), gene conversion, gene deletion, or point mutation. Observation of consistent cytogenetic rearrangements in other malignancies has led to demonstration of LOH in a number of other cancers (Table 14.2).

Function of Tumor Suppressor Genes

The Rb paradigm, where absence of the gene product in the homozygous state leads to the development of the tumor, indicates that

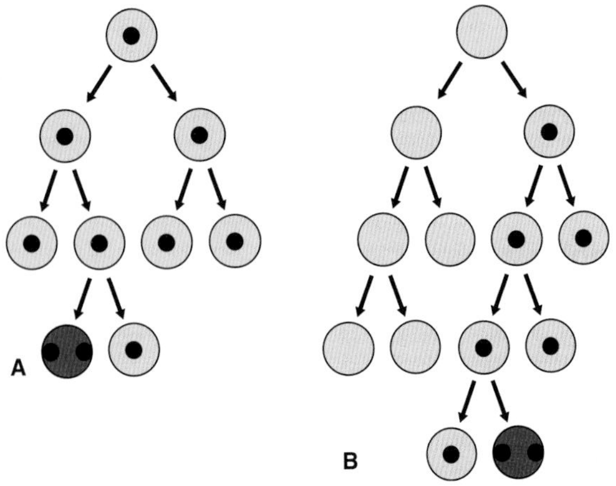

• **Fig. 14.7** Retinoblastoma and Knudson's "two-hit" hypothesis. All cells in the hereditary form (A) have one mutated copy of the *RB1* gene (i.e., the variant is in the *germline*). In the non-hereditary form (B) a variant in *RB1* arises as a postzygotic (*somatic*) event sometime early in development. The retinoblastoma tumor occurs only when both *RB1* genes are mutated—that is, after a(nother) somatic event, which is more likely to be earlier in life in the hereditary form compared with the non-hereditary form; it is also more likely to give rise to bilateral and multifocal tumors.

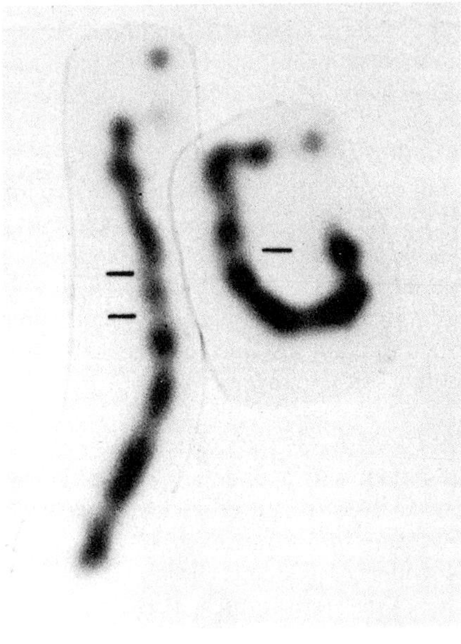

• **Fig. 14.8** Two homologues of chromosome 13 from a patient with retinoblastoma showing an interstitial deletion of 13q14 in the right-hand homologue, as indicated.

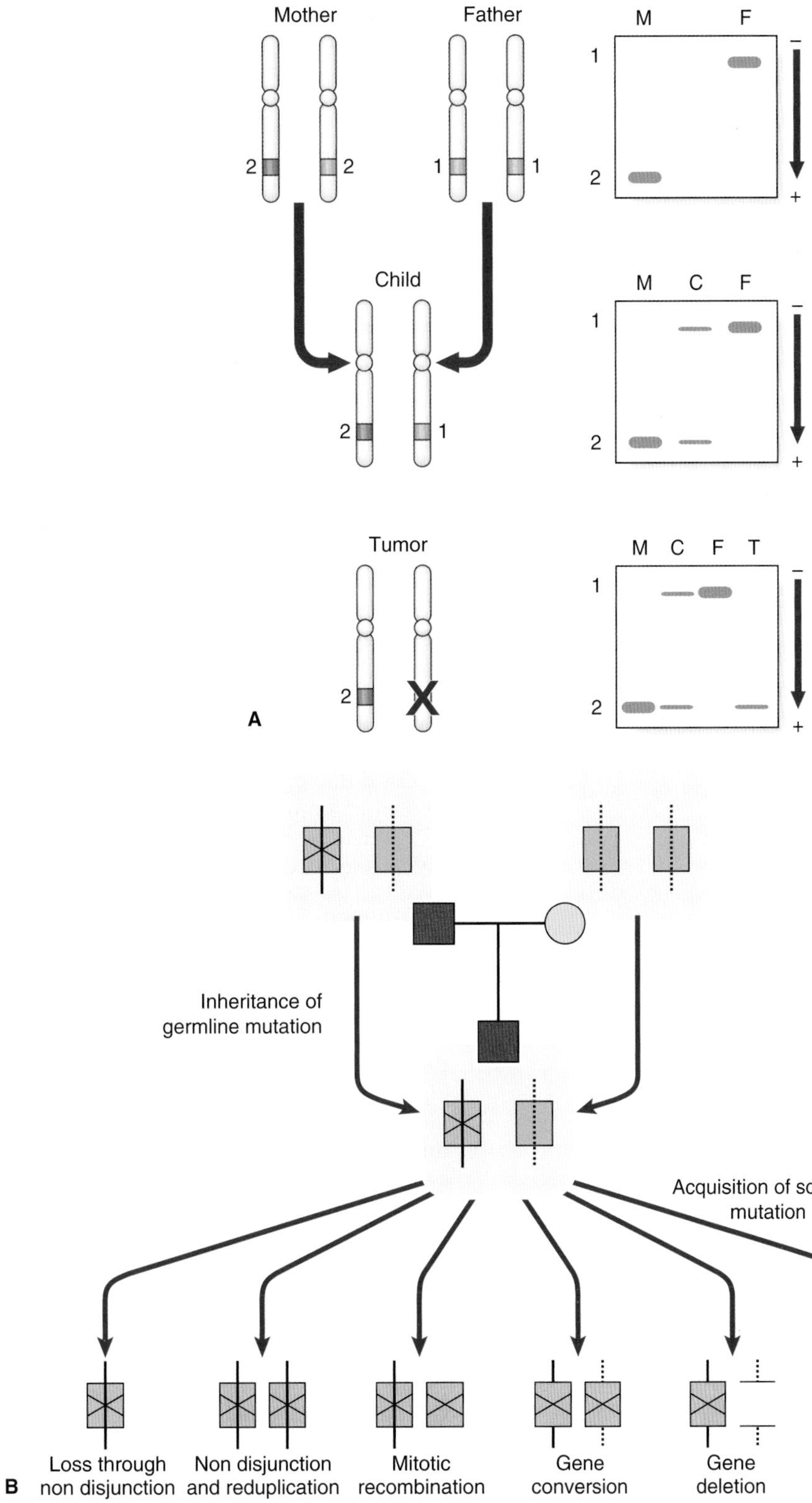

• **Fig. 14.9** (A) Diagrammatic representation of the loss of heterozygosity (LOH) in the development of a tumor. The mother (M) and father (F) are both homozygous for different alleles at the same locus, 2–2 and 1–1, respectively. The child (C) will therefore be constitutionally heterozygous, 1–2. If an analysis of DNA from a tumor at that locus reveals only a single allele, 2, this is consistent with LOH. (B) Diagrammatic representations of the mechanisms causing the "second hit" leading to the development of retinoblastoma.

the normal function of tumor suppressor genes is to suppress inappropriate cell proliferation. Further support for the *RB1* gene acting as a tumor suppressor comes from the observation that individuals with hereditary Rb have an increased risk of developing new malignancies later in life, including osteosarcoma, fibrosarcoma, and chondrosarcoma, as well as brain tumors and melanoma.

TABLE 14.2 Syndromes and cancers that show loss of heterozygosity, and their chromosomal locations

Syndrome or Cancer	Chromosomal Location
Retinoblastoma	13q14
Osteosarcoma	13q, 17p
Wilms tumor	11p13, 11p15, 16q
Renal carcinoma	3p25, 17p13
von Hippel–Lindau disease	3p25
Bladder carcinoma	9q21, 11p15, 17p13
Lung carcinoma	3p, 13q14, 17p
Breast carcinoma	11p15, 11q, 13q12, 13q14, 17p13, 17q21
Rhabdomyosarcoma	11p15, 17p13
Hepatoblastoma	5q, 11p15
Gastric cancer	1p, 5q, 7q, 11p, 13q, 17p, 18p
Familial adenomatous polyposis	5q21
Colorectal carcinoma	1p, 5q21, 8p, 17p13, 18q21
Neurofibromatosis I (von Recklinghausen disease)	17q
Neurofibromatosis II	22q
Meningioma	22q
Multiple endocrine neoplasia type I	11q
Melanoma	9p21, 17q
Ovarian	11q25, 16q, 17q
Pancreatic	9p21, 13q14, 17p13
Prostate cancer	1p36, 7q, 8p, 10q, 13q, 16q

The RB1 *Gene/p105-Rb Protein*

The *RB1* gene specifies a 4.7-kilobase (kb) transcript that encodes a nuclear protein called p105-Rb, which associates with DNA and is involved in the regulation of the cell cycle. The protein forms a complex with an oncogene-regulated inhibitor of a transcription factor called *E2F*, and the complex interferes with the ability of *E2F* to activate transcription of some key proteins required for DNA synthesis. When p105-Rb is hyperphosphorylated this complex does form, and the cell cycle proceeds to the S phase (p. 32). In the presence of abnormal p105-Rb, retinoblasts fail to differentiate normally. These findings highlight potentially complex mechanisms of interaction among oncogenes, tumor suppressor genes, and the cell cycle in cancer biology.

TP53

The p53 protein was first identified as a host cell protein bound to T antigen, the dominant transforming oncogene of the DNA tumor virus SV40. After the murine *p53* gene was cloned it was shown to be able to cooperate with activated *Ras* and act as an oncogene, transforming primary rodent cells *in vitro*, even though the rodent cells expressed the wild-type or normal *p53*. Subsequently, inactivation of *p53* was frequently found in murine Friend virus–induced erythroleukemia cells, which led to the proposal that the *Tp53* gene was, in fact, a tumor suppressor gene.

In humans, somatic variants in *TP53* are the most frequently reported of all known cancer genes across almost all tumor types. Somatic variants are seen in around 23% of breast cancers, where its presence appears to be a marker of poor prognosis, 43% of CRCs and up to 39% of cancers of the female genital tract. The *TP53* variants occur in different codons but are clustered in highly conserved regions in exons 5 to 8. This is in contrast to *TP53* variants in hepatocellular carcinoma, which occur in a "hotspot" at codon 249. The base change in this mutated codon, usually G to T, could be the result of an interaction with the carcinogen aflatoxin B_1, which is associated with liver cancer in China and South Africa, or with the hepatitis B virus that is also implicated as a risk factor in hepatomas. Aflatoxin B_1 is a ubiquitous food-contaminating aflatoxin in these areas and a mutagen in many animal species, inducing G to T substitutions in mutagenesis experiments.

Cancers frequently have a decreased cell death rate through altered **apoptosis**, and a major activator of apoptosis is *TP53*—thus p53 has been coined the "guardian of the genome." The p53 protein is a multimeric complex, and it functions as a checkpoint control site in the cell cycle at G_1 before the S phase, interacting with other factors, including cyclins and p21, preventing DNA damaged through normal "wear and tear" from being replicated. Mutant p53 protein monomers are more stable than the normal p53 proteins and can form complexes with the normal wild-type p53, acting in a dominant-negative manner to inactivate it.

Li-Fraumeni Syndrome

Because variants in *TP53* appear to be a common event in the genesis of many cancers, an inherited or germline pathogenic variant of *TP53* would be expected to have serious consequences, and indeed causes **Li-Fraumeni syndrome**. Members of families with this rare syndrome, inherited as an autosomal dominant trait, are highly susceptible to a variety of malignancies at an early age, including adrenal carcinomas, sarcomas, breast cancer, brain tumors and leukemia. This is a highly penetrant condition with an estimated cancer risk of 50% by age 30 years, and 90% by age 60 years. Many hundreds of variants have been reported in the gene, normally missense variants, although eight particular hotspot mutations are recognized which collectively account for around 28% of pathogenic variants. The R337H variant is particularly notable for its founder effect in the Brazilian population and high incidence of adrenocortical cancers in children.

Epigenetics and Cancer

Much of this chapter discusses familial cancer syndromes that follow mendelian inheritance, characterized by pathogenic variants in disease-specific genes. However, no discussion about cancer genetics is complete without considering epigenetic mechanisms. As discussed in Chapter 9 (p. 123–124), **epigenetics** refers to heritable changes to gene expression that are not owing to differences in the genetic code. Such gene expression can be transmitted stably through cell divisions, both mitosis and meiosis. In cancer, much is now known about alterations to the methylation status of the genome, both hypomethylation and hypermethylation, and in this section we also discuss telomere length and cancer.

DNA Methylation and Genomic Imprinting

The methylation of DNA is an **epigenetic** phenomenon (p. 124) and is the mechanism responsible for X-inactivation (p. 124–125) and genomic imprinting (p. 78). Methylation of DNA has the effect of silencing gene expression and maintaining stability of the genome, especially in areas where there is a vast quantity of repetitive DNA (heterochromatin) which might otherwise become erroneously involved in recombination events leading to altered regulation of adjacent genes. The relevance of this for cancer emerged in 1983 when studies showed that the genomes of cancer cells were hypomethylated compared with those of normal cells, primarily within repetitive DNA. This **loss of imprinting** (**LOI**) may lead to activation of an allele that is normally silent, and hence the high expression of a product that confers advantageous cellular growth. This appears to be an early event in many cancers and may correlate with disease severity. Chromosomal instability is strongly associated with increased tumor frequency, which is a feature of the "chromosome breakage" syndromes (p. 265–268), and is associated with a significant increased risk of developing cancers, particularly leukemia and lymphoma.

LOI and removal of normal gene silencing may lead to oncogene activation, and hence cancer risk. LOI has been studied extensively at the *IGF2*/*H19* locus on chromosome 11p15.5, as previously discussed in Chapter 6 (p. 80). The gene encoding insulin-like growth factor 2 *(IGF2)* and the *H19* gene are normally expressed from the paternal and maternal alleles, respectively (see Fig. 6.27), but reduced silencing of the maternal allele (i.e., hypomethylation) results in increased *IGF2* expression. This is a common LOI event across a wide range of common tumor types (e.g., lung, liver, colon, ovary), as well as Wilms tumor in which it was first identified.

Just as hypomethylation may lead to activation of oncogenes, the opposite effect of hypermethylation may also give rise to an increased cancer risk, in this case through silencing of tumor suppressor genes. Aberrant hypermethylation usually affects CpG nucleotide islands (C and G adjacent to each p, phosphodiester, bond), which are mostly unmethylated in somatic cells. This results in changes in chromatin structure (hypoacetylation of histone) that effectively silence transcription. When genes involved in cell regulatory activity are silenced, cells have a growth advantage. In clinical practice, hypermethylation is of particular relevance to CRC, where methylation of the *MLH1* promoter can be seen in association with sporadic bowel cancers. The effects of altered methylation leading to cancer are summarized in Fig. 14.10, although the mechanism(s) that initiate the processes are poorly understood.

Telomere Length and Cancer

Telomeres are specialized chromatin structures at the tips of chromosomes (p.26) and have a protective function. They consist of multiple double-stranded tandem repeats of the following specific DNA sequence: TTAGGG. This sequence is approximately 10 to 15 kb long in human cells and is bound by specific proteins. It is also the substrate for telomerase, an enzyme that can lengthen the telomeres in those cells in which it is expressed. The final stretch of DNA at the very tip of the telomere is a single-stranded overhang of 150 to 200 nucleotides. Telomerase recognizes the 3′ end of the overhang, allowing lengthening to proceed.

Every cell division appears to result in the loss of some TTAGGG repeats because conventional DNA polymerases cannot replicate a linear chromosome in its entirety, known as the "end-replication problem." This progressive loss of telomere length is a form of cellular clock believed to be linked to both aging and human disease. This relationship is displayed graphically in Fig. 14.11. When telomeres reach a critically short length, there is loss of protection, and a consequence is chromosomal, and therefore genomic, instability, which reduces cell viability. Short telomeres are a feature of the premature aging syndromes, such as ataxia telangiectasia, and other chromosome breakage disorders associated with early-onset cancer. It appears that the rate of telomere shortening is markedly increased in these conditions, so that cells and tissues literally "age" more quickly. However, some

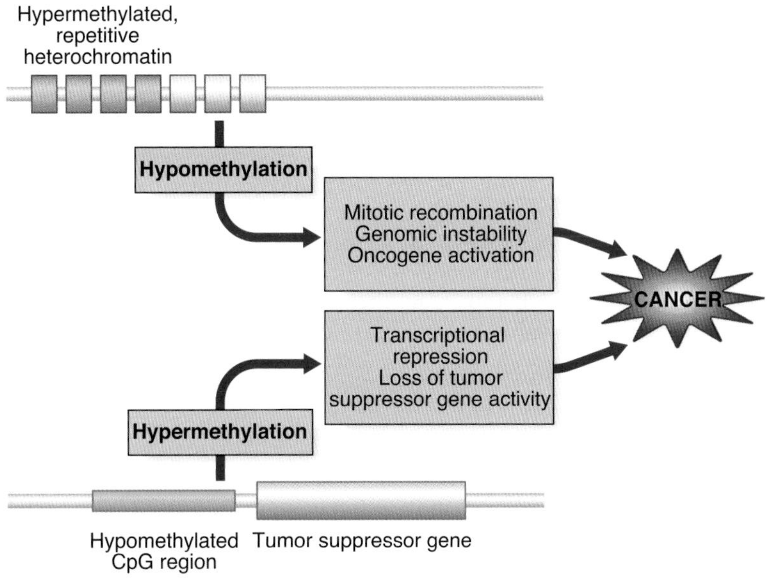

• **Fig. 14.10** Methylation of DNA and cancer. The top schema shows a region of hypermethylated repetitive DNA sequence (heterochromatin). When this loses its methylation imprint, chromosome instability may result, which may lead to activation of oncogene(s). In the lower schema, hypomethylated stretches of CpG sequence become methylated, resulting in transcriptional suppression of tumor suppressor and cell regulatory genes.

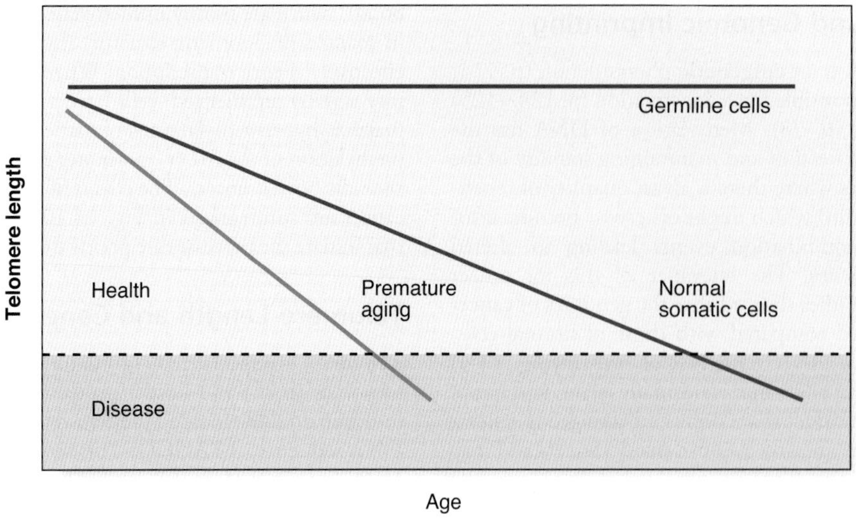

• **Fig. 14.11** Telomere length over age, in normal life, and in premature aging syndromes. The only cells in the body that maintain telomere length throughout life, and have high levels of telomerase, are those of the germline. Somatic cells, in the absence of disease, undergo a slowly progressive decrease in telomere length throughout life, so that disease and cancer become an increasing risk in the elderly. In premature aging syndromes, the process of telomere shortening is accelerated, and the risk of cancer becomes high from early adult life onward.

cancer cells express high levels of telomerase, thus maintaining cell viability. Most metastatic tissue contains telomerase-positive cells, suggesting that telomerase is required to sustain such growth, but cancer cells generally have relatively short telomeres. Thus, telomerase activation in cancer rescues short telomeres *and* perpetuates genomically unstable cells.

Genetics of Common Cancers

Approximately 5% to 10% of colorectal and breast cancers arise as a result of an inherited cancer susceptibility gene. A similar proportion of many other cancers are attributed to inherited predisposing genetic factors, but there are some notable exceptions in which only a very low incidence of a dominantly inherited predisposition is recorded. These include the lung and cervix, as well as leukemias, lymphomas and sarcomas. In these, external agents or stimuli, and/or stochastic genetic events, are presumed to be the main factors. Nevertheless, studies of the common cancers—colorectal and breast—have provided great insights into the genetics of cancer.

Colorectal Cancer

Approximately 1 in 20 people in the United Kingdom will develop CRC during their lifetime, and the highest incidence rates worldwide are seen across Australia, New Zealand, and Europe. An understanding of colorectal tumorigenesis has shed light on carcinogenesis more generally.

Multistage Process of Carcinogenesis

The majority of CRCs are thought to develop from "benign" adenomas, although only a small proportion of adenomas proceed to invasive cancer. Histologically, adenomatous polyps smaller than 1 cm in diameter rarely contain areas of carcinomatous change; however, polyp size is one of the most important risk factors for malignant transformation. The incidence of cancerous change in polyps is up to 40% in those greater than 2.5 cm, and up to 75% when they reach 3.5 cm in size. The transition from a small adenomatous polyp to an invasive cancer is thought to take between 5 and 10 years. Adenomatous polyps less than 1 cm in diameter have variants in the *RAS* gene in less than 10% of cases. As the size of the polyp increases to between 1 and 2 cm, the prevalence of *RAS* gene variants may reach 40%, rising to over 50% in full-blown CRCs.

Similarly, allele loss of chromosome 5 markers occurs in approximately 40% of adenomatous polyps and 70% of carcinomas. Deletions on chromosome 17p in the region containing the *TP53* gene occur in more than 75% of carcinomas, but this is an uncommon finding in small or intermediate-sized polyps. A region on 18q is deleted in approximately 10% of small adenomas, rising to almost 50% when the adenoma shows foci of invasive carcinoma, and in more than 70% of carcinomas (Fig. 14.12). Genes at this locus include deleted in colorectal cancer (*DCC*), *SMAD2* and *SMAD4*, the latter being part of the transforming growth factor-β (TGF-β) pathway (p. 108). In some CRCs variants in the *TGF-β* receptor gene have been identified. The *DCC* gene shows homology with the family of genes encoding cell adhesion molecules—and cell-cell and cell–basement membrane interactions are lost in overt malignancy. *DCC* is expressed in normal colonic mucosa, but its expression is either reduced or absent in CRCs.

It appears that variants of the *RAS* and *TP53* genes, and LOH on 5q and 18q, accumulate during the transition from a small "benign" adenoma to carcinoma. The accumulation of alterations, rather than the sequence, appears to be crucial. More than one of these four alterations are seen in only 7% of small, early adenomas. Two or more alterations are seen with increasing frequency when adenomas progress in size and show histological features of malignancy. More than 90% of carcinomas show two or more alterations, and approximately 40% show three.

The multistage process of the development of cancer is likely to be an oversimplification. The distinction between oncogenes and tumor suppressor genes (Table 14.3) has not always been clear-cut—for example, the *RET* oncogene and *MEN2* (p. 117). In addition, the same pathogenic variant in some of the inherited cancer syndromes (p. 197) can result in cancers at different sites in different individuals, which might be the consequence of variable somatic variants, variation in the background (germline) genetic make-up, or separate environmental exposures.

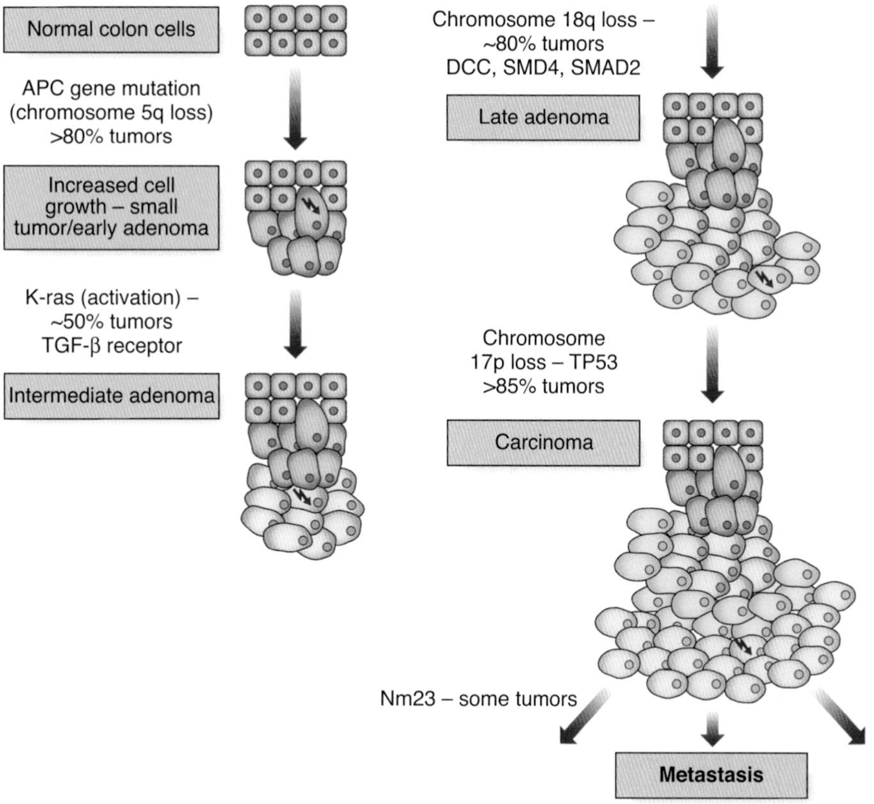

• **Fig. 14.12** The development of colorectal cancer is a multistage process of accumulating genetic errors in cells. The red arrows represent a new critical mutation event, followed by clonal expansion. At the stage of carcinoma, the proliferating cells contain all the genetic errors that have accumulated.

DNA Tumor Profiling, Mutational Signatures, and Tumor Mutational Burden

The advent of next-generation sequencing has dramatically enhanced our understanding of the genetic basis of cancer, and a global effort is underway to assemble big data on the cancer genome, curated through sites such as the Catalogue of Somatic Mutations in Cancer (COSMIC), which is currently the world's largest repository of somatic variation in cancer. Whereas cytogenetic and microarray-comparative genomic hybridization techniques highlighted the significance of multiple somatic, and often recurring, genetic events in tumorigenesis, such as disruptive chromosomal rearrangements and allele loss, tumor genome sequencing is vastly expanding knowledge of single-gene mutational events in cancer. The multiple mutational events that take place within a tumor can be schematically presented in the form of a circos plot, as depicted in Fig. 14.13.

We know that vast numbers (often thousands) of mutational events occur in tumor tissue when compared with analysis of germline DNA in an affected individual, and there are likely to be some similarities as well as many differences between the DNA profiles of tumors from two people, even though the histological diagnosis is the same. This has given rise to the notion of "signatures" of mutational processes—derived from the observation that different mutational processes appear to be associated with different combinations of mutation types. Many of the differences between the profiles of tumors comprise so-called "passenger" mutations, that is, variants that are generated but relatively non-contributory in driving cellular proliferation. Studying these variants led to the development of mutational signatures which provide information about the evolution and, in some cases, the molecular mechanism of a tumor.

Mutational signatures were originally established for the six classes of single base substitution (SBS)—C > A, C > G, C > T, T > A, T > C, and T > G. However, other classes of genetic variation can be incorporated into the genomic features that define a mutational signature, and doublet base substitutions (DBSs), for

TABLE 14.3 Some familial cancers or cancer syndromes caused by pathogenic variants in tumor suppressor genes

Disorder	Gene	Locus
Retinoblastoma	*RB1*	13q14
Familial adenomatous polyposis	*APC*	5q31
Li-Fraumeni syndrome	*Tp53*	17p13
von Hippel–Lindau syndrome	*VHL*	3p25-26
Multiple endocrine neoplasia type II	*RET*	10q11.2
Breast–ovarian cancer	*BRCA1*	17q21
Breast cancer	*BRCA2*	13q12-13
Gastric cancer	*CDH1*	16q22.1
Wilms tumor	*WT1*	11p13
Neurofibromatosis I	*NF1*	17q12-22

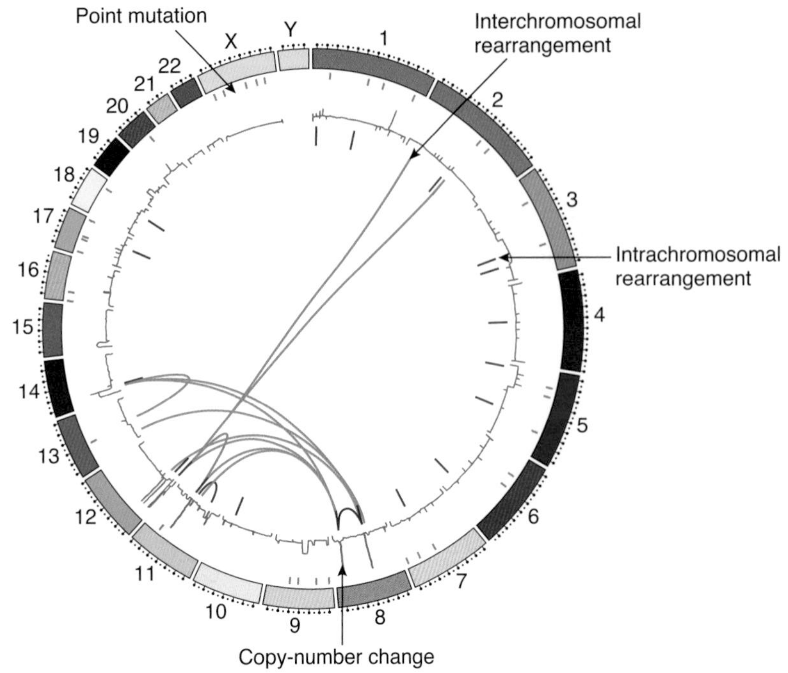

• **Fig. 14.13** A circos plot representation of somatic variation in a small-cell lung cancer. Individual chromosomes are depicted on the outer circle followed by concentric tracks for point mutation, copy number changes, and insertions/deletions. Chromosomal rearrangement data, that is, translocations/inversions, are represented in the center of the plot. Arrows indicate examples of the various types of somatic variation present in this cancer genome. (From Stratton MR, Campbell PJ, Futreal PA. The cancer genome. *Nature*. 2009;458:719–724. With permission.)

example, AC > GA, and small insertion and deletions (ID), are well-recognized genomic changes that produce specific mutational signatures. COSMIC currently lists 77 signatures based on SBS, DBS, and ID variants recorded in various cancer genomes, and two examples are shown in Fig. 14.14. As more is learned about molecular signatures, it is anticipated that they will play a greater role in the diagnostic pathway of cancers and have the potential to improve treatment options, for example, the use of poly-ADP-ribose polymerase (PARP) inhibitors in tumors exhibiting a signature consistent with a homologous recombination (HR) deficiency.

A further outcome of genomic testing in cancer is the quantification of tumor mutational burden, a measure of the total number of variants identified in a tumor genome sequence, which has already had an impact on treatments for some cancer types, bringing genomics into the realm of everyday medicine. In metastatic CRC, with a high mutational burden, patients have shown good response to immunological treatments in the form of checkpoint-inhibitors such as pembrolizumab or nivolumab. Many other tumor types are being studied, and it is likely that the benefit of such treatments will extend into other branches of oncology.

Precision Medicine

What is hopefully clear from understanding the outcomes of genomic sequencing in cancer is the potential it has to individualize cancer treatment. A greater understanding of cancer biology allows identification of key driver mutations which are potential targets for novel therapies. Although many of these therapies are yet to be discovered, one particularly noteworthy example, already in use, are the PARP inhibitors (e.g., olaparib, in ovarian cancer). Around 10% to 15% of patients with ovarian cancer will have a germline pathogenic variant in *BRCA1* or *BRCA2*, with a further 5% carrying a pathogenic somatic variant in one of these genes. In this group, PARP inhibition has shown excellent results in terms of progression-free survival, so much so that it is now licensed as a first-line treatment. PARP is an enzyme critical to the base excision repair (BER) pathway. Cells deficient in HR, as would be expected in *BRCA*-mutated cells, become dependent on PARP for DNA repair. PARP inhibitors work on the principle of synthetic lethality, thus a cell deficient in both HR and BER would not survive. PARP inhibition in BRCA-deficient ovarian cancer would lead to specific death of cancer cells, potentially avoiding the systemic effects of chemotherapy.

Although much research is ongoing, the impact of genomic technology in cancer diagnostics and treatment is likely to be significant as tumor genome analysis becomes part of routine testing for many types of cancer in the near future.

Circulating Tumor DNA

Another rapidly emerging application of next-generation sequencing in cancer genomics is the detection of circulating tumor DNA (ctDNA) in patients with cancer. Tumor DNA may be present in the plasma of a cancer patient as either circulating tumor cells (CTCs) or cell-free DNA. It has been shown that the frequency of CTCs and ctDNA in plasma correlates with the stage of cancer in the patient, that is, the more advanced the cancer, the higher the frequency of CTC and ctDNA; this also correlates with survival. This principle is well recognized in monitoring the response to treatment in CML (p. 187), whereby the presence and load of the specific chimeric *ABL* fusion product is monitored. However, massively parallel sequencing (MPS)—as opposed to some form of traditional PCR—facilitates the detection and monitoring of the numerous genetic alterations occurring in cancer tissue. The

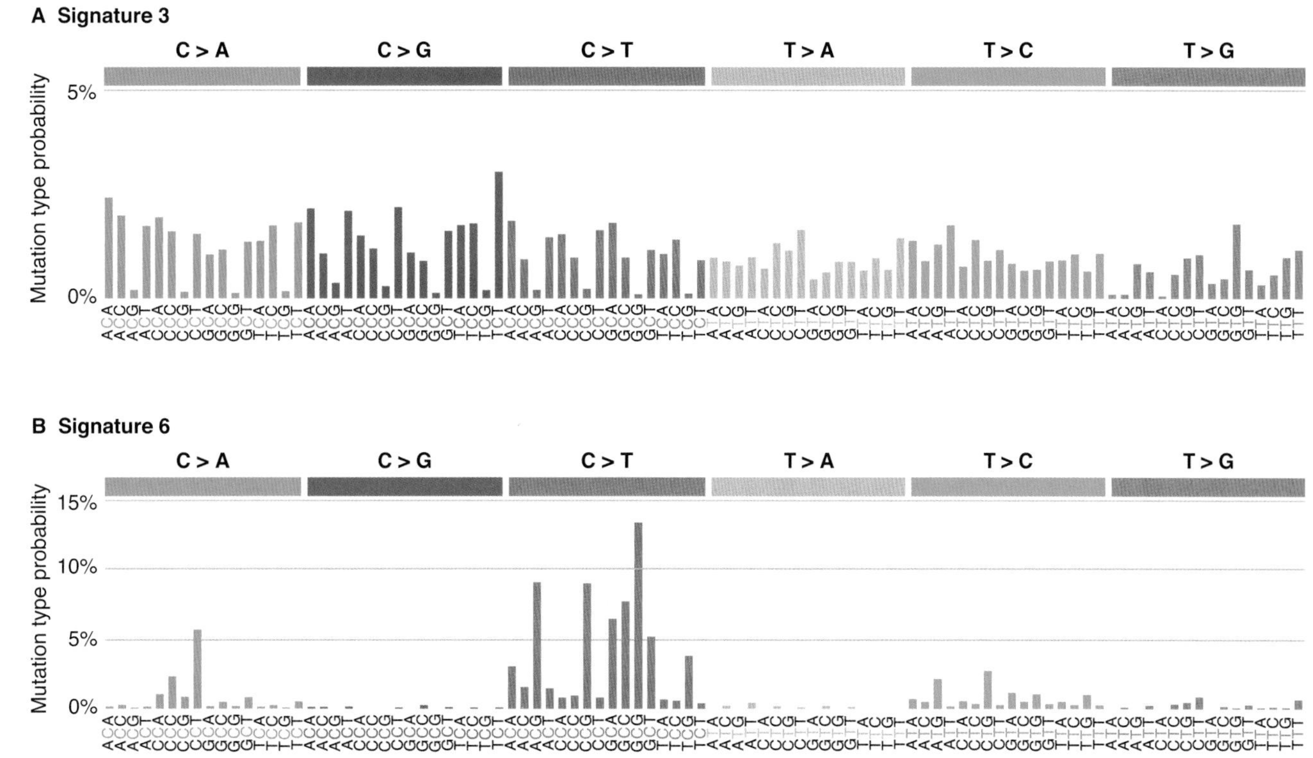

• **Fig. 14.14** Examples of mutational signatures based on single base substitutions. The display uses a 96 substitution classification defined by the substitution class and the sequence context immediately 3′ and 5′ to the mutated base. The probability for each of the six types of substitutions and the mutated bases, compared with the reference genome, are displayed in different colors as vertical bars. The variant types appear on the horizontal axis, and the percentage of variants attributed to a specific variant appears on the vertical axis. (A) **Signature 3**. Signature 3 is associated with failure of DNA-double stranded break repair because of defects in homologous recombination as seen in germline and somatic *BRCA1/BRCA2* variants. It is therefore frequently observed in breast, pancreatic and ovarian cancers. Large insertions and deletions (>3 base pairs [bp]) at breakpoint junctions are also associated. (B) **Signature 6**. Signature 6 has been reported in 17 cancer types but is most common in colorectal and uterine cancers, and is associated with defective DNA mismatch repair, as in microsatellite-unstable tumors. It is also associated with large numbers of small (<3-bp) insertions and deletions at mono/polynucleotide repeats. Signature 6 is one of four signatures associated with defective mismatch repair, with signature 15, 20 and 26 also seen. (Modified from Alexandrov LB, Nik-Zainal S, Wedge DC, et al. Signatures of mutational processes in human cancer. *Nature*. 2013;500:415–421, and COSMIC [http://cancer.sanger.ac.uk/cosmic/signatures].)

technical challenge derives from the fact that circulating DNA is present in fragments with an average length of 140 to 170 bp and just a few thousand amplifiable copies per milliliter of blood, and of these copies, only a fraction may be clinically relevant. A technique called tagged-amplicon deep sequencing (TAm-Seq) allows for the amplification and deep sequencing of genomic regions spanning thousands of bases, even from individual copies of fragmented DNA.

In a clinical setting one approach is to use MPS on solid tumor samples to initially identify specific genomic rearrangements and gene variants, which can then be identified in plasma; another is to use TAm-Seq to search for variants in genes commonly found in cancer, such as *TP53*, *EGFR*, *PIK3CA*, and *KRAS* in ovarian disease. An application of the technique can also detect and quantify commonly occurring deletions through targeting multiple single nucleotide polymorphisms (SNPs). These methods of characterizing and monitoring cancer have the potential advantage of providing a more comprehensive profile because individual tumors may harbor different clonal expansions of abnormal tissue which are not always captured in a biopsy. This exciting advance is set to change the way response to treatment is monitored (Fig. 14.15), as well as informing the treatment protocol.

A further application of ctDNA is cancer surveillance, where the so-called "liquid biopsy" could impact how we screen for cancer in those at increased risk, or perhaps at a population level. Research suggests that a test combining a panel of commonly mutated genes in cancer, as mentioned previously, with biomarkers, for example, Ca-125 and Ca 19-9, has potential as a non-invasive screening tool. The use of biomarkers aid localization of tumors as the gene variants tested are rarely tumor-specific. Screening in this way would be particularly advantageous for those cancers that prove difficult to detect at an early stage, for example ovarian or pancreatic cancers. Although further refinement is needed before this becomes part of routine screening protocols, it offers great hope, particularly for those with inherited cancer predisposition syndromes.

Inherited Cancer Syndromes

Familial cancer is a major component of the work of a clinical geneticist and comprises both common and rare conditions (Table 14.4). We begin with the condition which for many years was the best known example of an inherited cancer syndrome.

Familial Adenomatous Polyposis

Approximately 1% of persons who develop CRC do so through inheriting the altered gene for FAP. Affected individuals develop numerous polyps of the large bowel, often hundreds or thousands, which may involve the entirety of the bowel (Fig. 14.16). By the

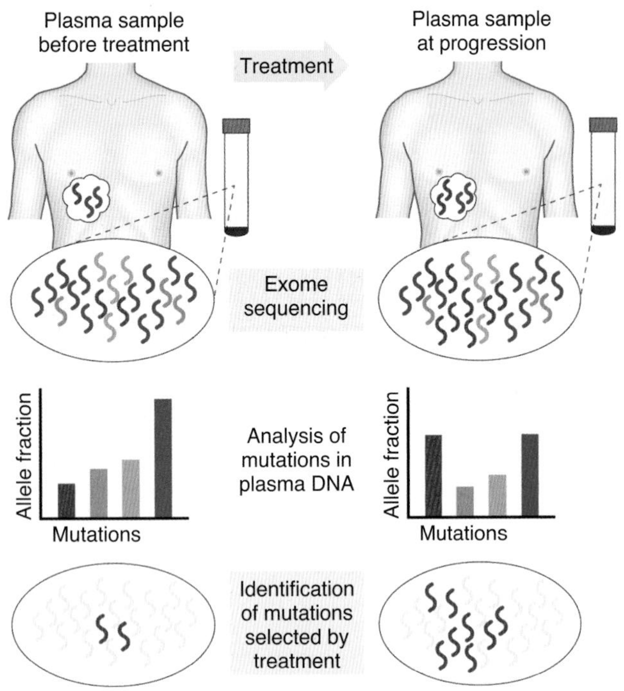

• **Fig. 14.15** Identification of treatment-associated mutational changes from exome sequencing of serial plasma samples. This diagram illustrates a study in which plasma was collected before treatment for advanced cancer and then at multiple timepoints during treatment. Exome sequencing was performed on circulating tumor DNA (ctDNA) from plasma, and germline DNA. The abundance (allele fraction) of variants in ctDNA at different time points was compared and showed that some variants significantly increased in abundance, which may indicate selection pressures associated with specific treatments. Some of the variants identified were known to promote tumor growth and drug resistance, whereas others were of unknown significance. Studies of this kind across large cohorts should lead to the identification of genes and pathways with recurrent variants.

age of 35 years, the vast majority of affected individuals will have many polyps in which there is a high risk of carcinomatous change, with 93% of untreated patients developing bowel cancer by the age of 50 years. Gastric and upper gastrointestinal cancer is also a significant risk in FAP, as we know from the improved survival of those who have had preventive colorectal surgery. They are also at risk of desmoid tumors, cutaneous sebaceous cysts, and lipomas.

Two forms of FAP exist, the classical form described and an attenuated version in which fewer polyps are seen alongside a later age of cancer diagnosis. Although both are caused by pathogenic variants in the same gene, the location of the variant is variable, and the differentiation between the two types has impact on clinical management.

The identification of an individual with FAP and an interstitial deletion of chromosome 5q21 led to the demonstration of linkage of FAP to DNA markers in that region, followed by isolation of the adenomatous polyposis coli *(APC)* gene. Analyses of *APC*-linked cancers from people with FAP have shown LOH, suggesting a similar mechanism of gene action at the cellular level. In non-hereditary CRC, LOH at 5q21 in the tumor material is common, with *APC* being deleted in 40% and 70% of sporadically occurring adenomas and carcinomas of the colon, respectively.

Lynch Syndrome

Approximately 5% of individuals with CRC have an underlying diagnosis of Lynch syndrome (LS), in which a small number of polyps are frequent, despite being previously referred to as hereditary non-polyposis colorectal cancer (HNPCC). Cancers are more frequently diagnosed in the proximal, or right, side of the colon, with an average age of onset in the mid-forties. A number of other cancers are associated with Lynch syndrome, including a significant risk of endometrial and ovarian cancers in women, as well as gastric, urothelial and hepatobiliary cancers. The risk of the associated cancers appears to vary depending upon the causative gene. LS is an autosomal dominant disorder caused by pathogenic variants in the mismatch repair genes.

DNA Mismatch Repair Genes

When looking for LOH, comparison of polymorphic microsatellite markers in tumor tissue and constitutional cells in persons with LS somewhat surprisingly revealed the presence of more, rather than fewer, alleles in the DNA from tumor tissue. In contrast to the site-specific chromosome rearrangements seen with certain malignancies (see Table 14.2), this phenomenon, known as **microsatellite instability (MSI)**, is generalized, occurring with all microsatellite markers analyzed, irrespective of their chromosomal location.

This phenomenon was recognized to be similar to that seen in association with variants in genes known as mutator genes, such as the *MutHLS* genes in yeast and *Escherichia coli.* In addition, the human homologue of the mutator genes were located in regions of the human chromosomes to which LS had previously been mapped, leading to rapid cloning of the genes responsible for LS in humans (Table 14.5). The mutator genes code for a system of "proofreading" enzymes and are known as **mismatch repair genes**, which detect mismatched base pairs arising through errors in DNA replication or acquired causes (e.g., mutagens). The location of the *EPCAM* gene, previously referred to as *TACSTD1*, is unusual. It lies directly upstream of *MSH2* and, when the last exons of the gene are deleted, transcription of *EPCAM* extends into *MSH2,* causing epigenetic inactivation of the *MSH2* allele. However, deletions in this gene appear to be a rare cause of LS.

Individuals who inherit a pathogenic variant in one of the mismatch repair genes are constitutionally heterozygous for a loss-of-function mutation (p. 22). Loss of function of the second copy through any of the mechanisms discussed in relation to LOH (p. 190, and Fig. 14.9) results in defective mismatch repair, leading to an increased mutation rate associated with an increased risk of developing malignancy. Certain germline pathogenic variants, however, seem to have dominant-negative effects (p. 22). Although LS accounts for a small proportion of CRC, estimated as 3% to 5% overall, approximately 15% of all CRCs exhibit MSI, the proportion being greater in tumors from persons who developed CRC at a younger age. Some of these individuals will have inherited constitutional variants in one of the mismatch repair genes in the absence of a family history of CRC. Analysis of tumor DNA for evidence of MSI is a standard test which can be used in cases where a diagnosis of LS is a possibility. High levels of MSI are suggestive of the presence of LS-related variants in the tumor, some of which will be somatic in origin, whereas in others there will be a pathogenic germline variant plus a "second hit" in the normal allele. However, the first-line test, which is now performed on all newly diagnosed CRCs as a standard population screen, is **immunohistochemistry (IHC)**. Using paraffin-embedded tumor tissue, loss of expression of specific mismatch repair genes can be tested using antibodies against the proteins hMSH2, hMLH1,

TABLE 14.4 **Inherited familial cancer syndromes, mode of inheritance, gene responsible, and chromosomal site**

Syndrome	Mode of Inheritance	Gene	Chromosomal Site	Main Tumor(s)
Breast/ovary families	AD	*BRCA1*	17q21	Breast, ovary, pancreatic
Breast/ovary families	AD	*BRCA2*	13q12	Breast, ovary, prostate, pancreatic
Familial adenomatous polyposis	AD	*APC*	5q21	Colorectal, duodenal, thyroid, brain[a]
Lynch syndrome	AD	*MLH1*	3p21	Colorectal, endometrial, urinary tract, ovarian, gastric, small bowel, hepatobiliary, brain[a]
		MSH2	2p22-21	
		MSH6	2p16	
		PMS2	7p22	
		EPCAM	2p21	
MYH polyposis	AR	*MYH*	1p33	Colorectal
Constitutional mismatch respair deficiency (CMMRD)	AR	*MLH1*	3p21	Childhood-onset colon/small bowel cancer, brain, hematological
		MSH2	2p22-21	
		MSH6	2p16	
		PMS2	7p22	
Juvenile polyposis	AD	*SMAD4*	18q21.1	Colorectal
		BMPR1A	10q22	
Peutz-Jegher syndrome	AD	*STK11*	19p13.3	Gastrointestinal, breast, uterus, ovary, cervix, testis
Cowden syndrome	AD	*PTEN*	10q23	Breast, thyroid (papillary), endometrial, testicular (seminoma), renal
Familial retinoblastoma	AD	*RB1*	13q14	Retinoblastoma, sarcoma, melanoma
Li-Fraumeni syndrome	AD	*TP53*	17p13	Sarcoma, breast, brain, leukemia, adrenal cortex
Multiple Endocrine Neoplasia (MEN)				
Type I (MEN1)	AD	*MEN1*	11q13	Parathyroid, anterior pituitary, gastro-entero-pancreatic (gastrinoma/insulinoma/glucagonoma/VIP-oma), adrenocortical
Type II (MEN2)	AD	*RET*	10q11.2	Thyroid (medullary), pheochromocytoma, parathyroid
von Hippel–Lindau disease	AD	*VHL*	3p25-26	CNS hemangioblastoma, renal, pancreatic (neuroendocrine), pheochromocytoma
Gorlin (nevoid basal cell carcinoma) syndrome	AD	*PTCH1*	9q22	Basal cell carcinoma, medulloblastoma, ovarian fibroma (odontogenic keratocysts)
Birt-Hogg-Dubé syndrome	AD	*FLCN*	17p11.2	Renal (oncocytoma/chromophobe), possible colorectal
Familial atypical multiple mole melanoma-pancreatic syndrome	AD	*CDKN2A*	9p21.3	Melanoma, pancreatic
Hereditary paraganglioma-pheochromocytoma syndromes	AD	*SDHA*	5p15.33	Paraganglioma, pheochromocytoma
		SDHB	1p36.13	
		SDHC	1q23.3	
		SDHD	11q23.1	
		SDHAF2	11q12.2	
		TMEM127	2q11.2	
		MAX	14q23.3	
BAP1 tumor predisposition syndrome	AD	*BAP1*	3p21.1	Atypical spitz, uveal melanoma, malignant mesothelioma, melanoma, renal, basal cell carcinoma
Hereditary leiomyomatosis and renal cell cancer	AD	*FH*	1q43	Renal, uterine leiomyosarcoma

AD, Autosomal dominant; *AR,* autosomal recessive; *CNS,* central nervous system; *VIP,* vasoactive intestinal peptide.

[a]Previously termed Turcot syndrome, although this term is now rarely used, and seen in both familial adenomatous polyposis and Lynch syndrome. A low-level risk is assumed in all patients with either condition.

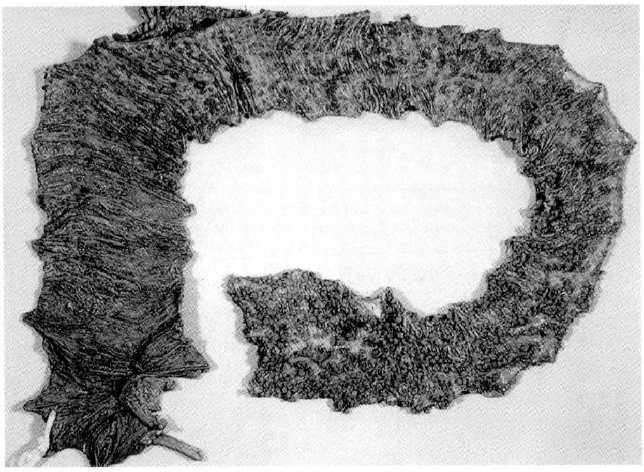

• **Fig. 14.16** Large bowel from a person with polyposis coli opened up to show multiple polyps throughout the colon. (Courtesy Mr P. Finan, Department of Surgery, General Infirmary, Leeds.)

TABLE 14.5 Mismatch repair genes associated with Lynch syndrome

Human Gene	Chromosomal Locus	*E. coli* Homologue	Lynch syndrome (%)
MSH2	2p22-21	*MutS*	40
MSH6	2p16	*MutS*	7–10
MLH1	3p21	*MutL*	50
PMS2	7p22	*MutL*	<5
EPCAM	2p21		~1–3

E. coli, Escherichia coli; HNPCC, hereditary non-polyposis colorectal cancer.

hMSH6 and hPMS2. Where tumor cells fail to stain (in contrast to surrounding normal cells), a loss of expression of that protein has occurred, and direct gene analysis and consultation with a clinical geneticist is likely to be required. Exceptions to this fall around the loss of MLH1/PMS2 expression, as this can be attributed to the presence of a somatic *BRAF* variant known as V600E. Loss of MLH1/PMS2 protein expression may also be a consequence of hypermethylation of the *MLH1* promoter; therefore further analysis may be indicated before proceeding to germline testing when IHC reveals a loss of MLH1/PMS2 expression.

Other Polyposis Syndromes

Although isolated intestinal polyps are common, occurring in approximately 1% of children, there are familial forms of multiple polyposis that are distinct from FAP but that show heterogeneity.

MYH Polyposis

In one large study, nearly 20% of familial polyposis cases showed neither dominant inheritance nor evidence of a pathogenic *APC* variant. Of these families, greater than 20% were found to have pathogenic variants in the *MYH* gene, and affected individuals were compound heterozygotes. In contrast to the other polyposis conditions described in the following section, MYH polyposis is an autosomal recessive trait, thus significantly affecting genetic counseling, as well as the need for screening in the wider family. The gene, located on chromosome band 1p33, is the human homolog of *mutY* in *E. coli*. The MutY bacterial mismatch repair protein operates in conjunction with MutM to correct A/G and A/C base pair mismatches. In tumors studied, an excess of G:C to T:A transversions was observed in the *APC* gene. Variants that effectively knock out the *MYH* gene therefore lead to defects in the base excision repair pathway; this is a form of DNA mismatch repair that, unusually, follows autosomal recessive inheritance.

Juvenile Polyposis Syndrome

Autosomal dominant transmission is well described for a rare form of juvenile polyposis that may present in a variety of ways, including bleeding with anemia, pain, intussusception, and failure to thrive. The polyps carry an approximate 13-fold increased cancer risk and, once diagnosed, regular surveillance (normally every 3 years) and polypectomy should be undertaken. The average age at diagnosis of cancer is in the third decade, although most affected individuals will have some detectable polyps by their 20s. Two genes have been identified as causative: *SMAD4* (18q) and *BMPR1A* (10q22). Both are components of the TGF-β signaling pathway (p. 108); *SMAD4* variants, which account for approximately 60% of cases, appear to carry a higher malignancy potential and the possibility of large numbers of gastric polyps for which upper gastrointestinal (GI) screening is required. In addition, 15% to 22% of patients with pathogenic *SMAD4* variants have a combined juvenile polyposis syndrome and hereditary hemorrhagic telangiectasia (p. 305) phenotype, common features of which include mucocutaneous telangiectasia, epistaxis, and pulmonary arteriovenous malformations, which are seen with relative high frequency in association with *SMAD4* variants and have important management implications.

Cowden Syndrome

Also known as **PTEN hamartoma tumor syndrome**, Cowden syndrome is autosomal dominant but very variable. Gastrointestinal polyps are found in the vast majority of cases and are generally benign hamartomas, although adenomas, juvenile polyps and ganglioneuromatous polyps have all been described. Multiple lipomas occur with high frequency, and the oral mucosa may have a "cobblestone" appearance (Fig. 14.17). Other dermatological findings may include trichilemmomas, facial papillomas, and palmoplantar keratoses. Significant macrocephaly is very common in this condition. Importantly, there is a high incidence of associated cancers for which surveillance is indicated. Females have an up to 85% lifetime risk of breast cancer, with a 50% penetrance by the age of 50 years. Thyroid disease is common, especially a benign multinodular goiter, but there is also a significant lifetime risk (35%) of follicular thyroid carcinoma. In addition, the lifetime risk of endometrial cancer is estimated at 28%, and the risk of renal cell carcinoma at 35%. There may also be increased incidence of CRC and melanoma, although these are at much lower levels than the other associated tumors. Pathogenic variants in the tumor suppressor gene *PTEN* on chromosome 10q23, encoding a tyrosine phosphatase, cause Cowden syndrome. A related phenotype with many overlapping features, which glories in the eponymous name of Bannayan-Riley-Ruvalcaba syndrome, has also been shown to be attributed to pathogenic variants in *PTEN* in a large proportion of cases.

Peutz-Jegher Syndrome

Also autosomal dominant, this condition is characterized by the presence of dark melanin spots on the lips, around the mouth

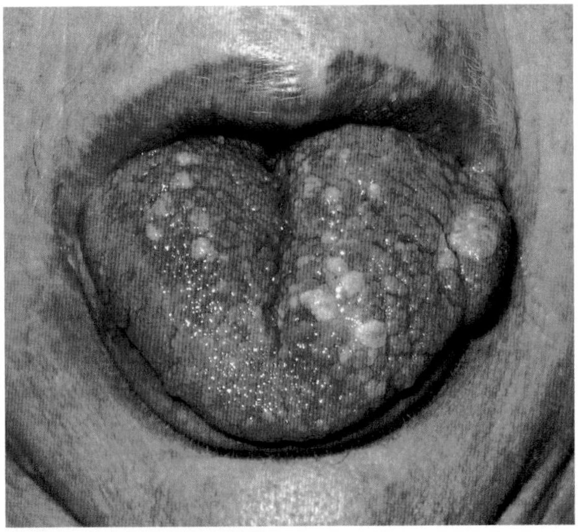

• **Fig. 14.17** Cowden disease. The so-called "cobblestone" appearance of the tongue.

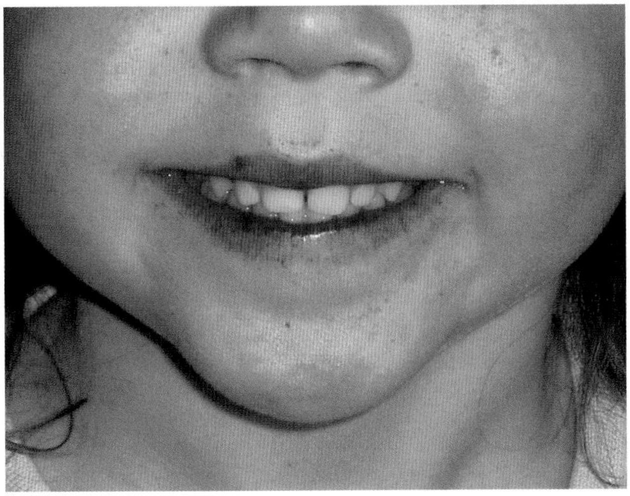

• **Fig. 14.18** Pigmented melanin spots affecting the oral mucosa of a child with Peutz-Jegher syndrome. These spots are usually more prominent in childhood compared with adult life. Affected individuals are at risk of multiple polypoid hamartomas throughout the gastrointestinal tract, which may undergo malignant change.

(Fig. 14.18), on the palms and plantar areas and on other extremities. These are usually present in childhood and can fade in adult life. Patients often present with colicky abdominal pain from childhood because of the development of multiple polyps that occur throughout the gastrointestinal tract, although they are most common in the small intestine. These are hamartomas, but there is a significant risk of malignant transformation. There is an increased risk of cancers at other sites, particularly breast, uterus, ovary, cervix, and testis, and these tend to occur in early adult life. Regular screening for cancers throughout adult life, often with a GI screen in childhood to detect and monitor polyp burden from an early age, is warranted; however, appropriate surveillance methods are not available for all tumor types. Pathogenic variants in a serine threonine kinase gene, *STK11* (19p13), cause Peutz-Jegher syndrome.

Breast Cancer

This is the most common cancer in women, with over 55,000 new diagnoses made annually in the United Kingdom—a quarter of a million new cases in the United States each year, and approximately 1 in 8 women in Western societies developing the disease in their lifetime. Some 15% to 20% of women with breast cancer have a positive family history of the disorder, and the risk to a female relative is greater when one or more of the following factors is present: (1) a clustering of cases in close female relatives; (2) early age (<50 years) at presentation; (3) the occurrence of bilateral disease; (4) the occurrence of ovarian cancer; and (5) a paternal (or close male relative) history of breast cancer.

Molecular studies of breast cancer tumors have revealed many regions of LOH, including (in descending order of frequency) 7q, 16q, 13q, 17p, 8p, 21q, 3p, 18q, 2q, and 19p, as well as several other regions with known candidate genes or fragile sites. With respect to cell growth and proliferation, the genes and pathways that are altered include the oncogenes *HER2*, c-*MYC*, and *RAS*, the estrogen receptor genes and the genes for cell cyclin D1 and E. An oncogene called *EMSY* (also known as *C11ORF30*) was found to be amplified in 13% of breast cancers and 17% of ovarian cancers, and was identified when looking for DNA sequences that interact with *BRCA2*—its normal function may be to switch off *BRCA2*. In addition, the tumor suppressor genes *RB*, *TP53*, and *PTEN* and the breast cancer susceptibility genes *BRCA1* and *BRCA2* are frequently implicated.

In practical terms, in a clinical pathological setting, the key protein markers evaluated are HER2, estrogen receptors and progesterone receptors. If these are all negative it means that tumor growth is not supported by the hormones estrogen and progesterone, so the tumors will not respond to therapies such as tamoxifen or Herceptin, and they tend to be more aggressive tumors. Some 10% to 20% of breast cancers are "triple negative" (TN), and at least one-third of the tumors in women who have *BRCA1* germline variants are TN. Although these tumors lack the normal hormone receptor targets for treatment, they are, understandably, a focus for research. For TN breast cancers, in the context of germline *BRCA1* variants, patients appear to have a better response to platinum-based chemotherapy compared with standard chemotherapy protocols. This platinum sensitivity is also well recognized in *BRCA*-associated ovarian cancers. For those breast cancers that exhibit a deficiency in homologous recombination, as would be expected in *BRCA*, PARP inhibitor use remains a hope for the future.

BRCA1 *and* BRCA2 *Genes*

Family studies of early-onset or premenopausal breast cancer showed that it behaved like a dominant trait in many families. Linkage analysis then mapped a locus to chromosome 17q, eventually leading to identification of the *BRCA1* gene. A proportion of families with early-onset breast cancer that did not show linkage to this region showed linkage to chromosome 13q, resulting in the identification of the *BRCA2* gene.

Pathogenic variants in *BRCA1* and *BRCA2* account for about 15% of cases of familial breast cancer. Carriers of pathogenic *BRCA1* variants have a 60% to 90% lifetime risk of developing the disease, as well as a 40% to 60% lifetime risk of ovarian cancer. The lifetime cancer risks for *BRCA2* gene mutation carriers are similar, with a breast cancer risk of 45% to 85% and a slightly lower ovarian cancer risk of 10% to 30%. Bearing in mind the population breast cancer risk of 1 in 8, and ovarian cancer risk of 1 in 50, the genes clearly carry a significantly elevated risk. In addition, male *BRCA2* gene carriers have lifetime prostate cancer risk of around 25%. Male breast cancer risk is elevated in carriers of both *BRCA1* and *BRCA2* mutations, although it is higher in *BRCA2* gene carriers.

Moderate Risk Breast Cancer Genes and Polygenic Risk Scores

As mentioned previously, variants in high-risk cancer genes, such as *BRCA1* and *BRCA2*, account for only a small proportion of cases of familial breast cancer. Thus from an early stage, it has been evident that other genetic factors, as well as lifestyle and environmental influences, must play an etiological role. Research has identified other genes which play a part in hereditary breast cancer risk, for example *PALB2* which is associated with a 30% to 60% lifetime risk of breast cancer; however genes such as this go only a small way towards understanding a person's individual risk since the vast majority of people will not carry a fault in a single high or moderate risk gene. Breast cancer screening is therefore offered on a population level, and at increased frequency dependent upon family history. A concern with this approach is the risk of screening itself; a drive to balance the risk-benefit of screening, alongside providing targeted surveillance for those at higher risk, has led to the development of **polygenic risk scores**.

An increasing number of common genetic variants, called SNPs, have been implicated in breast cancer risk although individually the effect size of each SNP is small. Looking at hundreds of SNPs simultaneously allows calculation of a polygenic score which, in turn, can be used to stratify patients into risk groups and refine surveillance programs for breast cancer.

Ovarian Cancer

More than 7000 new diagnoses of ovarian cancer are made annually in the United Kingdom, and approximately 1 in 50 women develop the disease, the incidence increasing with age. The majority of cases, approximately 90%, arise as a result of genetic alterations within the ovarian surface epithelium and are therefore referred to as epithelial ovarian cancer, which are mostly serous adenocarcinomas (rather than clear cell or mucinous) that are rapidly growing and aggressive. As with other cancers, a multistep process of genetic change and modification eventually leads to malignancy, although overall it is not well understood. What has become clear is that many of the ovarian cancers in patients with germline *BRCA* variants actually begin with in the fallopian tubes.

Approximately 5% of women with ovarian cancer have a family history of the disorder, and it is estimated that around 15% of all ovarian cancers are strongly predisposed for by single-gene variants, mainly variants in *BRCA1* and *BRCA2*, but less commonly in the genes responsible for LS (around 4% of cases). The age at presentation is 10 to 15 years earlier when predisposed by germline pathogenic variants in these genes. As with breast cancer, genes predisposing to a moderate ovarian cancer risk have been identified, and include *BRIP1*, *RAD51C*, and *RAD51D*. In families with two or more first-degree relatives affected with ovarian cancer, many genetics center offer gene panel testing to include the moderate risk genes alongside *BRCA1/2* and the mismatch repair genes. It is important to remember that a further approximately 5% of patients with ovarian cancer will have a somatic variant in *BRCA1* or *BRCA2*, therefore consideration of tumor testing is also relevant given that the result may have significant impact on management and potential use of PARP inhibition.

Prostate Cancer

Prostate cancer is the fourth most common cancer worldwide and is the most common cancer affecting men. It is increasingly common with age, and around 1 in 9 men will be diagnosed in their lifetime, although less than 3% will die as a consequence of their diagnosis. Enquiries into the family history of males presenting with prostate cancer have revealed a significant proportion (approximately 15%) to have a first-degree male relative with prostate cancer. Family studies have shown that first-degree male relatives of a man presenting with prostate cancer have between two and five times the population risk of developing prostate cancer.

Analysis of prostate cancer tumor material has revealed LOH at several chromosomal locations. Segregation analysis of family studies of prostate cancer suggested that a single dominant susceptibility locus could be responsible, accounting for 9% of all prostate cancers and up to 40% of early-onset prostate cancers (diagnosed before age 55 years). Linkage analysis studies identified two major susceptibility loci, *hereditary prostate cancer-1* and *-2* (*HPC1* and *HPC2*), and genome-wide association studies have highlighted a number of other susceptibility loci of variable significance. It is possible in due course that testing of multiple susceptibility loci will enable identification of high-risk individuals who can be offered surveillance, although this is not yet commonplace. Variants in the gene encoding ribonuclease L (*RNASEL*) were identified in two families showing linkage to the *HPC1* locus at 1q25. Variants have been found in the *ELAC2* gene at 17p11 and the *HPC2* locus, and variants in three genes—*PTEN*, *MXI1*, and *KAI1*—have been identified in a rare minority of families with familial prostate cancer. A small proportion of familial prostate cancer is associated with germline pathogenic variants in the *BRCA2* gene.

Although the majority of prostate cancers occur in men older than 65 years, individuals with a family history of prostate cancer, consistent with an inherited predisposition, are at increased risk of developing the disease at a relatively younger age (<55 years). Screening by measuring prostate-specific antigen levels is often offered, but problems with specificity and sensitivity mean that interpretation of results is often difficult, and further, potentially unnecessary, investigation may follow. It is possible that magnetic resonance imaging (MRI), with or without prostate biopsy, may become the screening modality of choice in the future.

Genetic Counseling in Familial Cancer

Recognition of individuals with an inherited susceptibility to cancer usually relies on taking a careful family history to document the presence or absence of other family members with similar or related cancers. The malignancies that develop in susceptible individuals are often the same as those that occur in the population in general. There are a number of other features that can suggest an inherited cancer susceptibility syndrome in a family (Box 14.1).

Inherited Cancer-Predisposing Syndromes

Although most cancers from an inherited cancer syndrome occur at a specific site, families have been described in which cancers occur at more than one site in an individual, or at different sites in various members of the family, more commonly than would be

• BOX 14.1 Features Suggestive of an Inherited Cancer Susceptibility Syndrome in a Family

Several close (first- or second-degree) relatives with a common cancer
Several close relatives with related cancers (e.g., breast and ovary or bowel and endometrial)
Two family members with the same rare cancer
An unusually early age of onset
Bilateral tumors in paired organs
Synchronous or successive tumors
Tumors in two different organ systems in one individual

expected. These families are referred to as having a **familial cancer-predisposing** syndrome. The majority of the rare inherited familial cancer-predisposing syndromes currently recognized are dominantly inherited, with offspring of affected individuals having a 50% chance of inheriting the gene and therefore of being at increased risk of developing cancer (see Table 14.4). For the clinician, awareness of the physical signs that may point to a diagnosis is important, for example, epidermoid cysts and desmoid disease in FAP, melanin spots around the mouth and lips in Peutz-Jegher syndrome (see Fig. 14.18), macrocephaly, lipomas and the cobblestone tongue in Cowden syndrome (see Fig. 14.17) and the dome-shaped skin papules, called trichodiscomas, over the face and neck in Birt-Hogg-Dubé syndrome (Fig. 14.19). In the latter condition pneumothorax may be a presenting feature. The **chromosomal breakage** syndromes (p. 265–268), which include ataxia telangiectasia and Bloom syndrome, also predispose to malignancy, and mostly follow autosomal recessive inheritance.

These cancer-predisposing syndromes carry a risk of a second primary tumor (multifocal or bilateral in the case of breast cancer) and generally present at a relatively young age compared with sporadic forms, and tumors may occur at different sites in the body, although one type of cancer usually predominates.

Inherited Susceptibility for the Common Cancers

The majority of people with a positive cancer family history do not, in fact, have a cancer-predisposing syndrome. The level of risk for persons with a family history of one of the common cancers, such as bowel or breast cancer, depends on the number of persons with cancer in the family, how closely related the at-risk person is to the affected relative, and the age of onset in affected family member(s). In most instances, where these criteria are not convincingly fulfilled, there is doubt about whether or not a cancer susceptibility gene is responsible. Here one relies on empirical data gained from epidemiological studies to provide risk estimates (Tables 14.6 and 14.7), although this may change with the future application of polygenic risk scores. With respect to mainly breast and ovarian cancers, the Manchester Scoring System (Table 14.8) has gained acceptance as a method of determining the likelihood of identifying a pathogenic *BRCA1* or *BRCA2* variant based on family history information and tumor markers.

The derived score discriminates the likelihood of finding a pathogenic germline variant in one of these genes, which may guide genetic testing—across the United Kingdom, a 10% threshold for testing is generally applied, which equates to a score of 15.

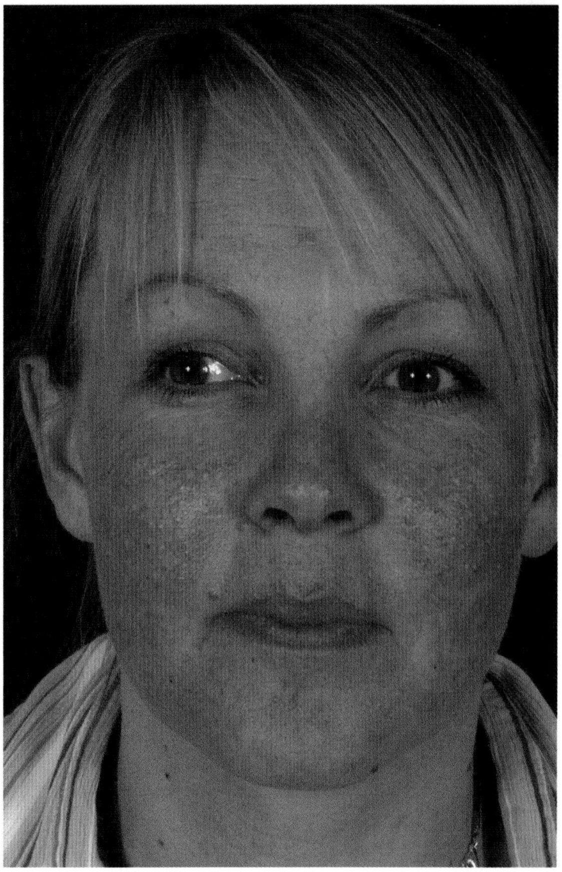

• **Fig. 14.19** Facial trichodiscomas—the pale, dome-shaped papules found on the head and neck of patients with Birt-Hogg-Dubé syndrome. Affected individuals are at risk of renal cell carcinoma, as well as colorectal cancer in some families.

Screening for Familial Cancer

Prevention or early detection of cancer is the ultimate goal of screening individuals at risk of familial cancer. The means of prevention for certain cancers can include a change in lifestyle or diet, drug therapy, prophylactic surgery, or screening.

TABLE 14.6 Lifetime risk of colorectal cancer for an individual according to the family history of colorectal cancer

Population risk	1 in 50
One first-degree relative affected	1 in 17
One first-degree relative and one second-degree relative affected	1 in 12
One relative younger than 45 years of age affected	1 in 10
Two first-degree relatives affected	1 in 6
Three or more first-degree relatives affected	1 in 2

(From Houlston RS, Murday V, Harocopos C, et al. Screening and genetic counseling for relatives of patients with colorectal cancer in a family screening clinic. *Br Med J.* 1990;301:366–368.)

TABLE 14.7 Lifetime risk of breast cancer in females according to the family history of breast cancer

Population risk	1 in 8
Sister diagnosed at 65–70 years of age	1 in 8
Sister diagnosed at younger than 40 years of age	1 in 4
Two first-degree relatives affected at younger than 40 years of age	1 in 3

Screening of those at risk of familial cancer is usually directed at detecting the phenotypic expression of the genotype (i.e., surveillance for a particular cancer or its precursor). Screening can also include diagnostic tests that indirectly reveal the genotype, looking for other clinical features that are evidence of the presence or absence of the gene. For example, individuals at risk of FAP can be screened for evidence of mutations in the *APC* gene by retinal examination, looking for areas of *c*ongenital *h*ypertrophy of the *r*etinal *p*igment *e*pithelium—known as *CHRPEs*. The finding of CHRPEs increases the likelihood of an individual at risk being heterozygous for a variant form of the *APC* gene, and therefore

TABLE 14.8 The Manchester Scoring System for predicting the likelihood that either a *BRCA1* or a *BRCA2* pathogenic variant will be identified, based on family history information

CANCER AND AGE AT DIAGNOSIS			
Female	**Male**	***BRCA1***	***BRCA2***
Breast <30		6	5
Breast 30–39		4	4
Breast 40–49		3	3
Breast 50–59		2	2
Breast >59		1	1
	Breast <60	5	8
	Breast >59	5	5
Ovarian <60		8	5
Ovarian >59		5	5
	Prostate <60	0	2
	Prostate >59	0	1
Pancreatic		0	1
Tumor Histology and Biomarkers in the Index Case			
Breast cancer adjustment		MODIFICATION TO SCORE	
Lobular		−2	0
DCIS only		−2	0
Grade 1		−2	0
Grade 3		+2	0
ER-positive		−1	0
ER-negative		+1	0
Triple negative		+4	0
HER2-positive		−6	0
Ovary: adjust for any cancer in family (as long as not >1 intervening unaffected female >60 years old)			
Mucinous germ cell or borderline tumors		0	0
High grade serous <60 years old		+2	0
Adopted, no known status in blood relatives		+2	+2

In bilateral breast cancer each tumor is counted separately, and ductal carcinoma *in situ* (DCIS) is included. Example: in the family the proband is a female diagnosed with breast cancer at age 28 (*BRCA1*, 6; *BRCA2*, 5); her mother had breast cancer at age 46 (*BRCA1*, 3; *BRCA2*, 3); a maternal aunt had breast cancer at age 54 (*BRCA1*, 2; *BRCA2*, 2); in addition, a paternal aunt had breast cancer at age 57 (*BRCA1*, 2; *BRCA2*, 2), but this is discounted because this does not provide the highest score in a direct lineage. The total score is therefore 21, which surpasses the 10% threshold (equal to a score of 15) for genetic testing. *DCIS*, Ductal carcinoma in situ; *ER*, estrogen receptor; *HER2*, human epidermal growth factor receptor.

developing polyposis and malignancy. CHRPEs are seen in persons with FAP when variants occur in the first part of the *APC* gene.

Presymptomatic, or predictive, genetic testing for a cancer-predisposing syndrome facilitates targeted surveillance screening—for example, renal cancer, central nervous system tumors and pheochromocytomas in von Hippel–Lindau disease (Table 14.9). Although the potential for prevention of cancer through screening those at high risk is considerable, it is important to remember that this does little to impact the overall rate of cancer in the population because these syndromes are relatively rare. Nevertheless, for many familial cancers there are now nationally (and internationally) agreed screening protocols. These must be evidence based and also deliver cost benefit to the health economy if possible (Box 14.2). In the United Kingdom, screening guidelines produced by the National Institute for Health and Clinical Excellence are seen as broadly determining what is available within the National Health Service, and these are continually evolving.

Who to Screen?

In the case of the rare familial cancer-predisposing syndromes such as FAP, von Hippel–Lindau, and MEN, those who should be screened can be identified on a simple mendelian basis. However, for Rb, for example, the situation is more complex. If no *RB1* variant has been identified (if the affected individual is not available or deceased), presymptomatic genetic testing cannot be offered. Some individuals with the non-hereditary form have bilateral tumors, whereas some with the hereditary form have no tumor (i.e., the condition is non-penetrant) or a unilateral tumor. It may be impossible to distinguish which form is present, and screening of second-degree, as well as first-degree, relatives may be appropriate given that early detection can successfully prevent blindness.

For those with a family history of the common cancers, such as bowel or breast, the risk levels at which screening is recommended, and below which screening is not likely to be of benefit, will vary. At each extreme of risk, the decision is usually straightforward, but with intermediate-level risks there may be doubt as to relative benefits and risks of screening.

What Age and How Often?

Screening programs must target those at highest risk, as well as cover those at moderate risk. The majority of cancer screening programs do not start until adulthood, although there are exceptions to this, for example in FAP where sigmoidoscopy to detect rectal polyps usually starts around the age of 12. The highest-risk age band for most inherited susceptibilities is 35 to 50 years, but because cancer can still develop in those at risk at a later age, screening is usually extended. In some families the age of onset of cancer can be especially early, and there may be scope to deviate from national guidelines in such cases. Childhood cancer risk, such as that for Rb or Wilms tumor, should obviously be dealt with very differently.

Screening intervals are determined from the natural history of the particular cancer. The development of CRC from an adenoma is believed to take place over a number of years, and in LS 18-monthly to 2-yearly screening is the recommended standard of care. Early diagnosis is critical in breast cancer care, so for those at high risk, for example *BRCA1* gene carriers, screening begins with annual breast MRI from 30 years of age, with the addition of mammograms from 40 years of age. For women with more moderately increased risk, annual mammography is recommended from 40 years of age.

> **• BOX 14.2 Requirements of a Screening Test for Persons at Risk for a Familial Cancer-Predisposing Syndrome or at Increased Risk for the Common Cancers**
>
> - The test should detect a malignant or premalignant condition at a stage before it is producing symptoms, with high sensitivity and specificity
> - The treatment of persons detected by screening should improve the prognosis
> - The benefit of early detection should outweigh potential harm from the screening test
> - The test should preferably be non-invasive, as most at-risk individuals require long-term surveillance
> - Adequate provision for prescreening counseling and follow-up should be available

Which Sites to Screen?

In conditions such as LS different sites are at risk of malignancy—mainly colorectal, of course, but also the endometrium, the ovaries, and others. Principles governing the sensitivity and specificity of screening apply here as elsewhere. Colonoscopy screening meets accepted criteria, but there is still no reliable screening modality for either endometrial or ovarian cancer. In some families with LS, specific screening of certain sites (e.g., stomach) may be offered if they appear to have unusually frequent manifestations of the disease. A similar, and more dramatic, example is Li-Fraumeni syndrome. Here a wide spectrum of cancers can occur, but, apart from regular breast MRI (from 20 years of age), no further screening is routinely recommended in adults (see Table 14.9). This is a topic of much discussion, particularly with reference to the childhood cancer risk associated with the condition. A United Kingdom consensus group has supported the use of annual whole-body MRI alongside 3- to 4-monthly abdominal ultrasound and clinical examination in children, although this is not yet routinely available nationwide.

Colorectal Cancer

CRC holds the greatest promise for prevention by screening. Endoscopy provides a sensitive and specific means of examination of the colorectal mucosa, and polypectomy can be carried out with relative ease so that screening, diagnosis, and treatment can take place concurrently. Colonoscopy requires a skilled operator because it is an invasive procedure and carries a small but consequent morbidity risk, especially in older people. For LS the screening protocol is well developed (see Table 14.9), but where this has not been proven the so-called **revised Amsterdam criteria** will help to determine what is offered to those at risk. These minimal criteria suggest a familial form of colonic cancer:

1. At least three relatives (related to each other) affected by an LS-related cancer, one a first-degree relative of the other two.
2. At least two successive generations affected.
3. LS-related cancer diagnosed before age 50 years in at least one relative.
4. FAP excluded.

In families fulfilling these criteria there is no debate about the appropriateness of genetic testing to look for a germline variant in one of the mismatch repair genes. However, a less obvious clustering of cases in many families should prompt consideration of tumor analysis to look for MSI and IHC. This is often decided on the strength of the **revised Bethesda guidelines**, as follows:

TABLE 14.9 Suggested screening guidelines for persons at significant risk of cancer: familial cancer-predisposing syndromes and common cancers

Condition/Cancer	Screening Test	Frequency	Starting Age (Y)
BREAST CANCER			
Moderate risk	Mammography	Annual	40–50 years then 3-yearly from 50 years
High risk (e.g., *BRCA1/BRCA2* mutations/ > 30% lifetime risk)	Breast MRI/mammography	Annual	MRI from 30–50 years Mammogram from 40–70 years
BREAST/OVARY			
Breast	MRI/mammography	Annual	As above, dependent on level of risk
Ovary	None recommended		Consider risk-reducing surgery when family complete
LYNCH SYNDROME (HNPCC)			
Colorectal	Colonoscopy	18-monthly to 2-yearly	25 years
Endometrial	None recommended		Consider risk-reducing surgery when family complete
Ovary	None recommended		Consider risk-reducing surgery when family complete
Gastric	Gastroscopy not routine, but all should be offered *H. pylori* screening ± eradication therapy		
Small bowel	None		
Hepatobiliary	None		
BOWEL CANCER			
High-moderate bowel cancer risk[c]	Colonoscopy	5-yearly	50–75
Low-moderate bowel cancer risk[c]	Colonoscopy	One-off	55
FAMILIAL ADENOMATOUS POLYPOSIS			
CHRPE[a]	Retinal examination		Childhood
Colorectal	Sigmoid/colonoscopy[a,d]	Annual	~12
Duodenal	Gastroscopy	3-yearly	30
LI–FRAUMENI[b]			
Breast	MRI	Annual	20
Sarcoma	Whole-body MRI	Annual	From birth
Brain	Brain MRI	Annual	From birth
Hematological	None		
Adrenal cortex	Abdominal USS	3- to 4-monthly	Birth–18
Skin	Dermatology review	Annual	18
MULTIPLE ENDOCRINE NEOPLASIA			
Type 1	Ca^{2+}, PTH, pituitary hormones, pancreatic hormones	Annual	8–50
Type 2	Calcitonin provocation test[a]	Annual	From diagnosis
Medullary thyroid	Thyroid US	Annual	Before thyroidectomy
Pheochromocytoma	Urinary VMA	Annual	8
Parathyroid adenoma	Ca^{2+}, PO_4, PTH	Annual	8
VON HIPPEL–LINDAU			
Retinal angioma	Retinal examination[a]	Annual	5

(Continued)

TABLE 14.9 Suggested screening guidelines for persons at significant risk of cancer: familial cancer-predisposing syndromes and common cancers—cont'd

Condition/Cancer	Screening Test	Frequency	Starting Age (Y)
Hemangioblastoma	MRI of brain/spine	3-yearly	16
Pheochromocytoma	Urinary/plasma metadrenalines	Annual	8
Renal	Abdominal USS (+MRI when lesions present)	Annual	16
GORLIN (NEVOID BASAL CELL CARCINOMA) SYNDROME			
BCCs	Clinical surveillance	Annual	Birth
Medulloblastoma	Parental surveillance		Birth
Odontogenic keratocysts	Dental review ± orthopantomography	Annual	Childhood
COWDEN (PTEN) SYNDROME (SUGGESTED)			
Breast	MRI and mammography	Annual	MRI from 30–50, mammography from 40–70
Thyroid	USS	Annual	16
Renal	USS/MRI	Annual	40
Endometrial	Not recommended		Gynecology review re: risk-reducing surgery
Colorectal	Colonoscopy		At 35 and 55 (+polyp follow-up if found)
BIRT-HOGG-DUBÉ SYNDROME (SUGGESTED)			
Renal	USS	Annual	18
Lungs (cysts)	Baseline CT	One-off	At diagnosis or 20
Colorectal (if positive family history)	Colonoscopy		45/50

BCC, Basal cell carcinoma; *CHRPE*, congenital hypertrophy of the retinal pigment epithelium; *CT*, computed tomography; *H. pylori*, *Helicobacter pylori*; *HNPCC*, hereditary non-polyposis colorectal cancer; *MRI*, magnetic resonance imaging; *PTEN*, phosphatase and tensin homologue; *PTH*, parathyroid hormone; *USS*, ultrasonography; *VMA*, vanillyl mandelic acid.

[a]Test to detect heterozygous state.

[b]Aside from breast screening, other suggested screening is not routinely available.

[c]As per British Society for Gastroenterology Guidelines.

[d]In individuals found to be affected, annual colonoscopy before colectomy and lifelong 4- to 6-monthly surveillance of the rectal stump after subtotal colectomy.

1. CRC diagnosed in an individual younger than 50 years of age.
2. Presence of synchronous, metachronous colorectal, or other Lynch tumors, regardless of age.
3. CRC with MSI-high histology (e.g., tumor-infiltrating lymphocytes) diagnosed in a patient younger than 60 years of age.
4. CRC diagnosed in one or more first-degree relatives with a Lynch-related tumor, with one of the tumors diagnosed at younger than 50 years of age.
5. CRC diagnosed in two or more first- or second-degree relatives with Lynch-related tumors, at any age.

For many cases, consideration of whom to offer tumor analysis to is no longer required because universal screening, with IHC testing on all newly diagnosed CRCs, has become standard care. It is also important to consider that, even in the presence of normal MSI/IHC testing, family members may still be eligible for increased surveillance on the basis of the family history.

Breast Cancer

In the United Kingdom screening of women age 50 years and older for breast cancer by regular mammography has become established as a national program as a result of studies demonstrating improved survival of women detected as having early breast cancer. For women with an increased risk of developing breast cancer because of their family history, there is conflicting evidence of the relative benefit of screening with respect to the frequency of mammography and the chance of developing breast cancer in the interval between the screening procedures (i.e., "interval" cancer). One reason is that cancer detection rates are lower in premenopausal breast tissue than in postmenopausal breast tissue.

It is also argued that the radiation exposure associated with annual mammography could be detrimental if started at an early age, leading to an increased risk of breast cancer through screening when carried out over a long period. Mammography is usually offered to women at moderately increased risk of breast cancer after the age of 40 years, because interpretation of mammograms is difficult before this age because of the density of the breasts. For most at high risk, MRI is used from 30 to 50 years of age (in addition to mammograms from 40 years of age), with the exception of Li-Fraumeni syndrome where MRI begins at 20 years, and mammograms are contraindicated because of the radiation exposure. Women should be taught breast self-examination to highlight concerns between screens.

Ovarian Cancer

Ovarian cancer, in the early stages, is frequently asymptomatic and often incurable by the time a woman presents with symptoms. The position of the ovaries within the pelvis and the lack of reliable screening modality make surveillance difficult. Ultrasonography and measurement of Ca-125 levels are not considered good diagnostic tests, especially as Ca-125 may not be elevated in all women with the disease, although it remains a useful tool for monitoring treatment response and progression.

The gold standard for management of woman at high risk of ovarian cancer is surgical with bilateral salpingoophrectomy (removal of the ovaries and fallopian tubes). The removal of the fallopian tubes is particularly relevant to *BRCA* because many *BRCA*-mutated ovarian cancers have been shown to originate in the fallopian tubes. The timing of surgery will, in part, be dependent upon the reason for the increased risk; for example, we know that in patients with pathogenic variants in *BRCA1* the risk of ovarian cancer climbs from 40 years. In patients with pathogenic variants in *BRCA2* this risk becomes more prominent from the age of 50 years. The timing of surgery needs to be carefully balanced with the risks of a premature menopause, although the use of hormone replacement therapy is acceptable until the age of a natural menopause provided the patient has not previously been diagnosed with an estrogen-positive breast cancer.

What Treatment Is Appropriate?

Surgical intervention is the treatment of choice for persons at risk for some of the familial cancer-predisposing syndromes—for example, prophylactic thyroidectomy in MEN type 2 (especially MEN2B) or colectomy in FAP. For those with a high risk from an inherited susceptibility for one of the common cancers (e.g., colon or breast/ovary), prophylactic surgery is also an accepted option, but the decision is more complex and dependent on the individual patient's choice. The option of prophylactic mastectomy in women at high risk of developing breast cancer is very appealing to some patients but totally abhorrent to others, and alternative management in the form of frequent surveillance may be preferred. Women with at least a moderate risk of breast cancer can also opt to take chemoprevention, commonly in the form of tamoxifen, which has been shown to reduce the incidence of breast cancer, although it is not without side effects. For patients at high risk of colonic cancer, dietary modification such as the use of non-digestible starch and a daily tablet of aspirin have some benefit (Table 14.10). Aspirin has shown particular benefit in patients with LS and, although the optimum dose remains to be determined, it is very likely to become part of the standard care of patients with this condition.

Those at an increased risk of developing cancer, especially those with single-gene dominantly inherited cancer-predisposing syndromes or one of the single-gene causes of the common cancers, find themselves in an unenviable situation concerning both their health and the possibility of transmitting the condition to their children. However, there is much hope that the future management and treatment of many forms of cancer will be transformed.

TABLE 14.10 Conditions in which prophylactic surgery is an accepted treatment, and the medical treatments in use, for the familial cancer-predisposing syndromes or individuals at increased risk for the common cancers

Disorder	Treatment
Surgical Treatment	
Familial adenomatous polyposis	Total colectomy
Lynch syndrome	Total hysterectomy ± oophrectomy
Ovarian cancer families/BRCA families	Bilateral salpingoophrectomy
High-risk breast cancer families	Bilateral mastectomy
MEN2	Total thyroidectomy (timing guided by genotype)
Medical Treatment	
Lynch syndrome	Aspirin—colorectal cancer risk reduction, optimum dose remains under investigation
Breast cancer families	Tamoxifen (when risk is at least moderate) Avoidance of long-term use of HRT (use until natural age of menopause is acceptable)
BRCA-associated cancers	PARP-inhibitors

HRT, Hormone replacement therapy; *MEN2*, multiple endocrine neoplasia type 2; *PARP*, poly-ADP-ribose polymerase.

ELEMENTS

1. Cancer has both genetic and environmental causes.
2. Genetic and environmental factors in the etiology of cancer can be differentiated by epidemiological studies, family and twin studies and analysis of disease, biochemical and viral associations.
3. Studies of tumor viruses have revealed genes present in humans known as oncogenes that are involved in carcinogenesis by altering cellular control mechanisms.
4. Study of rare, dominantly inherited tumors in humans, such as retinoblastoma, has led to the identification of tumor suppressor genes, consistent with the hypothesis that the development of cancer involves a minimum of two "hits." Persons at risk of familial cancer inherit the first "hit" in the germ cell, with the second "hit" occurring in somatic cells in mitosis. In persons with sporadically occurring cancer, both "hits" occur in somatic cells.
5. Genomic analysis of tumor DNA is transforming our understanding of cancer biology and the natural history of tumors. Knowledge of mutational signatures, the importance of mutational burden and the ability to identify variants driving carcinogenesis opens the door to precision, or personalized, medicine.
6. Similarly, the ability to detect and analyze circulating tumor DNA is likely to transform the way in which cancer is monitored, and screened for, in the future. This could be hugely significant for those cancers that normally present at a late stage.
7. Some 5% to 10% of the common cancers, such as breast and bowel cancer, arise as a result of an inherited cancer susceptibility. Familial susceptibility for cancer can occur as an inherited susceptibility for a single type of cancer or for a number of different types of cancer as part of a familial cancer-predisposing syndrome.
8. Persons at risk of an inherited cancer can be screened for associated features of a familial cancer-predisposing syndrome, or for particular associated cancers, and can be offered surgical risk management. These groups are also a focus for new treatments, for example, poly-ADP-ribose polymerase inhibitors in BRCA-associated ovarian cancer and aspirin use in Lynch syndrome.

CLINICAL SCENARIO 1

A 40-year-old woman presents to her GP with ascites. Further investigation confirms a diagnosis of high-grade serous ovarian cancer. She has no known family history of breast or ovarian cancer, but both her mother and her maternal aunt had hysterectomies and bilateral salpingooophrectomies at a young age.

What genetic investigations should be offered in this case, and might the results have any implications for treatment?

CLINICAL SCENARIO 2

A 43-year-old woman is referred to the genetics clinic with a diagnosis of chromophobe renal cancer. You note from the GP record that she has a past history of a multinodular goiter. There is no family history of cancer.

What are the key things to note from your history and examination? What, if any, genetic testing will you offer?

Further Reading

Alexandrov LB, Nik-Zainal S, Wedge DC, et al. Signatures of mutational processes in human cancer. *Nature*. 2013;500:415–421.

A technical but clear article introducing mutational signatures in cancer genomics.

Harris H, Miller OJ, Klein G, et al. Suppression of malignancy by cell fusion. *Nature*. 1969;350:377–378.

Study that eventually led to the concept of tumor suppressor genes.

Helleday T, Eshtad S, Nik-Zainal S. Mechanisms underlying mutational signatures in human cancers. *Nat Rev Genet*. 2014;15:585–598.

A technical article explaining the concept of mutational signatures in cancer.

Hodgson SV, Maher ER. *A Practical Guide to Human Cancer Genetics*. 3rd ed. Cambridge: Cambridge University Press; 2007.

An up-to-date second edition of this text covering the developing field of human cancer genetics.

Knudson AG. Mutation and cancer: statistical study of retinoblastoma. *PNAS*. 1971;68:820–823.

Proposal of the "two-hit" hypothesis for the development of retinoblastoma.

Lalloo F, Kerr B, Friedman J, Evans G. *Risk Assessment and Management in Cancer Genetics*. Oxford: Oxford University Press; 2005.

A comprehensive guide to the assessment and management of familal cancer with practical advice on genetic testing.

Li FP, Fraumeni JF. Soft tissue sarcomas, breast cancer, and other neoplasms: a familial syndrome? *Ann Intern Med*. 1969;71:747–752.

The original description of the Li-Fraumeni syndrome.

Lynch HT. "Cancer families": adenocarcinomas (endometrial and colon carcinoma) and multiple primary malignant neoplasms. *Recent Results Cancer Res*. 1967;12:125–142.

The description of the cancer family syndrome now known as Lynch syndrome.

Murtaza M, Dawson S, Tsui DWY, et al. Non-invasive analysis of acquired resistance to cancer therapy by sequencing of plasma DNA. *Nature*. 2013;497:108–112.

A frequently cited paper describing the monitoring of cancer genomics through treatment.

Stratton MR, Campbell PJ, Futreal A. The cancer genome. *Nature*. 2009;458:719–724.

An important overview of cancer genomics.

Volgelstein B, Kinzler KW. *The Genetic Basis of Human Cancer*. London: McGraw-Hill; 2002.

Very comprehensive book covering in detail the cellular biology of cancer and the clinical aspects of the familial cancer-predisposing syndromes and the common familial cancers.

Websites

Cancer Research UK:
https://www.cancerresearchuk.org.

Up-to-date on all aspects of cancer and user-friendly.

My Cancer Genome:
https://www.mycancergenome.org.

United States–based, aiming at a personalized approach related to genes and mutations.

National Institute for Health and Care Excellence (NICE):
https://www.nice.org.uk/.

The UK authority that issues numerous guidelines on drugs and screening.

COSMIC:
http://cancer.sanger.ac.uk/cosmic.

United Kingdom–based at the Sanger Centre; a wealth of information about cancer genomics is being assembled here.

Global Cancer Observatory:
https://gco.iarc.fr.

International Agency for Research on Cancer; presents global cancer statistics.

The Prospective Lynch Syndrome Database:
http://lscarisk.org.

Provides accurate estimates of cancer risks in Lynch syndrome according to age, gender, and genotype.

For variant interpretation:

InSiGHT Variant Database:
http://www.insight-database.org/classifications/.

The most comprehensive database of DNA variants in the genes that contribute to gastrointestinal cancer.

CanVar:
http://www.canvaruk.org.

An annotated cancer predisposition gene variant database.

15 Pharmacogenomics, Precision Medicine, and the Treatment of Genetic Disease

So little done. So much to do.

Alexander Graham Bell

If you can't fly then run, if you can't run then walk, if you can't walk then crawl, but whatever you do you have to keep moving forward.

Martin Luther King, Jr.

Pharmacogenomics

The world of human genetics/genomics has largely moved from using the term **pharmacogenetics** to **pharmacogenomics**. The difference in these terms, it must be said, is somewhat nuanced, but **pharmacogenomics** reflects the current emphasis on seeking to better understand how the entire genome is relevant to variation in individual sensitivity to the effects of a particular drug, especially the interaction between the drug and the whole genome. **Pharmacogenetics**, introduced by Vogel in 1959, is used to describe the influence of genes on the efficacy and side effects of drugs. The new term is therefore regarded by many as more inclusive. If polymorphic DNA sequence variation occurs in the coding portion or regulatory regions of genes, it is likely to result in variation in the gene product through alteration of function, activity, or level of expression. Automated analysis of genome-wide single nucleotide polymorphisms (p. 52) allows the possibility of identifying genes involved in drug metabolism, transport, and receptors that are likely to play a role in determining the variability in efficacy, side effects, and toxicity of a drug.

The possibility of utilising genome sequencing as a routine clinical diagnostic test opens up the possibility of creating an individual's own pharmacogenomics profile to provide information about optimal drug dosage or likelihood of adverse events.

It is important to appreciate that individual variation to drug sensitivity can be the result of factors that are not genetic. For example, both the young and the elderly are very sensitive to morphine and its derivatives, as are people with liver disease. However, individual differences in response to drugs in humans are often genetically determined. This whole field is important because adverse drug reactions are a major cause of morbidity and mortality, and form just part of the burden of iatrogenic disease which is so costly to health care.

The human genome influences the effects of drugs in at least three ways. Firstly, **pharmacokinetics** describes the metabolism of drugs, including the uptake of drugs, their conversion to active metabolites, and their detoxification or breakdown. Secondly, **pharmacodynamics** refers to the interaction between drugs and their molecular targets. An example would be the binding of a drug to its receptor. Thirdly, there is the way that the genome relates to palliative drugs that do not act directly on the cause of a disease, but rather on its symptoms. Analgesics, for example, do not influence the cause of pain, but merely the perception of pain in the brain.

Drug Metabolism

The metabolism of a drug usually follows a common sequence of events (Fig. 15.1). A drug is first absorbed from the gut, passes into the bloodstream, and becomes distributed and partitioned in the various tissues and tissue fluids. Only a small proportion of the total dose of a drug will be responsible for producing a specific pharmacological effect, with most of it being broken down or excreted unchanged.

Biochemical Modification

The actual breakdown process, which usually takes place in the liver, varies with different drugs. Some are oxidized completely to

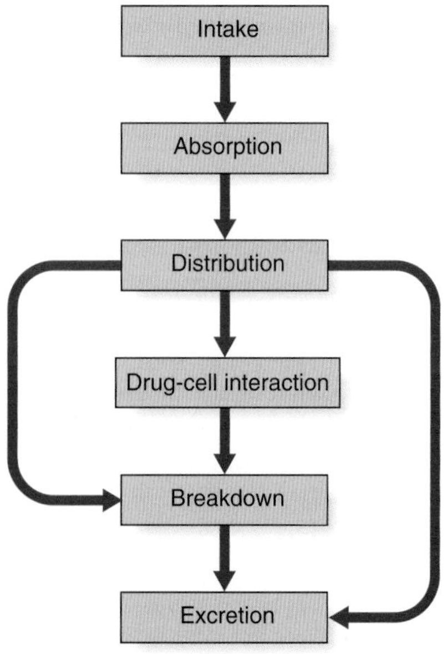

• **Fig. 15.1** Stages of metabolism of a drug.

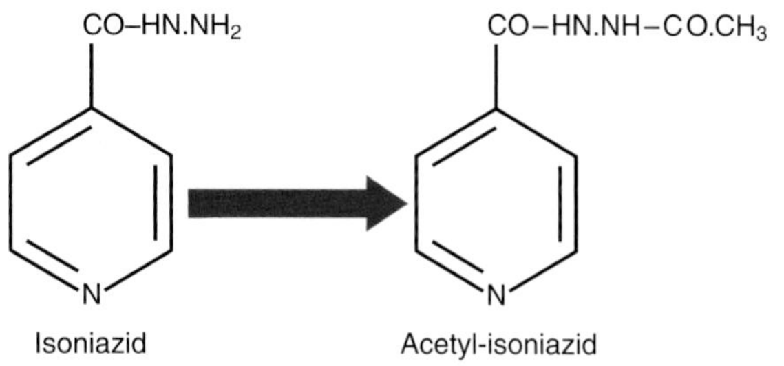

• **Fig. 15.2** Acetylation of the antituberculosis drug isoniazid.

carbon dioxide, which is exhaled through the lungs. Others are excreted in modified forms either via the kidneys into the urine, or by the liver into the bile, and thence the feces. Many drugs undergo biochemical modifications that increase their solubility, resulting in their being more readily excreted.

One important biochemical modification of many drugs is conjugation, which involves union with the carbohydrate glucuronic acid. Glucuronide conjugation occurs primarily in the liver. The elimination of morphine and its derivatives, such as codeine, is dependent almost entirely on this process. Isoniazid, used in the treatment of tuberculosis, and a number of other drugs, including the sulfonamides, are modified by the introduction of an acetyl group into the molecule, a process known as acetylation (Fig. 15.2).

Kinetics of Drug Metabolism

The study of the metabolism and effects of a particular drug usually involves giving a standard dose of the drug and then, after a suitable time interval, determining the response, measuring the amount of the drug circulating in the blood, or determining the rate at which it is metabolized. Such studies show that there is considerable variation in the way different individuals respond to certain drugs. This variability in response can be continuous or discontinuous.

If a dose–response test is carried out on a large number of subjects, their results can be plotted. A number of different possible responses can be seen (Fig. 15.3). In continuous variation, the results form a bell-shaped or unimodal distribution. With discontinuous variation the curve is bimodal, or sometimes even trimodal. A discontinuous response suggests that the metabolism of the drug is under monogenic control. For example, if the normal metabolism of a drug is controlled by a dominant gene, *R*, and if some people are unable to metabolize the drug because they are homozygous for a recessive gene, *r*, there will be three classes of individual: *RR*, *Rr*, and *rr*. If the responses of *RR* and *Rr* are indistinguishable, a bimodal distribution will result. If *RR* and *Rr* are distinguishable, a trimodal distribution will result, each peak or mode representing a different genotype. A unimodal distribution implies that the metabolism of the drug in question is under the control of many genes—that is, polygenic (p. 138).

Genetic Variations Revealed by the Effects of Drugs

Among the best-known examples of drugs that have been responsible for revealing genetic variation in response are isoniazid, primaquine, coumarin anticoagulants, certain anesthetic agents, the thiopurines, and debrisoquine.

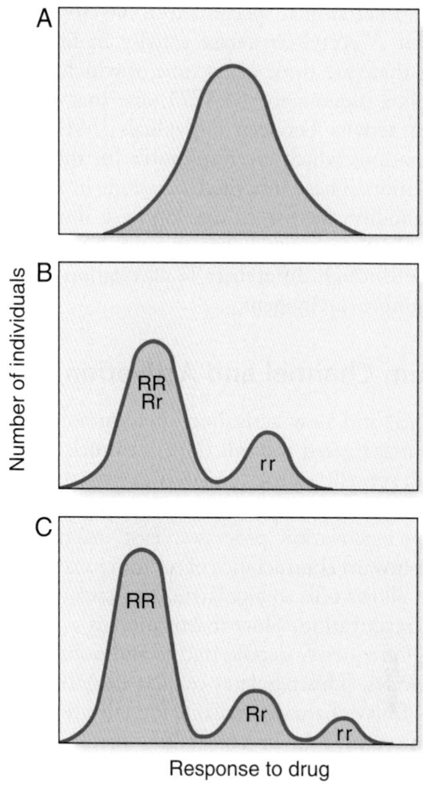

• **Fig. 15.3** Various types of response to different drugs consistent with polygenic and monogenic control of drug metabolism. **A**, Continuous variation, multifactorial control of drug metabolism. **B**, Discontinuous bimodal variation. **C**, Discontinuous trimodal variation.

N-Acetyltransferase Activity

Isoniazid is a first-line medication in prevention and treatment of tuberculosis. It is rapidly absorbed from the gut, resulting in an initial high blood level that is slowly reduced as the drug is inactivated and excreted. The metabolism of isoniazid allows two groups to be distinguished: rapid (or fast) and slow **inactivators**. In the former, blood levels of the drug fall rapidly after an oral dose; in the latter, blood levels remain high for some time. Family studies have shown that slow inactivators of isoniazid are homozygous for an autosomal recessive allele of the liver enzyme *N*-acetyltransferase, with lower activity levels. *N*-Acetyltransferase activity varies in different populations. In the United States and Western Europe, approximately 50% of the population are slow inactivators, in contrast with the Japanese, who are predominately rapid inactivators.

In some individuals, isoniazid can cause side effects such as polyneuritis, a systemic lupus erythematosus–like disorder, or liver damage. Blood levels of isoniazid remain higher for longer periods in slow inactivators than in rapid inactivators on equivalent doses. Slow inactivators have a significantly greater risk of developing side effects on the same doses that rapid inactivators require to ensure adequate blood levels for successful treatment of tuberculosis. Conversely, rapid inactivators have an increased risk of liver damage from isoniazid. Several other drugs are also metabolized by *N*-acetyltransferase, and therefore slow inactivators of isoniazid are also more likely to exhibit side effects. These drugs include hydralazine, which is an antihypertensive, and sulfasalazine, which is a sulfonamide derivative used to treat Crohn disease.

Studies in other animal species led to the cloning of the genes responsible for *N*-acetyltransferase activity in humans. This has revealed that there are three genes, one of which is not expressed and represents a pseudogene (*NATP*), one that does not exhibit differences in activity between individuals (*NAT1*), and a third (*NAT2*), mutations which are responsible for the inherited polymorphic variation. These inherited variations in *NAT2* have been reported to modify the risk of developing a number of cancers, including bladder, colorectal, breast, and lung cancer. This is thought to be through differences in acetylation of aromatic and heterocyclic amine carcinogens.

The Sodium Channel and Activation States

"Fast (or rapid) and slow activation" is terminology also used in relation to voltage-gated sodium (Nav) channels. These channels have essential, specialized roles in electrical signaling; rapid activation initiates the rising phase of the action potential, followed by fast and slow inactivation processes. Fast inactivation serves to attenuate the inward conductance of sodium ions (Na^+) in milliseconds, which allows cells to repolarize. Nav channels then become available for reactivation. Slow inactivation is a response to prolonged or high frequency depolarization and occurs over second to minute timescales. This regulates cellular excitability by reducing the number of Nav channels available for activation, and therefore plays an important role in controlling membrane excitability. Defective slow inactivation resulting from DNA variants in Nav channel genes is associated with several conditions of cell excitability, including hyperkalemic periodic paralysis, myotonia (p. 302), Brugada syndrome, and long-QT syndrome (p. 306). Sodium channel inhibitors, which include local anesthetics, anticonvulsants, antiarrhythmics, and analgesics, have the highest affinity for slow inactivated Nav channels and exert their effect by stabilizing an inactivated conformation of the channels (Fig. 15.4).

Glucose 6-Phosphate Dehydrogenase Variants

For many years, quinine was the drug of choice in the treatment of malaria. Although it has been very effective in acute attacks, it is not effective in preventing relapses. In 1926 primaquine was introduced and proved to be much better than quinine in preventing relapses. However, not long after primaquine was introduced, some people were found to be sensitive to the drug. The drug could be taken for a few days with no apparent ill effects, and then suddenly some individuals would begin to pass very dark, often black, urine. Jaundice developed, and the red cell count and hemoglobin concentration gradually fell as a consequence of hemolysis. Affected individuals usually recovered from such hemolytic episodes, but occasionally the destruction of the red cells was extensive enough to be fatal. The cause of such cases of primaquine sensitivity was subsequently shown to be a deficiency in the red cell enzyme glucose 6-phosphate dehydrogenase (G6PD).

G6PD deficiency is inherited as an X-linked recessive trait, rare in Caucasians but affecting approximately 10% of Afro-Caribbean males and relatively common in the Mediterranean. It is thought to be relatively common in these populations as a result of conferring increased resistance to the malarial parasite. These individuals are sensitive not only to primaquine, but also to many other compounds, including phenacetin, nitrofurantoin, and certain sulfonamides. G6PD deficiency is thought to be the first recognized pharmacogenetic disorder, having been described by Pythagoras around 500 BC.

Coumarin Metabolism by CYP2C9

Coumarin anticoagulant drugs, such as warfarin, are used in the treatment of a number of different disorders to prevent the blood from clotting (e.g., after a deep venous thrombosis). Warfarin is metabolized by the cytochrome P450 enzyme encoded by the *CYP2C9* gene, and two variants (CYP2C9*2 and CYP2C9*3) result in decreased metabolism. Consequently, these patients require a lower warfarin dose to maintain their target international normalized ratio range and may be at increased risk of bleeding.

Debrisoquine Metabolism by CYP2D6

Debrisoquine is a drug that was used frequently in the past for the treatment of hypertension. There is a bimodal distribution in the response to the drug in the general population. Approximately 5% to 10% of persons of European origin are poor metabolizers being homozygotes for an autosomal recessive gene with reduced hydroxylation activity.

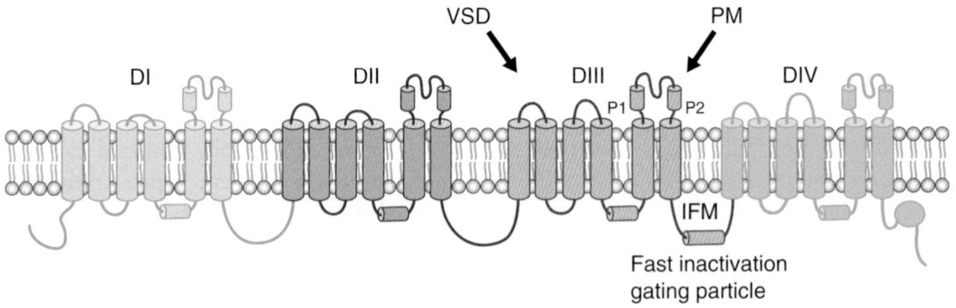

• **Fig. 15.4** Schematic view of a voltage-gated sodium (Nav) channel pore-forming α-subunit (β-subunit not shown). A pathogenic variant within the isoleucine-phenylalanine-methionine motif incapacitates fast inactivation but leaves slow inactivation intact. The mechanisms underlying slow inactivation are distinct from fast inactivation and involve other regions of the Nav channel, notably the P1 and P2 loops. *DI–DIV*, homologous domains; *IFM*, isoleucine-phenylalanine-methionine motif; *PM*, ion-conducting pore module; *VSD*, voltage-sensing domain. (Modified from Payandeh J. Progress in understanding slow inactivation speeds up. *J Gen Physiol.* 2018;150(9):1235–1238. Fig. 1.)

Molecular studies revealed that the gene involved in debrisoquine metabolism is one of the P450 family of genes on chromosome 22, known as *CYP2D6*. The variants responsible for the poor metabolizer phenotype are heterogeneous—at least 18 different variants have been reported.

CYP2D6 variation is important because the enzyme that this gene encodes is involved in the metabolism of more than 20% of prescribed drugs, including the β-blockers metoprolol and carvedilol, the antidepressants fluoxetine and imipramine, the antipsychotics thioridazine and haloperidol, the painkiller codeine, and the anticancer drug tamoxifen.

Malignant Hyperthermia

Malignant hyperthermia (MH) is a rare complication of anesthesia. Susceptible individuals develop muscle rigidity as well as excessive hyperthermia, often as high as 42.3° C (108° F), during anesthesia. This usually occurs when halothane is used as the anesthetic agent, particularly when succinylcholine is used as the muscle relaxant for intubation. If it is not recognized rapidly and treated with vigorous cooling, it often proves fatal.

MH susceptibility is inherited as an autosomal dominant trait affecting approximately 1 in 10,000 people. The most reliable prediction of an individual's susceptibility status requires a muscle biopsy with in vitro muscle contracture testing in response to exposure to halothane and caffeine.

MH is genetically heterogeneous, but the most common cause is a variant in the ryanodine receptor (*RYR1*) gene. Variants in other genes may influence susceptibility within individual families, which can explain the discordant results of the in vitro contracture test and the genotype in members of some families that segregate *RYR1* mutations.

Thiopurine Methyltransferase

A group of potentially toxic substances known as the thiopurines, which include 6-mercaptopurine, 6-thioguanine, and azathioprine, are used extensively in the treatment of leukemia to suppress the immune response in patients with autoimmune disorders such as systemic lupus erythematosus, and to prevent rejection of organ transplants. They are effective drugs clinically but have serious side effects, such as leukopenia and severe liver damage. Azathioprine is reported to cause toxicity in 10% to 15% of patients, and it is possible to predict those patients susceptible to side effects by measuring biochemical activity levels or analysing genetic variation within the thiopurine methyltransferase (*TPMT*) gene. This gene encodes an enzyme responsible for methylation of thiopurines, and approximately two-thirds of patients who experience toxicity have one or more variant alleles.

Dihydropyrimidine Dehydrogenase

Dihydropyrimidine dehydrogenase (DPYD) is the initial and rate-limiting enzyme in the catabolism of the chemotherapeutic drug 5-fluorouracil (5FU). Deficiency of DPYD is recognized as an important pharmacogenetic factor in the etiology of severe 5FU-associated toxicity. Measurement of DPYD activity in peripheral blood mononuclear cells or genetic testing for the most common *DPYD* gene mutation (a splice site mutation, IVS14 + 1G > A, which results in the deletion of exon 14) may be warranted in cancer patients before the administration of 5FU.

Precision Medicine

Using genetic or genomic information to select the most appropriate choice of pharmacological therapy at the correct dosage is a step towards **precision** medicine, a term which is used interchangeably with **personalized** or **individualized** medicine. Precision medicine, in a holistic sense, is a multidisciplinary approach to improving health care and health outcomes. During the past 10 years many examples of **stratified medicine** have emerged, where the treatment for a particular disease is dependent on the genetic subtype of the patient. These examples include monogenic subtypes of rare diseases where a different treatment is recommended for patients with variants in a specific gene, or stratification at the level of a tumor type based on its genetic characteristics. In other disorders, the treatment may depend on the subtype of variant, for example the new drugs developed to treat cystic fibrosis (CF) according to the effect of the variant. A genetic (or genomic) diagnosis is therefore an essential step towards the most appropriate treatment.

Maturity-Onset Diabetes of the Young

Maturity-onset diabetes of the young (MODY) is a monogenic form of diabetes characterized by young age of onset (often <25 years), dominant inheritance, and beta cell dysfunction. Many patients are misdiagnosed with type 1 diabetes and treated with insulin. The clinical observation of sensitivity to sulfonylurea treatment in a patient with a pathogenic *HNF1A* variant causing MODY led to a randomized crossover trial that showed a fourfold increased response to sulfonylureas in patients with *HNF1A* variants compared with a control group with type 2 diabetes (Fig. 15.5). For many patients a genetic diagnosis of *HNF1A* MODY means that they can transfer from insulin injections to sulfonylurea tablets.

Neonatal Diabetes

The most frequent cause of permanent neonatal diabetes is an activating variant in the *KCNJ11* or *ABCC8* genes, which encode the Kir6.2 and SUR1 subunits, respectively, of the adenosine

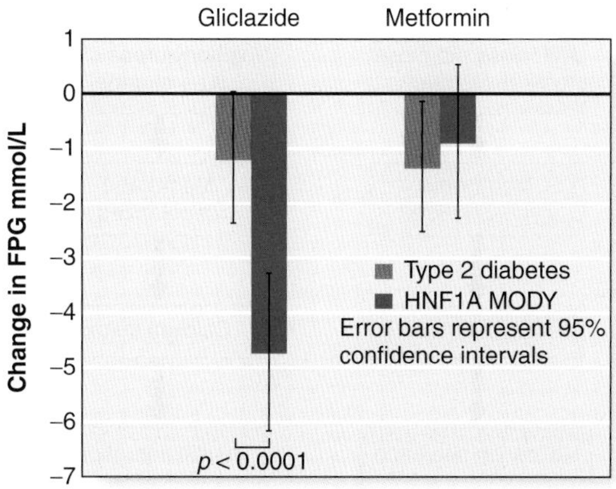

• **Fig. 15.5** Response to the sulphonylurea gliclazide and the type 2 diabetes drug metformin in patients with *HNF1A* maturity-onset diabetes of the young and type 2 diabetes. Patients (n = 18 in each group) were treated with each drug for 6 weeks in a randomized trial. *FPG*, Fasting plasma glucose. (Modified from Pearson ER, Starkey BJ, Powell RJ, et al. Genetic cause of hyperglycemia and response to treatment in diabetes. *Lancet*. 2003;362:1275–1281.)

triphosphate (ATP)-sensitive potassium (K_{ATP}) channel in the pancreatic beta cell. The effect of such variants is to prevent K_{ATP} channel closure by reducing the response to ATP. Because channel closure is the trigger for insulin secretion, these variants result in diabetes, and thus a requirement for lifelong insulin treatment. Defining the genetic etiology for this rare subtype of diabetes has led to improved treatment because most patients can be treated successfully with sulfonylurea tablets instead of insulin. These drugs bind to the sulfonylurea receptor subunits of the K_{ATP} channel to cause closure independently of ATP, thereby triggering insulin secretion (Fig. 15.6). High-dose sulfonylurea therapy results in improved glycemic control, which will reduce the risk of diabetic complications in later life. Some patients have a pathogenic variant that also affects the K_{ATP} channel function in the brain. Transfer from insulin to sulfonylureas can improve their motor and cognitive function, as well as control of their diabetes. International guidelines now recommend genetic testing for anyone diagnosed with diabetes in the first 6 months of life to identify those patients who will benefit from sulfonylurea treatment.

Adverse Events

It is estimated that approximately 15% of hospital inpatients will be affected by an adverse drug reaction. The objective of adverse-event pharmacogenomics is to identify a genetic profile that characterizes patients who are more likely to suffer such an adverse event. A well-known example is abacavir, a reverse transcriptase inhibitor used to treat human immunodeficiency virus (HIV) infection. Approximately 5% of patients show potentially fatal hypersensitivity to abacavir, and this limits its use. A strong association with the human leukocyte antigen allele B*5701 was proven in 2002. Testing for B*5701 is now routine practice before abacavir is prescribed.

At least 10% of Africans, North Americans, and Europeans are homozygous for a variant in the promoter of the *UGT1A1* gene (*UGT1A1**28) that results in reduced glucuronidation of irinotecan, a drug used to treat colorectal cancer, and increases the risk of severe neutropenia if exposed to the standard dose. A simple polymerase chain reaction–based test for *UGT1A1**28 can be used to determine the appropriate treatment dose.

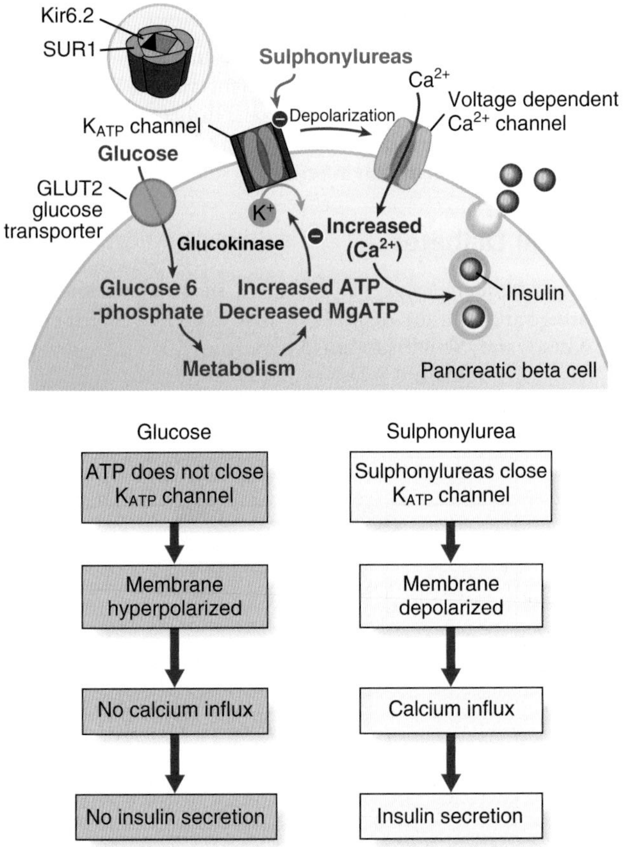

• **Fig. 15.6** Insulin secretion in the pancreatic beta cell. Activating mutations in the genes encoding the adenosine triphosphate–sensitive potassium channel subunits Kir6.2 and SUR1 prevent closure of the channel in the presence of glucose. Sulphonylureas bind to the SUR1 subunit to close the channel and restore insulin secretion. *ATP*, adenosine triphosphate. (From Professor A.T. Hattersley, University of Exeter Medical School, Exeter, UK.)

Efficacy

Apart from reducing morbidity and mortality from adverse events, it is hugely cost-effective to prescribe drugs only to those patients likely to respond to them. Several drugs developed for the treatment of various cancers have different efficacy depending on the molecular biology of the tumor (see Table 15.1). For example, trastuzumab (Herceptin) is an antibody that targets overexpression of HER2/neu protein observed in approximately one-third of patients with breast cancer. Consequently, patients are prescribed Herceptin only if their tumor has been shown to overexpress HER2/neu.

Imatinib is a protein tyrosine kinase inhibitor that has been used to treat chronic myeloid leukemia since 2001. It is a very effective treatment that works by binding the BCR-ABL fusion protein resulting from the t(9;22) translocation (p. 187). This is an example of effective drug design resulting from knowledge of the molecular etiology. It has also been shown to be effective in the treatment of gastrointestinal stromal tumors that harbor *KIT* mutations.

Approximately 13% of patients with non–small cell lung cancer have an activating *EGFR* mutation. These mutations increase the activity of the epidermal growth factor receptor tyrosine kinase domain so that the receptor is constitutionally active in the absence of epidermal growth factor. This leads to increased proliferation, angiogenesis, and metastasis. Drugs designed to block the EGFR tyrosine kinase domain and inhibit these effects have been developed. Patients with lung tumors harboring an activating *EGFR* mutation can show a dramatic response to treatment with these

TABLE 15.1 Examples of drugs effective for the treatment of specific cancers

Type of Cancer	Characteristic	Drug
Breast	*HER2* overexpression	Trastuzumab
Chronic myeloid leukemia	t(9;22) BCR-ABL fusion	Imatinib
Non–small cell lung cancer	*EGFR* activating mutation	Gefitinib or erlotinib
Gastrointestinal stromal tumor	*KIT* or *PDGFRA* activating mutation	Imatinib
Malignant melanoma	*BRAF* activating mutation	Vemurafenib

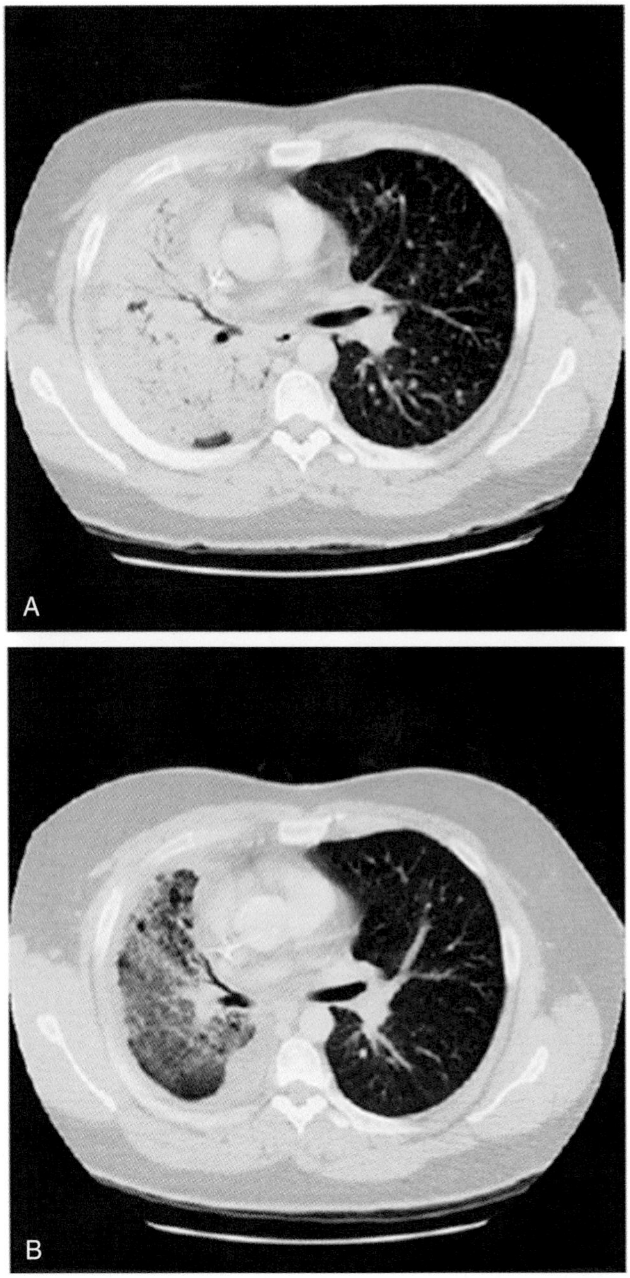

• **Fig. 15.7** Example of the response to gefitinib in a patient with non–small cell lung cancer and an activating epidermal growth factor receptor mutation. A computed tomographic scan of the chest shows a large mass in the right lung before treatment (**A**) and marked improvement 6 weeks after gefitinib was initiated (**B**). (From Lynch TJ, Bell DW, Sordella R, et al. Activating mutations in the epidermal growth factor receptor underlying responsiveness of non–small cell lung cancer to gefitinib. *N Engl J Med*. 2004;350:2129–2139. With permission.)

drugs (gefitinib and erlotinib), as shown in Fig. 15.7. Similarly, melanomas with activating *BRAF* mutations respond to the BRAF kinase inhibitor, vemurafenib, and targeted therapies are being developed for many other tumor types.

Treatment of Genetic Disease

Many genetic disorders are characterized by progressive disability or chronic ill health for which there is, at present, no effective treatment. In many cases disruption to normal processes occurs as a result of pathogenic variants in genes that are expressed for only a limited period in development, often very early in fetal life. Despite the undeniable challenges, one of the most exciting aspects of modern biotechnology is the prospect of new treatments mediated through gene transfer, RNA modification, or stem cell therapy. It is important, however, to keep a perspective on the limitations of these approaches for the immediate future and to consider, in the first instance, time-honored conventional approaches.

Conventional Approaches to Treatment of Genetic Disease

Most genetic disorders cannot be cured or even ameliorated using conventional methods of treatment, and, despite huge advances in gene discovery in rare disease, there are still disorders for which the underlying genetic cause is unknown, so there is little or no understanding of the basic defect. For some inborn errors of metabolism, however, it is sufficient to know the biochemistry to treat effectively. Examples include dietary restriction, as in phenylketonuria (p. 240); hormone replacement, as in congenital adrenal hyperplasia (p. 277); and supplementation with a vitamin or coenzyme that increases the activity of the defective enzyme, such as homocystinuria (p. 274) and some of the organic acidurias (p. 275) (Table 15.2).

Protein/Enzyme Replacement Therapy

For a genetic disorder found to result from deficiency or abnormality of a specific enzyme or protein, treatment could in theory involve replacement of the deficient or defective enzyme or protein. Successful examples are the use of factor VIII concentrate in the treatment of hemophilia A (p. 316) and C1-esterase inhibitor (plasma concentrate or recombinant) for attacks of hereditary angioneurotic edema.

For most inborn errors of metabolism for which an enzyme deficiency has been identified, recombinant DNA techniques may be used to biosynthesize the missing or defective gene product; however, protein replacement therapy (PRT) or enzyme replacement therapy (ERT) may not be successful if the metabolic processes involved are carried out within cells and the protein or enzyme is not normally transported into the cell. Modifications in β-glucocerebrosidase, as used in the treatment of Gaucher disease, enable it to enter the lysosomes, resulting in an effective form of treatment (p. 281). Another example is the modification of adenosine deaminase (ADA, p. 180) by an inert polymer, polyethylene glycol, to generate a replacement enzyme that is less immunogenic and has an extended half-life. Following attempted gene therapy for autosomal recessive dystrophic epidermolysis bullosa (Fig. 15.8), a more recent approach demonstrating promise has been both topically applied and intravenously administered human recombinant type VII collagen in mice.

In general, delivery of the protein or enzyme in its active form and to its precise site of action presents significant challenges. Many candidate compounds for monogenic PRT/ERT have received regulatory approval for clinical trials, notable among these being blood factors and lysosomal storage disorders, as well as other inborn errors of metabolism, alpha-1 antitrypsin deficiency, and specific mitochondrial diseases. The large majority relate to rare diseases, and the therapies therefore come into the category of "orphan drugs." Thus the numbers of patients for whom the treatment is targeted are relatively few, and consequently the cost of

TABLE 15.2 Examples of various methods for treating genetic disease

Treatment	Disorder
Enzyme Induction by Drugs	
Phenobarbitone	Congenital non-hemolytic jaundice
Replacement of Deficient Enzyme/Protein	
Blood transfusion	Thalassemia
Bone marrow transplantation	SCID resulting from adenosine deaminase deficiency; lysosomal storage disorders
Enzyme/Protein Preparations	
Trypsin	Trypsinogen deficiency
α_1-Antitrypsin	α_1-Antitrypsin deficiency
Collagen type VII	Autosomal recessive dystrophic epidermolysis bullosa
Cryoprecipitate/factor VIII	Hemophilia A
β-Glucosidase	Gaucher disease
α-Galactosidase	Fabry disease
C1-esterase inhibitor	Angioneurotic edema
Replacement of Deficient Vitamin or Coenzyme	
B_6	Homocystinuria
B_{12}	Methylmalonic acidemia
Biotin	Propionic acidemia
D	Vitamin D–resistant rickets
Replacement of Deficient Product	
Cortisone	Congenital adrenal hyperplasia
Thyroxine	Congenital hypothyroidism
Substrate Restriction in Diet	
AMINO ACIDS	
Phenylalanine	Phenylketonuria
Leucine, isoleucine, valine	Maple syrup urine disease
CARBOHYDRATE	
Galactose	Galactosemia
LIPID	
Cholesterol	Familial hypercholesterolemia
Protein	Urea cycle disorders
Drug Therapy	
Dantrolene	Malignant hyperthermia
Cholestyramine	Familial hypercholesterolemia
Everolimus	Tuberous sclerosis
Irbesartan / Losartan / β-blockers	Marfan syndrome
Pancreatic enzymes	Cystic fibrosis
Penicillamine	Wilson disease, cystinuria

(Continued)

TABLE 15.2 Examples of various methods for treating genetic disease—cont'd

Treatment	Disorder
Drug/Dietary Avoidance	
Sulfonamides	G6PD deficiency
Barbiturates	Porphyria
Replacement of Diseased Tissue	
Kidney transplantation	Adult-onset polycystic kidney disease, Fabry disease
Bone marrow transplantation	Lysosomal storage disorders, X-linked SCID, Wiskott-Aldrich syndrome
Removal of Diseased Tissue	
Colectomy	Familial adenomatous polyposis
Splenectomy	Hereditary spherocytosis

SCID, Severe combined immunodeficiency.

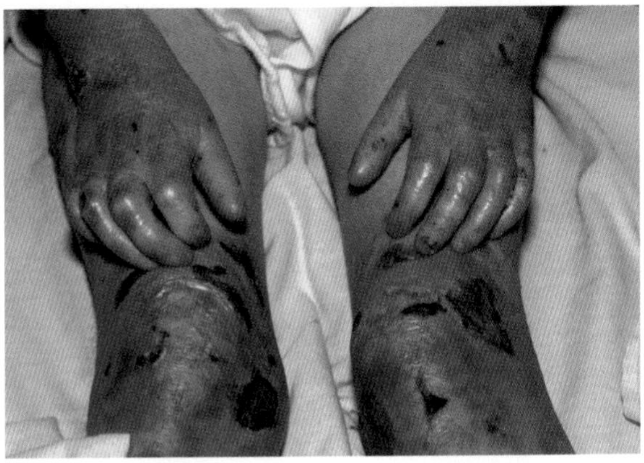

• **Fig. 15.8** Blistering skin in dystrophic epidermolysis bullosa, which has been the target of novel forms of protein replacement therapy aimed at restoring type VII collagen integrity. (From Joyce JC. Vesiculobullous Disorders. In: *Nelson Textbook of Pediatrics*. 21st ed. Kliegman RM, St Geme III JW, Blum NJ, et al., eds. Elsevier: Philadelphia; 2020: 3480–3491.e1.)

drug production per patient very high. However, legislation in the United States and European Union, as well as individual nations, provides incentives for the development of treatments for "orphan diseases."

Drug Treatment

In some genetic disorders, drug therapy is possible; for example, statins can help to lower cholesterol levels in familial hypercholesterolemia (p. 277). Statins function indirectly through the low-density lipoprotein (LDL) receptor by inhibiting endogenous cholesterol biosynthesis at the rate-limiting step that is mediated by hydroxymethyl glutaryl co-enzyme A reductase. This leads to upregulation of the LDL receptor and increased LDL clearance from plasma.

Recent years have seen the successful **repurposing** of drugs including sulfonylureas and rapamycin. The hypoglycemic effect of sulfonylureas was discovered in 1942, and these drugs have been used in tablet form to treat type 2 diabetes for nearly 70 years. Sulfonylureas work by binding to the K_{ATP} channels of the beta cell to depolarize the membrane and allow insulin release. When mutations in the genes encoding the K_{ATP} channel subunits were discovered to be the most common cause of neonatal diabetes it was possible to transfer these patients very quickly from insulin injections to sulfonylurea tablets and achieve better glycemic control. This was only possible because the rigorous safety testing required for new pharmaceutical products had been completed many decades earlier, and use in many thousands of patients had not revealed any safety issues.

Rapamycin was first discovered in 1975 in a soil sample on Easter Island (the island is also known as Rapa Nui, hence the name rapamycin). It is a macrolide, produced by the microorganism *Streptomyces hygroscopius*, and showed antifungal properties. Shortly after its discovery, immunosuppressive properties were detected, which later led to the establishment of rapamycin as an immunosuppressant. In the 1980s, it was also found to have anticancer activity, although the exact mechanism of action remained unknown until the 1990s when it was shown to inhibit cellular proliferation and cell cycle progression via the PI3K/AKT/mTOR pathway (Fig. 15.9). Rapamycin (sirolimus) has recently been used to treat congenital hyperinsulinism as an alternative to subtotal pancreatectomy, and the rapamycin derivative, everolimus, is used in patients with tuberous sclerosis who have subependymal giant cell astrocytomas.

Another group of drugs that act within signaling pathways are the well-known antihypertensive agents, angiotensin-converting enzyme (ACE) inhibitors such as losartan and irbesartan. These have a beneficial effect in limiting aortic root dilatation in Marfan syndrome (p. 308), which is caused by activating variants of the *fibrillin-1* gene that increase transforming growth factor-beta (TGFβ) signaling (p. 108). The ACE inhibitor drugs decrease TGFβ signaling by interfering with the step leading to the production of angiotensin II. They may not be more effective in this role than more traditional beta-blockers.

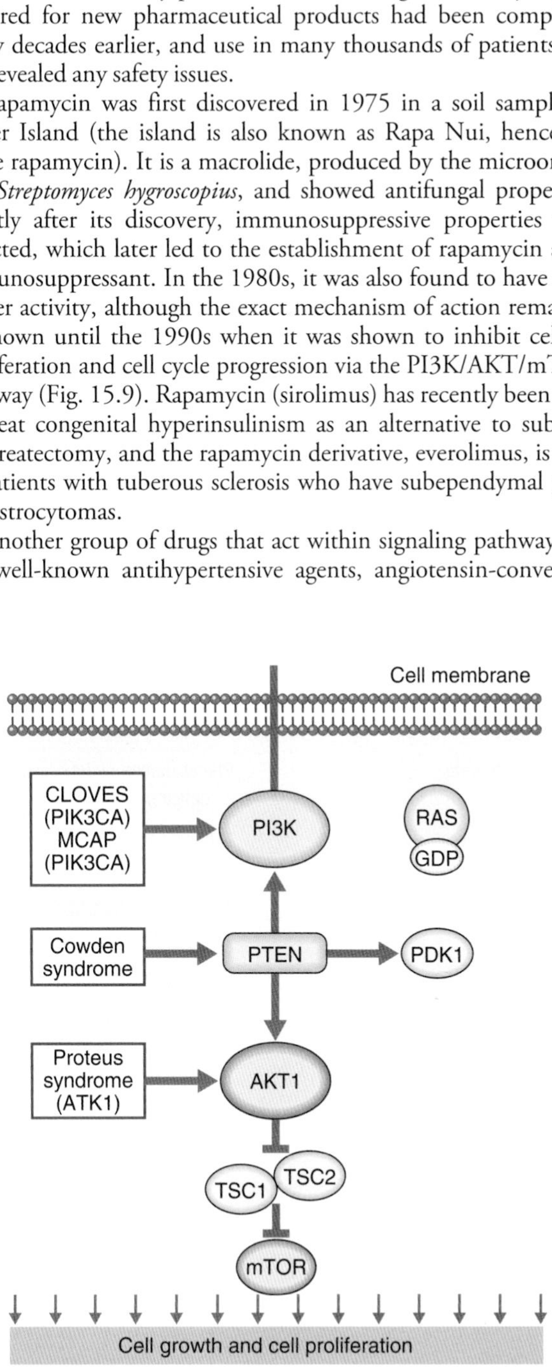

• **Fig. 15.9** The PI3K/AKT/mTOR pathway is an intracellular signaling pathway important in regulating the cell cycle. PI3K activation phosphorylates and activates AKT, localizing it in the plasma membrane. There are many known factors that enhance the PI3K/AKT pathway, including EGF, IGF-1, and insulin. The pathway is antagonized by various factors including PTEN. (Modified with permission from Eichenfield LF, Frieden I. Neonatal and Infant Dermatology. 3rd ed. Elsevier; 2014. With permission.)

Drug therapy might also be directed at a subset of patients according to their molecular defect. An example is the development of premature termination codon therapy (ataluren) for patients with nonsense mutations causing CF or Duchenne muscular dystrophy (DMD). Ataluren interacts with the ribosome to enable read-through of premature stop codons to produce full-length functional protein. It is now licensed in Europe for the treatment of DMD in boys aged 5 years and above. An alternative approach for treating DMD is to upregulate the dystrophin homolog, utrophin. Immune rejection is not a problem, and oral administration of the compound SMT022357 leads to increased utrophin expression in skeletal, respiratory, and cardiac muscles in the *mdx* mouse.

The cloning of the *CFTR* gene in 1989 gave great hope of a cure for CF through gene therapy. It was thought likely to be amenable to gene therapy because the level of functional protein sufficient to produce a clinical response might be as low as 5% to 10%, and the lung is a relatively accessible tissue. However, progress to date has been slow, and, although gene therapy can potentially correct the primary and secondary defects associated with CF, the extent and duration of gene expression has been inadequate, owing to the rapid turnover of lung epithelial cells.

The biggest breakthrough in the treatment of CF has come from the development of drugs designed to improve the function of the CFTR protein. The first drug, ivacaftor, is a CFTR potentiator that improves the transport of chloride ions through the ion channel by increasing the open probability of the channel. It was approved originally for the 4% of CF patients who have the p.Gly551Asp (G551D) mutation but is now also available for patients with nine other mutations that reduce channel activity. A second drug, lumacaftor, was developed to treat patients with the most common *CFTR* mutation, p.Phe508del. This mutation causes misfolding of the protein, and consequently the protein does not reach the cell surface. Lumacaftor, along with tezacaftor and elexacaftor, are correctors and designed to improve the folding of the protein in order for more protein to reach the cell surface. In 2015, combination therapy of ivacaftor with lumacaftor was shown to improve lung function for patients who are homozygous for the p.Phe508del *CFTR* mutation. These drugs were developed by Vertex pharmaceuticals in conjunction with the Cystic Fibrosis Foundation. Other combination therapies are now proving very successful, although they are very expensive drugs.

Tissue Transplantation. Replacement of diseased tissue has been a further option since the advent of tissue typing (p. 177). Examples are renal transplantation in adult polycystic kidney disease, lung transplantation in patients with CF, and bone marrow transplantation in a host of metabolic conditions.

Islet transplantation for treating type 1 diabetes mellitus was transformed in 2000 with development of the "Edmonton" protocol. Islet cells are prepared from donated pancreases (usually two per patient) and injected into the liver of the recipient: at 3 years posttransplant more than 80% of patients are still producing their own insulin.

Therapeutic Applications of Recombinant DNA Technology

The advent of recombinant DNA technology led to rapid progress in the availability of biosynthetic gene products. Insulin used in the treatment of diabetes mellitus was previously obtained from pig pancreases. It was purified very carefully, but even then occasionally produced sensitivity reactions in patients. Recombinant DNA technology enabled microorganisms to be used for the synthesis of large quantities of insulin from the human insulin gene.

Recombinant DNA technology is employed in the production of other biosynthetic products (Table 15.3). The biosynthesis of medically important peptides in this way is usually more expensive than obtaining the product from conventional sources because of the research and development involved. For example, the cost of treating one patient with Gaucher disease can exceed $150,000 per year. However, biosynthetically derived products have the dual advantages of providing a pure product that is unlikely to induce a sensitivity reaction, as well as being free of chemical or biological contamination. In the past, the use of growth hormone from human cadaver pituitaries was associated with the transmission of Creutzfeldt-Jakob disease, and HIV was a contaminant in cryoprecipitate containing factor VIII used in the treatment of hemophilia A (p. 316).

Gene Therapy

Gene therapy is the therapeutic delivery of nucleic acid polymers into a patient's cells as a drug to treat disease. It is defined by the UK Gene Therapy Advisory Committee ([GTAC], the UK Research Ethics Committee for gene therapy trials) as "the deliberate introduction of genetic material into human somatic cells for therapeutic, prophylactic, or diagnostic purposes." Gene therapy includes techniques for delivering synthetic or recombinant nucleic acids into humans; genetically modified biological vectors (such as viruses or plasmids), genetically modified stem cells, oncolytic viruses, nucleic acids associated with delivery vehicles, naked nucleic acids, antisense techniques (e.g., gene silencing, gene correction, or gene modification), genetic vaccines, DNA or RNA technologies such as RNA interference, and xenotransplantation of animal cells (but not solid organs).

Advances in molecular biology leading to the identification of many human disease genes and their protein products have raised the prospect of gene therapy for many monogenic (and nongenetic) disorders. The first human gene therapy trial began in 1990, but it is important to emphasize that, although it was heralded as the new panacea in medicine, progress has been slow, and there are still many practical difficulties to overcome before gene therapy can deliver its full potential. China undertook its first gene therapy trial in 2003 to treat head and neck squamous cell carcinoma, consisting of a modified virus carrying a gene which, when it reaches tumor cells, increases the expression of tumor-suppressing genes and immune response factors. Disorders that are possible candidates for gene therapy include both genetic and nongenetic diseases (Table 15.4).

TABLE 15.3 Proteins produced biosynthetically using recombinant DNA technology

Protein	Disease
Insulin	Diabetes mellitus
Growth hormone	Short stature resulting from growth hormone deficiency
Factor VIII	Hemophilia A
Factor IX	Hemophilia B
Erythropoietin	Anemia
α-Galactosidase A	Fabry disease (X-linked lysosomal storage disorder)
β-Interferon	Multiple sclerosis

TABLE 15.4 Diseases that can potentially be treated by gene therapy

Disorder	Defect
Immune deficiency	Adenosine deaminase deficiency
	Purine nucleoside phosphorylase deficiency
	Chronic granulomatous disease
Hypercholesterolemia	Low-density lipoprotein receptor abnormalities
Hemophilia	Factor VIII deficiency (A)
	Factor IX deficiency (B)
Gaucher disease	Glucocerebrosidase deficiency
Mucopolysaccharidosis VII	β-Glucuronidase deficiency
Emphysema	α_1-Antitrypsin deficiency
Cystic fibrosis	*CFTR* mutations
Phenylketonuria	Phenylalanine hydroxylase deficiency
Hyperammonemia	Ornithine transcarbamylase deficiency
Citrullinemia	Argininosuccinate synthetase deficiency
Muscular dystrophy	Dystrophin mutations
Spinal muscular atrophy	*SMN1* gene deletion
Thalassemia/sickle cell anemia	α- and β-globin mutations
Retinal diseases	RPE65, RPGR
Malignant melanoma	
Ovarian cancer	
Brain tumors	
Neuroblastoma	
Renal cancer	
Lung cancer	
Acquired immunodeficiency syndrome	
Cardiovascular diseases	
Rheumatoid arthritis	

Regulatory Requirements

There has been much publicity about the potential uses and abuses of gene therapy. Regulatory bodies have been established in several countries to oversee the technical, therapeutic, and safety aspects of gene therapy programs. There is universal agreement that **germline gene therapy**, in which genetic changes could be distributed to both somatic and germ cells, and thereby be transmitted to future generations, is morally and ethically unacceptable. Therefore programs are focusing only on **somatic cell gene therapy**, in which the alteration in genetic information is targeted to specific cells, tissues, or organs in which the disorder is manifest.

In the United States, the Human Gene Therapy Subcommittee of the National Institutes of Health has produced guidelines for protocols of trials of gene therapy that must be submitted for approval to both the US Food and Drug Administration (FDA) and the Recombinant DNA Advisory Committee, along with their institutional review boards. In the United Kingdom, the GTAC provides ethical oversight of proposals to conduct clinical trials involving gene or stem cell therapies in humans, taking account of the scientific merits, and the potential benefits and risks.

Some 3000 clinical trials of gene therapy have been approved for children and adults for a huge variety of genetic and non-genetic disorders, from inherited retinal/cone-rod dystrophies and neuromuscular conditions to cancer and heart failure (HF). Up until December 2019 there were 127 ongoing trials in the United Kingdom and approximately 1000 worldwide. Serious adverse events are rare, but the death in 1999 of a patient in a trial for ornithine transcarbamylase deficiency highlighted the risks of gene therapy and led to tighter regulation. There have also been three cases of leukemia in children, one of whom died, after receiving gene therapy for X-linked severe combined immunodeficiency (XL-SCID) (p. 180).

Technical Aspects

Prerequisites include that the genetic basis and pathophysiology of the disorder must be known, and the specific cells, tissue, or organ affected by the disease process must be accessible. The means by which the functional gene is introduced must be both efficient and safe. If gene therapy is to be considered as a realistic alternative to conventional treatments, there should be unequivocal evidence from trials of gene therapy carried out in animal models that the inserted gene functions adequately with appropriate regulatory, promoter, and enhancer sequences. In addition, it needs to be shown that the treated tissue or cell population has a reasonable lifespan, that the gene product continues to be expressed, and that the body does not react adversely to the gene product, for instance by producing antibodies to the protein product. Last, it is essential to demonstrate that introduction of the gene or DNA sequence has no deleterious effects, such as inadvertently leading to a malignancy or a mutagenic effect on either the somatic or the germ-cell lines, for example through mistakes arising as a result of the insertion of the gene or DNA sequence into the host DNA, or what is known as **insertional mutagenesis**. In two patients who developed leukemia after gene therapy for XL-SCID, the retrovirus used to deliver the γ-c *(IL2RG)* gene was shown to have inserted into the *LMO-2* oncogene on chromosome 11, which plays a role in some forms of childhood leukemia.

Gene Transfer

Gene transfer can be carried out either ex vivo by treatment of cells or tissue from an affected individual in culture, with reintroduction into the affected individual, or in vivo if cells cannot be cultured or replaced in the affected individual (Fig. 15.10). The ex vivo approach is limited to disorders in which the relevant cell population can be removed from the affected individual, modified genetically, and then replaced. The in vivo approach is the most direct strategy for gene transfer and can theoretically be used to treat many hereditary disorders.

Target Organs

Gene therapy is usually directed or limited to a particular organ, tissue, or body system.

Liver. Liver cells are susceptible to transfection by retroviruses in vitro. Cells removed from the liver by partial hepatectomy can be treated in vitro and then reinjected via the portal venous system, from which they seed in the liver. Hypercholesterolemia is a major cause of cardiovascular disease in the Western world. The most severe form, autosomal recessive familial hypercholesterolemia, is caused by biallelic variants in the LDL receptor (*LDLR*) gene. Patients are likely to require maintenance therapy with invasive LDL apheresis, and often die of myocardial infarction (MI) in their third decade of life. Gene therapy for lipid disorders has a high potential for success, but studies to date based on viral-mediated overexpression of *LDLR* cDNA have been unsuccessful, probably because vectors have lacked the sterol response elements that are required for regulated transcription.

Central Nervous System. Gene therapy for central nervous system disorders, such as Parkinson and Alzheimer diseases, requires delivery to the brain. Lentiviral vectors are particularly suitable because they integrate into the host genome of non-dividing cells and can

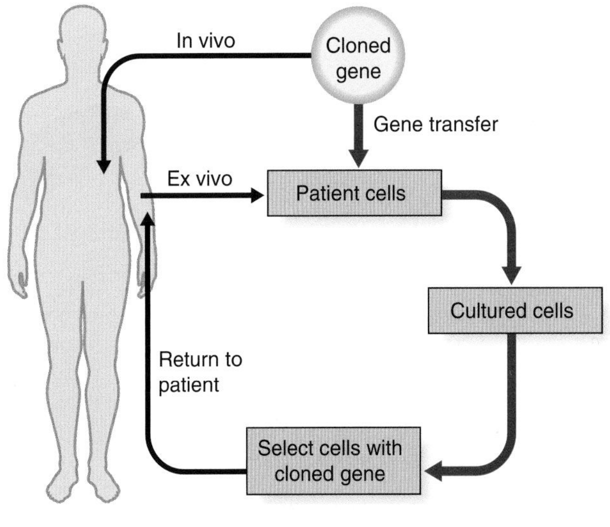

• **Fig. 15.10** In vivo and ex vivo gene therapy. In vivo gene therapy delivers genetically modified cells directly to the patient. An example is *CFTR* gene therapy using liposomes or adenovirus via nasal sprays. Ex vivo gene therapy removes cells from the patient, modifies them in vitro, and then returns them to the patient. An example is the treatment of fibroblasts from patients with hemophilia B by the addition of the factor IX gene. Modified fibroblasts are then injected into the stomach cavity.

potentially act as a delivery system for stable expression. Early clinical trials involving lentiviral delivery of three genes that encode enzymes that produce dopamine have yielded encouraging results. The first patients with advanced Parkinson disease to have this surgery have improved movement and better quality of life, and positron emission tomography scanning confirmed dopamine production in the brain.

Muscle. Unlike other tissues, direct injection of foreign DNA into muscle has been successful in terms of retention and expression of the foreign gene in the treated muscle. In 2012, the European Medicines Agency approved the first gene therapy treatment in either Europe or the United States. Alipogene tiparvovec is designed to restore lipoprotein lipase activity to clear fat-carrying chylomicron particles formed in the intestine after a fat-containing meal. It contains the human *LPL* gene packaged with a tissue-specific promoter in a non-replicating adeno-associated virus (AAV) vector. A naturally occurring variant of the gene is used that confers higher activity and is administered in a series of up to 60 intramuscular injections.

Heart. MI and HF are very common causes of morbidity and mortality worldwide. Massive loss of cardiomyocytes results from MI, with replacement by scar tissue because the adult mammalian heart has a low intrinsic regenerative capacity because of cell-cycle arrest; a frequent sequela is HF. The induction of cardiac regeneration by DNA-based or viral gene therapy approaches has met difficulties in the delivery of the introduced genes, and AAV vectors often trigger the production of neutralizing antibodies against the capsid. However, there is more hope from animal studies that modified mRNA (modRNA), which does not integrate into the host genome, will prove to be a safe, non-immunogenic treatment that is efficient, targeted and transient, but delivery remains a challenge.

In modRNA the naturally occurring uridine residue of mRNA is replaced by a modified nucleoside, pseudouridine. This change limits recognition by RNase (which cleaves mRNA) and the innate immune system via Toll-like receptors 7 and 8, which would otherwise lead to an increase in cytokine levels and toxicity, thus permitting enhanced translation (Fig. 15.11)

Bone Marrow. One of the first diseases for which gene therapy was attempted in humans is the inherited severe combined immunodeficiency disorder (SCID) caused by ADA deficiency (p. 180). The most successful conventional treatment for ADA deficiency is bone marrow transplantation from a matched sibling donor. The alternative is a twice weekly injection of the necessary enzyme, a life-long process that is very expensive and does not achieve optimal immune sufficiency.

A 4-year-old girl with ADA deficiency was the first patient ever to undergo gene therapy. The trial involved removal of white blood cells and correction with the *ADA* gene ex vivo before the cells were reinjected. This showed benefit, but the effect was temporary. In trials since 2009, patients have undergone autologous stem cell transplants with bone marrow cells corrected ex vivo using viral vectors. All treated children have developed their own new, fully functioning immune system and are now cured.

This approach has also been used in patients with beta thalassemia who have undergone ex vivo correction of their hematopoietic stem cells with a lentiviral vector containing the *HBB* gene and have not required blood transfusions since.

Eye. Leber congenital amaurosis is an autosomal recessive disorder caused by mutations in the *RPE65* gene and characterized by poor vision at birth with complete loss of vision in early adulthood. Early studies in a naturally occurring dog model (the Briard dog) showed that gene therapy by means of a single operation involving subretinal injection of an AAV vector carrying the full-length

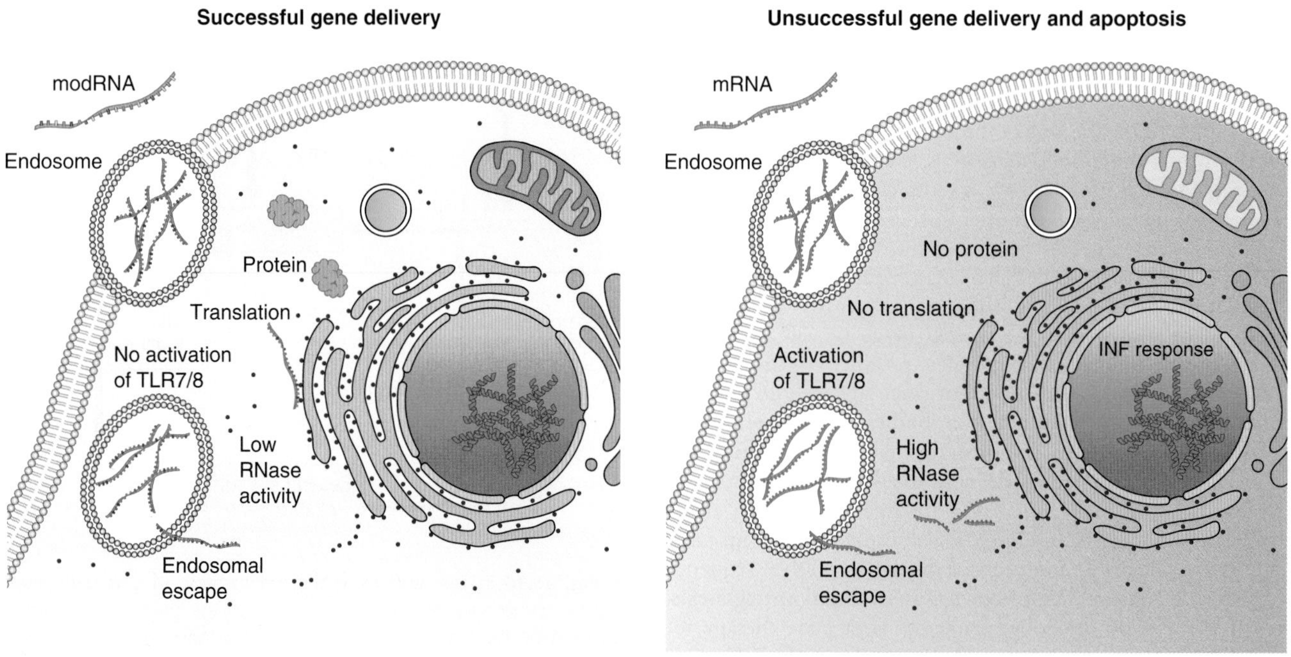

• **Fig. 15.11** The introduction of modified mRNA to the cell (left) largely avoids activation of the immune system via TLR7/8. mRNA would trigger such activation leading to degradation by RNase (right). (From Magadum A, Kaur K, Zangi L. mRNA-Based Protein Replacement Therapy for the Heart. *Mol Ther*. 2019;27:785–793. Fig. 2.)

RPE65 gene sequence was both safe and effective. Clinical trials in 2008 showed sustained improvement in 12 patients (aged 8–44 years) after treatment with an AAV vector containing the *RPE65* gene injected into the retinal pigment cells.

Another success is in treating choroidemia, caused by defects in the *CHM* gene. Lack of the REP-1 protein encoded by this gene means that cells in the retina stop working and slowly begin to die, causing blindness. Injection of an AAV vector carrying the *CHM* gene into the retina of six patients has shown improved vision. There is much excitement regarding the potential benefits for younger children whose loss of vision is not so far advanced. One obvious advantage for measuring the success of gene therapy in this condition is that a single eye can be treated whilst the other eye serves as a control. This research provides proof of principle that at least some forms of monogenic blindness may be reversed.

There are two main methods for delivering gene transfer, viral and non-viral.

Viral Agents

A number of different viruses can be used to transport foreign genetic material into cells, and the most successful viral agents are described in the following sections.

Lentiviruses. The lentivirus family includes HIV. Lentiviruses are complex viruses that infect macrophages and lymphocytes, but their main advantage is that they can be integrated into non-dividing cells. They may, therefore, be useful in the treatment of neurological conditions.

Adenoviruses. Adenoviruses can be used as vectors in gene therapy, as they infect a wide variety of cell types. They are stable, can infect non-dividing cells, and can carry up to 36 kilobases (kb) of foreign DNA. In addition, they are suitable for targeted treatment of specific tissues such as the respiratory tract, and have been extensively used in gene therapy trials for the treatment of CF.

Adenoviruses do not integrate into the host genome, thereby avoiding the possibility of insertional mutagenesis but having the disadvantage that expression of the introduced gene is usually unstable and often transient. They also contain genes known to be involved in the process of malignant transformation, so there is a potential risk that they could inadvertently induce malignancy. By virtue of their infectivity, they can produce adverse effects secondary to infection and by stimulating the host immune response. This was demonstrated by a vector-related death following intravascular administration of high doses (3.8×10^{13}) of adenovirus particles to a patient with ornithine transcarbamylase deficiency.

Adeno-Associated Viruses. AAVs are non-pathogenic parvoviruses in humans that require coinfection with helper adenoviruses or certain members of the herpes virus family to achieve infection. In the absence of the helper virus, the AAV DNA integrates into chromosomal DNA at a specific site on the long arm of chromosome 19 (19q13.3-qter). Subsequent infection with an adenovirus activates the integrated AAV DNA-producing virions. They have the advantages of being able to infect a wide variety of cell types, exhibiting long-term gene expression and not generating an immune response to transduced cells. The safety of AAVs as vectors occurs by virtue of their site-specific integration, but unfortunately, this is often impaired with the inclusion of foreign DNA in the virus. The disadvantages of AAVs include the fact that they can be activated by any adenovirus infection and that, although 95% of the vector genome is removed, they can take inserts of foreign DNA of only up to 5 kb in size.

Non-viral Methods

There are a number of different non-viral methods of gene therapy, but the most popular is liposome-mediated DNA transfer. This has the theoretical advantage of not eliciting an immune response, being safer and simpler to use, and allowing large-scale production, but efficacy is limited.

Liposomes. Liposomes are lipid bilayers surrounding an aqueous vesicle that can facilitate the introduction of foreign DNA into a target cell (Fig. 15.12). A disadvantage of liposomes is that they are not very efficient in gene transfer, and the expression of the foreign gene is transient, so that the treatment has to be repeated. An advantage of liposome-mediated gene transfer is that a much larger DNA sequence can be introduced into the target cells or tissues than with viral vector systems.

RNA Modification

RNA modification therapy targets mRNA, either by suppressing mRNA levels or by correcting/adding function to the mRNA.

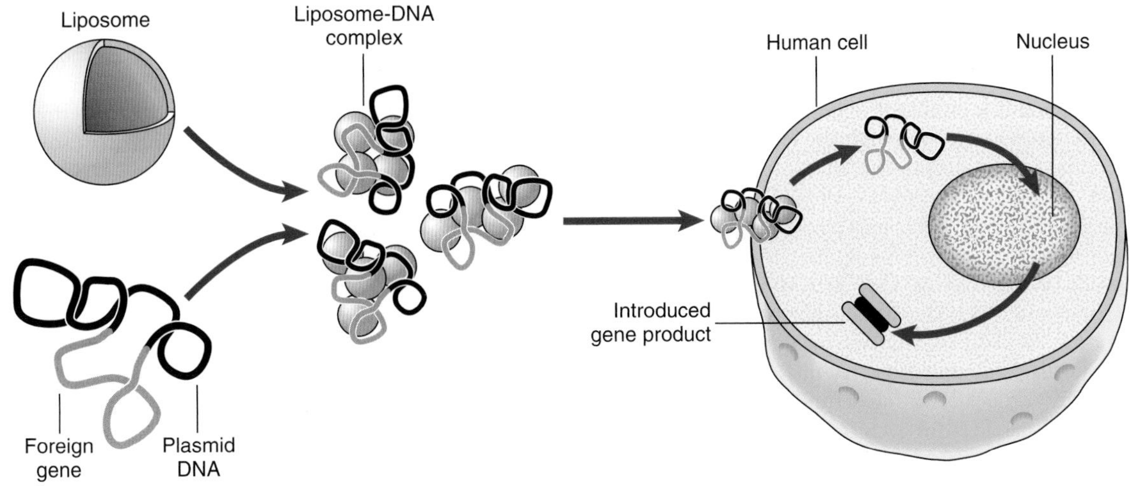

• **Fig. 15.12** Diagrammatic representation of liposome-mediated gene therapy.

Antisense Oligonucleotides

Antisense therapy may be used to modulate the expression of genes associated with monogenic disorders. The principle of antisense technology is the sequence-specific binding of an antisense oligonucleotide (typically 18 to 30 bases in length) to a target mRNA that results in inhibition of gene expression at the protein level.

Antisense oligonucleotides can be used to force exon skipping and convert out-of-frame deletions that cause DMD to in-frame deletions usually associated with the milder Becker muscular dystrophy phenotype. This approach could be successful for up to 70% of patients with DMD. The first clinical trial involved four patients who underwent intramuscular injection of an antisense oligonucleotide targeted to the specific skipping of exon 51, using eteplirsen (*aka* Exondys 51). Dystrophin was restored in the vast majority of muscle fibers at levels between 17% and 35%, without any adverse effects. However, the results from a phase III trial in 2013 were disappointing. Whereas the boys who received 48 weeks' treatment with the antisense drug, drisapersen, were able to walk approximately 10 meters further than those who received the placebo, this difference was not statistically significant.

One key hurdle in the use of antisense oligonucleotide therapy is the fact that each different antisense is considered a new drug and requires separate regulatory approval. This makes their development more expensive and not feasible for low-prevalence mutations for which there would be insufficient patients for clinical trials. In 2017 to 2018 a young patient with Batten disease (caused by biallelic pathogenic variants in *CLN7*) was treated with a bespoke 22-nucleotide antisense oligonucleotide, milasen. There was measurable benefit in the reduction of seizure frequency.

The potential for antisense therapy is perhaps greater in spinal muscular atrophy (p. 294) where the non-expressed *SMN2* gene could be converted to generate functional SMN1 protein in virtually all patients, using an FDA-approved antisense oligonucleotide drug, nusinersen. Trials have shown extended survival in infants, and use of the therapy in clinical practice is drawing closer. An antisense approach is also under trial for Huntington disease (p. 289), using intraspinal injections of a drug named ISIS-HTT designed to bind with mRNA produced from the expanded allele and encourage the toxic protein to be eliminated.

RNA Interference

This technique also has broad therapeutic application, as any gene may be a potential target for silencing by RNA interference. In contrast to antisense oligonucleotide therapy, where the target mRNA is bound, as a result of RNA interference the target mRNA is cleaved, and it is estimated to be up to 1000-fold more active. RNA interference works through the targeted degradation of mRNAs containing homologous sequences to synthetic double-stranded RNA molecules known as small interfering RNAs (siRNAs) (Fig. 15.13). The siRNAs may be delivered in drug form using strategies developed to stabilize antisense oligonucleotides, or from plasmids or viral vectors. One such compound is ALN-TTR02 (*aka* patisiran), which targets transthyretin (TTR) amyloid deposits. These are the cause of familial amyloidotic polyneuropathy in patients with *TTR* mutations. A phase I study showed approximately 85% knockdown of serum TTR protein and neurological disease stabilized or even improved over 6 months. However, more conventional therapy is also proving effective because stabilization of the correctly folded tetrameric form of TTR is possible through a pharmacological chaperone called tafamidis, which binds in one of the two thyroxine-binding sites of the tetramer.

Another success for siRNA therapy has been achieved using once-monthly subcutaneous injections of givosiran in patients with acute intermittent porphyria (AIP, p. 282). AIP is caused by induction of delta aminolevulinic acid synthase 1 (*ALAS1*) gene expression. Patients in the treatment arm of the trial showed reductions in induced *ALAS1* mRNA levels, as well as the neurotoxic intermediates, delta aminolevulinic acid and porphobilinogen, and a lower rate of porphyria attacks occurred compared with those in the placebo arm. Some low-grade adverse events were reported.

Targeted Gene Correction

The repair of genes in situ through the cellular DNA repair machinery (p. 23) is promising. Proof of principle has been demonstrated in an animal model of Pompe disease (p. 277). The point mutation was targeted by chimeric double-stranded DNA-RNA oligonucleotides containing the correct nucleotide sequence. Repair was demonstrated at the DNA level, and normal enzyme activity was restored.

Homologous recombination can be stimulated by the use of engineered zinc-finger nucleases (ZFNs). Targeted cleavage of DNA is achieved by zinc-finger proteins designed to recognize unique chromosomal sites and fuse to the nonspecific DNA cleavage domain of a restriction enzyme. A double-strand break induced by the resulting ZFNs can create specific changes in the genome by stimulating homology-directed DNA repair between the locus of interest and an extrachromosomal molecule. One report describes ZFN-driven gene correction in bone marrow stem cells from patients with sickle cell disease that resulted in the production of wild-type hemoglobin tetramers.

In the future, CRISPR/Cas9 technology (p. 47) offers great potential for genome editing to treat genetic disease. Early approaches will harvest patient hematopoietic stem cells and correct the genetic defect *ex vivo* before returning the cells to the patient's bone marrow.

Stem Cell Therapy

Stem cells are unspecialized cells that are defined by their capacity for self-renewal and the ability to differentiate into specialized cells along many lineages. Embryonic stem cells are pluripotent, which means they can give rise to derivatives of all three germ layers (i.e., all cell types that are found in the adult organism). Somatic stem cells can only differentiate into the cell types found in the tissue from which they are derived (Fig. 15.14), but can be isolated from any human, whatever their age. Nowadays the term **induced pluripotent stem cell** (**iPS cell**) is used rather than **somatic** or **adult stem cell**.

Bone-marrow transplantation is a form of somatic stem cell therapy that has been used for more than 40 years. During the past 5 years, cord blood stem cells have emerged as an alternative source. Although these transplants can be an effective treatment for a number of genetic disorders, including ADA deficiency, SCID, X-linked adrenoleukodystrophy, lysosomal storage diseases, and Fanconi anemia, the associated risks of infection caused by immunosuppression and graft-versus-host disease are high. The main limitation is the lack of a suitable bone-marrow donor or availability of matched cord blood stem cells.

Transplantation of stem cells (e.g., pluripotent hematopoietic stem cells) in utero offers the prospect of a novel mode of treatment

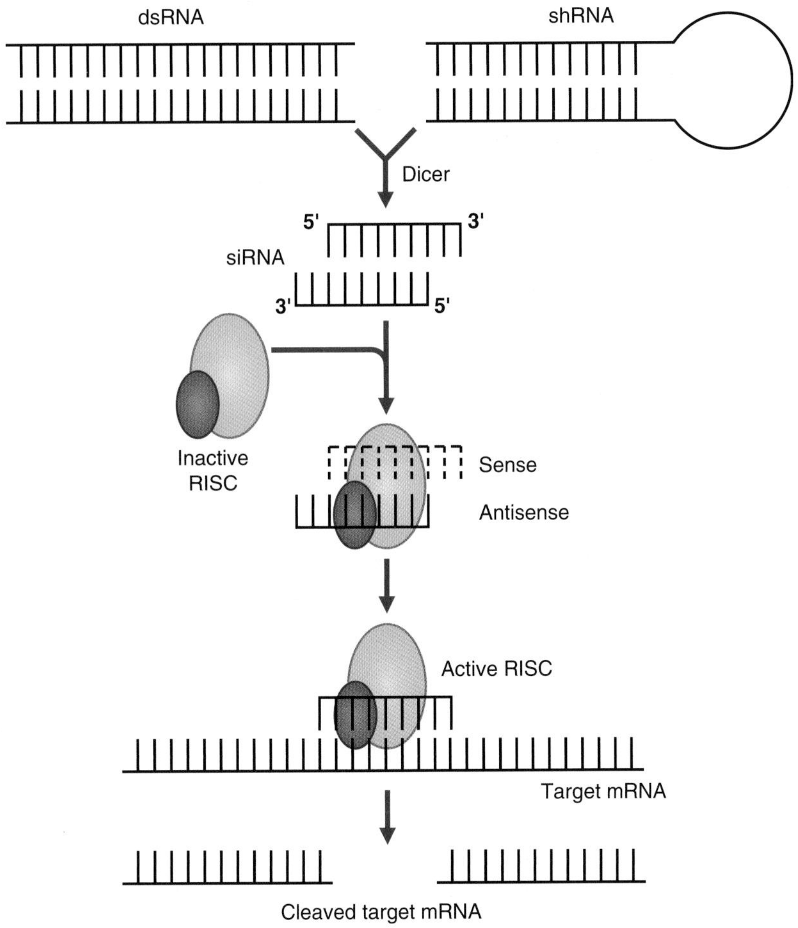

• **Fig. 15.13** Mechanism of RNA interference. Double-stranded (ds) RNAs are processed by Dicer, in an adenosine triphosphate (ATP)-dependent process, to produce small interfering RNAs (*siRNAs*) of about 21–23 nucleotides in length with two-nucleotide overhangs at each end. Short hairpin RNAs, either produced endogenously or expressed from viral vectors, are also processed by Dicer into siRNA. An ATP-dependent helicase is required to unwind the dsRNA, allowing one strand to bind to the RNA-induced silencing complex (*RISC*). Binding of the antisense RNA strand activates the RISC to cleave mRNAs containing a homologous sequence. (From Lieberman J, Song E, Lee SK, Shankar P. Interfering with disease: opportunities and roadblocks to harnessing RNA interference. *Trends Mol Med*. 2003;9:397–403. With permission.)

for genetic disorders with a congenital onset. The immaturity of the fetal immune system means that the fetus will be tolerant of foreign cells, so that there is no need to match the donor cells with those of the fetus. A small number of trials have been performed, but engraftment has so far only been successful in cases of SCID.

Embryonic Stem Cell Therapy

Teratomas (benign) and teratocarcinomas (malignant) are tumors that are found most commonly in the gonads. Their name is derived from the Greek word "teratos" (monster); it describes their appearance well, as these tumors contain teeth, pieces of bone, muscles, skin, and hair. A key experiment demonstrated that if a single cell is removed from one of these tumors and injected intraperitoneally, it acts as a stem cell by producing all the cell types found in a teratocarcinoma.

Mouse embryonic stem cells were first isolated and cultured 30 years ago. Studies of human embryonic stem cells have lagged behind, but the pace of research increased exponentially following the achievement in 1998 of the first cultured human embryonic stem cells.

Embryonic Stem Cells for Transplantation

The ability of an embryonic stem cell (ESC) to differentiate into any type of cell means that the potential applications of ESC therapy are vast. One approach involves the differentiation of ESCs in vitro to provide specialized cells for transplantation. For example, it is possible to culture mouse ESCs to generate dopamine-producing neurons. When these neural cells were transplanted into a mouse model for Parkinson disease, the dopamine-producing neurons showed long-term survival and ultimately corrected the phenotype. This "therapeutic cloning" strategy has been proposed as a future therapy for other brain disorders such as stroke and neurodegenerative diseases. However, after many encouraging small studies of fetal cell transplantation for Parkinson disease, three randomized, double-blind, placebo-controlled studies found no net benefit. Also, patients in two of the studies developed dyskinesias that persisted despite reductions in medication. Further research is needed to understand and overcome the dual problems of unpredictable benefit and troublesome dyskinesias after dopaminergic cell transplantation. In addition, postmortem analysis of patients who received fetal brain cell transplantation revealed that implanted cells are prone to degeneration just like endogenous

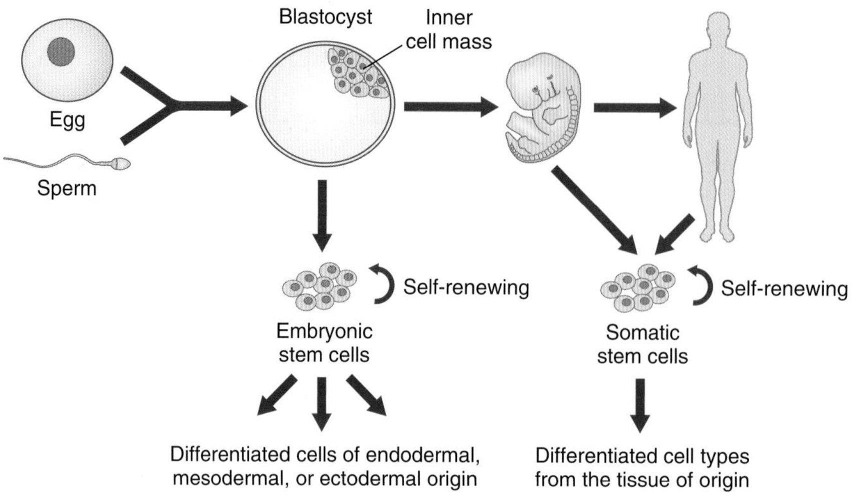

• **Fig. 15.14** Generation of embryonic and somatic stem cells. The fusion of the sperm and egg during fertilization establishes a diploid zygote that divides to create the blastocyst. Embryonic stem cells (ESCs) are derived from the inner cell mass of the blastocyst. ESCs in culture are capable of self-renewal without differentiation and are able to differentiate into all cell types of the endoderm, mesoderm, and ectoderm lineages using appropriate signals. Somatic stem cells are also capable of self-renewal and, with appropriate signals, differentiate into various cell types from the tissue from which they are derived.

neurons in the same pathological area, indicating that long-term efficacy of cell therapy of Parkinson disease needs to overcome the degenerative environment in the brain.

Gene Therapy Using Embryonic Stem Cells

An alternate strategy is to use ESCs as delivery vehicles for genes that mediate phenotype correction through gene-transfer technology. One potential barrier to using human ESCs to treat genetic disorders is immunorejection of the transplanted cells by the host. This obstacle might be overcome by using gene transfer with the relevant normal gene to autologous cells (such as cultured skin fibroblasts), transfer of the corrected nucleus to an enucleated egg from an unrelated donor, development of "corrected" ESCs and, finally, differentiation and transplantation of the corrected relevant cells to the same patient (Fig. 15.15).

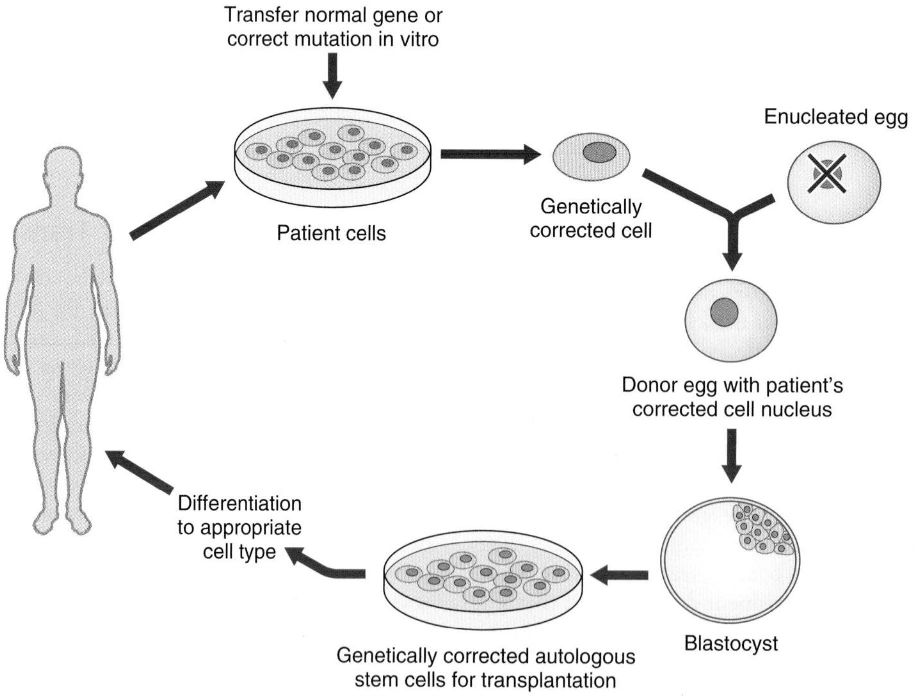

• **Fig. 15.15** Embryonic stem cells for gene therapy. The strategy depicted starts with removing cells (e.g., fibroblasts) from a patient with a monogenic disorder and then transferring the normal gene using a vector (or perhaps by correcting the mutation in vitro). The nucleus from a corrected cell is then transferred to an enucleated egg obtained from an unrelated donor by somatic cell nuclear transfer. The egg, now containing the genetically corrected genome of the patient, is activated to develop into a blastocyst in vitro, and corrected autologous stem cells are derived from the inner cell mass. The stem cells are then directed to differentiate into a specific cell type and transferred to the patient, thereby correcting the disorder.

A crucial component of future clinical applications of this strategy is the ability to derive "personalized" human ESC lines using the nuclear transfer technique. Although research on this technology has been controversial, the efficient transfer of somatic cell nuclei to enucleated oocytes from unrelated donors, and the subsequent derivation of human ESC lines from the resulting blastocysts, is a technical hurdle that has been overcome.

There has been much debate around the ethical issues of using ESCs, and it seems that embryonic stem cells may not be an essential prerequisite, as iPS cells have been found in many more tissues than was once thought possible. Hence iPS cells might be used for transplantation.

Induced Pluripotent Stem Cell Therapy

Certain kinds of somatic stem cell appear to have the ability to differentiate into a number of different cell types, given the right conditions. Recent progress in stem cell biology has shown that iPS-derived cells can be used to successfully treat rodent Parkinson disease models, thus solving the problem of immunorejection and paving the way for future autologous transplantations for treating this disease and others.

Mesenchymal Stem Cells

Mesenchymal stem cell (MSC) therapy, through its promise of repair and regeneration of cardiac tissue, represents an exciting avenue of treatment for a range of cardiovascular diseases. Cardiovascular disease is the leading cause of death in developed countries. Although cardiomyocytes retain limited plasticity following maturation, the heart is grossly unable to recover from structural damage.

MSCs are relatively immunoprivileged, lacking both major histocompatibility II and T-cell co-stimulatory signal expression, and possess the unique ability to home into sites of myocardial damage when delivered systemically. They are obtained either from the bone marrow of healthy adult volunteers or from the patients themselves and cultured in vitro with appropriate factors before being delivered to the damaged heart. Animal studies have shown therapeutic benefit via several distinct mechanisms, the most important of which appears to be the abundant secretion of paracrine factors that promote local regeneration. Clinical trials have shown that this approach is safe, and the results of further trials are awaited to see if there will be clear clinical benefit.

The genetic disorder retinitis pigmentosa (p. 339) results in the loss of photoreceptors, leading to visual symptoms in the teens and blindness by 40 to 50 years of age. Systemic administration of pluripotent bone marrow-derived MSCs in a rat model has demonstrated improved visual function, and trials are in progress to test this approach in humans. This is a potentially exciting development for the future treatment of other forms of retinal degeneration and other ocular vascular diseases such as diabetic retinopathy.

A third application of MSC therapy is in bone repair and metabolic bone diseases such as osteogenesis imperfecta (p. 77) and hypophosphatasia, because MSCs can also differentiate to form bone and cartilage.

Limbal Stem Cells

The corneal limbus harbors corneal epithelial stem cells known as **limbal stem cells** (**LSC**s). Corneal conditions, such as infections, tumors immunological disorders, trauma, and chemical burns, often lead to the deficiency of the corneal stem cells and subsequent vision loss. Treatment of limbal stem cell deficiency (LSCD) has been achieved in eight patients who had complete LSCD in one eye. A small sample of the limbal epithelium of the patient's healthy eye was removed and grown in cell culture using the patient's own serum and donated amniotic cells to provide the required conditioning medium. Twelve days later, the LSCs were transplanted onto the patients' unhealthy eye, and the group was followed for around 18 months. Overall, all patients had a decrease in pain and an increase in visual acuity.

Stem cell therapy has now progressed from preclinical (animal studies) to clinical trials for a variety of disorders. In general, these studies have shown enormous potential in the animal models but more limited success in humans so far. Aside from participation in regulated trials, patients should be advised that stem cell therapy is at an early stage and discouraged from undergoing forms of treatment whose safety and efficacy is not yet proven. An unwanted spin-off from stem cell research has been the development of so-called stem cell tourism. Patients have traveled to countries where stem cell–based treatment is not regulated to receive expensive treatments that are scientifically unproven. These treatments are at best, ineffective, and at worst, dangerous.

ELEMENTS

1. Pharmacogenomics is defined as the study of the interaction of an individual's genetic makeup and response to a drug. The key distinction between pharmacogenetics and pharmacogenomics is that the former describes the study of variability in drug responses attributed to individual genes and the latter describes the study of the entire genome related to drug response.
2. Knowledge regarding the genetic etiology and pathophysiology of the disease process can lead to stratified treatments. Examples of so-called personalized or precision medicine include sulfonylurea therapy for certain monogenic subtypes of diabetes, ivacaftor and lumacaftor for CF, trastuzumab for breast cancers showing *HER2* overexpression, imatinib for chronic myeloid leukemia, and gefitinib for non–small cell lung cancers with activating *EGFR* mutations. Testing for B*5701 status before prescribing abacavir is now routine for patients with human immunodeficiency virus infection to reduce the risk of potentially fatal hypersensitivity.
3. Gene therapy is the therapeutic delivery of genetic material into a patient's cells as a drug to treat disease. It requires that the gene involved must be characterized, the particular cell type or tissue to be targeted must be identified, an efficient, reliable, and safe vector system that results in stable continued expression of the introduced gene has to be developed, and the safety and effectiveness of the particular modality of gene therapy has to be demonstrated. Some success has been achieved by delivering a functional copy of the relevant gene, or through modifying gene expression through antisense therapy, but gene therapy is still in its infancy despite the regulatory approval of many trials.
4. Germline gene therapy is universally viewed as ethically unacceptable, whereas somatic cell gene therapy is generally viewed as being acceptable, because this is seen as similar to existing treatments such as organ transplantation.
5. Embryonic or induced pluripotent stem cells might be used therapeutically in a regenerative approach in which they are differentiated *in vitro* to specialized cell types (or progenitors of the target specialized cells), and then transplanted *in vivo* to replace diseased cells or tissues. Alternatively they could be used as delivery vehicles for gene-transfer technology.

Further Reading

Aartsma-Rus A, van Ommen GJB. Progress in therapeutic antisense applications for neuromuscular disease. *Eur J Hum Genet.* 2010;18: 146–153.

A review of antisense oligonucleotide therapy for Duchenne muscular dystrophy, spinal muscular atrophy, and myotonic dystrophy.

Belmonte JCI, Ellis J, Hochedlinger K, Yamanaka S. Induced pluripotent stem cells and reprogramming: seeing the science through the hype. *Nat Rev Genet.* 2009;10:878–883.

An overview of the advantages and disadvantages of embryonic stem cell vs. induced pluripotent stem cell therapy.

Brown BD, Naldini L. Exploiting and antagonizing microRNA regulation for therapeutic and experimental applications. *Nat Rev Genet.* 2009;10:578–585.

Article describing the potential applications of RNA interference.

Goldstein DB, Tate SK, Sisodiya SM. Pharmacogenetics goes genomic. *Nat Rev Genet.* 2003;4:937–947.

Review of pharmacogenetics/genomics.

Kim J, Hu C, El Achkar CM, et al. Patient-customized oligonucleotide therapy for a rare genetic disease. *N Engl J Med.* 2019;381: 1644–1652.

Case report of antisense oligonucleotide treatment of Batten disease.

Lim KRQ, Maruyama R, Yokota T. Eteplirsen in the treatment of Duchenne muscular dystrophy. *Drug Des Devel Ther.* 2017;11: 533–545.

A report of the use of exon-skipping therapy for Duchenne muscular dystrophy.

Newman W, Payne K. Removing barriers to a clinical pharmacogenetics service. *Per Med.* 2008;5:471–480.

A review article describing the application of pharmacogenetics to current clinical practice.

Pearson ER, Flechtner I, Njolstad PR, et al. Switching from insulin to oral sulfonylureas in patients with diabetes due to Kir6.2 mutations. *N Engl J Med.* 2006;355:467–477.

Pharmacogenetic treatment of monogenic diabetes.

Pennisi E. The CRISPR craze. *Science.* 2013;341:833–836.

The discovery and promise of CRISPR technology.

Sardh E, Harper P, Balwani M, et al. Phase 1 trial of an RNA interference therapy for acute intermittent porphyria. *N Engl J Med.* 2019; 380:549–558.

Therapy using small interfering RNA.

Yamanaka S. Induced pluripotent stem cells: Past, present and future. *Cell Stem Cell.* 2012;10:678–684.

The fascinating history and future of stem cell research, with insights into the future applications of induced pluripotent stem cells.

16 Congenital Abnormalities, Dysmorphic Syndromes, and Intellectual Disability

They certainly give very strange names to diseases.

Plato

The formation of a human being, sometimes called **morphogenesis**, involves extremely complicated cell biology and, although still not fully elucidated, has begun to yield its mysteries (see Chapter 9). Given the complexity, it is not surprising that on occasion it goes wrong. Nor is it surprising that in many congenital abnormalities genetic factors can clearly be implicated. More than 5000 dysmorphic, multiple congenital anomaly and intellectual disability (ID) syndromes are described in the London Dysmorphology Database, covering single-gene (mendelian) disorders and sporadic and nongenetic conditions, as well those caused by teratogenic agents. For most of those attributed to single-gene pathogenic variants the cause is now known, and next-generation sequencing technology has the power to uncover the underlying reason in many of the rest. We cannot do justice to this vast field in a limited space, and many examples feature elsewhere (e.g., Chapters 9 and 17), but in this chapter we consider the overall impact of abnormalities in morphogenesis by reviewing:

1. The incidence of abnormalities at various stages from conception onwards.
2. Their nature and the ways in which they can be classified.
3. Their causes, when known, with particular emphasis on the role of genetics.

Incidence

Spontaneous First-Trimester Pregnancy Loss

It has been estimated that approximately 50% of all human conceptions are lost either before implantation at 5 to 6 days postconception or shortly afterwards, that is, before the woman realizes she is pregnant. Among recognized pregnancies, at least 15% end in spontaneous miscarriage before 12 weeks' gestation. Even when material from the abortus can be obtained, it is often very difficult to establish why a pregnancy loss has occurred. However, careful study of large numbers of spontaneously aborted embryos has shown that gross structural abnormalities are present in 80% to 85%. These abnormalities vary from complete absence of an embryo in the developing pregnancy sac—a **blighted ovum**—to a very distorted body shape, or a specific abnormality in one body system.

Chromosome abnormalities such as trisomy, monosomy, or triploidy are found in approximately 50% of all spontaneous abortions. This incidence rises to 60% when a gross structural abnormality is present, and it is very likely that submicroscopic or *de novo* single-gene abnormalities account for a proportion of the remainder.

Congenital Abnormalities and Perinatal Mortality

Perinatal mortality figures include all infants who are stillborn after 28 weeks' gestation plus deaths during the first week of life. Of all perinatal deaths, 25% to 30% occur as a result of a serious structural abnormality, and in 80% of these cases genetic factors can be implicated. The relative contribution of structural abnormalities to perinatal mortality is lower in developing countries, where environmental factors and health care provision play a much greater role.

Newborn Infants

Surveys reviewing the incidence of both major and minor anomalies in newborn infants have been undertaken in many countries. A major anomaly can be defined as one that has an adverse outcome on either the function or the social acceptability of the individual (Table 16.1). In contrast, minor abnormalities are of neither medical nor cosmetic importance (Box 16.1). However, the division between major and minor abnormalities is not always straightforward; for instance, an inguinal hernia occasionally leads to strangulation of bowel and always requires surgical correction, so there is a risk of serious sequelae.

Surveys consistently show that 2% to 3% of all newborns have at least one major abnormality apparent at birth. The true incidence, taking into account abnormalities that present later in life, such as brain malformations, is probably around 5%. Minor abnormalities are found in approximately 10% of all newborns. If two or more minor abnormalities are present in a newborn, there is a 10% to 20% risk that the baby will also have a major malformation.

The long-term outlook for a baby with a major abnormality obviously depends on the nature of the specific birth defect and whether it can be treated. The overall prognosis for this group of newborns is relatively poor, with up to 25% dying in early infancy, 25% having subsequent mental or physical disability, and the remaining 50% having a fair or good outlook after treatment.

Childhood Mortality

Congenital abnormalities make a significant contribution to mortality throughout childhood. During infancy, approximately 25%

TABLE 16.1 Examples of major congenital structural abnormalities

System and Abnormality	Incidence per 1000 Births
Cardiovascular	***10***
Ventricular septal defect	2.5
Atrial septal defect	1
Patent ductus arteriosus	1
Tetralogy of Fallot	1
Central Nervous System	***10***
Anencephaly	1
Hydrocephaly	1
Microcephaly	1
Lumbosacral spina bifida	2
Gastrointestinal	***4***
Cleft lip/palate	1.5
Diaphragmatic hernia	0.5
Esophageal atresia	0.3
Imperforate anus	0.2
Limb	***2***
Transverse amputation	0.2
Urogenital	***4***
Bilateral renal agenesis	2
Polycystic kidneys (infantile)	0.02
Bladder exstrophy	0.03

of all deaths are the result of major structural abnormalities, falling to 20% between 1 and 10 years of age and to approximately 7.5% between 10 and 15 years.

Collating the incidence data on abnormalities noted in early spontaneous miscarriages and newborns, at least 15% of all recognized human conceptions are structurally abnormal (Table 16.2), and genetic factors are implicated in probably at least 50% of these.

Definition and Classification of Birth Defects

So far in this chapter the terms 'congenital abnormality' and 'birth defect' have been used in a general sense to describe all types of structural abnormality that can occur in an embryo, fetus or newborn infant. Although these terms are perfectly acceptable for the purpose of lumping together all these abnormalities when studying their overall incidence, they do not provide any insight into possible underlying mechanisms. More specific definitions have been devised that have the added advantage of providing a combined clinical and etiological classification.

• BOX 16.1 Examples of Minor Congenital Structural Abnormalities

Preauricular pit or tag
Epicanthic folds
Lacrimal duct stenosis
Brushfield spots in the iris
Lip pits
Single palmar crease
Fifth finger clinodactyly
Syndactyly between second and third toes
Supernumerary nipple
Umbilical hernia
Hydrocele
Sacral pit or dimple

TABLE 16.2 Incidence of structural abnormalities

Incidence	(%)
Spontaneous Miscarriages	
First trimester	80–85
Second trimester	25
All Babies	
Major abnormality apparent at birth	2–3
Major abnormality apparent later	2
Minor abnormality	10
Death in perinatal period	25
Death in first year of life	25
Death at 1–9 years	20
Death at 10–14 years	7.5

Single Abnormalities

Single abnormalities may have a genetic or non-genetic basis. The system of terms used helps us to understand the different mechanisms that might be implicated, and these can be illustrated in schematic form (Fig. 16.1).

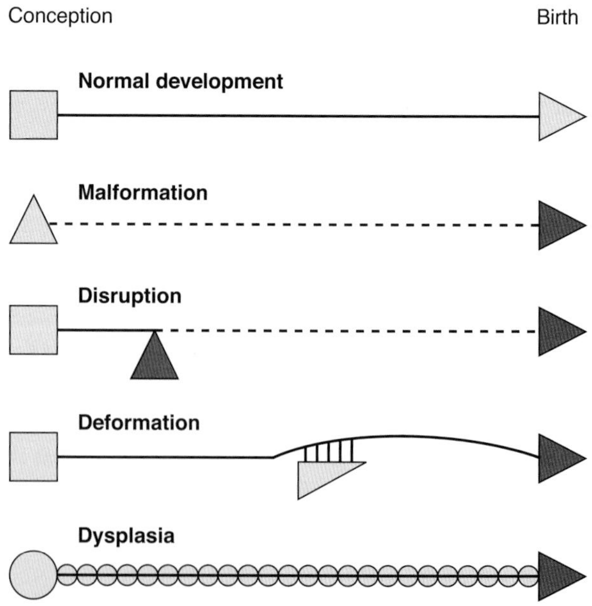

• **Fig. 16.1** Schematic representation of the different mechanisms in morphogenesis. For malformation, disruption and dysplasia, the broken line symbolizes developmental potential rather than timing of the manifestation of the defect, which might be late in embryogenesis. (Modified from Spranger J, Benirschke K, Hall JG, et al. Errors of morphogenesis: concepts and terms. *J Pediatr*. 1982;100:160–165.)

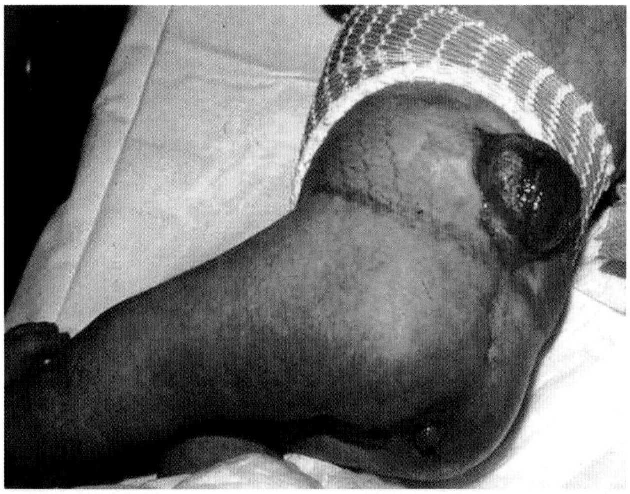

• **Fig. 16.2** Child with a large thoracolumbar myelomeningocele consisting of protruding spinal cord covered by meninges.

Malformation

A **malformation** is a primary structural defect of an organ, or part of an organ, that results from an inherent abnormality in development. This used to be known as a primary or intrinsic malformation. The presence of a malformation implies that the early development of a particular tissue or organ has been arrested or misdirected. Common examples include congenital heart abnormalities such as ventricular or atrial septal defects, cleft lip, and/or palate or neural tube defects (Fig. 16.2). Most malformations involving only a single organ show multifactorial inheritance, implying an interaction of gene(s) with other factors (see Chapter 10). Multiple malformations are more likely to be as a result of chromosomal abnormalities but may be caused by single gene pathogenic variants.

Disruption

The term **disruption** refers to an abnormal structure of an organ or tissue as a result of external factors disturbing the normal developmental process. This used to be known as a secondary or extrinsic malformation, and includes ischemia, infection, and trauma. An example of a disruption is the effect seen on limb development when a strand, or band, of amnion becomes entwined around a baby's limb or digits (Fig. 16.3). By definition a disruption is not genetic, although occasionally genetic factors can predispose to disruptive events. For example, a small proportion of amniotic bands are caused by an underlying genetically determined defect in collagen that weakens the amnion, making it more liable to tear or rupture spontaneously.

Deformation

A **deformation** is a defect resulting from an abnormal mechanical force that distorts an otherwise normal structure. Examples include dislocation of the hip and mild positional talipes, or clubfoot (Fig. 16.4), resulting from reduced amniotic fluid (oligohydramnios), intrauterine crowding from twinning, or a structurally abnormal uterus. Deformations usually occur late in pregnancy and carry a good prognosis with appropriate treatment—for instance, gentle splinting for talipes—because the underlying organ is fundamentally normal in structure.

Dysplasia

A **dysplasia** is an abnormal organization or assembly of cells into tissue. The effects are usually seen wherever that particular tissue is

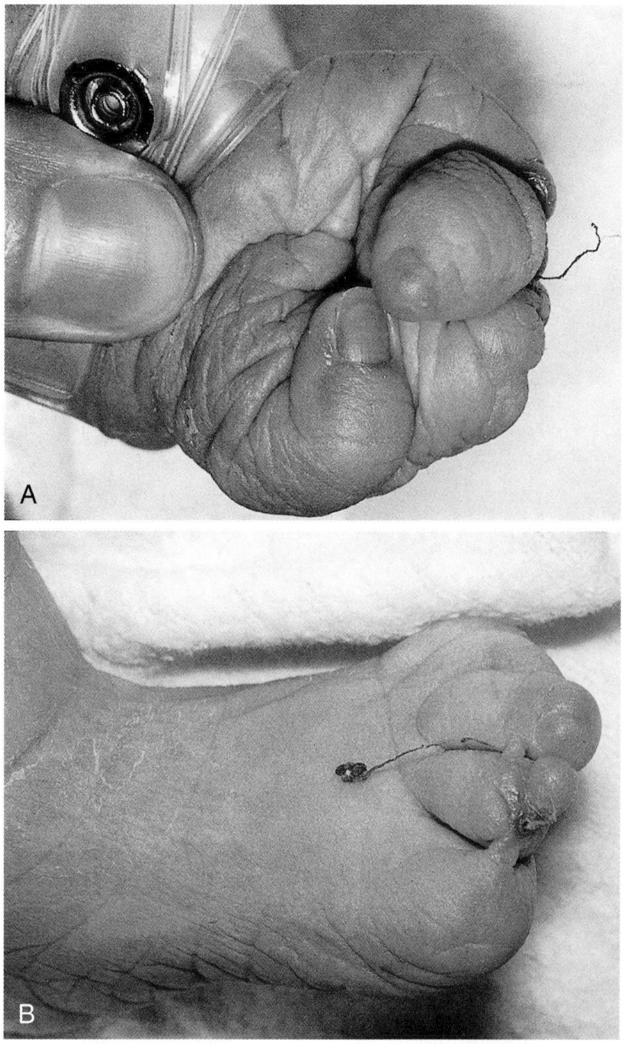

• **Fig. 16.3** Hand (A) and foot (B) of a baby with digital amputations resulting from amniotic bands showing residual strands of amnion. (Courtesy Dr Una MacFadyen, Leicester Royal Infirmary, UK.)

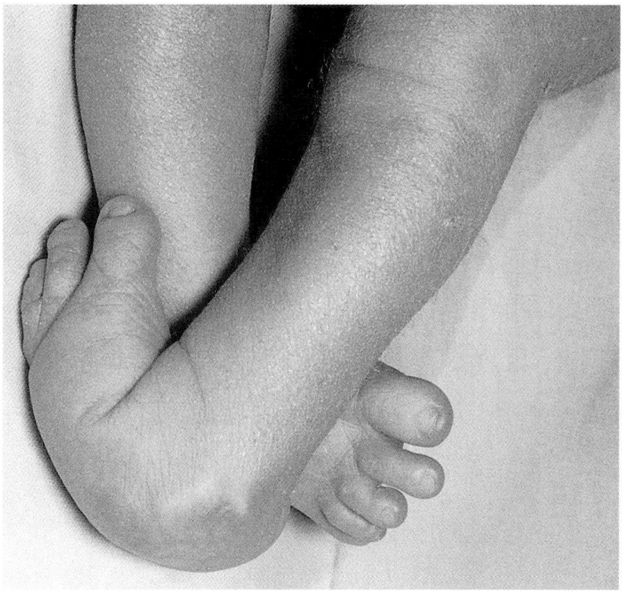

• **Fig. 16.4** Lower limbs of a baby with talipes equinovarus.

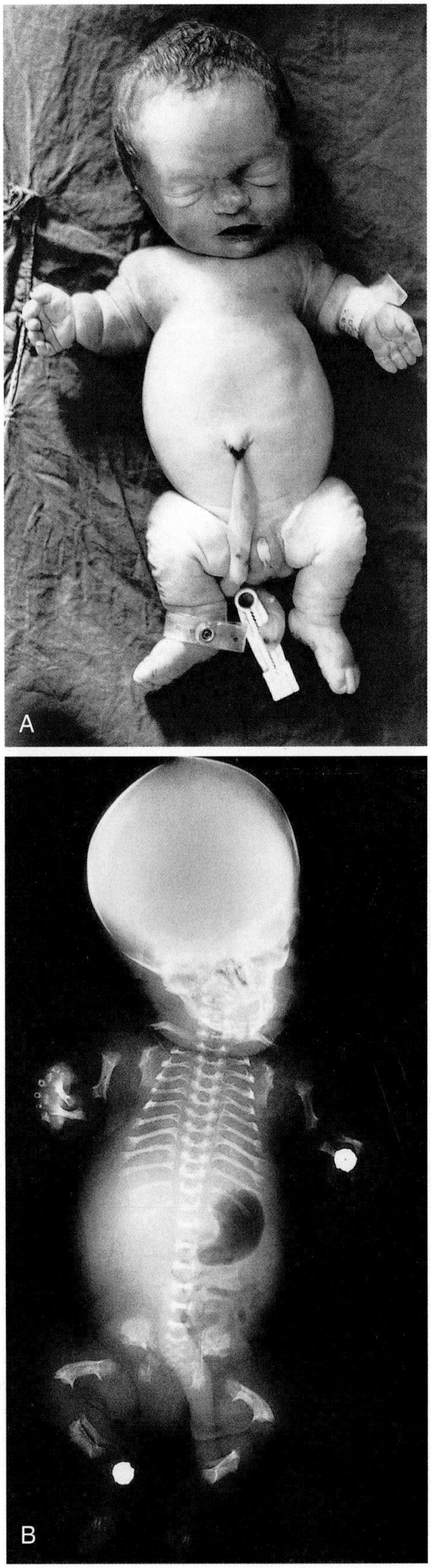

• **Fig. 16.5** (A) Infant with thanatophoric dysplasia. (B) Radiograph of the infant showing short ribs, flat vertebral bodies, and curved femora.

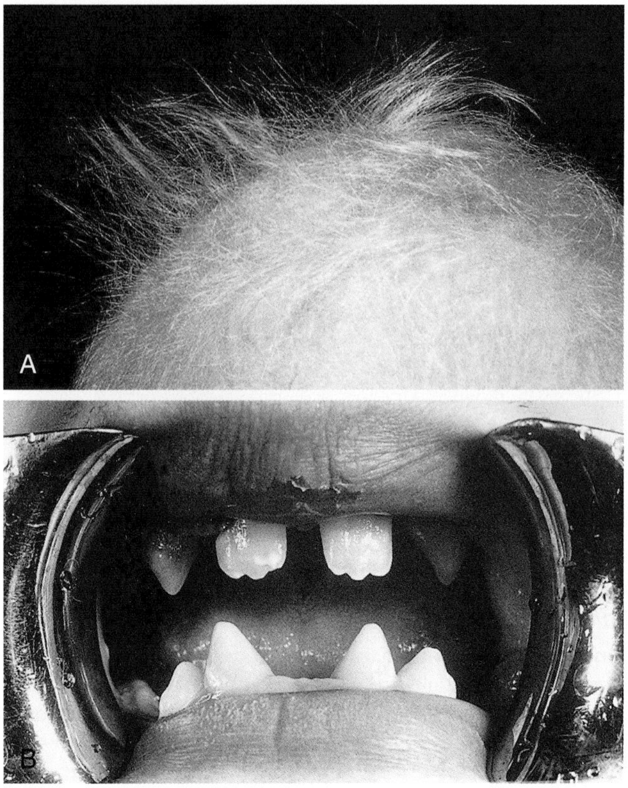

• **Fig. 16.6** Hair (A) and teeth (B) of a male with ectodermal dysplasia.

present. For example, in thanatophoric dysplasia, a skeletal dysplasia caused by a variant in *FGFR3* (p. 118), almost all bones are affected (Fig. 16.5). Similarly, in an ectodermal dysplasia, widely dispersed tissues of ectodermal origin, such as hair, teeth, skin, and nails, are involved (Fig. 16.6). Most dysplasias are caused by single gene variants and may be associated with high recurrence risks for siblings and/or offspring.

Multiple Abnormalities

Sequence

This concept describes the findings that occur as a consequence of a cascade of events initiated by a single primary factor and may result in a single organ malformation. In the "Potter" sequence, chronic leakage of amniotic fluid or defective fetal urinary output results in oligohydramnios (Fig. 16.7). This in turn leads to fetal compression, resulting in flattened facial features, dislocation of the hips, talipes, and pulmonary hypoplasia (Fig. 16.8), usually resulting in neonatal death from respiratory failure.

Syndrome

In practice the term **syndrome** is used very loosely (e.g., the amniotic band "syndrome"), but in theory it should be reserved for consistent and recognizable patterns of abnormalities for which there is often a known underlying cause. These underlying causes can include chromosome abnormalities, as in Down syndrome, or single-gene defects, as in the Van der Woude syndrome, in which cleft lip and/or palate occurs in association with pits in the lower lip (Fig. 16.9).

The clinical study of malformation syndromes is the discipline of **dysmorphology**. Clinical diagnosis has been greatly helped by

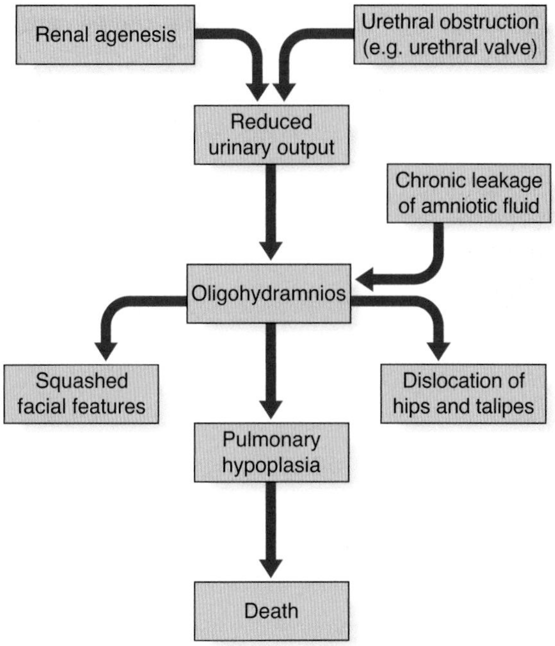

• **Fig. 16.7** The "Potter" sequence showing the cascade of events leading to and resulting from oligohydramnios (reduced volume of amniotic fluid).

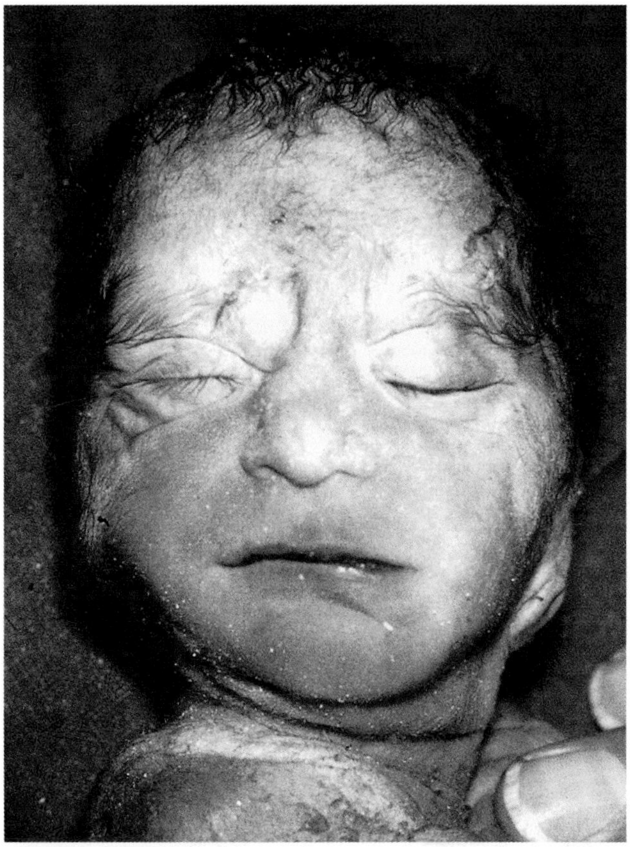

• **Fig. 16.8** Facial appearance of a baby with Potter sequence from oligohydramnios as a consequence of bilateral renal agenesis. Note the squashed appearance caused by *in utero* compression.

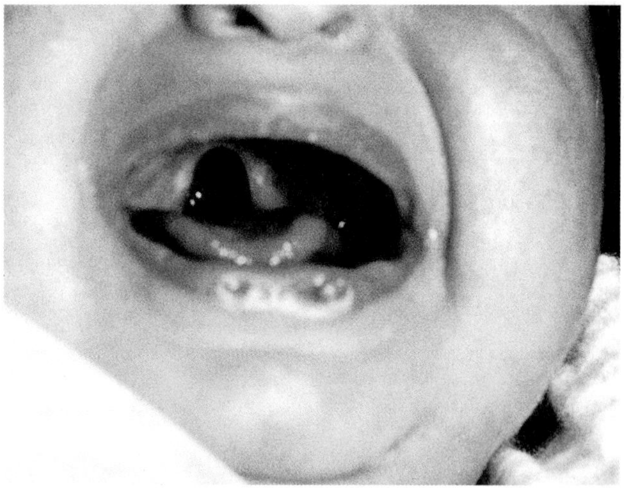

• **Fig. 16.9** Posterior cleft palate and lower lip pits in a child with Van der Woude syndrome.

the development of computerized and online resources (see Appendix) with a search facility based on key features. Even with the help of these extremely valuable tools there are many dysmorphic children for whom no diagnosis is reached, so it may be very difficult to provide accurate information about the likely prognosis and recurrence risk. Chromosome microarray (CMA) technology and next-generation sequencing (p. 76) have made phenomenal inroads into this large group of undiagnosed patients and will continue to do so.

Association

The term **association** was introduced in recognition of the fact that certain malformations tend to occur together more often than would be expected by chance, yet this non-random occurrence of abnormalities cannot be easily explained on the basis of a sequence or a syndrome. The main differences from a syndrome are the lack of consistency of abnormalities from one affected individual to another and the absence of a satisfactory underlying explanation. The names of associations are often acronyms; for example, the VACTERL association features *v*ertebral, *a*nal, *c*ardiac, *t*racheo*e*sophageal, *r*enal, and *l*imb abnormalities. Associations generally convey a low risk of recurrence and are thought not to be genetic in most cases. However, heterogeneity is likely, and at least a proportion of cases probably have a genetic basis. In VACTERL, for example, rare cases have been described with a variant in the XL gene *ZIC3*, which is also a cause of XL laterality (heterotaxy) defects. This is turn has led to the suggestion that VACTERL may be a condition related to defective laterality processing in early development.

This classification of birth defects is not perfect—it is far from being either fully comprehensive or mutually exclusive. For example, bladder outflow obstruction caused by a primary malformation such as a urethral valve will result in the oligohydramnios or Potter sequence, leading to secondary deformations such as dislocation of the hip and talipes. To complicate matters further, the absence of both kidneys, which will result in the same sequence of events, is usually erroneously referred to as Potter syndrome. Despite this semantic confusion, classifications can aid understanding of causes and recurrence risks (Chapter 8), and most parents are comforted by having a name for their child's condition.

TABLE 16.3 Causes of congenital abnormalities

Cause	%
Genetic	***30–40***
Chromosomal	6
Single-gene	7.5
Multifactorial	20–30
Environmental	***5–10***
Drugs and chemicals	2
Infections	2
Maternal illness	2
Physical agents	1
Unknown	***50***
Total	100

Genetic Causes of Malformations

There are multiple causes of congenital abnormalities, and the relative contribution of different mechanisms varies depending on ascertainment and the prevailing public health issues in diverse societies around the world. Table 16.3 gives a rough breakdown of the different contributing factors.

Chromosome Abnormalities

These account for approximately 6% of all recognized congenital abnormalities, or more if CMA-positive cases are included. As a rule, any perceptible degree of autosomal imbalance, such as duplication, deletion, trisomy, or monosomy, will result in significant structural and developmental problems, which may lead to early miscarriage. Common chromosome syndromes are described in Chapter 17. It is not known whether malformations caused by a significant chromosome abnormality such as a trisomy are the result of dosage effects of the individual genes involved ("additive" model) or general developmental instability caused by a large number of abnormal developmental gene products ("interactive" model).

Single-Gene Defects

These account for up to 10% of all congenital abnormalities. Some of these are isolated—that is, they involve only one organ or system (Table 16.4). Other single gene defects result in multiple congenital abnormality syndromes involving many organs or systems that do not have any obvious underlying embryological relationship. For example, ectrodactyly, also known as split-hand/foot malformation (Fig. 16.10), in isolation can be inherited as an apparent autosomal dominant (AD) trait with reduced penetrance when caused by microduplications at 10q24 or 17p13.3, microdeletions at 2q31.1, or subtle imbalances at 7q21.3 (p. 107). Occasionally, autosomal recessive (AR) inheritance has been reported as a result of biallelic variants in *DLX5* (7q21.3). It can also occur as one manifestation of the EEC syndrome (*e*ctodermal dysplasia, *e*ctrodactyly, and *c*left lip/palate), which follows AD inheritance and is

TABLE 16.4 Congenital abnormalities that can be caused by single-gene defects

	Inheritance	Abnormalities
Isolated		
CENTRAL NERVOUS SYSTEM		
Hydrocephalus	XR	
Megalencephaly	AD	
Microcephaly	AD/AR	
OCULAR		
Aniridia	AD	
Cataracts	AD/AR	
Microphthalmia	AD/AR	
LIMB		
Brachydactyly	AD	
Ectrodactyly	AD/AR	
Polydactyly	AD	
OTHER		
Infantile polycystic kidneys	AR	
Syndromes		
Apert	AD	Craniosynostosis, syndactyly
EEC	AD	Ectodermal dysplasia, ectrodactyly, cleft lip/palate
Meckel	AR	Encephalocele, polydactyly, polycystic kidneys
Roberts	AR	Cleft lip/palate, phocomelia
Van der Woude	AD	Cleft lip/palate, lip pits

AD, Autosomal dominant; *AR*, autosomal recessive; EEC, *e*ctodermal dysplasia, *e*ctrodactyly and *c*left lip/palate; *XR*, X-linked recessive.

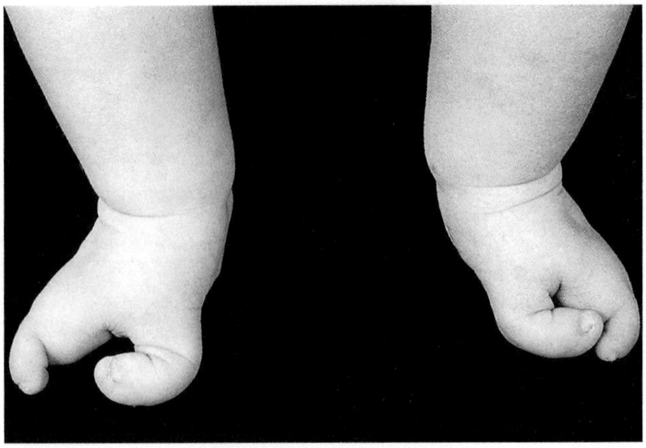

• **Fig. 16.10** Appearance of the feet in a child with ectrodactyly.

caused by mutations in *TP63*. Therefore different variants, allelic or non-allelic, can cause similar or identical malformations.

The importance of determining a cause for a congenital abnormality, particularly if it has a single gene basis, lies in the need for accurate genetic counseling for the immediate and wider family. In addition, from a research perspective single gene causes can provide clues to susceptibility loci for similar malformations and phenotypes that appear to show multifactorial inheritance.

From the many examples of progress in identifying the genes that cause congenital abnormalities and dysmorphic syndromes, two are now illustrated from the field of pediatric genetics. In both, the gene function in relation to widespread expression in many tissues has yet to be determined.

Noonan Syndrome and the "RAS-opathies"

First described by Noonan and Ehmke in 1963, this well-known condition has an incidence that may be as high as 1:2000 births, with an equal sex ratio. The features resemble those of Turner syndrome in females—short stature, neck webbing, increased carrying angle at the elbow and congenital heart disease. Pulmonary stenosis is the most common lesion, but atrial septal defect, ventricular septal defect, and sometimes hypertrophic cardiomyopathy occur. A characteristic mild pectus deformity may be seen, and the face shows hypertelorism, down-slanting palpebral fissures, and low-set ears (Fig. 16.11). Some patients have a mild bleeding diathesis, and mild ID occurs in approximately one-quarter.

In a three-generation Dutch family, Noonan syndrome (NS) was mapped to 12q22 in 1994, but it was not until 2001 that variants were identified in the protein tyrosine phosphatase, non-receptor-type 11 *(PTPN11)* gene. Attention has turned rapidly to phenotype-genotype correlation, and variant-positive cases have a much higher frequency of pulmonary stenosis than variant-negative cases, whereas few variants have been found in patients with cardiomyopathy. However, facial features are similar, whether or not a variant is found. Pathogenic variants in *PTPN11* account for approximately half of all cases of NS. Variants in the *SOS1*, *SHOC2*, *KRAS*, *RIT1*, and *MAPZK1* genes have been found in a proportion of *PTPN11* variant−negative cases. NS caused by a pathogenic variant in *SHOC2* is illustrated in Fig. 16.12. These genes belong to the same pathway, known as RAS-MAPK (Fig. 16.13). The protein product of *PTPN11* is SHP-2, which, together with SOS1, positively transduces signals to Ras-GTP, a downstream effector. The *KRAS* variants in NS appear to lead to K-ras proteins with impaired responsiveness to GTPase activating proteins (p. 188). Neurofibromatosis, the most common disorder of this group, is dealt with in Chapter 19 (p. 296).

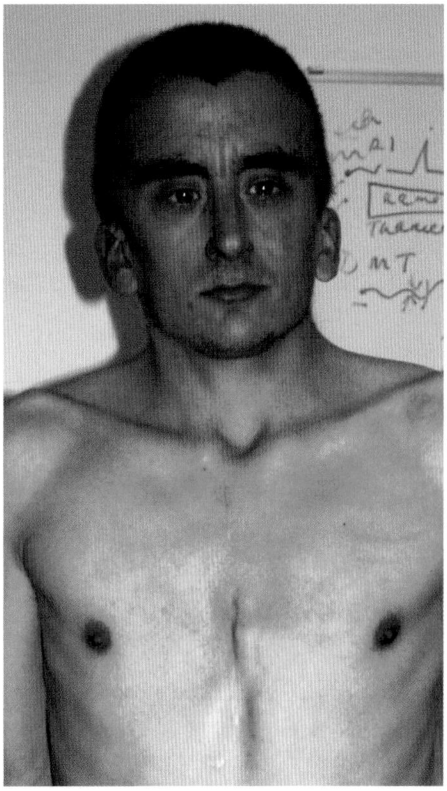

• **Fig. 16.12** Noonan syndrome in an adult male caused by a pathogenic variant in the *SHOC2* gene. His facial features are subtle but he has a mild pectus excavatum deformity.

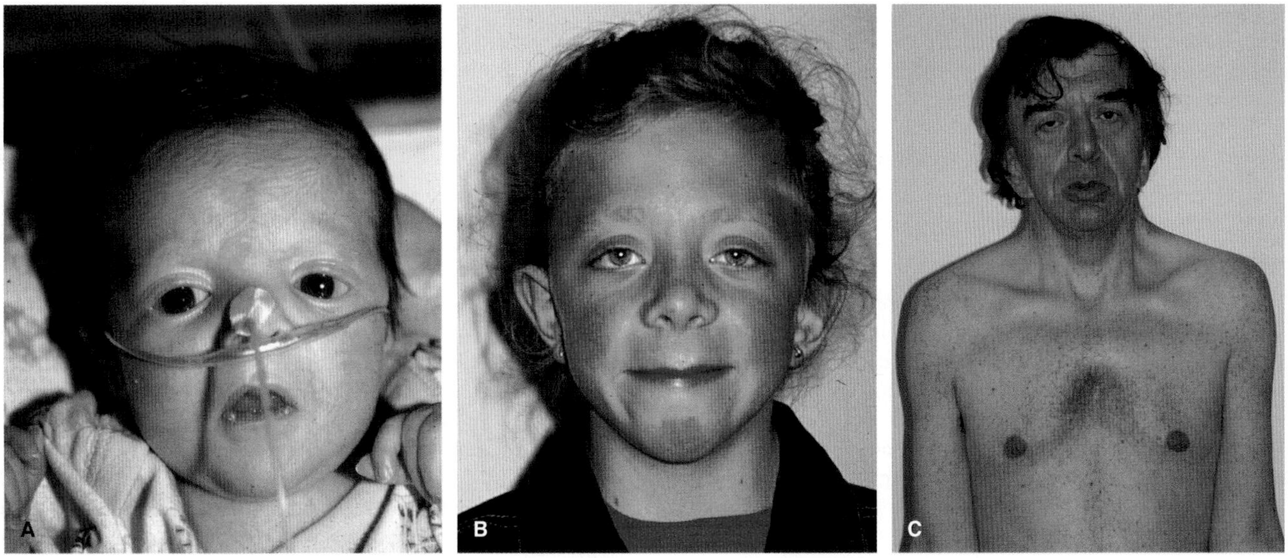

• **Fig. 16.11** Noonan syndrome: (A) in a baby presenting with cardiomyopathy at birth (which later resolved); (B) in a child; and (C) in a 57-year-old man.

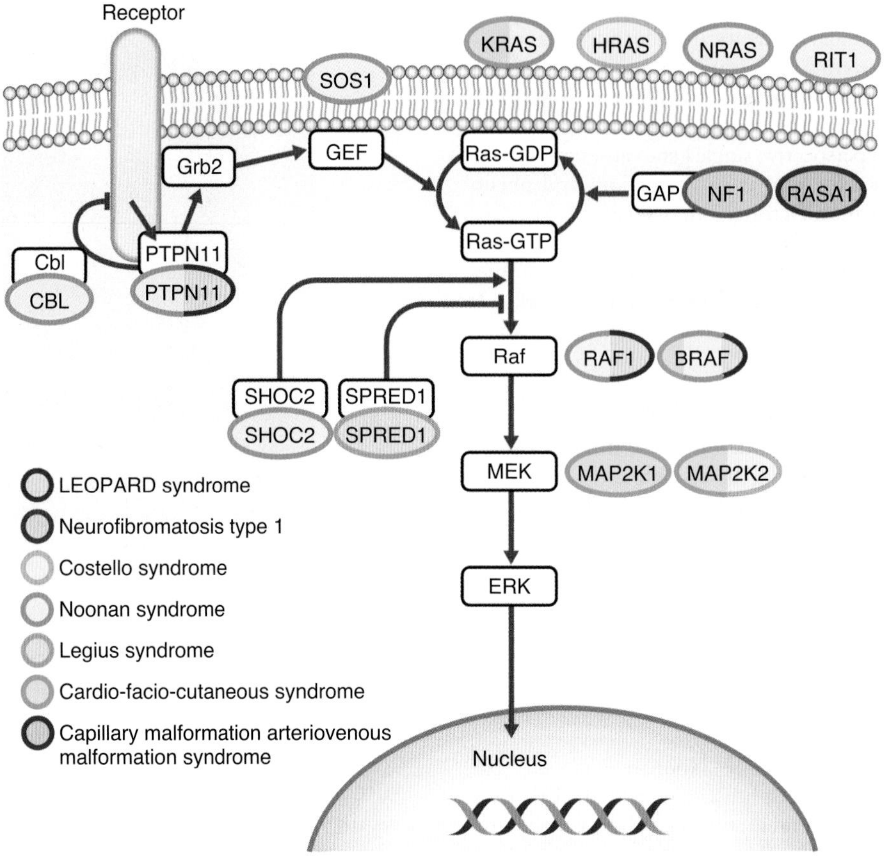

• **Fig. 16.13** The RAS-MAPK pathway. HRAS and KRAS are activated by PTPN11 and SOS1. The pathway is dysregulated by variants in key components, resulting in the distinct but related phenotypes of Noonan syndrome, cardio-facio-cutaneous syndrome, Costello syndrome, and neurofibromatosis type 1 (see Table 16.5). Neurofibromin is a GTPase-activating protein (*GAP*) that functions as a tumor suppressor. Mutant RAS proteins display impaired GTPase activity and are resistant to GAPs. The effect is for RAS to bind GTP, which results in activation of the pathway (gain of function). *NF1*, Neurofibromatosis type 1.

For years dysmorphologists recognized overlapping features between NS and the rarer conditions known as cardio-facio-cutaneous (Fig. 16.14) and Costello (Fig. 16.15A,B) syndromes. These conditions are now recognized to form part of a spectrum of disorders explained by variants in different components of the RAS-MAPK pathway, with each syndrome displaying considerable genetic heterogeneity (Table 16.5). Many are gain-of-function missense variants, which may explain the increase in solid tumors in Costello syndrome, as well as cellular proliferation in some tissues in cardio-facio-cutaneous syndrome (e.g., hyperkeratosis). The effect is for RAS to bind GTP, which results in activation of the pathway (gain-of-function). Neurofibromin is a GTPase activating protein, and functions as a tumor suppressor.

Sotos Syndrome

First described in 1964, this is one of the "overgrowth" syndromes, previously known as cerebral gigantism. Birth weight is usually increased, and macrocephaly noted. Early feeding difficulties and hypotonia may prompt many investigations, and there is often motor delay and ataxia. Height progresses along the top of, or above, the normal centile lines, but final adult height is always markedly increased. Advanced bone age may be present, as well as large hands and feet, and the cerebral ventricles may be mildly dilated on imaging. The face is characteristic (Fig. 16.16), with a high prominent forehead, hypertelorism with down-slanting palpebral fissures, a characteristic nose in early childhood, and a long, pointed chin. Scoliosis develops in some cases during adolescence. Parent-child transmission is rare, probably because most patients have ID, but mild cases can occur, with the result that the condition may occasionally be traced over several generations.

Among patients with Sotos syndrome reported to have balanced chromosome translocations were two with breakpoints at 5q35. From these crucial patients a Japanese group in 2002 went on to identify a 2.2-megabase deletion in a series of Sotos syndrome cases. The deletion takes out a gene called *NSD1*, which contains 23 exons and encodes an androgen receptor-associated co-regulator. The Japanese group found a small number of frameshift variants in their patients, but, interestingly, a study of European cases found that variants were far more common than deletions. For the large majority of cases the variants and deletions occur *de novo*.

Multifactorial Inheritance

This accounts for the majority of congenital abnormalities in which genetic factors can clearly be implicated. These include most isolated ("non-syndromal") malformations involving the heart, central nervous system, and kidneys (Box 16.2). For many of these conditions, empirical risks have been derived (p. 102) based on large epidemiological family studies, so that it is usually possible to provide the parents of an affected child with a clear indication of the likelihood that a future child will be similarly affected. Risks to the offspring of patients who were themselves treated

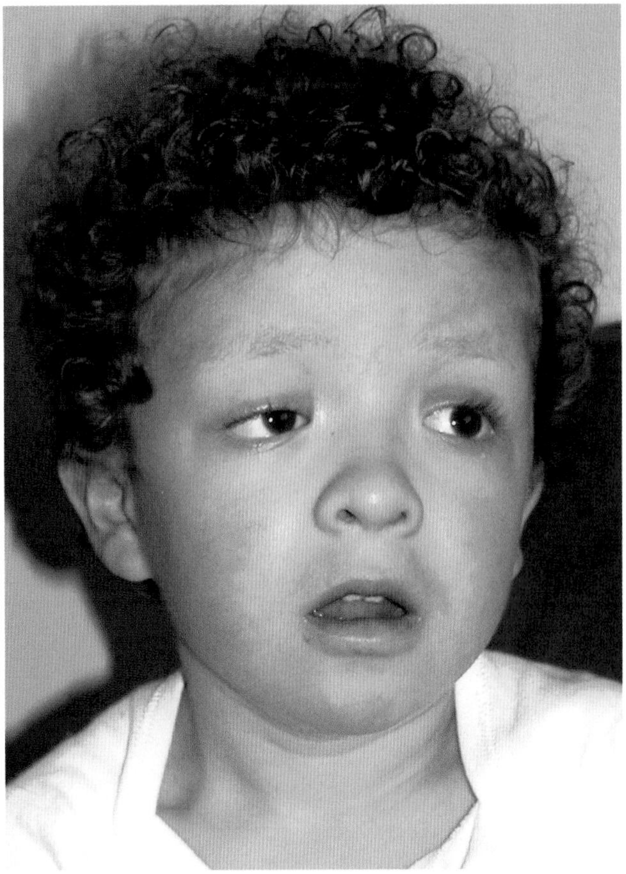

• **Fig. 16.14** A child with cardio-facio-cutaneous syndrome caused by a mutation in the *BRAF1* gene. Note the unusually curly hair.

successfully in childhood are becoming available, particularly for congenital heart disease. These are usually similar to the risks that apply to siblings, as would be predicted by the multifactorial model (see Chapter 10).

Genetic Heterogeneity

It has long been recognized that specific congenital malformations can have many different causes, hence the importance of trying to distinguish between syndromal and isolated cases. This causal diversity has become increasingly apparent as developments in molecular biology have led to the identification of highly conserved families of genes that play crucial roles in early embryogenesis.

This subject is discussed at length in Chapter 9. In the current chapter, two specific malformations, holoprosencephaly and neural tube defects, will be considered to demonstrate the rate of progress in this field and the extent of the challenge that lies ahead.

Holoprosencephaly

This severe and often fatal malformation is caused by a failure of cleavage of the embryonic forebrain or prosencephalon. Normally this divides transversely into the telencephalon and the diencephalon. The telencephalon divides in the sagittal plane to form the cerebral hemispheres and the olfactory tracts and bulbs. The diencephalon develops to form the thalamic nuclei, the pineal gland, the optic chiasm, and the optic nerves. In holoprosencephaly, there is incomplete or partial failure of these developmental processes, and in the severe alobar form this results in an abnormal facial

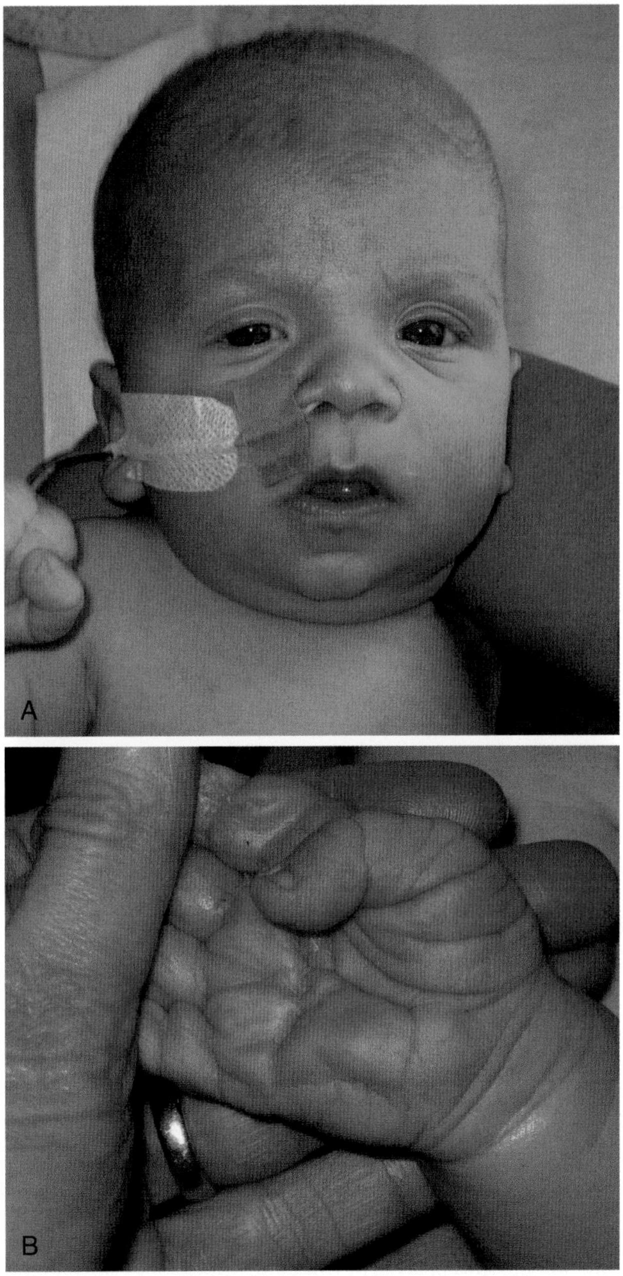

• **Fig. 16.15** A baby (A) with Costello syndrome caused by a pathogenic variant in *HRAS* gene. The palmar creases (B) are unusually deep (picture taken in the neonatal period).

appearance (see Fig. 9.10, p. 112) with profound neurodevelopmental impairment.

Etiologically, holoprosencephaly can be classified as chromosomal, syndromal, or isolated. Chromosomal causes account for approximately 30% to 40% of cases, with the most common abnormality being trisomy 13 (p. 253). Other chromosomal causes include deletions of 18p, 2p21, 7q36, and 21q22.3, duplication of 3p24-pter, duplication or deletion of 13q, and triploidy (p. 253). Syndromal causes of holoprosencephaly are numerous and include relatively well-known conditions such as the deletion of 22q11 (DiGeorge syndrome) (p. 259) and a host of much rarer multiple malformation syndromes, some of which show AR

TABLE 16.5 Genes of the RAS-MAPK pathway and associated syndromes

Gene	Noonan Syndrome	Cardio-Facio-Cutaneous Syndrome	Costello Syndrome
PTPN11	Common: ≤ 50% Also accounts for most cases of LEOPARD syndrome	—	—
RIT1	~5%	—	—
KRAS	Rare	Rare	Rare
HRAS	—	—	Common: > 50%
SHOC2	Rare	—	—
SOS1	Rare	—	—
BRAF	—	Common: ≤ 50%	Some
MAP2K1	Rare	Some	Some
MAP2K2	—	Rare	—

LEOPARD, Lentigines, electrocardiogram, ocular, pulmonary stenosis, abnormal genitalia, retardation of growth, deafness.

inheritance. One of these, Smith-Lemli-Opitz syndrome (pp. 111, 284), is associated with low levels of cholesterol and is as a result of a defect in the early part of the Sonic hedgehog pathway (p. 110).

The third group, isolated holoprosencephaly, is sometimes explained by heterozygous variants in three genes. The effects can be very variable, ranging from very mild with minimal features such as anosmia, to the full-blown, lethal, alobar form. The genes implicated are *Sonic hedgehog* (*SHH*) at 7q36, *ZIC2* at 13q32, and *SIX3* at 2p21. Of these, *SHH* is thought to make the greatest contribution, accounting for up to 20% of all familial cases and between 1% and 10% of isolated cases. Some sibling recurrences of holoprosencephaly, not as a result of AR Smith-Lemli-Opitz syndrome, have been shown to be caused by germline variants in these genes.

That so many familial cases remain unexplained indicates that more holoprosencephaly genes await identification. Causal heterogeneity is further illustrated by its association with poorly controlled maternal diabetes mellitus (p. 240).

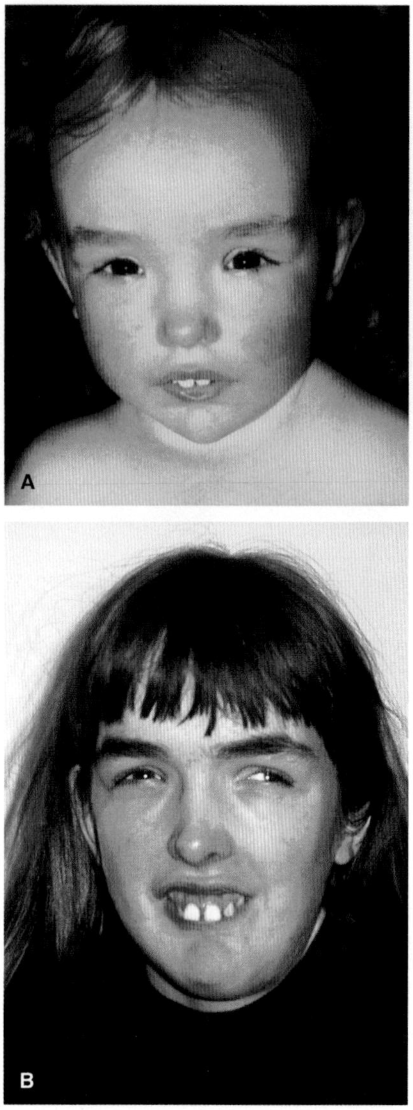

• **Fig. 16.16** Sotos syndrome. (A) A young child who has the typical high forehead, large head, and characteristic tip to the nose. (B) The same individual at age 18 years, with intellectual disability and a spinal curvature (scoliosis).

Neural Tube Defects

Neural tube defects (NTDs) such as spina bifida and anencephaly illustrate many of the underlying principles of multifactorial inheritance and emphasize the importance of trying to identify possible adverse environmental factors. These conditions result from defective closure of the developing neural tube during the first month of embryonic life. A defect occurring at the upper end of the developing neural tube results in either exencephaly/anencephaly or an encephalocele (Fig. 16.17). A defect occurring at the lower end of the developing neural tube leads to a spinal lesion such as a lumbosacral meningocele or myelomeningocele (see Fig. 16.2), and a defect involving the head plus cervical and thoracic spine leads to craniorachischisis. These different entities relate to the different embryological closure points of the neural tube. Most NTDs have serious consequences. Anencephaly and craniorachischisis are not compatible with survival for more than a few hours after birth. Large lumbosacral lesions usually cause partial or complete paralysis of the lower limbs with impaired bladder and bowel continence.

As with many malformations, NTDs can be classified etiologically under the headings of chromosomal, syndromal, and isolated. Chromosomal causes include trisomy 13 and trisomy 18, and both of these NTDs show an incidence of approximately 5% to 10%. Syndromal causes include the relatively rare AR disorder Meckel-Gruber syndrome, which is characterized by encephalocele in association with polycystic kidneys and polydactyly. However, most NTDs represent isolated malformations in otherwise normal infants, and appear to show multifactorial inheritance.

The empiric recurrence risks to first-degree relatives (siblings and offspring) vary according to the local population incidence and are as high as 4% to 5% in areas where NTDs are common. The incidence in the United Kingdom is highest in people of Celtic origin. If such individuals move from their country of origin to another part of the world, the incidence in their offspring

• BOX 16.2 Isolated (Non-syndromal) Malformations That Show Multifactorial Inheritance

Cardiac

Atrial septal defect
Tetralogy of Fallot
Patent ductus arteriosus
Ventricular septal defect

Central Nervous System

Anencephaly
Encephalocele
Spina bifida

Genitourinary

Hypospadias
Renal agenesis
Renal dysgenesis

Other

Cleft lip/palate
Congenital dislocation of hips
Talipes

declines but remains higher than among the indigenous population. These observations suggest the presence of susceptibility genes in Celtic populations.

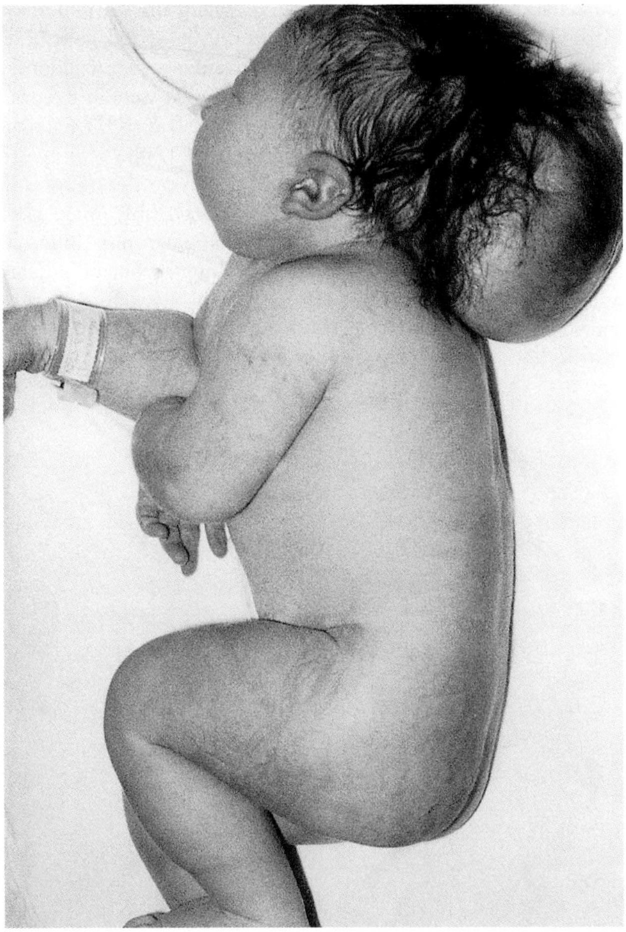

• **Fig. 16.17** A baby with a large occipital encephalocele.

No single NTD susceptibility gene has been identified in humans, although there is some evidence that the common 677C > T polymorphism in the *methylenetetrahydrofolate reductase* (*MTHFR*) gene can be a susceptibility factor in some populations. Reduction in MTHFR activity results in decreased plasma folate levels, which are known to be causally associated with NTDs (see the following section). Research efforts have also focused on developmental genes, such as genes belonging to the *PAX* family (p. 113), which are expressed in the embryonic neural tube and vertebral column. In mouse models, approximately 80 genes have been linked to exencephaly, approximately 20 genes to lumbosacral myelomeningocele, and approximately five genes to craniorachischisis. One example is an interaction between mutations of *PAX1* and the *platelet-derived growth factor* α gene (*PDGFRA*) that results in severe NTDs in 100% of double-mutant embryos. This rare example of digenic inheritance (p. 76) serves as a useful illustration of the difficulties posed by a search for susceptibility genes in a multifactorial disorder. However, to date there have been no equivalent breakthroughs in understanding the processes in human NTDs.

Environmental factors include poor socioeconomic status, multiparity, and valproic acid (VPA) exposure (p. 240, Fig. 16.20). Firm evidence has also emerged that periconceptional multivitamin supplementation reduces the risk of recurrence by a factor of 70% to 75% when a woman has had one affected child. Studies have shown that folic acid is likely to be the effective constituent in multivitamin preparations, and the World Health Organization recommends periconceptional folate supplementation of 400 μg/day, which is adopted in some form by most nations. In some countries, including the United States, bread is fortified with folic acid. Many nations officially recommend that all women who have previously had a child with an NTD should take 4 to 5 mg of folic acid daily, both before conceiving and throughout the first trimester.

Environmental Agents (Teratogens)

An agent that can cause a birth defect by interfering with normal embryonic or fetal development is known as a teratogen. Many teratogens have been identified, and exhaustive tests are now undertaken before any new drug is approved for use by pregnant women. The potential effects of any particular teratogen usually depend on the dosage and timing of administration during pregnancy, along with the susceptibility of both the mother and fetus.

An agent that conveys a high risk of teratogenesis, such as the rubella virus or thalidomide, can usually be identified relatively quickly. Unfortunately, it is much more difficult to detect a low-grade teratogen that causes an abnormality in only a small proportion of cases. This is because of the relatively high background incidence of congenital abnormalities, and also because many pregnant women take medication at some time in pregnancy, often for a poorly-defined "flu-like" illness. Despite extensive study, controversy still surrounds the use of a number of drugs in pregnancy. The antinausea drug Debendox was the subject of successful litigation in the United States despite a lack of firm evidence to support a definite teratogenic effect. A group of drugs under scrutiny more recently is the selective serotonin reuptake inhibitors. These are commonly prescribed antidepressants, and in Europe some 3% of pregnant women take antidepressants, rising to approximately 8% in the United States. Despite concerns about a teratogenic potential, particularly congenital heart disease, several large studies have failed to demonstrate a significant difference in the frequency of birth defects.

TABLE 16.6 Drugs with a proven teratogenic effect in humans

Drug	Effects
ACE inhibitors	Renal dysplasia
Alcohol	Cardiac defects, microcephaly, characteristic facies, neurodevelopment
Chloroquine	Chorioretinitis, deafness
Diethylstilbestrol	Uterine malformations, vaginal adenocarcinoma
Ethinylestradiol/norethisterone (hormone pregnancy test, eg Primidos)	Effects: limb defects, VACTERL spectrum
Lithium	Cardiac defects (Ebstein anomaly)
Phenytoin	Cardiac defects, cleft palate, digital hypoplasia
Retinoids	Ear and eye defects, hydrocephalus
Streptomycin	Deafness
Tetracycline	Dental enamel hypoplasia
Thalidomide	Phocomelia, cardiac and ear abnormalities
Valproic acid	Neural tube defects, clefting, limb defects, characteristic facies, neurodevelopment
Warfarin	Nasal hypoplasia, stippled epiphyses

ACE, Angiotensin-converting enzyme.

Drugs and Chemicals

Drugs and chemicals with a proven teratogenic effect in humans are listed in Table 16.6. These may account for approximately 2% of all congenital abnormalities. Many drugs have been proposed as possible teratogens, but because these drugs are taken only rarely in pregnancy, and reported cases are even rarer, it has been difficult to confirm a damaging effect. This applies to many anticancer drugs, including methotrexate. Although still controversial, case reports suggest a methotrexate embryopathy can occur, including growth deficiency, microcephaly, various craniofacial abnormalities, limb anomalies, and deficiencies and possibly tetralogy of Fallot. Controversy always surrounds the use of agents deployed in warfare, such as dioxin (Agent Orange) in Vietnam and various nerve gases in the Gulf War.

The Thalidomide Tragedy

Thalidomide was used widely in Europe during 1958 to 1962 as a sedative. In 1961 an association with severe limb anomalies in babies whose mothers had taken the drug during the first trimester was recognized, and the drug was subsequently withdrawn from use. It is possible that more than 10,000 babies were damaged over this period. Review of these babies' records indicated that the critical period for fetal damage was between 20 and 35 days postconception (i.e., 34–50 days after the beginning of the last menstrual period). Unfortunately, thalidomide was reintroduced in Brazil as a treatment for leprosy, and, despite warnings about its teratogenicity, a significant cohort of younger "thalidomiders" now exists.

The most characteristic abnormality caused by thalidomide was phocomelia (Fig. 16.18). This is the name given to a limb that is malformed because of absence of some or all of the long bones, with retention of digits giving a "flipper" or "seal-like" appearance. Other external abnormalities included ear defects, microphthalmia, and cleft lip/palate. In addition, approximately 40% died in early infancy from severe internal abnormalities affecting the heart, kidneys, or gastrointestinal tract. Many thalidomiders have grown up and had children of their own, and in some cases these offspring have also had similar defects. It is therefore most likely, not surprisingly, that thalidomide was wrongly blamed in a proportion of cases that were in fact from single-gene conditions following AD inheritance (e.g., *SALL4* variants [see Fig. 9.26C, p. 126] in Okihiro syndrome [p. 120]).

The thalidomide tragedy focused attention on the importance of avoiding all drugs in pregnancy as far as is possible unless absolute safety has been established. Drug manufacturers undertake extensive research trials before releasing a drug for general use, and invariably urge caution about the use of any new drug in pregnancy. Monitoring systems, in the form of congenital abnormality registers, have been set up in most Western countries in the hope

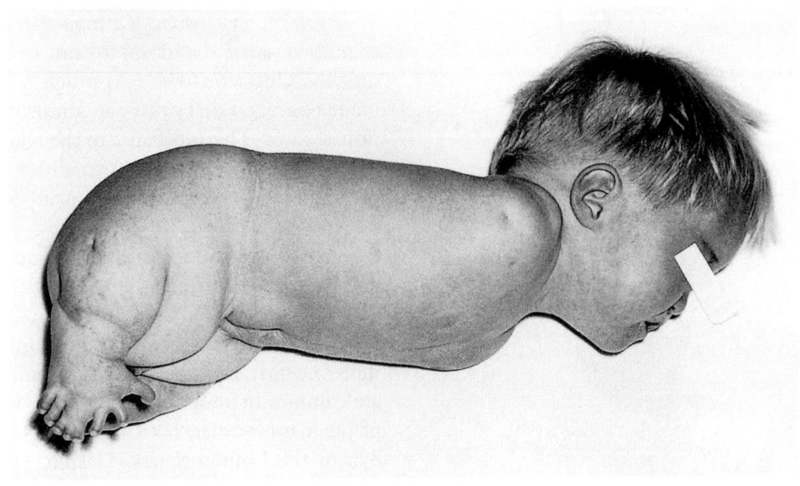

• **Fig. 16.18** A child with thalidomide embryopathy. There is absence of the upper limbs (amelia). The lower limbs show phocomelia and polydactyly. (Courtesy Emeritus Professor R. W. Smithells, University of Leeds, UK.)

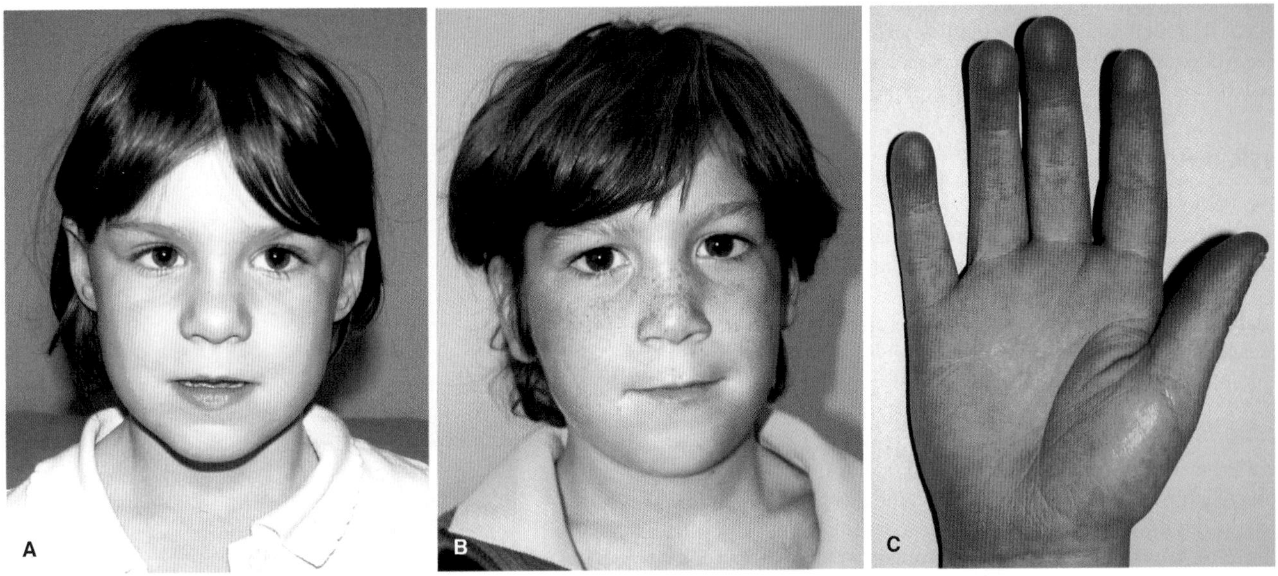

• **Fig. 16.19** (A) and (B) Two children with fetal alcohol syndrome, showing short palpebral fissures, a long smooth philtrum, and a thin upper lip. Although unrelated to each other, they bear a close resemblance. (C) A "hockey-stick" crease of the palm extending into the interdigital space between the index and middle fingers.

that an "epidemic" on the scale of the thalidomide tragedy could never happen again.

Fetal Alcohol Syndrome

Children born to mothers who have consistently consumed large quantities of alcohol during pregnancy tend to have a small head circumference, a distinctive facial appearance with short palpebral fissures, a smooth philtrum, and a thin upper lip (Fig.16.19A,B). The ear helix may show a "railroad" configuration of the folds, and in the hands a "hockey-stick" crease may be present (see Fig. 16.19C). These children also show developmental delay with hyperactivity and a reduced sense of moral responsibility, resulting in altercations with civil authorities as they grow older. This may be referred to as "fetal alcohol spectrum disorder," and if the physical aspects are lacking, "alcohol-related neurodevelopmental defects" may be applied. There is uncertainty about the "safe" level of alcohol consumption in pregnancy, and there is evidence that mild-to-moderate ingestion can be harmful. Thus total abstinence is advised throughout pregnancy.

TABLE 16.7 Infectious teratogenic agents

Infection	Effects
Viral	
Cytomegalovirus	Chorioretinitis, deafness, microcephaly
Herpes simplex	Microcephaly, microphthalmia
Rubella	Microcephaly, cataracts, retinitis, cardiac defects
Varicella zoster	Microcephaly, chorioretinitis, skin defects
Bacterial	
Syphilis	Hydrocephalus, osteitis, rhinitis
Parasitic	
Toxoplasmosis	Hydrocephalus, microcephaly, cataracts, chorioretinitis, deafness

Maternal Infections

Several infectious agents can interfere with embryogenesis and fetal development (Table 16.7), with the developing brain, eyes, and ears being particularly susceptible to damage.

Rubella

The rubella virus, which damages 15% to 25% of all babies infected during the first trimester, causes cardiovascular malformations such as patent ductus arteriosus and peripheral pulmonary artery stenosis. Congenital rubella infection can be prevented by the widespread use of immunization programs based on administration of either the measles, mumps, and rubella vaccine in early childhood, or the rubella vaccine alone to young adult women.

Cytomegalovirus

At present no immunization is available against cytomegalovirus (CMV), even though trials have been undertaken on a wide range of vaccines. Studies indicate that between 1 in 200 and 1 in 30 newborns are infected by CMV transmission from the mother. The risk of abnormality is greatest when infection occurs during the first trimester. The risk and severity also depend on the mother's status for CMV—infections carry the worst prognosis when the mother is seronegative, but maternal seropositivity does not necessarily protect the fetus from serious consequences.

Toxoplasmosis

Maternal infection with the parasite *Toxoplasma gondii* conveys a risk of 20% that the fetus will be infected during the first trimester, rising to 75% in the second and third trimesters. Vaccines are not available, but there is interest in the human equivalent of a vaccine delivered by nasal spray that appears to protect mice and sheep.

Investigation for possible congenital infection can be made by sampling fetal blood to look for specific immunoglobulin-M antibodies. Fetal blood analysis can also reveal generalized evidence of infection, such as abnormal liver function and thrombocytopenia.

There is some evidence to suggest that maternal infection with *Listeria*, contracted from contaminated food, can cause miscarriage, stillbirth, and premature labor, but a pattern of birth defects has not emerged. Maternal listeriosis can result in neonatal sepsis and meningitis. Maternal infection with *parvovirus* can cause severe anemia in the fetus, resulting in hydrops fetalis and pregnancy loss.

Physical Agents

Women who have had babies with congenital abnormalities usually scrutinize their own history in great detail and ask about exposure to agents such as radio waves, ultrasound, magnetic fields, and various chemicals and medicines, as well as minor trauma. It is invariably impossible to prove or disprove causal link, but there is some evidence that two specific physical agents, ionizing radiation and prolonged hyperthermia, can have teratogenic effects.

Ionising Radiation

Heavy doses of ionizing radiation, far in excess of those used in routine diagnostic radiography, can cause microcephaly and ocular defects in the developing fetus. The most sensitive time of exposure is 2 to 5 weeks postconception. Ionizing radiation can also have mutagenic and carcinogenic effects and, although the risks associated with low-dose diagnostic procedures are minimal, radiography should be avoided during pregnancy if possible.

Prolonged Hyperthermia

There is evidence that prolonged hyperthermia in early pregnancy can cause microcephaly and microphthalmia, as well as neuronal migration defects. Consequently, it is recommended that care should be taken to avoid excessive use of hot baths and saunas during the first trimester.

Maternal Illness

Several maternal illnesses are associated with an increased risk of an untoward pregnancy outcome.

Diabetes Mellitus

Maternal diabetes mellitus is associated with a two- to threefold increase in the incidence of congenital abnormalities in offspring. Malformations that occur most commonly in such infants include congenital heart disease, neural tube defects, vertebral segmentation defects and sacral agenesis, femoral hypoplasia, holoprosencephaly, and sirenomelia ("mermaidism"). The likelihood of an abnormality is inversely related to the control of the mother's blood glucose levels during early pregnancy, which should be regularly monitored by testing plasma glucose and glycosylated hemoglobin levels.

Phenylketonuria

Another maternal metabolic condition that conveys a risk to the fetus is untreated phenylketonuria (p. 271). A high serum level of phenylalanine in a pregnant woman with phenylketonuria will almost invariably result in serious damage (e.g., ID). Structural abnormalities may include microcephaly and congenital heart defects. All women with phenylketonuria should be strongly advised to adhere to a strict and closely monitored low phenylalanine diet before and throughout pregnancy.

Maternal Epilepsy

There is a large body of literature devoted to the question of maternal epilepsy, the link with congenital abnormalities, and the teratogenic effects of antiepileptic drugs (AEDs). The largest and best-controlled studies suggest that maternal epilepsy itself is not associated with an increased risk of congenital abnormalities. However, all studies have shown an increased incidence of birth defects in babies exposed to AEDs. The risks are in the region of 5% to 10%, which is 2 to 4 times the background population risk. These figures apply mainly to single-drug therapy but may be higher if the fetus is exposed to more than one AED. Some drugs are more teratogenic than others, with the highest risks applying to sodium valproate (VPA). The range of abnormalities occurring in the "fetal valproate syndrome" (FVS), also known as "fetal valproate spectrum disorder," is wide, including neural tube defect (up to 2%), oral clefting, genitourinary abnormalities such as hypospadias, congenital heart disease, and both major and minor limb defects. The abnormalities themselves are not specific to FVS, making a diagnosis in an individual case therefore difficult. Characteristic facial features may also be present in FVS (Fig. 16.20), which strongly supports a clinical diagnosis.

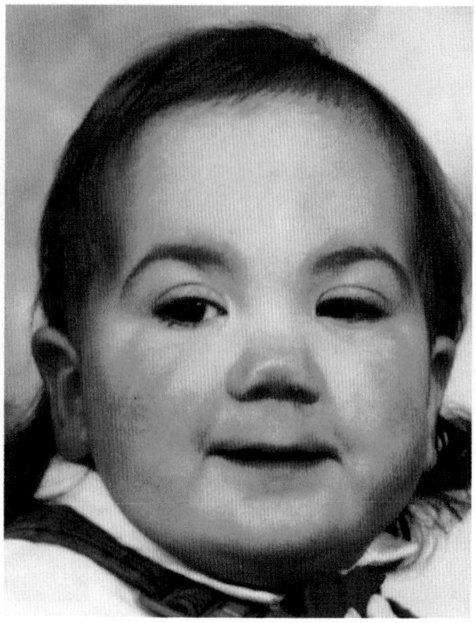

• **Fig. 16.20** A child with fetal valproate syndrome. She has a broad nasal root, blunt nasal tip, and thin upper lip.

The most controversial aspect of AEDs and FVS has been the risk of ID and behavioral problems. However, well-controlled prospective studies have provided convincing evidence that prenatal exposure to VPA carries a significant risk of neurodevelopmental and behavioral sequelae. But potential risks to the fetus must be weighed against the dangers of stopping AED treatment and risking seizures during pregnancy. If the patient has been seizure-free for at least 2 years, she can be offered withdrawal of anticonvulsant medication before proceeding with a pregnancy. If therapy is essential, then single-drug treatment is much preferred, and VPA should be avoided if possible.

Malformations of Unknown Cause

In approximately 50% of all congenital abnormalities no clear cause can be established. This applies to many relatively common conditions such as orofacial clefting, congenital heart disease, isolated diaphragmatic hernia, tracheoesophageal fistula, anal atresia and limb anomalies. For an isolated limb reduction defect, such as absence of a hand, disruption of vascular supply at a critical time during the development of the limb bud can lead to developmental arrest, perhaps with the formation of only vestigial digits. This mechanism may sometimes apply to other organ malformations, although is usually less certain.

Symmetry and Asymmetry

When trying to assess whether a birth defect is genetic or non-genetic, it may be helpful to consider aspects of symmetry. As a very broad generalization, symmetrical and midline abnormalities frequently have a genetic basis. Asymmetrical defects are less likely to have a genetic basis. In the examples shown in Fig. 16.21, the child with cleidocranial dysplasia (see Fig. 16.21A) has symmetrical defects (absent or hypoplastic clavicles) and other features indicating a generalized tissue disorder that is overwhelmingly likely to have a genetic basis. The striking asymmetry of the limb deformities in Fig. 16.21B is likely to have a non-genetic basis. Caution is important, however, as split-hand/foot malformation (ectrodactyly) is virtually always genetic but shows very variable expression —sometimes only one extremity manifesting an anomaly.

Counseling

In cases where the precise diagnosis is uncertain, an assessment of symmetry and midline involvement may be helpful for genetic counseling. Although it may be very frustrating that no detailed explanation is possible, in many cases reassurance about a low recurrence risk in a future pregnancy can be given, based on empirical data. It is worth noting that this does not necessarily mean genetic factors are irrelevant. Some "unexplained" malformations and syndromes could well be attributed to *de novo* heterozygous pathogenic variants, microdeletions (p. 258) or uniparental disomy (p. 77). All of these would convey negligible recurrence risks to future siblings, although with new variants or microdeletions a significant risk (usually 50%) applies to the offspring of affected individuals. Increasingly, as discussed elsewhere, next generation sequencing methods, particularly whole-exome sequencing, are providing answers to many of these difficult cases, especially where moderate or severe learning disability is the principle feature of the syndrome.

Intellectual Disability

ID is a huge part of clinical genetic practice, and the numerous causes are woven into many other chapters of this book, for example, chromosome disorders (Chapter 17), developmental genetics (Chapter 9), and inborn errors of metabolism (Chapter 18). The genetic basis of ID, especially at the severe end of the spectrum, is increasingly being identified through CMA and next-generation sequencing techniques, but there are many non-genetic causes such as cerebral palsy and teratogens, as discussed in this chapter. Clinical geneticists tend to view ID in the context of a syndrome or its genetic cause, but for the patients themselves, their families and carers, and other professionals, the issues of daily life, support, and managing difficult circumstances are all-consuming. Having a child with ID may bring a parent's career and earning capacity to an end, with significant long-term consequences.

The terminology of ID generates much discussion because there is increasing sensitivity about political correctness and a concern to enhance the value of individuals with any sort of disability to help them fight discrimination, a process to which clinical geneticists can contribute significantly. Approximately 2% to 3% of the population has mild to moderate ID, and 0.5% to 1% has ID in the moderate to severe range. The measurement of intelligence quotient (IQ) is problematic but across the population follows a normal distribution, with the mean conventionally set at 100. Mild ID is defined as an IQ of 50 to 70, moderate 35 to 49, severe 20 to 34, and profound ID (formerly mental retardation)

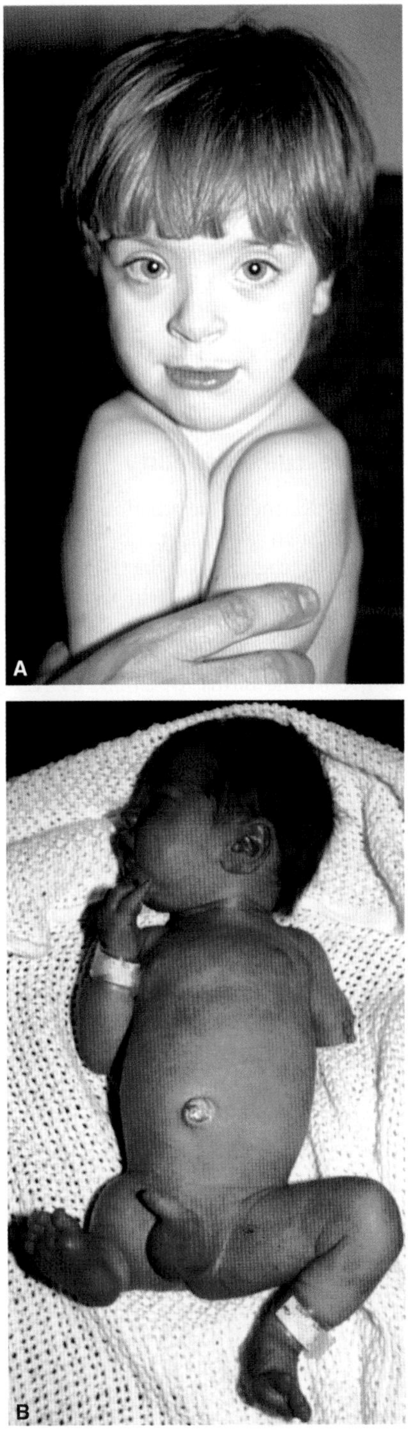

• **Fig. 16.21** (A) A boy with cleidocranial dysplasia in whom the clavicles have failed to develop, hence the remarkable mobility of his shoulders. He also has a relatively large head with widely spaced eyes (hypertelorism). He presented with ear problems—conductive deafness is a recognized feature. Skeletal dysplasias usually manifest in one main tissue and are symmetrical, suggesting a genetic basis. (B) A child with congenital limb deformities from amniotic bands. The marked asymmetry suggests a non-genetic cause.

less than 20. However, there are many types of ID, and much academic effort has been invested in developing classification systems, as well as the tools to dissect and describe the many different specific disabilities, although for many patients with genetic conditions the term "global developmental delay" often applies.

In the absence of a family history of ID, emerging data indicate that the risk of a non-consanguineous couple having a child with ID ranges from 1 in 400 for a young couple around 20 years of age to 1 in 200 for an older couple around 40 years of age. Much of the increased risk for an older couple is attributable to *de novo* variants generated during spermatogenesis. The majority of cases of ID occurring in the offspring of non-consanguineous parents are caused by *de novo* heterozygous pathogenic variants, with AR causes accounting for just 1 in 30 cases.

X-Linked Intellectual Disability

Previously known as XL mental retardation, X-linked ID (XLID) refers to ID associated with genetic variants on the X-chromosome. It was recognized in the 1930s that there was a 25% excess of males with severe ID in institutions, and it was later calculated in British Columbia that the incidence of XLID was 1.83 per 1000 live male births, with a carrier frequency of 2.44 per 1000 live female births. By 2006, 24 XL genes associated with ID, both syndromic and non-syndromic, were identified, but that figure now exceeds 100. One rare but well-known example is the *RPS6KA3* gene, for which pathogenic variants cause Coffin-Lowry syndrome (Fig. 16.22A,B,C). Individually these conditions are rare, with the exception of fragile-X syndrome, which is covered in Chapter 17. They also include a proportion of genes implicated in XL dominant conditions, which very often occur as *de novo* mutations, of which Rett syndrome is the best known, but many others are well recognized.

Autistic Spectrum Disorder

In 1943 Dr Leo Kanner provided the first succinct description of autism when he wrote: *"These children come into the world with the innate inability to form the usual biologically provided affective contact with people ... an inability to relate themselves in the ordinary way to people and situations from the beginning of life ..."* and *"There is from the start an extreme autistic aloneness that, whenever possible, disregards, ignores, shuts out anything that comes into the child from the outside."* A year later Dr. Hans Asperger noted that *"... in every instance where it is possible to make a close study similar traits were to be found in some degree in parents and other relatives."* These elegant observations encompass the key features of autistic spectrum disorder (ASD), namely impaired development of: (1) selective **social** attachments; (2) expressive or receptive language used for social **communication**; and (3) functional or symbolic play **behavior**—as well, of course, as the issue of **heritability**.

Today the diagnostic criteria for ASD are detailed, and the assessment lengthy and sophisticated (Box 16.3), and ASD is sometimes classified with other so-called "pervasive developmental disorders." The epidemiological aspects of ASD are shown in Box 16.4. There is also a paternal age–related effect: for children born to a father aged 45 years or older the risk of developing ASD is 3 to 4 times higher than for children born to fathers aged 20 to 24. Evidence for heritability is incontrovertible, and twin studies have been key to showing this. For classical autism, monozygotic (MZ) twins demonstrate a concordance rate of approximately 60%, whereas the rate for dizygotic (DZ) twins is 0%. When the broader phenotype is examined, this becomes approximately 92% for MZ twins and approximately 10% for DZ twins. The sibling recurrence risk for the broad ASD phenotype is up to 6%. Overall, the heritability of ASD is estimated to be greater than 90%.

The data are convincing, but the search for precise genetic causative factors using genome-wide association studies has been far from fruitful, despite the combined efforts of large consortia worldwide. Multiple different loci have been implicated, indicating extreme genetic heterogeneity. The exception to this otherwise confusing picture has been the clear association with various copy number variants identified through CMA analysis, giving rise to new microdeletion and microduplication syndromes, some of which are described in Chapter 17.

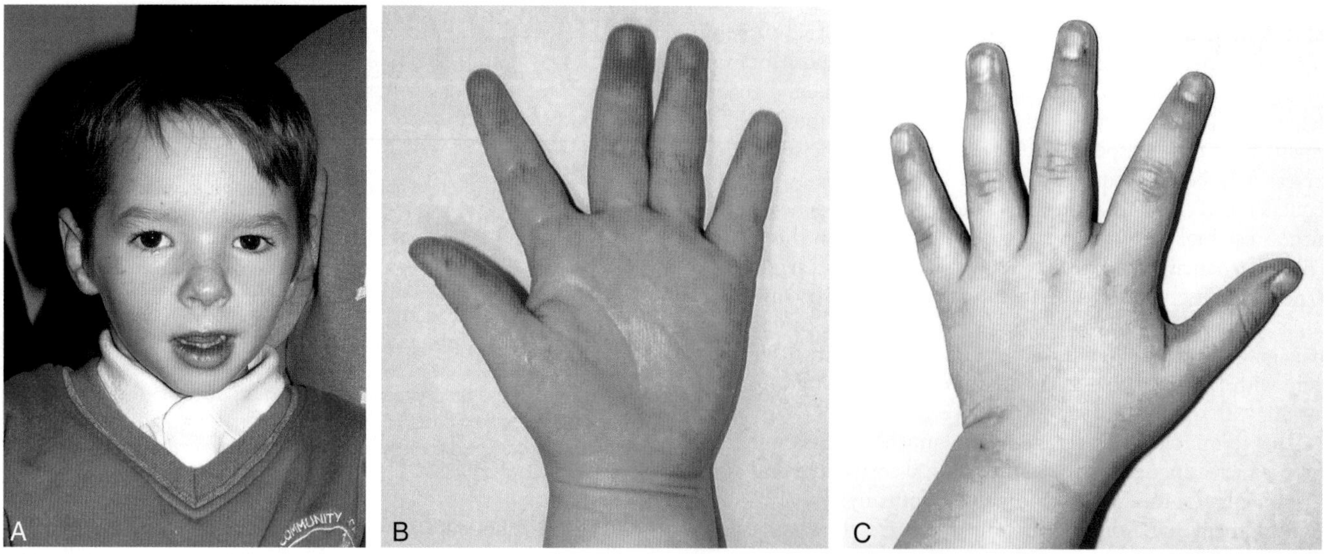

• **Fig. 16.22** (A) A child with X-linked Coffin-Lowry syndrome due to a pathogenic variant in the *RPS6KA3* gene. He has a characteristic facial appearance. (B) The same child showing the typical "straight" ulnar border of the hand. (C) The same child showing typical fingers–proximally broad and tapering.

• BOX 16.3 Diagnostic Criteria for Autistic Spectrum Disorder

Abnormal or impaired development at less than 3 years of age in one or more of the following:

- Development of selective **social** attachments
- Expressive or receptive language used for social **communication**
- Functional or symbolic play—**behavior**

For a diagnosis the child must have six or more of the following:

Social (≥ 2)
Failure of eye-to-eye gaze
Failure of peer relationships—interests, activities, emotions
Failure to recognize social norms
Failure to share enjoyment

Communication (≥ 1)
Speech delay and failure to compensate by gesture
Failure to sustain conversation or reciprocate
Stereotypic/repetitive use of language
Lack of make-believe imitative play

Behavior (≥ 1)
Preoccupations—restricted patterns of interest
Compulsivity
Stereotypic/repetitive motor mannerisms (e.g., hand flapping)
Preoccupations with nonfunctional elements (e.g., odor, touch)

Some Classic and New Intellectual Disability Syndromes

This is a vast area of clinical genetics, and for many classic ID syndromes the reader must explore other chapters of this book. This section highlights some that are not covered elsewhere, as well as a small number of newer conditions identified through cohort studies using trio whole-exome sequencing.

Cornelia de Lange Syndrome

This distinctive condition owes its name to the observations of the outstanding Dutch pediatrician in Amsterdam, Cornelia de Lange, in 1933, although was earlier reported by Brachmann in 1916, hence it is also known as Brachmann-de Lange syndrome. The facial features are very recognizable when classically present, consisting of characteristic eyebrows—neat, arched and meeting in the middle (synophrys), a crescent-shaped mouth with thin lips, and a long philtrum (Fig. 16.23A,B). In addition, the hands can help to confirm or refute a clinical diagnosis—individuals with this condition have short tapering fingers, especially the fifth, with clinodactyly, and the thumbs are usually small and proximally placed (Fig. 16.23C). In approximately one-quarter of cases there may be a severe upper limb deficiency, often unilateral, such that monodactyly arises from a short forearm. ID is profound in up to half of all affected individuals, as well as behavior problems such as self-injury and aggression, but can be very mild in perhaps 10%, so marked variability occurs. Congenital heart disease, diaphragmatic hernia, and intestinal malrotation may be present, and feeding difficulties are a common management issue.

In 2004 heterozygous variants were found in the first (and main) gene for Cornelia de Lange syndrome (CdLS), namely *NIPBL*, a homologue of Drosophila *Nipped-B*, which encodes a "cohesin" protein. The associated protein complex is required for normal sister chromatid cohesion in cell division. Since then variants have been found in other genes in patients with CdLS-like features, including *SMC3* and XL *SMC1A* (see below), which may account for approximately 5% of cases.

• BOX 16.4 Epidemiology of Autistic Spectrum Disorder

Frequency:	
Classical autism (severe):	1.7 in 1000
Autism, Asperger and pervasive developmental disorders:	3.4–6.3 in 1000
Male:Female Ratio:	
Overall:	4:1
Asperger syndrome:	8:1
Severe autism:	1:1 (approx.)
Twin and sibling studies (broad ASD phenotype):	
Monozygotic twin concordance:	approximately 92%
Dizygotic twin concordance:	approximately 10%
Sibling recurrence risk:	3% to 6% (25 × background risk)

Other features:
Epilepsy occurs in 25% to 30%, suggesting an underlying neurodevelopmental disorder
Head circumference is in the upper centiles in approximately 25%

CHARGE Syndrome

CHARGE used to be considered an association and is an acronym for *c*oloboma of iris or retina, congenital *h*eart defects, *a*tresia of the choanae, *r*etardation of growth and development, *g*enital anomalies (males), and *e*ar abnormalities (including deafness), although not all patients manifest all features. Tracheoesophageal fistula is an occasional complication, as well as clefting and facial asymmetry (Fig. 16.24). ID can range from severe to mild, and occasional parent-child transmission has been reported.

Since the finding of heterozygous variants in the *CHD7* (*KIAA1416*) gene the condition is now regarded as a syndrome rather than an association, and a second gene, *SEMA3E* (*KIAA0331*), has been implicated. *CHD7* is a positive regulator of the production of ribosomal RNA in the nucleolus.

Kabuki Syndrome

First described in 1981 in Japan, this condition was so named because patients' faces resembled the make-up worn by actors of the traditional Japanese Kabuki theater. Indeed, for some time it was known as "Kabuki make-up" syndrome, as well as Niikawa-Kuroki syndrome after the scientists who first described it. Apart from the distinctive facies (Fig.16.25A,B) and mild to moderate ID, patients are typically hypermobile and hypotonic, may have congenital heart disease—particularly of the left outflow tract—suffer sensorineural hearing impairment, show digital anomalies (Fig. 16.25C) including persistent fetal finger pads, have renal tract anomalies, and occasionally exhibit diaphragmatic hernia. Some present in the neonatal period with hypoglycemia secondary to hyperinsulinism.

After a number of false trails looking for the cause of Kabuki syndrome, variants in the gene *KMT2D* (previously *MLL2*), encoding a histone methyltransferase, were confirmed as the cause in many patients in 2010. Subsequently, in 2013, heterozygous variants in the XL gene *KDM6A*, encoding a histone demethylase, were also found to cause the Kabuki syndrome phenotype in a proportion of patients. Both of these genes are chromatin modifiers, and the clue to their involvement came from patients that had chromosomal imbalances at the respective loci. *KDM6A* is unusual because it escapes X-inactivation at Xp11.3, and haploinsufficiency is probably the pathogenic basis. Up to 30% of Kabuki syndrome cases remain unexplained.

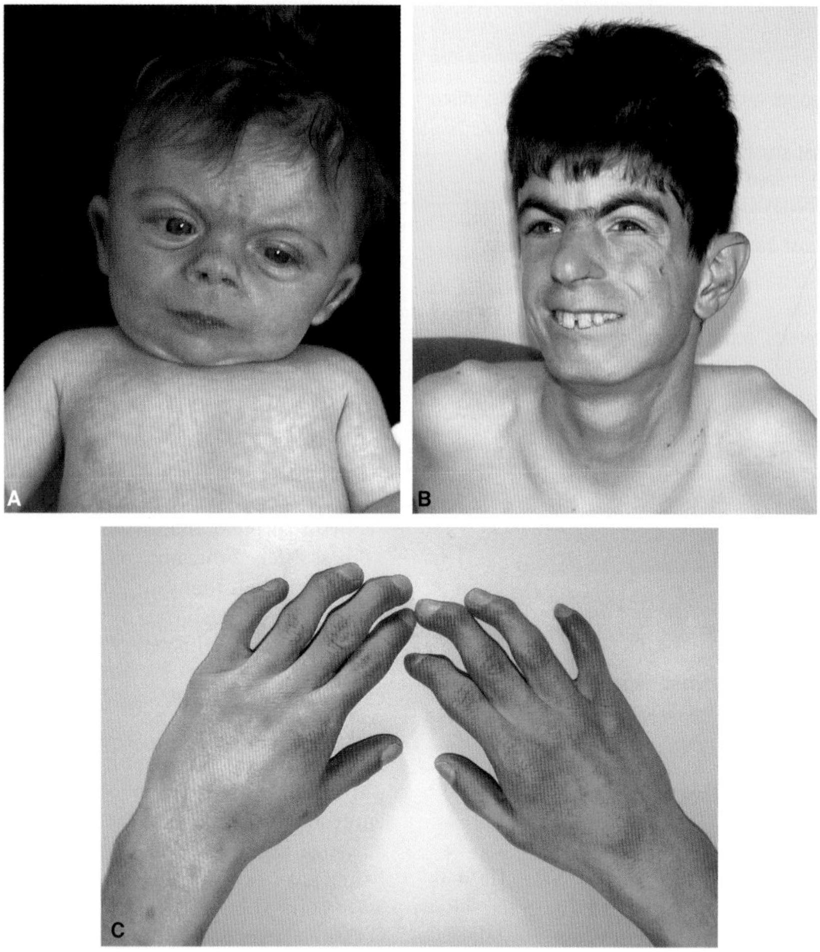

• **Fig. 16.23** (A) A child aged 2 months with typical Cornelia de Lange Syndrome (CdLS). (B) A young adult with CdLS and (C) his hands showing small thumbs, fifth fingers, and short nails.

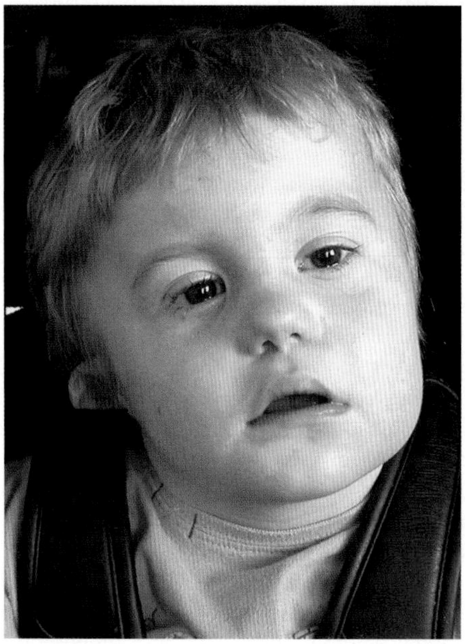

• **Fig. 16.24** A young child with CHARGE (*c*oloboma of iris or retina, congenital *h*eart defects, *a*tresia of the choanae, *r*etardation of growth and development, *g*enital anomalies (males) and *e*ar abnormalities) syndrome and a mutation in the *CHD7* gene.

Mowat-Wilson Syndrome

This condition also has distinctive facial features (Fig. 16.26) and finally emerged as a discrete entity in 2003 after a few earlier reports had gathered together similar patients with severe ID, Hirschsprung disease, microcephaly, absent speech, and agenesis of the corpus callosum. Congenital heart disease, particularly right outflow tract anomalies, may occur, as well as microphthalmia, hypospadias in males and seizures.

Chromosome imbalances were again the clue to the genetic locus at 2q22; indeed, some cases are the result of microdeletions, whilst others are caused by heterozygous variants in *ZEB2* (previously *SIP-1*, or *ZFHX1B*). The gene encodes a DNA-binding transcriptional repressor that interacts with the histone deacetylation complex via SMADs and the TGF-β signaling pathway (p. 108).

Pitt-Hopkins Syndrome

In 1978 Pitt and Hopkins reported patients with severe ID, macrostomia, and episodes of overbreathing. These patients also have microcephaly, sometimes agenesis of the corpus callosum and cerebellar hypoplasia. They may have seizures, constipation, or frank Hirschsprung disease and hypogenitalism in males.

Through a microdeletion at 18q21 detected in one patient through CMA, heterozygous variants in *TCF4* were identified as the cause. *TCF4* encodes a basic helix-loop-helix transcription factor. An affected child is shown in Fig. 16.27.

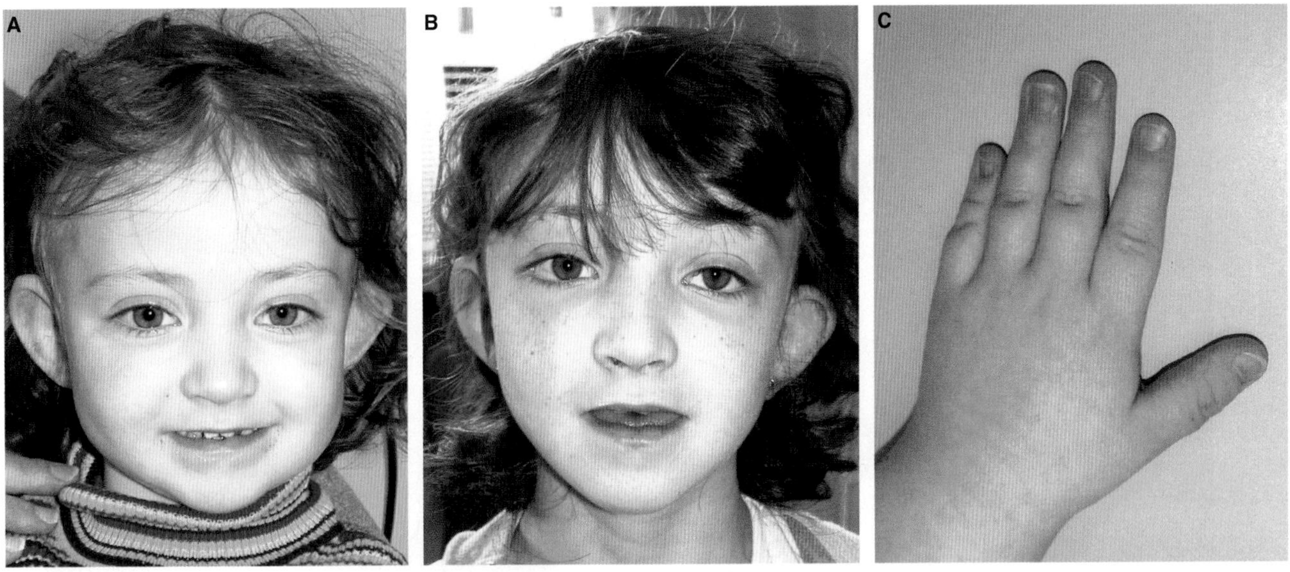

• **Fig. 16.25** (A) A 2-year-old child with Kabuki syndrome, and (B) the same child aged 8 years. Note interrupted eyebrows, prominent ears and everted lateral third of the lower eyelid. (C) The left hand of the same child, showing some shortening and tapering of the fingers, especially the fifth, which also has a small nail.

Wiedemann-Steiner Syndrome

Originally reported in 1985 and 2000 without much follow-up, this syndrome burst on the scene, so to speak, in 2012 with the finding of heterozygous variants in the *MLL1* gene, now reassigned as *KMT2A*. Like *MLL2* (*KMT2D*, Kabuki syndrome), this gene encodes a lysine-specific methyltransferase, a DNA-binding protein which in this case methylates histone H3.

The syndrome itself is characterized by ID to a variable degree, significant feeding difficulties, hypotonia and constipation in early childhood, and quite striking hypertrichosis of the back and forearms. The eyebrows tend to be thick and sometimes meet in the middle (synophrys), the eyelashes are long, the palpebral fissures are narrow and slightly down-slanting, the nasal bridge is broad, and there may be hypertelorism (Fig. 16.28). Stature tends to be short, and autistic features are part of the behavior disorder.

Genitopatellar Syndrome

Along with the so-called Say-Barber-Biesecker-Young-Simpson variant of Ohdo syndrome, genitopatellar syndrome is the other major phenotype caused by heterozygous variants in the *KAT6B* gene, which encodes a histone acetyltransferase. Both conditions, like the one previously discussed, suddenly had a high profile in

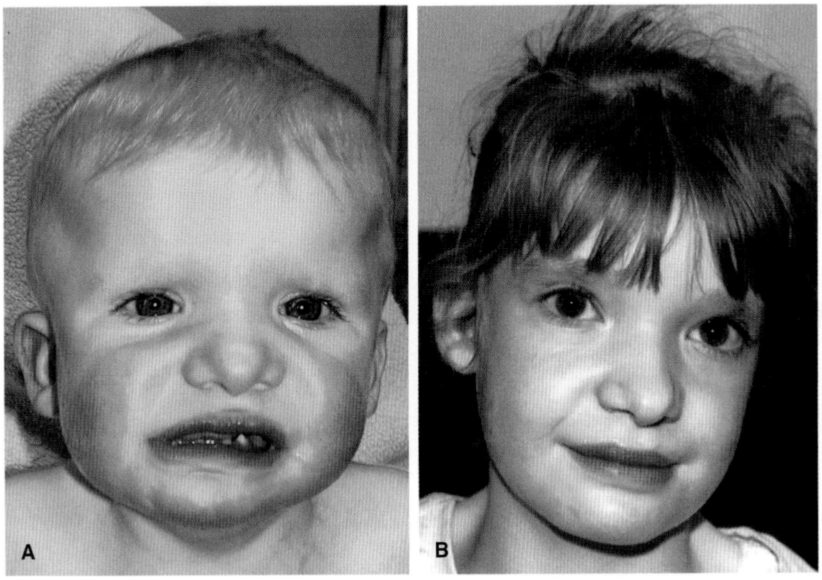

• **Fig. 16.26** Mowat-Wilson syndrome. (A) A young child aged 1 year. Note the prominent supra-orbital ridges, deep-set eyes and prominent mandible. (B) The same child aged 7 years.

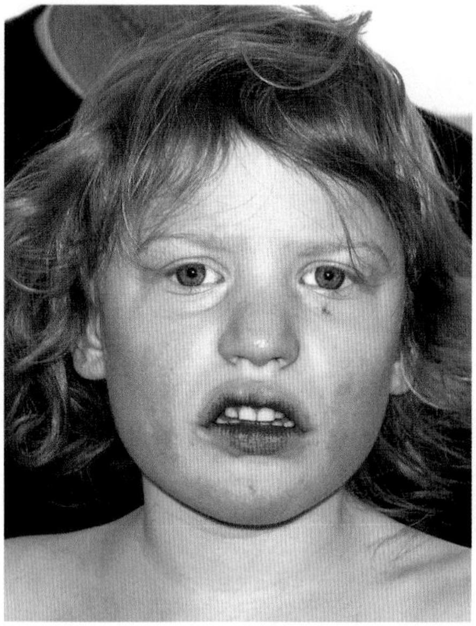

• **Fig. 16.27** A child with Pitt-Hopkins syndrome. Note the macrostomia.

2011 to 2012 when next-generation sequencing linked them to the gene.

Genitopatellar syndrome is characterized by severe ID, microcephaly, agenesis of the corpus callosum and neuronal migration defects, small patellae, hypogenitalism in males, renal tract anomalies, occasional dextrocardia and intestinal malrotation, and osteoporosis with consequent fractures. Facial features include hypertelorism (Fig. 16.29A), and the thumbs and great toes are typically long (see Fig. 16.29B,C).

Coffin-Siris Syndrome

Coffin-Siris syndrome is sufficiently variable that it is hard to believe some patients are grouped with others under the same label, and it is also genetically heterogeneous, with at least six genes implicated in those with the diagnosis—*ARID1A*,

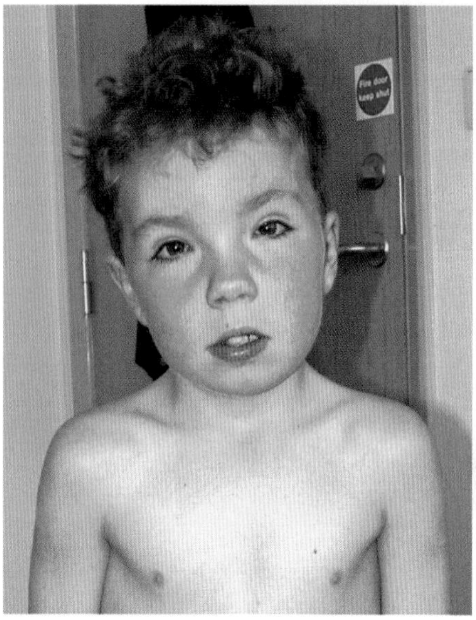

• **Fig. 16.28** A child with Wiedemann-Steiner syndrome. Note the broad nasal bridge and mild hypertelorism.

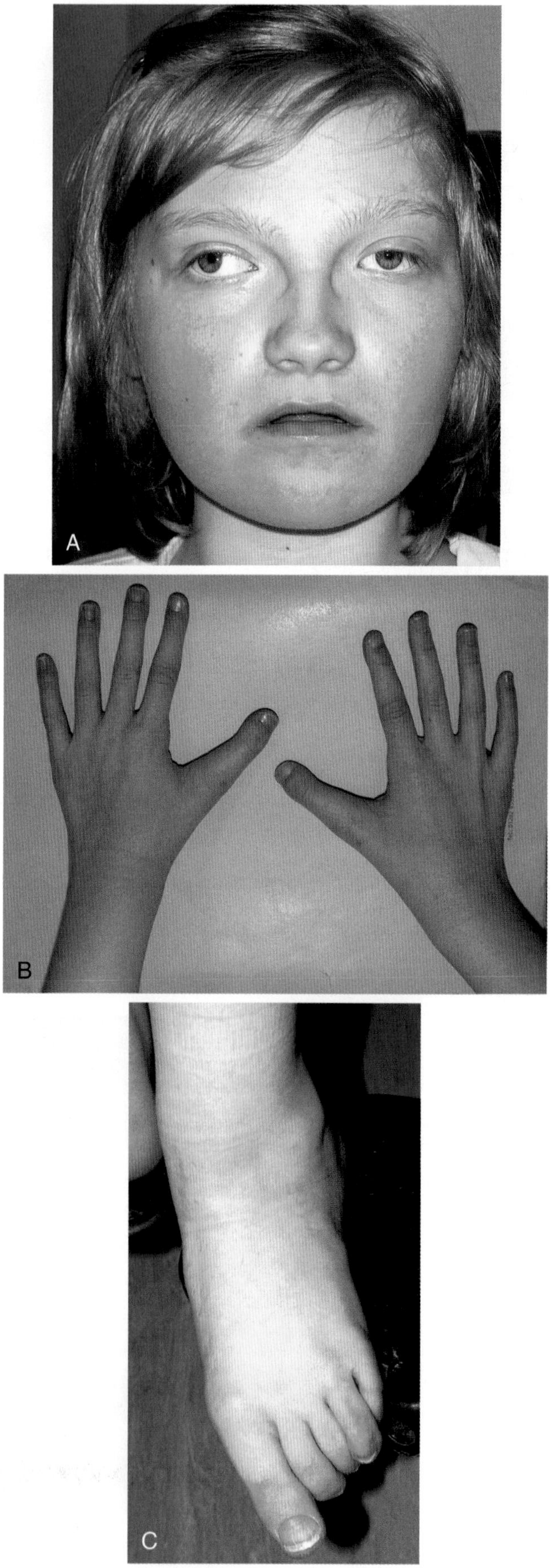

• **Fig. 16.29** A girl with genitopatellar syndrome. (A) Soft dysmorphic features, especially a broad nasal root. (B) and (C) The thumbs and great toes are unusually long.

ARID1B, *ARID2*, *SMARCA4*, *SMARCB1*, and *SMARCE1*. Conventionally, the key clinical features are ID, which can range from mild to severe and include very limited language development, hypoplasia of the fifth digit distal phalanx and nail, and rather coarse facies with hirsute features affecting the eyebrows, eyelashes and hairline, a flat nasal bridge, ptosis, and a broad oral stoma with thick lips (Fig. 16.30). Agenesis of the corpus callosum may be present, as well as congenital heart disease, and hypotonia/laxity in early childhood can be pronounced. However, the concept of Coffin-Siris syndrome as a distinct entity is in question and likely to evolve.

ARID1B has turned out to be a relatively common gene implicated in ID, accounting for up to 1% of cases in some cohorts. Heterozygous deletions and point mutations may cause the phenotype. To illustrate the difficulties with delineation, not all cases have fifth fingernail abnormalities, and not all individuals with pathogenic variants have typical facial features. The gene, which is also designated *KIAA1235*, encodes a protein which forms a subunit of a complex that remodels chromatin through regulation of gene expression.

SETD5-*Associated Mental Retardation*

This is an example of one of the newly reported ID disorders reported in 2014 caused by variants in *SETD5*, also designated *KIAA1757*, which is believed to encode a methyltransferase. In common with many of the newly delineated ID conditions, this disorder does not yet have a name other than being known by its gene. Moderate to severe ID occurs together with autistic features, and the facial features are subtle but probably recognizable with experience (Fig.16.31). The gene is located at 3p25, and not surprisingly there are overlapping features with the corresponding microdeletion 3p25 syndrome.

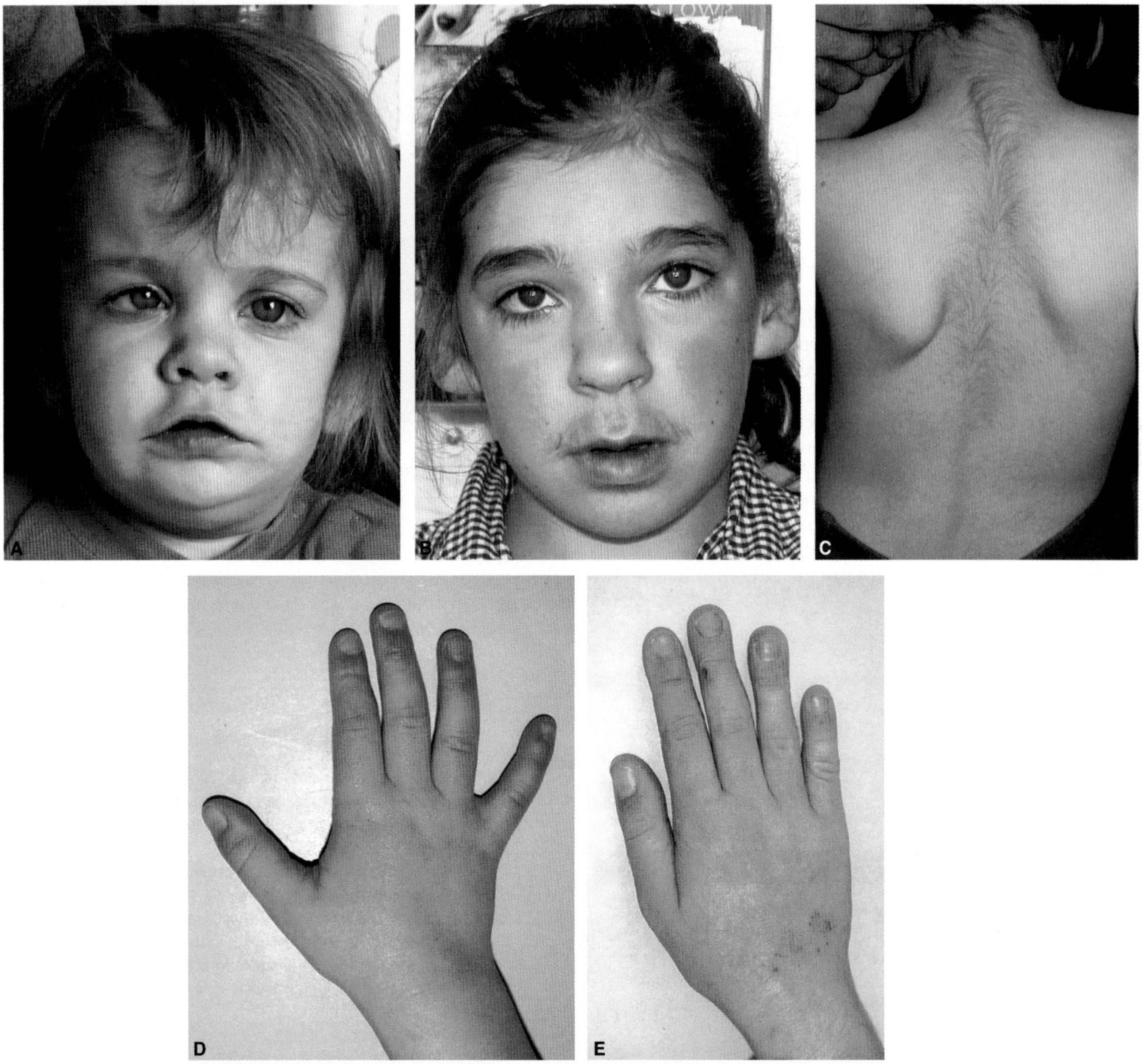

• **Fig. 16.30** A toddler and an older child with Coffin-Siris syndrome due to a variant (A) and deletion (B) of the *ARID1B* gene. Note the broad nasal root, broad nose, flat nasal tip, hirsute features, and fleshy ears. (C) The hirsute back of the child in (B). (D) and (E) The hands of the children shown in (A) and (B), respectively, showing slightly spatulate digits and slightly short fifth fingers with small nails.

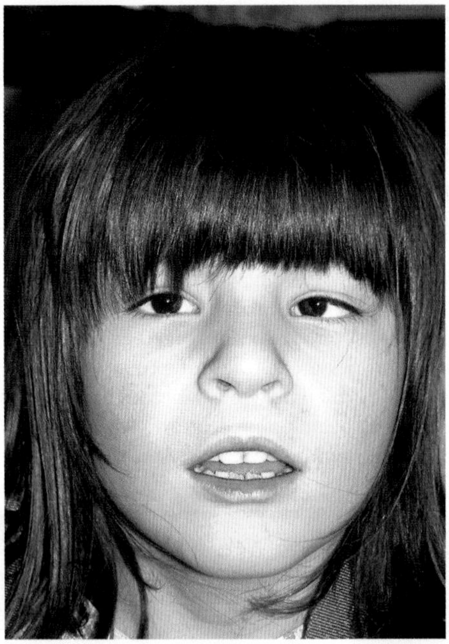

• **Fig. 16.31** A child with a *de novo* mutation in *SETD5*, giving rise to soft dysmorphic features and significant learning disability.

KCNQ2-*Associated Early Infantile Epileptic Encephalopathy*

Heterozygous *de novo* variants in *KCNQ2* cause one of the many varieties of early infantile epileptic encephalopathy (EIEE). The group of disorders is characterized by very early–onset epilepsy which can be very difficult to bring under control, although it sometimes improves over several years. Severe ID accompanies the disorder and is most likely a primary aspect rather than secondary to multiple seizures. Genes such as *SCN1A*, *SCN2A*, *ARX* and *CDKL5* (both XL), *STXBP1*, and many others, are associated with specific subtypes, although they are virtually impossible to distinguish clinically. The term **Ohtahara syndrome** is sometimes used. A child with severe developmental delay and early seizures is shown in Fig. 16.32A.

SMC1A-*Associated EIEE*

To conclude this chapter, and bring this section full circle, we return to the gene implicated in a rare form of CdLS, that is, XL *SMC1A* (p. 243). It emerged, in 2015 to 2016, that novel frameshift mutations can cause a form of EIEE more or less indistinguishable from the others and, notably, not accompanied by features of CdLS. An affected child is shown in Fig. 16.32B.

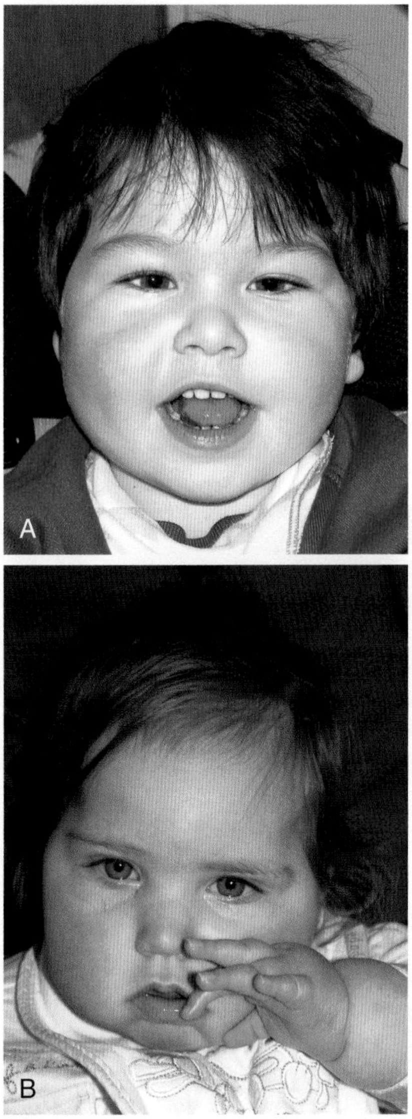

• **Fig. 16.32** Two children with early infantile epileptic encephalopathy due to a *de novo* variant in *KCNQ2* (A) and a *de novo* frameshift variant in the XL gene *SMC1A* (B) (without features of Cornelia de Lange syndrome).

ELEMENTS

1. Congenital abnormalities are apparent at birth in 1 in 40 of all newborn infants. They account for 20% to 25% of all deaths occurring in the perinatal period and in childhood up to the age of 10 years.
2. A single abnormality can be classified as a malformation, a deformation, a dysplasia, or a disruption. Multiple abnormalities can be classified as a sequence, a syndrome, or an association.
3. Congenital abnormalities can be caused by chromosome imbalance, single gene defects, multifactorial inheritance, or non-genetic factors. Many isolated malformations, including isolated congenital heart defects and neural tube defects, show multifactorial inheritance, whereas most dysplasias have a single gene etiology.
4. Many congenital malformations, including cleft lip/palate, congenital heart defects and neural tube defects, show etiological heterogeneity, so that when counseling patients it is important to establish whether these malformations are isolated or are associated with other abnormalities.
5. Many environmental agents have been shown to have a teratogenic effect with lifelong physical and neurodevelopmental implications, for example, alcohol, which should be avoided in pregnancy.
6. Intellectual disability is a huge part of clinical genetic practice and is often part of a syndrome; chromosome microarray and next generation sequencing are enabling great advances to be made in understanding the genetic causes.
7. For non-consanguineous couples, the risk of having a child with intellectual disability ranges from 1 in 400 for those around 20 years of age to 1 in 200 for those around 40 years of age. The majority of cases are attributed to *de novo* heterozygous pathogenic variants, with autosomal recessive causes accounting for 1 in 30 cases.

CLINICAL SCENARIO 1

You see a family affected by split-hand/foot malformation, also known as ectrodactyly. You draw the family pedigree, and two individuals are affected—II.5, an adult of 30 years, and III.1, a child of 3 years, both male. No other family member is affected. II.5 has relatively severe manifestations with both hands and one foot involved; III.1 has just one hand involved, with the other extremities normal.

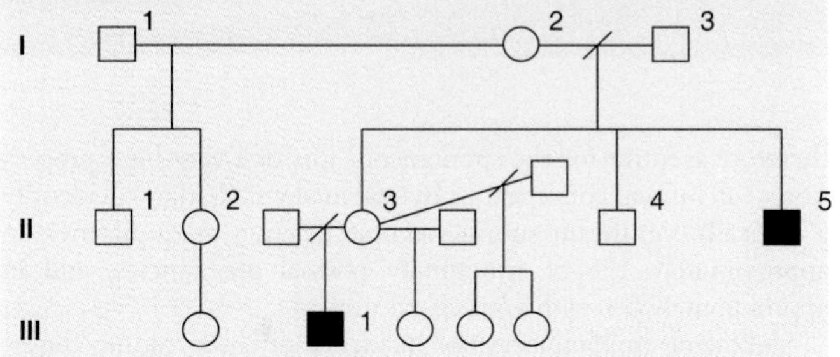

How might this pattern of ectrodactyly in the family be explained?

CLINICAL SCENARIO 2

A neonate is born with a very severe eye malformation—anophthalmia affecting one eye and severe microphthalmia in the other. Examination is otherwise unremarkable at this stage.

A sample of DNA from the baby is sent to a research group which is focused on identifying anophthalmia/microphthalmia genes. No positive result is forthcoming, and the child is lost to follow-up in Clinical Genetics.

Years later the same child is referred back to Clinical Genetics as a 19-year-old young man. He has been followed by pediatricians for many years and has severe intellectual disability besides being registered blind. He was found on magnetic resonance imaging scan to have partial agenesis of the corpus callosum, and he has had seizures which are reasonably well controlled. He has a history of loss of consciousness, with several recorded episodes of hypoglycemia. He also appears to have been prone to infections in recent years. His chromosome microarray analysis, undertaken by a pediatrician, was normal.

Your examination finds that he has a head circumference in the 3rd centile, somewhat large and prominent ears, minor digital anomalies of his hands, oligodontia, and dislocatable patellae.

How would you continue investigations in this young man?

Further Reading

Aase J. *Diagnostic Dysmorphology*. London: Plenum; 1990.

A detailed text of the art and science of dysmorphology.

Clayton-Smith J, Bromley R, Dean J, et al. Diagnosis and management of individuals with fetal valproate spectrum disorder; a consensus statement from the European Reference Network for Congenital Malformations and Intellectual Disability. *Orphanet J Rare Dis*. 2019;14:180.

The outcome of a working group set up to develop new diagnostic guidelines and clinical practice recommendations related to valproic acid embryopathy.

Jones KL, Jones MC, del Campo M. *Smith's Recognisable Patterns of Human Malformation*. 7th ed. Elsevier; 2013.

The standard pediatric textbook guide to syndromes.

Stevenson RE, Hall JG, Everman DB, Solomon BD. *Human Malformations and Related Anomalies*. 3rd ed. New York: Oxford University Press; 2015.

The definitive guide, in two volumes, to human malformations.

17

Chromosome Disorders

If chromosomes are broken by various means, the broken ends appear to be adhesive and tend to fuse with one another 2-by-2.

Barbara McClintock (1902-92, botanist, cytogeneticist, and Nobel Laureate)

The development of a reliable technique for chromosome analysis in 1956 soon led to the discovery that several previously described conditions were caused by an abnormality in chromosome number. Within 3 years, the causes of Down syndrome (47,XX + 21/47,XY + 21), Klinefelter syndrome (47,XXY), and Turner syndrome (45,X) had been established. Shortly after, other autosomal trisomy syndromes were recognized, and over the ensuing years many other multiple malformation syndromes were described in which there was loss or gain of chromosome material.

Presently, there are tens of thousands of chromosome abnormalities registered in laboratory databases, and the disciplines of cytogenetics and molecular genetics have merged through the development of chromosome microarray (CMA), also known as microarray comparative genomic hybridization (microarray-CGH), technology (pp. 62, 259). When very small genomic imbalances are detected by these techniques, we may be unsure whether it is appropriate to classify them as "chromosome disorders." Individually, most conditions are very rare, but together they make a major contribution to human morbidity and mortality. Chromosome abnormalities account for a large proportion of spontaneous pregnancy loss and childhood disability, and also contribute to malignancy throughout life as a consequence of acquired translocations and other aberrations.

In Chapter 3, the basic principles of chromosome structure, function and behavior during cell division were described, together with an account of chromosome abnormalities and how they can arise and be transmitted in families. In this chapter, the medical aspects of chromosome abnormalities, and some of their specific syndromes, are described.

Incidence of Chromosome Abnormalities

Chromosome abnormalities are present in at least 10% of all spermatozoa and 25% of mature oocytes. Some 15% to 20% of all recognized pregnancies end in spontaneous miscarriage, and many more zygotes and embryos are so abnormal that survival beyond the first few days or weeks after fertilization is not possible. Approximately 50% of all spontaneous miscarriages have a chromosome abnormality (Table 17.1), and the incidence of chromosome abnormalities in morphologically normal embryos is approximately 20%. Using high-resolution techniques, as many as 80% of embryos generated for *in vitro* fertilization can be identified as possibly having genomic imbalances. Chromosome anomalies therefore account for the spontaneous loss of a very high proportion of all human conceptions. In fetal medicine CMA will identify a clinically significant submicroscopic deletion or duplication in approximately 1% of structurally normal pregnancies, and in approximately 6% with a structural anomaly.

Following implantation the incidence of chromosome abnormalities falls rapidly. By birth it has declined to a level of 0.5% to 1%, although the total is higher (5%) in stillborn infants. Table 17.2 lists the incidence figures for chromosome abnormalities based on newborn surveys. It is notable that, among the commonly recognized aneuploidy syndromes, there is also a high proportion of spontaneous pregnancy loss (Table 17.3). This is illustrated by comparison of the incidence of conditions such as Down syndrome at the time of chorionic villus sampling (11 to 12 weeks), amniocentesis (16 weeks), and term (Fig. 17.1).

Down Syndrome (Trisomy 21)

This condition derives its name from Dr. Langdon Down, who first described it in the Clinical Lecture Reports of the London Hospital in 1866. The chromosomal basis of Down syndrome was not established until 1959 by Lejeune and colleagues in Paris.

Incidence

The overall birth incidence, when adjusted for the increasingly widespread impact of antenatal screening, is approximately 1:1000 in the United Kingdom, which has a national register. In the

TABLE 17.1 Chromosome abnormalities in spontaneous abortions (percentage values relate to total of chromosomally abnormal abortuses)

Abnormality	Incidence (%)
Trisomy 13	2
Trisomy 16	15
Trisomy 18	3
Trisomy 21	5
Other trisomy	25
Monosomy X	20
Triploidy	15
Tetraploidy	5
Other	10

TABLE 17.2 Incidence of chromosome abnormalities in the newborn

Abnormality	Incidence per 10,000 Births
Autosomes	
Trisomy 13	2
Trisomy 18	3
Trisomy 21	15
Sex Chromosomes	
Female Births	
45,X	1–2
47,XXX	10
Male Births	
47,XXY	10
47,XYY	10
Other unbalanced rearrangements	10
Balanced rearrangements	30
Total	90

TABLE 17.3 Spontaneous pregnancy loss in commonly recognized aneuploidy syndromes

Disorder	Proportion Undergoing Spontaneous Pregnancy Loss (%)
Trisomy 13	95
Trisomy 18	95
Trisomy 21	80
Monosomy X	98

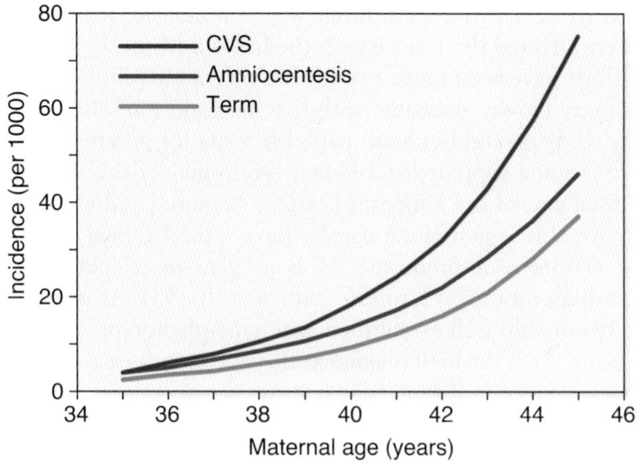

• **Fig. 17.1** Approximate incidence of trisomy 21 at the time of chorionic villus sampling (CVS) (11–12 weeks), amniocentesis (16 weeks) and delivery. (From Hook EB, Cross PK, Jackson L, et al. Maternal age-specific rates of 47, +21 and other cytogenetic abnormalities diagnosed in the first trimester of pregnancy in chorionic villus biopsy specimens. *Am J Hum Genet*. 1988;42:797–807; and Cuckle HS, Wald NJ, Thompson SG. Estimating a woman's risk of having a pregnancy associated with Down syndrome using her age and serum alpha-fetoprotein level. *Br J Obstet Gynaecol*. 1987;94:387–402.)

TABLE 17.4 Incidence of Down syndrome in relation to maternal age

Maternal Age at Delivery (Years)	Incidence of Down Syndrome
20	1 in 1500
25	1 in 1350
30	1 in 900
35	1 in 400
36	1 in 300
37	1 in 250
38	1 in 200
39	1 in 150
40	1 in 100
41	1 in 85
42	1 in 65
43	1 in 50
44	1 in 40
45	1 in 30

(Modified from Cuckle HS, Wald NJ, Thompson SG. Estimating a woman's risk of having a pregnancy associated with Down syndrome using her age and serum alpha-fetoprotein level. *Br J Obstet Gynaecol.* 1987;94:387–402.)

United States, the birth incidence has been estimated at approximately 1:800. In the United Kingdom, approximately 60% of Down syndrome cases are detected prenatally. There is a strong association between the incidence of Down syndrome and advancing maternal age (Table 17.4).

Clinical Features

These are summarized in Box 17.1. The most common finding in the newborn period is significant hypotonia. Usually the facial characteristics of upward sloping palpebral fissures, small ears, and protruding tongue (Figs. 17.2 and 17.3) prompt rapid suspicion of

• BOX 17.1 Common Findings in Down Syndrome

Newborn period

Hypotonia, sleepy, excess nuchal skin

Craniofacial

Brachycephaly, epicanthic folds, protruding tongue, small ears, upward sloping palpebral fissures

Limbs

Single palmar crease, small middle phalanx of fifth finger, wide gap between first and second toes

Cardiac

Atrial and ventricular septal defects, common atrioventricular canal, patent ductus arteriosus

Other

Anal atresia, duodenal atresia, Hirschsprung disease, short stature, strabismus

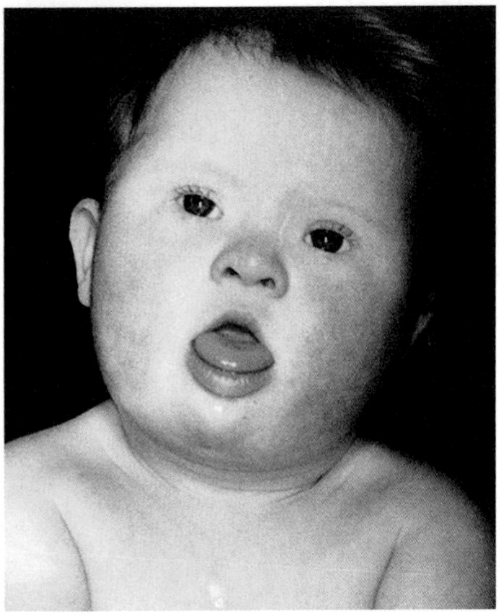

• **Fig. 17.2** A child with Down syndrome.

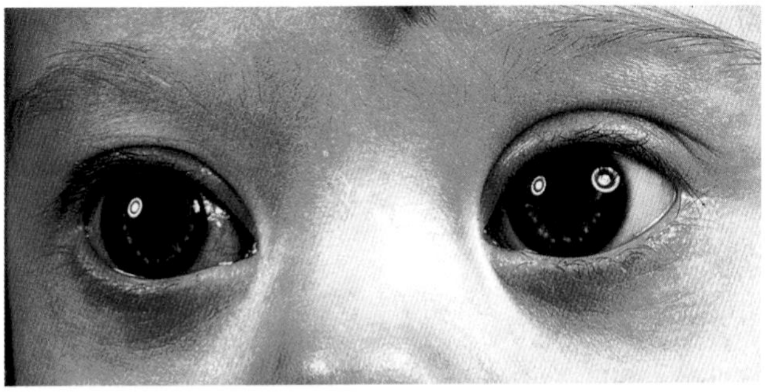

• **Fig. 17.3** Close-up view of the eyes and nasal bridge of a child with Down syndrome showing upward sloping palpebral fissures, Brushfield spots, and bilateral epicanthic folds.

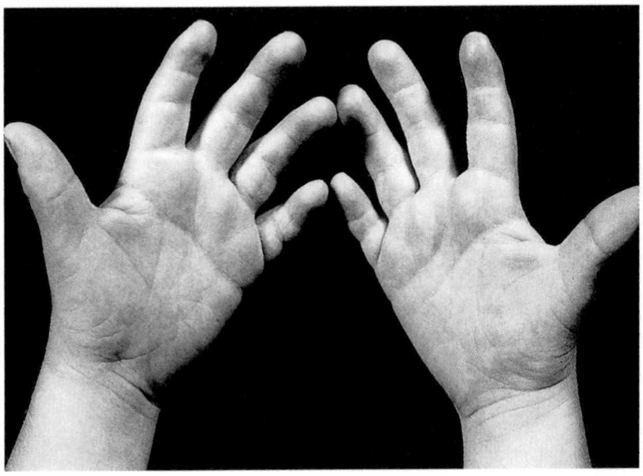

• **Fig. 17.4** The hands of an adult with Down syndrome. Note the single palmar crease in the left hand plus bilateral short curved fifth fingers (clinodactyly).

the diagnosis, although this can be delayed in very small or premature babies. Single palmar creases are found in 50% of children with Down syndrome (Fig. 17.4), in contrast to between 2% and 3% of the general population, and congenital cardiac defects in 40% to 45%, the four most common lesions being atrioventricular canal defects, ventricular septal defects, patent ductus arteriosus, and tetralogy of Fallot.

TABLE 17.5 Chromosome abnormalities in Down syndrome

Abnormality	Frequency (%)
Trisomy	95
Translocation	4
Mosaicism	1

Natural History

Affected children show a broad range of intellectual ability, with intelligence quotient (IQ) scores ranging from 25 to 75. The average IQ of young adults is around 40 to 45. Social skills are relatively well advanced, and most children are happy and very affectionate. Adult height is approximately 150 cm. In the absence of a severe cardiac anomaly, which despite modern surgery and intensive care leads to early death in 15% to 20% of cases, average life expectancy is 50 to 60 years. Overall, about 90% of live-born individuals with Down syndrome reach 20 years of age. Most affected adults develop Alzheimer disease in later life, possibly because of a gene dosage effect—the amyloid precursor protein (*APP*) gene is on chromosome 21. This gene is known to be implicated in some familial cases of Alzheimer disease (Chapter 19, p. 291).

Chromosome Findings

These are listed in Table 17.5. In cases resulting from trisomy 21, the additional chromosome is maternal in origin in more than 90% of cases, and DNA studies have shown that this arises most commonly as a result of nondisjunction in maternal meiosis I (p. 32). Robertsonian translocations (p. 38) account for approximately 4% of all cases, in roughly one-third of which a parent is found to be a carrier. Children with mosaicism are often less severely affected than those with the full syndrome.

Efforts have been made to correlate the various clinical features in trisomy Down syndrome with specific regions of chromosome 21 by studying children with partial trisomy for different regions. There is some support for a Down syndrome "critical region" at the distal end of the long arm (21q22) because children with trisomy for this region alone usually have typical Down syndrome facial features. Chromosome 21 is a "gene-poor" chromosome with a high ratio of AT to GC sequences (p. 53). At present the only reasonably well established genotype-phenotype correlation in trisomy 21 is the high incidence of Alzheimer disease (*APP* gene dosage).

Recurrence Risk

For straightforward trisomy 21, the recurrence risk is related to maternal age (variable) and the simple fact that trisomy has already occurred (approximately 1%). The combined recurrence risk is usually between 1:200 and 1:100. In translocation cases, similar figures apply if neither parent is a carrier. In familial translocation cases, the recurrence risks vary from 1% to 3% for male carriers and up to 10% to 15% for female carriers, with the exception of very rare carriers of a 21q21q translocation, for whom the recurrence risk is 100% (p. 39).

Prenatal diagnosis can be offered based on analysis of chorionic villi or cultured amniotic cells. Prenatal screening programs have been introduced based on the so-called triple or quadruple tests of maternal serum at 16 weeks' gestation (p. 323).

Patau Syndrome (Trisomy 13) and Edwards Syndrome (Trisomy 18)

These very severe conditions were first described in 1960 and share some features in common (Figs. 17.5 and 17.6). The incidence of Edwards syndrome is approximately 1:6000, Patau syndrome is two or three times less frequent, and prognosis is very poor, with most infants dying during the first days or weeks of life, although most cases are now detected prenatally with intrauterine growth retardation and some abnormal fetal ultrasound features, often leading to termination. In the unusual event of longer-term survival, there is severe intellectual disability (ID). Cardiac abnormalities occur in at least 90% of cases. The facial features in trisomy 13 are characteristic, often with clefting, and affected infants frequently have scalp defects, exomphalos, and postaxial polydactyly. Trisomy 18 is characterized by poor growth, microcephaly, micrognathia, clenched hands and "rocker bottom" feet.

Chromosome analysis usually reveals straightforward trisomy. Both disorders occur more frequently with advanced maternal age, the additional chromosome being of maternal origin (see Table 3.4, p. 36). Approximately 10% of cases are caused by mosaicism or unbalanced rearrangements, particularly Robertsonian translocations in Patau syndrome.

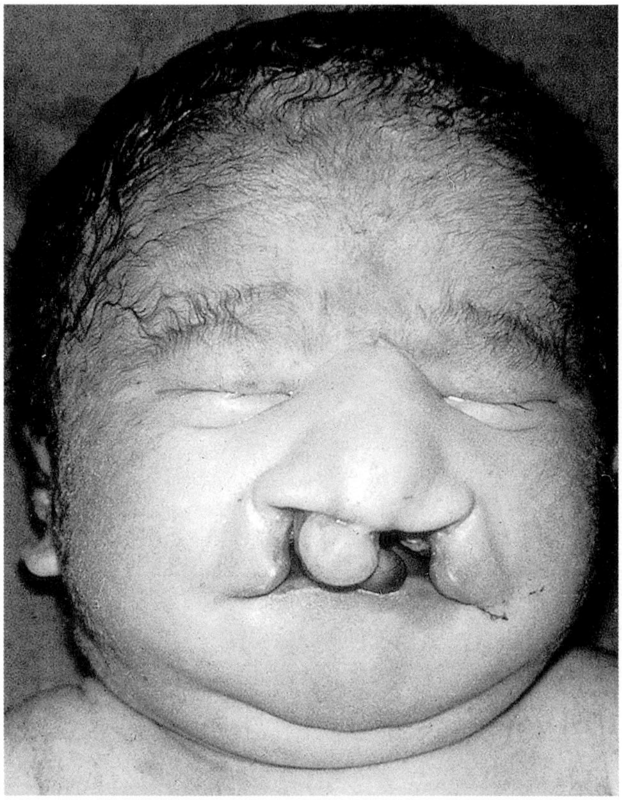

• **Fig. 17.5** Facial view of a child with trisomy 13 showing severe bilateral cleft lip and palate, and a typical broad nose.

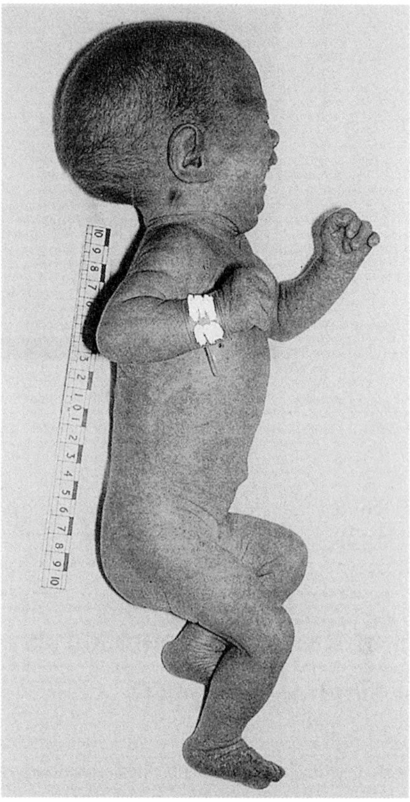

• **Fig. 17.6** A baby with trisomy 18. Note the prominent occiput and tightly clenched hands.

Triploidy

Triploidy (69,XXX, 69,XXY, 69,XYY) is a relatively common finding in material cultured from spontaneous abortions but is seen only rarely in a live-born infant. Such a child almost always shows severe intrauterine growth retardation with relative preservation of head growth at the expense of a small, narrow trunk. Syndactyly involving the third and fourth fingers and/or the second and third toes is a common finding. Cases of triploidy resulting from a double paternal contribution usually miscarry in early to midpregnancy and are associated with partial hydatidiform changes in the placenta (p. 122). Cases with a double maternal contribution survive for longer but rarely beyond the early neonatal period.

Hypomelanosis of Ito

Several children with mosaicism for diploidy/triploidy have been identified. These can demonstrate the clinical picture seen in full triploidy but in a milder form. An alternative presentation occurs as the condition known as hypomelanosis of Ito. In this curious disorder the skin shows alternating patterns of normally pigmented and depigmented streaks that correspond to the embryological developmental lines of the skin known as Blaschko lines (Fig. 17.7). Most children with hypomelanosis of Ito have moderate ID and convulsions that can be particularly difficult to treat. There is increasing evidence that this clinical picture represents a nonspecific embryological response to cell or tissue mosaicism. A similar pattern of skin pigmentation is sometimes seen in women with one of the rare XL dominant disorders (p. 75) with skin involvement, such as incontinentia pigmenti (see Fig. 6.18,

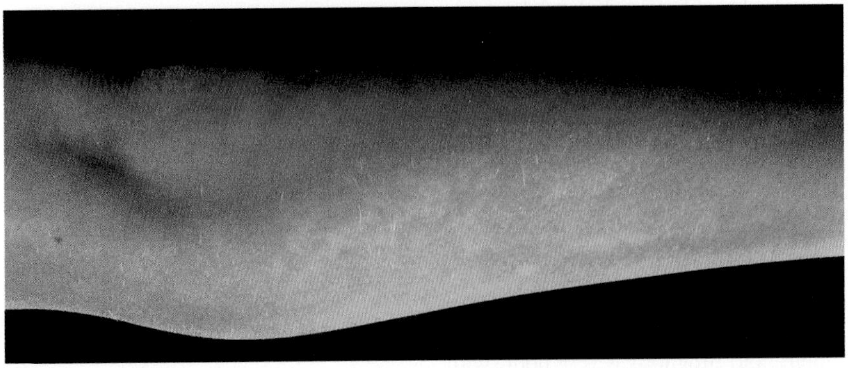

• **Fig. 17.7** Mosaic pattern of skin pigmentation on the arm of a child with hypomelanosis of Ito. (From Jenkins D, Martin K, Young ID. Hypomelanosis of Ito associated with mosaicism for trisomy 7 and apparent "pseudomosaicism" at amniocentesis. *J Med Genet*. 1993;30:783–784. With permission.)

p. 75). Such women are essentially mosaic because some cells express the normal gene, whereas others express only the mutated gene.

Disorders of the Sex Chromosomes

Klinefelter Syndrome (47,XXY)

First described clinically in 1942, this relatively common condition with an incidence of 1:1000 live male births was shown in 1959 to be caused by the presence of an additional X chromosome.

Clinical Features

In childhood the presentation may be with clumsiness or mild ID, particularly in relation to verbal skills. The overall verbal IQ is reduced by 10 to 20 points below unaffected siblings and controls, and children can be rather self-obsessed in their behavior. Adults tend to be slightly taller than average, with long lower limbs. Approximately 30% show moderately severe gynecomastia (breast enlargement), and all are infertile as a result of azoospermia, with small, soft testes. Fertility has been achieved for a small number of affected males using the techniques of testicular sperm aspiration and intracytoplasmic sperm injection. There is an increased incidence of leg ulcers, osteoporosis, and carcinoma of the breast in adult life. Treatment with testosterone from puberty onward is beneficial for the development of secondary sexual characteristics and the long-term prevention of osteoporosis.

Chromosome Findings

Usually the karyotype shows an additional X chromosome. Molecular studies have shown that there is a roughly equal chance that this is maternal or paternal in origin. The maternally derived cases are associated with advanced maternal age. A small proportion of cases show mosaicism (e.g., 46,XY/47,XXY). Rarely, a male with more than two X chromosomes is encountered, for example 48,XXXY or 49,XXXXY. These individuals usually have quite severe ID and also share physical characteristics with Klinefelter men, often to a more marked degree.

Turner Syndrome (45,X)

This condition was first described clinically in 1938. The absence of a Barr body, consistent with the presence of only one X chromosome, was noted in 1954, and cytogenetic confirmation was realized in 1959. Although common at conception and in spontaneous abortions (see Table 17.1), the incidence in live-born female infants is low, with estimates ranging from 1:5000 to 1:10,000.

Clinical Features

Presentation can be at any time from pregnancy to adult life. Increasingly, Turner syndrome is detected during the second trimester through routine ultrasonography, showing either generalized edema (hydrops) or swelling localized to the neck (nuchal cyst or thickened nuchal pad) (Fig. 17.8). At birth many babies with Turner syndrome look entirely normal. Others show the residue of intrauterine edema, with puffy extremities (Fig. 17.9), and neck webbing. Other findings may include a low posterior hairline, increased carrying angles at the elbows, short fourth metacarpals, widely spaced nipples, and coarctation of the aorta, which is present in approximately 15% of cases.

Intelligence in Turner syndrome is within the normal range. However, studies have shown mild differences in social cognition and higher order executive function skills according to whether the X chromosome was paternal or maternal in origin. Those with a paternal X chromosome scored better, from which the existence of

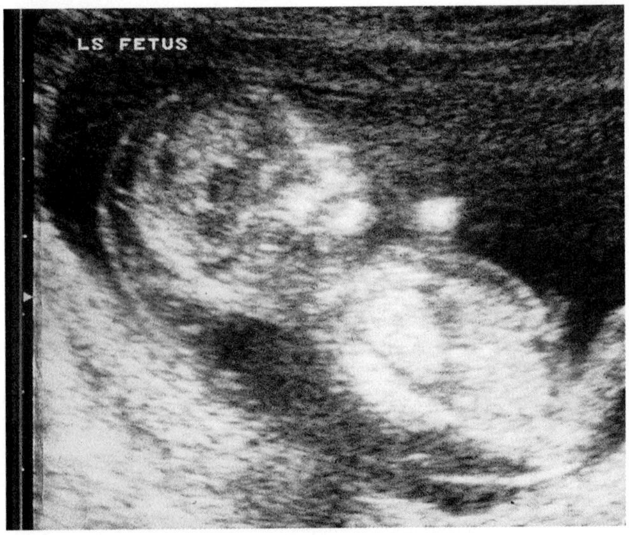

• **Fig. 17.8** Ultrasonographic scan at 18 weeks' gestation showing hydrops fetalis. Note the halo of fluid surrounding the fetus. (Courtesy Dr D. Rose, City Hospital, Nottingham, UK.)

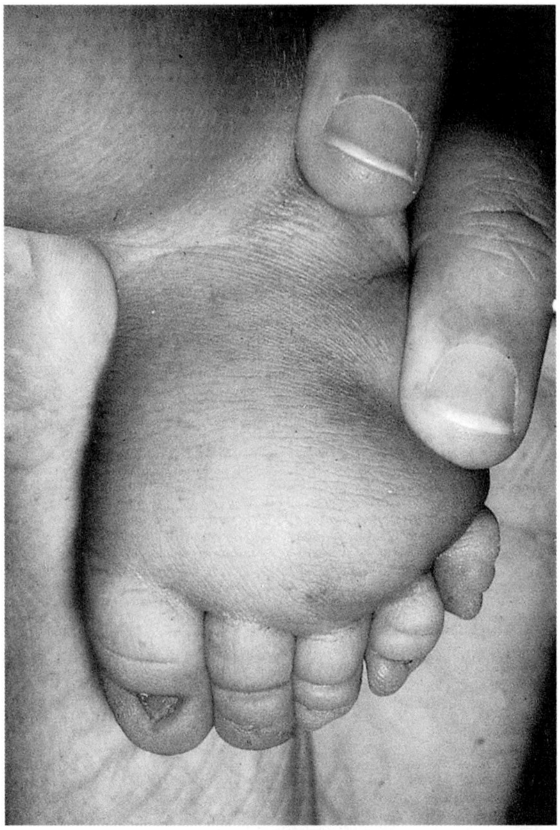

• **Fig. 17.9** The foot of an infant with Turner syndrome showing edema and small nails.

a locus for social cognition on the X chromosome can be postulated. If such a locus is not expressed from the maternal X, this could provide at least part of the explanation for the excess difficulty with language and social skills observed in 46,XY males, as their X is always maternal in origin.

The two main medical problems are short stature and ovarian failure. Short stature becomes apparent by mid-childhood, and without growth hormone treatment the average adult height is 145 cm. This is due, at least in part, to haploinsufficiency for the *SHOX* gene, which is located in the pseudoautosomal region (p. 125). Ovarian failure commences during the second half of intrauterine life and almost invariably leads to primary amenorrhea and infertility. Estrogen replacement therapy should be initiated at adolescence for the development of secondary sexual characteristics and long-term prevention of osteoporosis. *In vitro* fertilization using donor eggs offers the prospect of pregnancy for women with Turner syndrome.

Chromosome Findings

These are summarized in Table 17.6. The most common finding is 45,X. In 80% of cases, it arises through loss of a sex chromosome (X or Y) at paternal meiosis. In a significant proportion of cases, there is chromosome mosaicism, and those with a normal cell line (46,XX) have a chance of being fertile. Some cases with a 46,XY cell line are phenotypically male, and all cases with some Y-chromosome material in their second cell line must be investigated for possible gonadal dysgenesis—intracellular male gonads can occasionally become malignant and require surgical removal.

TABLE 17.6 Chromosome findings in Turner syndrome

Karyotype	Frequency (%)
Monosomy X: 45,X	50
Mosaicism (e.g., 45,X/46,XX)	20
Isochromosome: 46,X,i(Xq)	15
Ring: 46,X,r(X)	5
Deletion: 46,X,del(Xp)	5
Other	5

XXX Females

Birth surveys have shown that approximately 0.1% of all females have a 47,XXX karyotype. These women usually have no obvious physical abnormalities (though head circumference is usually in the lower centiles) but can show a mild reduction of 10 to 20 points in intellectual skills and sometimes quite oppositional behavior. This is rarely of sufficient severity to require special education. Studies have shown that the additional X chromosome is of maternal origin in 95% of cases and usually arises from an error in meiosis I. Adults are usually fertile and have children with normal karyotypes.

As with males who have more than two X chromosomes, women with more than three X chromosomes show a high incidence of ID, the severity being directly related to the number of X chromosomes.

The 46,Xr(X) Phenotype

A 46,Xr(X) karyotype—a ring chromosome X—is found in some women with typical features of Turner syndrome. This is consistent with the ring lacking X-chromosome sequences, which are normally not inactivated and which are needed for a normal phenotype. Curiously, a few 46,Xr(X) women have congenital abnormalities and show intellectual impairment. In these women it has been shown that *XIST* is not expressed on the ring X, so their relatively severe phenotype is likely to be caused by functional disomy for genes present on their ring X chromosome.

XYY Males

This condition shows an incidence of about 1:1000 in males in newborn surveys but is found in 2% to 3% of males who are in institutions because of ID or antisocial criminal behavior. However, it is important to stress that most 47,XYY men have neither learning difficulty nor a criminal record, although they can show emotional immaturity and impulsive behavior. Fertility is normal.

Physical appearance is normal, and stature is usually above average. Intelligence is mildly impaired, with an overall IQ score of 10 to 20 points below controls. The additional Y chromosome must arise either as a result of nondisjunction in paternal meiosis II or as a postzygotic event.

Fragile-X Syndrome

Fragile-X syndrome (FXS), which could equally well be classified as a single-gene disorder rather than a chromosome abnormality, has the unique distinction of being one of the most common inherited causes of ID and the first disorder in which a dynamic mutation (triplet repeat expansion) was identified (p. 20) in 1991. It affects approximately 1:5000 males and accounts for 4% to 8% of all males with ID. As such it would fit equally well in Chapter 16. Martin and Bell described the condition in the 1940s before the chromosome era, and hence it has also been known as Martin-Bell syndrome. The chromosome abnormality was first described in 1969, but the significance not fully realized until 1977.

Clinical Features

Older boys and adult males usually have a recognizable facial appearance with high forehead, large ears, long face, and prominent jaw (Fig. 17.10A,B). After puberty most affected males have large testes (macro-orchidism). There may also be evidence of connective tissue weakness, with hyperextensible joints, stretch marks on the skin (striae), and mitral valve prolapse. ID is moderate to severe, and many show autistic features and/or hyperactive behavior. Speech tends to be halting and repetitive. Female carriers can show some of the facial features, and approximately 50% of women with the full mutation show mild to moderate ID.

The Fragile-X Chromosome

The syndrome takes its name from the appearance of the X chromosome, which shows a so-called fragile site close to the telomere at the end of the long arm at Xq27.3 (Fig. 17.11). A fragile site is a non-staining gap usually involving both chromatids at a point at which the chromosome is liable to break. Detection involves the use of special culture techniques such as folate or thymidine depletion, which can result in the fragile site being detectable in up to 50% of cells from affected males. Demonstration in female carriers is much more difficult by cytogenetics, although a positive result confirms carrier status. The absence of the fragile site does not exclude a woman from being a carrier and, of course, diagnosis is now much easier by DNA analysis.

The Molecular Defect

The fragile-X locus is known as *FRAXA*, and the pathogenic variant consists of an increase in the size of a region in the 5′ untranslated region of the *FMR1* gene. This region contains a long CGG trinucleotide repeat sequence with the normal range between 5 and 44 copies, and these alleles are inherited in a stable manner. However, a small increase to between 55 and 200 copies renders this repeat sequence unstable, a condition referred to as a **premutation**. Alleles containing 45 to 54 copies are referred to as **intermediate**.

A man who carries a premutation used to be known as a "normal transmitting male," but premutation carriers are at increased risk of a late-onset neurological condition called **fragile-X–associated tremor/ataxia syndrome** (FXTAS). Roughly half of male permutation carriers will be affected by their 70s. All the daughters of these males will inherit the premutation and have normal intelligence,

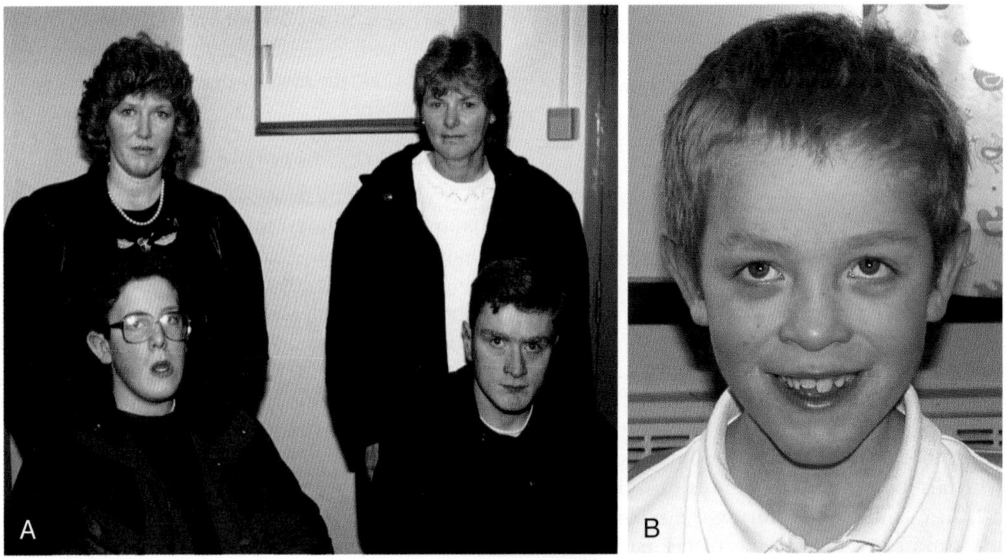

• **Fig. 17.10** (A) A family affected by fragile-X syndrome. Two sisters, both carriers of a small *FRAXA* mutation inherited from their father, have had affected sons with different degrees of learning difficulty. (B) A young boy with typical facial features of fragile-X syndrome, showing the long face, long ears, and slightly large head.

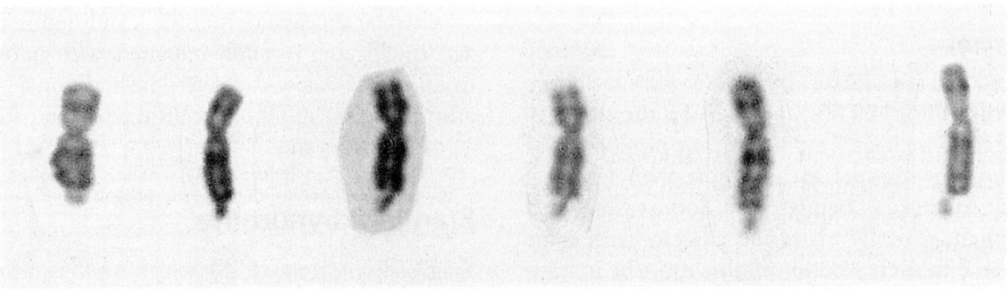

• **Fig. 17.11** X chromosome from several males with fragile X syndrome. (Courtesy Ashley Wilkinson, City Hospital, Nottingham, UK.)

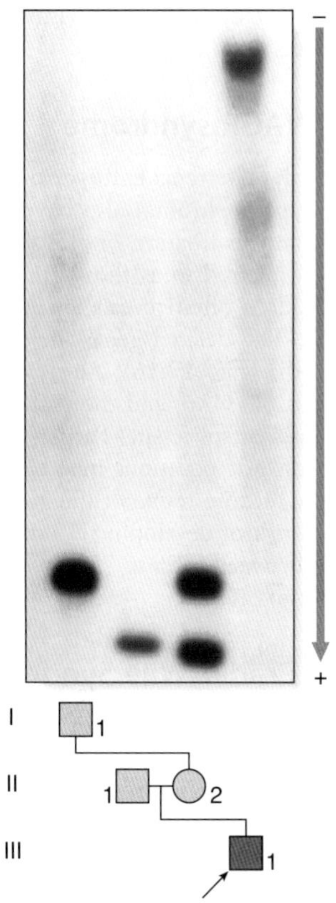

• **Fig. 17.12** Southern blot of DNA from a family showing expansion of the CGG triplet repeat being passed from a normal transmitting male (I1) through his obligate carrier daughter (II2) to her son (III1) with fragile-X intellectual disability. (Courtesy Dr G. Taylor, St. James's Hospital, Leeds, UK.)

but they are also at small risk of FXTAS in later years. When they have sons, there is a significant risk that the premutation will undergo a further increase in size during meiosis, and if this exceeds 200 CGG repeats it becomes a full mutation. The third FMR1 disorder after FXS and FXTAS is ***FMR1* primary ovarian insufficiency**. This is a form of hypergonadotropic hypogonadism occurring before age 40 years and affects approximately 20% of women who carry a premutation allele compared with approximately 1% of women in the general population.

The full mutation is unstable not only during female meiosis but also in somatic mitotic divisions. Consequently, in an affected male gel electrophoresis shows a "smear" of DNA consisting of a range of different-sized alleles rather than a single band (Fig. 17.12). Note that a normal allele and premutation can be identified by polymerase chain reaction (PCR), whereas Southern blotting is necessary to detect full mutations because the long CGG expansion is often refractory to PCR amplification. At the molecular level, a full mutation suppresses transcription of the *FMR1* gene by hypermethylation, and this in turn is thought to be responsible for the clinical features seen in males, as well as some females with a large expansion (Table 17.7). The *FMR1* gene contains 17 exons encoding a cytoplasmic protein that plays a crucial role in the development and function of cerebral neurons. The FMR1 protein can be detected in blood using specific monoclonal antibodies.

Another fragile site adjacent to *FRAXA* has been identified at Xq28. This is known as *FRAXE*. The expansion mutations at *FRAXE* also involve CGG triplet repeats but are much rarer than *FRAXA* mutations. Some males with these mutations have mild learning difficulties, whereas others are just as severely affected as men with pathogenic *FRAXA* variants. *FRAXE* may show up as a fragile site cytogenetically, but the PCR test is separate. A third fragile site, *FRAXF*, has been identified close to *FRAXA* and *FRAXE*. This does not seem to cause any clinical abnormality.

Genetic Counseling and the Fragile-X Syndrome

This common cause of ID presents a major counseling problem. Inheritance can be regarded as modified or atypical XL. All of the daughters of a normal transmitting male will carry the premutation. Their male offspring are at risk of inheriting either the premutation or a full mutation. This risk is dependent on the size of the premutation in the mother, with mutations greater than 100 CGG repeats usually increasing in size to become full mutations.

For a woman who carries a full mutation there is a 50% risk that each of her sons will be affected with the full syndrome and that each of her daughters will inherit the full mutation. Because approximately 50% of females with the full mutation have mild ID, the risk that a female carrier of a full mutation will have a daughter with ID equals 1/2 × 1/2 (i.e., 1/4). Prenatal diagnosis can be offered based on analysis of DNA from chorionic villi, but in the event of a female fetus with a full mutation an accurate prediction of ID cannot be made.

TABLE 17.7 Fragile-X syndrome: genotype-phenotype correlations

Number of Triplet Repeats (Normal Range 5–44)	Fragile Site	Intelligence Detectable
Males		
45–54 (intermediate alleles)		
55–200 (premutation)	No	Normal (normal transmitting male)
200–2000 (full mutation)	Yes (in up to 50% of cells)	Moderate-to-severe intellectual disability (ID)
Females		
45–54 (intermediate alleles)		
55–200 (premutation)	No	Normal
200–2000 (full mutation)	Yes (usually <10% of cells)	50% normal, 50% mild ID

"Classic" Chromosome Deletion Syndromes

Deletion 4p and 5p Syndromes

Microscopically visible deletions of the terminal portions of chromosomes 4 and 5 cause the Wolf-Hirschhorn (4p−) (Fig. 17.13) and cri-du-chat (5p−) (Fig. 17.14) syndromes, respectively. In both conditions severe ID is usual, often with failure to thrive. However, there is considerable variability, particularly in Wolf-Hirschhorn syndrome, and no clear correlation of the phenotype with the precise loss of chromosomal material. Cri-du-chat syndrome derives its name from the characteristic cat-like cry of affected neonates—a consequence of underdevelopment of the larynx. Both conditions are rare, with estimated incidences of approximately 1:50,000 births. Not all cases have cytogenetically visible chromosome deletions, but CMA detects them all.

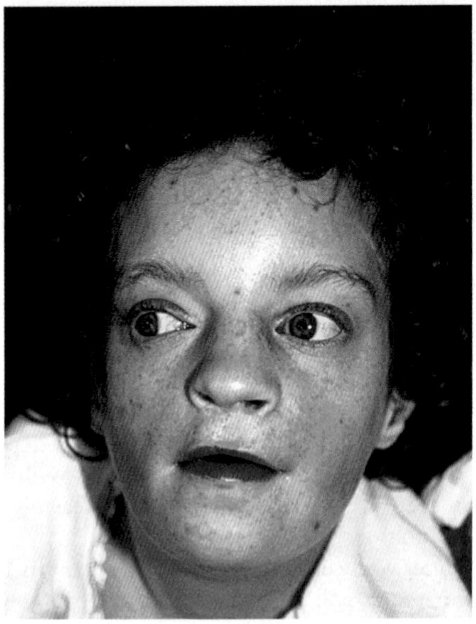

• **Fig. 17.13** A child with deletion 4p syndrome; Wolf-Hirschhorn syndrome.

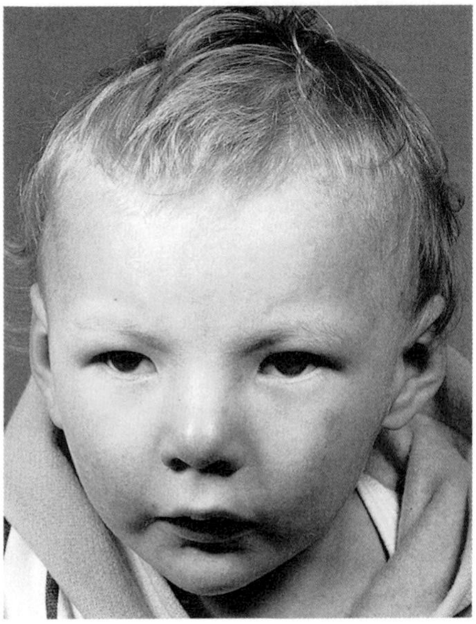

• **Fig. 17.14** Facial view of a 2-year-old boy with cri-du-chat syndrome.

Wilms Tumor/WAGR syndrome

Some children with the rare renal embryonal neoplasm known as Wilms tumor (or hypernephroma) also have *a*niridia, *g*enitourinary abnormalities, and *r*etardation of growth and development. This combination is referred to as the WAGR syndrome. CMA analysis in these children often reveals an interstitial deletion of 11p13 (Fig. 17.15). The deleted genes include *PAX6*, which is responsible for aniridia (Fig. 17.16). Aniridia alone will prompt targeted gene analysis of *PAX6*, and the pathogenic variants may be nonsense, missense, or splice site. Partial- or whole-gene deletions occur, which on rare occasions may be telomeric to *PAX6* without affecting the reading frame of the gene itself. Loss of the *WT1* gene confers a risk of developing Wilms tumor (see also p. 192, Table 14.2) of between 50% to 75%, which will manifest by 4 years of age in 90% of cases.

Angelman and Prader-Willi Syndromes

These two conditions have a special place in medical genetics as a paradigm for genomic imprinting. Children with Angelman syndrome (see Fig. 6.24, p. 80) have inappropriate laughter, convulsions, poor coordination (ataxia), and severe learning difficulties. Children with Prader-Willi syndrome (see Fig. 6.22, p. 79) are very hypotonic with poor feeding in infancy, and later develop hyperphagia and obesity, with mild to moderate ID. A large proportion of children with these disorders have a microdeletion involving 15q11−13, which is always the paternally derived chromosome 15 in Prader-Willi syndrome. In contrast, a deletion occurring at the same region on the maternally inherited chromosome 15 causes Angelman syndrome. Non-deletion cases also exist and are often as a result of uniparental disomy (p. 77), with both number 15 chromosomes being paternal in origin in Angelman syndrome, and maternal in origin in Prader-Willi syndrome. These parent-of-origin effects are explained by imprinting (see Fig. 6.23, p. 79).

Contiguous Gene Syndromes

CMA is currently the most widely used technique to diagnose submicroscopic losses of genomic material, that is, microdeletions. Some microdeletions involve loss of several genes at closely adjacent loci, resulting in **contiguous gene syndromes**. For example, several boys with Duchenne muscular dystrophy (DMD) have been described who also have other XL disorders, such as retinitis pigmentosa and glycerol kinase deficiency. The loci for these disorders are very close to the DMD locus on Xp21. Many, even most, microdeletions give rise to contiguous gene syndromes because, in general, the larger the deletion the more likely it is that affected individuals will have multiple medical and developmental problems. Examples of well-known microdeletion syndromes are given in Table 17.8, together with the key gene within the locus where appropriate. Most of them are relatively rare.

Deletion Xp22.3

As with the rare example already described in relation to Xp21, a microdeletion at Xp22.3 is a classic contiguous gene syndrome. The locus incorporates XL recessive chondrodysplasia punctata (aryl sulfatase-E, *ARSE*, gene), mental retardation (*VCX-A* gene), ichthyosis (steroid sulfatase, *STS*, gene), and Kallmann syndrome (*KAL1* gene).

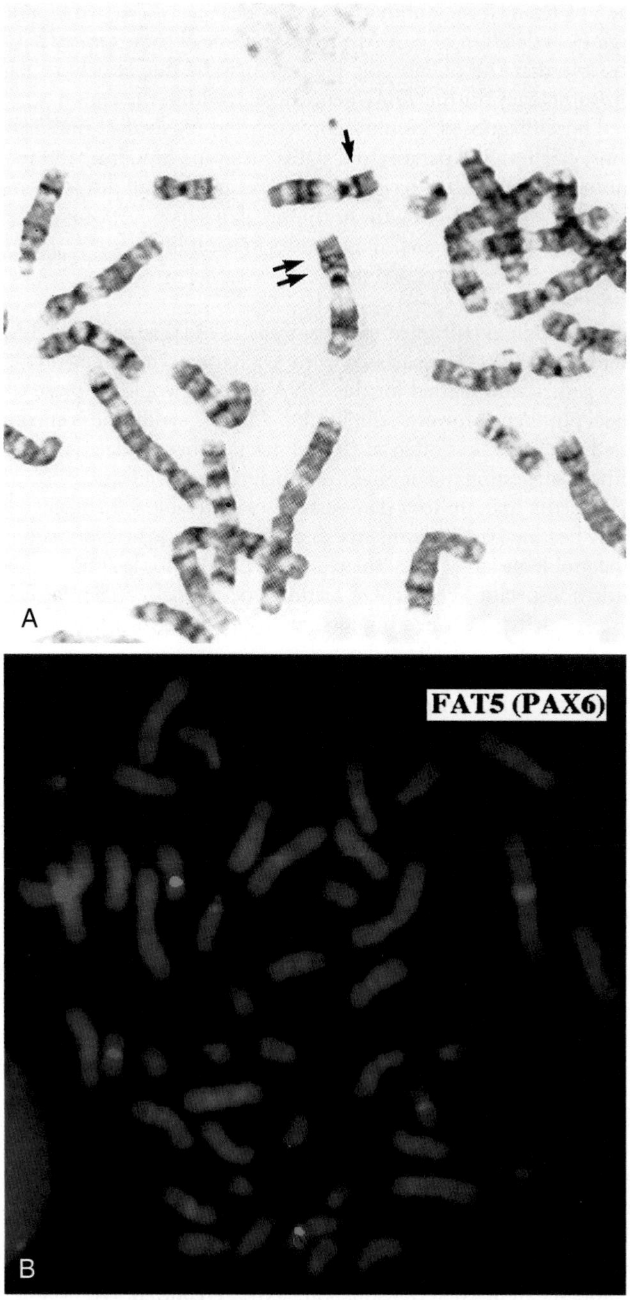

• **Fig. 17.15** (A) Metaphase spread showing the number 11 chromosomes (*double arrows*). The chromosome indicated by the *single arrow* has an interstitial deletion in the short arm. See Figs. 17.11 and 17.12. (Courtesy Meg Heath, City Hospital, Nottingham, UK.) (B) Fluorescence *in situ* hybridization showing failure of a *PAX6* locus specific probe (*red*) to hybridize to the deleted number 11 chromosome shown in (A) from a child with WAGR syndrome. The *green* probe acts as a marker for the centromere of each number 11 chromosome. (Courtesy Dr John Crolla, Salisbury, UK and Dr Veronica van Heyningen, Edinburgh, UK.)

Short stature also usually occurs because of loss of the short stature homeobox-containing gene (*SHOX*), which when mutated on its own gives rise to Leri-Weill dyschondrosteosis (p. 126). Depending on the size and extent of the deletion, therefore, individuals may present variably with short stature, a flat face and small nose with a flat nasal tip, short digits, dry skin and hair, hypogonadotropic hypogonadism, anosmia, and ID.

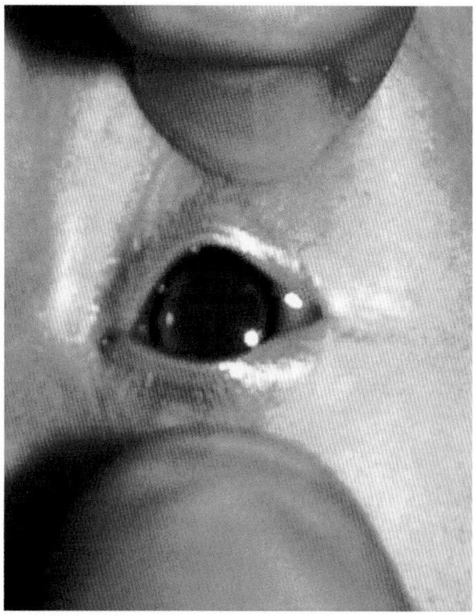

• **Fig. 17.16** A baby with deletion 11p13 presenting with aniridia on routine neonatal examination.

Retinoblastoma

It was originally observed that approximately 5% of children presenting with retinoblastoma had other abnormalities, including ID. In some of these, a constitutional interstitial deletion of a region of chromosome 13q was identified. The smallest region of overlap was 13q14, which was subsequently shown to be the position of the locus for the autosomal dominant form of retinoblastoma because of mutations in the *RB1* gene (p. 189).

Chromosome Microarray/Microarray-Comparative Genomic Hybridization

The 1990s witnessed the development of fluorescence *in situ* hybridization (FISH)–based analysis of all chromosome telomeres using subtelomeric probes. This led to the diagnosis of some cases of ID/dysmorphic patients, not detected by multiplex ligation-dependent probe amplification (p. 62). From around 2005 this has been rapidly superseded by extensive CMA testing (p. 62), and a significant number of new microdeletion (and to a lesser extent microduplication) syndromes have emerged. At high resolution, this technology yields significant results in about 20% of cases of well-selected, previously unknown dysmorphic patients with developmental delay/learning disability. This compares to a positive pick-up rate of 4% to 5% from standard karyotyping of patients considered likely to have a chromosome disorder. Examples of these new syndromes are shown in the following section.

Microdeletion and Microduplication Syndromes: "Old" and "New"

DiGeorge/Sedláčková/Velocardiofacial Syndrome

DiGeorge syndrome affects approximately 1:4000 births, is usually sporadic, and is characterized by heart malformations (particularly those involving the cardiac outflow tract), thymic and parathyroid

TABLE 17.8 **Well-known microdeletion syndromes**

Syndrome	Chromosome	Key Gene(s)
Deletion 1p36	1p36	
Deletion 2q37	2q37	
Wisconsin	3q24-q25	*MBNL1*
Wolf-Hirschhorn	4p	
Cri-du-chat	5p	
Williams (Williams-Beuren)	7q11.23	*ELN* (Supravalvular aortic stenosis) *LIMK1* (Neurological features)
Langer—Giedion	8q24.11	*TRPS1* (Trichorhinophalangeal features) *EXT1* (Exostoses)
Kleefstra	9q34.3	*EHMT1*
WAGR	11p13	*RB1, WT1*
Jacobsen	11q23	
Angelman	15q11.2	*UBE3A*
Prader-Willi	15q11.2	*SNRPN*
Deletion 16p11.2	16p11.2	*TBX6* (Scoliosis)
Rubinstein-Taybi	16p13.3	*CREBBP*
Miller-Dieker	17p13.3	*LIS1*
Smith-Magenis	17p11.2	*RAI1*
Koolen-de Vries	17q21.31	*KANSL1*
DiGeorge/Sedláčková/velocardiofacial	22q11.2	*TBX1*
Phelan-McDermid	22q13	*SHANK3*

WAGR, Wilms tumor, aniridia, genitourinary malformations and retardation of growth and development.

hypoplasia, cleft palate and typical facies. The molecular defect is a 3-megabase (Mb) microdeletion on chromosome 22 (22q11.2). Dr. Eva Sedláčková from Prague reported a large series of children with a congenitally short palate in 1955, 10 years earlier than DiGeorge, and these patients clearly had the same condition. A similar phenotype was described by Shprintzen and was referred to as velocardiofacial syndrome. Because of the confusion of eponyms and other terms given to this condition over the years, "deletion 22q11 syndrome" now has the most widespread acceptance (at the molecular level the deleted DNA segment is still often called the DiGeorge Critical Region). Fig. 17.17 shows individuals with deletion 22q11.2 at different ages. Because it is the most common of the microdeletion syndromes, it has been intensely researched. It is variable, and many affected individuals are able to reproduce, so the condition follows autosomal dominant (AD) inheritance in some families. The 3-Mb deletion occurs because this region is flanked by two identical sequences of DNA, known as low-copy repeats (LCRs), of the type that occur frequently throughout the genome. At meiosis the chromosomes can be "confused" when they align, such that the downstream DNA sequence aligns with the upstream. If recombination occurs between these two flanking regions, a deletion of ~3 Mb results on one chromosome 22. It is possible that the phenotypic features may be due largely to haploinsufficiency for the *TBX1* gene that lies within the region.

Those diagnosed should be investigated for cardiac malformations, calcium and parathyroid status, immune function, and renal anomalies. About half have short stature, and a small proportion of these have partial growth hormone deficiency. Approximately 25% have schizophrenia-like episodes in adult life.

Duplication 22q11.2

The misaligned pairing at meiosis of the LCRs that flank the 3 Mb region at 22q11.2, associated with DiGeorge syndrome, predicts that gametes duplicated for this DNA segment would be present in equal numbers. However, duplication 22q11.2 syndrome is encountered somewhat less often in clinical practice than its deletion counterpart, suggesting that it might be subclinical in its effects.

Patients that are seen demonstrate considerable variability, with some bearing passing similarity to the deletion 22q11.2 phenotype. The problems range from isolated mild ID to multiple abnormalities with nonspecific dysmorphic features, occasional congenital heart disease, cleft palate, hearing loss, and postnatal growth deficiency. Fig. 17.18 shows an affected patient.

Williams Syndrome

Williams syndrome (WS) occurs because of a microdeletion at chromosome 7q11.23 and diagnosis is made and/or confirmed by CMA. The clinical phenotype was first reported by Williams in 1961 and later expanded by Beuren (hence, sometimes, Williams-Beuren syndrome). Hypocalcemia is a variable feature in childhood and sometimes persists, whereas supravalvular aortic stenosis (SVAS) and peripheral pulmonary artery stenosis are congenital abnormalities of the great vessels. Haploinsufficiency at 7q11.23 leads to loss of one copy of the gene that encodes elastin, a component of connective tissue. This is probably the key factor causing SVAS and the vascular problems that are more common in later life. Patients with pathogenic variants in elastin have a variety of congenital heart defects, sometimes complex and severe. WS individuals have a characteristic appearance (Fig. 17.19) with mild short stature, a full lower lip, and sloping shoulders. Equally characteristic is their behavior. They are typically very outgoing in childhood—having a "cocktail party manner"—but become withdrawn and sensitive as adults. All are intellectually impaired to the extent that they cannot lead independent lives, and the majority do not reproduce, although parent-child transmission has been reported.

Smith-Magenis Syndrome

This microdeletion syndrome is caused by loss of chromosome material at 17p.11.2, often visible cytogenetically. As with DiGeorge syndrome, the deletion mechanism in many cases involves homologous recombination between flanking LCRs. The physical characteristics are not highly distinctive (Fig. 17.20), but congenital heart disease occurs in one-third, scoliosis develops in late childhood in more than one-half, and hearing impairment occurs in about two-thirds. The syndrome is most likely to be recognized by the behavioral characteristics: as children, patients exhibit self-harming (head-banging, pulling out nails, and inserting objects into orifices), a persistently disturbed sleep pattern and characteristic "self-hugging." ID is the norm and is usually moderate-severe. The sleep pattern can often be managed by judicious use of melatonin. The same phenotype may be caused by a mutation in the *RAI1* gene, which is located within the deleted segment.

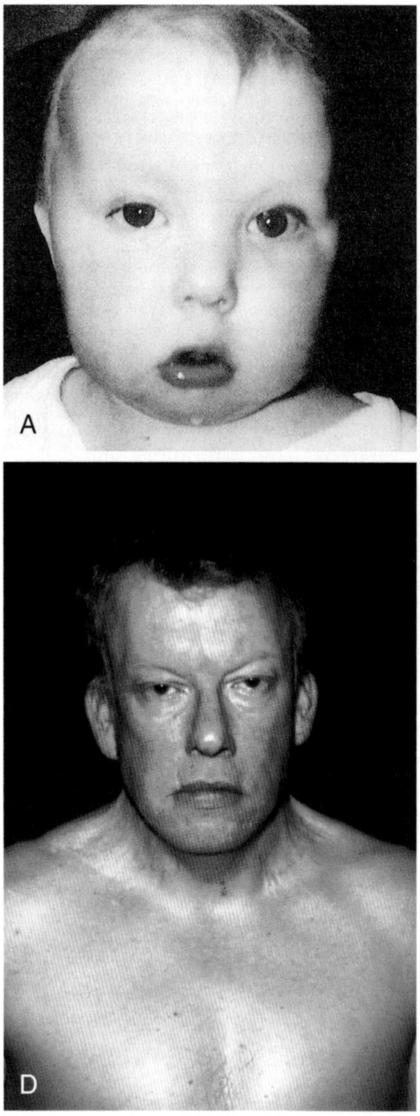
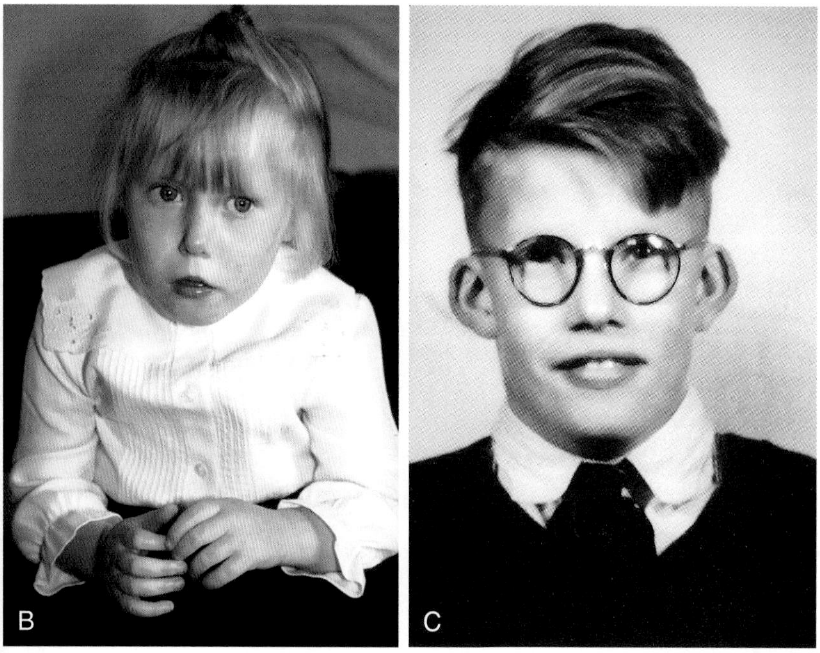

• **Fig. 17.17** Deletion 22q11.2 (DiGeorge/Sedláčková/velocardiofacial) syndrome. (A) A young infant. (B) A young child. (C) An older child. (C) The same individual shown in (C) as an adult aged 49 years.

Deletion 1p36 Syndrome

This microdeletion syndrome emerged through improved cytogenetic techniques and the use of FISH in the 1990s. In keeping with the modern approach to nomenclature, deletion 1p36 syndrome has no eponym. The features are hypotonia, microcephaly, growth delay, severe learning difficulties, epilepsy (including infantile spasms), characteristically straight eyebrows with slightly deep-set eyes, and midface hypoplasia (Fig. 17.21). Some cases develop dilated cardiomyopathy.

Deletion 9q34 (Kleefstra) Syndrome

Another of the relatively new microdeletion syndromes, this was first reported as a condition featuring significant ID, hypotonia, obesity, brachycephaly, arched eyebrows, synophrys, anteverted nostrils, prognathism, sleep disturbances, and behavioral problems. Many patients have severe speech delay, and not all manifest obesity. The case pictured in Fig. 17.22 bears a passing resemblance to Angelman syndrome. As with some of the other microdeletion syndromes (e.g., Smith-Magenis), some patients with the phenotypic features but no microdeletion have been shown to have mutations in the euchromatin histone methyl transferase 1 *(EHMT1)* gene, which lies within the region. The syndrome might therefore be mainly caused by haploinsufficiency for this gene.

Deletion 17q21.31 (Koolen-de Vries) Syndrome

This was one of the first new deletion syndromes delineated through CMA, has a prevalence of approximately 1:16,000 and is probably significantly underdiagnosed. The main features are severe ID, hypotonia and characteristic facial dysmorphisms including a long face with a high forehead and tubular or pear-shaped nose, a bulbous nasal tip, large ears, and everted lower lip (Fig. 17.23). Individuals tend to be friendly. Other clinically important features include epilepsy, heart defects, kidney anomalies, and long, slender fingers. The *KANSL1* gene is key, and there are patients with pathogenic variants who do not have CMA-detectable deletions.

Deletion 22q13 (Phelan-McDermid) Syndrome

Understanding of this condition, which is distinct from the better-known deletion 22q11.2 (DiGeorge) syndrome, predated the CMA era as cases with cytogenetically visible deletions were

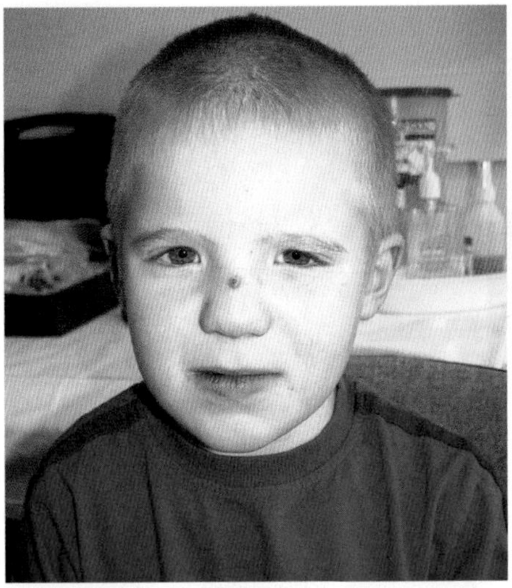

• **Fig. 17.18** A patient with duplication 22q11.2. The features are variable and not as recognizable as in deletion 22q11.2, and it is diagnosed less often.

identified. Before diagnosis some patients were considered to possibly have Angelman syndrome because of the very poor speech acquisition and happy affect. Small deletions are associated with mild difficulties, but overall the features are not highly specific. They consist of hypotonia, significant speech delay or absent speech, general ID, behavior problems that do not strictly meet the criteria for autistic spectrum disorder and soft, dysmorphic features. There is a recurrent breakpoint on distal 22q which disrupts the *SHANK3* gene, and indeed patients have been identified with pathogenic variants in this gene without deletions (Fig. 17.24).

Deletion 1q21.1 Syndrome

This condition was first identified in three individuals from a cohort of 505 with congenital heart disease. The phenotype is broad and includes mild-moderate ID, small head size, growth retardation, heart defects, cataracts, hand deformities, and skeletal problems, seizures and autism. However, some individuals with the deletion are only mildly affected, and sometimes apparently unaffected. A mother and her child, both with the deletion, are shown in Fig. 17.25. Variable penetrance and lack of highly

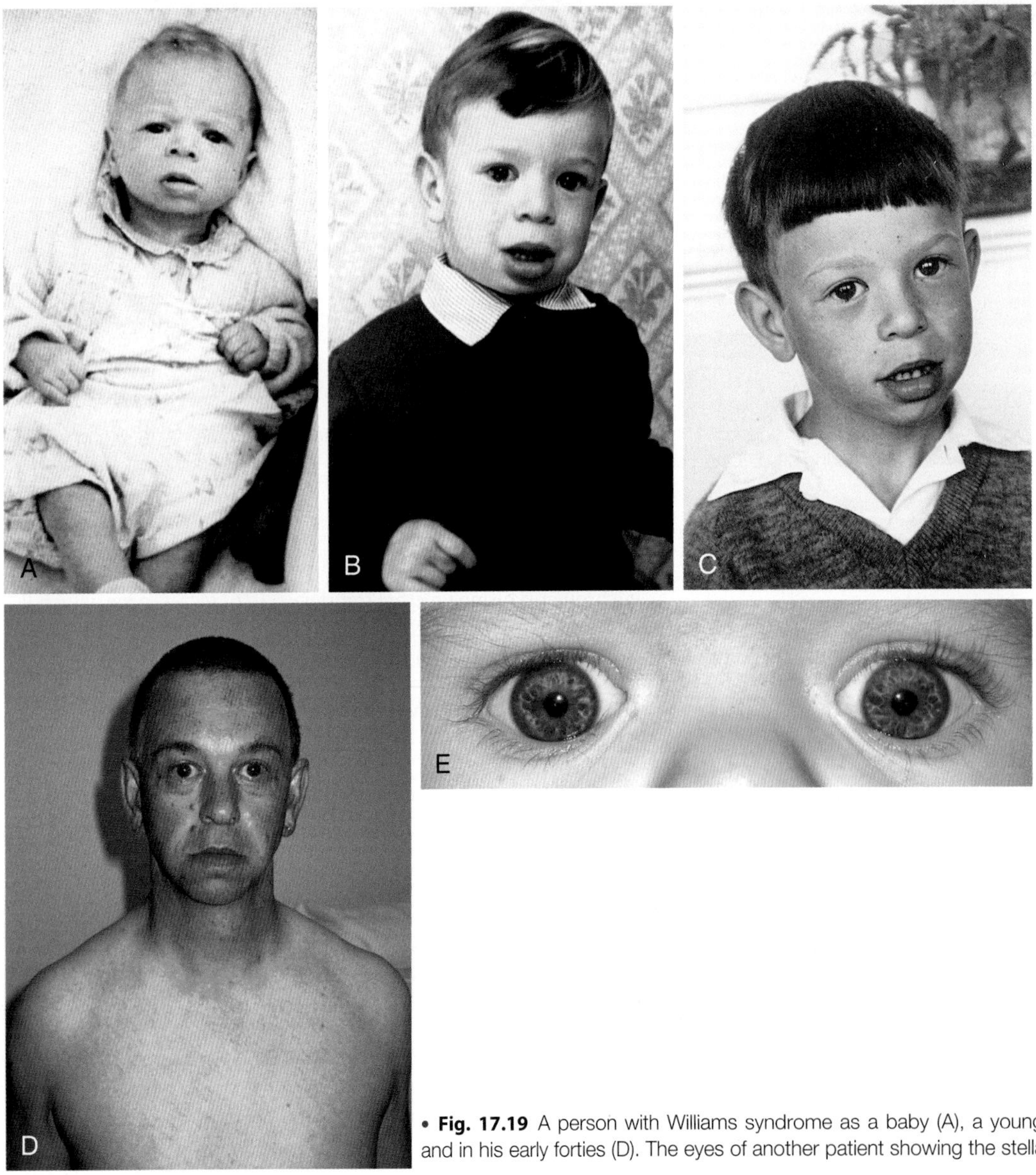

• **Fig. 17.19** A person with Williams syndrome as a baby (A), a young child (B) and an older child (C), and in his early forties (D). The eyes of another patient showing the stellate irides (E).

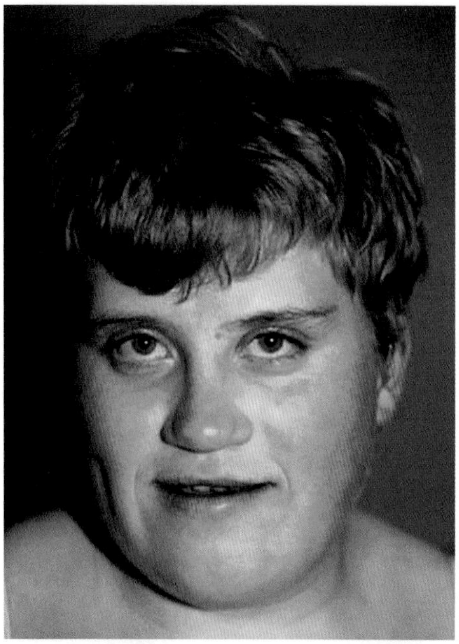

• **Fig. 17.20** A young person with Smith-Magenis syndrome; the facial features are not highly distinctive, but the philtrum is usually short. As babies, chromosome studies are often requested because the possibility of Down syndrome is raised.

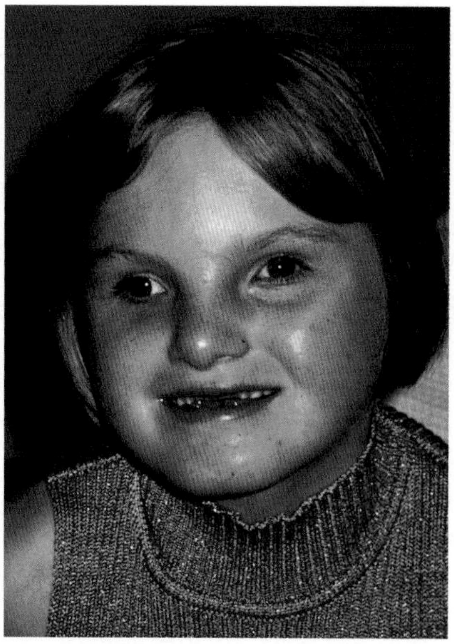

• **Fig. 17.22** A child with deletion 9q34 syndrome. She has arched eyebrows, narrow upslanting palpebral fissures, brachycephaly, prognathism, and severe intellectual disability. She was initially investigated for possible Angelman syndrome.

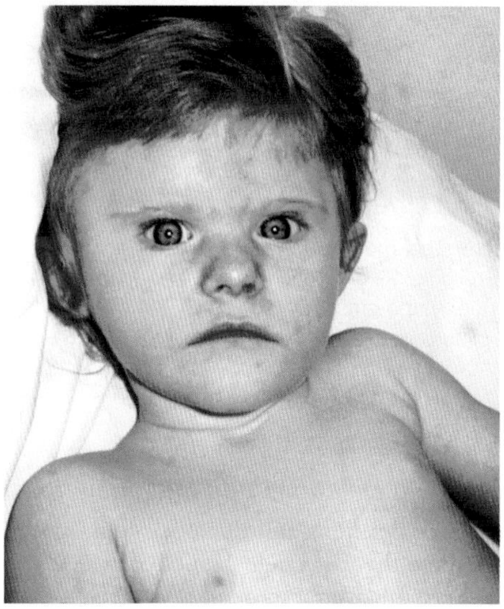

• **Fig. 17.21** A child with deletion 1p36 syndrome; very straight eyebrows, epilepsy, and learning difficulties.

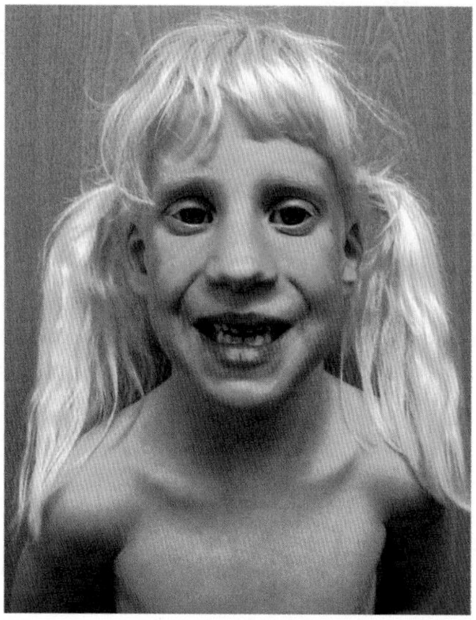

• **Fig. 17.23** This child shows the characteristic facial features of deletion 17q21.31 syndrome. The face is long and the nose somewhat tubular or pear-shaped, and the nasal tip bulbous. There is developmental delay. (Courtesy Dr David Koolen, Nijmegen, Netherlands.)

distinctive features make genetic counseling for this genomic imbalance highly problematic.

This locus is now known for its role in determining the thrombocytopenia-absent radius (TAR) syndrome (Fig. 17.26). In addition to thrombocytopenia the condition is defined by the absence of the radius but preservation of the thumb. In cohort studies, a common 200-kilobase (kb) microdeletion of 1q21.1 (adjacent to, but distinct from, the 1q21.1 microdeletion already described) was found in all affected individuals and one-third of unaffected family members, suggesting that the deletion alone is not sufficient to cause the phenotype. When it was found that a small number of TAR patients did not have a 1q21.1 microdeletion, but rather a truncating mutation of the *RBM8A* gene at the same locus, further studies showed that the non-deleted allele always harbored one of two low-frequency single nucleotide polymorphisms in regulatory elements of *RBM8A*. TAR is therefore a syndrome caused by compound heterozygosity at this locus, usually with a typical microdeletion on one allele.

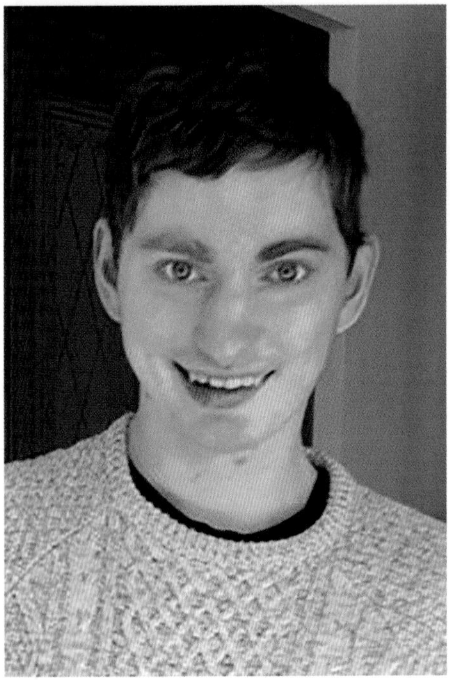

• **Fig. 17.24** A young adult with a pathogenic variant in the *SHANK3* gene, giving rise to features consistent with a severe form of Phelan-McDermid syndrome—moderate-severe intellectual disability and absent speech. The nose is rather bulbous, and many individuals with this syndrome have only soft, dysmorphic features.

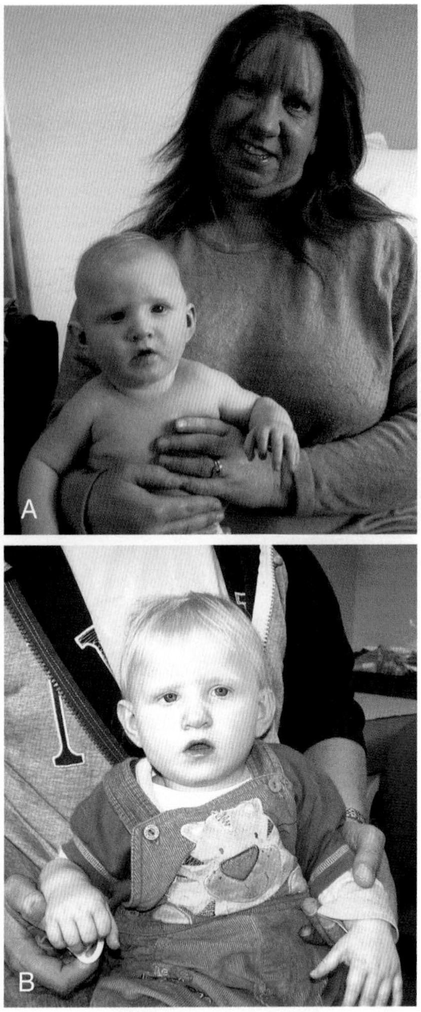

• **Fig. 17.25** (A) This mother and child have deletion 1q21.1 syndrome. They bear a resemblance to each other, and there is evidence of mild development delay and small head size. (B) The same child nearly 1 year after the first picture was taken.

Deletion 16p11.2 Syndrome

The CMA era since 2006 has yielded a significant number of new microdeletion and microduplication syndromes, and more such conditions will continue to be delineated. One of the most common imbalances seen in clinical practice occurs at 16p11.2. The microdeletion condition (Fig. 17.27) is very variable clinically, and the precise extent and position of the loss of genomic material tends to be related to the severity. So-called "type 1" deletion cases are most likely to give rise to the recognizable features, characterized by low muscle tone, delay in speech and in language development, mild ID, susceptibility to autism/autistic spectrum disorder and seizures, minor facial dysmorphisms, and a tendency to both be overweight and have an enlarged head circumference. Some individuals show no unusual features or neurodevelopmental problems, and, when familial, there may be marked variation between those with the deletion. Overall, del16p11.2 is found in approximately 1% of children with autism, and around three in 10,000 people from the general population.

Duplication 16p11.2

The reciprocal imbalance at 16p11.2, the microduplication, probably occurs at roughly the same frequency as the microdeletion both in the general population and in autistic spectrum disorder. The features overlap considerably regarding mild ID and language delay, susceptibility to both seizures and mental health problems, and the presence of minor facial dysmorphisms. It is also very variable. If anything, there is a tendency to display the opposite physical characteristics compared with deletion cases, that is, individuals are more likely to have mild short stature, be underweight and have a small head circumference (Fig. 17.28).

Chromosome 15q Deletions and Microdeletions

The complexity of deletions and microdeletions affecting chromosome 15q illustrate the vast range of molecular cytogenetic aberrations that has been uncovered through CMA technology, which as a consequence has stimulated a wealth of medical genetic research with important clinical application. Deletions can occur anywhere on 15q, and, in general, the larger the deletion the more severe the phenotype and clinical problems. However, the proximal 15q region (Fig. 17.29) has been an area of particular interest, largely because of its association with Prader-Willi and Angelman syndromes.

As discussed more fully elsewhere (pp. 79, 258), a relatively large deletion encompassing 15q11-q13 will give rise to Prader-Willi syndrome when this occurs on the paternally derived chromosome 15, and Angelman syndrome when the maternally derived 15 is deleted. In terms of the DNA structure, the region contains a number of LCRs, and these regions of repetitive sequence are susceptible to rearrangements with several identified "breakpoints"—bp1, bp2 and bp3 (see Fig. 17.29). Deletions between bp1 and bp2, approximately 500 kb (0.5 Mb) in size,

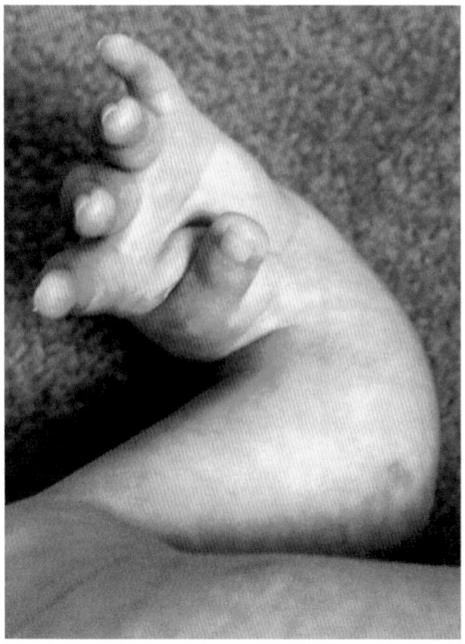

• **Fig. 17.26** A child with thrombocytopenia-absent radius syndrome. In this limb malformation the thumb is preserved. (From Goldfarb CA, Wustrack R, Pratt JA, et al. Thumb function and appearance in thrombocytopenia: absent radius syndrome. *J Hand Surg*. 2007;32: 157–161. With permission.)

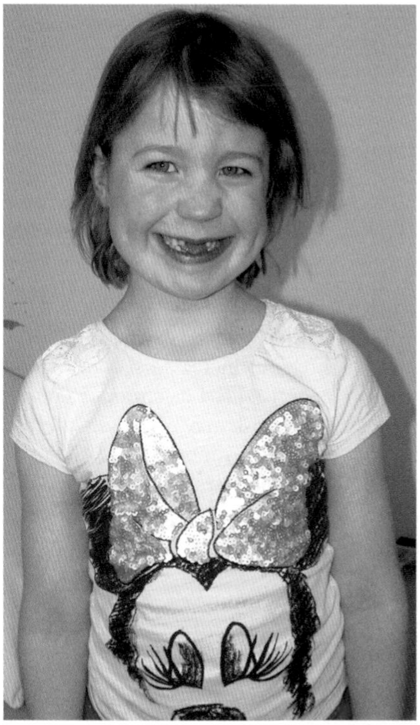

• **Fig. 17.27** A child with deletion 16p11.2. The phenotype is not highly distinctive, and dysmorphic features are "soft." Apart from mild neurodevelopmental problems there is a tendency towards being overweight and having a relatively large head.

give rise to deletion 15p11.2 syndrome. This is associated with a variable phenotype, or sometimes none at all. Mostly, however, the pattern is one of mild ID, behavioral and emotional problems with short attention span and autistic spectrum disorder, mild

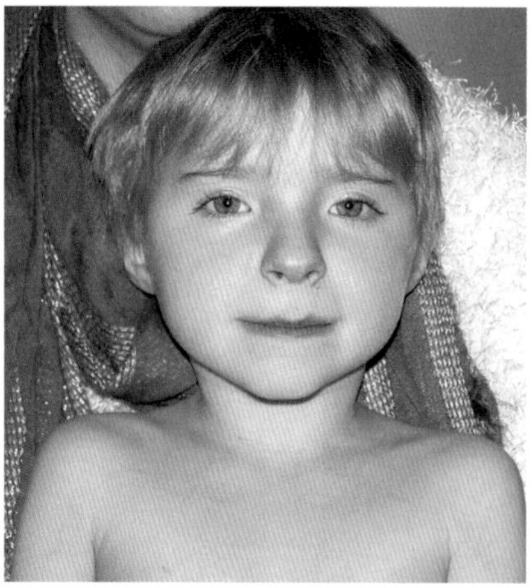

• **Fig. 17.28** A child with duplication 16p11.2. Apart from mild neurodevelopmental problems and soft dysmporphic features, there is a tendency towards small stature and a relatively small head.

speech delay and a possible increased risk of seizures. Birth defects are unusual. The role of the particular genes that are deleted (see Fig. 17.29) has not been fully elucidated.

Virtually the same pattern of fairly nonspecific neurodevelopmental problems affects children and older individuals with a deletion of 15q13.3, and it may have been transmitted by a parent who is essentially unaffected.

Chromosome Disorders and Behavioral Phenotypes

The distinctive behavior of children with WS—their outgoing "cocktail party manner"—has been recognized as part of the condition for a long time. As the microdeletion conditions have emerged, it has been increasingly clear that patterns of behavior can reliably be attributed to certain disorders. This is very striking in Smith-Magenis syndrome, but also apparent to a lesser extent in deletion 22q11, cri-du-chat, Angelman, and Prader-Willi syndromes. It is also apparent in the aneuploidies (Down and Klinefelter syndromes), as well as in 47,XXX and 47,XYY and fragile-X syndromes. Behavioral phenotypes have therefore become an area of considerable interest to clinical scientists, and the observations lend support to the belief that behavior, to a greater or lesser extent, is genetically determined. In studying chromosome disorders we are of course looking at genetically abnormal situations, and from this we cannot necessarily extrapolate directly to "normal" situations. For the latter, twin studies have provided substantial and valuable information. This field of study remains complex and understandably controversial. However, most now accept that behavior is a complex interaction of genetic background, physical influences during early development (e.g., fetal wellbeing), nurturing experiences, family size, culture, and belief systems.

Chromosome Breakage Syndromes

A small number of hereditary disorders are characterized by an excess of chromosome breaks and gaps, as well as an increased susceptibility to neoplasia. The chromosome breakages that are acquired, that is, occur as somatic events and predispose to malignancy, are considered in Chapter 14.

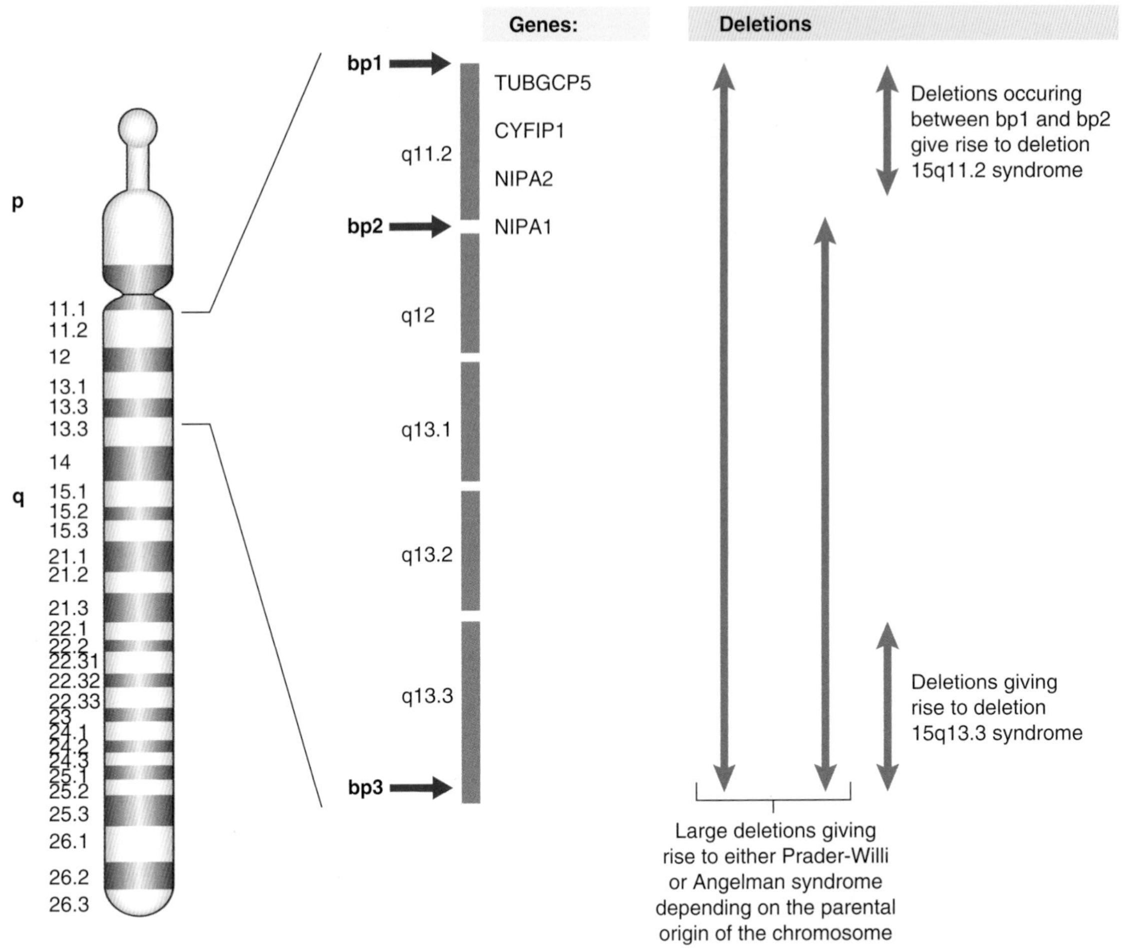

• **Fig. 17.29** The complexity of deletions occurring at the proximal chromosome 15q region. Large proximal deletions of 15q11-q13 give rise to Prader-Willi or Angelman syndromes depending on the parental origin of the deleted chromosome; deletions between bp1 and bp2 give rise to deletion 15q11.2; and deletions of 15q13.3 also occur.

Ataxia Telangiectasia

This autosomal recessive (AR) disorder presents in early childhood with ataxia, oculocutaneous telangiectasia (Fig. 17.30), radiation sensitivity and susceptibility to sinus and pulmonary infection (p. 181). The risk of neoplasia developing is in the region of 35% to 40%, of which approximately 85% are leukemias or B-cell lymphomas. The risk of other cancers is increased several-fold, for example, a two- to threefold increased risk of breast cancer. The ataxia telangiectasia gene is *ATM* at chromosome region 11q23. However, the breast cancer risk may be variant-specific, as a significant association has emerged with c.7271 T > G (p.Val2424Gly). Cells from patients show an increase in spontaneous chromosome abnormalities, such as chromatid gaps and breaks, which are enhanced by radiation. The protein product is thought to act as a "checkpoint" protein kinase, which interacts with the *TP53* and *BRCA1* gene products to arrest cell division and thereby allow repair of radiation-induced chromosome breaks before the S phase in the cell cycle (p. 32).

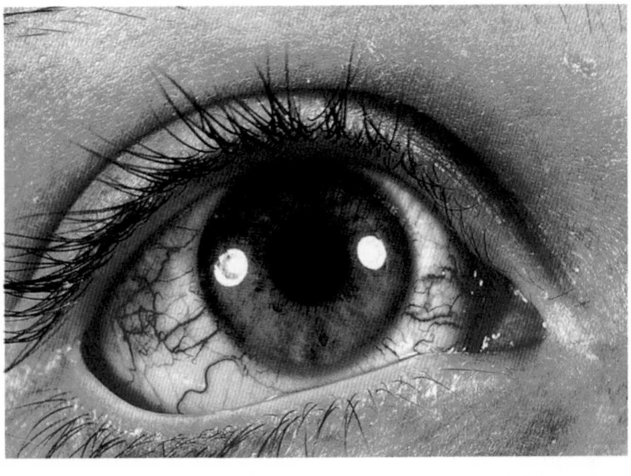

• **Fig. 17.30** Ocular telangiectasia in a child with ataxia telangiectasia.

Bloom Syndrome

Children with this AR disorder are small, with a light-sensitive facial rash and reduced immunoglobulin (IgA and IgM) levels. The risk of lymphoreticular malignancy is approximately 20%. Cultured cells show an increased frequency of chromosome breaks, particularly if they are exposed *in vitro* to ultraviolet light. The gene for Bloom syndrome, *RECQL3*, is at chromosome region 15q26, and encodes one member of a group of enzymes called the DNA helicases. These are responsible for unwinding double-stranded DNA before replication, repair, and recombination (p. 23).

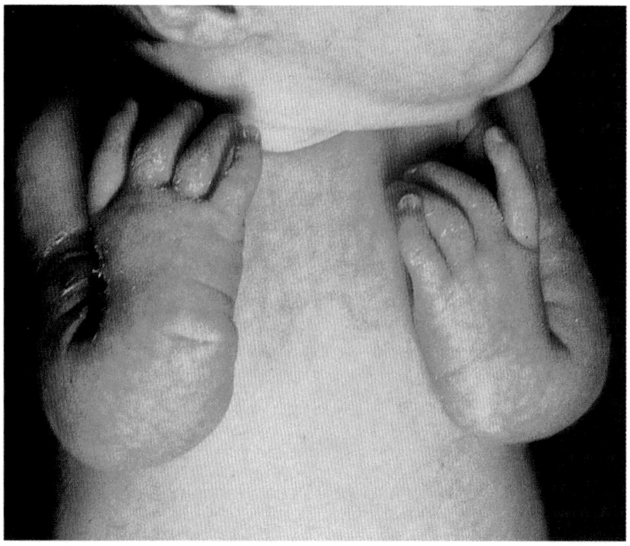

• **Fig. 17.31** Bilateral radial aplasia with absent thumbs in an infant with Fanconi anemia.

Normally *RECQL3* plays a major role in maintaining genome stability. When defective in the homozygous state, DNA repair is impaired, and the rate of recombination between sister chromatids is increased dramatically. This can be demonstrated by looking for sister chromatid exchanges.

TABLE 17.9 The subtypes of Fanconi anemia: genes and loci

Fanconi Subtype	Fanconi Gene	Chromosome Locus
FANCA	*FANCA*	16q24.3
FANCB	*FANCB*	Xp22
FANCC	*FANCC*	9q22
FANCD1	*BRCA2*	13q12
FANCD2	*FANCD2*	3p25
FANCE	*FANCE*	6p22
FANCF	*FANCF*	11p15
FANCG	*XRCC9*	9p13
FANCI	*FANCI*	15q25
FANCJ	*BRIP1*	17q22
FANCL	*PHF9*	2p16
FANCN	*PALB2*	16p12
FANCO	*RAD51C*	17q22
FANCP	*SLX4*	16p13
FANCQ	*ERCC4*	16p13
FANCT	*UBE2T*	1q31

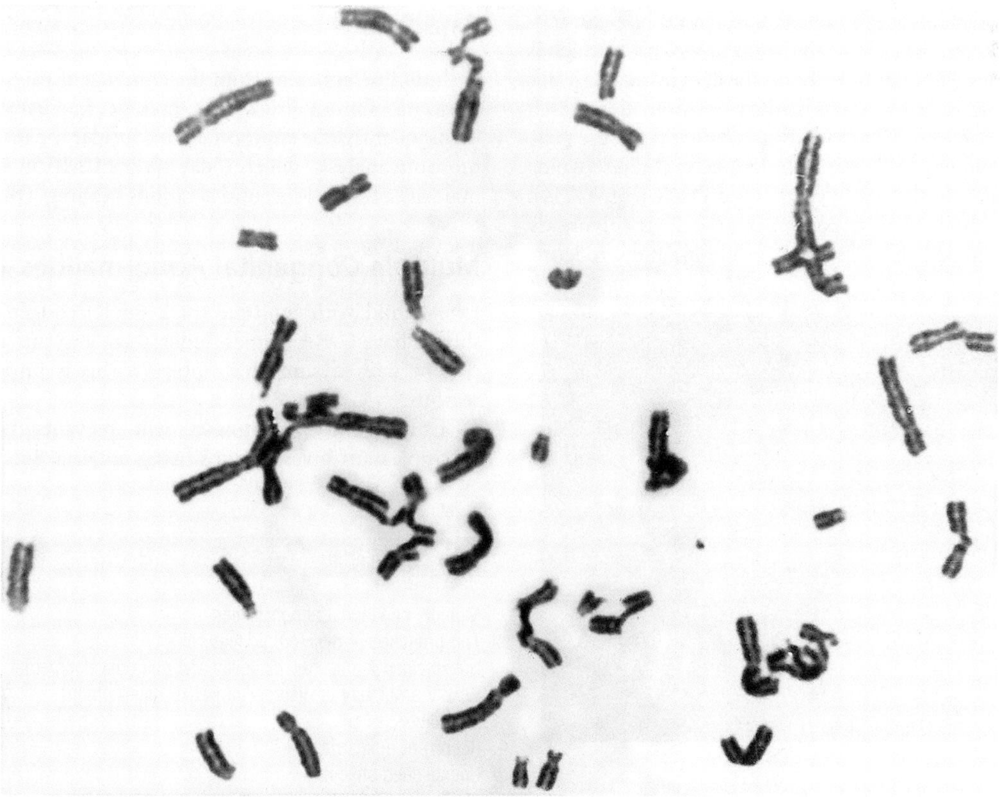

• **Fig. 17.32** Multiple chromosome breaks and gaps in a metaphase spread prepared from a child with Fanconi anemia.

Fanconi Anemia

This AR disorder is associated with upper limb abnormalities involving the radius and thumb (Fig. 17.31), increased pigmentation and bone marrow failure leading to deficiency of all types of blood cells (i.e., pancytopenia). There is also an increased risk of neoplasia, particularly leukemia, lymphoma, and hepatic carcinoma. Multiple chromosomal breaks are observed in cultured cells (Fig. 17.32), and the basic defect lies in the repair of DNA strand cross-links. There are at least 16 known subtypes of Fanconi anemia, each caused by variants at different autosomal loci (Table 17.9), the most common of which is type A.

Xeroderma Pigmentosum

This exists in at least seven different forms, all of which follow AR inheritance. Patients present with a light-sensitive pigmented rash and usually die from skin malignancy in sun-exposed areas before the age of 20 years (Fig. 17.33). Cells cultured from these patients show chromosome abnormalities only after exposure to ultraviolet (UV) light. These disorders are caused by defects in the nucleotide excision repair pathway, which involves endonuclease cleavage 5′ and 3′ to each damaged nucleotide, excision of the damaged nucleotide(s), and finally restoration of the damaged strand using the intact opposite strand as a template.

Chromosome Breakage and Sister Chromatid Exchange

Strong evidence of increased **chromosome instability** is provided by the demonstration of an increased number of **sister chromatid exchanges (SCEs)** in cultured cells. An SCE is an exchange (crossing over) of genetic material between the two chromatids of a chromosome in mitosis, in contrast to recombination in meiosis I, which is between homologous chromatids. SCEs can be demonstrated by differences in the uptake of certain stains by the two chromatids of each metaphase chromosome after two rounds of cell division in the presence of the thymidine analogue, 5-bromodeoxyuridine, which becomes incorporated in the newly synthesized DNA (Fig. 17.34). There are normally about 10 SCEs per cell, but the number is greatly increased in cells from patients with Bloom syndrome and xeroderma

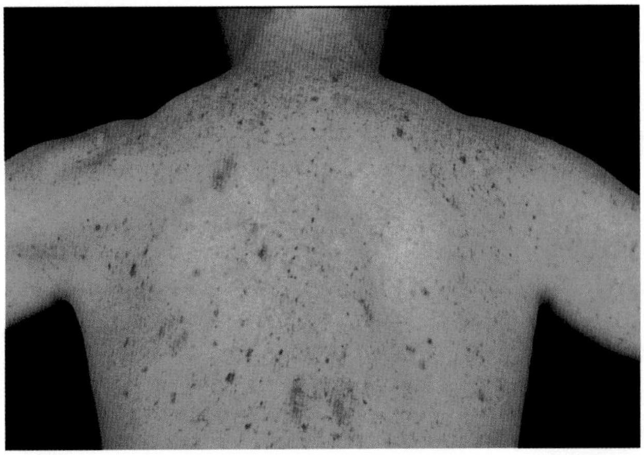

• **Fig. 17.33** Xeroderma pigmentosum: skin features with multiple melanomas and non-melanoma skin cancers. (Courtesy of Dr. Hiva Fassihi, London.)

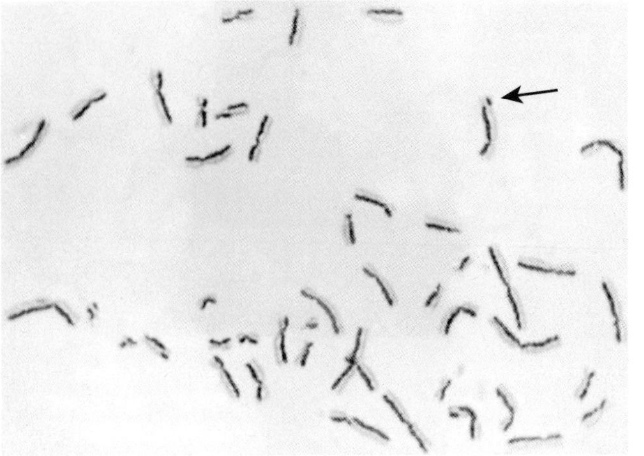

• **Fig. 17.34** Chromosome preparation showing sister chromatid exchanges (*arrow*).

pigmentosa. In the latter condition this is apparent only after the cells have been exposed to UV light.

It is not clear how SCEs relate to the increased chromosome breakage observed in these two disorders, but it is thought that the explanation could involve one of the steps in DNA replication. It is also of interest that the number of SCEs in normal cells is increased on exposure to certain carcinogens and chemical mutagens. For this reason the frequency of SCEs in cells in culture can be used as an *in vitro* test of the carcinogenicity and mutagenicity of chemical compounds (p. 23).

Indications for Chromosome Microarray Analysis

It should be apparent from the contents of this chapter that chromosome abnormalities can present in many different ways. Consequently it is appropriate to consider the indications for chromosome analysis, which today means **CMA** in the overwhelming majority of situations, under various headings (Box 17.2).

Multiple Congenital Abnormalities

Every child with multiple (or a single) congenital abnormalities should have CMA studies undertaken, and this also applies to any patient with dysmorphic features. This is important for several reasons:

1. Establishing a diagnosis will prevent further potentially unpleasant investigations being undertaken.

• BOX 17.2 Indications for Chromosome Analysis

Multiple congenital abnormalities
The presence of dysmorphic features
Unexplained intellectual disability and neurodevelopmental disorders
Sexual ambiguity or disorder of sexual development
Infertility
Recurrent miscarriage
Unexplained stillbirth
Malignancy and chromosome breakage syndromes

2. Information about the prognosis can be provided, along with details of the relevant support group and an offer of contact with other families (assuming other cases are known).
3. A diagnosis should facilitate accurate genetic risk counseling.

Although it can be very distressing for parents to be told that their child has a chromosome imbalance, they will often be relieved that an explanation for their child's problems has been found.

Unexplained Intellectual Disability and Neurodevelopmental Disorders

Chromosome anomalies, including microdeletions, and microduplications, cause at least one-third of the 50% of learning difficulties that are attributable to genetic factors. Although many children with a chromosome imbalance have other features such as growth retardation and physical anomalies, this is not always so. Along with CMA studies it is important not to forget that fragile-X syndrome might be a possibility, and this requires specific molecular analysis.

Sexual Ambiguity

The birth of a child with ambiguous genitalia—a form of disorder of sex development (DSD, Chapter 9)—should be regarded as a medical emergency, not only because of the inevitable parental anxiety, but also because of the importance of ruling out the potentially life-threatening diagnosis of salt-losing congenital adrenal hyperplasia (p. 277).

DSDs presenting in later life, with problems such as delayed puberty, primary amenorrhea, or male gynecomastia, are also mandatory indications for CMA analysis as a first-line investigation. This can provide a diagnosis such as Turner (45,X) or Klinefelter (47,XXY) syndromes. Alternatively, a normal CMA result will stimulate a search for other possible explanations, such as an endocrine abnormality, although mosaicism detectable in another tissue may also need to be considered.

Infertility and Recurrent Miscarriage

Unexplained involuntary infertility should prompt a request for chromosome and CMA studies, particularly if investigations reveal evidence of azoospermia in the male partner. At least 5% of such men are found to have Klinefelter syndrome. More rarely a complex chromosome rearrangement such as a translocation can cause such severe mechanical disruption in meiosis that complete failure of gametogenesis ensues.

Some couples experience recurrent pregnancy loss—usually defined as more than three spontaneous miscarriages. Often no explanation is found, and many such couples go on to have successful pregnancies. However, in 3% to 6% of cases one partner is found to carry a chromosome rearrangement that predisposes to severe imbalance through malsegregation at meiosis (p. 32). Consequently it is now standard practice to offer chromosome analysis to all such couples.

Unexplained Stillbirth/Neonatal Death

The presence of growth retardation and at least one congenital abnormality in a stillbirth or neonatal death is an indication for CMA studies based on analysis of blood or skin collected from the baby before or as soon after death as possible. Skin fibroblasts continue to be viable for several days after demise. In cases of stillbirth and neonatal death where the infant has no congenital anomaly or dysmorphic features, the chance of a positive finding on CMA is small, and attention is increasingly turning to exome sequencing in this group.

Malignancy and Chromosome Breakage Syndromes

Certain types of leukemia and many solid tumors, such as retinoblastoma (pp. 189, 259) and Wilms tumor (192, 258), are associated with specific chromosome imbalances and rearrangements that can be of both diagnostic and prognostic value. Clinical features suggestive of a chromosome breakage syndrome (p. 265), such as a combination of photosensitivity and short stature, should also lead to appropriate chromosome fragility studies, such as analysis of sister chromatid exchanges.

ELEMENTS

1. Chromosome abnormalities account for 50% of all spontaneous miscarriages and are present in 0.5% to 1.0% of all newborn infants.
2. Down syndrome is the most common autosomal chromosome syndrome, with a strong association between increasing incidence and advancing maternal age. Some 95% of all cases are caused by trisomy 21. Chromosome studies are necessary in all cases so that the rare but important cases caused by unbalanced familial Robertsonian translocations can be identified.
3. An ever-expanding number of chromosome microdeletion and microduplication syndromes are being recognized. These have helped in gene mapping and in enhancing understanding of underlying genetic mechanisms, monogenic disorders and imprinting. Microdeletions of chromosome 15q are found in both Angelman and Prader-Willi syndromes, depending on whether the chromosome is maternally or paternally derived, respectively.
4. Triploidy is a common finding in spontaneously aborted products of conception but is rare in a live-born infant. Some children with diploidy/triploidy mosaicism present with intellectual disability and areas of depigmentation, a condition known as hypomelanosis of Ito.
5. Sex chromosome abnormalities include Klinefelter (47,XXY), Turner (45,X), XYY (47,XYY), and triple X (47,XXX) syndromes. In all of these conditions, intellectual ability is either normal or only mildly impaired. Infertility is the rule in Klinefelter and Turner syndromes. Fertility is normal in the XYY and the triple X syndrome.
6. The fragile-X syndrome is the most common inherited cause of intellectual disability (ID). It is associated with a fragile site on the long arm of the X chromosome and shows modified X-linked inheritance. Affected males have moderate to severe ID; carrier females can show mild ID. At the molecular level there is expansion of a CGG triplet repeat, which can exist as an intermediate allele, a premutation or a full mutation.
7. The chromosome breakage syndromes are rare autosomal recessive disorders characterized by increased chromosome breakage in cultured cells and an increased tendency to neoplasia, such as leukemia and lymphoma. They are caused by underlying defects in DNA repair.
8. Standard karyotyping still has a place in genetic investigations but the technique has been largely superseded by chromosome microarray (CMA), that is, molecular cytogenetics. Current developments in next-generation sequencing technology are likely to replace CMA in due course.

CLINICAL SCENARIO 1

You examine a 6-year-old boy who has profound intellectual disability with very late motor milestones but is now walking independently. He has a history of prolonged seizures from infancy which are now reasonably well controlled on an antiepileptic medication, his speech consists of approximately 10 single words, he has soft dysmorphic features with a head circumference on the 5th centile and he has probable hypogenitalism (very small penis, but testes have been identified as present). His behavior is extremely difficult at home.

The result of chromosome microarray (CMA) reveals a microdeletion at 15q11.2. Testing of the parents reveals that this was paternally inherited, and the boy's father had some educational difficulties within a mainstream school environment. He never had seizures and is able to maintain employment as a gardener.

How do you interpret this CMA finding in the family?

CLINICAL SCENARIO 2

You meet a 10-year-old girl in clinic with her parents. She is one of the shortest children in her school class but is making reasonable educational progress with no major concerns. She is not obviously dysmorphic.

The parents explain that her chromosomes were tested at the age of 2½ years because of concern about her growth. This revealed a karyotype of 47,XXX. The parents were told that she might have some behavioral difficulties but would be expected to progress satisfactorily through school. She would most likely be tall for her age eventually and would be able to have children normally. Furthermore, there is no particular risk that her children would have a chromosome abnormality.

You offer her a buccal smear test or skin biopsy to look at chromosome analysis in a tissue other than blood. What is the rationale for this, and what might be found?

Further Reading

Levy B, Wapner R. Prenatal diagnosis by chromosomal microarray analysis. *Fertil Steril.* 2018;109(2):201–212.

A paper reviewing the use of chromosomal microarray after its introduction in prenatal testing.

McKinlay Gardner RJ, Amor DJ. *Gardner and Sutherland's Chromosome Abnormalities and Genetic Counseling (Oxford Monographs on Medical Genetics).* Oxford University Press, Oxford; 2018.

A superb guide to all aspects of chromosome disorders and related genetic counseling.

Miller DT, Adam MP, Aradhya S, et al. Consensus statement: chromosomal microarray is a first-tier clinical diagnostic test for individuals with developmental disabilities or congenital anomalies. *Am J Hum Genet.* 2010;86:749–764.

An important early review of chromosomal microarray after the first few years of use.

Ratcliffe S. Long-term outcome in children of sex chromosome abnormalities. *Arch Dis Child.* 1999;80:192–195.

A very useful and clear description of the cognitive and social outcomes of long-term follow-up studies of sex chromosome aneuploidies.

Unique—The Rare Chromosome Disorder Support Group. https://www.rarechromo.org/

Unique produces an excellent series of guides for specific chromosome disorders that can be downloaded free of charge.

18
Inborn Errors of Metabolism

Life . . . is a relationship between molecules.

Linus Pauling

The existence of chemical individuality follows of necessity from that of chemical specificity, but we should expect the differences between individuals to be still more subtle and difficult of detection.

Archibald Garrod (1908)

In this chapter we consider single-gene biochemical, or metabolic, diseases, often known as **inborn errors of metabolism** (IEMs), including **mitochondrial disorders**. The range of known disorders is vast, so only an overview is possible. At the beginning of the 20th century, Garrod introduced the concept of "chemical individuality," leading in turn to the concept of IEMs. Beadle and Tatum, some 30 years later, developed the idea that metabolic processes, whether in humans or any other organism, proceed by steps. They proposed that each step was controlled by a particular enzyme that was, in turn, the product of a particular gene. This was referred to as the **one gene–one enzyme (or protein)** concept.

In excess of 600 IEMs are known that can be grouped by the main class of metabolite, metabolic pathway, enzyme function, or cellular organelle involved; Table 18.1 shows an adaptation of the classification of the Society for the Study of IEMs. In a substantial longitudinal study of children with IEMs in British Columbia, published in 2000, the overall incidence of IEMs in the population was approximately 40 per 100,000 live births, and this was estimated to make up approximately 15% of all single-gene disorders in their population. Most IEMs follow autosomal recessive (AR) or X-linked (XL) recessive inheritance, whereas a few follow autosomal dominant (AD) inheritance, and those attributed to mitochondrial mutations follow matrilinear inheritance. In autosomal IEMs the defective protein in most cases is a diffusible enzyme, and there is usually sufficient residual activity in the heterozygous state (loss-of-function, see pp. 22, 121) for the enzyme to function normally in most situations. If, however, the reaction catalyzed by an enzyme is rate limiting (haploinsufficiency, see p. 22) or the gene product is part of a multimeric complex (dominant-negative, see p. 22), the disorder can manifest in the heterozygous state and follow AD inheritance.

Because there is great similarity in the clinical presentation of many IEMs, investigation of early onset lethargy, vomiting, hypotonia, neurodevelopmental delay, and seizures, is usually focused on a "metabolic screen." This involves measurement of basic blood chemistry and electrolytes including glucose and lactate, liver, renal and thyroid function tests, amino acids, glycosaminoglycans (GAGs) (see Mucopolyssacharidoses, p. 278), and lysosomal (white cell) enzymes. Increasingly this is backed up by direct gene or whole-exome/-genome sequencing (WES/WGS) analysis. There is inevitably great interest in newborn screening by WES/WGS where this is available, precisely for the reason that early diagnosis in a range of rare metabolic conditions (that might not be covered by local newborn bloodspot screening) can lead to early dietary intervention and prevention, or at least amelioration, of long-term sequelae. This approach has to be undertaken with caution because of the difficulty of interpreting variants of uncertain significance, and in the area of IEMs confirmatory biochemical testing will continue to have a vital role.

Disorders of Amino Acid and Peptide Metabolism

This large group of IEMs has many subdivisions (see Table 18.1), and we consider the more well-known groups.

Disorders of Phenylalanine or Tyrosine Metabolism

Phenylketonuria

Children with phenylketonuria (PKU), if untreated, are severely intellectually impaired and often develop seizures. There is a deficiency of the enzyme required for the conversion of phenylalanine to tyrosine, phenylalanine hydroxylase (PAH)—causing a "genetic block" in the metabolic pathway (Fig. 18.1).

PKU was the first genetic disorder in humans shown to be caused by a specific enzyme deficiency, by Jervis in 1953. As a result of the enzyme defect, phenylalanine accumulates and is converted into phenylpyruvic acid and other metabolites that are excreted in the urine. The enzyme block leads to a deficiency of tyrosine, with a consequent reduction in melanin formation, and children therefore often have blond hair and blue eyes (Fig. 18.2). In addition, areas of the brain that are usually pigmented, such as the substantia nigra, may also lack pigment.

Treatment of Phenylketonuria. An obvious method of treating children with PKU would be to replace the missing enzyme, but this is not easily achievable. Bickel, just 1 year after the enzyme deficiency had been identified, suggested that PKU could be treated by removal of phenylalanine from the diet, and this has proved effective. If PKU is detected early enough in infancy, intellectual impairment can be prevented by giving a phenylalanine-restricted diet. Phenylalanine is an essential amino acid and therefore cannot be removed entirely from the diet. By monitoring the level of phenylalanine in the blood, it is possible to supply sufficient amounts to meet normal requirements while avoiding toxic levels leading to brain damage. After brain development is complete, dietary restriction can be relaxed—from adolescence onward.

TABLE 18.1 Classification of inborn errors of metabolism

1	Disorders of Amino Acid and Peptide Metabolism	
	1.1	Urea cycle disorders and inherited hyperammonemias
	1.2	Organic acidurias
	1.3	Metabolism of branched-chain amino acids (not organic acidurias)
	1.4	Phenylalanine or tyrosine metabolism
	1.5	Metabolism of sulfur amino acids
	1.6	Histidine, tryptophan, or lysine metabolism
	1.7	Serine, glycine, or glycerate metabolism
	1.8	Ornithine or proline metabolism
	1.9	Amino acid transport
	1.10	Amino acid metabolism
	1.11	Gamma-glutamyl cycle
	1.12	Other peptide metabolism
2	Disorders of Carbohydrate Metabolism	
	2.1	Galactose metabolism
	2.2	Fructose metabolism
	2.3	Pentose metabolism
	2.4	Glycerol metabolism
	2.5	Glyoxylate metabolism
	2.6	Glucose transport
	2.7	Gluconeogenesis
	2.8	Glycogen storage disorders
	2.9	Other carbohydrate disorders
3	Disorders of Fatty Acid and Ketone Body Metabolism	
	3.1	Lipolysis
	3.2	Carnitine transport and the carnitine cycle
	3.3	Mitochondrial fatty acid oxidation
	3.4	Ketone body metabolism
	3.5	Other fatty acid and ketone body metabolism
4	Disorders of Energy Metabolism	
	4.1	Pyruvate metabolism
	4.2	Citric acid cycle
	4.3	Mitochondrial respiratory chain
	4.4	Mitochondrial membrane transport
	4.5	Unspecified mitochondrial disorders
	4.6	Creatine metabolism
	4.7	Other energy metabolism
5	Disorders in the Metabolism of Purines, Pyrimidines, and Nucleotides	
	5.1	Purine metabolism
	5.2	Pyrimidine metabolism
	5.3	Nucleotide metabolism
6	Disorders of the Metabolism of Sterols	
	6.1	Sterol biosynthesis
	6.2	Bile acid biosynthesis
	6.3	Bile acid metabolism and transport
	6.4	Other metabolism of sterols
7	Disorders of Porphyrin and Heme Metabolism	
8	Disorders of Lipid and Lipoprotein Metabolism	
	8.1	Inherited hypercholesterolemias
	8.2	Inherited hypertriglyceridemias
	8.3	Inherited mixed hyperlipidemias
	8.4	High-density lipoprotein metabolism
	8.5	Inherited hypolipidemias
	8.6	Other lipid and lipoprotein metabolism
	8.7	Unspecified disorders of lipid and lipoprotein metabolism
9	Congenital Disorders of Glycosylation and Other Disorders of Protein Modification	
	9.1	Protein N-glycosylation
	9.2	Protein O-glycosylation
	9.3	Glycosphingolipid and glycosylphosphatidylinositol anchor glycosylation
	9.4	Multiple glycosylation and other glycosylation pathways
	9.5	Protein ubiquitinylation
	9.6	Other disorders of protein modification
10	Lysosomal Disorders	
	10.1	Mucopolysaccharidoses
	10.2	Oligosaccharidoses
	10.3	Sphingolipidoses
	10.4	Ceroid lipofuscinoses, neuronal
	10.5	Lysosomal export disorders
	10.6	Other lysosomal disorders
11	Peroxisomal Disorders	
	11.1	Peroxisome biogenesis
	11.2	Rhizomelic chondrodysplasia punctata
	11.3	Peroxisomal alpha-, beta-, and omega-oxidation
	11.4	Other peroxisomal disorders
12	Disorders of Neurotransmitter Metabolism	
	12.1	Metabolism of biogenic amines
	12.2	Metabolism of gamma-aminobutyrate
13	Disorders in the Metabolism of Vitamins and (Non-protein) Cofactors	
	13.1	Folate metabolism and transport
	13.2	Cobalamin absorption, transport, and metabolism
	13.3	Pterin metabolism
	13.4	Vitamin D metabolism and transport
	13.5	Biotin metabolism
	13.6	Pyridoxine metabolism
	13.7	Thiamine metabolism
	13.8	Molybdenum cofactor metabolism
	13.9	Other vitamins and cofactors
14	Disorders in the Metabolism of Trace Elements and Metals	
	14.1	Copper metabolism
	14.2	Iron metabolism
	14.3	Zinc metabolism
	14.4	Phosphate, calcium, and vitamin D metabolism
	14.5	Magnesium metabolism
	14.6	Other trace elements and metals
15	Disorders and Variants in the Metabolism of Xenobiotics	
	15.1	Cytochrome P450–mediated oxidation
	15.2	Other enzymes that oxidize xenobiotics
	15.3	Xenobiotics conjugation
	15.4	Xenobiotics transport

(*Continued*)

TABLE 18.1 Classification of inborn errors of metabolism—cont'd

(Modified from Society for the Study of IEMs, 2011.)

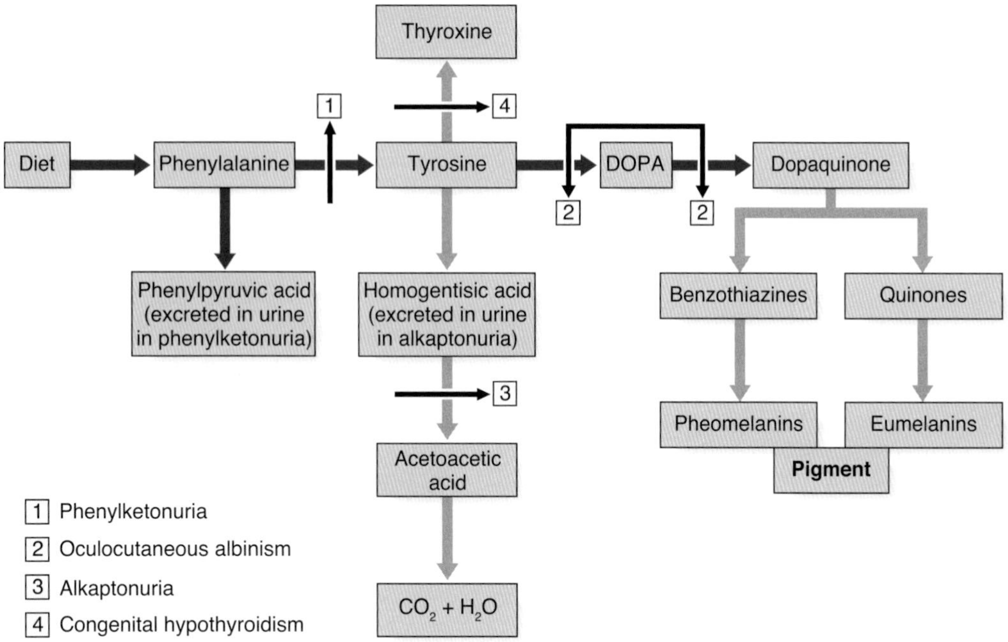

• **Fig. 18.1** Sites of "biochemical block" in phenylketonuria, alkaptonuria, congenital hypothyroidism, and oculocutaneous albinism.

The intellectual impairment seen in children with PKU is likely caused by toxic levels of phenylalanine, and/or its metabolites, rather than a deficiency of tyrosine, of which adequate amounts are present in a normal diet. Both prenatal and postnatal factors may be responsible for developmental delay in untreated PKU.

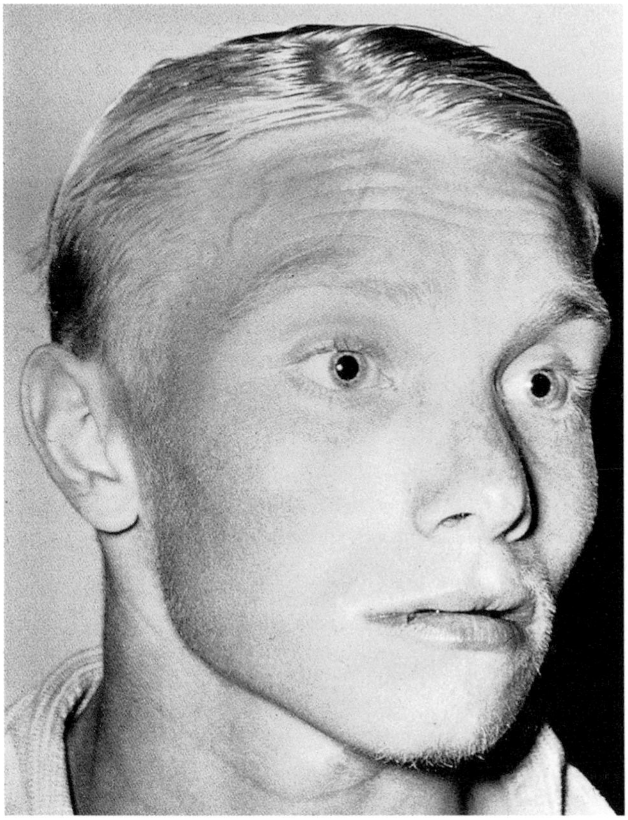

• **Fig. 18.2** Face of a male with phenylketonuria; he has a fair complexion.

Diagnosis of Phenylketonuria. PKU affects approximately 1 in 10,000 people in Western Europe and was the first IEM routinely screened for in newborns (Chapter 11; p. 157). The test detects the presence of the metabolite of phenylalanine—phenylpyruvic acid—in the urine by its reaction with ferric chloride, or through increased levels of phenylalanine in the blood. The latter, originally known as the Guthrie test and now known as newborn bloodspot screening, involved analyzing blood from newborns and comparing the amount of growth induced by the sample, against standards, in a strain of the bacterium *Bacillus subtilis*, which requires phenylalanine for growth. This has been replaced by the use of a variety of biochemical assays of phenylalanine levels.

Heterogeneity of Hyperphenylalaninemia. Raised phenylalanine levels in the newborn period may be attributed to causes other than PKU. Rarely, newborns have a condition called benign hyperphenylalaninemia, caused by a transient immaturity of liver cells to metabolize phenylalanine. Treatment is not necessary, because these children are not at risk of developing learning disability. Two rare but serious causes of hyperphenylalaninemia, in which levels of the enzyme PAH are normal, are deficiency of: (1) dihydropteridine reductase, and (2) dihydrobiopterin synthase. These two enzymes help synthesize tetrahydrobiopterin, a cofactor necessary for normal activity of PAH. They are more serious than classic PKU because of a high risk of mental retardation despite satisfactory management of phenylalanine levels.

Mutational Basis of Phenylketonuria. Hundreds of pathogenic variants in the *PAH* gene have been identified. Some are more prevalent in specific population groups, and in western Europeans with PKU they are found on the background of a limited number of DNA haplotypes. However, a variety of different individual variants has been found in association with some of these haplotypes.

Maternal Phenylketonuria. Children born to mothers with PKU may have an increased risk of learning disability even when their mothers are on closely controlled dietary restriction, suggesting that the reduced ability of the mother with PKU to deliver an appropriate amount of tyrosine to her fetus *in utero* may cause reduced fetal brain growth. Commencing dietary restriction preconception is important.

Alkaptonuria

Alkaptonuria was the original AR IEM described by Garrod. Here there is a block in the breakdown of homogentisic acid, a metabolite of tyrosine, because of a deficiency of the enzyme homogentisate 1,2-dioxygenase, encoded by the *HGD* gene (see Fig. 18.1). As a consequence, homogentisic acid accumulates and is excreted in the urine, which then darkens upon exposure to air. Dark pigment is also deposited in certain tissues, such as the ear wax, cartilage, and joints, where it is known as ochronosis, which in joints can lead to arthritis later in life.

Oculocutaneous Albinism

Oculocutaneous albinism (OCA) follows AR inheritance and results from deficiency of the enzyme tyrosinase, which catalyzes the formation of melanin from tyrosine (see Fig. 18.1). In OCA the skin, hair, iris, and ocular fundus lack pigment (Fig. 18.3), and the lack of eye pigment results in poor visual acuity (usually in the range of 20/100 to 20/400) and uncontrolled pendular eye movements—nystagmus. Reduced fundal pigmentation leads to underdevelopment of the part of the retina for fine vision—the fovea—and misrouting of the optic nerve fiber radiations at the chiasm, resulting in strabismus, reduced stereoscopic vision and altered (crossed) visually evoked potentials.

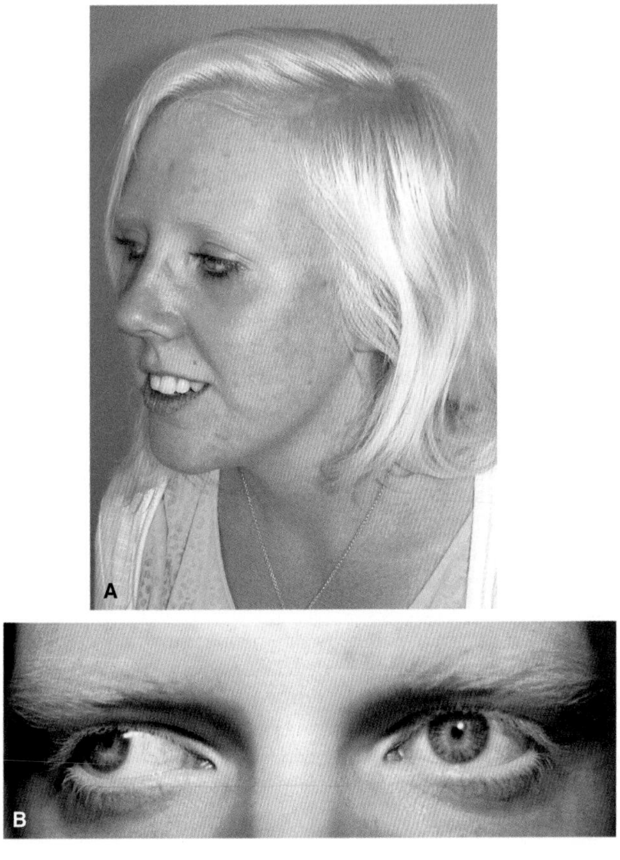

• **Fig. 18.3** Oculocutaneous albinism type 1. (A) A young Caucasian woman. She has a small amount of pigment production because her hair is not absolutely white; (B) the eyes of another patient: note the white eyebrows and lashes, strabismus, and transillumination of the iris.

Heterogeneity of Oculocutaneous Albinism. OCA is genetically and biochemically heterogeneous. Cells from those with classic albinism have no measurable tyrosinase activity, the so-called **tyrosinase-negative** form. However, cells from some persons with albinism show reduced but residual tyrosinase activity and are termed **tyrosinase-positive**. This is usually reflected clinically by variable development of pigmentation of the hair and skin with age. Both types are known as **tyrosinase gene–related OCA type 1**.

OCA type 1 is caused by variants in the tyrosinase (*TYR*) gene on chromosome 11q, but linkage studies in some families with tyrosinase-positive OCA excluded this gene. Some have variants in the *P* gene, the human homologue of a mouse gene called pink-eyed dilution, or "pink-eye," located on chromosome 15q. This has been termed **OCA type 2. OCA3** is attributed to variants in the gene encoding tyrosinase-related protein-1 (*TYRP1*), chromosome 9p23, as well as four further loci at which the causative genes have been identified. These tend to be mild forms of albinism.

Urea Cycle Disorders

The urea cycle is a five-step metabolic pathway that takes place primarily in liver cells for the removal of waste nitrogen from the amino groups of amino acids arising from the normal turnover of protein. It converts two molecules of ammonia and one of bicarbonate into urea (Fig. 18.4). Deficiencies of enzymes in the urea cycle result in intolerance to protein from the accumulation of ammonia in the body—hyperammonemia. Increased ammonia levels are toxic to the central nervous system and can lead to coma and, with some untreated urea cycle disorders, death—in infancy in severe cases. They are collectively and individually rare and, with the exception of XL ornithine transcarbamylase deficiency, inherited as AR traits. Other conditions in the group are citrullinemia, arginosuccinic aciduria and hyperammonemia-hyperornithinemia-homocitrullinuria syndrome.

Disorders of the Metabolism of Sulphur Amino Acids

Homocystinuria

Homocystinuria is a sulfur amino-acid IEM caused by deficiency of cystathionine β-synthase, and follows AR inheritance. It is characterized by learning disability, seizures, thrombophilia, osteoporosis, scoliosis, pectus excavatum, long fingers and toes (arachnodactyly) (Fig. 18.5), and a tendency to dislocation of the lenses. The somatic features therefore resemble the AD disorder Marfan syndrome (p. 308).

Screening for homocystinuria is possible by means of the cyanide nitroprusside test, which detects the presence of increased levels of urinary homocystine. The diagnosis is confirmed by raised plasma homocystine levels and variant analysis of the *CBS* gene. Treatment involves a low-methionine diet with cystine supplementation. A proportion of individuals with homocystinuria are responsive to the enzyme cofactor pyridoxine (i.e., the pyridoxine-responsive form). Some affected individuals have variants in genes

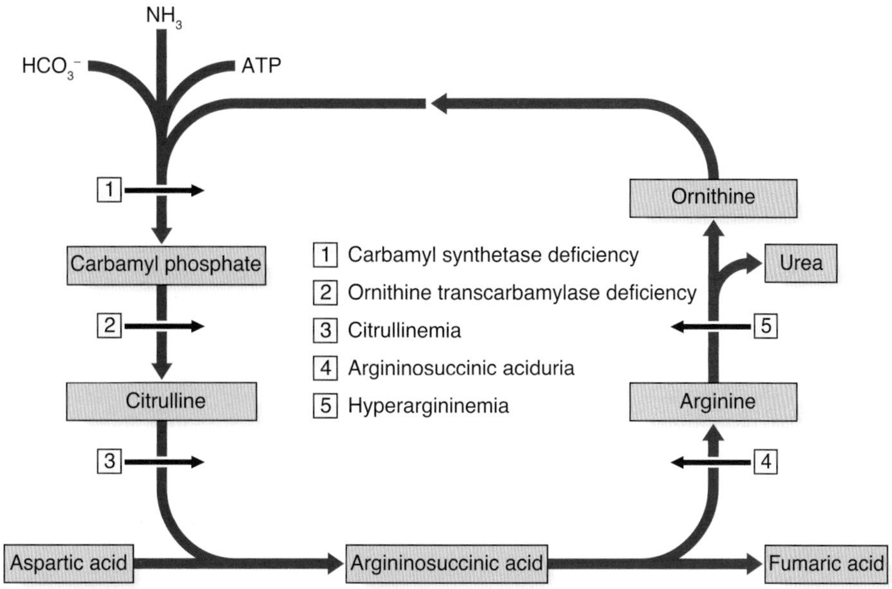

• **Fig. 18.4** Diagram indicating the position of the various inborn errors of the urea cycle.

leading to deficiencies of enzymes involved in the synthesis of cofactors for cystathionine β-synthase.

Organic Acidurias

Glutaric Aciduria I

Glutaric aciduria type I (glutaryl-CoA dehydrogenase deficiency) and II (multiple acyl-CoA dehydrogenase deficiency) are included as examples of an organic aciduria that is intermediate in fatty-acid oxidation (see later under mitochondrial disorders). Macrocephaly is present at birth, and infants suffer episodes of encephalopathy with spasticity, dystonia, seizures, and developmental delay. Treatment is by dietary restriction of glutarigenic amino acids—lysine, tryptophan, and hydroxylysine. Because this condition is common among the Old Order Amish of Pennsylvania, neonatal screening has been introduced in the area.

Methylmalonic and Propionic Acidurias

These two disorders are caused by deficiency of the enzymes methylmalonyl-CoA mutase and propionyl-CoA carboxylase,

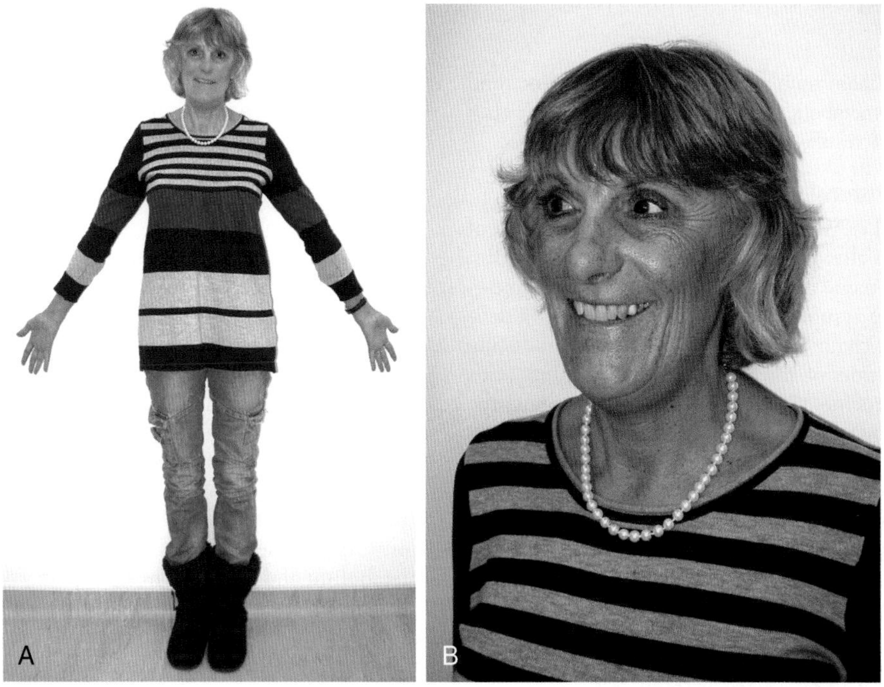

• **Fig. 18.5** A lady with homocystinuria who presented with ectopia lentis from a young age and for many years was thought to have Marfan syndrome. (A) Her apparently Marfanoid habitus (long arms and legs); (B) her facial features, which may also resemble Marfan syndrome.

respectively. The enzyme deficiency results in accumulation of the toxic organic-acid metabolites derived from deamination of certain amino acids, specific long-chain fatty acids and cholesterol side chains. Children present with periodic episodes of poor feeding, vomiting, and lethargy in association with a severe metabolic acidosis, low white cell (neutropenia) and platelet (thrombocytopenia) counts, low blood sugar (hypoglycemia), and high blood ammonia levels (hyperammonemia). These episodes are often precipitated by intercurrent illness or increased protein intake, and after such an episode affected children can lose developmental skills. During these episodes there are high plasma levels of glycine (hyperglycinemia).

Therapy for the acute episode involves the treatment of any infection, fluid replacement, correction of the metabolic acidosis and cessation of protein intake. Long-term prophylactic treatment involves restriction of protein intake and rapid recognition and management of any intercurrent illness. A proportion of individuals affected with propionic acidemia are responsive to biotin, whereas some with methylmalonic acidemia are sensitive to vitamin B12.

Methylglutaconic Aciduria (Barth Syndrome)

Barth syndrome, strictly speaking "3-methylglutaconic aciduria type II," which is also known as XL cardioskeletal myopathy, is characterized by congenital dilated cardiomyopathy, including endocardial fibroelastosis. It is also a generalized myopathy, with skeletal muscle showing increased lipid levels, and growth retardation, and neutropenia occur. A five- to 20-fold increase in urinary 3-methylglutaconic acid (3-MGC), as well as moderately raised urinary 3-methylglutaric acid and 2-ethylhydracrylic acid, is usually present. However, levels of 3-MGC, as well as neutropenia, can fluctuate, although they are useful in achieving a diagnosis. Pathogenic variants occur in the *G4.5* (*TAZ*) gene at Xq28, and it is thought that cardiolipin remodeling within the inner mitochondrial membrane is the pathological consequence.

Disorders of Branched-Chain Amino Acid Metabolism

The essential branched-chain amino acids leucine, isoleucine, and valine, have part of their metabolic pathways in common. Deficiency of the enzyme involved results in maple syrup urine disease.

Maple Syrup Urine Disease

Newborn infants with this AR disorder present in the first week of life with vomiting, then alternating tone, leading to death within weeks if untreated. The name derives from the odor of the urine—likened to that of maple syrup. The disorder is caused by a deficiency of the branched-chain ketoacid decarboxylase, producing increased urinary excretion of the branched-chain amino acids valine, leucine and isoleucine, the presence of which suggests the diagnosis, confirmed by demonstration of the three essential branched-chain amino acids in blood. Treatment involves dietary restriction of these three amino acids to the amounts necessary for growth. Affected individuals are particularly susceptible to deterioration, particularly in association with intercurrent illnesses leading to catabolic protein degradation.

Disorders of Carbohydrate Metabolism

The inborn errors of carbohydrate metabolism are subdivided into many categories (see Table 18.1) and include well-known intolerances such as that for lactose and a rare disorder of intolerance for disaccharides. We describe the better-known conditions within the disorders of galactose and fructose metabolism before considering the large group of glycogen storage disorders.

Classic Galactosemia

Galactosemia is an AR disorder resulting from deficiency of the enzyme galactose 1-phosphate uridyl transferase, necessary for the metabolism of the dietary sugar galactose. Newborns with galactosemia present with vomiting, lethargy, failure to thrive, and jaundice in the second week of life. If untreated, they develop complications that include intellectual disability, cataracts, and liver cirrhosis. Complications can be prevented by early diagnosis and feeding infants with milk substitutes that do not contain galactose or lactose—the sugar found in milk that is broken down into galactose. Early diagnosis is essential, and galactosemia can be screened for by the presence of reducing substances in the urine with specific testing for galactose.

Hereditary Fructose Intolerance

Hereditary fructose intolerance is an AR disorder resulting from a deficiency of the enzyme fructose 1-phosphate aldolase. Dietary fructose is present in honey, fruit, and certain vegetables, and in combination with glucose in the disaccharide sucrose in cane sugar. Individuals with hereditary fructose intolerance present at different ages, depending on when fructose is introduced into the diet. Symptoms can be minimal but might also be as severe as those seen in galactosemia, which include failure to thrive, vomiting, jaundice, and seizures. The diagnosis is confirmed by the presence of fructose in the urine and enzyme assay on an intestinal mucosal or liver biopsy sample. Dietary restriction of fructose is associated with a good long-term prognosis.

Glycogen Storage Disorders

Glycogen is the form in which the sugar glucose is stored in muscle and liver as a polymer, acting as a reserve energy source. In the glycogen storage disorders (GSDs) glycogen accumulates in excessive amounts in skeletal muscle, cardiac muscle and/or liver because of a variety of inborn errors of the enzymes involved in synthesis and degradation of glycogen. In addition, because of the metabolic block, glycogen is unavailable as a normal glucose source. This can result in hypoglycemia, impairment of liver function, and neurological abnormalities.

In all, there are now around 30 different GSD entities identified, but we briefly describe six major types, virtually all following AR inheritance (see GSD VI). Each has a specific enzyme defect involving one of the steps in glycogen synthesis or degradation. Although listed by their numerical place in the classification, types II (Pompe) and V (McArdle) primarily affect muscle, whilst the others primarily affect the liver. Among the rare types not discussed are Fanconi-Bickel syndrome (GSD type XI) and aldolase A deficiency.

von Gierke Disease (GSD I)

von Gierke disease was the first described disorder of glycogen metabolism and results from a deficiency of the enzyme glucose-6-phosphatase, which is responsible for degradation of liver glycogen to release glucose. Infants present with an enlarged liver (hepatomegaly) and/or sweating and a fast heart rate because of hypoglycemia, which can occur after fasting of only 3 to 4 hours' duration. Treatment is simple—frequent feeding and avoidance of fasting to maintain the blood sugar concentration.

Pompe Disease (GSD II)

Infants with Pompe disease usually present in the first few months of life with floppiness (hypotonia) and delay in the gross motor milestones because of muscle weakness. They then develop an enlarged heart and die from cardiac failure in the first or second year. Voluntary and cardiac muscle accumulates glycogen because of deficiency of the lysosomal enzyme α-1,4-glucosidase, which is needed to break down glycogen. The diagnosis can be confirmed by enzyme assay of white blood cells or fibroblasts. Early reports of enzyme replacement therapy appear promising.

Cori Disease (GSD III)

Cori disease is caused by deficiency of the enzyme amylo-1,6-glucosidase, which is also known as the debrancher enzyme. Deficiency results in glycogen accumulation in the liver and other tissues because of the inability to cleave the "branching" links of the glycogen polymer. Infants may present with hepatomegaly because of glycogen accumulation, and/or muscle weakness. Treatment involves avoiding hypoglycemia by frequent feeding and avoiding prolonged periods of fasting.

Andersen Disease (GSD IV)

Anderson disease results from deficiency of glycogen brancher enzyme leading to the formation of abnormal glycogen consisting of long chains with few branches that cannot be broken down by the enzymes normally responsible for glycogen degradation. Infants present with hypotonia and abnormal liver function in their first year, progressing rapidly to liver failure. No effective treatment is available apart from the possibility of a liver transplant.

McArdle Disease (GSD V)

Individuals with McArdle disease present with muscle cramps during exercise in the teenage years. The condition is caused by a deficiency of muscle phosphorylase, which is necessary for degradation of muscle glycogen. There is no effective treatment, although in some the muscle cramps tend to decline if exercise is continued, probably as a result of other energy sources becoming available from alternative metabolic pathways.

Hepatic Glycogen Phosphorylase Deficiency (GSD VI)

Hepatic phosphorylase is a multimeric enzyme complex with subunits coded for by both autosomal and XL genes. Deficiency of hepatic phosphorylase obstructs glycogen degradation, which results in children presenting in the first 2 years of life with hepatomegaly, hypoglycemia, and failure to thrive. Treatment is with carbohydrate supplementation.

Disorders of Steroid Metabolism

The disorders of steroid metabolism include a number of AR inborn errors of the biosynthetic pathways of cortisol. Virilization of a female fetus may occur together with salt loss in infants of either sex from a deficiency of the hormone aldosterone. In addition, defects of the androgen receptor result in lack of virilization of chromosomally male individuals (Fig. 18.6).

Congenital Adrenal Hyperplasia

The diagnosis of congenital adrenal hyperplasia (CAH) should be considered in any newborn female infant presenting with virilization of the external genitalia, because this is the most common cause of ambiguous genitalia in female newborns (see Fig. 9.35, p. 132) (Fig. 18.7) (see Chapter 9 for more detail of Sex Determination and Disorders of Sex Development). A deficiency of 21-hydroxylase accounts for more than 90% of cases. Approximately 25% have the salt-losing form, presenting in the second or third week of life with circulatory collapse, hyponatremia and hyperkalemia. Less commonly, CAH is a result of deficiency of the enzymes 11β-hydroxylase or 3β-dehydrogenase, and very rarely as a result of deficiencies of enzymes 17α-hydroxylase and 17,20-lyase. Desmolase deficiency is very rare, with all pathways blocked, causing a reversed phenotype of ambiguous genitalia in males and severe Addisonian crises. Males with the rare 5α-reductase deficiency are significantly under-masculinized but do not suffer other metabolic problems and are raised as females during childhood. At puberty, however, the surge in androgen production is sufficient to stimulate growth of the phallus, and these individuals are then visibly male. In the inbred communities where the problem recurs and is well accepted, "switching" to male gender in every respect is possible, even routine.

Affected females with classic CAH are virilized from accumulation of the adrenocortical steroids proximal to the enzyme block in the steroid biosynthetic pathway, many of which have testosterone-like activity (see Fig. 18.6). However, they have normal Müllerian-derived internal organs. The possibility of CAH should not be forgotten, of course, in male infants presenting with circulatory collapse in the first few weeks of life.

Affected infants, in addition to requiring urgent correct assignment of gender, are treated with replacement cortisol, along with fludrocortisone if they have the salt-losing form. Virilized females may require plastic surgery later. Steroid replacement is life-long and should be increased during intercurrent illness or stress, such as surgery. Menarche in girls with salt-losing CAH is late, menstruation irregular, and they are subfertile.

Disorders of Lipid and Lipoprotein Metabolism

This group of disorders embraces a variety of disorders affecting cholesterol, triglycerides, and lipoproteins, and is important because of the consequences for cardiovascular disease. Additional coverage is given in Chapter 10; this group of disorders is associated with high morbidity and mortality rates through premature coronary artery disease.

Familial Hypercholesterolemia

Familial hypercholesterolemia (FH) is the most common autosomal dominant single-gene disorder in Western society. Individuals have raised cholesterol levels without symptoms but carry a significant risk of developing premature coronary artery disease, leading to significant morbidity and increased mortality rates. They can present in childhood or adolescence with subcutaneous deposition of lipid, known as xanthomata (Fig. 18.8). Starting with families who presented with early coronary artery disease, Brown and Goldstein unraveled the biology of the low-density lipoprotein (LDL) receptor (Fig. 18.9) and the pathological basis of FH.

Cells normally derive cholesterol from either endogenous synthesis or dietary uptake from LDL receptors on the cell surface. Intracellular cholesterol levels are maintained by a feedback system, with free cholesterol inhibiting LDL receptor synthesis, as well as reducing the level of *de novo* endogenous synthesis.

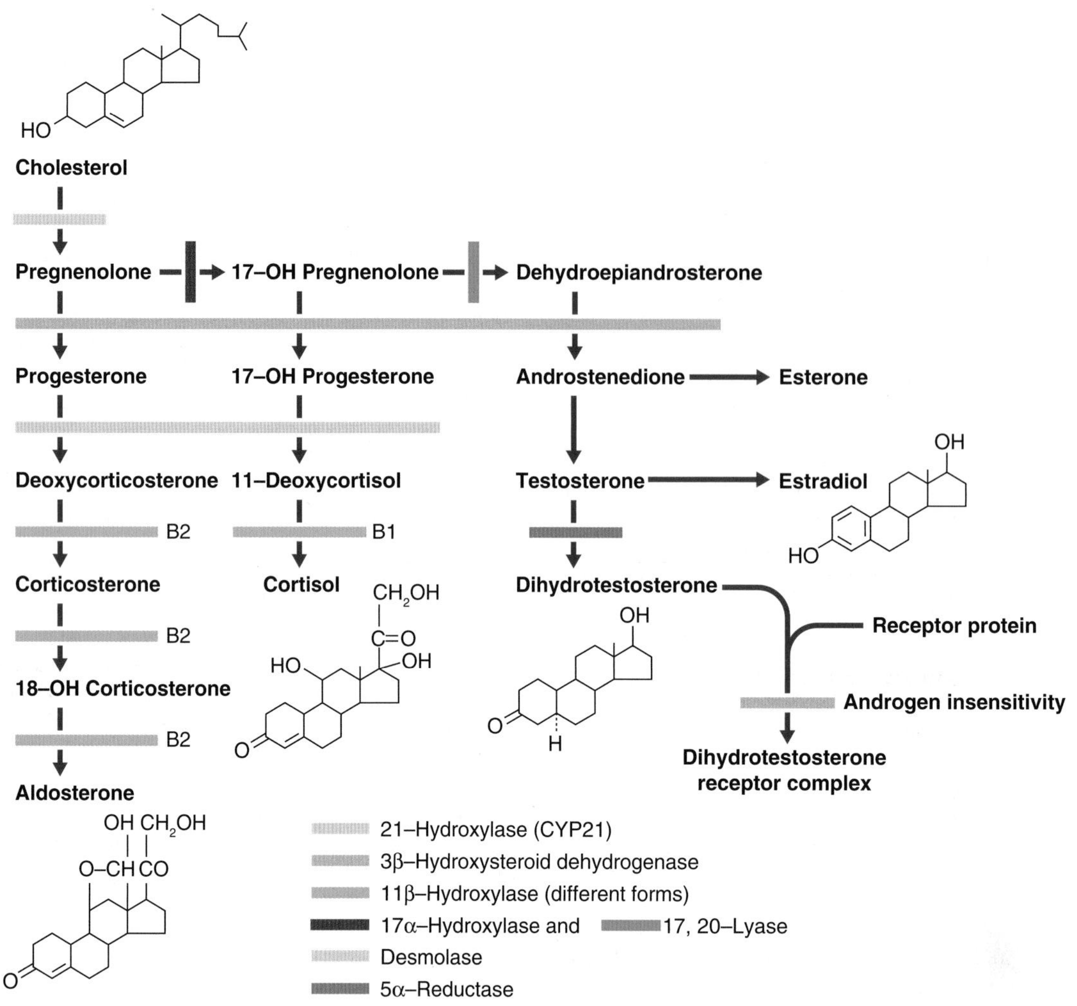

• **Fig. 18.6** Steroid biosynthesis indicating the site of the common inborn errors of steroid biosynthesis.

High cholesterol levels in FH are caused by deficient or defective function of the LDL receptors leading to increased levels of endogenous cholesterol synthesis. Four main classes of variants in the LDL receptor have been identified: (1) reduced or defective biosynthesis of the receptor; (2) reduced or defective transport of the receptor from the endoplasmic reticulum to the Golgi apparatus; (3) abnormal binding of LDL by the receptor; and (4) abnormal internalization of LDL by the receptor. Specific mutations are more prevalent in certain ethnic groups because of founder effects (46, 89).

The mainstay of management is dietary restriction of cholesterol intake and drug treatment with "statins" that reduce the endogenous synthesis of cholesterol by inhibiting the enzyme 3-hydroxy-3-methylglutaryl coenzyme A reductase. Cholesterol levels in affected families are variable, and lipid assays do not necessarily identify those with variants. There is, therefore, interest in the introduction of widespread genetic testing, although most variants are missense, which may pose problems of interpretation.

Lysosomal Storage Disorders

In addition to the IEMs in which an enzyme defect leads to deficiency of an essential metabolite and accumulation of intermediate metabolic precursors, there are a number of disorders in which deficiency of a lysosomal enzyme involved in the degradation of complex macromolecules leads to their accumulation. This accumulation occurs because macromolecules are normally in a constant state of flux, with a delicate balance between their rates of synthesis and breakdown. Children born with lysosomal storage diseases are usually normal initially but with the passage of time commence a downhill course of variable duration owing to the accumulation of one or more of a variety or type of macromolecules.

Mucopolysaccharidoses

Children with one of the mucopolysaccharidoses (MPSs) present with skeletal, vascular, or central nervous system findings along with coarsening of the facial features. These features are attributed to progressive accumulation of sulfated polysaccharides (GAGs) caused by defective degradation of the carbohydrate side-chain of acid mucopolysaccharide.

Six different MPSs are recognized, based on clinical and genetic differences. Each specific MPS type has a characteristic pattern of excretion in the urine of the glycosaminoglycans, dermatan, heparan, keratan, and chondroitin sulfate. Subsequent biochemical investigation has revealed the various types to be caused by deficiency of different individual enzymes. All but Hunter syndrome, which is XL, are AR disorders.

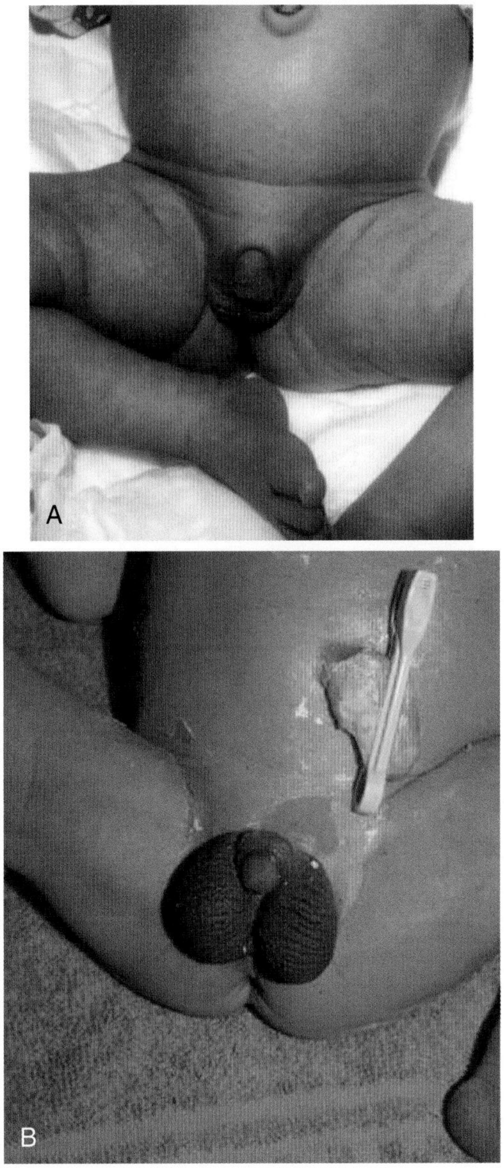

• **Fig. 18.7** (A) Virilized external genitalia in a female with congenital adrenal hyperplasia. (B) A male baby with hypospadias who clearly has testes in the scrotal sacs.

Hurler Syndrome (MPS I)

Hurler syndrome is the most severe MPS. Infants present in the first year with corneal clouding, a characteristic curvature of the lower spine and subsequent poor growth. They develop hearing loss, coarse facial features, an enlarged liver and spleen, joint stiffness, and vertebral changes in the second year. These features progress together with mental deterioration and eventually death by mid-adolescence from a combination of cardiac failure and respiratory infections.

The diagnosis of Hurler syndrome was initially made by demonstrating the presence of metachromatic granules in the cells (i.e., lysosomes distended by the storage material that is primarily dermatan sulfate). Increased urinary excretion of dermatan and heparan sulfate (GAGs) is commonly used as a screening test, but confirmation of the diagnosis involves demonstration of reduced activity of the lysosomal hydrolase, α-L-iduronidase, and direct gene (*IDUA*) analysis. Less severe allelic forms of Hurler syndrome caused by varying levels of residual α-L-iduronidase activity were previously classified separately as Scheie disease (MPS-I S) and Hurler/Scheie disease (MPS-I H/S).

Hunter Syndrome (MPS II)

Males with Hunter syndrome usually present between age 2 and 5 years with hearing loss, recurrent infections, diarrhea, and poor growth. Facial features are characteristic, with coarsening (Fig. 18.10), the liver and spleen are enlarged, and joint stiffness ensues. Spinal radiographs show abnormal vertebral shape. Progressive physical and mental deterioration occur, with death usually in adolescence.

The diagnosis is confirmed by the presence of excess amounts of dermatan and heparan sulfate in the urine, deficient or decreased activity of the enzyme iduronate sulfate sulfatase in serum or white blood cells and direct gene (*IDS*) analysis.

Sanfilippo Syndrome (MPS III)

Sanfilippo syndrome is the most common MPS. Affected individuals may present in childhood with mild coarsening of features, and skeletal changes, but these somatic features are subtle. Over time there is progressive intellectual loss with behavioral problems, seizures and death in early adult life. The diagnosis is confirmed by the presence of increased urinary heparan and chondroitin sulfate excretion, and deficiency of one of four enzymes involved in the degradation of heparan sulfate: N-sulphoglucosamine sulphohydrolase (MPS-IIIA, *SGSH* gene), α-N-acetylglucosaminidase (MPS-IIIB, *NAGLU* gene), heparan-α-glucosaminide N-acetyltransferase (MPS-IIIC, *HGSNAT* gene), and N-acetylglucosamine-6-sulfatase (MPS-IIID, *GNS* gene). Types A and B together account for 90% of cases, but the four subtypes cannot be distinguished clinically. The diagnostic pick-up through targeted gene testing or WES/WGS has significantly improved.

Morquio Syndrome (MPS IV)

Children with Morquio syndrome present at age 2 to 3 years with short stature, thoracic deformity and spinal curvature (kyphoscoliosis). Intelligence is normal, and survival is long-term, but there is a risk of spinal cord compression from progression of the skeletal

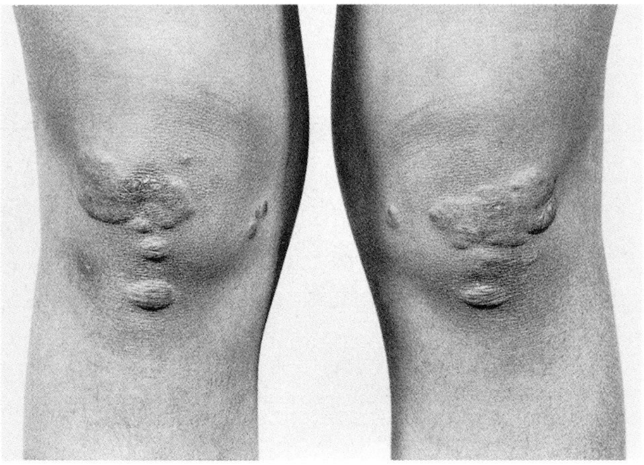

• **Fig. 18.8** Legs of a person homozygous for familial hypercholesterolemia, showing multiple xanthomata. (Courtesy Dr E. Wraith, Royal Manchester Children's Hospital, Manchester, UK.)

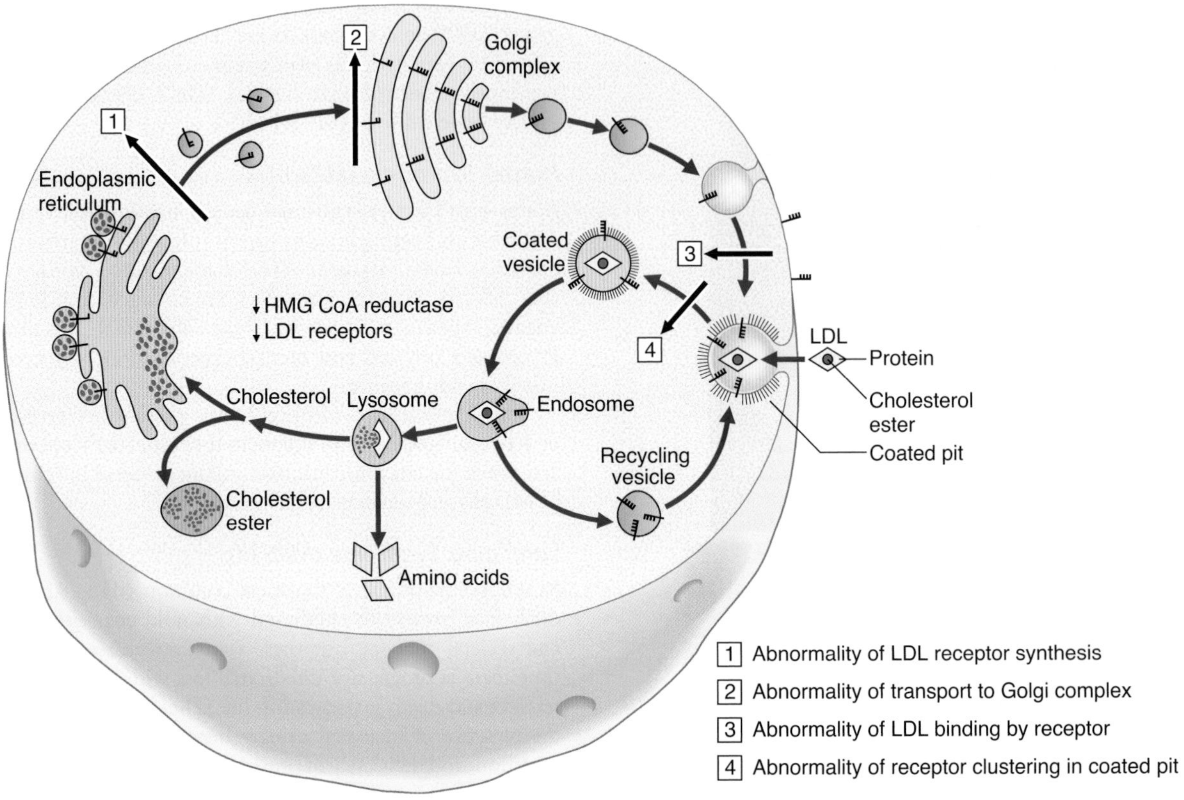

• **Fig. 18.9** Stages in cholesterol biosynthesis and in the metabolism of low-density lipoprotein receptors, indicating the types of mutation in familial hypercholesterolemia. *LDL*, Low-density lipoprotein. (Modified from Brown MS, Goldstein JL. A receptor-mediated pathway for cholesterol homeostasis. *Science*. 1986;232:34–47.)

involvement, as well as odontoid hypoplasia and cervical instability. The diagnosis is confirmed by the presence of keratan sulfate in the urine and deficiency of either galactosamine-6-sulphatase (MPS-IVA, *GALNS* gene) or β-galactosidase (MPS-IVB, *GLB1* gene).

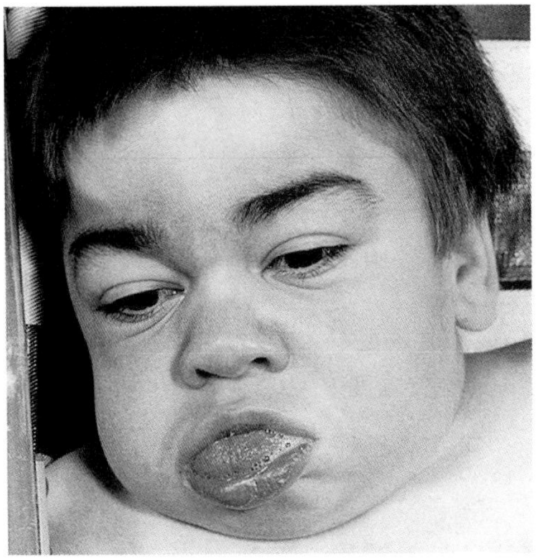

• **Fig. 18.10** Face of a male with the mucopolysaccharidosis, Hunter syndrome. (Courtesy Dr E. Wraith, Royal Manchester Children's Hospital, Manchester, UK.)

Maroteaux-Lamy Syndrome (MPS VI)

This MPS presents with Hurler-like features in early childhood, including coarse facial features, short stature with thoracic deformity, kyphosis, and restriction of joint mobility. In addition, corneal clouding and cardiac valve abnormalities develop; intelligence is normal. A milder form presents later, with survival into late adulthood, in contrast to the severe form in which survival is usually only to the third decade. The diagnosis is confirmed by the presence of increased urinary dermatan sulfate excretion and arylsulfatase B deficiency in white blood cells or fibroblasts, as well as direct gene (*ARSB*) analysis.

Sly Syndrome (MPS VII)

This is an extremely variable MPS. Presentation ranges from skeletal features that include mild kyphoscoliosis and hip dysplasia to coarse facial features, hepatosplenomegaly, corneal clouding, cardiac abnormalities, and mental retardation, with death in childhood or adolescence. Increased urinary glycosaminoglycans excretion and β-glucuronidase deficiency in serum, white blood cells, or fibroblasts confirm the diagnosis, together with direct gene (*GUSD*) analysis.

Treatment of the MPS Disorders. Treatment of these conditions by enzyme replacement (p. 215) is partially successful and inevitably very expensive. Similarly, bone marrow transplantation has had varying success biochemically and clinically, in relation to the skeletal and cerebral aspects of disease.

Sphingolipidoses

In the sphingolipidoses, there is an inability to degrade sphingolipid, resulting in the progressive deposition of lipid or glycolipid, primarily in the brain, liver, and spleen. Central nervous system involvement results in progressive mental deterioration, often with seizures, leading to death in childhood. There are at least 16 different types, with specific enzyme deficiencies—Tay-Sachs, Gaucher, metachromatic leukodystrophy, Fabry, and Niemann-Pick diseases are the most common.

Tay-Sachs Disease

This well-known sphingolipidosis has an incidence of approximately 1:3600 in Ashkenazi Jews (p. 151). Infants usually present by 6 months of age with poor feeding, lethargy, and floppiness. Developmental regression usually becomes apparent in late infancy, feeding becomes increasingly difficult, and the infant progressively deteriorates, with deafness, visual impairment and spasticity, which progresses to rigidity. Death usually occurs by 3 years from respiratory infection. Less severe juvenile, adult, and chronic forms are reported.

The diagnosis is supported clinically by the presence of a "cherry-red" spot in the centre of the macula of the fundus. Biochemical confirmation of Tay-Sachs disease is by demonstration of reduced hexosaminidase A levels in serum, white blood cells, or cultured fibroblasts, and direct gene (*HEXA*) analysis is available. Reduced hexosaminidase A activity is caused by deficiency of a subunit of the enzyme β-hexosaminidase that leads to accumulation of the sphingolipid GM_2 ganglioside. This deficiency leads to reduced activity of the isozyme hexosaminidase B, causing the other GM_2 gangliosidosis, Sandhoff disease, which presents with similar clinical features.

Gaucher Disease

This is the most common sphingolipidosis and, as with Tay-Sachs, is relatively more frequent among Ashkenazi Jews. There are two main types based on the age of onset.

Type I, with adult onset, is the more common form and presents with febrile episodes, pain in limbs, joints, or trunk and a tendency to pathological fractures. Clinical examination usually reveals hepatosplenomegaly, and investigations show mild anemia and radiological changes in the vertebrae and proximal femora. The central nervous system is spared.

In type II, infantile Gaucher disease, central nervous system involvement is a major feature and presents at age 3 to 6 months with failure to thrive and hepatosplenomegaly. By 6 months, developmental regression and neurological deterioration occur, with spasticity and seizures. Recurrent pulmonary infections cause death in the second year.

The diagnosis is confirmed by reduced activity of the enzyme glucosylceramide β-glucosidase in white blood cells or cultured fibroblasts, and direct gene (*GBA*) analysis.

Treatment in type 1 involves symptomatic analgesia, and sometimes splenectomy to prevent premature sequestration of red blood cells (hypersplenism). Initial attempts to treat adults by enzyme replacement therapy met with little success because of difficulty in obtaining sufficient quantities of enzyme and in targeting the appropriate sites. However, modification of β-glucosidase by the addition of mannose 6-phosphate, which targets the enzyme to macrophage lysosomes, has led to dramatic alleviation of symptoms and regression of organomegaly. The treatment is expensive, and regimens using lower doses and alternative methods to target the enzyme may be more rational.

Metachromatic Leukodystrophy

Metachromatic leukodystrophy (MLD) is also referred to as arylsulfatase A deficiency (ARSA); following AR inheritance, this condition is variable; although it tends to breed true within a family. Three basic forms are recognized: late-infantile (50%–60%), juvenile (20%–30%), and adult (15%–20%). The earlier the age of onset, the more progressive the illness.

The late-infantile form presents during the second year of life with weakness, hypotonia, unsteadiness and falls, toe walking, and slurred speech. Neurodevelopment regresses, leading to increased tone, seizures, and eventually decerebrate posturing and lack of awareness. Death ensues from 3 to 10 years after the onset. The juvenile form begins between 4 years of age and early puberty. The presentation is more insidious, but eventual cognitive and neurological decline ensues in a similar way (although more slowly). The adult form, starting from puberty onwards, and sometimes well into adulthood, may present with decline in performance, personality change, and progressive neurological problems including seizures. The disease course may be around 30 years.

The diagnosis of MLD is established by demonstration of ARSA enzyme deficiency, often in a child showing evidence of leukodystrophy on magnetic resonance imaging, elevated urinary excretion of sulfatides, and/or direct gene (*ARSA*) analysis.

Fabry Disease

Fabry disease is XL and caused by deficiency of α-galactosidase, encoded by the *GLA* gene, resulting in progressive lysosomal deposition of globotriaosylceramide in body cells and tissues. The severe form begins in childhood or adolescence with episodes of very unpleasant pain in the extremities. In due course, vascular cutaneous angiokeratomas develop, sweating abnormalities are common, and characteristic corneal and lenticular opacities occur. Hematuria and deteriorating renal function leading to end-stage renal disease may occur in men in their 20s to 40s. Fabry disease is a cause of hypertrophic cardiomyopathy (HCM) (p. 308) and early cerebrovascular disease. α-Galactosidase activity is a routine screening test in males with HCM where there is no evidence of male-male transmission, and if positive is followed up by *GLA* gene analysis. Some heterozygous females develop milder symptoms and have a later age of onset than their male counterparts.

Niemann-Pick Disease

Infants with Niemann-Pick disease type A present with failure to thrive and hepatomegaly, and a cherry-red spot may be found on their macula. Developmental regression progresses rapidly by the end of the first year, with death by 4 years of age. A characteristic finding is the presence of what are called foam cells in the bone marrow from sphingomyelin accumulation. Confirmation of the diagnosis is by demonstration of deficiency of the enzyme acid sphingomyelinase and/or sequencing of the *SMPD1* gene. A less severe form (type B) without neurological involvement is allelic. As with Tay-Sachs and Gaucher diseases, it is more common in Ashkenazi Jews from eastern Europe.

Niemann-Pick type C, also known as the Nova Scotian type, is early-onset like type A, and genetically distinct, because of variants in the *NPC1* gene.

Disorders in the Metabolism of Purines, Pyrimidines, and Nucleotides

Disorders of Purine Metabolism

Primary Idiopathic Gout

Gout is the classic disorder of abnormal purine metabolism. Joint pain, swelling, and tenderness are a result of the inflammatory response of the body to deposits of crystals of a salt of uric acid. In fact, only a minority of persons with gout have an IEM. The condition in most instances results from a combination of genetic and environmental factors; however, it is always important to consider disorders that can result in an increased turnover of purines (e.g., a malignancy such as leukemia) or reduced secretion of the metabolites (e.g., renal impairment) as a possible underlying precipitating cause.

Lesch-Nyhan Syndrome

This is a particularly disabling disorder of purine metabolism, follows XL inheritance, and is caused by the deficiency of the enzyme hypoxanthine guanine phosphoribosyltransferase, encoded by *HPRT1*, which results in increased levels of phosphoribosylpyrophosphate. The latter is normally a rate-limiting chemical in the synthesis of purines. Excess amounts lead to an increased rate of purine synthesis and accumulation of uric acid and some of its metabolic precursors. The main effect is neurological, with uncontrolled movements, spasticity, mental retardation, and compulsive self-mutilation. Although drugs such as allopurinol, which inhibit uric acid formation, can lower uric acid levels, none is highly satisfactory.

Adenosine Deaminase Deficiency

About half of all children with the AR form of severe combined immunodeficiency with impaired B- and T-cell function (p. 180) have deficiency of the enzyme adenosine deaminase (ADA). Presentation is in infancy with recurrent viral and bacterial infections which, if untreated, soon cause death from overwhelming infection. The diagnosis is confirmed by deficient red blood cell ADA activity, as well as other cell types, together with biallelic variants in the *ADA* gene. Bone marrow transplantation has been successful—even for the fetus *in utero*—and experimental gene therapy has been underway for approximately 20 years using various viral vectors.

Purine Nucleoside Phosphorylase Deficiency

A proportion of children susceptible to severe, recurrent and potentially fatal viral infections with isolated impaired T-cell function have been shown to have a deficiency of the enzyme purine nucleoside phosphorylase. Treatment with irradiated red blood cells may result in a temporary improvement in immune function.

Disorders of Pyrimidine and Nucleotide Metabolism

Within this group of disorders, those affecting pyrimidine metabolism and nucleotide metabolism are rarer. The pyrimidine group includes orotic aciduria, and the nucleotide group includes Aicardi-Goutières syndrome.

Orotic Aciduria

In orotic aciduria, following AR inheritance and attributed to variants in the *UMPS* gene, some degree of learning disability occurs in addition to megaloblastic anemia, with hypochromic, microcytic circulating erythrocytes that are unresponsive to vitamin B12 and folic acid. Substantial quantities of orotic acid are present in the urine. The problems usually respond to pyrimidine replacement therapy, and thus most cases have a good prognosis. Some cases have additional features, including immune deficiencies and congenital malformations.

Disorders of Porphyrin and Heme Metabolism

There are several different disorders of porphyrin metabolism that are from a deficiency of enzymes in the biosynthetic pathway of the iron-containing group in hemoglobin—heme (see Chapter 12) (Fig. 18.11). They follow AD inheritance, with the exception of AR congenital erythropoietic porphyria and an XL form of erythropoietic protoporphyria. This is because the enzymes are rate-limiting (p. 22), so that haploinsufficiency results in clinical disease.

The different types of porphyria are variably associated with neurological or visceral involvement and cutaneous photosensitivity from an accumulation of the different porphyrin precursors in those organs. The porphyrias are divided into two types depending on whether the excess production of porphyrins occurs predominantly in the liver or in the erythropoietic system.

Hepatic Porphyrias

Acute Intermittent Porphyria

Acute intermittent porphyria (AIP) is characterized by attacks of abdominal pain, weakness, vomiting, and mental disturbance in the form of confusion, emotional upset, or hallucinations. Even coma may occur, and women are more severely affected than men, with symptoms sometimes associated with the menstrual cycle. Attacks can also be precipitated by the administration of certain drugs, such as exogenous steroids, anticonvulsants, and barbiturates. It is caused by a partial deficiency of the enzyme uroporphyrinogen synthase (*aka* porphobilinogen deaminase) leading to increased excretion of the porphyrin precursors porphobilinogen and δ-aminolevulinic acid in urine. Diagnosis can be confirmed by direct gene (*HMBS*, aka *PBGD*) analysis.

Hereditary Coproporphyria

In hereditary coproporphyria, a related condition also inherited as an AD trait, there is partial deficiency of the enzyme coproporphyrinogen oxidase, encoded by the *CPOX* gene. The disorder is clinically indistinguishable from acute intermittent porphyria, although approximately one-third of affected persons also have photosensitivity of the skin.

Porphyria Variegata

People with this form of porphyria, particularly prevalent in South African Afrikaners (p. 67), have variable skin photosensitivity with neurological and visceral features that can also be triggered by drugs. Increased fecal excretion of the porphyrin precursors protoporphyrin and coproporphyrin can be demonstrated, and the disorder has been shown to be caused by deficiency of the enzyme protoporphyrinogen oxidase, encoded by the *PPOX* gene.

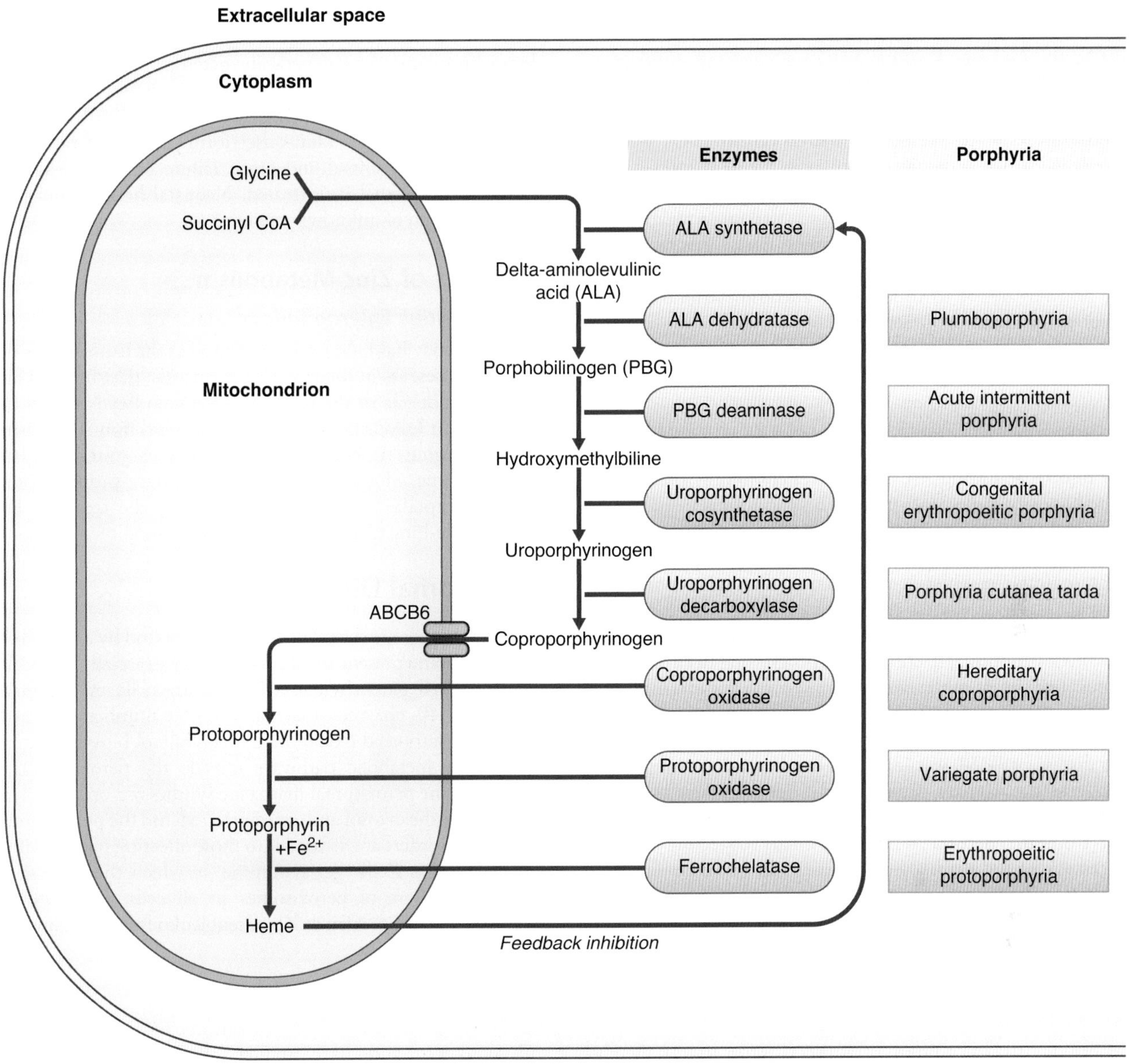

• **Fig. 18.11** The porhyrin-heme biosynthetic pathway, highlighting the enzymes involved in the various different forms of porphyria.

Erythropoietic Porphyrias

Congenital Erythropoietic Porphyria

The only member of this group following AR inheritance, congenital erythropoietic porphyria (CEP) manifests an extreme photosensitivity with blistering of the skin leading to extensive scarring, to the extent that most affected people are unable to go out in normal daylight. In addition, many have a hemolytic anemia requiring regular blood transfusion and frequently splenectomy. Affected individuals have red-brown discoloration of the teeth, which show red fluorescence under ultraviolet light. CEP is caused by deficiency of the enzyme uroporphyrinogen III synthase, encoded by the *UROS* gene.

Erythropoietic Protoporphyria

Erythropoietic protoporphyria is from a deficiency of the enzyme ferrochelatase, encoded by *EPP1*, which is responsible for the insertion of ferrous iron into the porphyrin precursor to form heme. Affected persons have photosensitivity and sometimes develop chronic liver disease. Successful treatment of the photosensitivity has been reported with β-carotene.

The XL form of this condition is caused by gain-of-function variants in the *ALAS2* gene (loss-of-function variants in this gene cause XL sideroblastic anemia).

Disorders in the Metabolism of Trace Elements and Metals

Within this group there are many rare entities, but we focus on the disorders involving copper, iron, and zinc.

Disorders of Copper Metabolism

There are two distinct IEMs involving copper metabolism: Menkes disease and Wilson disease.

Menkes Disease

Menkes disease is an XL recessive disorder in which affected males present in the first few months of life with feeding difficulties, vomiting, and poor weight gain. Subsequently, hypotonia, seizures, and progressive neurological deterioration ensue, with death from recurrent respiratory infection usually occurring by 3 years. A characteristic feature is the hair, which lacks pigment and is kinky and brittle. This was noted to resemble the wool of sheep suffering from copper deficiency. Serum copper and ceruloplasmin levels are very low. Cloning of the gene for Menkes disease was facilitated through an affected female with an X-autosome translocation (p. 74) and revealed it to code for an adenosine triphosphatase (ATPase) cation transport protein for copper (Cu^{++}-transporting ATPase, alpha polypeptide, encoded by *ATP7A*). Treatment regimens with different exogenous copper sources have had limited benefit to date.

Wilson Disease

Wilson disease, following AR inheritance, commonly presents in childhood or early adolescence with fits and abnormal neurological findings, including deteriorating coordination, involuntary movements, abnormal tone, dysarthria, dysphagia, and changes in behavior or frank psychiatric disturbance. Clinical examination may reveal "Kayser-Fleischer rings," which are golden brown or greenish collarettes at the corneal margins. Investigation can reveal the presence of abnormal liver function, progressing to cirrhosis.

High copper levels in the liver, decreased serum concentrations of the copper transport protein ceruloplasmin and abnormal copper loading test results are suggestive of the diagnosis. The gene for Wilson disease, *ATP7B*, was identified on the basis of anticipated homology to the Menkes gene, and the gene product has been shown to be an ATPase cation transport protein involved in copper transfer from the hepatocytes to the biliary collecting system. Improvement of the neurological features can be achieved using chelating agents such as D-penicillamine.

Disorders of Iron Metabolism

Hemochromatosis

Hemochromatosis is a common late-onset disorder of iron metabolism that results in accumulation of iron, with symptoms emerging between 40 and 60 years. The liver is the most commonly damaged tissue, with iron deposition leading to cirrhosis and liver failure. Patients are at increased risk of hepatocellular carcinoma. Other organs that may be affected include the pancreas, heart, pituitary gland, skin, and joints. The iron overload is easily treated by venesection, and this is very effective at reducing morbidity and mortality. The ratio of affected males to females is 5:1, and the disease is underdiagnosed in the general population but overdiagnosed in patients with secondary iron overload.

The *HFE* gene is close to the HLA region on chromosome 6p21. Between 85% and 100% (depending on population) of affected individuals are homozygous for the *C282Y* variant, and the carrier frequency in Northern Europe is approximately 1 in 10. The variant *H63D* is more common in the general population, and homozygosity is associated with only a modest (approximately four-fold) increase in risk of hemochromatosis. Compound heterozygosity for *C282Y* and *H63D* is associated with reduced penetrance—only 1% of compound heterozygotes are thought likely to develop symptoms. Up to 50% of C282Y homozygotes develop iron overload, and up to a third may develop symptoms related to iron overload. End organ damage—cirrhosis, diabetes, cardiomyopathy—is much more common in males compared with females. Hemochromatosis is a genetically heterogeneous disorder, with mutations also reported in the transferrin receptor 2 (*TFR2*) gene and the *SLC40A1* gene, which encodes ferroportin. In addition to the common recessive adult-onset form, there is a rare juvenile form with iron overload and organ failure before the age of 30 years, which is lethal if untreated. Neonatal hemochromatosis is severe and often of unknown etiology.

Disorders of Zinc Metabolism

Acrodermatitis Enteropathica

Zinc deficiency has long been recognized as the cause of this disorder which presents in infancy with dermatitis, diarrhea and failure to thrive. Alopecia of the scalp, eyebrows, and eyelashes is usual, with the skin lesions being bullous. The condition is predisposed by homozygous or compound heterozygous mutations in the *SLC39A4* gene, which encodes a transmembrane protein that facilitates zinc uptake. Fortunately it is one of the treatable IEMs, requiring life-long dietary zinc supplementation.

Peroxisomal Disorders

The peroxisomes are subcellular organelles bound by a single bilayer lipid membrane present in all cells; they are especially abundant in liver and renal parenchymal cells. The organelle matrix contains more than 40 enzymes that carry out a number of reactions involved in fatty-acid oxidation and cholesterol biosynthesis interacting with metabolic pathways outside the peroxisomes. The enzymes of the peroxisomal matrix are synthesized on the polyribosomes, enter the cytosol and are transferred into the peroxisomes.

These disorders are divided into those affecting peroxisome biogenesis, such as Zellweger syndrome, in which there are severely reduced numbers of peroxisomes in all cells, those involving defects in oxidation, such as XL adrenoleukodystrophy, and chondrodysplasia punctata.

Zellweger Syndrome

Newborn infants with Zellweger syndrome present with hypotonia and weakness and have mildly dysmorphic facial features (Fig. 18.12) consisting of a prominent forehead and a large anterior fontanelle. They may also have cataracts and an enlarged liver. They generally go on to have fits with developmental regression and usually die by 1 year of age. Investigations can reveal renal cysts and abnormal calcification in the cartilaginous growing ends of the long bones (Fig. 18.13). There is a range of severity of this disorder, with different clinical diagnoses being given to the less severe types. The diagnosis can be confirmed by raised levels of plasma long-chain fatty acids and gene analysis. It is genetically heterogeneous, because of any one of several *PEX* genes crucial to peroxisome biogenesis.

It is unusual for IEMs to give rise to a dysmorphic syndrome, but another is Smith-Lemli-Opitz syndrome (p. 111), an inborn error of cholesterol biosynthesis from a mutation in the sterol delta-7-reductase (*DHCR7*) gene, as well as some of the MPS group (p. 278).

X-Linked Adrenoleukodystrophy

Males with the X-linked disorder adrenoleukodystrophy (ALD) classically present in late childhood with deteriorating school performance, although presentation may occur at any age, and carrier

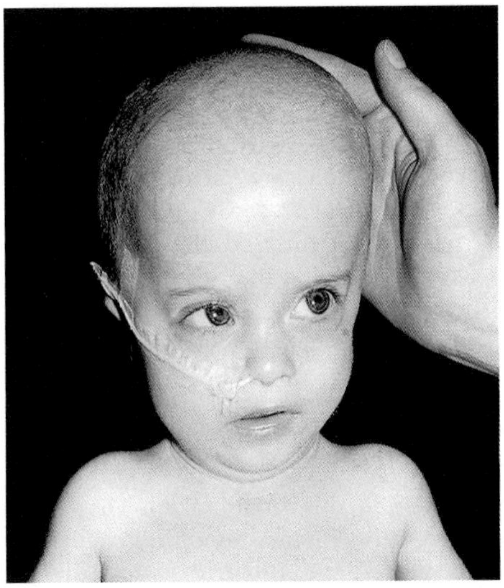

• **Fig. 18.12** Face of an infant with Zellweger syndrome showing a prominent forehead.

females may sometimes develop symptoms; occasionally, there are no symptoms. Some males present in adult life with less severe neurological features and adrenal insufficiency, so-called adrenomyeloneuropathy. ALD has been shown to be associated with a deficiency of the enzyme very long-chain fatty acid CoA synthase, but is secondary to deficiency of a peroxisomal membrane protein, owing to mutation in the *ABCD1* gene.

Treatment of ALD with a diet that uses an oil with low levels of very long-chain fatty acids—"Lorenzo"s oil'—has proved disappointing.

Rhizomelic Chondrodysplasia Punctata

Chondrodysplasia punctata describes the particular radiological feature of bony stippling, or punctate calcifications, usually around the joints, in the early newborn period, and there are a variety of causes. Rhizomelic chondrodysplasia punctata type 1 (RCDP1), however, is a specific entity and a disorder of peroxisome biogenesis. The proximal humerus and sometimes femur are relatively short (rhizomelia), and coronal clefts occur in the vertebral bodies. Cataracts are usually present at birth or appear soon afterwards. Growth deficiency ensues, intellectual disability is severe, and seizures usually develop. Most children succumb by 10 years, some much earlier. A milder form does occur, often consisting of congenital cataracts, minimal skeletal problems, and much less severe intellectual disability. Biochemically, plasmalogens are deficient in red blood cells, phytanic acid is elevated in plasma, and very long-chain fatty acids are normal. The sole mutated gene associated with RCDP1 is *PEX7*, encoding the receptor for a subset of peroxisomal matrix enzymes.

• **Fig. 18.13** Radiograph of the knee of a newborn infant with Zellweger syndrome showing abnormal punctate calcification of the distal femoral epiphyses.

Disorders of Fatty Acid and Ketone Body Metabolism

This group of disorders includes the various defects in carnitine transport and carnitine cycle. The carnitine cycle is a biochemical pathway required for the transport of long-chain fatty acids into the mitochondrial matrix, and those less than 10 carbons in length are then activated to form acyl-CoA esters. The carnitine cycle is one part of the pathway of mitochondrial β-oxidation that plays a major role in energy production, especially during periods of fasting. Carnitine deficiency is a secondary feature of the β-oxidation disorders, with the exception of the carnitine transport defect where it is primary, and this rare condition responds dramatically to carnitine replacement. The more common fatty-acid oxidation disorders are outlined—the conditions caused by faulty "chain acyl CoA dehydrogenase" enzymes—which can be broadly grouped under disorders of mitochondrial function.

Disorders of Mitochondrial Fatty Acid Oxidation

Medium-Chain Acyl-CoA Dehydrogenase Deficiency

Medium-chain acyl-CoA dehydrogenase (MCAD) deficiency is the most common of this group of disorders, presenting most frequently as episodic hypoketotic hypoglycemia provoked by fasting. The metabolic defect means that adipose cannot be broken down fast enough to meet the body's needs, especially in stressful episodes when energy demands are higher than normal, such as intercurrent illness—when calorie intake is often reduced. Hepatomegaly and liver dysfunction may be present in an acute episode. The onset is often in the first 2 years of life and, tragically, is occasionally fatal, resembling sudden infant death syndrome. Management rests on maintaining adequate caloric intake and avoiding fasting, which can be challenging in young children when ill. An AR disorder resulting from variants in the *ACADM* gene, 90% of alleles resulting from a single point mutation, and neonatal population screening is now routine in many countries.

Long-Chain and Short-Chain Acyl-CoA and Long-Chain 3-Hydroxyacyl-CoA Dehydrogenase Deficiencies

These rare AR conditions present early in life with a variable combination of skeletal features and cardiomyopathy, hepatocellular dysfunction with hepatomegaly, and encephalopathy. Treatment revolves around nutritional maintenance and avoidance of fasting but is not very rewarding in short-chain acyl-CoA deficiencies.

Multiple Acyl CoA Dehydrogenase Deficiency, or Glutaric Aciduria II

Type II glutaric aciduria is variable, with two severe forms having neonatal onset, one of these including urogenital anomalies. In both of these severe types, hypotonia, hepatomegaly, metabolic acidosis, and hypoketotic hypoglycemia occur. The late-onset form may present in early childhood, rather than the neonatal period, with failure to thrive, metabolic acidosis, hypoglycemia, and encephalopathy. Treatment of the severe forms is supportive only, but in the milder form riboflavin, carnitine, and diets low in protein and fat have been more successful.

Disorders of Energy Metabolism

This broad group of conditions includes the various disorders affecting the pyruvate dehydrogenase complex, which includes an XL form, as well as the vast and important disorders of the mitochondrial respiratory chain.

Mitochondrial Respiratory Chain Disorders

Mitochondrial disease was first identified in 1962 in a patient whose mitochondria showed structural abnormalities and loss of coupling between oxidation and phosphorylation, although it was not until 20 years later that the relevance of mutated mitochondrial DNA (mtDNA) to human disease began to be appreciated. The small, circular, double-stranded mtDNA (see Fig. 2.7, p. 15) contains genes coding for ribosomal RNA (rRNA) production and various transfer RNAs (tRNA) required for mitochondrial protein biosynthesis, as well as some of the proteins involved in electron transport. There are 5523 codons and a total of 37 gene products. Guanine and cytosine nucleotides are asymmetrically distributed between the two mtDNA strands—the guanine-rich strand being called the heavy (H) strand, and the cytosine-rich the light (L) strand. Replication and transcription is controlled by a 1122−base pair (bp) sequence of mtDNA known as the displacement loop (D-loop). Oxidative phosphorylation (OXPHOS) is the biochemical process responsible for generating much of the ATP required for cellular energy. The process is mediated by five intramitochondrial enzyme **complexes**, referred to as complexes I to V, and the mtDNA encodes 13 OXPHOS subunits, 22 tRNAs, and two rRNAs.

The "complexes" are aptly named (Fig. 18.14)! Analysis of complex I, for example, has revealed approximately 45 different subunits thus far—38 nuclear-encoded and seven mitochondrial-encoded subunits—variants in any of which can affect function. Most affected individuals have a phenotype of **Leber hereditary optic neuropathy** (LHON) or **Leigh syndrome**. Complex V comprises 12 or 13 subunits, of which two, ATPase 6 and 8, are encoded by mtDNA. Maximal activity of complex V appears to require tight linking with cardiolipin (see Barth syndrome, p. 276), encoded by nuclear DNA.

Because most mitochondrial proteins, including subunits involved in electron transport, are encoded by nuclear genes, these most often follow AR inheritance, but AD and XL forms also occur. As with other metabolic AR diseases, disorders resulting from variants in these genes tend to breed true. However, the disorders resulting from variants in mtDNA are extremely variable owing to the phenomenon of heteroplasmy (see Fig. 6.30, p. 82). The clinical features are mainly a combination of neurological signs (encephalopathy, dementia, ataxia, dystonia, neuropathy, and seizures) and myopathic signs (hypotonia, weakness, and cardiomyopathy with conduction defects). Other symptoms and signs may include deafness, diabetes mellitus and retinal pigmentation, and acidosis may occur. The clinical manifestations are so variable that a mitochondrial cytopathy should be considered as a possibility at any age when the presenting illness has a neurological or myopathic component. Several distinct clinical entities have been determined and, although some of them overlap considerably, there is a degree of genotype-phenotype correlation.

Myoclonic Epilepsy and Ragged Red Fiber Disease

Myoclonic epilepsy and ragged red fiber (MERRF) disease was first described in 1973 and so called because Gomori's trichrome staining of muscle revealed abnormal deposits of mitochondria as "ragged red." In 1988 it was determined that the condition was maternally inherited. The classic picture is of progressive myoclonic epilepsy, myopathy, and slowly progressive dementia. Optic atrophy is frequently present, and the electroencephalogram is characteristically abnormal. Postmortem brain examination reveals widespread neurodegeneration. In 1990 it was reported that MERRF results from a single-bp variant in the gene for lysine tRNA.

Mitochondrial Encephalomyopathy, Lactic Acidosis, and Stroke-Like Episodes

First delineated in 1984, this condition, known as MELAS, is now recognized as one of the most common mitochondrial disorders. Short stature may be a feature, but it is stroke-like episodes that mark out this particular disorder, although these episodes do not necessarily occur in all affected family members. When they do occur, they may manifest as vomiting, headache, or visual disturbance, and sometimes lead to transient hemiplegia, or hemianopia. A common presenting feature is type 2 diabetes mellitus, plus sensorineural hearing loss (described as maternally inherited diabetes and deafness [MIDD]). These latter clinical features are associated with the most common variant, an A > G substitution at nucleotide m.3243, which affects tRNA leucine^{UUR}. This is found in approximately 80% of patients, followed by a T > C transition at nucleotide m.3271, also affecting tRNA leucine^{UUR}.

Neurodegeneration, Ataxia, and Retinitis Pigmentosa

The early presenting feature is night blindness, which may be followed years later by neurological symptoms. Dementia may occur in older patients, but seizures can present at almost any age, and younger patients show developmental delay. The majority of cases are caused by a single-bp variant—the T > G substitution at nucleotide m.8993, which occurs in the coding region of subunit 6 of ATPase. This change is often referred to as the NARP (neurodegeneration, ataxia, and retinitis pigmentosa) mutation.

Leigh Disease

This condition is characterized by its neuropathology, consisting of typical spongiform lesions of the basal ganglia, thalamus, substantia nigra, and tegmental brainstem. In its severe form, death occurs in infancy or early childhood, and it was in such a patient that the m.8993 T > G NARP mutation was first identified. In effect, therefore, one form of Leigh disease is simply a severe form of NARP, and higher proportions of mutant mtDNA have been reported in these cases. However, variability is again sometimes marked, which between first-degree relatives might range from death in early childhood to slow recovery from a general anesthetic.

The same or very similar pathology, and a similar clinical course, has now been described in patients with a range of different molecular defects. Cytochrome *c* deficiency was reported in patients shown to have variants in *SURF1*, a nuclear gene encoding a putative maintenance factor for cytochrome *c* that is vital for complex IV integrity. A dozen or so genes encoding various crucial subunits of cytochrome *c* have been identified, the number continues to grow, and they follow AR inheritance. Leigh disease is therefore genetically heterogeneous, and also includes an XL form (*NDUFA1* gene) linked to complex 1 deficiency.

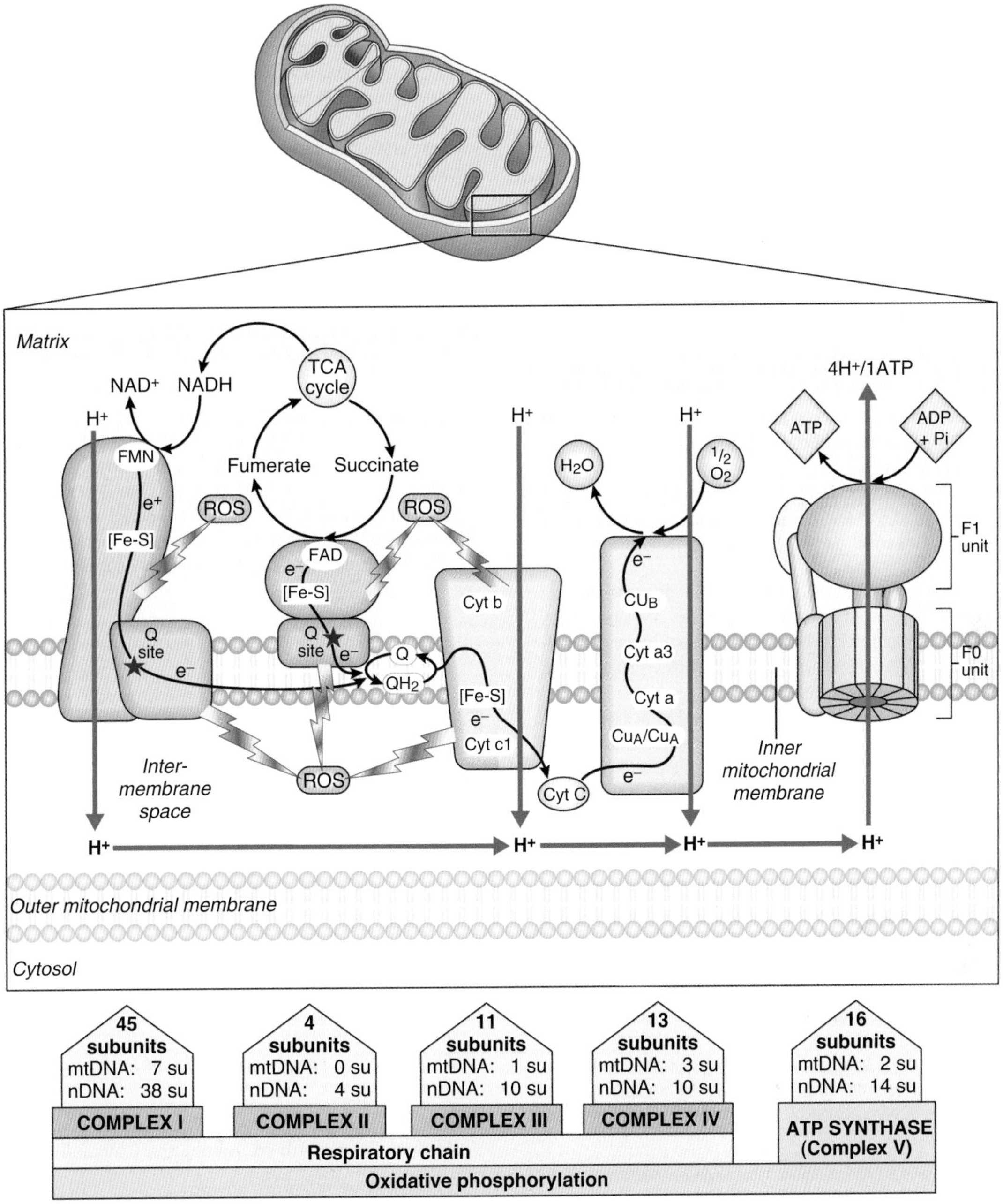

• **Fig. 18.14** Representation of the mitochondrial respiratory chain complexes and the oxidative phosphorylation system. The four complexes of the respiratory chain and the adenosine triphosphate synthase (complex V) are schematized, and the electron/proton pathways along these complexes are indicated. *ADP*, adenosine diphosphate; *ATP*, adenosine triphosphate; *FAD*, flavin adenine dinucleotide; *FMN*, flavin mononucleotide; *ROS*, reactive oxygen species; *TCA*, tricarboxylic (citric) acid cycle.

Leber Hereditary Optic Neuropathy

LHON was the first human disease to be shown to result from a mtDNA single-bp variant; some 18 different pathogenic variants have now been described. The most common occurs at nucleotide m.11,778 (*MTND4*), accounting for up to 70% of cases in Europe and more than 90% of cases in Japan. It presents with acute, or subacute, loss of central visual acuity without pain, which typically occurs between 12 and 30 years of age. Males in affected pedigrees are much more likely to develop visual loss than females. In some LHON pedigrees, additional neurological problems occur.

Prenatal Diagnosis of Inborn Errors of Metabolism

For the majority of IEMs in which an abnormal or deficient gene product can be identified, prenatal diagnosis is possible. Biochemical analysis of cultured amniocytes obtained at midtrimester amniocentesis is possible but has largely given way to earlier testing using direct or cultured chorionic villi (CV), which allows a diagnosis to be made by 12 to 14 weeks' gestation (p. 324). For most conditions direct DNA analysis has superseded biochemical analysis. This avoids the inherent delay of culturing CV tissue and is of particular value for inborn errors for which the biochemical basis is not clearly identified, or where the enzyme is not expressed in amniocytes or CV.

Prenatal diagnosis of mitochondrial disorders from mtDNA mutations presents particular difficulties because of the problem of heteroplasmy and the inability to predict the outcome for any result obtained, whether positive or negative for the mutation in question. This presents challenging counseling issues and also raises consideration of other reproductive options, such as ovum donation. The possibility of donated mitochondria using nuclear transfer technology is also becoming a reality (see Chapter 20).

ELEMENTS

1. Metabolic processes in all species occur in steps, each controlled by a particular enzyme which is the product of a specific gene, leading to the one gene–one enzyme concept.
2. A block in a metabolic pathway results in the accumulation of metabolic intermediates and/or a deficiency of the end-product of the particular metabolic pathway concerned, giving rise to an "inborn error of metabolism."
3. The majority of the inborn errors of metabolism are inherited as autosomal recessive or X-linked recessive traits. A few are inherited as autosomal dominant disorders involving rate-limiting enzymes, cell-surface receptors, or multimeric enzymes through haploinsufficiency, or dominant negative pathogenic variants.
4. A wide range of inborn errors of metabolism are screened for in the newborn period and treated successfully by dietary restriction or supplementation.
5. Whole-exome or whole-genome sequencing is increasingly being employed as one of the early investigations for infants and children presenting with suspected metabolic conditions, especially as early diagnosis may help prevent long-term sequelae where a treatment exists.
6. Prenatal diagnosis of many inborn errors of metabolism is increasingly undertaken by direct analysis of the pathogenic variants for which the fetus is at risk, rather than conventional biochemical methods.
7. Mitochondrial diseases present in similar ways to inborn errors of metabolism and usually follow matrilinear (mitochondrial) or autosomal recessive inheritance, although some follow autosomal dominant, and rarely X-linked recessive, inheritance.
8. Because of the problem of heteroplasmy and vary variable degrees of severity, prenatal diagnosis for disease caused by variants in the mitochondrial genome is complicated by great difficulty in predicting the phenotype.

CLINICAL SCENARIO 1

The parents of a 2½-year-old boy, their 4th child, are worried about him. When he has an upper respiratory infection with pyrexia he has episodes of significant lethargy, drowsiness, and vomiting he can be much more ill compared with other children at his nursery when they have colds, although he does not seem to suffer more infectious episodes than other children. On one occasion 6 months ago, they thought he might have had a seizure, but it was transient. In general his growth and development appear entirely satisfactory. Examination in clinic confirms that he is not dysmorphic, and nothing abnormal is found.

The parents lost their first child to a cot death at 4 months of age after a short prodromal illness, and went on to have two more children who are healthy and doing well at school.

1. What does the history suggest?
2. What investigations would you perform?

CLINICAL SCENARIO 2

A 9-year-old girl gives a history of poor exercise tolerance and increasing muscle weakness, and her performance at school has declined. Her mother, aged 44, has increasing fatigue, although she had a small stroke episode at the age of 40. She has also suffered a significant decline in her hearing over a period of 5 to 10 years. The 9-year-old's maternal grandmother had strokes in her 50s and developed dementia by the age of 60, dying aged 63. The family history is otherwise unremarkable.

What does the clinical and family history suggest?

Further Reading

Applegarth DA, Toone JR, Lowry RB. Incidence of inborn errors of metabolism in British Columbia, 1969–1996. *Pediatrics.* 2000;105:e10.

A large population study of inborn errors of metabolism, providing good epidemiological data.

Garrod AE. Inborn errors of metabolism. *Lancet.* 1908; 2:1-7, 73-79, 142-148, 214-220.

Reports of the first inborn errors of metabolism.

Nyhan WL, Ozand PT. *Atlas of Metabolic Diseases.* London: Chapman & Hall; 1998.

A detailed text but very readable and full of excellent illustrations and clinical images.

Rimoin DL, Connor JM, Pyeritz RE, Korf BR. *Principles and Practice of Medical Genetics.* 4th ed. Edinburgh: Churchill Livingstone; 2001.

The section on metabolic disorders includes 13 chapters covering in succinct detail the various groups of metabolic disorders.

Scriver CR, Beaudet AL, Sly WS, Valle D. *The Metabolic and Molecular Bases of Inherited Disease.* 8th ed. New York, NY: McGraw-Hill; 2001.

A huge multiauthor three-volume comprehensive detailed text on inborn errors of metabolism. This has now become: The Online Metabolic and Molecular Bases of Inherited Disease. David Valle (Editor-in-Chief), et al. https://ommbid.mhmedical.com/book.aspx?bookID = 2709.

19

Mainstream Monogenic Disorders

In the history of medicine, there are few instances in which a disease has been more accurately, more graphically or more briefly described.

Sir William Osler, in reference to 'On Chorea' (1872) by George Huntington

More than 10,000 single-gene, or monogenic, traits and disorders are known. Most are individually rare, but together they affect between 1% and 2% of the general population at any one time. The diagnosis, investigation, and family management of these disorders present the major workload challenge in clinical genetics. Many uncommon or rare monogenic disorders have been covered in other chapters, (e.g., Chapters 6, 9, 12, 13, 14, 16, and 18), but here we attempt an overview of those conditions that are traditionally better known to physicians in mainstream medicine. For many of these, as with rare disorders, there have been significant genetic and clinical advances in recent times.

Neurological Disorders

Adult-onset inherited neurological disorders have lent themselves to genetic research by virtue of the fact that large affected families, with normal biological fitness, are often encountered, thus greatly facilitating successful linkage analysis and subsequent gene identification—many of these disorders were among the first to yield their molecular genetic secrets.

Huntington Disease

Huntington disease (HD) derives its eponymous title from Dr George Huntington, who described multiple affected individuals in a large North American kindred in 1872. His paper, published in the Philadelphia journal *The Medical and Surgical Reporter*, gave a graphic description of the progressive neurological disability that continues to evoke apprehension and fear. The natural history is characterized by slowly progressive selective cell death in the CNS, and only recently is there a significant prospect of amelioration through antisense oligonucleotide trials (Chapter 15, p. 222). The prevalence in most parts of the world is approximately 1:10,000, although it is higher in some areas, such as Tasmania and the Lake Maracaibo region of Venezuela. The onset is mostly between 30 and 60 years, but it can start at virtually any age, including a rare juvenile form with different clinical features. The variable age of onset is explained, at least in part, by the underlying molecular defect.

Clinical Features

The disease is characterized by a slowly progressive movement disorder—chorea—and insidious impairment of intellectual function with psychiatric disturbance and eventual dementia (Fig. 19.1). The mean duration of the illness is between 15 and 25 years. Chorea movements are involuntary, consisting of facial grimacing, twitching of the face and limbs, folding of the arms, crossing of the legs, and progressively unsteady gait and unclear speech.

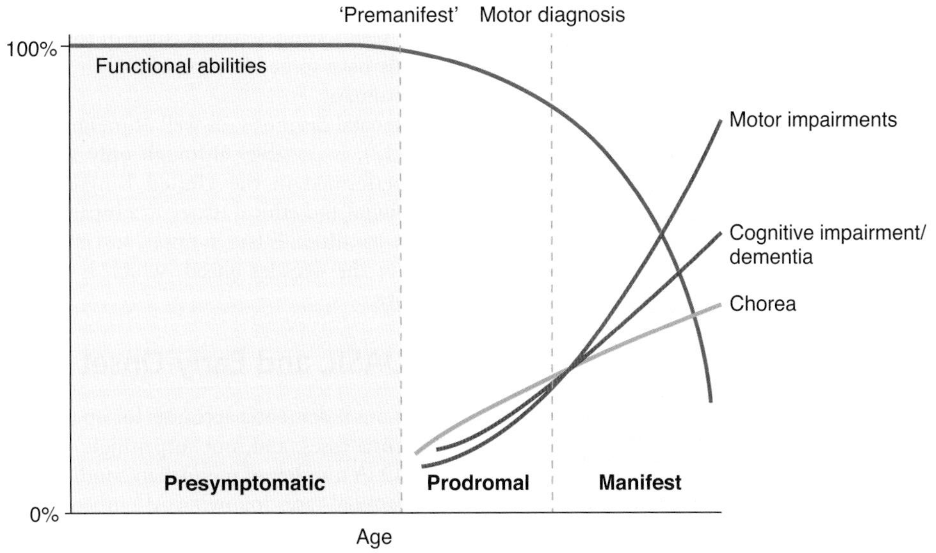

• **Figure 19.1** The natural history of Huntington disease. Clinical diagnosis is usually made on the basis of the movement disorder (i.e., chorea). However, other neurological problems are also typically part of the prodromal phase.

Intellectual changes in the early stages of HD include memory impairment and poor concentration span. Anxiety and panic attacks, mood changes and depression, aggressive behavior, paranoia, irrationality, increased libido, and alcohol abuse can also occur. There is a gradual deterioration in intellectual function, leading eventually to total incapacitation and dementia.

Up to 5% of HD cases present before the age of 20 years, when the term **juvenile HD** is used, and instead of chorea there is rigidity, with slowing of voluntary movement and clumsiness. A decline in school performance heralds the onset of a severe progressive dementia, often in association with epileptic seizures. The average duration of the illness is 10 to 15 years.

Genetics

HD follows autosomal dominant (AD) inheritance, has a variable age of onset, has almost full penetrance, and demonstrates anticipation (p. 76), sometimes markedly so through *paternal* transmission, hence sometimes giving rise to juvenile HD. The new mutation rate is very low.

HD was one of the first disorders to be mapped by linkage analysis, greatly assisted by studying the huge Venezuelan pedigree, and the nature of the mutation was discovered in 1993. This is a highly polymorphic CAG (polyglutamine) trinucleotide repeat sequence located in the 5′ region of the *huntingtin* gene (*HTT*; also known as *IT15*). The messenger RNA (mRNA) codes for a protein of approximately 350 kDa, known as HTT, which is expressed in many different cells throughout the CNS, as well as in other tissues. Four categories of CAG repeat length are recognized according to their clinical implications (Table 19.1).

Normal alleles contain 26 or fewer CAG repeats, are not associated with disease manifestations and are stable in meiosis. Allele sizes of 27 to 35 CAG repeats do not cause disease but occasionally show meiotic instability with a potential to increase or decrease in size, and are therefore **mutable**, constituting the reservoir from which larger, pathogenic alleles arise. When an apparently new mutation case of HD occurs, it usually transpires that the father carries a mutable allele, and there is evidence that the expansion occurs on the background of a particular haplotype DNA pattern, suggesting that certain haplotypes are more mutable than others.

Reduced penetrance alleles consist of 36 to 39 CAG repeats. These are associated with either late-onset disease or sometimes complete absence of disease expression, that is, non-penetrance.

Disease alleles contain 40 or more CAG repeats. These are invariably associated with disease, although sometimes late in onset. Statistically, there is a direct relationship between length of CAG repeat and disease expression, with the average age of onset for allele sizes of 40, 45, and 50 repeats being 57, 37, and 26 years, respectively. Most affected adults have repeat sizes of between 36 and 50, whereas juvenile cases often have an expansion greater than 55 repeats.

TABLE 19.1 Comparison of genetic aspects of Huntington disease and myotonic dystrophy

	Huntington Disease	Myotonic Dystrophy
Inheritance	Autosomal dominant	Autosomal dominant
Chromosome locus	4p16.3	19q13.3
Trinucleotide repeat	CAG in 5′ translated region	CTG in 3′ untranslated region
Repeat sizes	Normal ≤26	Normal <37
	Mutable 27–35	
	Reduced penetrance	Full mutation
	36–39	50–2000 +
	Fully penetrant ≥40	
Protein product	Huntingtin	Dystrophia myotonica protein kinase
Early-onset form	Juvenile	Congenital
	Usually paternally transmitted	Usually maternally transmitted

Parent of Origin Effect. The risk to offspring is 50% regardless of whether the affected parent is male or female, according to AD inheritance. However, for reasons that are not clear, meiotic instability is greater in spermatogenesis than in oogenesis. This is reflected in anticipation, occurring mainly when the mutant allele is transmitted by a male. Juveniles with the rigid form of HD have almost always inherited the mutant allele from their more mildly affected father.

Explanations for this include the possibility that expansion is caused by **slippage** of DNA polymerase (p. 51), simply reflecting the number of mitoses undergone during gametogenesis (p. 320). An alternative possibility is based on the observation that *HTT* is expressed in oocytes, so there could be selection against oocytes with large expansions as a consequence of preferential apoptosis.

Predictive and Prenatal Testing. HD has provided the paradigm for predictive presymptomatic testing in inherited disease, which is part of routine clinical genetic practice, but there is universal agreement that this should be offered only as part of a careful counseling package. Experience indicates that more women than men opt for this, and the psychological disturbance in those given positive results is low. Some 60% of candidates test negative (i.e., they receive good news), although the reasons for the departure from the expected 50% is unclear. It could be that more of the "worried well" seek testing, whereas some of those destined to develop HD already have some blunting of their insight before being obviously symptomatic.

Prenatal diagnosis, as well as preimplantation genetic diagnosis (p. 332), is possible, although only approximately 25 such tests are performed in the United Kingdom annually. Considerable emotional and ethical issues accompany termination of pregnancy —the condition is late in onset, and effective therapy may be available in the decades ahead, which is an area of intense research activity.

CADASIL and Early-Onset Dementia

Early-onset dementia accounts for up to 5% of the total number of dementia cases, and, not surprisingly, the causes are not confined to HD. A number of mendelian conditions are well Characterized, and familial cases following AD inheritance are much more likely in the early-onset group, although approximately 20% of late-onset dementia and Alzheimer disease is recognized to demonstrate clustering in families. It is important to consider this in context— the majority of common, late-onset dementia does not follow mendelian inheritance and is the result of the accumulation of various risk factors, both known and unknown, genetic as well as environmental (see Chapter 10).

CADASIL

CADASIL is easier to say and remember than "cerebral autosomal dominant arteriopathy with subcortical infarcts and leucoencephalopathy," and is the most common inherited cause of stroke and vascular dementia. It is essentially a microangiopathy affecting mainly the brain, due to pathogenic variants in *NOTCH3*, a membrane-bound receptor of the Notch signaling pathway (p. 109). The condition is characterized by a history of migraine accompanied by aura in approximately 30% to 40% of individuals, occurring between 30 to 60 years of age. This is accompanied by the premature onset of cerebrovascular disease, mood disturbance, apathy, depression, and cognitive disturbance progressing to dementia, all worsened by the occurrence of strokes. The profile of the main clinical features with age is shown in Fig. 19.2. Brain magnetic resonance imaging (MRI) scanning highlights diffuse white matter lesions and subcortical infarcts, and it is usually the combination of these findings with a migraine history that suggests the diagnosis. Transient ischemic attacks may occur over a wide age range (20–70 years).

Most *NOTCH3* gene variants are located in exon 4, followed by exons 3, 5, 6, and 11, and mutations are found in more than 90% of cases. Geographic variations have been described, showing exon 3 to be the second most common variant site in the French, British, and German populations, whereas mutations in exon 11 are more frequently seen in the Dutch. For individuals strongly suspected to have CADASIL, but who test negative on *NOTCH3* sequencing, a skin biopsy may show electron-dense granules in the media of arterioles on electron microscopy, which is pathognomonic.

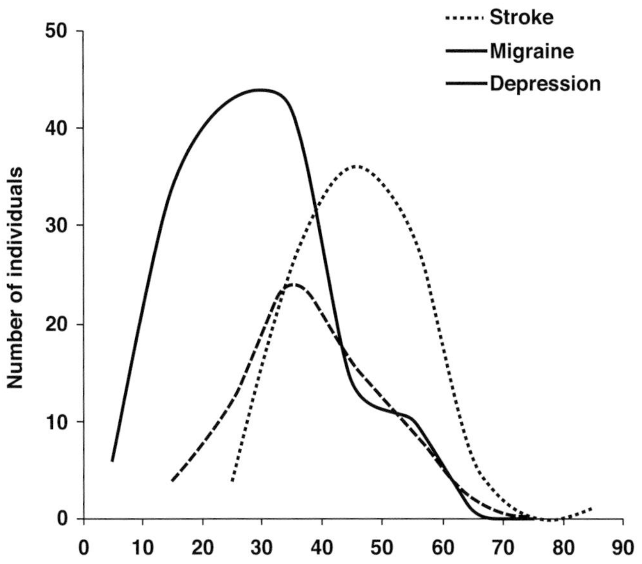

• **Figure 19.2** The profile of the main clinical features of CADASIL (cerebral autosomal dominant arteriopathy with subcortical infarcts and leukoencephalopathy) with age (in years on the *x*-axis), that is, migraine, depression and stroke. (From Adib-Samii P, Brice G, Martin RJ, et al. Clinical spectrum of CADASIL and effect of cardiovascular risk factors on phenotype. Study on 200 consecutively recruited individuals. *Stroke.* 2010;41:630–634. With permission of the American Heart Association.)

Immunostaining of *NOTCH3* is also sensitive and specific and may be more easily performed than electron microscopy.

Early-Onset Dementia

Alzheimer disease is the most common form of progressive dementia in the elderly, characterized by the accumulation of extracellular amyloid plaques and intracellular neurofibrillary tangles in regions of the brain, and the "presenile" form, starting at younger than 60 to 65 years of age, is identical. The clinical presentation includes memory impairment, poor judgment, agitation, withdrawal, confusion, language difficulties, and occasionally Parkinsonian features and seizures, all culminating in gradual decline leading to death. The duration may be more than 20 years, but is wide, and severe early-onset dementia (EOD), for example, beginning in the patient's 30s, may demonstrate rapid progression and death within 5 years.

The highly penetrant genes linked to early-onset Alzheimer disease, following AD inheritance, are *APP* (amyloid precursor protein), accounting for up to approximately 15% of cases; *PSEN1* (more common); and *PSEN2* (relatively rare). The latter two, like *NOTCH3*, are part of the Notch signaling pathway. APP is located on chromosome 22, and overexpression is thought to explain why individuals with Down syndrome almost invariably show signs of Alzheimer's from their 40s.

Other forms of EOD show overlap with **frontotemporal dementia** (FTD), sometimes referred to as **Pick disease**, although purists might argue that the term can be used only when "Pick *bodies*" are seen on neuropathological investigation. These are argyrophilic, intraneuronal inclusions; "Pick *cells*" are enlarged neurons. Genes linked to FTD are *MAPT*, *GRN*, and *C9orf72* (also linked to **amyotrophic lateral sclerosis** [ALS], see p. 295).

The Hereditary Ataxias

This is a hugely diverse group of progressive conditions characterized by a poorly coordinated, wide-based gait, often accompanied by dysarthria, abnormal eye movements (nystagmus), and poor upper limb coordination. Abnormal cerebellar structure and/or function is usually present. There are many non-genetic causes of ataxia, but the hereditary forms may follow any of the main patterns of inheritance—AD, autosomal recessive (AR), and X-linked (XL). Mitochondrial disorders may also feature ataxia among other clinical signs and symptoms. Here we cover the most common disorders only.

Spinocerebellar Ataxias

This large group of disorders is essentially equivalent to the hereditary ataxias following AD inheritance (even though recessively inherited forms are described), and approximately 40 different types are recognized, based on the specific genes that are implicated, or in some cases the gene locus only. Prevalence may be up to 5:100,000. The onset is usually some time in adulthood, and the different types can be difficult or impossible to distinguish clinically. Cognitive decline and dementia occur in several forms, and in some there are additional features, for example, visual loss with retinopathy in spinocerebellar ataxia (SCA) type 7 (*ATXN7* gene), which also tends to be rapidly progressive and life-shortening. In most surveys SCA type 3 (*ATXN3* gene), also known as Machado-Joseph disease, is the most commonly encountered form and also tends to be life-shortening. Some types, for example, SCA1, 2, and

4, may manifest features of peripheral neuropathy. One rare type of ataxia that mimics HD and, strictly speaking, is not classified as a subtype of SCA is dentatorubral-pallidolysian atrophy (DRPLA), caused by mutated *ATN1*.

Genetics

The majority of SCA types, as well as DRPLA, like HD, are caused by particular trinucleotide expansions in the coding regions of their respective genes, in most cases the CAG triplet (see Table 2.5). As such they may demonstrate anticipation over several generations (in SCA7 and DRPLA the CAG repeat is particularly unstable), potentially more marked as a result of paternal transmission.

Episodic Ataxias

These conditions follow AD inheritance and are characterized by intermittent periods, or paroxysms, of unsteady gait, perhaps lasting several hours, with nystagmus and dysarthria. Approximately seven subtypes are currently recognized, episodic ataxias (EA)1 and EA2 being caused by mutations in *KCNA1* and *CACNA1A*, respectively. The symptom of vertigo in EA2 may distinguish it clinically from EA1, as well as the finding of cerebellar vermis hypoplasia on MRI scan. In both cases the finding of a pathogenic heterozygous variant will confirm the diagnosis, and *CACNA1A* is the same gene implicated in both SCA6 and familial hemiplegic migraine; indeed, aspects of these clinical phenotypes may be seen among affected members of the same family.

Friedreich Ataxia

Of the many ataxias following AR inheritance Friedreich ataxia (FRDA) is probably the best known, as well as being the most common, but there are a variety of other disorders that may need to be considered at presentation, including the various forms of Joubert and pontocerebellar syndromes, metabolic diseases such as disorders of glycosylation and peroxisomal biogenesis, and ataxia telangiectasia (pp. 181, 266). In adulthood a variety of rare ataxias following AR inheritance may be encountered, including cerebrotendinous xanthomatosis, which is characterized by the finding of xanthoma lesions (e.g., around the Achilles tendon).

In FRDA the onset is usually in late childhood or early adolescence, and a slowly progressive ataxia ensues. There is absence of lower limb reflexes (in contrast to the finding in SCA) and loss of position and vibration sense. Approximately two-thirds of cases go on to develop hypertrophic cardiomyopathy (sometimes "dilated" later on), and one-third diabetes mellitus. Dysarthria, dysphagia, and scoliosis are all common features, as well as autonomic dysfunction. Optic nerve atrophy may be seen in approximately 25% of cases.

Genetics

FDRA is another triplet repeat disease, but in this case the triplet is GAA (see Table 2.5) and it occurs in an intronic region of the *FXN* gene. Pathogenic alleles number in the hundreds, and, as a recessively inherited condition, anticipation is not seen. However, there is broad inverse correlation of the age of onset with the numbers of GAA repeats, although not to the extent that the age of onset or severity can be predicted from the molecular findings.

Inherited Peripheral Neuropathies

This is another group of conditions that has become increasingly complex from a genetic viewpoint and incorporates hereditary sensory neuropathies, various forms of **familial dysautonomia** (FD), as well as the better-known hereditary motor and sensory neuropathies (HMSNs), which are synonymous with Charcot-Marie-Tooth (CMT) disease. In addition, the astute clinician has to be very aware that peripheral neuropathy symptoms can be a presenting feature of other disorders, for example, neurofibromatosis type 2 and metabolic disorders such as Fabry disease (p. 281), XL adrenoleukodystrophy (p. 284), and others.

Hereditary Motor and Sensory Neuropathies/Charcot-Marie-Tooth Disease

The HMSNs, also known as **CMT disease** and **peroneal muscular atrophy**, are clinically and genetically heterogeneous, with at least 70 different genes or loci identified (Fig. 19.3), but all are basically characterized by slowly progressive distal muscle weakness and wasting. Their overall incidence is approximately 1:3000.

Clinical classification on the basis of motor nerve conduction velocity (MNCV) is still useful. HMSN type 1 is "**demyelinating**," accompanied by hypertrophic changes with "onion bulb" formation if a nerve biopsy is undertaken, and the MNCV is reduced to

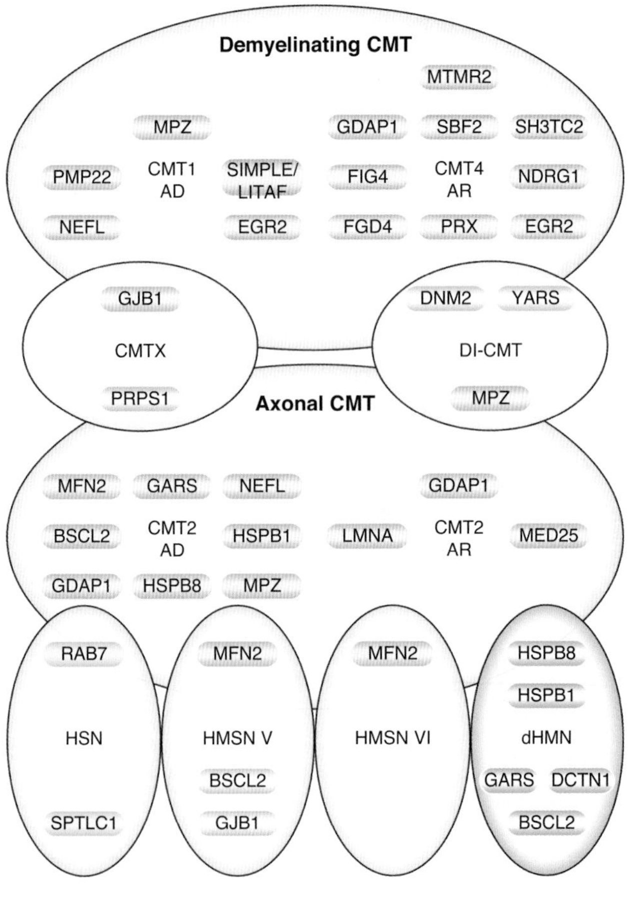

• **Figure 19.3** The different forms of Charcot-Marie-Tooth disease, or hereditary motor and sensory neuropathy, and their associated genes, highlighting the clinical and genetic overlap. The most commonly encountered genes are highlighted in red. *dHMN*, Distal hereditary motor neuropathy; *DI*, dominant intermediate; *HSN*, hereditary sensory neuropathy. (Modified from Pareyson D, Marchesi C. Diagnosis, natural history, and management of Charcot-Marie-Tooth disease. *Lancet Neurol*. 2009;8:654–667.)

5 to 30 m/sec (normal: >40–45 m/sec). HMSN type 2 is "**axonal**" (non, demyelinating), and the MNCV is normal or only slightly reduced, in the range 35 to 48 m/sec, and a nerve biopsy shows axonal degeneration. Although many patients can be categorized as type 1 or 2 on this basis, some genetic varieties of HMSN demonstrate a mixed picture and/or variability between different affected family members.

Clinical Features

In AD HMSN1a—the most common form—the onset occurs as slowly progressive distal muscle weakness and wasting in the lower limbs between the ages of 10 and 30 years, followed later by the upper limbs in many patients, often with associated ataxia and tremor. The appearance of the lower limbs has been likened to that of an "inverted champagne bottle" (Fig. 19.4), and peripheral nerve reflexes are absent or greatly diminished. Over time, locomotion becomes more difficult, and the feet tend to show exaggeration of their normal arch, known as "pes cavus." Many patients may retain reasonable muscle strength and not be badly disabled, although others may be significantly restricted. Vision, hearing, and intellect are not impaired. Palpable thickening of peripheral nerves can sometimes be detected.

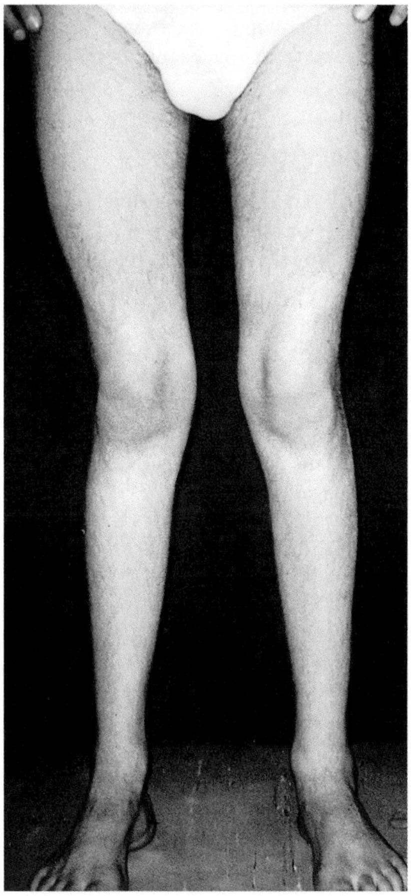

• **Figure 19.4** Lower limbs of a male with hereditary motor and sensory neuropathy showing severe muscle wasting below the knees.

The clinical features in other forms of HMSN are similar but may differ in the age of onset, rate of progression, and presence of other neurological involvement. For example, the onset in HMSN2 is usually later and the disease course milder than type 1, and peripheral reflexes may be relatively preserved. In some of the rarer forms of HMSN additional neurological features (e.g., optic atrophy) may be present.

Genetics

HMSN may show AD, AR, or XL inheritance, although AD forms are by far the most common. Rarely, mitochondrial inheritance may apply, for example, in neuropathy, ataxia, and retinitis pigmentosa syndrome (NARP, p. 286). Some 75% of cases of HMSN1 (type a) are caused by a DNA **duplication** of 1.5 megabases (Mb) on chromosome 17p that harbors the peripheral myelin protein-22 (*PMP22*) gene, whose glycoprotein product is present in the myelin membranes of peripheral nerves, where it helps to arrest Schwann cell division. HMSN1a is therefore the result of a *PMP22* dosage effect, and the duplication is generated by misalignment and subsequent recombination between homologous sequences that flank the *PMP22* gene (Fig. 19.5); this event usually occurs in male gametogenesis. The reciprocal **deletion** product of this misaligned recombination event, giving rise to haploinsufficiency, causes a relatively mild disorder known as **hereditary neuropathy with liability to pressure palsies**. Minor nerve trauma, such as pressure from prolonged sitting on a long-haul flight, causes focal numbness and weakness. The same misalignment recombination mechanism occurs in Hb Lepore and anti-Lepore (see Fig. 12.3; p. 163), congenital adrenal hyperplasia (p. 277), and deletion 22q11 syndrome (p. 259), to name but a few.

In a small proportion of HMSN1 cases another myelin protein, **myelin protein zero** (encoded by the *MPZ* gene), is implicated. This plays a crucial role as an adhesion molecule in the compaction of myelin in peripheral nerves, and in fact variants in this gene lead to a mixed, or intermediate, type of demyelination and

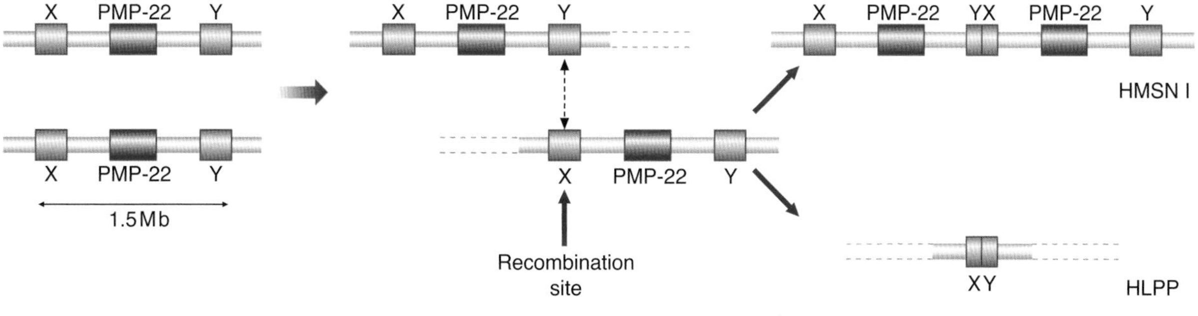

• **Figure 19.5** Mechanism by which misalignment and recombination with unequal crossing over lead to formation of the duplication and deletion that cause hereditary motor and sensory neuropathy type I and hereditary neuropathy with liability to pressure palsies. X and Y represent homologous sequences flanking the *PMP22* gene.

axonal neuropathy. The many other genetic varieties of HMSN1 are rare.

HMSN2 is genetically heterogeneous, and a genetic diagnosis is achieved less often compared with type 1. Some 20% of cases are attributed to variants in the nuclear gene *MFN2* encoding defective Mitofusin 2, which produces abnormal mitochondrial fusion/fission (HMSN2a). The other genes in which pathogenic variants are seen occasionally in CMT2 are *NEFL*, *GDAP1*, *GARS*, and *YARS*, and intermediate demyelinating/axonal effects are again seen.

HMSN type 4, or **CMT4**, is a group of rare demyelinating and axonal peripheral neuropathies that are set apart from the others purely by the fact that they follow AR inheritance. Otherwise they may be clinically indistinguishable, and their causation determined only by genetic testing.

The main XL form of HMSN, **CMTX1**, may account for 5% to 10% of HMSN cases overall, is caused by mutated *GJB1* (previously *connexin 32*), and shows XL *dominant* inheritance. Both sexes are usually affected, although males have typical features, with females relatively mildly affected.

Hereditary Sensory and Autonomic Neuropathies

Hereditary sensory and autonomic neuropathies (HSANs) are a group of axonal neuropathies, usually following AD inheritance, where symptoms are primarily sensory, with little or no motor involvement. The most common form, HSAN1, is caused by mutations in *SPTLC1*, and affected patients describe very unpleasant and disabling "burning feet," and may develop ulceration on pressure points, and potentially neuropathic arthropathy. Another gene implicated is *ATL3*.

The HSAN group includes **FD**, or HSAN III, which is an early-onset, debilitating, and progressive condition whereby the development and survival of sensory, sympathetic, and parasympathetic neurons is greatly affected. The diagnosis can be difficult, as affected individuals have gastrointestinal dysfunction with vomiting crises, recurrent pneumonia, impaired pain and temperature sensitivity, and cardiovascular instability. Life expectancy is greatly reduced, but early diagnosis and supportive treatment improves the outlook. It is recessively inherited, attributed to mutated *IKBKAP*, and more common in Ashkenazi Jews, where one founder mutation accounts for the majority of cases.

HSAN IV is **congenital insensitivity to pain with anhydrosis**, which may closely resemble FD. Typically, high fevers occur, which may be life-threatening, and multiple unrecognized injuries can result in mutilating effects. Also recessively inherited, it is caused by mutated *NTRK1*.

Hereditary Spastic Paraparesis

Hereditary spastic paraparesis (HSP) is also known as hereditary spastic paraplegia, and sometimes Strumpell disease. This large group of disorders (> 80 different types to date) is characterized by lower limb spasticity and weakness, the onset varying from infancy to adulthood, and both progressive and non-progressive forms exist. The spasticity and gait closely resemble the pattern seen in spastic diplegic cerebral palsy. In "uncomplicated" cases the effects are limited to the lower limbs with hyperreflexia, although urinary urgency and paraesthesia may occur. With few exceptions, cognitive impairment and/or dysarthria do not occur. Where pathology is established, the cause is axonal degeneration affecting the distal ends of the corticospinal tracts. Complex, syndromic forms may be seen, which may include cognitive decline, seizures, and peripheral neuropathy.

In clinical practice the most commonly encountered forms of HSP follow AD inheritance, with the *SPAST* (*SPG4*), *ATL1* (*SPG3A*), and *REEP1* (*SPG31*) genes most often implicated. AR forms are seen much less often, and include HSP type 7 caused by mutated *SPG7*, and clinically there may be optic disc pallor, an axonal neuropathy, and occasionally intellectual disability.

XL forms also exist, and these are complicated forms of HSP that include the *L1CAM* (*SPG1*) gene, also implicated in **X-linked hydrocephalus**, and the *PLP1* (*SPG2*) gene, associated with a broader phenotype known as **Pelizaeus-Merzbacher disease**, with characteristic white matter changes on MRI and peripheral neuropathy.

Spinal Muscular Atrophy

There are a variety of rare disorders classified under "spinal muscular atrophy (SMA)," but the best-known and most common concerns molecular pathology at the *SMN1* gene locus. This is recessively inherited and characterized by degeneration of the anterior horn cells of the spinal cord, leading to progressive muscle weakness and ultimately death. Three common childhood forms and one adult-onset form (Box 19.1) are recognized, with an incidence, collectively, of approximately 1:10,000. The carrier frequency is therefore close to 1:50. In fact, although three childhood types are described, the molecular pathology overlaps, and they constitute a continuum.

Clinical Features

SMA type I, also known as **Werdnig-Hoffmann disease**, presents before 6 months of age, often within days of birth, with significant hypotonia and poverty of movement. Fetal movements may have been reduced. Affected children show normal development otherwise, but profound muscle weakness leads to death within the first 2 years of life, often before 12 months. Electromyography has been superseded by genetic testing to make the diagnosis, and there is currently no effective treatment.

SMA type II is less severe than type I, with onset between 6 and 12 months, although the main presenting features are also muscle weakness and hypotonia. Affected children sit unaided but never achieve independent locomotion, and the rate of progression is slow, with survival into early adulthood.

SMA type III, also known as **Kugelberg-Welander disease**, presents after 12 months, and limited walking is achieved. Slow progression leads to the use of a wheelchair by early adult life, and long-term survival can be compromised by recurrent respiratory infection and the development of scoliosis.

• BOX 19.1 Definition of the Different Forms of Spinal Muscular Atrophy

- Spinal muscular atrophy (SMA) I: onset before 6 months of age
- SMA II: onset between 6 and 12 months of age
- SMA III: onset after 12 months of age and ability to walk ≥25 meters (current or historical)
- SMA IV: adult onset

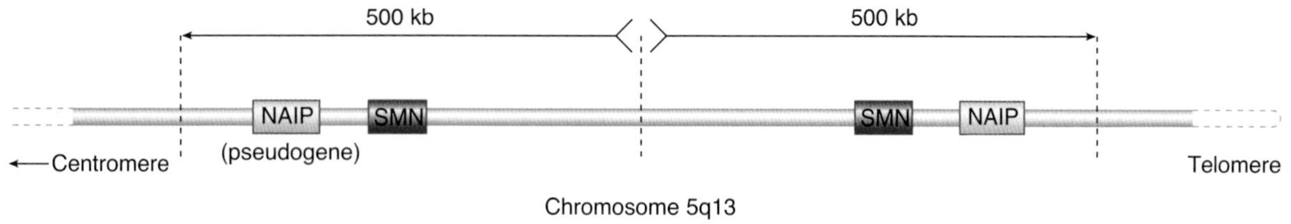

• **Figure 19.6** The inverted duplication with the *SMN* and *NAIP* genes. Spinal muscular atrophy occurs when both copies of the *SMN1* gene are mutated (autosomal recessive inheritance); in 95% to 98% this is a deletion of exons 7 to 8, and point mutations account for the remainder. *SMN*, Survival motor neuron; *NAIP*, neuronal apoptosis-inhibitory protein.

Genetics

SMA follows AR inheritance, with the exception of some rarer forms, where dominant and XL inheritance may apply (e.g., spinal and bulbar muscular atrophy, also known as Kennedy disease, see Fig. 2.5). SMA type I as described, attributed to variants in *SMN1*, generally shows a high degree of intrafamilial concordance, with affected siblings showing an almost identical clinical course, although in types II and III more intrafamilial variation occurs.

SMN1 is located on chromosome 5q in a region that is noted for its instability, and at this locus an inverted, duplicated segment occurs (Fig. 19.6). There are also a relatively large number of pseudogenes (p. 14). The *SMN* genes are now referred to as *SMN1* and *SMN2* (the pseudogene of *SMN1* that shares approximately 99% homology). *SMN1* shows homozygous deletion of exons 7 to 8 in 95% to 98% of all patients with childhood-onset SMA. Point mutations in *SMN1* have been identified in 1% to 2% of patients with childhood SMA, where one allele is not deleted for exons 7 to 8. The number of copies of *SMN2*, arranged in tandem in *cis* configuration on each chromosome, varies between zero and five. It produces a similar transcript to *SMN1*, but this is not sufficient to fully compensate. Nevertheless, the presence of copies of *SMN2* modifies the phenotype, and there is a broad inverse correlation between the number of copies of *SMN2* and the severity.

SMN1 is always mutated in SMA, in the vast majority by deletion of exons 7 to 8, and in the remainder by point mutation. Diagnostic testing is therefore very reliable, and prenatal testing is an option for those couples who request it, assuming both parents are carriers. Carrier detection is based on determining the number of exon 7–containing *SMN1* gene copies present in an individual. However, results can be difficult to interpret because some carriers have the normal number of *SMN1* gene copies caused by the presence either of two *SMN1* gene copies in *cis* configuration on one chromosome, or of a *SMN1* point mutation. Approximately 4% of the general population has two copies of *SMN1* on a single chromosome. Furthermore, 2% of individuals with SMA have one *de novo* mutation, meaning that only one parent is a carrier. Because of these difficulties, SMA carrier testing should be provided in the context of formal, expert genetic counseling.

There is great interest in gene therapy for SMA designed to deliver a functional copy of the *SMN1* gene to motor neurons. A normal copy of the *SMN1* gene, that is, not deleted for exons 7 to 8, is delivered in a "capsid," the shell of a genetically engineered adeno-associated virus. Early trials have been promising.

Motor Neurone Disease

Each year up to 3 individuals per 100,000 of the population are diagnosed with motor neurone disease (MND), which is the same as **amyotrophic lateral sclerosis** (ALS), also known as **Lou Gehrig disease**. It follows on neatly from SMA because adult-onset SMA is part of the differential diagnosis of ALS, and is a progressive neurodegenerative condition of both upper and lower motor neurons. The presentation may be with focal and asymmetric weakness in the extremities or with bulbar signs such as dysphagia or dysarthria. The basic diagnostic criteria are shown in Box 19.2. The average age of onset is approximately 56, and most patients live only 1 to 5 years from diagnosis to death as they become increasingly weak and respiratory function declines. Some aspects of cognitive function are affected in approximately one-third of sufferers.

• **BOX 19.2 Diagnostic Criteria for Amyotrophic Lateral Sclerosis (Motor Neurone Disease)**

- Evidence of (all three):
  1. Lower motor neuron degeneration—clinically, electrophysiologically or by neuropathology assessment
  2. Upper motor neuron degeneration—clinically
  3. Progressive spread of symptoms or signs—within a region or to other regions
- Absence of evidence of:
  1. Other disease or processes to explain the neurological signs—electrophysiologically or by pathology
  2. Other disease processes—by neuroimaging

Roughly 10% of ALS is familial—FALS—and in this group the average age of onset is approximately 46 years. As with so many other inherited neurological disorders, FALS is proving to be genetically heterogeneous, with rapid recent progress in our understanding owing to the power of next-generation sequencing. Most cases follow AD inheritance, but some rare recessive forms have been reported. For many years we knew of only one gene for FALS, namely *SOD1*, but this accounts for only approximately 20% of cases of FALS. Some *SOD1* variants are associated with "mild" ALS and a slowly progressive course up to 20 years. A slightly larger proportion of cases are now known to be caused by variants in *C9orf72*, which is also implicated in familial FTD. The pathogenic variant is a heterozygous expansion of a non-coding GGGGCC hexanucleotide repeat, which leads to the loss of one alternatively spliced transcript of *C9orf72*. Approximately 4% of cases of FALS are associated with a mutation in the *FUS* gene, and a similar proportion with mutation of the *TARDBP* gene.

Neurocutaneous Disorders

This group of neurological disorders is diverse, but the common clinical feature is the presence of disease manifestations in skin, which in some conditions is crucial to the diagnosis. We cover only the better-known ones here.

Neurofibromatosis Type 1

Neurofibromatosis type 1 (NF1) and NF2 have some overlapping features but in truth are distinct conditions and hence dealt with separately. NF1 has a birth incidence of approximately 1:3000, and references to the clinical features first appeared in 18th-century medical literature. Historically, however, the disorder is associated with Von Recklinghausen, a German pathologist who coined the term "neurofibroma" in 1882. It is one of the most common genetic disorders in humans and gained a public profile when it was suggested that Joseph Merrick, the "Elephant Man," might have been affected. However, it is now thought he had **Proteus syndrome**.

Clinical Features

The most notable features of NF1 are small pigmented skin lesions, known as **café-au-lait** (CAL) spots, and small, soft, fleshy growths known as **neurofibromata** (Fig. 19.7A). CAL spots first appear in early childhood (Fig. 19.7B) and continue to increase in both size and number until puberty. A minimum of six CAL spots at least 5 mm in diameter is required to support the diagnosis in childhood, and an additional feature such as axillary and/or inguinal freckling should be present. Neurofibromata are benign tumors that arise most commonly in the skin, usually appearing in adolescence or adult life and increasing in number with age. However, large **plexiform** neurofibromata (Fig. 19.7C) may occur and be deep-seated and/or cutaneous. As well as being cosmetically unsightly, they can interfere with function, depending on their location.

Other clinical findings include relative macrocephaly and Lisch nodules. The latter are small harmless raised pigmented hamartomata of the iris (Fig. 19.8). The most common complication, occurring in one-third of childhood cases, is mild developmental delay characterized by a nonverbal learning disorder. For many, significant improvement is seen through the school years. Most individuals with NF1 enjoy a normal life and are not unduly inconvenienced by their condition. However, a small number of patients develop one or more major complications, such as epilepsy, a CNS tumor, or scoliosis. Renal artery stenosis and pheochromocytoma are rare associations.

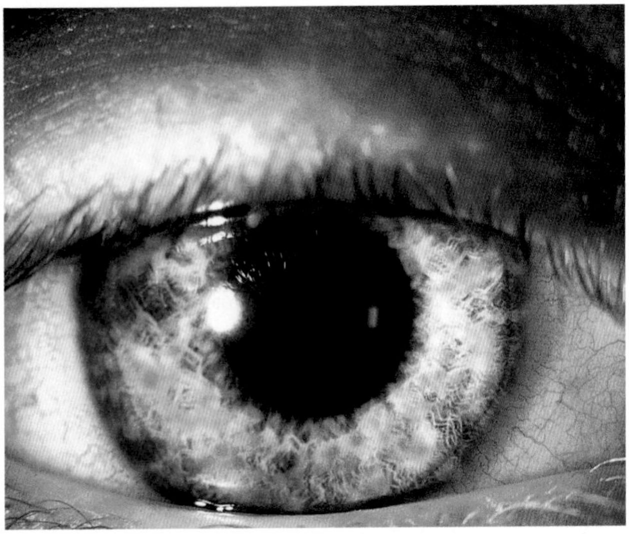

• **Figure 19.8** Lisch nodules seen in neurofibromatosis type I. *(Courtesy Mr R. Doran, Department of Ophthalmology, General Infirmary, Leeds, UK.)*

Genetics

NF1 shows AD inheritance, with virtually 100% penetrance by age 5 years. Variability and striking differences in disease severity can be seen within affected families, although monozygotic twins are usually very similar. Approximately 50% of cases are caused by new

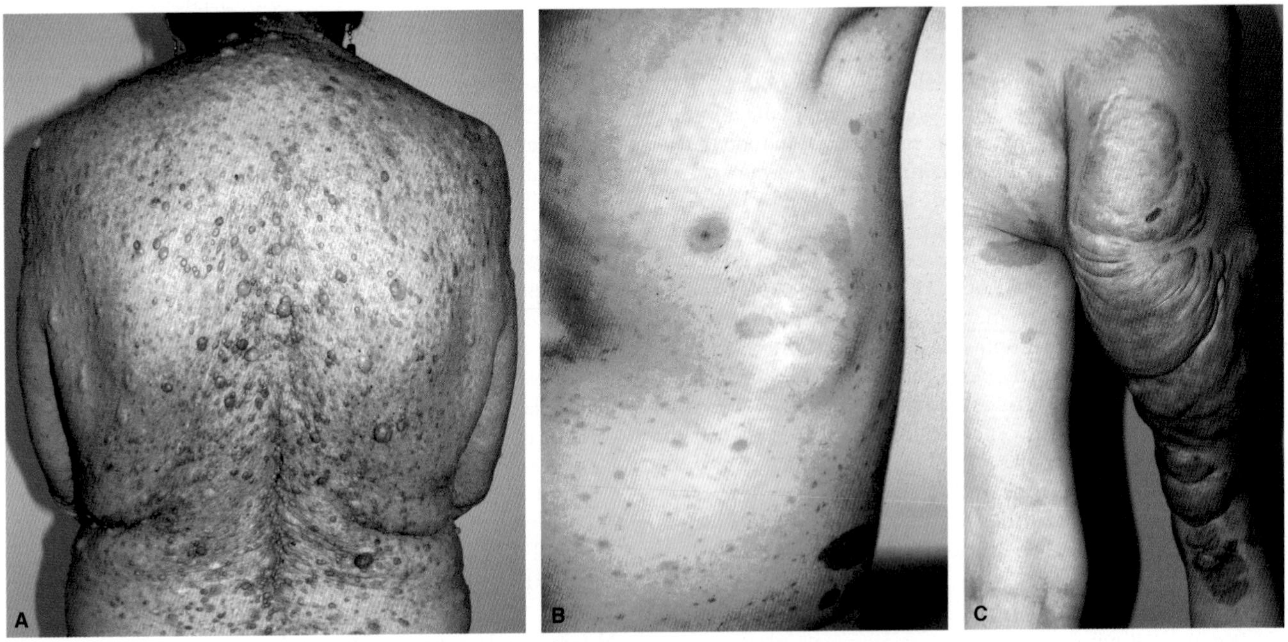

• **Figure 19.7** Neurofibromatosis type 1. (A) A patient with neurofibromatosis type I showing truncal freckling and multiple neurofibromata. (B) Café-au-lait spots on the chest of a child, axillary freckling and a subcutaneous plexiform neurofibroma below and lateral to the left nipple. (C) A large and unsightly plexiform neurofibroma affecting the left buttock and leg.

mutations, with the estimated mutation rate being approximately 1 per 10,000 gametes. This is approximately 100 times greater than the average mutation rate per generation per locus in humans.

Where more than one affected child is born to unaffected parents, this is almost always the result of gonadal mosaicism (p. 77), usually paternal in origin. Somatic mosaicism in NF1 can manifest with features limited to a particular part of the body, referred to as **segmental NF**.

The NF1 gene, *neurofibromin-1*, mapped in 1987 following the identification of two patients with balanced translocations involving a breakpoint at 17q11.2, is large, spanning more than 350 kilobases (kb) of genomic DNA and comprising 61 exons. Three distinct genes lie within a single intron of *neurofibromin-1*, where they are transcribed in the opposite direction (p. 11). The neurofibromin protein encoded by this gene shows structural homology to the guanosine triphosphatase (GTPase)-activating protein (GAP), which is important in signal transduction owing to its role in downregulating *RAS* activity. The place of neurofibromin in the RAS-MAPK pathway is shown in Fig. 16.13, highlighting the link with Noonan syndrome and other rasopathy conditions (p. 234). Loss of heterozygosity (p. 190) for chromosome 17 markers has been observed in several malignant tumors in patients with NF1, as well as in a small number of benign neurofibromata, indicating that the gene is a tumor suppressor (p. 190), and it contains a GAP-related domain (GRD), which interacts with the *RAS* proto-oncogene product. An mRNA editing site exists in the *neurofibromin-1* gene, and the edited transcript encodes a truncated GRD protein, which inactivates the tumor suppressor function. A higher range of editing is seen in more malignant tumors.

Other genes, including *TP53* (p. 192) on the short arm of chromosome 17, are also involved in tumor development and progression in NF1. Conversely, it is also known that the *neurofibromin-1* gene is implicated in the development of sporadic tumors not associated with NF, including carcinoma of the colon, neuroblastoma, and malignant melanoma, confirming that it plays an important role in cell growth and differentiation.

Many different pathogenic variants have been identified in *neurofibromin-1*, including deletions, insertions, duplications, and point substitutions (p. 19). Most lead to severe truncation of the protein or complete absence of gene expression. There is little evidence for a genotype-phenotype relationship, with the exception of one specific mutation, a 3-bp in-frame deletion in exon 17, which has recurred in different cases and families, and affected individuals do not appear to develop cutaneous neurofibromata. Generally, NF1 shows quite striking intrafamilial variation, suggesting the possibility of modifier genes. Patients with large deletions encompassing the entire *neurofibromin-1* gene tend to be more severely affected, with significant intellectual impairment, a somewhat marfanoid habitus, and a larger than average number of cutaneous neurofibromata.

Legius Syndrome

This fairly rare condition is the closest known "phenocopy" to NF1; indeed, it may be very difficult to distinguish from NF1 clinically. The features are multiple CAL macules (although patients lack neurofibromas and other tumors such as optic nerve glioma, as well as Lisch nodules and sphenoid wing dysplasia). They may have mild macrocephaly, intertriginous freckling, lipomas, and mild learning disabilities or attention deficit hyperactivity disorder, all of which mimic NF1. It is associated with variants in the *SPRED1* gene, which is also part of the RAS-MAPK signal transduction pathway (see Fig. 16.13), in which it functions as a negative regulator.

Neurofibromatosis Type 2

NF2 is rare compared with NF1, with a birth incidence of approximately 1:35,000 and a prevalence of approximately 1:60,000. Both CAL spots and neurofibromata can occur, but much less commonly than in NF1. The cardinal feature is the development in early adult life of tumors involving the 8th cranial nerves—**vestibular schwannomas** (still sometimes called **acoustic neuromas**), which are best treated early (if possible) by stereotactic radiotherapy. Several other central nervous system (CNS) tumors occur frequently (e.g., meningioma), although more than half remain asymptomatic. An ophthalmic feature seen in NF2, but not NF1, is cataracts, which are frequent but often subclinical. Spinal and peripheral schwannomas without vestibular schwannomas, following AD inheritance, represent an entity known as **schwannomatosis**, and is due to variants in *SMARCB1*.

The *NF2*, or *neurofibromin-2*, gene on chromosome 22q was identified in 1993 and is thought to be a cytoskeleton protein that acts as a tumor suppressor. Deletions and point mutations in the gene give rise to the condition, although in contrast to *NF1*, deletion cases tend to be mild rather than severe compared with point mutations. The frequency of somatic mosaicism in NF2 is significant but generally associated with a low offspring risk.

NF2 is one condition where therapeutic options have become a reality recently. Administration of the angiogenesis inhibitor bevacizumab has been demonstrated to reduce the size of spinal tumors. This is a recombinant monoclonal antibody that exerts its negative effects on angiogenesis by inhibiting vascular endothelial growth factor A, a chemical that aberrantly promotes angiogenesis.

Tuberous Sclerosis

The incidence of this well-known multisystem, dominantly inherited, and very variable neurocutaneous disorder is approximately 1:6000. It has already been used (Fig. 6.5) to illustrate patterns of inheritance because a high proportion of cases (~80%) occur *de novo*, but it may also demonstrate variable penetrance to the extent that it sometimes appears to "skip" a generation. Furthermore, clinical geneticists have to be very aware of the risk of gonadal mosaicism (p. 77). Although this is usually quoted as approximately 1% to 2%, there has been debate about this over the years, and sibling recurrences may occur because of subclinical somatic mosaicism in one of the parents.

Clinical Features

The facial rash of tuberous sclerosis (TSC), angiofibromas, or "adenoma sebaceum" (Fig. 19.9; Fig. 6.5A), can vary from being florid to virtually nonexistent and is one of several classic skin features. The others are hypomelanotic macules (Fig, 19.10), shagreen

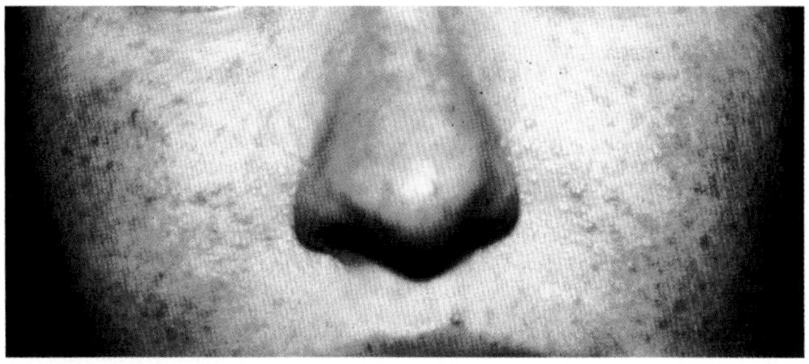

• **Figure 19.9** Tuberous sclerosis—facial angiofibromas, or "adenoma sebaceum."

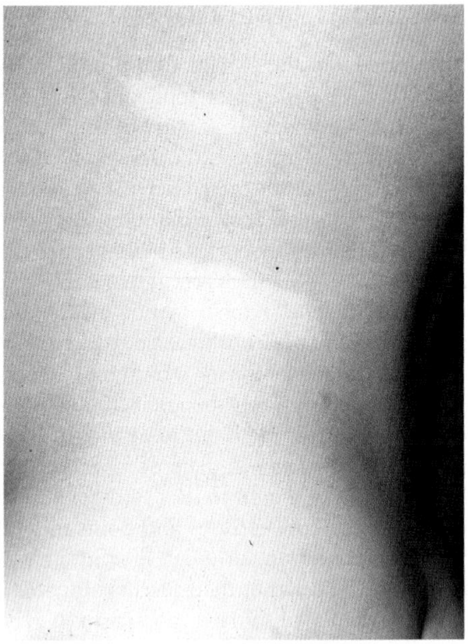

• **Figure 19.10** Tuberous sclerosis—depigmented "ash leaf" patches on the trunk.

• BOX 19.3 The Clinical Features of Tuberous Sclerosis

Skin
Facial angiofibromas
Hypopigmented macules
Shagreen patches
Ungual fibromas

Eye
Retinal nodular hamartomas
Achromic patches

Brain
Subependymal nodules
Cortical dysplasias, including "tubers"
Subependymal giant cell astrocytomas

Kidney
Benign angiomyolipomas (common)
Renal cysts
Malignant angiomyolipomas and renal cell carcinoma (rare)

Heart
Rhabdomyomas

Lung
Lymphangioleiomyomatosis
Multifocal micronodular pneumonocyte hyperplasia

Central nervous system-related manifestations
- Seizures
- Autistic spectrum disorder/attention deficit hyperactivity disorder
- Learning disability
- Disruptive behavior

patches and ungual fibromas (Fig. 6.5B, p. 69), which appear after 10 years of age. Examination of the eye may reveal multiple retinal nodular hamartomas or achromic patches and, internally, the organs typically affected are the brain, kidney, heart, and lung (Box 19.3). Almost 100% of patients have a cutaneous manifestation of TSC, a renal abnormality on ultrasound scan is present in approximately 80% by age 10 years, CNS pathology is present in approximately 90%, seizures in approximately 80%, and learning disability in greater than 50%. Cardiac rhabdomyomas occur in up to two-thirds of cases, are particularly evident early in life, and, when seen on fetal ultrasound, are an important marker for TSC. They usually regress by adulthood.

Management and treatment options for TSC now include the group of drugs known as mTOR inhibitors, including rapamycin and everolimus, and Fig. 19.11 shows the signaling pathway, their site of action, and the conditions linked to components of the pathway.

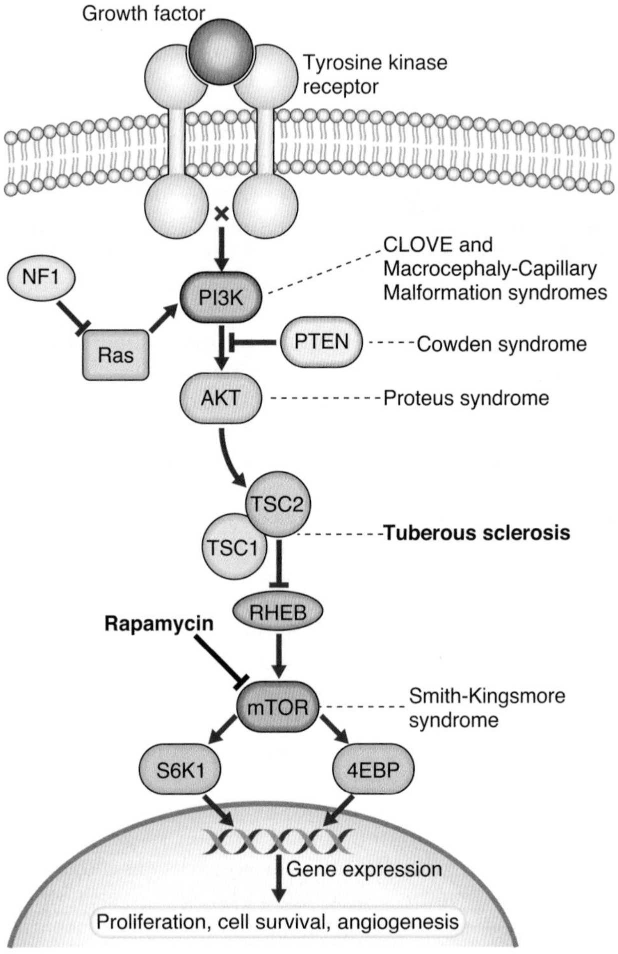

• **Figure 19.11** The mTOR signaling pathway. Also known as the PI3K/AKT/mTOR pathway, this is an important intracellular pathway in regulating the cell cycle. Activation of the pathway by growth factors controls protein synthesis at the level of translation initiation and ribosome biogenesis, ultimately leading to cell growth, proliferation, and survival. Alterations in control of the pathway, for example, through mutations of the genes encoding these proteins, can result in cellular transformation. The agent rapamycin inhibits mTOR activity and therefore blocks AKT-induced tumorigenesis. Altered proteins in the pathway (and the genes encoding them) are linked to genetic conditions as indicated, with particular attention drawn here to tuberous sclerosis. Pathogenic variants in *mTOR* have been found to cause Smith-Kingsmore syndrome—macrocephaly with frontal bossing and dysmorphic features, intellectual disability, and seizures.

Genetics

Heterozygous variants in two genes, *TSC1* and *TSC2*, cause TSC, and overall pathogenic variants are found in approximately 90% of patients meeting the clinical criteria for a diagnosis. The *TSC2* gene lies adjacent to the *PKD1* gene (for AD polycystic kidney disease, see later), so that a contiguous gene deletion affecting both occasionally occurs. Generally speaking, pathogenic variants in *TSC2* tend to give rise to a more severe phenotype than pathogenic variants in *TSC1*, for example, in terms of the risk for renal malignancy, learning disability, and behavior disorders. Among *de novo* cases, *TSC2* variants are approximately four times more prevalent compared with *TSC1*. However, among familial TSC cases, the prevalence of *TSC1* and *TSC2* variants is roughly equal.

Muscular Dystrophies

Because there are at least 100 muscular dystrophies, we can cover only those most likely to be encountered in clinical practice, and collectively they have a hugely important place in human and medical genetics, the history of which has been superbly documented by Professor Alan Emery. Fig. 19.12 shows the principle muscle groups affected in the more common dystrophies, four of which are covered in the text.

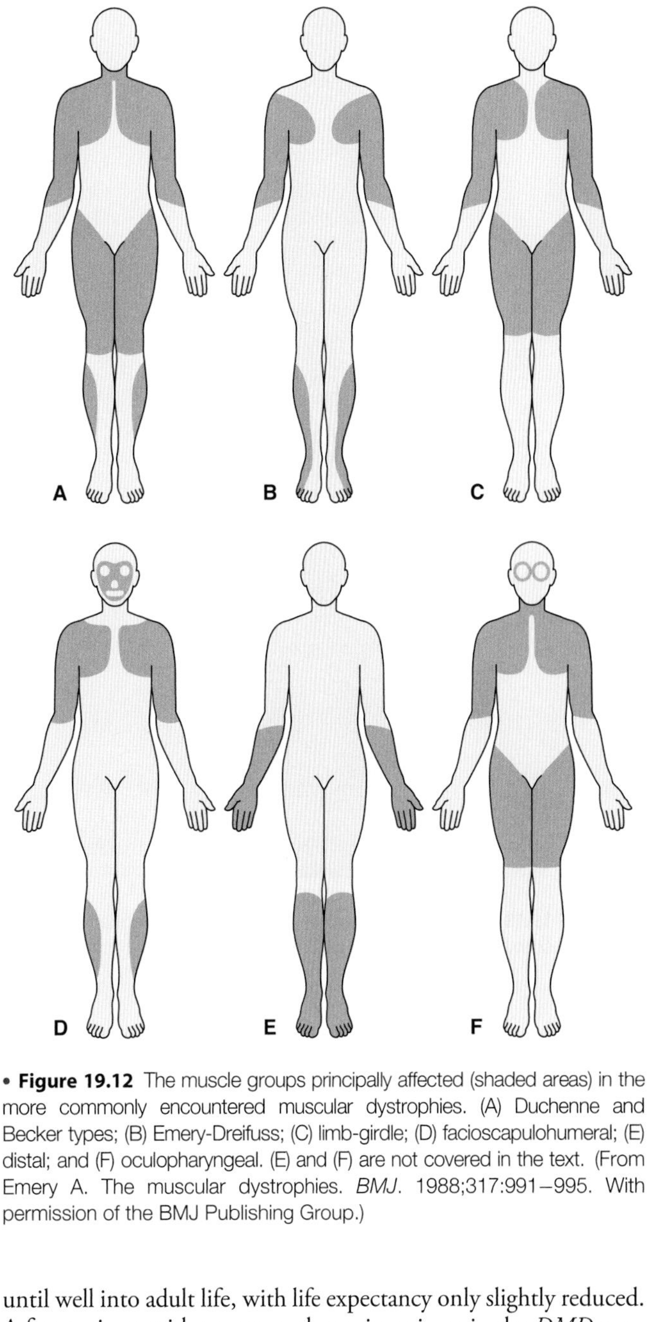

• **Figure 19.12** The muscle groups principally affected (shaded areas) in the more commonly encountered muscular dystrophies. (A) Duchenne and Becker types; (B) Emery-Dreifuss; (C) limb-girdle; (D) facioscapulohumeral; (E) distal; and (F) oculopharyngeal. (E) and (F) are not covered in the text. (From Emery A. The muscular dystrophies. *BMJ*. 1988;317:991–995. With permission of the BMJ Publishing Group.)

Duchenne and Becker Muscular Dystrophies—Xp21

Duchenne muscular dystrophy (DMD) and Becker muscular dystrophy (BMD) together are sometimes referred to as Xp21-dystrophies on account of the genetic basis being variants in the *DMD* gene, which encodes dystrophin, at this locus. DMD is the most common severe form of muscular dystrophy, and BMD its much milder "companion." The French neurologist Guillaume Duchenne described a case in 1861, but Edward Meryon, an English physician, had documented it a decade earlier, as championed by Alan and Marcia Emery. The incidences of DMD and BMD are approximately 1:3500 males and 1:20,000 males, respectively.

Clinical Features

Males with DMD usually present between the ages of 2 and 4 years with slowly progressive muscle weakness resulting in an awkward gait, inability to run quickly, and difficulty in rising from the floor, which can be achieved only by pushing on, or "climbing up," the legs and thighs (Gowers' sign). Most affected boys require a wheelchair by the age of 11 because of severe proximal weakness. Subsequent deterioration leads to lumbar lordosis, joint contractures, and cardiorespiratory failure, resulting in death at approximately 20 years without supportive measures, although life expectancy has been improving as a result of some treatment options and careful management, such as steroids and respiratory support in the form of continuous positive airways pressure (CPAP).

Males with either DMD or BMD show an apparent increase in the size of the calf muscles, but this is because of replacement of muscle fibers by fat and connective tissue—referred to as **pseudohypertrophy** (Fig.6.14; Fig. 19.13). In addition, approximately one-third of boys with DMD show mild-moderate intellectual impairment, with the mean intelligence quotient of approximately 83. BMD is similar but runs a much less aggressive course. The mean age of onset is 11 years, and many patients remain ambulant until well into adult life, with life expectancy only slightly reduced. A few patients with proven pathogenic variants in the *DMD* gene have been asymptomatic into their fifth or sixth decade.

Genetics

These are classic XL recessive diseases, and, because males with DMD rarely if ever reproduce, the genetic fitness is zero. The mutation rate equals the incidence of affected males divided by three (p. 88), which approximates to 1:10,000—one of the highest known mutation rates in humans. Identification of the *DMD* gene in 1987 represented a major scientific achievement at the time, because of a successfully applied positional cloning strategy. Clues to the DMD locus were provided by reports of females affected with DMD who had balanced X-autosome translocations—the breakpoint in common being at Xp21. In such cases, those cells in which the derivative X chromosome is randomly inactivated are greatly disadvantaged because of inactivation of the autosomal segment (Fig. 6.16; p. 74), which would most likely be

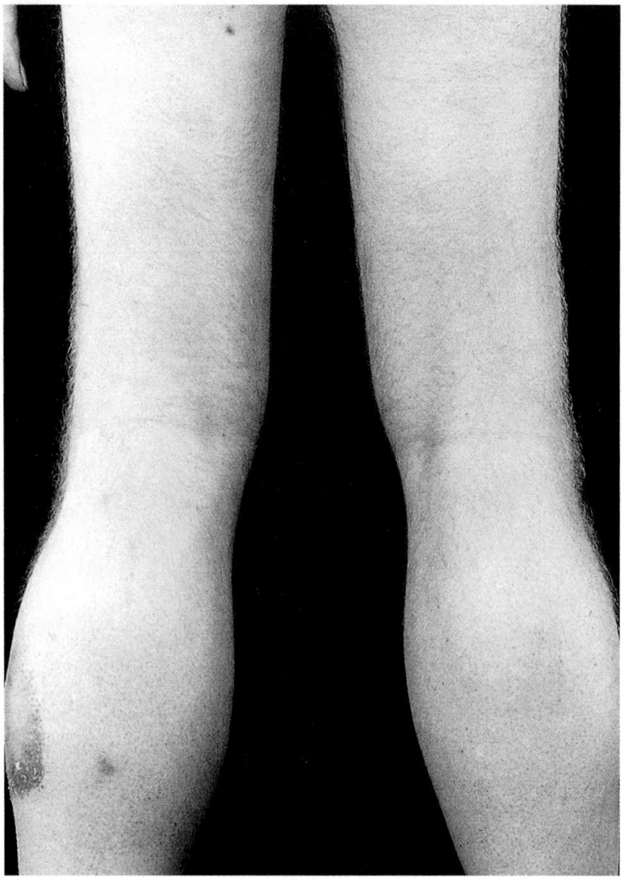

• **Figure 19.13** Lower limbs of an adult male with Becker muscular dystrophy showing proximal wasting and calf pseudohypertrophy.

developmentally catastrophic. Consequently, cells in which the normal X chromosome has been randomly inactivated are more likely to survive. The net result is that the derivative X-autosome is active in most cell lines, and if the breakpoint has damaged an important gene, in this case *DMD*, the individual will be affected by the disease that otherwise is almost always seen in males. Additional clues emerged from affected males with small cytogenetically visible deletions incorporating Xp21, followed by the identification of conserved sequences in muscle complementary DNA libraries that were shown to be exons from the gene itself.

The *DMD* gene is huge in molecular terms, possibly explaining the high mutation rate, consisting of 79 exons and spanning 2.3 Mb of genomic DNA, of which only 14 kb are transcribed into mRNA. It is transcribed in brain as well as muscle, explaining why some boys with DMD show learning difficulties. **Deletions** of various sizes, and at almost any location, account for two-thirds of all *DMD* pathogenic variants and arise almost exclusively in maternal meiosis, probably because of unequal crossing over. Some affected males have **duplications.** Deletion "hotspots" occur in the first 20 exons and exons 45 through 53. One of the deletion breakpoint hotspots in intron 7 contains a cluster of transposon-like repetitive DNA sequences that could facilitate misalignment in meiosis, with a subsequent crossover leading to deletion and duplication products.

Deletions causing DMD usually disturb the translational reading frame (p. 15) whereas those seen in males with BMD usually do not alter the reading frame (i.e., they are "in-frame"). This means that the amino-acid sequence of the protein product downstream of the deletion is normal, explaining the milder features in BMD. Occasionally in-frame deletions are entirely benign; the males are asymptomatic with normal creatine kinase (CK) levels. Pathogenic variants in the other one-third of boys with DMD include stop codons, frameshift mutations, altered splicing signals, and promoter mutations, most leading to premature translational termination and little, if any, protein product. In contrast to deletions, point mutations in *DMD* often arise in *paternal* meiosis, most probably because of a copy error in DNA replication. Full sequencing of *DMD* has transformed molecular diagnosis of DMD, BMD, and carrier detection.

The 427-kDa dystrophin protein is located close to the muscle membrane, where it links intracellular actin with extracellular laminin. Absence of dystrophin, as in DMD, leads gradually to muscle cell degeneration. The presence of dystrophin in a muscle biopsy sample can be assessed by immunofluorescence, and levels less than 3% are diagnostic. In muscle biopsies from males with BMD, the dystrophin shows qualitative rather than gross quantitative abnormalities.

Dystrophin binds to a glycoprotein complex in the muscle membrane through its C-terminal domain (Fig. 19.14). This glycoprotein complex consists of several subunits, abnormalities of which cause other rare genetic muscle disorders, including several

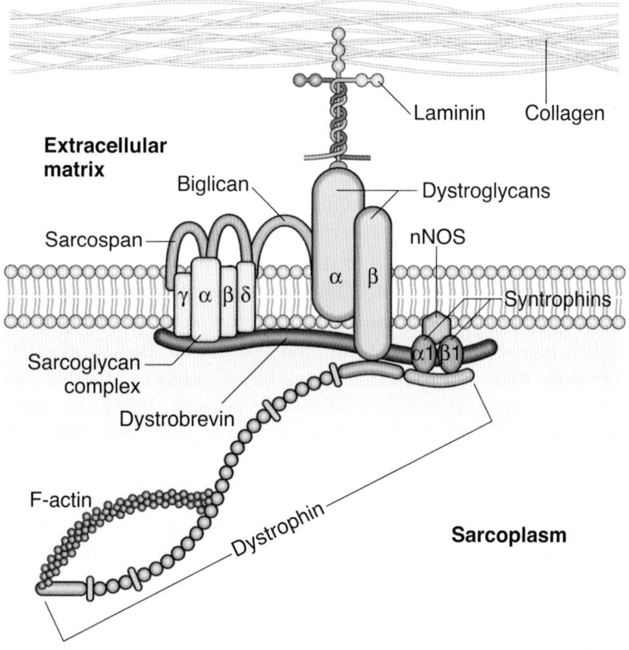

• **Figure 19.14** The dystrophin-associated protein complex (DAPC). Dystrophin lies beneath the basal lamina and extends through the sarcoplasm, binding cytoskeletal F-actin through its N-terminus domain and the DAPC through its C-terminus. It therefore links the internal cytoskeleton and extracellular matrix. The central rod domain (blue circles) is formed by triple-helical segments, interrupted by four hinge regions. The C-terminal region binds β-dystroglycan, as well as the syntrophins and α-dystrobrevin. In addition, dystrobrevin links dystrophin with the sarcoglycan-sarcospan complex, which is also indirectly linked to dystrophin through the dystroglycan complex (α-dystroglycan and β-dystroglycan). The individual sarcoglycan subunits are each implicated in different forms of limb-girdle muscular dystrophy. (From Fairclough RJ, Wood MJ, Davies KE. Therapy for Duchenne muscular dystrophy: renewed optimism from genetic approaches. *Nat. Rev. Genet.* 2013;14:373–378; and Rahimov F, Kunkel LM. The cell biology of disease: cellular and molecular mechanisms underlying muscular dystrophy. *J. Cell Biol.* 2013;201:499–510.)

different types of AR limb girdle muscular dystrophy, as well as congenital muscular dystrophy.

Before DNA analysis, determination of carrier status was based on pedigree information combined with serum CK assay. CK levels are grossly increased in boys with DMD, and marginally raised in approximately two-thirds of all carriers (see Fig. 11.2; p. 152). CK levels are only occasionally useful today because DMD can be fully sequenced. Family linkage studies are sometimes undertaken where no DNA is available from a deceased affected male, but DNA from normal males can help to build an informative picture—each situation has to be individually assessed. The interpretation of linkage data must take account of the high recombination rate of 12% across the *DMD* gene.

At present, there is no cure for DMD or BMD, although aggressive support through physiotherapy, the use of steroids, and CPAP is improving life expectancy by a few years. Gene therapy approaches may offer hope in the long term. Using transgenic and naturally occurring dystrophin-negative mutant mice, direct injection of recombinant DNA, myoblast implantation, and transfection with retroviral or adenoviral vectors carrying a *DMD* minigene (containing only those sequences that code for important functional domains) have all been tried. Another approach is antisense technology (p. 222) to block an exon-splicing enhancer sequence—"exon-skipping"—to generate a protein with an in-frame deletion that encodes a protein with residual function, that is, a BMD rather than a DMD phenotype. The latest technique offering hope—"gene editing"—using a molecular approach called CRISPR/Cas9 (p. 47) has similar aims and relies on a sequence of RNA to steer the enzyme Cas9 to the mutation site in *DMD*. Cas9 excises the faulty exon and repairs the DNA sequence to produce a shortened, functional version of the gene. This has been shown to improve performance in mice injected in multiple muscle sites with a viral vector.

Limb-Girdle Muscular Dystrophies

This broad group of muscular dystrophies are rarer than their dystrophinopathy counterparts, but a number of them are biologically related by virtue of the common mechanistic link and interaction of membrane-bound muscle proteins (see Fig. 19.13)—the sarcoglycan complex. Clinically, the pattern of weakness and wasting is mostly confined to the limbs, with proximal groups more severely affected than distal ones. The age of onset, progression, and natural history vary greatly according to the genetic subtype. Serum CK is usually elevated but to nowhere near the extent seen in males with DMD, and a muscle biopsy shows degeneration and regeneration (dystrophic) changes. Once an XL dystrophinopathy has been ruled out, specific immunostaining or immunblotting can be performed on muscle tissue to help reach a more precise diagnosis, specifically a sarcoglycanopathy, calpainopathy, dysferlinopathy, or even dystroglycanopathy (O-linked glycosylation defects). Where staining points to a particular protein abnormality, mutation studies of the corresponding gene can be performed.

Regarding subtypes, limb-girdle muscular dystrophy (LGMD) type 1 is the designation reserved for those entities following AD inheritance, whereas LGMD2 covers the AR forms. The latter incorporates the sarcoglycanopathies as well as calpain and dysferlin, and cardiac involvement is sometimes present. The dystroglycanopathies cover most of the congenital muscular dystrophies, (e.g., the *FKRP*, *FKTN*, *POMT1*, and *POMT2* genes). LGMD1 incorporates defects of caveolin (LGMD1C; *CAV3* gene)—the so-called "rippling muscle disease"—and desmin (LGMD1D; *DES* gene), which can also include cardiac conduction problems and a form of dilated cardiomyopathy. LGMD1B defines the condition because of mutations in *LMNA*, in which cardiac conduction defects are also important. The *LMNA* gene is known for its extremely pleiotropic associated phenotypes (p. 69), but in this context it is synonymous with the autosomal variety of Emery-Dreifuss muscular dystrophy (EDMD), and both dominant and, rarely, recessive forms occur.

The XL recessive EDMD is worthy of mention here, not only because it is an important differential diagnosis of the LGMD group but also because of the pioneering work of the geneticist after whom both the condition and this book are named. Muscle weakness and wasting are progressive and seen first in a humero-peroneal distribution, later extending to the scapular and pelvic girdle muscles. This is accompanied by the onset of contractures of the elbow joints and Achilles tendons in childhood, and cardiac involvement including arrhythmia and later congestive heart failure. The *EMD* gene encodes the protein emerin, which localizes to the inner nuclear membrane and functions in anchorage of the membrane to the cytoskeleton.

Facioscapulohumeral Muscular Dystrophy

Facioscapulohumeral muscular dystrophy (FSHD), occuring in up to 10 individuals per 100,000 members of the population, follows AD inheritance and is characterized, as the name helpfully indicates, by muscle weakness involving the face, scapular muscles, and upper arm. In addition, the peroneal and hip girdle muscles of the leg are involved. It is very variable but usually presents in adolescence and is progressive, with approximately 20% of sufferers requiring a wheelchair by mid-life. Winging of the scapulae is evident (Fig. 19.15), and facial weakness can be assessed by asking the patient to attempt to smile (Fig. 19.16), whistle, pout the lips, and grimace, all of which are limited. Eyelid weakness is present, and some sufferers are noted to sleep with their eyes open. Approximately half of patients have a peripheral retinal vasculopathy, although this does not affect vision, and at least half develop a high-tone sensorineural hearing loss (SNHL).

The genetics of FSHD are intriguing, and two types are now recognized. The chromosome 4q35 subtelomeric region contains a microsatellite repeat called *D4Z4*, within which is located a double homeobox gene, *DUX4*. Both FSHD1 and FSHD2 result from inappropriate expression of *DUX4*. Normal *D4Z4* alleles contain between 11 and 100 repeats, each approximately 3.3 kb in size,

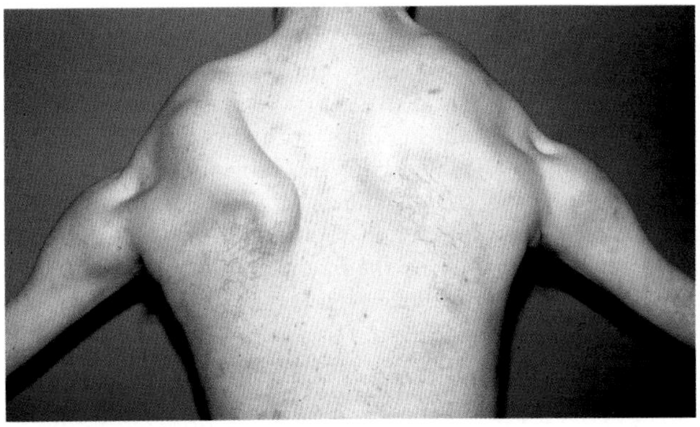

• **Figure 19.15** Facioscapulohumeral dystrophy. Winging, or prominence, of the scapulae.

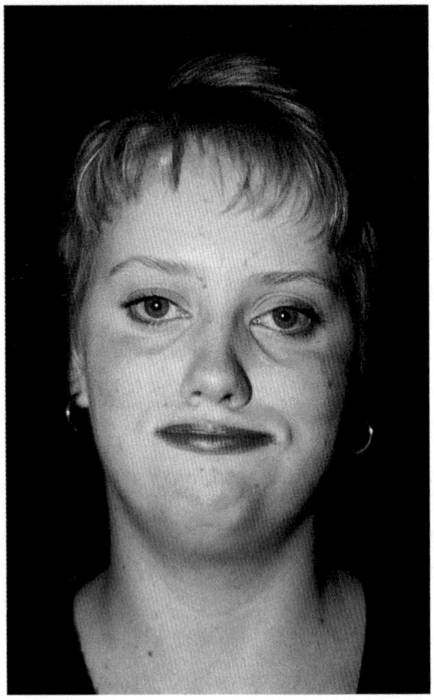

• **Figure 19.16** Facioscapulohumeral dystrophy. Facial muscle weakness—the patient is attempting to smile broadly.

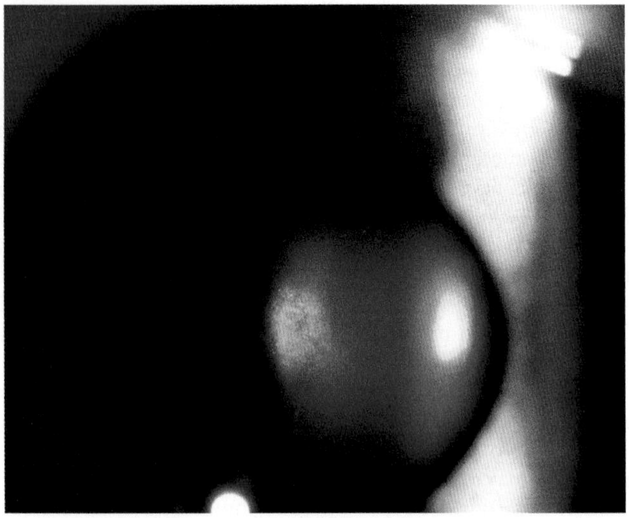

• **Figure 19.17** Refractile lens opacities in an asymptomatic person with myotonic dystrophy. (Courtesy of R. Doran and M. Geall, Department of Ophthalmology, General Infirmary, Leeds, UK.)

but in FSHD1 contraction of *D4Z4* occurs such that the repeat number is reduced to between 1 and 10 units. This contraction leads to relaxation, or opening, of the chromatin structure, including the *DUX4* promoter, which in turn causes *derepression* of *DUX4*. FSHD1 therefore follows AD inheritance, as these changes are heterozygous at 4q35 and account for approximately 95% of FSHD overall. However, the genetics are more complicated, because: (1) the *D4Z4* contraction is pathogenic only on the background of a particular haplotype; and (2) a repeat sequence almost identical to *D4Z4* is present on 10q26 (and therefore readily detected by standard molecular testing), but the *DUX4*-like gene at this locus does not transcribe to a stable product.

In FSHD2, chromatin relaxation at the *D4Z4* locus also occurs, but not because of the contraction of units. Instead, this occurs because of loss of CpG methylation caused by heterozygous mutations in the *SMCHD1* gene (at chromosome 18p11), although again requires the permissive 4q35 haplotype. FSHD2 is therefore an example of digenic inheritance (p. 76).

Myotonic Dystrophy Type 1

Myotonic dystrophy type 1 (MD1) is the most common form of muscular dystrophy seen in adults, with an overall incidence of approximately 1:8000. Like HD (see Table 19.1), it shows AD inheritance with anticipation, and an early-onset form with different clinical features. However, in MD the early-onset form is transmitted almost exclusively by the mother and presents at birth, in contrast to juvenile HD, which is generally paternally transmitted with an age of onset in the teens.

Clinical Features

Individuals with MD usually present in adult life with slowly progressive weakness and myotonia—which refers to tonic muscle spasm with prolonged relaxation. This can manifest as a delay in releasing the grip on shaking hands. However, MD1 is a multisystem disorder, and other clinical features include cataracts (Fig. 19.17), cardiac conduction defects, disturbed gastrointestinal peristalsis (dysphagia, constipation, diarrhea), weak sphincters, increased risk of diabetes mellitus and gallstones, somnolence, frontal balding, and testicular atrophy. Delayed recovery from general anesthesia may also occur. The age of onset is very variable, and in its mildest form the condition usually runs a relatively benign course. However, as the age of onset becomes earlier, the clinical symptoms increase in severity, and more body systems are involved. In the "congenital" form, affected babies present at birth with hypotonia, talipes, and respiratory distress that can prove life threatening (see Fig. 6.19). Children who survive have a facial myopathy with delayed motor development and intellectual disability (Fig. 19.18). Important components of the management of MD1 include regular surveillance for cardiac conduction defects and the provision of information about risks associated with general anesthesia.

Presymptomatic genetic testing and prenatal diagnosis can be offered where appropriate and acceptable, accompanied by a full explanation and support. This is particularly relevant for couples at risk of having a child with the severe congenital form.

Genetics

It follows AD inheritance with increasing severity in succeeding generations—**anticipation** (p. 76). This was once believed to reflect ascertainment bias, but clinical studies in the 1980s confirmed anticipation to be a real phenomenon, and the molecular basis provides the explanation. In 1992, the mutational basis was shown to be instability in a CTG repeat sequence present in the 3′ untranslated region of a protein kinase gene, now named dystrophia myotonica protein kinase *(DMPK)*. In unaffected persons the CTG sequence lying 3′ to the *DMPK* gene consists of up to 37 repeats (see Table 19.1). Affected individuals have an expansion of at least 50 CTG repeats. There is a close correlation between disease severity and the size of the expansion, which can exceed 2000 repeats or more. The severe congenital cases show the largest repeat copy number, with almost invariable inheritance from the mother. Thus meiotic or germline instability is greater in the female for

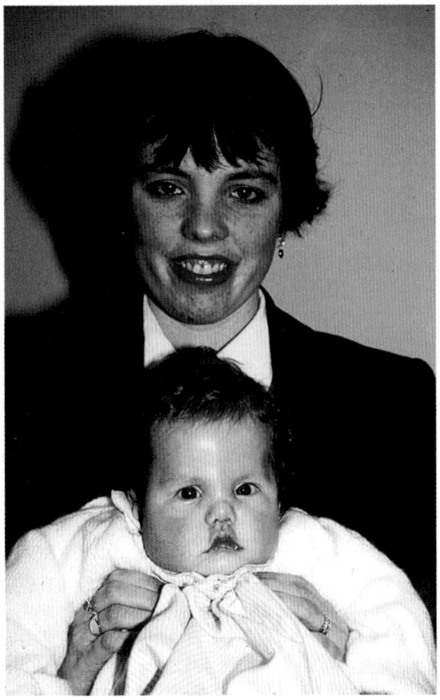

• **Figure 19.18** A mother and child with myotonic dystrophy. The child has clear features of facial myopathy and suffers from the congenital form; the mother has only mild facial myopathy. The marked generational difference in the severity of disease illustrates the phenomenon of anticipation.

alleles containing large sequences. Expansion of a relatively small number of repeats appears to occur more commonly in males, and most MD mutations are thought to have originated during spermatogenesis. One possible explanation for these observations is that mature spermatozoa can carry only small expansions, whereas ova can accommodate much larger expansions.

A curious feature of MD1 is the reported tendency for healthy individuals, heterozygous for MD alleles in the normal size range, to preferentially transmit alleles greater than 19 CTG repeats in size. This possible example of meiotic drive (p. 89) might explain the constant replenishment of a reservoir of potential MD mutations.

Perhaps surprisingly, it may be that *DMPK* is not directly responsible for muscle symptoms—mice with both overexpression and underexpression of *Dmpk* show neither myotonia nor other typical clinical features of MD. We now know that the RNA produced by expanded *DMPK* alleles interferes with the cellular processing of RNA produced by a variety of other genes. Expanded *DMPK* transcripts accumulate in the cell nuclei and are believed to have a gain-of-function effect through binding with a CUG RNA-binding protein (CUG-BP) that has been identified. Excess CUG-BP has been shown to interfere with a number of genes relevant to MD, and CUG repeats are known to exist in various alternately spliced muscle-specific enzymes.

Myotonic Dystrophy Type 2

Some families with a variable presentation of similar features to MD1, but without the $(CTG)_n$ expansion of *DMPK*, have a genetically distinct condition linked to 3q21. Originally referred to as **proximal myotonic myopathy**, these cases are designated MD type 2. The molecular defect has been shown to be a $(CCTG)_n$ expansion mutation in intron 1 of a gene called *ZNF9*, and the protein that it encodes is thought to bind RNA. Most families are of German descent, and haplotype studies suggest a single founder mutation occurring between 200 and 500 generations ago.

Respiratory Disorders

Cystic Fibrosis

Cystic fibrosis (CF) was first recognized as a discrete entity in 1936 and was known as "mucoviscidosis" because of the accumulation of thick mucus secretions that lead to blockage of the airways and secondary infection. Although physiotherapy, antibiotics, and pancreatic supplementation have been very effective in improving life expectancy from less than 5 years in 1955 to at least 30 years, CF remains a significant cause of chronic ill health and premature death. CF is the most common severe AR disorder in western Europe, the incidence varying from 1 in 2000 to 1 in 3000. The incidence is slightly lower in eastern and southern European populations, and much lower in both African (1 in 15,000) and Asian (1 in 31,000) Americans.

Clinical Features

The organs most commonly affected in CF are the lungs and pancreas. Chronic lung disease caused by recurrent infection eventually leads to fibrotic changes with secondary cardiac failure, that is, **cor pulmonale**. At this stage only a successful heart-lung transplant will provide long term benefit.

In 85% of CF sufferers, pancreatic function is impaired with reduced enzyme secretion from blockage of the pancreatic ducts by inspissated secretions leading to malabsorption and an increase in the fat content of stools. However, it is satisfactorily treated with oral pancreatic enzyme supplements. Other problems commonly encountered in CF include nasal polyps, rectal prolapse, cirrhosis, and diabetes mellitus. A small percentage of children with CF present in the newborn period with **meconium ileus**—obstruction of the small bowel from thickened meconium.

Almost all males with CF are infertile because of congenital bilateral absence of the vas deferens (CBAVD). On occasion CBAVD is the only feature of CF, and one can debate whether CF is the correct designation. Other rare presentations include chronic pancreatitis, diffuse bronchiectasis and bronchopulmonary allergic aspergillosis.

Genetics

As indicated, CF follows AR inheritance and is relatively common. Possible explanations for the high incidence include a high mutation rate, meiotic drive, and heterozygote advantage. The latter explanation, possibly mediated by increased heterozygote resistance to chloride-secreting bacterially induced diarrhea, is sometimes favored, although does not explain why CF is rare in tropical regions where diarrheal diseases are common. The mapping and isolation of the CF gene was a celebrated milestone in human molecular genetics, and it is easy to forget how very difficult and time consuming such progress was 30 years ago. The CF locus was mapped to chromosome 7q31 in 1985 by the demonstration of a series of linkages to a number of markers. The gene was eventually cloned by two groups of scientists in North America in 1989 by a combination of chromosome jumping, physical mapping, isolation of exon sequences and variant analysis. It was named the CF transmembrane conductance regulator *(CFTR)* gene (or alternatively *ABCC7*), spans a genomic region of

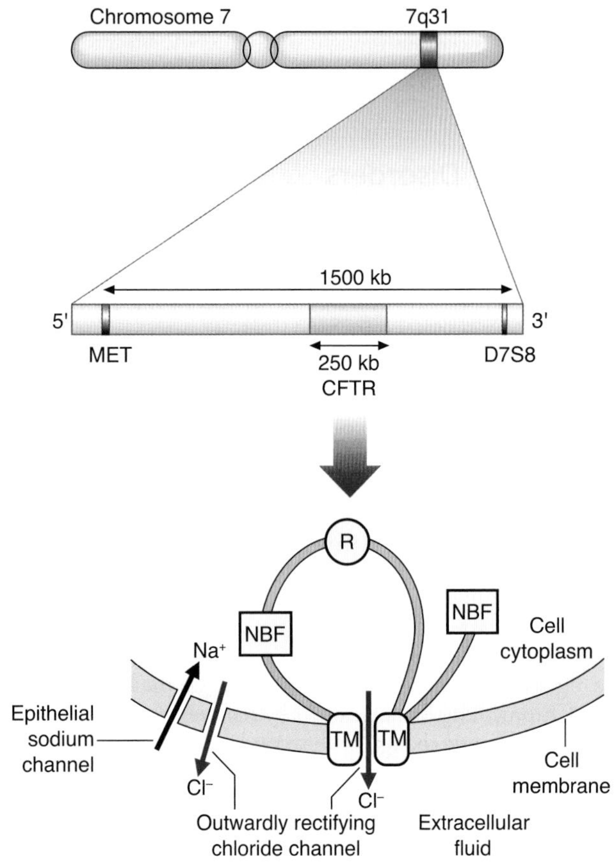

• **Figure 19.19** The cystic fibrosis locus, gene and protein product, which influences closely adjacent epithelial sodium and outwardly rectifying chloride channels. *CFTR*, Cystic fibrosis transmembrane conductance regulator; *R*, regulatory domain; *NBF*, nucleotide binding fold; *TM*, transmembrane domain.

approximately 250 kb and contains 27 exons. In due course one particular CF variant was found to be associated with one particular haplotype pattern in more than 80% of cases, consistent with a single ancestral variant having occurred and thus responsible for a large proportion of CF.

The CFTR protein contains 1480 amino acids and has a molecular weight of 168 kDa. It consists of two transmembrane domains that anchor it to the cell membrane, two nucleotide binding folds (NBFs) that bind ATP, and a regulatory domain, which is phosphorylated by protein kinase A (Fig. 19.19). The primary function of the CFTR protein is to act as a chloride channel. Activation by phosphorylation of the regulatory domain, followed by binding of ATP to the NBF domains, opens the outwardly rectifying chloride channel and exerts a negative effect on intracellular sodium absorption by closure of the epithelial sodium channel. The net effect is to reduce the level of intracellular sodium chloride, which improves the quality of cellular mucus secretions.

The first pathogenic variant to be identified in *CFTR* was a deletion of three adjacent base pairs at the 508th codon, which results in the loss of a phenylalanine residue. Technically, this variant is **c.1521_1523delCTT**, **p.Phe508del** or **F508del** (though the first designation, "deltaF508," is still used by many), and accounts for approximately 70% of all mutations in *CFTR*, the highest incidence occurring in Denmark at 88% (Table 19.2). More than 2000 other variants in the *CFTR* gene have been identified. These include missense, frameshift, splice-site, nonsense, and deletion variants (p. 19). The vast majority are extremely uncommon, although a few can account for a small but significant proportion overall in a particular population. For example, the G542X and G551D variants account for 12% and 3%, respectively, of all CF variants in the Ashkenazi Jewish and North American Caucasian populations. Commercial multiplex polymerase chain reaction-based kits detect approximately 90% of all carriers, and using these can reduce the carrier risk for a healthy individual from 1 in 25 (population risk) to less than 1 in 200.

TABLE 19.2 Contribution of Phe508del mutation to all cystic fibrosis mutations

Country	%
Denmark	88
Netherlands	79
United Kingdom	78
Ireland	75
France	75
United States	66
Germany	65
Poland	55
Italy	50
Turkey	30

(Data from European Working Group on CF Genetics gradient of distribution in Europe of the major CF mutation and of its associated haplotype. *Hum Genet.* 1990; 85:436–445, and Worldwide survey of the Phe508del mutation—report from the Cystic Fibrosis Genetic Analysis Consortium. *Am J Hum Genet.* 1990;47:354–359.)

Variants in *CFTR* can influence the function of the protein product by:

1. Causing a complete or partial reduction in its synthesis—for example, G542X and IVS8-6(5T)
2. Preventing it from reaching the epithelial membrane—for example, Phe508del
3. Causing it to function incorrectly when it reaches its final location—for example, G551D and R117H.

The net effect is to reduce the normal functional activity of the CFTR protein, reduced protein activity, and transmembrane movement of chloride, correlates well with the clinical phenotype. Levels of less than 3% are associated with severe, or "classic," CF, sometimes referred to as the **PI** type because of associated pancreatic insufficiency (PI). Activity levels between 3% and 8% cause a milder "atypical" form of CF in which there is respiratory disease but relatively normal pancreatic function. This is referred to as the pancreatic sufficient (**PS**) form. Finally, levels of activity between 8% and 12% cause the mildest CF phenotype, in which virtually the only clinical abnormality is CBAVD in males.

The genotype-phenotype relationship is complex; homozygotes for Phe508del almost invariably have severe classic CF, as do compound heterozygotes with Phe508del and G551D or G542X. The outcome for other compound heterozygote combinations can be much more difficult to predict.

The complexity of the interaction between *CFTR* alleles is illustrated by the IVS8-6 poly T variant. This contains a polythymidine tract in intron 8 that influences the splicing efficiency of exon 9, resulting in reduced synthesis of normal CFTR protein. Three variants consisting of 5T, 7T, and 9T have been identified. The 9T variant is associated with normal activity, but the 5T allele leads to a reduction in the number of transcripts containing exon 9. The 5T variant has a population frequency of approximately 5%, but is more often found in patients with CBAVD (40%–50%) or disseminated bronchiectasis (30%). Curiously, it has been shown that the number of thymidine residues influences the effect of another mutation, R117H. When R117H is in *cis* with 5T, it causes the PS form of CF when another CF mutation is present on the other allele. However, in compound heterozygotes, for example, Phe508del/R117H, where R117H is in *cis* with 7T, it can result in a milder but variable phenotype, ranging from CBAVD to PS CF. A mild phenotype is likely to result from the expression of higher levels of full-length R117H protein with some residual activity. The increasing number of *CFTR* variants and the clinical variability provoke the question that a label of CF may be inappropriate for patients with milder symptoms.

Prenatal testing, as well as preimplantation genetic diagnosis, can be offered to couples at risk of having a child with CF (see Chapter 20). Carrier testing of the relatives of those who are carriers, or affected with known mutations, is standard practice in many countries—known as **cascade screening**. Population screening aimed at identifying CF carriers (p. 159) and neonatal screening aimed at identifying CF homozygotes (p. 158) have been widely implemented.

CF is a prime candidate for gene therapy because of the relative accessibility of the main target organs—the lungs. Several clinical trials in small groups of volunteer patients with CF, using viral vectors in an attempt to deliver a normal copy of *CFTR*, have been disappointing. A new drug treatment approved by the US Food and Drug Administration in 2012—**Orkambi**—is attracting much attention because it appears to slow the progression of lung disease in CF. It is expensive, not surprisingly, and suitable only for Phe508del homozygotes. It contains two component drugs—*lumacaftor* enables more CFTR protein to the reach the cell surface, while *ivacaftor* opens the ion channel, thus enabling CFTR to function (see also Chapter 15, p. 217).

Alpha-1 Antitrypsin Deficiency

Alpha-1 antitrypsin deficiency (AATD) is an important cause of chronic obstructive pulmonary disease (COPD), with emphysema being the most likely manifestation, but also chronic bronchitis and bronchiectasis, with the onset of symptoms in early middle life in smokers and slightly later in non-smokers. In addition, liver disease may present at almost any age, including obstructive jaundice in infancy. It is inherited as an AR trait with a frequency of 1:1500 or greater, making disease alleles more common in the population than those of CF. However, as a later-onset condition with reduced penetrance, it is not perceived as being as serious as CF.

The diagnosis relies on biochemical assay of alpha-1 antitrypsin (AAT) levels, and, unlike many genetic conditions, variant analysis of the gene, *SERPINA1*, is unlikely to supersede well-established and reliable clinical chemistry. Levels of AAT are low in carriers and very low in homozygotes. Once these low levels have been determined, further characterization—"phenotyping"—of the abnormal protein—the **protease inhibitor (Pi)**—is usually performed. The normal function of this protein is to block the damaging action of the body's protease enzymes. "Pi typing" uses the technique of polyacrylamide gel isoelectric focusing (IEF) electrophoresis, with the different protein variants, or isoforms, designated by letters according to their migration pattern. The normal protein is "M"—hence the allele is known as Pi*M, and most of the population are therefore PiMM. The most pathogenic allele, and the slowest moving on IEF, is "Z," followed by "S," which shows reduced penetrance, and between them these alleles account for approximately 95% of AATD. Roughly 1:50 people in the general population are PiMZ, and approximately 1:20 are PiMS.

The emphysema risk for ZZ individuals is greater than 80%, for SZ up to 50%, and for SS there is little difference to the background risk. Childhood liver disease in AATD is confined to the ZZ phenotype and may occur in up to 20%, being severe in approximately 2%. Between 15% and 20% of ZZ adults aged over 50 years develop liver cirrhosis, with lower risks at younger ages. It is recognized, however, that these risks are higher where a sibling is relatively severely affected, which applies at all ages. The treatment and management of AATD centers on prevention and monitoring. Avoidance or cessation of smoking is crucial, and very good advice for carriers too, and alcohol intake should be minimal, if at all. COPD is managed in the standard way, and in severe cases transplantation surgery (lungs and liver) may be indicated.

Pulmonary Arterial Hypertension

In clinical practice pulmonary arterial hypertension (PAH) is an important cause of morbidity, and the symptoms are nonspecific, ranging from none to dyspnea (most commonly), general fatigue, syncope, palpitations, and chest pain. The majority of cases are secondary to other causes, such as heart disease (including congenital heart disease, cardiomyopathies, valve disease), advanced lung disease (including CF), pulmonary embolism, and hereditary hemorrhagic telangiectasia (HHT—see later). The diagnosis may be suspected clinically and from various non-invasive investigations, such as electrocardiogram (ECG) or echocardiography (providing evidence of right ventricular hypertrophy or strain), but may require confirmation by the invasive procedure of cardiac catheterisation and direct measurement of pulmonary artery pressure.

PAH has a place here because of the relatively uncommon heritable form, which is obviously suspected when two or more family members have been affected and other more common causes have been excluded—and used to be known as primary pulmonary hypertension. The heritable form follows AD inheritance and is clinically indistinguishable from other causes of PAH. Roughly 75% of cases are caused by a pathogenic variant in the *BMPR2* gene but rarely pathogenic variants have been identified in other genes, including *ACVRL1*, *ENG*, *KCNK3*, *CAV1*, *SMAD9*, and *BMPR1B*. Both *ACVRL1* and *ENG* are important genes in HHT, and PAH-associated genes in general are members of the transforming growth factor β (TGF-β) superfamily of cell-signaling molecules (p. 108).

Medical treatment of PAH does not alter the underlying pathology significantly, but lung transplantation improves survival—though the limited availability of donors and the magnitude of the surgery greatly restrict this option.

Hereditary Hemorrhagic Telangiectasia

HHT, also known as Osler-Weber-Rendu disease, has almost certainly been underdiagnosed in the past, despite its place in medical history. Like hereditary PAH, it is essentially a genetically determined disorder of vasculature, and the genes implicated are part of

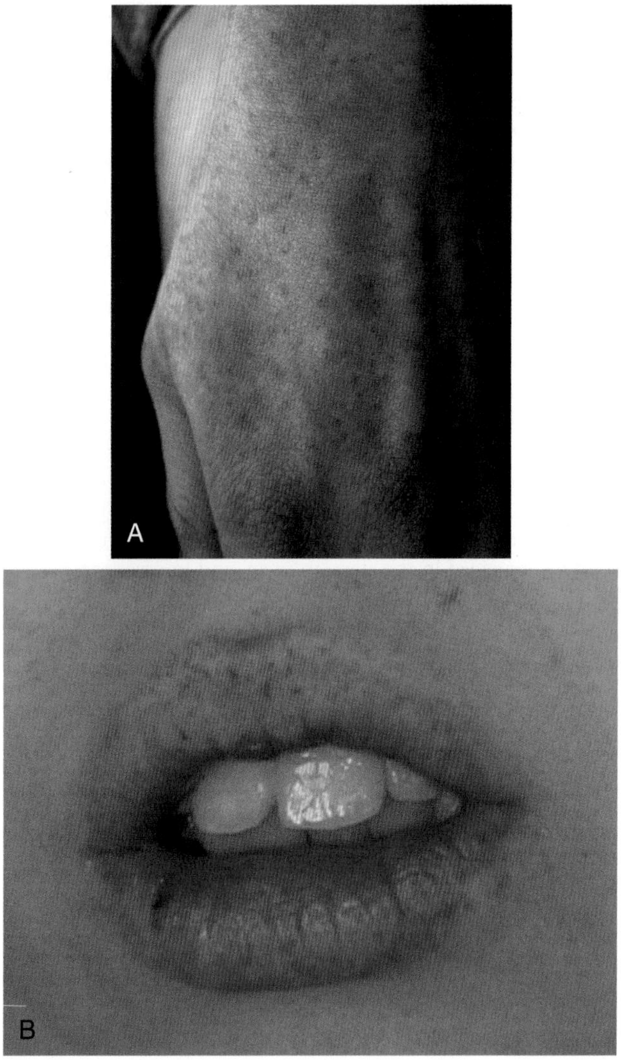

• **Figure 19.20** Hereditary hemorrhagic telangiectasia. Characteristic mucocutaneous telangiectasia on (A) the hands and (B) the lips.

the TGF-β/BMP signaling cascade (p. 108). The key features are quite distinctive, namely spontaneous and recurrent nosebleeds (epistaxis), multiple mucocutaneous telangiectases seen on the hands (Fig. 19.20A), nose, lips, and mouth (Fig. 19.20B) and arteriovenous malformations (AVMs) affecting primarily the lungs but also the gastrointestinal tract, liver, and cerebral circulation.

Occasionally, hemorrhage from an AVM can be prolonged, and hence serious and life threatening, simply from extensive blood loss. Hemorrhage from a cerebral AVM, present in approximately 10% of HHT patients, carries a high risk of neurological sequelae, and there is ongoing debate regarding the merits of actively scanning patients with HHT to identify such lesions. There is a consensus that pregnant women should have a spinal scan to ascertain whether asymptomatic AVMs are located in the lumbar spinal canal, which would contraindicate having an epidural or spinal anesthetic. There is also a clear consensus to actively screen for pulmonary AVMs, which occur in up to half of affected patients, by contrast echocardiography. If large and untreated, these can lead to high-output heart failure, and the migration of emboli to the cerebral circulation can give rise to blood vessel occlusion and cerebral abscess. These pulmonary AVMs are treated by embolization, and prophylactic antibiotic cover is recommended for dental procedures.

HHT is an AD condition with several known associated genes—*ENG*, *ACVRL1* (which together account for the majority of mutation-positive cases), *SMAD4*, and *GDF2*. In addition, there are believed to be at least two more loci as yet unidentified.

Inherited Cardiac Conditions

In approximately 4% of sudden cardiac death in persons aged 16 to 64 years no explanation is evident. In England this equates to approximately 200 such deaths annually, each one enormously traumatic for the family left behind. Understandably, there can be great anxiety when this is familial and affects young people. The terms **sudden cardiac death**, **inherited cardiac condition** (**ICC**), and (less often now) **sudden adult death syndrome** are used.

Inherited Arrhythmias

This group of conditions includes the **long QT syndromes** (**LQTSs**), **Brugada syndrome**, and **catecholaminergic** (stress-induced) **polymorphic ventricular tachycardia** (**CPVT**). LQTS and Brugada syndrome are sodium and potassium **ion channelopathies**. Calcium channel defects include **CPVT**, **Timothy syndrome**, and **arrhythmogenic right ventricular cardiomyopathy** (**ARVC**), the latter usually considered under "inherited cardiomyopathies." Overlap between arrhythmogenic disorders and cardiomyopathies is also evident in the XL (*EMD* gene) and autosomal (*LMNA* gene) forms of **Emery-Dreifuss muscular dystrophy**, the **desminopathies** and the **caveolinopathies** (mentioned earlier under "Limb-Girdle Muscular Dystrophies," p. 301).

When sudden unexplained death occurs, a careful review of the postmortem findings and an exploration of the history of the deceased, as well as the family history, are indicated. Most who die are young males, and death may occur during sleep or while inactive. In a proportion of cases, death occurs while swimming, especially in LQTS type 1. Emotional stress can be a trigger, especially in LQTS2, and cardiac events are more likely in sleep for LQTS2 and LQTS3. Careful investigation and questioning may reveal an antecedent history of episodes of syncope, palpitation, chest discomfort, and dyspnea, and these symptoms should be explored in the relatives in relation to possible triggers. If the deceased had a 12-lead ECG, this may hold some key evidence; however, a normal ECG is present in approximately 30% of proven cases of LQTS, and possibly in a higher proportion of Brugada syndrome cases.

In LQTS, also known as **Romano-Ward syndrome**, the ECG findings are dominated by—as the name suggests—a QT interval outside the normal limits, remaining long when the heart rate increases. They are classified according to the gene involved (Table 19.3). The inheritance is overwhelmingly AD, but a rare recessive form exists combined with sensorineural deafness, which is known as **Jervell and Lange-Nielsen syndrome**. The ECG changes may be evident from a young age, and a cardiac event occurs by age 10 years in approximately 50%, and by age 20 years in 90%. First cardiac events tend to be later in LQTS2 and LQTS3. Predictive genetic testing, where possible, is helpful to identify those at risk in affected families, and decisions about prophylactic β-blockade can be made. β-Blockers are particularly useful in LQTS1 but less so in LQTS2 and LQTS3—indeed, it is possible that β-blockers may be harmful in LQTS3. Overall, LQTS1 and LQTS2 account for approximately one-third of all LQTSs, LQTS3 for 5% to 10%, and LQTS4 to LQTS15 for less

TABLE 19.3 The inherited cardiac arrhythmias

Arrhythmia Locus	Onset	Triggers/Other Features	Gene	Locus
LQTS1 (Romano-Ward)	90% by age 20 years	Exercise (swimming)	*KCNQ1*	11p15
LQTS2	Early adult life	Stress/sleep	*KCNH2*	7q35
LQTS3	Early adult life	Stress/sleep	*SCN5A*	3p21
LQTS4	Adulthood		*Ankyrin-B*	4q25
LQTS5	Childhood		*KCNE1*	21q22
LQTS6	Adulthood		*KCNE2*	21q22
LQTS7 (Andersen-Tawil syndrome)	Adulthood	Muscle weakness, periodic paralysis, mandibular hypoplasia	*KCNJ2*	17q23
LQTS8 (Timothy syndrome)	Childhood	Syndactyly, learning disability, autism	*CACNA1C*	12p13
LQTS9	Childhood		*CAV3*	3p25
LQTS10	Any age		*SCN4B*	11q23
LQTS11	Childhood		*AKAP9*	7q21
LQTS12	Childhood		*SNTA1*	20q11
LQTS13	Adulthood		*KCNJ5*	11q24
LQTS14	Childhood		*CAML1*	14q32
LQTS15	Childhood		*CALM2*	2p21
Brugada syndrome	Adulthood		*SCN5A*	3p21
CPVT	Childhood/adolescence	Stress	*RYR2*	1q42
ARVC1	Childhood/adolescence		*TGFB3*	14q23
ARVC2	Childhood/adolescence		*RYR2*	1q42
ARVC3, 4, 6	Childhood/adolescence			14q12, 2q32, 10p14
ARVC5	Childhood/adolescence		*TMEM43*	3p25
ARVC7 (Myofibrillar myopathy)	Childhood/adolescence		*DES*	2q35
ARVC8	Childhood/adolescence		*Desmoplakin*	6p24
ARVC9	Childhood/adolescence		*PKP2—plakophilin-2*	12p11
ARVC10	Childhood/adolescence		*DSG2*	
ARVC11	Childhood/adolescence		*DSC2*	
ARVC12 (Naxos disease, autosomal recessive)	Childhood		*JUP—plakoglobin*	17q21

ARVC, Arrhythmogenic right ventricular cardiomyopathy; *CPVT*, catecholaminergic polymorphic ventricular tachycardia; *LQTS*, long QT syndromes.

than 1%. Molecular testing is negative in approximately 20%. In perhaps 5% of cases digenic inheritance is seen, usually giving rise to a severe phenotype.

Brugada syndrome, like LQTS, follows AD inheritance, and was first described in 1992. The cardiac event is characterized by a proneness to idiopathic ventricular tachycardia (VT), and there may be abnormal ST-wave elevation in the right chest leads with incomplete right bundle branch block. In at-risk family members with a normal ECG the characteristic abnormalities can usually be unmasked by the administration of potent sodium channel blockers such as flecainide. The condition is relatively common in Southeast Asia, with a male:female ratio of 8:1. The average age of arrhythmic events is 40, but very-early-onset cases occasionally occur. The definitive treatment is an implantable defibrillator, and exercise is not a particular risk factor. Pathogenic variants in the *SCN5A* gene are found in approximately 20% of Brugada syndrome patients, as well as some cases of LQTS3 (see Table 19.3). In some families both arrhythmias occur. Variants in at least

23 genes are currently implicated in Brugada syndrome, but apart from those in *SCN5A*, all are rare.

In **CPVT**, also known as **Coumel's VT**, individuals with CPVT present with syncopal events, often in childhood or adolescence, and reproducible stress-induced VT, without a prolonged QT interval. At rest the ECG is normal, and the heart is also structurally normal. *RYR2* is the gene most commonly implicated in CPVT—approximately 50% of cases—and heterozygous variants cause a dominantly inherited form, as do variants in *CALM1*, rarely. Homozygosity or compound heterozygosity for variants in *CASQ2* cause an AR form of CPVT, as do variants in *TRDN* (rare).

Inherited Cardiomyopathies

Hypertrophic cardiomyopathy (HCM) is genetically heterogeneous, and the large majority of cases follow AD inheritance. The group includes asymmetric septal hypertrophy, hypertrophic subaortic stenosis, and ventricular hypertrophy. In general, septal hypertrophy of 15 mm in isolated cases, and 13 mm in the context of an affected family, is diagnostic of HCM. Sudden death can occur, especially in young athletes. The two most common single genes involved are *MYH7* (14q11) and *MYBPC3* (11p11), which encode the cardiac β-myosin heavy chain and myosin-binding protein C-cardiac type, respectively. The next significant contribution is from *TNNT2* (1q32) and *TNNI3* (19q13), encoding the "T" and "I" isoforms of cardiac troponin, respectively, but there are many other genes implicated, most of them very rare. The variant detection rate from gene panel tests is approximately 60% when HCM is clearly familial. Cardiomyopathy associated with *TNNT2* in particular may appear to be mild and with subclinical hypertrophy, but there is nevertheless a high incidence of sudden death. Mutations in this and some other genes are sometimes implicated in dilated cardiomyopathy, left ventricular non-compaction, and secondary arrhythmias.

Clinically, when assessing a family, it is important to look for male-male transmission of HCM in the pedigree because this excludes Fabry disease (p. 281) as a cause and is easily ruled out by a biochemical assay of alpha-galactosidase in males (Table 15.2; p. 216). Enzyme replacement therapy is available. The astute clinician should also be aware that Noonan syndrome (p. 233) can include HCM as a feature.

Dilated cardiomyopathy (DCM) is characterized by cardiac dilatation and reduced systolic function. Causes include myocarditis, coronary artery disease, systemic and metabolic diseases, and toxins. When these are excluded, the prevalence of idiopathic DCM is 35 to 40 per 100,000, and familial cases account for approximately 25% of cases. As with the inherited cardiac arrhythmias, they are genetically heterogeneous but nearly always follow AD inheritance. They are also very variable, and within the same family affected members may show symptoms in childhood at one end of the spectrum and very late onset of symptoms at the other. As with HCM, many genes and loci are implicated in DCM, the most common (up to 20%) being *TTN* (2q31), encoding titin, which may also cause a generalized proximal myopathy. DCM may also result from variants in the *LMNA* gene (1q22), which encodes lamin A/C and is noted for its pleiotropic effects (p. 69). Overall, because there are several non-genetic causes of DCM, the mutation detection rate from gene panel tests is considerably lower than with HCM.

ARVC usually follows AD inheritance and is characterized by localized or diffuse atrophy and fatty infiltration of the right ventricular myocardium. It can lead to VT and sudden cardiac death in young people, especially athletes with apparently normal hearts. The ECG shows right precordial T-wave inversion and prolongation of the QRS complex. ARVC demonstrates substantial genetic heterogeneity (see Table 19.3), with at least 13 genes identified, one of which, *junction plakoglobin* (*JUP*), is implicated in the rare recessive form found on the island of Naxos. As in CPVT, the *RYR2* gene accounts for a proportion of cases (type 2), although *PKP2* is the most common overall, with considerable geographical variation.

Genetic testing is routine, but genetic heterogeneity means the pick-up rate for pathogenic variants is approximately 50%. Furthermore, digenic inheritance may account for a significant proportion of cases, and estimates vary widely. After a diagnosis has been made in an index case, a detailed family history is indicated, and investigation of first-degree relatives by ECG, echocardiogram, and cardiac MRI should be offered. Screening may need to continue well into adult life.

Connective Tissue Disorders

This very broad group of conditions includes, at one end of the spectrum, several hundred rare skeletal dysplasias. However, we concentrate on the "mainstream" entities for consistency and include Marfan syndrome (MFS) and related conditions, although for practical clinical purposes these are often grouped with the ICCs.

Marfan Syndrome

The original patient described by the French pediatrician Antoine-Bernard Marfan in 1896 probably had the similar but rarer condition now known as **Beal syndrome**, or **congenital contractual arachnodactyly** (p. 309). In clinical practice physicians often consider the diagnosis of MFS for any patient who is tall with subjective features of long limbs and fingers. However, it is essential to be objective in clinical assessment because a number of conditions have "marfanoid" features, and many tall, thin people simply have constitutional tall stature. Detailed diagnostic criteria, known as the **Ghent criteria**, are in general use by geneticists. In the modern era clinical criteria were published in 1986 (Berlin) and brought up to date in 1996 (Ghent; Table 19.4), and the latter underwent revision in 2010 (Table 19.5).

Clinical Features

MFS is a disorder of fibrous connective tissue, specifically a defect in **fibrillin type 1**, a glycoprotein encoded by the *FBN1* gene. In the classic presentation affected individuals are tall compared with unaffected family members, have joint laxity, a span:height ratio greater than 1.05, a reduced upper to lower segment body ratio, pectus deformity (Fig. 19.21), and scoliosis. The connective tissue defect gives rise to ectopia lentis (lens subluxation) in a proportion of families (but not all) and, very importantly, dilatation of the ascending aorta, which can lead to dissection. The latter complication is obviously life threatening, and for this reason alone care must be taken over the diagnosis. Aortic dilatation may be progressive, but the rate of change can be reduced by β-adrenergic blockade (if tolerated) and angiotensin-II receptor antagonists (similar properties to angiotensin-converting enzyme inhibitors). Surgical replacement should be undertaken if the diameter reaches 50 to 55 mm. Pregnancy is a risk factor for a woman with MFS who already has some dilatation of the aorta, and monitoring is very important.

TABLE 19.4 Ghent criteria for making a diagnosis of Marfan syndrome

Diagnostic Criteria Interpretation

INDEX CASE (NO CONTRIBUTORY FAMILY HISTORY):

- Major criteria should be present in at least two different organ systems, plus involvement of a third organ system
- If a known pathogenic mutation is present, one major criterion in an organ system plus involvement of a second organ system

RELATIVE OF AN INDEX CASE:

- Presence of a major criterion in the family history, and in the relative one major criterion in an organ system plus involvement of a second organ system

Organ System	Major Criteria	Minor Criteria
Skeletal	*Four of these should be present:* Pectus carinatum Pectus excavatum requiring surgery Reduced upper to lower segment body ratio or span:height ratio >1.05 Hypermobility of wrist and thumbs Medial displacement of medial malleolus Radiological protrusio acetabulae	Pectus excavatum Joint hypermobility High arched palate with dental crowding Facial features, including downslanting palpebral fissures causing pes planus
Ocular	Ectopia lentis	Flat cornea Increased axial length of the globe Hypoplastic iris
Cardiovascular	Dilatation of the ascending aorta	Mitral valve prolapse
	Dissection of the ascending aorta	Dilatation or dissection of descending thoracic or abdominal aorta under the age of 50 years
Pulmonary	None	Spontaneous pneumothorax Apical blebs
Skin/connective tissue	Lumbosacral dural ectasia	None
Family history/genetics	First-degree relative who meets criteria	None
	Presence of *FBN1* mutation, or high-risk haplotype in Marfan syndrome family	None

(From De Paepe A, Devereux RB, Dietz HC, et al. Revised diagnostic criteria for the Marfan syndrome. *Am J Med Genet.* 1996;62(4):417–426. With permission.)

A diagnosis of MFS requires careful clinical assessment, body measurements looking for evidence of disproportion, echocardiography, ophthalmic evaluation, and, in some doubtful cases, lumbar MRI to look for evidence of dural ectasia. Neither the metacarpophalangeal index, a radiological measurement of the ratio of these hand bone lengths, nor high-arched palate is considered to have any diagnostic value. Where the family history is non-contributory, a positive diagnosis is made when the patient has a minimum of two major criteria plus involvement of a third organ system in the Ghent criteria (see Table 19.4), but a slightly different system of assessment is proposed in the revised Ghent criteria (see Table 19.5).

Genetics

MFS follows AD inheritance, and the majority of cases are linked to the large *FBN1* gene on 15q21, with 65 exons spanning 200 kb and containing five distinct domains. The largest of these, occupying approximately 75% of the gene, comprises approximately 46 epidermal growth factor repeats (pp. 188, 214). Finding pathogenic variants in affected patients was initially very difficult, but hundreds have now been reported. Most are missense and have a dominant-negative effect, resulting in less than 35% of the expected amount of fibrillin-1 in the extracellular matrix. Variants have also occasionally been found in related phenotypes such as neonatal MFS, familial ectopia lentis, Shrintzen-Goldberg syndrome, and the MASS phenotype (mitral valve prolapse, myopia, borderline aortic enlargement, nonspecific skin and skeletal findings).

Congenital Contractural Arachnodactyly—Beal Syndrome

Congenital contractual arachnodactyly (CCA)—Beal syndome—was probably the condition originally described by Antoine-Bernard Marfan in 1896. Many features overlap with MFS, but there is less risk of aortic dilatation and its catastrophic consequences. Individuals have congenital contractures of their digits, a crumpled ear helix, and sometimes marked scoliosis. It is because of mutated **fibrillin type 2** (*FBN2*), which shares the same organizational structure as fibrillin-1 and maps to 5q23.

Loeys-Dietz Syndrome

Familial aortic aneurysm is not confined to MFS, and the most important "Marfan-like" condition is Loeys-Dietz syndrome (LDS).

TABLE 19.5 Revised Ghent criteria for making a diagnosis of Marfan syndrome

For a Diagnosis of Marfan Syndrome (MFS) (With No Family History):

(1) Aortic root dilatation (Z score ≥ 2) plus ectopia lentis
(2) Aortic root dilatation (Z score ≥ 2) plus pathogenic *FBN1* mutation
(3) Aortic root dilatation (Z score ≥ 2) plus Systemic Score ≥ 7 points (below)
(4) Ectopia lentis plus pathogenic *FBN1* mutation with known aortic root diameter

If Family History (FH) Present:

(5) Ectopia lentis plus FH of MFS, as defined above
(6) Systemic Score (≥ 7 points) plus FH of MFS
(7) Aortic root dilatation (Z score ≥ 2 above 20 years old; ≥ 3 below 20 years old) plus FH of MFS

Systemic Score Feature	Points
Wrist and thumb sign	3
Wrist or thumb sign	1
Pectus carinatum deformity	2
Pectus excavatum or chest asymmetry	1
Hindfoot deformity	2
Plain pes planus	1
Pneumothorax	2
Dural ectasia	2
Protrusio acetabuli	2
Reduced upper segment/lower segment ratio and increased arm/height ratio (and no severe scoliosis)	1
Scoliosis or thoracolumbar kyphosis	1
Reduced elbow extension	1
Facial features (3/5 should be present): dolichocephaly, enophthalmos, downslanting palpebral fissures, malar hypoplasia, retrognathia	1
Skin striae	1
Myopia >3 diopters	1
Mitral valve prolapse (all types)	1

(From Loeys BL, Dietz HC, Braverman AC, et al. The revised Ghent nosology for the Marfan syndrome. *J Med Genet.* 2010;47:476–485. With permission.)

This also follows AD inheritance, and aneurysms can be aggressive and occur before major aortic dilatation—thus surgery is usually recommended when the measurement at the sinus of Valsalva reaches 4.5cm. Additional findings may include cleft palate or bifid uvula, craniosynostosis, mild learning disability, and generalized arterial tortuosity, with aneurysms occurring elsewhere in the circulation. Some individuals have features overlapping with MFS—indeed many of these patients were assumed to have MFS before genetic testing—but they do not fully satisfy the accepted Ghent diagnostic criteria. Affected patients are more prone to simple hernias, as well as having thin, atrophic scars indistinguishable from the type seen in Ehlers-Danlos syndrome (EDS). They do not, however, develop ectopia lentis. An unusual feature, and one that can be helpful in making a clinical diagnosis, is the presence of facial milia (Fig. 19.22). These are small, pearly-white, keratin-filled cysts very similar to "milk spots" seen in newborns (which are not permanent). In cases/families negative for *FBN1* testing, the gene for LDS was identified through a candidate approach. Transforming growth factor (TGF) signaling (p. 108) had been shown to be important in vascular and craniofacial development in mouse models, which led Loeys and colleagues to sequence the TGF-β receptor 2 gene (*TGFBR2*) in a number of families. Heterozygous variants were found in most of these, and in the others missense variants were found in the related gene, *TGFBR1*.

Familial Thoracic Aortic Aneurysm Disease

Clinical geneticists are commonly asked to assess patients with aortic root dilatation, aneurysm, or dissection for features of MFS, especially if they are relatively young. Approximately 20% of individuals with thoracic aortic aneurysm disease (TAAD) have an affected first-degree relative, and sometimes multiple affected relatives. In approximately 5% of TAAD cases an associated finding is the presence of a bicuspid aortic valve (BAV), and BAV is common in the general population—to the extent of approximately 1%—and is frequently familial in its own right—approximately 20% of those requiring surgery have a positive family history.

Overall, barely a quarter of all familial thoracic aortic aneurysm disease (FTAAD) is accounted for by variants in known genes, and in the era of next-generation sequencing regular progress is being made in finding more. It is important to point out that abdominal aortic aneurysm is nearly always caused by a combination of other factors such as age, smoking, hypertension, and atherosclerosis, although in younger people the possibility of vascular Ehlers-Danlos syndrome (vEDS—type IV) should be considered. Common to all cases, however, is degeneration and breakdown of elastic fibers and loss of smooth muscle cells—so-called "medial necrosis."

The age of onset of FTAAD is very variable and may well be asymptomatic until a sudden catastrophic event such as dissection occurs. When suspected, therefore, regular screening of first-degree relatives by echocardiography, MRI, or computed tomography scan is indicated, and a judgment may be necessary about the timing of aortic root replacement surgery. After MFS, CCA, LDS, and vEDS are excluded, genetic testing in FTAAD is not at present very rewarding but is expected to improve. Variants in *ACTA2* are occasionally seen where FTAAD is associated with BAV, and there are also reports of the *NOTCH1* gene being implicated in this scenario. A variant of the *MYH11* gene, encoding a smooth muscle myosin heavy-chain protein, is occasionally seen, and this is important because its locus is 16p13.11, and microdeletions affecting this region are associated with an increased risk of aortic dilatation. Variants in *SMAD3* give rise to a syndromic form of FTAAD that resembles LDS—Loeys-Dietz syndrome type 3—including early-onset osteoarthritis, especially in the knees, spine, and thumb base.

Ehlers-Danlos Syndrome

EDS is a family of connective tissue conditions typically characterized by the triad of joint hypermobility, skin hyperextensibility, and abnormal and delayed wound healing. When all aspects of this triad are florid in their manifestations, the patient usually has EDS—classical type (cEDS), but a wide range of genetically distinct disorders are embraced within the EDS family (Table 19.6).

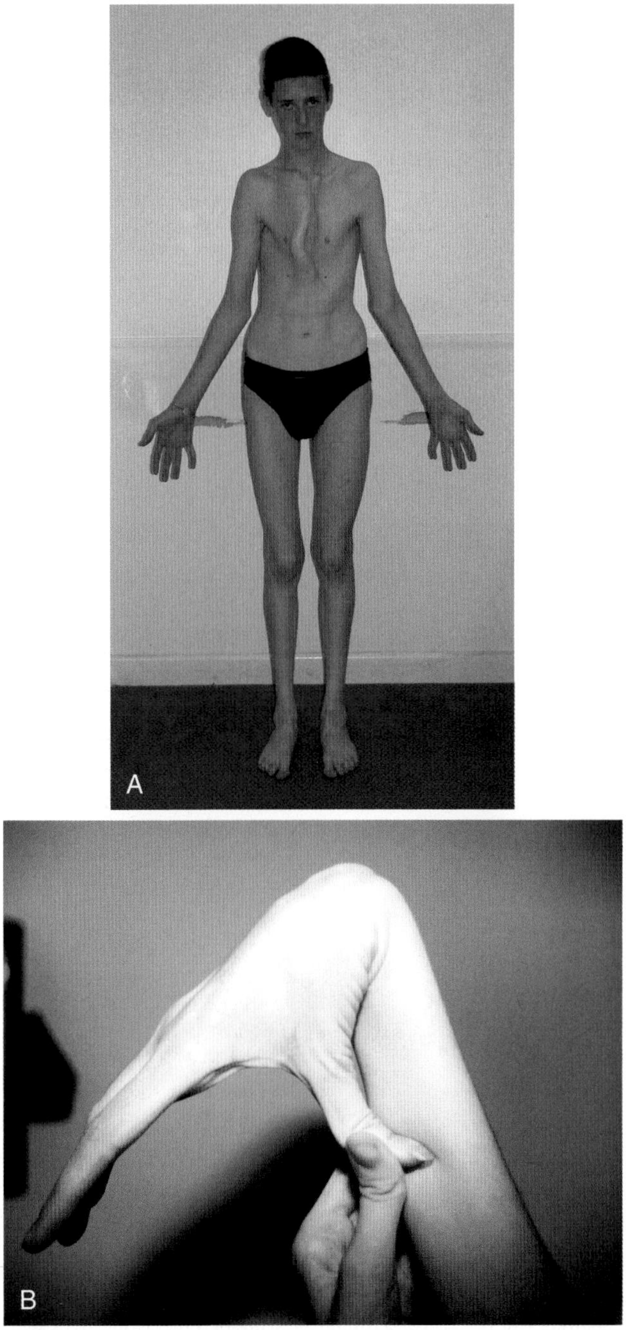

• **Figure 19.21** (A) An adolescent with Marfan syndrome showing disproportionately long limbs (arachnodactyly) and a very extreme example of chest bone deformity; he also has a dilated aortic root. (B) Joint hypermobility at the wrist in a woman with Marfan syndrome; this appearance might also be seen in other joint-laxity conditions, such as Ehlers-Danlos syndrome.

Hyperextensible skin is illustrated in Fig. 21.1, joint (wrist) hypermobility in Fig. 19.21B, and skin features in Fig. 19.23, specifically loose skin, abnormal scars, and subcutaneous spheroids, which comprise calcified fibro-fatty lumps and may be seen in the classical type (but not usually the hypermobile type).

It is not possible here to do justice to the huge range of clinical features and complications that may occur as a consequence of these various tissue laxity/fragility disorders. It is important, however, to appreciate the following:

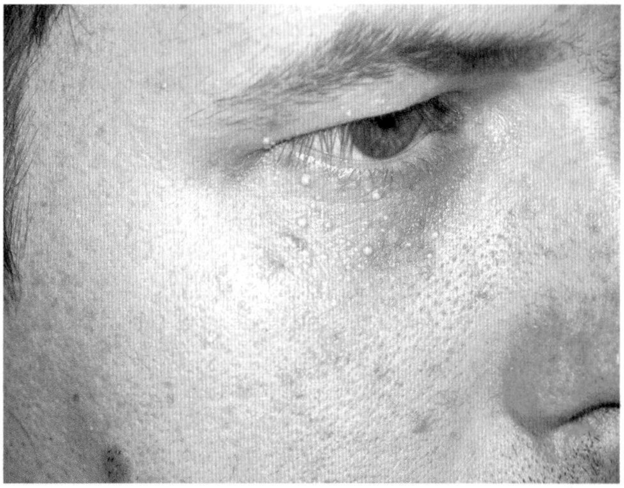

• **Figure 19.22** Loeys-Dietz syndrome (LDS). A cluster of permanent raised white spots seen below the right eyelid. These occur frequently in LDS and can be helpful in making a clinical diagnosis in conjunction with other features.

- Joint laxity is common in the general population, affecting perhaps 10% of adults and one-third of children, but only when there are no accompanying problems or symptoms is it justified to diagnose 'benign joint hypermobility syndrome'.
- Joint hypermobility is assessed using the Beighton score (Table 19.7), which has been shown to be reproducible and reliable, although it does not include all joints (e.g., shoulders, ankles).
- In clinical practice EDS-hypermobile type (hEDS, formerly EDS III, and also known as 'joint hypermobility syndrome') is the most common entity encountered, and all other types of EDS are relatively rare.

Management of this group of disorders is far from easy, and clinicians should be aware of the following:

- Where delayed healing and atrophic scarring is part of the disorder (e.g., cEDS) additional measures are required to ensure wound healing after trauma or surgery, that is, sutures to remain for a longer period.
- hEDS is usually accompanied, to a variable degree, by generalized chronic pain affecting the musculoskeletal system, chronic fatigue, and a range of autonomic nervous system dysfunction such as postural orthostatic tachycardia syndrome, reflux and irritable bowel syndrome, and poor thermoregulation (dysthermia); in addition, local anesthesia for dental procedures and pain management in labor is often only partially effective. Unfortunately, these aspects are not reflected in the diagnostic terms used.
- Vascular EDS (vEDS, previously known as EDS type IV) carries life-threatening risks because of major arterial or organ rupture, and surgical management should be very carefully evaluated.

Pseudoxanthoma Elasticum

Pseudoxanthoma elasticum (PXE) is a specific connective tissue disorder, primarily affecting elastic tissue, which may present in a variety of ways because manifestations occur in the skin, eyes, and cardiovascular and gastrointestinal systems. Most commonly, clusters

TABLE 19.6 **The 2017 international classification of the Ehlers-Danlos syndromes**

Type (With some key features)	Abbreviation	Inheritance	Gene(S)	Previously Known As:
Classical Hyperextensible skin Atrophic scars Joint hypermobility	cEDS	AD	*COL5A1, COL5A2* (>90%) *COL1A1*; c.934C > T (rare)	Type I (and Type II when milder)
Classical-like	clEDS	AR	*TNXB*	
Cardiac-valvular	cvEDS	AR	*COL1A2* {biallelic)	
Vascular Thin, translucent skin Arterial/intestinal/uterine fragility or rupture Extensive bruising Characteristic facial features ('acrogeric')	vEDS	AD	*COL3A1* *COL1A1*; c.934C > T; c.1720C > T; c.3227C > T (rare)	Type IV
Hypermobile Smooth, velvety skin (+/− hyperextensible) Joint hypermobility (+/− recurrent subluxations/dislocations) Wider symptom complex/dysautonomia	hEDS	AD	*n/k*	Type III
Arthrochalasia Joint hypermobility (+/− recurrent subluxations/dislocations) Congenital bilateral hip dislocation	aEDS	AD	*COL1A1, COL1A2*	Type VII
Dermatosparaxis Severe skin fragility Redundant, sagging skin	dEDS	AR	*ADAMTS2*	
Kyphoscoliotic Congenital and progressive scoliosis Scleral fragility, rupture of the ocular globe Joint hypermobility Hypotonia	kEDS	AR	*PLOD1, FKBP14*	Type VI
Brittle Cornea syndrome	BCS	AR	*ZNF469, PRDM5*	
Spondylo-dysplastic	spEDS	AR	*B4GALT7, B3GALT6, SLC39A13*	
Musculo-contractural	mcEDS	AR	*CHST14, DSE*	
Myopathic	mEDS	AD/AR	*COL12A1*	
Periodontal	pEDS	AD	*C1R, C1S*	Type VIII

Adapted from:Malfait F, Francomano C, Byers P, et al. The 2017 international classification of the Ehlers-Danlos syndromes. Am J Med Genet C Semin Med Genet. 2017 Mar;175(1):8-26.

of papules—xanthoma-like lesions—occur in the neck and flexural regions (Fig. 19.24A), and angioid streaks may be seen on routine retinal examination (Fig. 19.24B). It is normally diagnosed in adulthood, and life expectancy is probably not reduced, although patients may suffer intermittent claudication pain and/or angina, gastrointestinal bleeding, and sometimes vision loss because of secondary retinal complications such as hemorrhage and scarring.

Skin biopsy shows calcification of fragmented elastic fibers. The condition follows AR inheritance, and only one gene is implicated, namely *ABCC6* (16p13.1), which encodes an ATP-binding cassette protein.

Renal Disorders

The kidney is very frequently involved in genetic and hereditary disease, whether at the gross structural, ultrastructural, or metabolic level. Basic tests of renal function are conducted routinely in pediatric and adult medicine, and there is also usually a low threshold for performing imaging studies—ultrasonography initially. Renal involvement should therefore be considered in almost any setting when an unusual syndrome is diagnosed, and, conversely, the diagnosis of an underlying syndrome should be considered when the primary presentation is renal.

Dysmorphic Syndromes and Renal Involvement

All varieties of structural anomaly may occur across a very wide range of conditions. Renal agenesis may be part of branchio-oculo-facial (p. 119 and Fig. 9.23, p. 122), deletion 22q11.2/DiGeorge (p. 259), Goldenhar (also known as oculo-auriculo-vertebral spectrum, see Table 9.5, p. 121), and Kallmann (p. 258) syndromes, as well as diabetic embryopathy (p. 240). Ectopic or supernumerary kidneys have been reported in Baller-Gerold, Floating-Harbor, Peters plus, Schinzel-Giedion, and CHARGE (p. 243) syndromes. Syndromic multiple cysts and/or dysplasia are a feature of TSC (p. 297), von Hippel-Lindau disease (see Table 14.4, p. 199), and

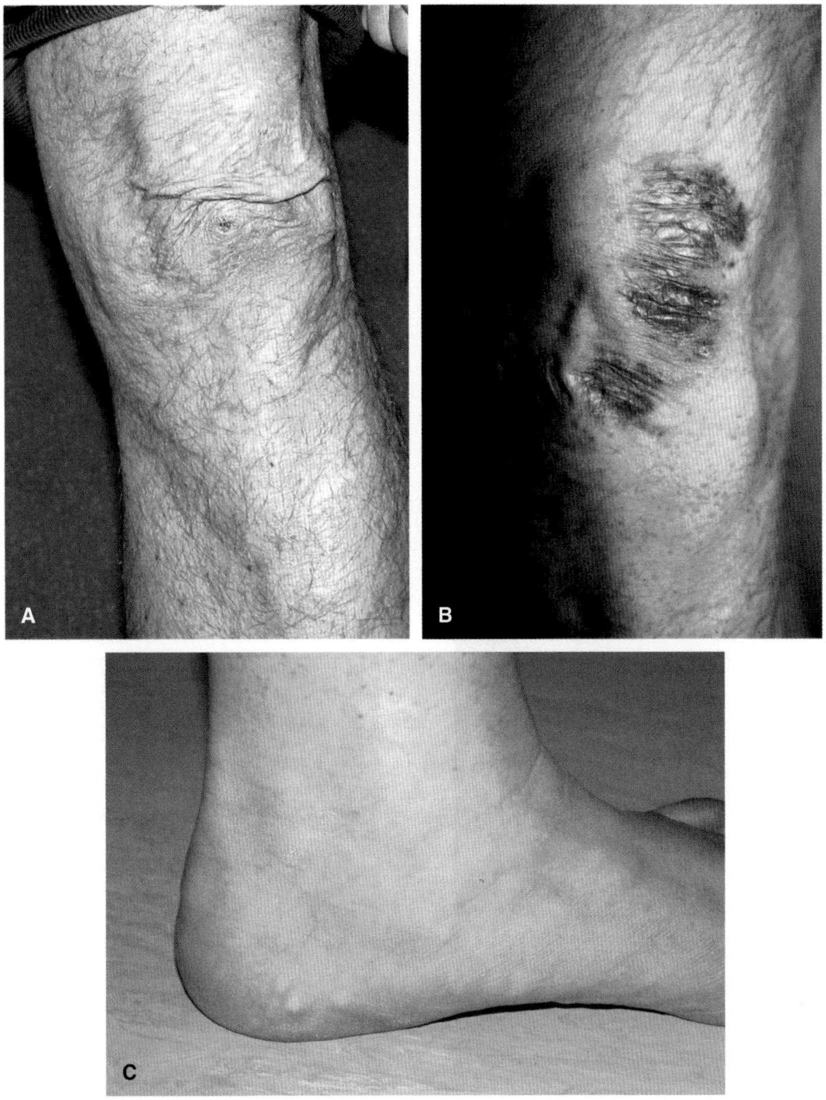

• **Figure 19.23** Ehlers-Danlos syndrome. (A) Loose skin over a knee joint; (B) thin, wide, atrophic scars, also over a knee joint; (C) subcutaneous spheroids on the medial aspect of this patient's heel.

TABLE 19.7 The Beighton score for assessing joint hypermobility

Feature/Range of Movement	Negative	Unilateral	Bilateral
Passive dorsiflexion of fifth finger >90 degrees	0	1	2
Passive flexion of thumbs to the forearm	0	1	2
Hyperextension of elbows >190 degrees	0	1	2
Hyperextension of knees >190 degrees	0	1	2
Flexion of trunk, knees fully extended, palms resting on floor	0	1	

A score of ≥5 indicates significant hypermobility.

renal cysts and diabetes (RCAD). Among the rarer conditions with cysts are Alagille (p. 110), Kaufman-McKusick, Meckel, Simpson-Golabi-Behmel (SGB), and Beckwith-Wiedemann (BWS) syndromes, as well as various ciliopathies (p. 119) such as Bardet-Biedl, Jeune, and the short-rib polydactyly syndromes; metabolic conditions including Zellweger syndrome and glutaric aciduria type II should not be forgotten. Enlarged kidneys may be part of BWS (p. 80), SGB, Perlman and Proteus syndromes, as well as a number

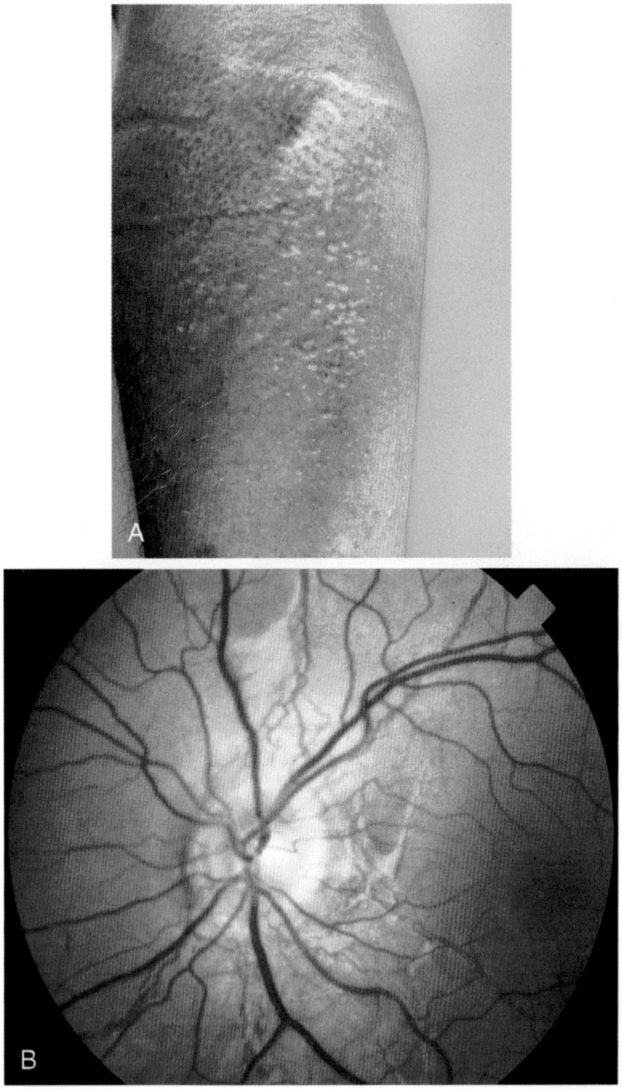

• **Figure 19.24** Pseudoxanthoma elasticum. (A) Xanthoma-like lesions cluster in flexural areas such as the elbow and neck; (B) angioid streaks are seen in the retinal fundus.

of metabolic disorders such as galactosialidosis, glutaric aciduria type II, and glycogen storage disease type 1 (p. 276).

It is important to appreciate, however, that there is great variability and overlap in these renal manifestations across different disorders; any combination of structural anomalies, multiple cysts/dysplasia, and ectopic kidneys may occur in, for example, branchio-oto-renal (see Table 9.5, p. 121), Pallister-Hall (p. 114), oral-facial digital, Townes-Brocks, and RCAD syndromes, as well as the vertebral, anal, tracheoesophageal, radial, and renal anomalies (VATER), vertebral defects, anal atresia, cardiac defects, tracheo-esophageal fistula, renal anomalies, and limb abnormalities (VACTERL) (p. 231), and Müllerian duct aplasia, renal aplasia, and cervicothoracic somite dysplasia (MURCS) associations. Therefore, with a few exceptions, as a general rule there is little specificity or sensitivity in these structural anomalies, and the findings on renal imaging, whether by ultrasound or MRI, can be challenging for the radiologist. However, the angiomyolipomas of TSC can usually be distinguished (see Fig. 11.4, p. 154), as well as the multiple cysts of AD polycystic kidney disease (ADPKD), for example. It is also possible to distinguish cystic disease from the entity known as renal cystic dysplasia, which in most cases is probably a consequence of disruption events in early development, although occasional families showing AD inheritance have been described.

Autosomal Dominant Polycystic Kidney Disease

ADPKD is a common single-gene disorder, probably affecting at least 1 in 1000 people and, because it leads to end-stage renal disease (ESRD) by middle age ($\sim$50% by age 60 years), constitutes a significant burden on dialysis and transplantation services. The key feature is the progressive development and enlargement of bilateral renal cysts (Fig. 19.25), detectable by ultrasound in at least 90% of sufferers by age 20 years. The development of hypertension and progression to ESRD is very variable, and indeed may not occur at all. It is also a multisystem disorder with hepatic and pancreatic cysts, intracranial arterial aneurysms, and sometimes mitral valve prolapse and aortic root dilatation occurring. There is a significant risk of subarachnoid hemorrhage, highlighting the importance of treating hypertension effectively.

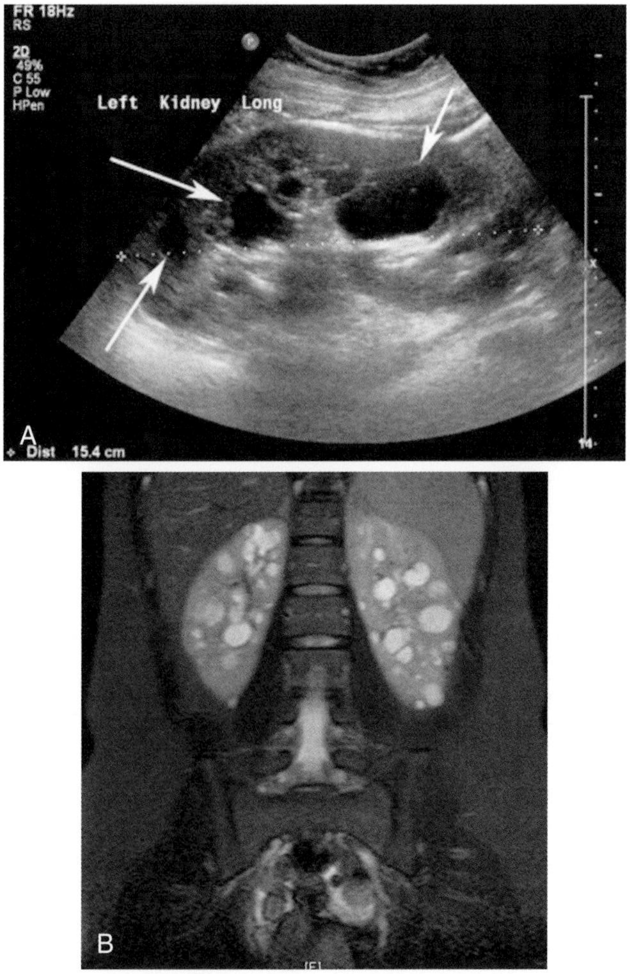

• **Figure 19.25** Autosomal dominant polycystic kidney disease. (A) Ultrasound of an enlarged left kidney in a child, showing multiple simple cysts (arrows) of varying size. (B) In the same patient, a coronal T2 gradient echo image showing multiple renal cysts throughout both kidneys. (Reproduced from Allan PL, Baxter GM, Weston MJ. *Clinical Ultrasound*. 3rd ed. Elsevier: 2011.)

Two genes are associated with ADPKD—*PKD1* (16p13.3) and *PKD2* (4q22.1). Pathogenic variants in *PKD1* account for approximately 85% of cases and, overall, are associated with more severe disease, and greater likelihood of ESRD, than variants in *PKD2*. In clinical practice genetic testing is infrequent, although it is increasing with the availability of next-generation sequencing. This is partly because variants tend to be "private" to individual families, but mainly because ultrasound is usually an effective diagnostic modality, especially in the context of a family history. *PKD1* happens to be very close at 16p13.3 to the *TSC2* gene (for tuberous sclerosis), and a contiguous gene deletion involving both gives rise to TSC with severe polycystic kidneys, sometimes detectable *in utero*.

Autosomal Recessive Polycystic Kidney Disease

As might be predicted, autosomal recessive polycystic kidney disease (ARPKD) is much rarer than ADPKD and also much more severe. It may present antenatally with oligohydramnios, which carries a significant risk of pulmonary hypoplasia and respiratory distress after delivery, but the majority of children are diagnosed in the neonatal period. Mortality in the first year is up to one-third, but survival rates are much better for those who reach the second year of life. ESRD affects approximately 50% of children in the first decade. Apart from the renal aspects, hepatobiliary disease is very common, giving rise to hepatosplenomegaly and eventually progressive portal hypertension because of periportal fibrosis. These long-term complications are becoming more apparent as renal disease is more effectively managed (e.g., by transplantation, in survivors).

The kidneys are usually very enlarged so that ultrasonography is highly sensitive; it is also very specific with increased echogenicity and poor corticomedullary differentiation. These findings, together with evidence of hepatobiliary involvement, are diagnostic. Until recently only one gene was associated with ARPKD—*PKHD1* (6p21). Recent studies appear to have identified a second gene—*DZIP1L*. When the classic criteria are met, molecular genetic testing is not essential for diagnosis but may be useful in mild cases where there is doubt, and would be essential for parents requesting prenatal diagnosis.

Nephronophthisis and Medullary Cystic Kidney Disease

Nephronophthisis (NPHP) type 1 is an early-onset disease and the most common genetic cause of renal failure in childhood; it follows AR inheritance, is caused by variants in *NPHP1* (2q13) and is characterized by fibrosis and formation of cysts at the medullary or corticomedullary junction (Fig. 19.26). In fact, however, a host of loci for disorders featuring NPHP are known; when this occurs in combination with retinitis pigmentosa, this describes Senior-Loken syndrome, with cerebellar vermis hypoplasia Joubert syndrome (see Table 9.6, p. 124), and with encephalocele and polydactyly Meckel-Gruber syndrome (p. 236). As most of the proteins altered by the different genes localize to the cilium, these disorders are rightly classed as ciliopathies (p. 119).

Adult-onset medullary cystic kidney disease (MCKD) was once thought to be a late-onset form of the same condition that we now know as NPHP, but although there are overlapping features on renal ultrasound, it is a separate entity caused by variants in *MUC1* (1q22). It can give rise to hypertension, hyperuricemia, and gout, and ESRD may supervene around age 60 years.

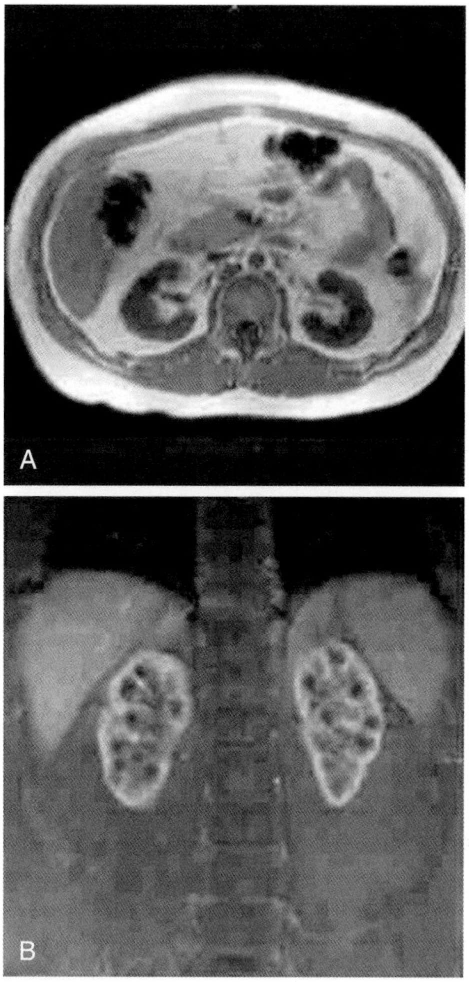

• **Figure 19.26** Nephronophthisis and medullary cystic kidney disease. Magnetic resonance tomography of the kidneys in a patient with nephronophthisis type 1, showing multiple cysts at the corticomedullary junction. (A) Axial view; (B) coronal view. (From Geary DF, Schaefer F. *Comprehensive Pediatric Nephrology*. 1st ed. Philadelphia: Mosby Elsevier; 2008.)

Alport Syndrome

Alport syndrome (AS) is a thin basement membrane nephropathy because of abnormalities in type IV collagen, and renal biopsy with electron microscopy is required to diagnose the features at an ultrastructural level. Renal disease is progressive, starting with microscopic hematuria, followed by proteinuria, deteriorating renal function, and ESRD. Progressive high-tone SNHL also occurs, usually symptomatic by late childhood or early adolescence. In the eye, a virtually pathognomonic form of anterior lenticonus, as well as maculopathy and corneal changes, is evident.

Type IV collagen comprises six different chains, each encoded by its own gene. Abnormalities in three—*COL4A3*, *COL4A4*, and *COL4A5*—are implicated in AS. Of these, *COL4A5* is XL (XLAS) and accounts for approximately 80% of AS, with the rest split almost equally between the other two (both on chromosome 2). XLAS is a serious disorder because all affected males eventually develop ESRD—approximately 90% by age 40 years—and approximately 90% develop SNHL. The hallmark in the early stage is persistent microscopic hematuria. "Carrier" females are also significantly at risk, with more than 90% showing microhematuria, and approximately one-third develop ESRD by age 60 years. Screening of those at risk, by urine testing, should commence in mid, childhood.

For the 20% of AS cases caused by mutated *COL4A3* or *COL4A4*, AR inheritance (ARAS) is approximately three times as common as AD, and the latter tends to follow a milder and more slowly progressive course. It is potentially confusing, however, that approximately 50% of carriers of ARAS will show microhematuria, so this test may not be helpful in trying to establish the pattern of inheritance.

Renal Tubular Disorders

This encompasses a wide range of disorders affecting all aspects of mineral, ion, water, and acid-base balance for which kidney function is key—indeed, a lot has been learned about normal renal physiology through their understanding. Individually, these various disorders are rare, but awareness is important because many can be managed satisfactorily. A basic knowledge of normal renal ultrastructure is essential—from glomerulus to proximal tubule, to loop of Henle, to distal tubule, and finally to collecting duct.

For one group of disorders in particular—those related to salt homeostasis—there is a vital interaction with the endocrine system, namely the adrenal gland, and these are included as they encompass most monogenic causes of hypertension. Salt-wasting disorders are distinct. The disorders of water balance—failure of reabsorption—are known as nephrogenic diabetes insipidus, with 90% of cases being the XL form. The kidney is unable to respond to vasopressin, resulting in polyuria, polydipsia, failure to thrive, and growth retardation—presenting in infancy usually. When the collecting duct fails to remove excess circulating acid into the urine, this describes renal tubular acidosis, which is heterogeneous and sometimes a secondary consequence of various drugs. In addition to these conditions there are a number of different inherited, metabolic, stone-forming disorders, which include Dent disease and cystinuria, although the genetics of the latter is complex.

Although not an exhaustive list of conditions, the most important are summarized in Table 19.8.

Blood Disorders

The hemoglobinopathies have been covered elsewhere in Chapter 12. There are of course numerous other rare inherited blood disorders affecting different components and coagulation factors, and to conclude this chapter we confine ourselves to the one most well known.

Hemophilia

There are two forms of hemophilia: A and B. **Hemophilia A** is the most common severe inherited coagulation disorder, with an incidence of approximately 1:5000 males, and is caused by a deficiency of factor VIII. This factor, together with factor IX, plays a critical role in the intrinsic pathway activation of prothrombin to thrombin. Thrombin then converts fibrinogen to fibrin, which forms the

TABLE 19.8 Monogenic renal tubular disorders

Condition	Gene(s) (Chromosome)	Inheritance	Biochemical Effect(s)	Clinical Effect(s)	Treatment
Hypertensive/Salt-Retaining Disorders					
Glucocorticoid-remediable aldosteronism	*CYP11B2/CYP11B1* chimera (8q24)	AD	↑ Aldosterone ↓ Renin Mild ↓ potassium	Risk of cerebrovascular accident	Dexamethasone Spironolactone Amiloride
11-β hydroxylase deficiency	*CYP11B1* (8q24)	AR	Suppressed aldosterone ↓ Potassium ↑ Sex steroids	Virilisation	Dexamethasone
17-α hydroxylase deficiency	*CYP17A1* (10q24)	AR	Suppressed aldosterone ↓ Potassium ↓ Sex steroids	Primary amenorrhea Sexual infantilism	Dexamethasone
Liddle syndrome	*Β* or *γ ENaC* (16p12)	AD	Suppressed aldosterone ↓ Renin Mild ↓ potassium	Mild hypertension	Amiloride
Pseudo-hypoaldosteronism type 2 (PHA2; Gordon syndrome)	Chrom. 7 [PHA2A] *WNK4* (17q21) [PHA2B] *WNK1* (12p13) [PHA2C] *KLHL3* (5q31) [PHA2D] *CUL3* (2q36) [PHA2E]	AD	↑ Potassium ↑ Chloride Acidosis	Short stature Dental anomalies	Thiazide diuretics
Salt-Wasting Disorders					
Pseudo-hypoaldosteronism type 1A	*NR3C2* (4q31)	AD	↑ Potassium ↓ Sodium ↑ Aldosterone ↑ Renin Mild acidosis	Neonatal vomiting/dehydration	Symptomatic (improves with age)

(*Continued*)

TABLE 19.8 Monogenic renal tubular disorders—cont'd

Condition	Gene(s) (Chromosome)	Inheritance	Biochemical Effect(s)	Clinical Effect(s)	Treatment
Pseudo-hypoaldosteronism type 1B	*ENaC* (16p12)	AD	↑ Potassium ↓ Sodium ↑ Aldosterone ↑ Renin Acidosis	Neonatal vomiting/ dehydration (severe)	Aggressive symptomatic (may persist)
Gitelman syndrome	*SLC12A3* (16q13)	AR	↓ Potassium ↓ Magnesium ↓ Chloride Hypocalciuria Alkalosis	Weakness Tetany (Asymptomatic)	Magnesium and potassium supplements Thiazide diuretics
Bartter syndrome	*SLC12A1* (15q21) [Type 1] *KCNJ1* (11q21) [Type 2] *CLCNKB* (1p36) [Type 3] *BSND* (1p32) [Type 4A] Simultaneous *CLCNKA* and *CLCNKB* (1p36)	AR	↓ Potassium ↓ Chloride ↑ Aldosterone ↑ Renin Hypercalciuria (hypocalciuria in type 3) Alkalosis	Types 1 and 2: antenatal presentation with polyhydramnios Dehydration Failure to thrive Deafness in Type 4	Aggressive replacement of sodium and potassium Indomethacin
Disorders of Water Balance					
Nephrogenic diabetes insipidus	*AVPR2* (Xq28) *AQP2* (12q13)	XL AR, AD (rare)	↑ Sodium	Polyuria Polydipsia Vomiting Failure to thrive	Thiazide diuretics Amiloride Low sodium diet
Renal Tubular Acidosis (RTA)					
RTA type 1, distal	*SLC4A1* (17q21)	AD	↑ Chloride Mild ↓ potassium Mild acidosis	Late onset Nephrolithiasis Nephrocalcinosis Mineral bone loss (Asymptomatic)	Citrate Bicarbonate
RTA type 2, proximal	*SLC4A4* (4q13)	AR	↑ Chloride Mild ↓ potassium Severe acidosis	Early onset Growth retardation Learning disability Corneal opacities	Bicarbonate +
RTA with deafness	*ATP6B1* (2p13)	AR	↑ Chloride ↓ Potassium Severe acidosis	Infancy or childhood Growth failure Vomiting/dehydration Progressive SNHL Rickets Nephrolithiasis	Citrate Bicarbonate
RTA with late-onset deafness	*ATP6V0A4* (7q34)	AR	↑ Chloride ↓ Potassium Severe acidosis	Infancy or childhood Growth failure Vomiting/dehydration Progressive SNHL Rickets Nephrolithiasis	Citrate Bicarbonate
Osteopetrosis with RTA	*CA2* (8q21)	AR	↑ Acid phosphatase Mild acidosis	Learning disability Short stature Features of osteopetrosis	Bicarbonate
Renal Stone–Forming Disorders					
Dent Disease	*CLCN5* (Xp11)	XL	Hypercalciuria	Nephrolithiasis	Increased fluid intake Supportive measures
Cystinuria	*SLC3A1* (2p21) [Type A] *SLC7A9* (19q13) [Type B] *SLC3A1* & *SLC7A9* [Type AB]	AR, AD	Aminoaciduria—defective transport of cysteine and other dibasic amino acids in the proximal tubule	Nephrolithiasis	Increased fluid intake Dietary restriction of methionine and sodium Citrate Bicarbonate

structural framework of clotted blood. Historically, hemophilia was recognized in the Jewish Talmud, and 2000 years ago the religious authorities excused from circumcision the sons of the sisters of a mother who had given birth to an affected boy. Queen Victoria was a carrier, and, as well as having an affected son—Leopold, Duke of Albany—she transmitted the disorder through two of her daughters to most of the royal families of Europe (Fig. 19.27).

Hemophilia B affects approximately 1:40,000 males and is caused by factor IX deficiency. It is also known as **Christmas disease** (after the first boy diagnosed at Oxford in 1952), whereas hemophilia A is sometimes referred to as "classic hemophilia."

Clinical Features

These are similar in both forms of hemophilia and vary from mild bleeding following major trauma or surgery to spontaneous hemorrhage into muscles and joints. The clinical severity correlates closely with the reduction in factor VIII or IX activity. Levels below 1% are usually associated with a severe hemorrhagic tendency from birth. Hemorrhage into joints causes severe pain and swelling that, if recurrent, causes a progressive arthropathy with severe disability (Fig. 19.28). Within families males with the disorder are generally affected to a similar degree of severity.

The mainstay of treatment for both hemophilia A and B is replacement therapy. Clotting factor concentrates can be made from donated human blood, but the purification process must be robust to prevent the transmission of viruses such as human immunodeficiency virus, which has been a problem in the past. A major difficulty, however, is that antibodies can develop that destroy the clotting factor(s) from the outset. These antibodies, called inhibitors, develop in approximately a quarter of severe hemophilia A sufferers and up to 5% of those with hemophilia B.

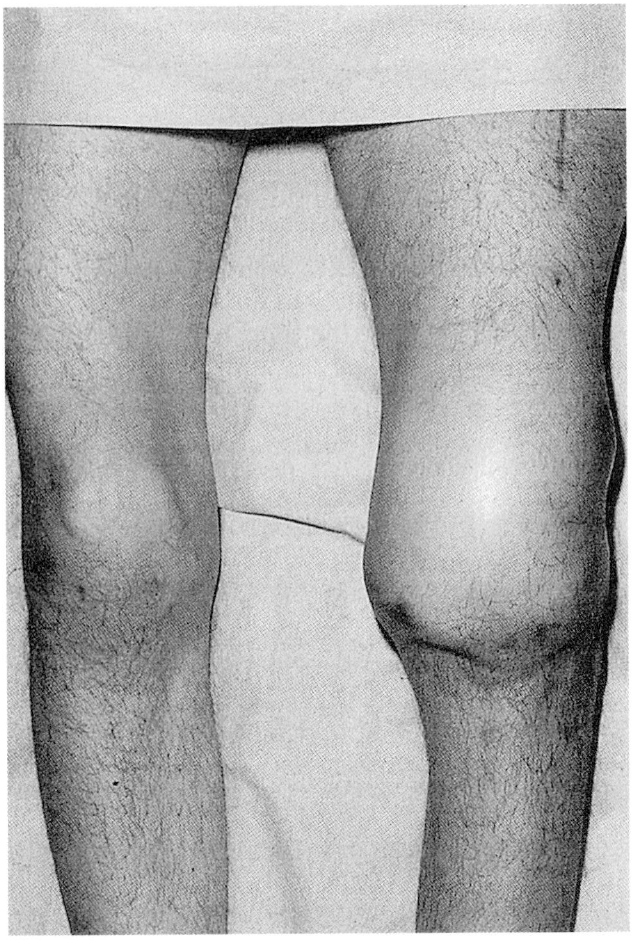

• **Figure 19.28** Lower limbs of a male with hemophilia showing the effect of recurrent hemorrhage into the knees. (Courtesy Dr G. Dolan, University Hospital, Nottingham, UK.)

Genetics

Both forms of hemophilia show XL recessive inheritance, and the loci are close—Factor VIII (*F8* gene) at Xq28 and Factor IX (*F9* gene) at Xq27.1.

Hemophilia A. The *F8* gene comprises 26 exons and spans 186 kb, with a 9-kb mRNA transcript. Deletions account for approximately 5% of all cases and usually cause complete absence of *F8* expression. In addition, hundreds of frameshift, nonsense, and missense variants have been described, besides insertions and

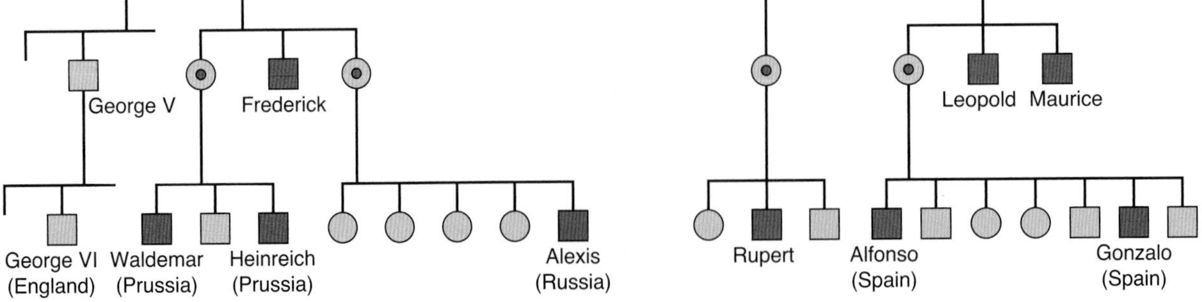

• **Figure 19.27** Pedigree showing the segregation of hemophilia among Queen Victoria's descendants.

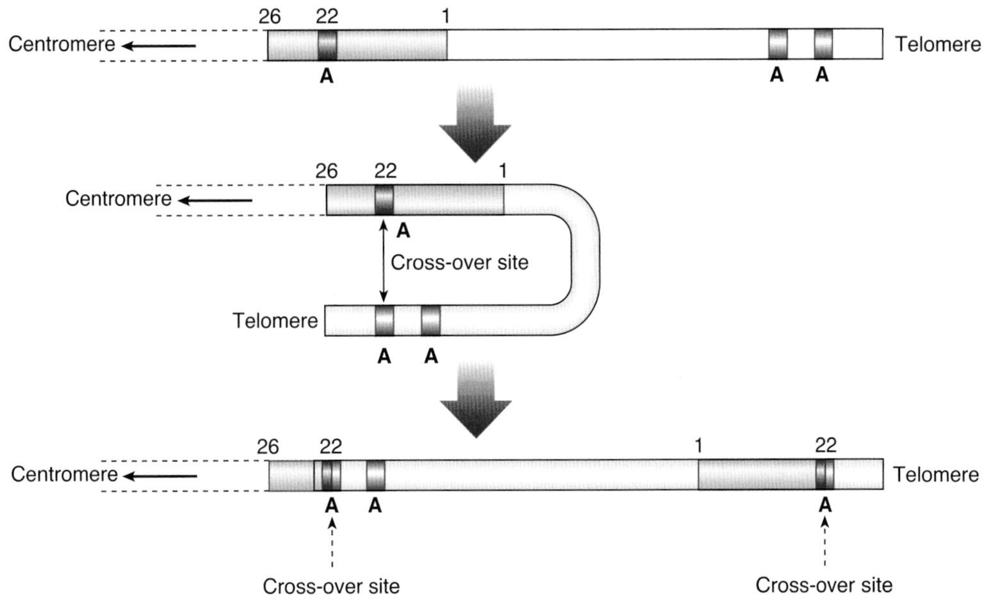

• **Figure 19.29** How intrachromosomal recombination causes the "flip" inversion, which is the most common mutation found in severe hemophilia A. (Modified from Lakich D, Kazazian HH, Antonarakis SE, Gitschier J. Inversions disrupting the factor VIII gene are a common cause of severe hemophilia A. *Nat Genet*. 1993;5:236–241.)

an inversion of intron 22, which accounts for approximately one-sixth of all pathogenic variants and nearly 40% of variants in severe cases (UK population). This is caused by recombination between a small gene called *F8A* located within intron 22 and homologous sequences upstream of *F8* (Fig. 19.29). The inversion disrupts *F8*, resulting in very low factor VIII activity. The genetic test is straightforward, but detection of the numerous other mutations requires direct sequencing.

As in DMD, point mutations usually originate in spermatogenesis, whereas deletions arise mainly in oogenesis. The intron 22 inversion shows a greater than tenfold higher mutation rate in male compared with female germ cells, probably because Xq does not pair with a homologous chromosome in male meiosis—so that there is much greater opportunity for **intrachromosomal** recombination to occur via looping of distal Xq (see Fig. 19.29).

Factor VIII levels are approximately 50% of normal in carrier females, many of whom show a bleeding predisposition. Carrier detection used to be based on assay of the ratio of factor VIII coagulant activity to the level of factor VIII antigen but, as with the CK assay in DMD (Fig. 11.2), this is not always discriminatory. Direct gene sequencing is now routine. Linkage analysis may occasionally be helpful in resolving carrier status.

Hemophilia B. The *F9* gene comprises 8 exons and is 34 kb long. More than 800 different point mutations, deletions, and insertions have been reported, but analysis of only 2.2 kb of the gene detects the mutation in 96% of cases. A rare variant form known as **hemophilia B Leyden** shows the extremely unusual characteristic of age-dependent expression. During childhood the disease is very severe, with factor IX levels of less than 1%. After puberty the levels rise to between 40% and 80% of normal, and the condition resolves. Hemophilia B Leyden is caused by mutations in the promoter, and this so-called Leyden-specific region (LSR) has been narrowed to approximately 50 bp between nucleotides −34 and +19, that is, in the 5′ untranslated region of the *F9* gene. The mutations disrupt binding sites for certain enhancers/transcription factors, but the LSR also contains an androgen-responsive element, and with the onset of puberty *F9* expression resumes, and the effects of the mutation are bypassed.

The mainstay of treatment is enzyme replacement therapy, but these two forms of hemophilia are prime candidates for the development of novel treatments such as gene therapy (see Chapter 15), and trials are under way aimed at delivering a functioning copy of the *F8* gene (and for hemophilia B, the *F9* gene) via a modified virus to liver cells where the proteins are naturally produced.

ELEMENTS

1. Single-gene "mendelian" conditions have formed a very important part of mainstream medicine for centuries, with detailed descriptions of many diseases in the early medical literature. Huntington disease, characterized by choreiform movements and progressive dementia, is a classic example of a late-onset dominantly inherited disorder that evokes fear and foreboding because there is no satisfactory treatment. Predictive and prenatal genetic testing for HD has become a paradigm for appropriate genetic counseling in many other conditions.
2. Genetic testing by next-generation sequencing, using gene panels, is transforming diagnostics in mainstream medicine, given that many clinical presentations, for example hereditary motor and sensory neuropathy (HMSN), could be the result of pathogenic variants in any one of numerous genes now identified. HMSN-Ia, the most common form, is due to a duplication of the *PMP22* gene on chromosome 17p, which encodes a transmembrane myelin protein. The reciprocal deletion product of the unequal crossover leads to a mild disorder known as hereditary liability to pressure palsies.
3. The childhood forms of spinal muscular atrophy are characterized by hypotonia and progressive muscle weakness and follow autosomal recessive inheritance. The *SMN* gene locus is at 5q13, and the majority of cases are caused by a deletion of exons 7 to 8 in the *SMN1* gene. However, the severity of the condition is determined by the number of copies of a pseudogene, *SMN2*.
4. Neurofibromatosis type I shows autosomal dominant inheritance with a high spontaneous mutation rate and complete penetrance but variable expression. It is one of the most common mendelian diseases and one

of the neurocutaneous disorders. The involved protein, neurofibromin, acts as a tumor suppressor by inactivating the RAS-mediated signal transduction of mitogenic signaling.

5. Duchenne muscular dystrophy (DMD) shows X-linked recessive inheritance, with most carriers being healthy. The DMD locus lies at chromosome Xp21 and is the largest known human gene. The involved protein, dystrophin, links intracellular actin with extracellular laminin. The most common mutational mechanism is a deletion that disturbs the translational reading frame. Deletions that maintain the reading frame cause the milder Becker form of muscular dystrophy.
6. Myotonic dystrophy shows autosomal dominant inheritance with anticipation and is characterized by slowly progressive weakness, myotonia, and multisystem involvement. The *DMPK* gene at 19q harbors an unstable CTG triple repeat sequence in the 3' untranslated region, which has the potential to massively expand. The range of meiotic expansion is greater in females, almost certainly accounting for the near-exclusive maternal inheritance of the severe "congenital" form.
7. Cystic fibrosis (CF) shows autosomal recessive inheritance and is characterized by recurrent chest infection, malabsorption, and male infertility. The *CFTR* gene encodes the CF transmembrane receptor protein that functions as a chloride channel and controls the level of intracellular sodium chloride, which in turn influences the viscosity of mucus secretions. Aggressive management has greatly improved prognosis, and novel therapies are being trialed.
8. Inherited cardiac conditions are a major area of clinical activity among geneticists and cardiologists. Sudden cardiac death can be caused by a cardiomyopathy, an inherited arrhythmia, or a connective tissue condition such as Marfan or Loeys-Dietz syndromes. In every case assessment and investigation of the immediate relatives are indicated.
9. Autosomal dominant polycystic kidney disease is one of the most common single-gene conditions. Diagnosis by ultrasound imaging is usually specific, and genetic testing is infrequent in routine practice but increasing. Besides the significant long-term risk for a patient developing end-stage renal disease, it is important to control blood pressure because of the risk of subarachnoid hemorrhage from rupture of a cerebral aneurysm.
10. Hemophilia A is the most common severe inherited coagulation disorder in humans. It shows X-linked recessive inheritance and is caused by a deficiency of factor VIII. The most common pathogenic variant is an inversion that disrupts the *F8* gene at intron 22. Treatment with factor VIII replacement therapy is generally very effective, and gene therapy trials are under way.

CLINICAL SCENARIO 1

In the pedigree diagram the two affected males in the bottom generation, who are cousins through their mothers, have a diagnosis of Duchenne muscular dystrophy (DMD). They are both found to have a pathogenic variant in the *DMD* gene, which is a point mutation, thus confirming the diagnosis.

The affected boys' mothers are confirmed as carriers of DMD through genetic testing, as expected. Initially it is assumed the boys' maternal grandmother is a carrier for DMD. She is tested because of the potential risk to members of her wider family; however, she tests negative for the *DMD* pathogenic variant.

What is the usual interpretation of this negative result in the grandmother?

Haplotype analysis at the *DMD* locus is then undertaken for the affected boys, the unaffected brother, and their mothers. The haplotype patterns within and around the *DMD* gene locus are represented by colored bars—blue, red, green.

What does this haplotype pattern show, and how do you interpret the transmission of DMD in this family?

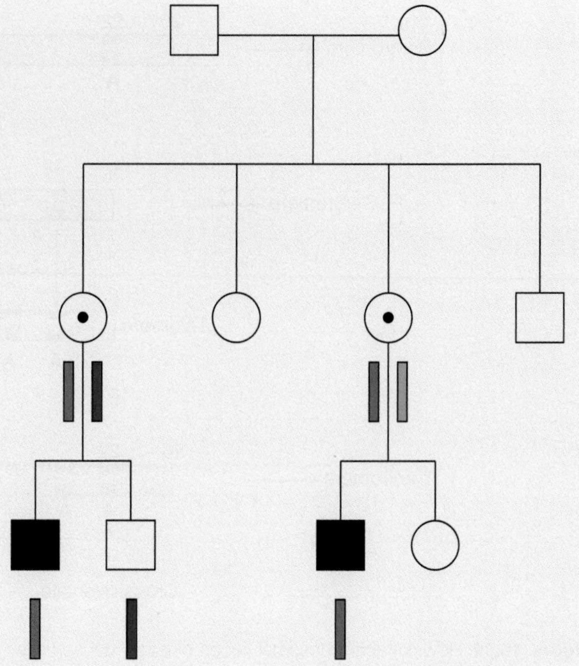

CLINICAL SCENARIO 2

A 25-year-old man collapses while participating in a strenuous team sport. Emergency medical staff are unable to revive him, and he is pronounced dead at the scene. A postmortem examination is performed, but no abnormalities are detected in the heart, nor in any other systems. A toxicology screen did not identify any suspicious substances in his blood. No DNA sample is obtained for storage, as this is not a legal requirement.

Six weeks later the healthy parents of the deceased are referred to your genetic clinic. They tell you that their 21-year-old daughter is healthy but had two unexplained transient losses of consciousness within the last 3 to 4 years, which were ascribed to her partying lifestyle by one doctor and possible petit mal absences by another.

How will you investigate and advise this family?

Further Reading

Bates G, Harper PS, Jones L. *Huntington's Disease*. 3rd ed. Oxford: Oxford University Press; 2002.

A comprehensive review of the clinical and genetic aspects of Huntington disease.

Emery AEH. The muscular dystrophies. *Lancet*. 2002;359:687–695.

An excellent and succinct overview of the commonly encountered muscular dystrophies.

Emery AEH, Emery MLH. *The History of a Genetic Disease: Duchenne Muscular Dystrophy or Meryon's Disease*. 2nd ed. Oxford: Oxford University Press; 2011.

The definitive history of the first descriptions of Duchenne muscular dystrophy.

Emery AEH, Muntoni F. *Duchenne Muscular Dystrophy*. 3rd ed. Oxford: Oxford University Press; 2003.

A detailed monograph reviewing the history, clinical features, and genetics of Duchenne and Becker muscular dystrophy.

Ferner RE, Huson S, Evans DGR. *Neurofibromatoses in Clinical Practice*. Springer-Verlag London Limited; 2011.

A very thorough description of the different types of neurofibromatosis.

Flinter F, Maher E, Saggar-Malik A. *The Genetics of Renal Disease*. Oxford: Oxford University Press; 2003.

A thorough and wide-ranging multiauthor text.

Harper PS. *Myotonic Dystrophy (The Facts)*. 2nd ed. Oxford: Oxford University Press; 2009.

A comprehensive review of the clinical and genetic aspects of myotonic dystrophy.

Loeys BL, Dietz HC, Braverman AC, et al. The revised Ghent nosology for the Marfan syndrome. *J Med Genet*. 2010;2010(47):476–485.

Essential reading for those seeking to make a diagnosis of Marfan syndrome using up-to-date criteria.

20

Prenatal Testing and Reproductive Genetics

The more alternatives, the more difficult the choice.

Abbe Dallavalle

Until relatively recently, couples at high risk of having a child with a genetic disorder had to choose between taking the risk or considering the options of long-term contraception, sterilization or termination of pregnancy (TOP). Other alternatives included adoption or long-term fostering, and donor insemination (DI). But since the mid-1960s, when it first became possible to perform a karyotype on the unborn child, prenatal diagnosis, the ability to detect abnormalities in the fetus, has become a highly developed specialty—fetal medicine. The expert contribution of clinical geneticists in both diagnosis and counseling is now well established, although for all the advancement in medical science the decision to terminate a pregnancy is no less painful for the couple emotionally. The ethical issues in this field are considered in Chapter 22 (p. 347), whereas here the focus is on the practice of prenatal and reproductive genetics.

Techniques Used in Prenatal Diagnosis

Several techniques and procedures are available for the prenatal diagnosis of fetal abnormalities and genetic disorders (Table 20.1).

Ultrasonography

Ultrasonography (USS) is useful not only for obstetric indications, such as placental localization and the diagnosis of multiple pregnancies, but also for assessment of fetal size and the prenatal diagnosis of structural abnormalities. It is non-invasive and carries no known risk to the fetus or mother. Highly advanced equipment in the hands of a skilled and experienced operator is increasingly sensitive. For example, polydactyly may be detected, which might be part of a multiple abnormality syndrome such as one of the autosomal recessive short-rib polydactyly syndromes associated with severe pulmonary hypoplasia—often lethal (Fig. 20.1). Similarly, a scan can reveal that the fetus has a small jaw, which can be associated with a posterior cleft palate and other more serious abnormalities in several single-gene syndromes (Fig. 20.2).

Today, routine scanning is offered at around 12 weeks' gestation as part of early pregnancy assessment, including confirmation of the gestational age, and the fetal heart can be seen beating. An early view of body proportions provides clues to fetal wellbeing, and a particular focus of attention is assessment of nuchal pad thickness, or **nuchal translucency** (NT). Increased NT is seen in fetuses with Down syndrome, as well as other trisomies, and the measurement of the NT (Fig. 20.3) in the first trimester is

TABLE 20.1 Standard techniques used in prenatal diagnosis

Technique	Optimal Time (Weeks)	Disorders Diagnosed
Non-invasive		
MATERNAL SERUM SCREENING		
Combined test	10–14	Down syndrome, Edwards syndrome, Patau syndrome
Ultrasound	18–20	Structural abnormalities (e.g., central nervous system, heart, kidneys, limbs)
Invasive		
Amniocentesis	15 +	Chromosome abnormalities, metabolic disorders, molecular defects
Chorionic villus sampling	11–13 + 6	Chromosome abnormalities, metabolic disorders, molecular defects
Fetoscopy (rarely used in prenatal diagnosis)		
Blood (cordocentesis)		Chromosome abnormalities, hematological disorders, congenital infection
Liver		Metabolic disorders (e.g., ornithine transcarbamylase deficiency)
Skin		Hereditary skin disorders (e.g., epidermolysis bullosa)

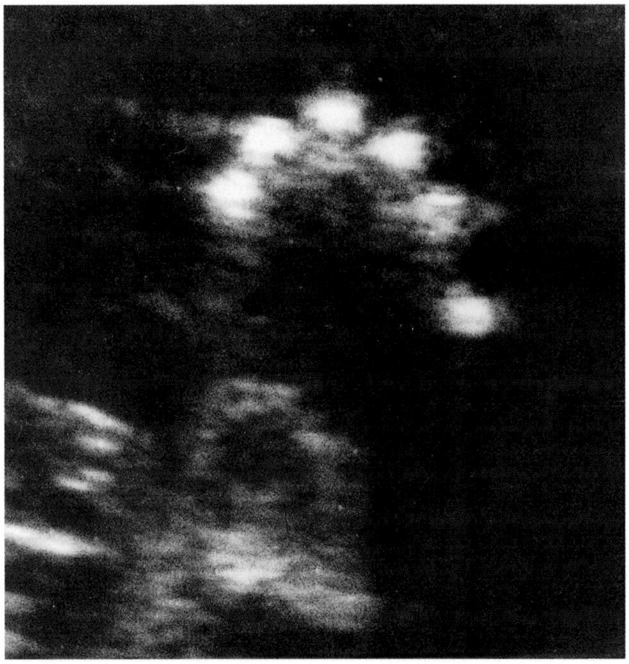

• **Fig. 20.1** Ultrasonographic image of a transverse section of the hand of a fetus showing polydactyly.

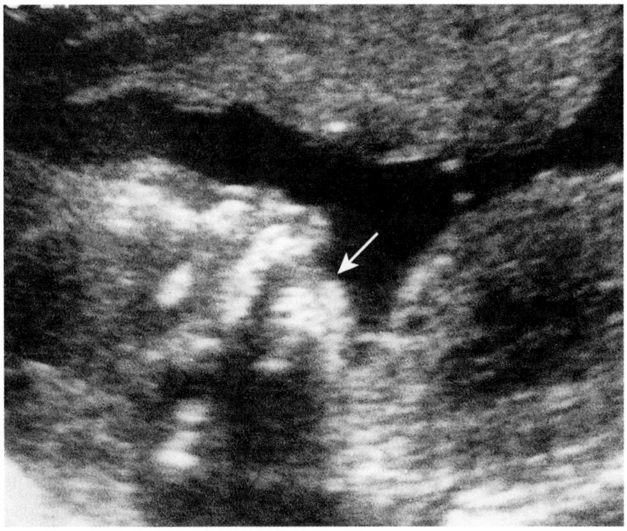

• **Fig. 20.2** Longitudinal sagittal ultrasonographic image of the head and upper chest of a fetus showing micrognathia (small jaw) (*arrow*).

incorporated into the combined screening test offered for Down syndrome (p. 250–253), Edwards syndrome, and Patau syndrome. A raised NT measurement is not specific and may be seen in various chromosomal anomalies, as well as in isolated congenital heart disease. USS at this early stage can detect a significant neural tube defect (NTD) and other major anomalies. Thereafter, USS is offered routinely to all pregnant women at around 20 weeks' gestation as further screening for structural abnormalities because the fetus has grown to a size that makes detailed visualization possible.

Advancements in fetal scanning now allow three-dimensional imaging and magnetic resonance imaging (MRI), which is particularly useful for visualizing abnormalities of the fetal brain. However, detection of abnormalities of the developing brain may not be possible until beyond 24 weeks' gestation, which is late for making a decision about the pregnancy. However, for those severe malformations thought to have poor prognosis, late TOP can be offered. Although fetal MRI will enable the unborn baby to be visualized in far greater detail, it will also generate bigger challenges for the dysmorphologist, who might be expected to diagnose serious disorders on the basis of very subtle features. In reality a whole team of people, including fetal medicine specialists and neuroradiologists, would be involved in these discussions and conclude on the prognosis for the unborn child regardless of whether a genetic diagnosis can be confirmed within the time scale of the pregnancy.

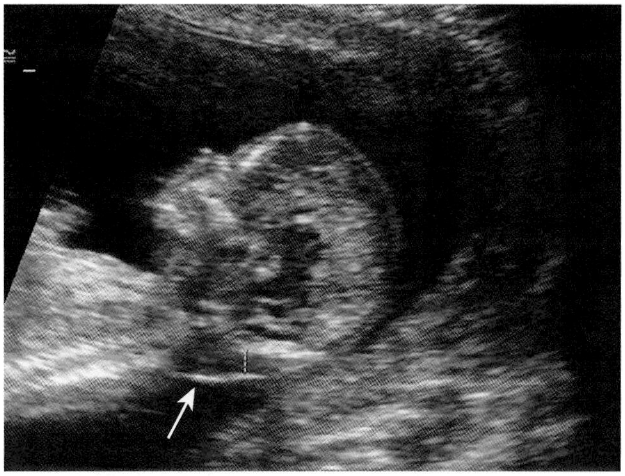

• **Fig. 20.3** Nuchal thickening—an accumulation of fluid at the back of the neck. The greater the thickness, the more likely there will be a chromosomal abnormality (e.g., Down syndrome) and/or cardiac anomaly. This finding leads to detailed fetal heart scanning and, usually, invasive testing (quantitative fluorescent-polymerase chain reaction and array-comparative genomic hybridization). (Courtesy Dr Helen Liversedge, Exeter, UK.)

Amniocentesis

In amniocentesis 10 to 20 mL of amniotic fluid is aspirated through the abdominal wall under ultrasonographic guidance (Fig. 20.4), from the 15th week of gestation. The sample is spun down to yield a pellet of cells and supernatant fluid. The fluid was previously used to assay α-fetoprotein to diagnose NTDs (p. 326), but USS has superseded this method. The cell pellet is resuspended in culture medium to stimulate cell growth. Most cells in the amniotic fluid have been shed from the amnion, fetal skin and urinary tract epithelium and are non-viable, but some will grow. After approximately 14 days, there are usually sufficient cells for chromosome analysis, although a longer period may be required before enough cells are obtained for biochemical assays. Direct DNA analysis using quantitative fluorescent-polymerase chain reaction (QF-PCR) is performed, before completion of cell cultures, as a rapid test for aneuploidies of chromosomes 13, 18, 21, X, and Y. The assay uses fluorescently labeled primers to analyze up to five short tandem repeat markers from each chromosome after fragment length separation in capillary gel electrophoresis. The amount of fluorescence and the size of the DNA fragments are quantified, and the ratios are presented graphically (Fig. 20.5), thus showing how many copies of the chromosomes are present.

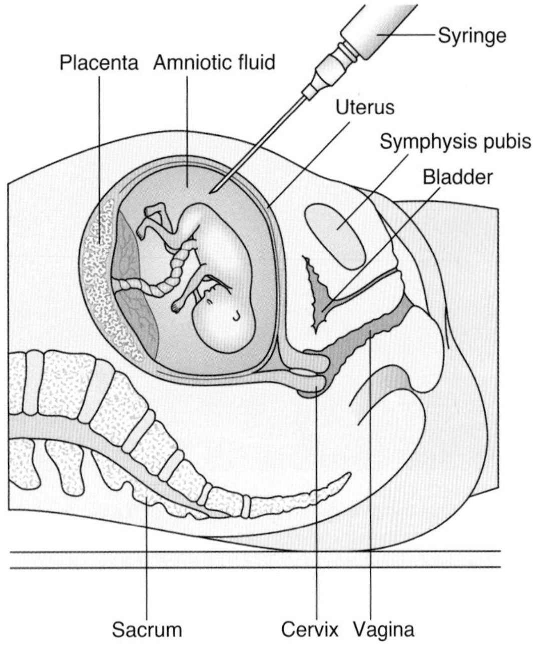

• **Fig. 20.4** Diagram of the technique of amniocentesis.

This rapid method of detecting common aneuploidies may also detect abnormalities such as triploidy well before the karyotype is ready. A full karyotype is mostly only needed to confirm the results of an abnormal QF-PCR, with array-comparative genomic hybridization (CGH) testing now being the standard method of chromosome analysis when invasive testing is indicated. If a couple have opted to have amniocentesis to look for a known single-gene disorder for which the unborn child is at risk, this too is performed as a direct DNA analysis. Both this, and QF-PCR testing, usually produce results within 3 days.

When a couple is considering amniocentesis, they should be informed of the 0.5% to 1% risk of miscarriage associated with the procedure and that if the result is abnormal they will face the possibility of a midtrimester TOP that usually involves induction of labor, although some providers now offer surgical termination up to 24 weeks' gestation. The Royal College of Obstetricians and Gynecologists recommends that feticide is offered for any TOP from 22 weeks' gestation onwards, which undoubtedly adds to the emotional burden of such a decision.

Trials of amniocentesis earlier in pregnancy, at 12 to 14 weeks' gestation, yielded comparable rates of success in obtaining results, with a similar risk of miscarriage. However, the volume of amniotic fluid at this early stage of pregnancy is low, and early amniocentesis is not widely practiced. Although it would provide an earlier result, a midtrimester TOP is still a potential if the fetus is affected.

Chorionic Villus Sampling

In contrast to amniocentesis, chorionic villus sampling (CVS), first developed in China, enables prenatal diagnosis to be undertaken during the first trimester. This procedure is usually carried out at 11 to 13 + 6 weeks' gestation under ultrasonographic guidance by either transcervical or, more usually, transabdominal aspiration of chorionic villus (CV) tissue (Fig. 20.6). This tissue is fetal in origin, being derived from the outer cell layer of the blastocyst (i.e., the trophoblast), and goes on to form the placenta. Maternal decidua, usually present in the biopsy sample, must be removed before the sample is analyzed. **Placental biopsy** is the term used when the procedure is carried out at later stages of pregnancy. The CV sample is divided, and one part is set up in culture. From the other, DNA is extracted for analysis of the genetic disorder for which the fetus is at risk, that is, a direct mutation test or, on occasion, a high-risk set of haplotype markers. QF-PCR for the common aneuploidies is also usually performed, as discussed. Array-CGH is now the standard chromosome analysis for cases meeting criteria for testing, and a full karyotype analysis may be required after culture, for example to confirm a suspected unbalanced translocation in the fetus, although this is no longer a standard test. Sometimes the analysis is biochemical (e.g., for inborn errors of metabolism). This can usually be performed on the tissue sample but, if too small, will be undertaken after culture.

The risk of miscarriage from the procedure is usually quoted at 1%, although in practice, with experienced operators, is usually lower.

Fetoscopy

Fetoscopy involves visualization of the fetus by means of an endoscope. To a very large extent this technique has been superseded by detailed USS, other imaging techniques and genetic testing to achieve a diagnosis. Fetoscopy is used when surgical interventions in the developing baby may prevent irreversible damage, for example the insertion of a drain in the urinary tract to prevent secondary damage from posterior urethral valves, and the treatment of amniotic bands and twin-to-twin transfusion syndrome. It could be used to take specific biopsy samples to aid diagnosis; however, the procedure is not without significant risk of fetal loss or preterm delivery. Therefore, any such intervention needs to be carefully considered in terms of its risks and benefits for both the baby and the mother. Any such procedures would be performed only in specialized centers.

Cordocentesis

Fetoscopy was previously used to obtain a small sample of fetal blood from one of the umbilical cord vessels in the procedure known as cordocentesis, but this is rarely required with the visualization now provided by modern USS. Fetal blood sampling is possible from around 20 weeks' gestation and is used routinely in the management of Rhesus isoimmunization (p. 182), as well as some cases of non-immune fetal hydrops where a hemoglobinopathy (see Chapter 12) is suspected. Occasionally, a sample for chromosome analysis may help to resolve problems associated with possible mosaicism in CV or amniocentesis samples.

Radiography

The fetal skeleton can be visualized by radiography from 10 weeks onwards, and this technique has been used in the past to diagnose inherited skeletal dysplasias. It may still be useful on occasion, despite the widespread availability of high-resolution USS.

Antenatal and Prenatal Screening

The history of widespread antenatal screening really began with the finding, in the early 1970s, of an association between raised maternal serum α-fetoprotein (AFP) and NTDs. Estimation of AFP levels was gradually introduced into clinical service, and the next significant development was USS, followed in the 1980s by

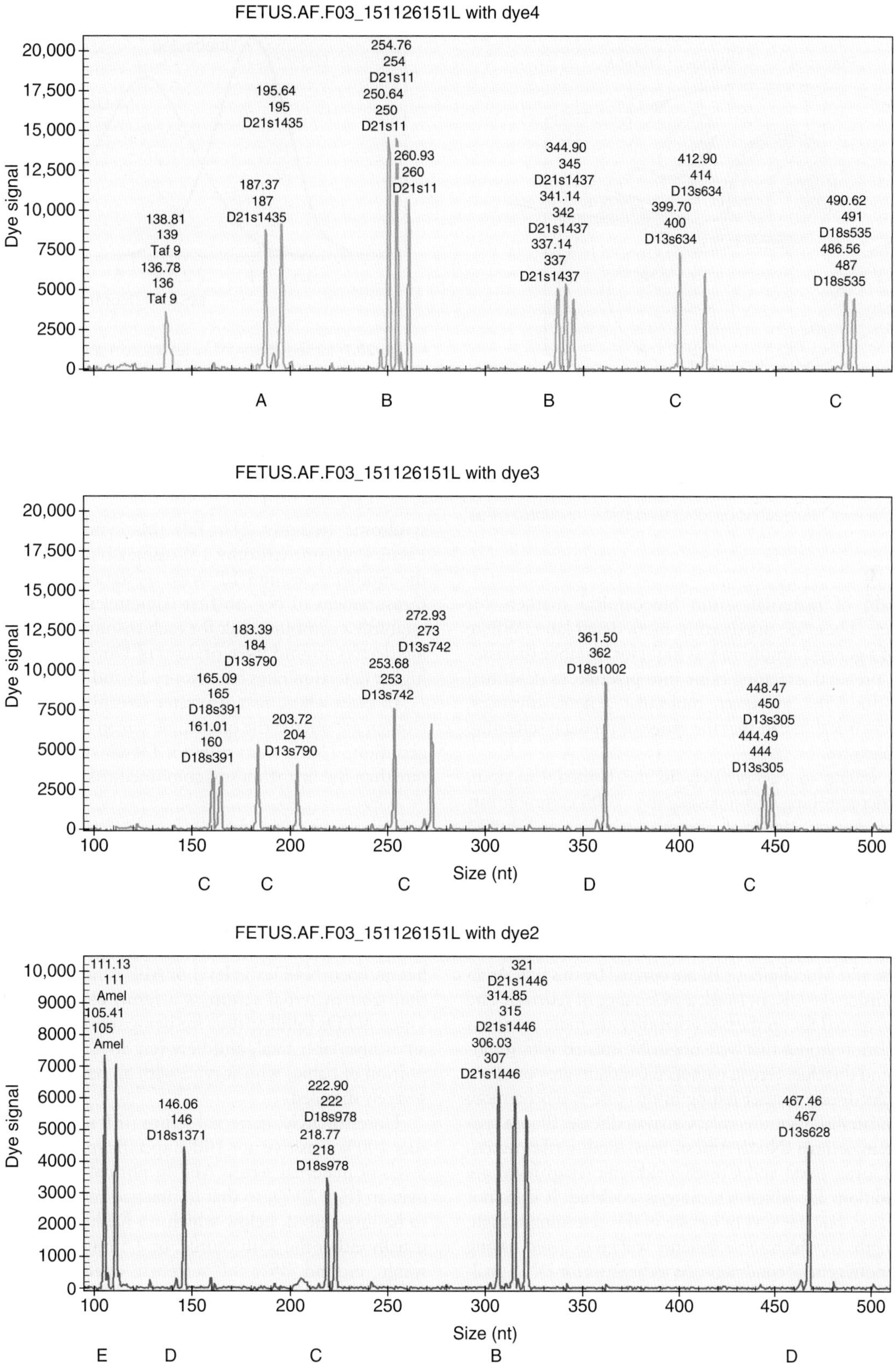

• **Fig. 20.5** A quantitative fluorescent-polymerase chain reaction result for a fetus with Down syndrome, trisomy 21. (A) A biallelic marker for chromosome 21, with one peak twice the height of the other; (B) triallelic markers confirming a diagnosis of trisomy 21; (C) biallelic markers for chromosomes 13 and 18; (D), chromosome 18 markers—large peaks indicating two copies of this chromosome; (E) sex chromosome markers (at Xp22 and Yp11) to determine sex (male in this case). (Courtesy of Bristol Genetics Laboratory.)

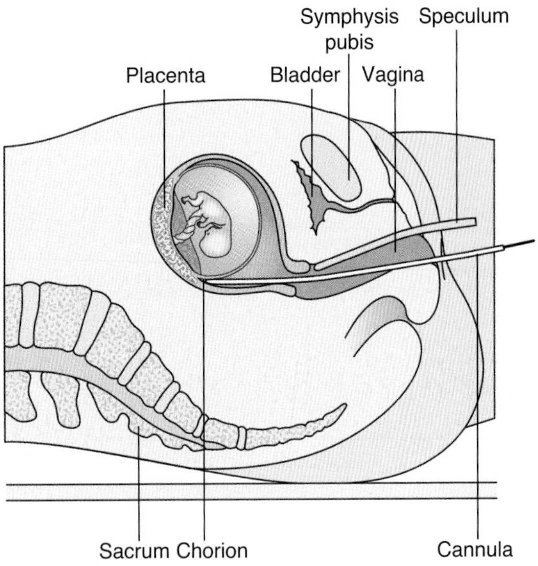

• **Fig. 20.6** Diagram of the technique of transcervical chorionic villus sampling.

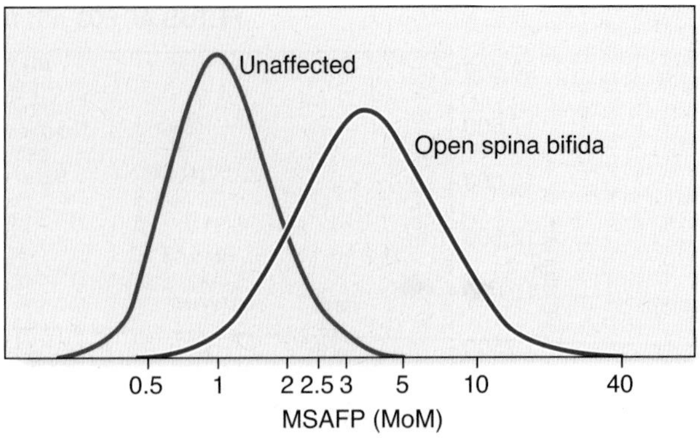

• **Fig. 20.7** Maternal serum α-fetoprotein (*MSAFP*) levels at 16 weeks' gestation plotted on a logarithmic scale as multiples of the median (*MoMs*). Women with a value of 2.5 MoMs or above are offered further investigations. (Modified from Brock DJH, Rodeck CH, Ferguson-Smith MA, eds. *Prenatal diagnosis and screening*. Edinburgh: Churchill Livingstone; 1992.)

the identification of maternal serum biochemical markers for Down syndrome. These are discussed in more detail later. Where the incidence of a genetic condition was high, for instance thalassemia in Cyprus, prenatal screening came into practice, as described in Chapter 11 (p. 158). However, molecular genetic advances, rather than biochemical, mean that the range of prenatal screening is continuing to evolve.

For couples willing to pay privately in the United Kingdom, "panethnic" carrier screening encompassing over 2000 common variants seen in 250 diseases, largely of autosomal recessive or X-linked recessive inheritance, can be arranged. A more focused screen for nine common conditions seen in the Ashkenazi Jewish population is also available, partly funded by a charity called Jnetics; Tay-Sachs disease, cystic fibrosis, familial dysautonomia, Canavan disease, glycogen storage disorder type 1a, Fanconi anemia, Niemann-Pick disease type A, Bloom syndrome and Mucolipidosis IV are covered by this test. As an example from outside the UK, in Israel, a wide range of relatively rare diseases can be screened for on the basis that they are more common in specific population groups that were originally isolated with multiple inbreeding, and therefore certain pathogenic variants are prevalent. Besides Tay-Sachs disease (carrier testing in this case is biochemical; see Chapter 11); familial dysautonomia, Canavan disease, Bloom syndrome, ataxia telangiectasia (North African Jews), limb-girdle muscular dystrophy (Libyan Jews) and Costeff syndrome (Iraqi Jews) are among the conditions for which screening is available. It does not come free of charge, but the level of uptake of this screening is high, revealing the lengths to which some societies will go to avoid having children with serious genetic conditions. As techniques for DNA analysis develop and become affordable it is inevitable that screening will evolve, as the introduction of non-invasive methods of cell-free fetal DNA from the maternal circulation demonstrate (see later).

Maternal Serum Screening

It has been government policy in the United Kingdom since 2001 that antenatal Down syndrome screening be available to all women, although it was introduced in the late 1980s. Where it is standard practice, maternal serum screening is offered for Down syndrome (trisomy 21), Edwards syndrome (trisomy 18) and Patau syndrome (trisomy 13) using a blood sample obtained from the mother at around 12 weeks' gestation. This is combined with measurement of NT on first trimester scan and maternal age, to establish a combined risk for each trisomy. This method of screening detects around 90% of cases of Down syndrome, with slightly higher detection rates for trisomy 13 and 18.

In cases where first trimester screening has not been possible, women are offered the quadruple screen between 14 and 20 weeks' gestation. This screens only for Down syndrome and is less accurate than the first trimester combined risk.

Neural Tube Defects

In 1972 it was recognized that many pregnancies in which the baby had an open NTD (p. 229) could be detected at 16 weeks' gestation by assay of AFP in maternal serum. AFP is the fetal equivalent of albumin and is the major protein in fetal blood. If the fetus has an open NTD, the level of AFP is raised in both the amniotic fluid and maternal serum as a result of leakage from the defect. Open NTDs fulfill criteria for being serious disorders as anencephaly is invariably fatal, and between 80% to 90% of the small proportion of babies who survive with an open lumbosacral lesion are severely disabled.

Unfortunately, maternal serum AFP screening for NTDs is neither 100% sensitive nor 100% specific (p. 155). The curves for the levels of maternal serum AFP in normal and affected pregnancies overlap (Fig. 20.7), so that in practice an arbitrary cut-off level has to be introduced, below which no further action is taken. This is usually either the 95th centile, or 2.5 multiples of the median; as a result, around 75% of screened open spina bifida cases are detected. Because most women now have fetal anomaly USS scanning at around 20 weeks, this is usually sufficient to visualize and diagnose NTDs, provided the sonographer can get satisfactory views of the brain, spine, and overlying skin. USS scanning has therefore superseded maternal serum screening for NTD. Anencephaly shows a dramatic deficiency in the cranium (Fig. 20.8), and an open myelomeningocele is almost invariably associated with herniation of the cerebellar tonsils through the foramen magnum. This deforms the cerebellar hemispheres, which then have a curved appearance known as the "banana sign"; the

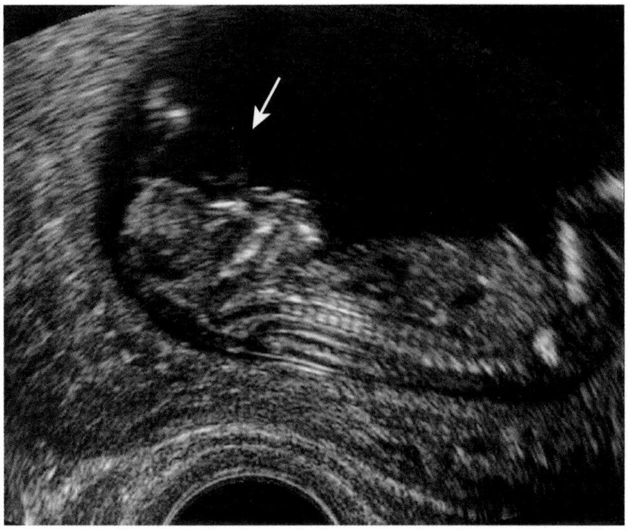

• **Fig. 20.8** Anencephaly (*arrow*). There is no cranium, and this form of neural tube defect is incompatible with life. (Courtesy Dr Helen Liversedge, Exeter, UK.)

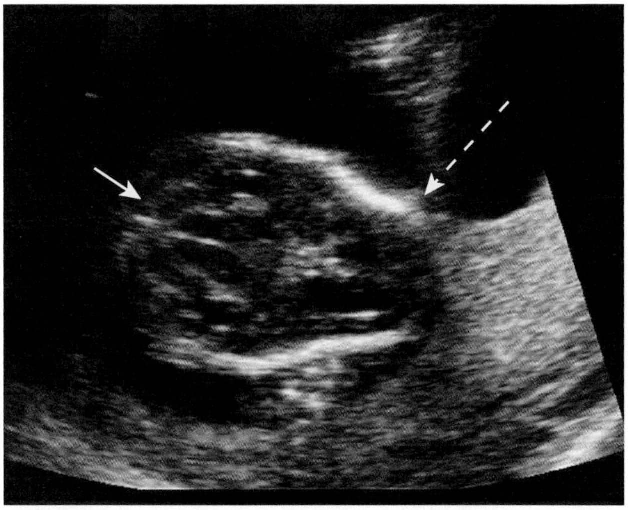

• **Fig. 20.9** The so-called banana sign showing the distortion of the cerebellar hemispheres into a curved structure (*solid arrow*). The forehead is also distorted into a shape referred to as the "lemon sign" (*broken arrow*). (Courtesy Dr Helen Liversedge, Exeter, UK.)

forehead is also distorted, giving rise to a shape referred to as the "lemon sign" (Fig. 20.9). A posterior encephalocele is readily visualized as a sac in the occipital region (Fig. 20.10) and always prompts a search for additional anomalies that might help diagnose a recognizable condition, for example Meckel-Gruber syndrome.

A raised maternal serum AFP concentration is not specific for open NTDs (Box 20.1). Other causes include threatened miscarriage, twin pregnancy, and a fetal abnormality such as exomphalos, in which there is a protrusion of abdominal contents through the umbilicus.

As a result of these screening modalities, the birth incidence of open NTDs, which was 1 in 250 in 1973 in the United Kingdom, has dramatically fallen. Other contributory factors have been a general improvement in diet and the introduction of periconceptional folic acid supplementation (p. 237).

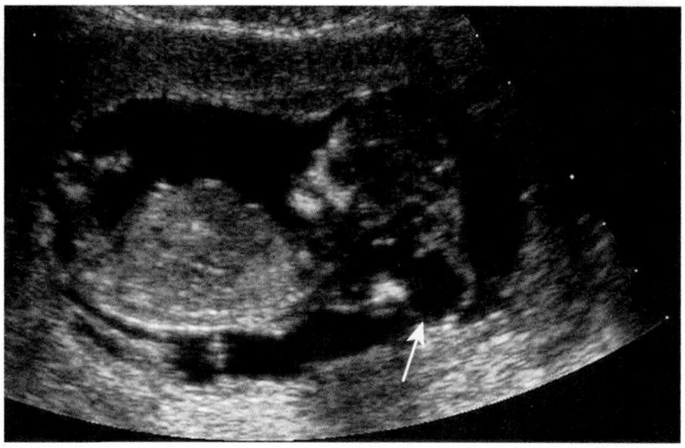

• **Fig. 20.10** Posterior encephalocele (*arrow*), a rare form of neural tube defect. This may be an isolated finding or associated with polydactyly and cystic renal changes in Meckel-Gruber syndrome. (Courtesy Dr Helen Liversedge, Exeter, UK.)

• BOX 20.1 Causes of Raised Maternal Serum A-Fetoprotein Level

Anencephaly
Open spina bifida
Incorrect gestational age
Intrauterine fetal bleed
Threatened miscarriage
Multiple pregnancy
Congenital nephrotic syndrome
Abdominal wall defect

Down Syndrome and Other Chromosome Abnormalities

The Combined Test

Confirmation of a chromosome abnormality in an unborn baby requires cytogenetic or molecular studies using material obtained by an invasive procedure such as CVS or amniocentesis (p. 323–324). However, chromosome abnormalities, in particular Down syndrome, Edwards syndrome, and Patau syndrome, can be screened for in pregnancy by taking into account risk factors such as maternal age, the levels of biochemical markers in maternal serum (Table 20.2) and NT.

The use of biochemical markers in antenatal screening was based on the discovery that, at 16 weeks' gestation, maternal serum AFP, and unconjugated estriol levels tended to be lower in Down syndrome pregnancies compared with normal, whereas the level of maternal serum human chorionic gonadotropin (hCG) was usually raised. Further research confirmed biochemical markers able to add to quantification of risk in the first trimester, which in turn led to the combined screen widely used today. The combined first trimester test measures beta-hCG and pregnancy-associated plasma protein-A (PAPP-A) levels in maternal serum. PAPP-A is produced by the placenta and is thought to regulate multiple factors responsible for placental growth. Low levels in the first trimester are associated with all three trisomies. The biochemical results are combined with maternal age and gestational age (based on crown-rump length) to calculate the overall probability that the unborn

TABLE 20.2 Maternal risk factors for Down syndrome

Advanced Age (≥35 years) Maternal Serum	MoM[a]
α-Fetoprotein	(0.75)
Unconjugated estriol	(0.73)
Human chorionic gonadotropin	(2.05)
Inhibin-A	(2.10)

[a]Values in parentheses refer to the mean values in affected pregnancies, expressed as multiples of the median (MoMs) in normal pregnancies.

baby is affected with trisomy 21, 18, or 13. This is expressed as a probability, with any risk exceeding 1 in 150 being offered additional testing. This may be in the form of CVS, but in some centers non-invasive prenatal testing (NIPT) would now be offered. This technique, using free fetal DNA in the maternal circulation, is not a diagnostic test; however, if risk is low on NIPT, further invasive testing can be avoided.

A large UK prospective study showed that the combined test had a detection rate of 90% or greater for trisomies 21, 18, and 13, with a false positive rate of 4%. This was the detection rate at a risk level of 1 in 150 at term, or when invasive testing is recommended in the United Kingdom. In addition, the test also identified nearly all cases of monosomy X (Turner syndrome) and triploidy, as well as more than 50% of other chromosome abnormalities. Incorporating measurement of fetal heart rate into the algorithm for combined risk improved the detection rate for Down syndrome, although it had no effect on the detection of other trisomies and is not a standard part of this test.

NIPT holds further potential for improving first-trimester screening. NIPT has demonstrated higher detection rates for trisomy 21 (99%), trisomy 18 (96%), and trisomy 13 (91%), with a much lower false positive rate of 0.35%. Universal screening with NIPT would improve detection rates for the three trisomies; however, it would be expensive to implement for all pregnancies, and benefits of the current antenatal screening program would be lost, for example the ability to detect other chromosome abnormalities and major fetal defects. A more appropriate solution would be to combine the two screening tests, as mentioned above, reserving the use of NIPT for those at certain levels of risk. In doing so, screening will become increasingly accurate, and the need for invasive prenatal testing will continue to decline.

The Quadruple Test

For those women who book late in pregnancy, or where NT measurement is not possible in the first trimester, the quadruple screen is offered. This combines four biochemical markers: AFP, hCG, unconjugated oestriol (uE3) and inhibin-A, to produce an assessment of risk for trisomy 21 only. Low levels of uE3 and elevated levels of inhibin-A are associated with Down syndrome in the second trimester. As with the combined test, the result is combined with maternal age, and dating of the pregnancy is required, this time by fetal head circumference measurement rather than crown-rump length. If the fetal head measures 101 mm or more, the test can be offered. This method of screening has a lower trisomy 21 detection rate, and higher rate of positive screen results, than the combined test, but is the recommended screening test, if needed, in the second trimester.

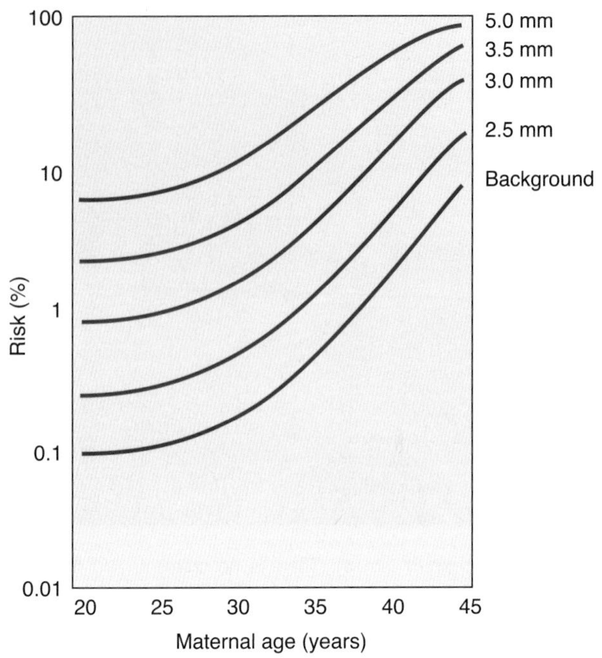

• **Fig. 20.11** Risk for trisomy 21 (Down syndrome) by maternal age, for different absolute values of nuchal translucency at 12 weeks' gestation.

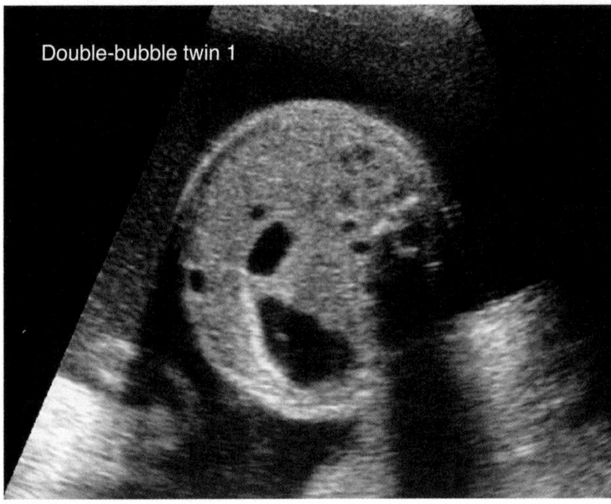

• **Fig. 20.12** The "double-bubble sign," suggestive of duodenal atresia, sometimes associated with Down syndrome. (Courtesy Dr Helen Liversedge, Exeter, UK.)

Ultrasonography

A routine "dating" scan at around 12 weeks' gestation provides an opportunity to look for the abnormal accumulation of fluid behind the baby's neck—increased fetal NT (see Fig. 20.3). This applies to Down syndrome, the other autosomal trisomy syndromes (trisomies 13 and 18; p. 253), Turner syndrome and triploidy, as well as a wide range of other fetal abnormalities and rare syndromes. The risk for Down syndrome correlates with absolute values of NT as well as maternal age (Fig. 20.11), but, because NT also increases with gestational age, it is more usual now to relate the risk to the percentile value for any given gestational age. In one study, for example, 80% of Down syndrome fetuses had NT above the 95th percentile. Some babies with Down syndrome have duodenal atresia, which shows up as a "double-bubble sign" on later USS of the fetal abdomen (Fig. 20.12).

Fetal anomaly scanning, usually undertaken on all pregnancies around 20 weeks' gestation, may raise suspicion of chromosomal abnormalities, for example if exomphalos (Fig. 20.13) or a rocker-bottom foot (Fig.20.14) (Table 20.3) is seen. A chromosome abnormality is found in 50% of fetuses with exomphalos identified at 18 weeks, and a rocker-bottom foot is characteristic, although not specific, for trisomy 18, in which growth retardation is invariable. The use of other ultrasonographic "soft markers" in identifying chromosome abnormalities in pregnancy is discussed in the following section (p. 332).

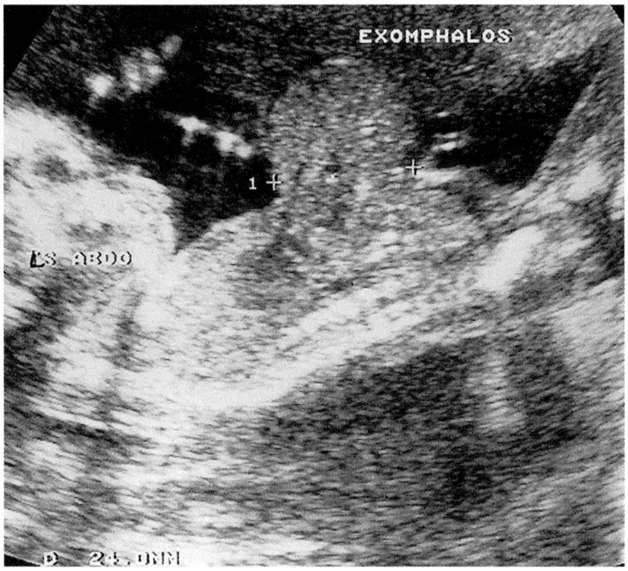

• **Fig. 20.13** Ultrasonogram at 18 weeks showing exomphalos. (Courtesy Dr D. Rose, City Hospital, Nottingham, UK.)

Indications for Prenatal Testing

Couples at high or increased prior risk of having a baby with a serious genetic condition are usually offered prenatal testing, and ideally they should come forward and be assessed before embarking on a pregnancy to allow for unrushed counseling and decision making. Certain orthodox Jewish communities are extremely well organized in this respect in relation to Tay-Sachs disease, as described in Chapter 11 (p. 158). In real life, all too often, many couples at increased risk because of their wider family history, or their own previous reproductive history, do not come forward, or are not referred, until pregnancy is underway. In some cases, it may be too late to undertake the most thorough clinical and laboratory work-up in preparation for prenatal diagnosis.

TABLE 20.3 Prenatal ultrasonographic findings suggestive of a chromosome abnormality

Feature	Chromosome Abnormality
Cardiac defect (especially common atrioventricular canal)	Trisomy 13, 18, 21
Clenched overlapping fingers	Trisomy 18
Cystic hygroma or fetal hydrops	Trisomy 13, 18, 21
Duodenal atresia	45,X (Turner syndrome) Trisomy 21
Exomphalos	Trisomy 13, 18
Rocker-bottom foot	Trisomy 18

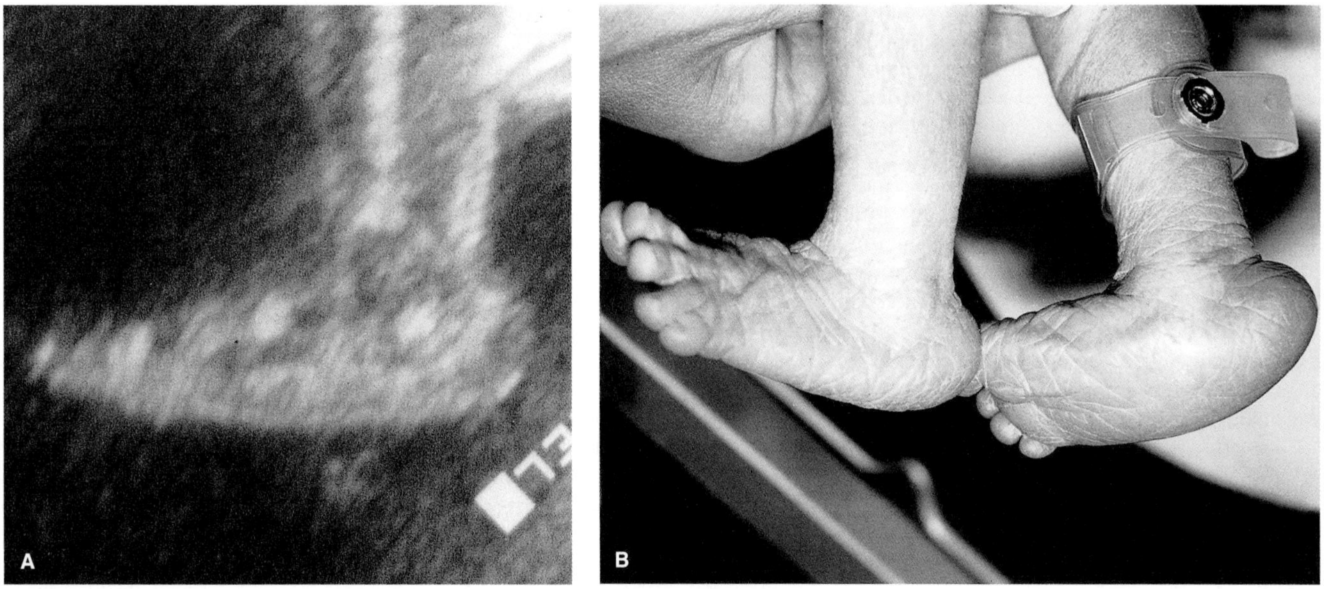

• **Fig. 20.14** (A) Ultrasonogram at 18 weeks showing a rocker-bottom foot in a fetus subsequently found to have trisomy 18. (B) Photograph of the feet of a newborn with trisomy 18. (Courtesy Dr D. Rose, City Hospital, Nottingham, UK.)

Advanced Maternal Age

This has been a common indication for offering prenatal testing on account of the well-recognized association between advancing maternal age and the risk of having a child with Down syndrome (see Table 17.4; p. 251), as well as other autosomal trisomies. However, given the high detection rates of antenatal screening, advanced maternal age ($>$ 35 years) alone is not considered an indication for invasive testing in the United Kingdom, although it is still an accepted criterion in some countries. Interestingly, despite advances in screening, the absolute numbers of Down syndrome births has changed very little over the period of 1990 to 2010, although the number of prenatal diagnoses made has increased, which is attributed to the slightly older age at which women now have children (National Down Syndrome Cytogenetic Register). There may also be an increasing willingness to raise a child with the condition, and individuals with Down syndrome are living longer.

Previous Child With a Chromosome Abnormality

Although there are a number of series with slightly different recurrence risk figures, for couples who have had a child with Down syndrome because of nondisjunction or a *de novo* unbalanced Robertsonian translocation, the risk in a subsequent pregnancy is usually given as the mother's age-related risk plus approximately 1%. If one of the parents has been found to carry a balanced chromosomal rearrangement, such as a chromosomal translocation (p. 37–39) or pericentric inversion (p. 39), that has caused a previous child to be born with serious problems because of an unbalanced chromosome abnormality, the recurrence risk is likely to be between 1% to 2% and 15% to 20%. The precise risk depends on the nature of the rearrangement of the parental chromosomes and the specific segments of the individual chromosomes involved.

Family History of a Chromosome Abnormality

Couples may be referred because of a family history of a chromosome abnormality, for example, Down syndrome in the offspring of a sibling, or a balanced chromosome rearrangement in a sibling. Because most cases of trisomy 21 will have arisen as a result of nondisjunction, rather than as a result of a familial translocation, most couples would have no greater risk than the general population, and invasive prenatal testing would not be indicated. However, each situation should be evaluated carefully, either by confirming the nature of the chromosome abnormality in the affected individual or, if this is not possible, by urgent chromosome analysis of the parent at risk. Where there is a known balanced chromosome rearrangement in a family member, analysis is easily offered to others at risk, which may need to be arranged on an urgent basis should a pregnancy already be ongoing. If a parent is found to carry a rearrangement, invasive testing in pregnancy can be offered.

Family History of a Single-Gene Disorder

If prospective parents have already had an affected child, or if one of the parents is affected or has a positive family history of a single-gene disorder that conveys a significant offspring risk, then the option of prenatal testing should be discussed with them. As prenatal testing comes with a small miscarriage risk, most couples would not choose this path unless they would end an affected pregnancy. Therefore, testing for single-gene disorders in pregnancy would generally be performed only for genetic conditions with serious or life-limiting consequences.

Family History of, or Previous Child With, Congenital Structural Abnormalities

In keeping with standard clinical genetic practice, a carefully constructed family pedigree is fundamental and should enable a risk evaluation derived from the results of empiric studies. If the risk to a pregnancy is increased, and no genetic test can be offered, detailed fetal USS can be offered from around 16 weeks' gestation onwards. USS and dedicated fetal echo will detect most serious cranial, cardiac, renal, and limb malformations. A positive finding does not always mean TOP but allows a couple to prepare for the future and allows medical teams to plan the postnatal management of the child. This approach could equally apply to couples who have had a child, perhaps with a serious heart, brain, or multiple malformation condition, where genetic testing has not identified a diagnosis, but where one is thought likely, and hence a recurrence risk may apply. Even with extensive testing, often including exome sequencing, reaching a diagnosis is not always possible. In this setting, detailed scanning, fetal echo, or brain MRI may be used to look for signs of recurrence.

Family History of Undiagnosed Learning Difficulty

An increasingly common scenario is the urgent referral of a pregnant couple who already has a child, or close relative, with an undiagnosed learning difficulty, with or without dysmorphic features. This will usually lead to urgent array-CGH (p. 55–56, Figure 5.7) testing of the index case, and fragile-X syndrome testing if appropriate. Increasingly, next-generation sequencing technology will be used in this scenario where the array-CGH test is normal and a single-gene cause of learning difficulty is suspected. Where the couple already have a child with severe learning difficulty, for example, they may be desperate to know whether the recurrence risk is 1 in 4 because the condition follows autosomal recessive inheritance, or very low because of a *de novo* gene variant.

Abnormalities Identified in Pregnancy

The widespread introduction of prenatal screening has meant that many couples are faced with diagnostic uncertainty during the pregnancy. Indications for invasive testing include raised first-trimester combined risk, raised risk following NIPT (p. 334), raised risk on second trimester biochemical screening and abnormal scan findings (e.g., structural abnormalities or an NT $\geq$ 3.5 mm). These are an indication for fetal QF-PCR (p. 62) and array-CGH analysis. The finding of a serious and generally nonviable chromosome abnormality, such as trisomy 18 or triploidy (p. 253), usually leads to termination of the pregnancy. It is more usual, however, for such a decision to be very difficult because of the uncertainty of the long-term outcome depending on the diagnosis or anomaly identified. The close involvement and expertise of clinical geneticists and genetic counselors through this process, in providing prognostic information and associated counseling, must be emphasized.

Other High-Risk Factors

These factors include parental consanguinity, a poor obstetric history, and certain maternal illnesses. Parental consanguinity increases the risk that a child will have a hereditary disorder or congenital abnormality (p. 341). Consequently, if the parents are concerned, it is appropriate to offer detailed USS to try to exclude a serious structural abnormality. It may also be appropriate to consider carrier testing for any common recessive conditions relevant to a couple's ethnicity and family history. A poor obstetric history, such as recurrent miscarriage or a previous unexplained stillbirth, is also an indication for monitoring future pregnancies, including detailed USS. A history of three or more unexplained miscarriages should prompt genetic analysis to look for a chromosomal rearrangement such as a translocation or inversion (p. 37–40). It is now recommended by the Royal College of Obstetricians and Gynaecologists (RCOG) that this analysis is performed on products of conception, with parental follow-up if the results suggest a parent may carry a balanced chromosome rearrangement. As with prenatal testing, this testing normally comprises a QF-PCR followed by array-CGH. Maternal illnesses, such as poorly controlled diabetes mellitus (p. 145, 240) or epilepsy treated with anticonvulsant medications such as sodium valproate (p. 240), are also indications for detailed USS because of the increased risk of structural fetal abnormalities.

Special Problems in Prenatal Diagnosis

The significance of the result of a prenatal test is often clear-cut, but situations can arise that pose major problems of interpretation. Problems also occur when the diagnostic investigation is unsuccessful or an unexpected result is obtained.

Failure to Obtain a Sample or Culture Failure

It is important that every woman undergoing one of these invasive procedures is alerted to the possibility that, on occasion, it can prove impossible to obtain a suitable sample, or the cells obtained subsequently fail to grow. Fortunately, the risk of either of these events occurring is less than 1%.

An Ambiguous Chromosome Result

In approximately 1% of cases, CVS shows evidence of apparent chromosome mosaicism—that is, the presence of two or more cell lines with different chromosome constitutions (p. 42). This can occur for several reasons:

1. The sample is contaminated by maternal cells. This is more likely to be seen in cultured cells than direct preparations.
2. The mosaicism is a **culture artifact**. Usually, more than one cell culture is established at the time of the procedure to help resolve this problem rapidly. If mosaicism is present in only one culture then it is probably an artifact, not reflecting the true fetal karyotype.
3. The mosaicism is limited to a portion of the placenta, or what is known as **confined placental mosaicism** (CPM). This arises because of an error in mitosis during the formation and development of the trophoblast. Although this is of no consequence to the chromosome status of the fetus, it can impact upon the pregnancy because the placenta may not function as effectively, leading to growth restriction in the second and third trimesters.
4. There is **true fetal mosaicism**.

In the case of amniocentesis, in most laboratories it is routine for more than one separate culture to be established. If a single abnormal cell is identified in only one culture, this is assumed to be a culture artefact, or what is termed **level 1 mosaicism**, or **pseudomosaicism**. If the mosaicism extends to two or more cells in two or more cultures this is taken as evidence of true mosaicism, or what is known as **level 3 mosaicism**. The most difficult situation to interpret is when mosaicism is present in two or more cells in only one culture, termed **level 2 mosaicism**. This is most likely to represent a culture artifact, but there is up to a 20% chance of true fetal mosaicism.

To resolve the uncertainty of chromosomal mosaicism in cultured CV tissue it may be necessary to proceed to amniocentesis. If the latter test yields a normal chromosomal result, then it is usually concluded that the earlier result represented CPM.

Counseling in this situation may be extremely difficult. If true mosaicism is confirmed, it is extremely difficult to predict the phenotypic outcome for the baby, which would be dependent on the level of mosaicism in different tissues. In theory, fetal blood sampling could be performed for further chromosome analysis, although this would give limited additional information and would rarely be performed given the associated risks. Whatever option the parents choose, it is important that tissue (blood, skin or placenta) is obtained at the time of delivery, whether the couple elects to terminate or continue with the pregnancy, to resolve the significance of the prenatal findings.

An Unexpected Chromosome Result

Four different types of unexpected chromosome results may occur, each of which usually necessitates specialized and detailed genetic counseling.

A Different Numerical Chromosomal Abnormality

Although most invasive procedures (i.e., CVS and amniocentesis) are carried out because of an increased risk of trisomy (13, 18, or 21) identified as a result of first-trimester screening, a chromosomal abnormality other than these three trisomies may be found, for example a sex chromosome aneuploidy (45,X, 47,XXX, 47, XXY or 47,XYY). The sex chromosome aneuploidies present counseling challenges. It is very difficult to cover all the possible outcomes of the test at the time of the procedure—even the more common ones—so when a result such as Turner syndrome (45,X; p. 254–255) or Klinefelter syndrome (47,XXY; p. 254) is obtained it is essential that the parents are given full details of the nature and consequences of the diagnosis. When objective and informed counseling is available, less than 50% of the parents of a fetus with an "incidental" diagnosis of a sex chromosome abnormality opt for termination of the pregnancy.

A Structural Chromosomal Rearrangement

A second difficult situation is the discovery of an apparently balanced chromosome rearrangement in the fetus, such as an inversion or translocation. If analysis of parental chromosomes shows that one of the parents has the same structural chromosomal rearrangement, they can be reassured that this is very unlikely to cause problems in the child. If, however, this is a *de novo* event in the fetus, there is a 5% to 10% chance that the fetus has a subtle, unbalanced rearrangement with resulting physical abnormalities and/or developmental delay. This problem should largely be eliminated by the use of array-CGH in place of karyotype in the prenatal setting. Array-CGH will not detect a balanced rearrangement but would identify the products of an unbalanced rearrangement triggering further parental testing. The extended family should be investigated if a rearrangement is found in one of the parents.

The Presence of a Marker Chromosome

Another difficult situation is the finding of a small additional "marker" chromosome, that is, a small chromosomal fragment for which the specific identity cannot be determined by conventional cytogenetic techniques (p. 29). If this is found to be present in one of the parents, then it is unlikely to be of any significance to the fetus, but if *de novo* there is up to a 15% chance that the fetus will be phenotypically abnormal. The risk is lower when the marker chromosome contains satellite material (p. 14) or is made up largely of heterochromatin (p. 27) than when it does not have satellites and is mostly made up of euchromatin (p. 27). The availability of fluorescence *in situ* hybridization (p. 29) and array-CGH (p. 55, Figure 5.7) means that the origin of the marker chromosome can often be determined more specifically, which may help prognostic interpretation. The most common single abnormality of this kind is a marker chromosome 15.

An Incidental Finding

Clear guidelines are in place for the reporting of prenatal array-CGH, and certain findings, neurosusceptiblity loci (e.g., 15q11 deletions) being a good example, would not be routinely reported in the prenatal setting. However, there are occasions when findings deemed to be relevant to the fetus or the family would be reported even if they are not the explanation for the abnormality that triggered invasive testing. A good example is identifying an X-chromosome deletion involving the dystrophin gene in a female fetus, thus confirming Duchenne muscular dystrophy (DMD) carrier status. Reporting this allows testing of the mother, which may be relevant for future male pregnancies, allows cardiac screening in carrier females and is of relevance when the child has children of their own.

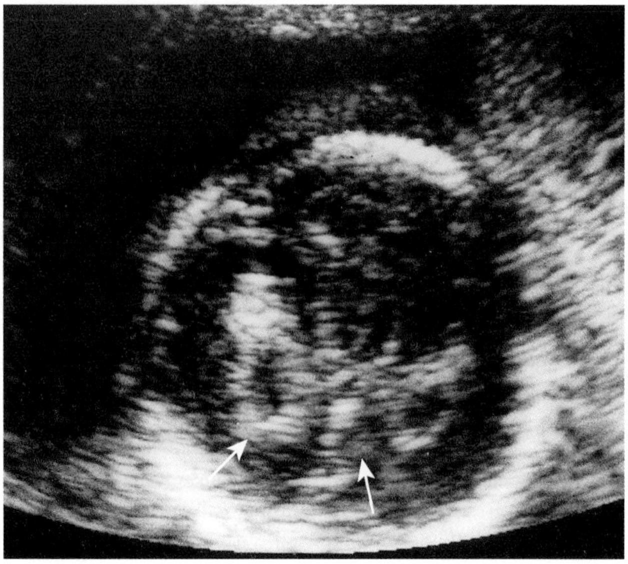

• **Fig. 20.15** Ultrasonogram of a fetal brain showing bilateral choroid plexus cysts (*arrows*).

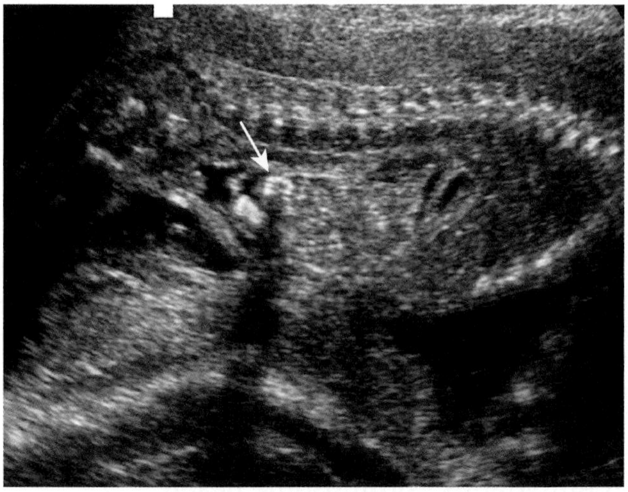

• **Fig. 20.16** Echogenic bowel. Regions of the bowel showing unusually high signal (*arrow*). This is occasionally a sign of meconium ileus seen in cystic fibrosis. (Courtesy Dr. Helen Liversedge, Exeter, UK.)

Ultrasonographic "Soft" Markers

Sophisticated USS has resulted in the identification of subtle anomalies in the fetus, the significance of which are not always clear. For example, choroid plexus cysts are sometimes seen in the developing cerebral ventricles in midtrimester (Fig. 20.15). Initially, it was thought that these were invariably associated with the fetus having trisomy 18, but in fact they occur frequently in normal fetuses, although if large and not spontaneously resolving they may be associated with a chromosome abnormality.

Increased echogenicity of the fetal bowel (Fig. 20.16) has been reported in association with cystic fibrosis (CF)—the prenatal equivalent of meconium ileus (p. 303). Initial reports suggested this finding could convey a risk as high as 10% for the fetus having CF, but it is now clear that this risk is probably no greater than 1% to 2%. Novel ultrasonographic findings of this kind are often called **soft markers**, and a cautious approach to interpretation is appropriate, including serial scans.

Termination of Pregnancy

The presence of a serious abnormality in a fetus in the majority of developed countries is an acceptable legal indication for TOP. However, this is often far from an easy choice. All couples undergoing a prenatal test, whether invasive or non-invasive, should be provided with information about the practical aspects of TOP before the procedure is carried out. This should include an explanation of both medical and surgical termination. Traditionally, surgical termination (via vacuum aspiration), performed under general anesthesia, was available only in the first trimester. This is now generally available until 15 weeks, although it varies between services. Increasingly, surgical terminations are being offered into the second trimester with a procedure called dilatation and evacuation. Medical termination uses mifepristone and misoprostol as a means of inducing labor and is the most frequent method used in the United Kingdom. The RCOG recommend the use of feticide before termination at 22 weeks' gestation and beyond.

Preimplantation Genetic Diagnosis

For many couples, prenatal testing on an established pregnancy, with a view to possible termination, is too difficult to contemplate. For some of these, **preimplantation genetic diagnosis** (PGD) provides an acceptable alternative. The second largest group of

PGD users are those with subfertility or infertility who wish to combine assisted reproduction with genetic testing of the early embryo. In the procedure, the female partner is given hormones to induce hyperovulation, and oocytes are then harvested transcervically, under sedation and ultrasonographic guidance. Motile sperm from a semen sample are added to the oocytes in culture (***in vitro* fertilization** [IVF]—the same technique as developed for infertility) and incubated to allow fertilization to occur—or, commonly, fertilization is achieved using **intracytoplasmic sperm injection** (ICSI).

At the eight-cell stage (blastocyst), the early embryo is biopsied, and one, or sometimes two, cells (blastomeres) are removed for analysis. Whatever genetic analysis is undertaken, it is essential that this is a practical possibility on genomic material from a single cell, and in many cases an analysis using a genome amplification method called **multiple displacement amplification** and haplotype markers—**preimplantation genetic haplotyping**—which was pioneered in 2006 is the method of choice. The technique reveals the parental origin of inherited alleles and reduces the vulnerability to contamination by extraneous DNA, as well as the problem of allele dropout, thus significantly improving efficiency. From the embryos tested, one or two that are both healthy and unaffected by the disorder from which they are at risk are reintroduced into the mother's uterus. Implantation must then occur for a successful pregnancy, and this is a major hurdle—the success rate for the procedure is only about 30% per cycle of treatment, even in the best centers, although this continues to improve. A variation of the technique is removal of the first, and often second, polar bodies from the unfertilized oocyte, which lie under the zona pellucida. Because the first polar body degenerates quite rapidly, analysis is necessary within 6 hours of retrieval. Analysis of polar bodies is an indirect method of genotyping because the oocyte and first polar body divide from each other during meiosis I and therefore contain different members of each pair of homologous chromosomes.

In the United Kingdom, centers must be licensed to practice PGD and are regulated by the Human Fertilization and Embryology Authority (HFEA). In numerical terms, the impact of PGD has been small to date. The United Kingdom's largest center, licensed since 1997 and performing more than 60% of the United Kingdom's PGD cycles, has had over 1000 babies born following successful PGD (2018 data) and tests for over 300 genetic conditions, examples of which are shown in Table 20.4. Each condition requires an HFEA license for PGD, over 600 of which are currently in place. The most common referral reasons for single-gene disorders are CF, myotonic dystrophy, Huntington disease, β-thalassemia, spinal muscular atrophy, and fragile-X syndrome. The technique for identifying normal and abnormal alleles in these conditions and for performing DNA linkage analysis, where appropriate, is PCR (p. 51). Sex selection in the case of serious X-linked conditions is permitted where single-gene analysis is not possible. The biggest group of referrals for PGD, however, is chromosome abnormalities—reciprocal and Robertsonian translocations in particular (p. 37–38).

In recent years, PGD has on rare occasions been used not only to select embryos unaffected for the genetic disorder for which the pregnancy is at risk, but also to provide a human leucocyte antigen tissue-type match so that the new child can act as a bone marrow donor for an older sibling affected by, for example, Fanconi anemia. The ethical debate surrounding these so-called "savior sibling" cases is discussed further in Chapter 22.

A further development using micromanipulation methods has attracted a lot of attention. To circumvent the problem of devastating genetic disease resulting from a pathogenic variant in the mitochondrial genome (where the recurrence risk may be as high as 100%), the nucleus of the oocyte from the genetic mother (carrying the mitochondrial variant) can be removed and inserted into a donor oocyte from which the nucleus has been removed. This is cell nuclear replacement technology, similar to that used in reproductive cloning experiments in animals ("Dolly" the sheep; see p. 352), and was legalized in the United Kingdom in 2015. The ethical controversy has been fuelled by the media soundbite "three-parent babies," even though the donor DNA amounts to 0.005% of the total. Part of the concern relates to the potential for matrilinear transmission of the donor mitochondria to future generations.

TABLE 20.4 Some of the conditions for which preimplantation genetic diagnosis has been used and is available

Mode of Inheritance	Disease
Autosomal dominant	Charcot-Marie-Tooth
	Familial adenomatous polyposis
	Huntington disease
	Marfan syndrome
	Myotonic dystrophy
	Neurofibromatosis
	Osteogenesis imperfecta
	Tuberous sclerosis
	BRCA1 + BRCA2
Autosomal recessive	β-Thalassemia
	Cystic fibrosis
	Epidermolysis bullosa
	Gaucher disease
	Sickle-cell disease
	Spinal muscular atrophy
	Tay-Sachs disease
X-linked	Alport syndrome
	Duchenne muscular dystrophy (DMD)
	Hunter syndrome
	Kennedy syndrome
	Fragile-X syndrome
X-linked: sexing only	DMD
	Ornithine transcarbamylase deficiency
	Incontinentia pigmenti
Mitochondrial	MELAS
Chromosomal	Robertsonian translocations
	Reciprocal translocations
	Inversions, deletions

MELAS, Mitochondrial myopathy encephalopathy, lactic acidosis, stroke.

Assisted Conception and Implications for Genetic Disease

In Vitro Fertilization

Many millions of babies worldwide have been born by IVF since 1978 when the technique led to the first live birth. The indication for the treatment in most cases is subfertility, which now affects one in seven couples. In some Western countries, 1% to 3% of all births are the result of assisted reproductive technologies (ARTs). The cohort of offspring conceived in this way is therefore large, and evidence is gathering that the risk of birth defects is increased by 30% to 40% compared with the general population conceived naturally, with about 50% more children likely to be small for gestational age (SGA). Specifically, a small increase in certain epigenetic conditions because of defective genomic imprinting (p. 78) has been observed—Beckwith-Wiedemann (p. 80) and Angelman (p. 79) syndromes, and "hypomethylation" syndrome, although the possible mechanisms are unclear. In cases studied, loss of imprinting was observed at the *KCNQ1OT1* locus (see Fig. 6.27; p. 81) in the case of Beckwith-Wiedemann syndrome and at the *SNRPN* locus (see Fig. 6.23; p. 79) in the case of Angelman syndrome. No apparent imprinting differences explain the increase in SGA babies conceived by ICSI.

Epigenetic events around the time of fertilization and implantation are crucial for normal development (p. 123). If there is a definite increased risk of conditions from abnormal imprinting after ARTs, this may relate, in part, to the extended culture time of embryos, which has become a trend in infertility clinics. Instead of transferring cleavage-stage embryos, it is now more routine to transfer blastocysts, which allows the healthier-looking embryos to be selected. However, in animal models it has been shown that *in vitro* culture affects the extent of imprinting and gene expression, and therefore the potential for normal development.

Intracytoplasmic Sperm Injection

As mentioned, this technique is commonly used as part of IVF when combined with PGD, but the main indication for directly injecting sperm into the egg is male subfertility because of low sperm count, poor sperm motility, abnormal sperm morphology, or mechanical blockage to the passage of sperm along the vas deferens. Chromosomal abnormalities or rearrangements have been found in about 5% of men for whom ICSI is suitable, and 10% to 12% of those with azoospermia or severe oligospermia. Examples include the Robertsonian 13:14 translocation and Y-chromosome deletions. For men with azoospermia or severe oligospermia the karyotype should be checked, including the application of molecular techniques looking for submicroscopic Y deletions. In those with mechanical blockage because of congenital bilateral absence of the vas deferens (CBAVD), a significant proportion have CF variants. ICSI offers hope to men with CBAVD, as well as those with Klinefelter syndrome, following testicular aspiration of sperm.

Some of the chromosomal abnormalities in the men may be heritable—especially those involving the sex chromosomes—and there is a small but definite increase in chromosomal abnormalities in the offspring (1.6%).

Donor Insemination

As a means of assisted conception to treat male infertility, or to circumvent the risk of a genetic disease, **donor insemination (DI)** has been used since the 1950s. Only relatively recently, however, has awareness of medical genetic issues been incorporated into practice. Following the cases of children conceived by DI who were subsequently discovered to have balanced or unbalanced chromosome disorders, or in some cases CF (indicating that the sperm donor was a carrier for CF), screening of sperm donors for CF variants and chromosome rearrangements has become routine practice in many countries. This was recommended only as recently as 2000 by the British Andrology Society. In the Netherlands, a donor whose sperm was used to father 18 offspring developed an AD late-onset neurodegenerative disorder (one of the spinocerebellar ataxias), thus indicating that all 18 offspring conceived were at 50% risk. This led to a ruling that the sperm from one donor should be used no more than 10 times, as against 25 before this experience. In the United Kingdom, men older than 40 years cannot be donors because of the small but increasing risk of new germline variants arising in sperm with advancing paternal age.

Of course, it is not possible to screen the donor for all eventualities, but these cases have served to highlight the potential conflict between treating infertility (or genetic disease) by DI and maintaining a high level of concern for the welfare of the child conceived. More high profile in this respect is the ongoing debate about how much information DI children should be allowed about their genetic fathers, and the law varies across the world. The issues apply equally to women who donate their ova.

Assisted Conception and the Law

In the United States, no federal law exists to regulate the practice of assisted conception other than the requirement that outcomes of IVF and ICSI must be reported. In the United Kingdom, strict regulation operates through the HFEA based on the Human Fertilisation and Embryology Act 1990 (updated in 2008). The HFEA reports to the Secretary of State for Health, issues licenses and arranges inspections of registered centers. The different licenses granted are for treatment (Box 20.2), storage (gametes and embryos) and research (on human embryos *in vitro*). A register of all treatment cycles, the children born by IVF and the use of donated gametes must be kept. The research permitted under license covers treatment of infertility, increase in knowledge regarding birth defects, miscarriage, genetic testing in embryos, the development of the early embryo, and potential treatment of serious disease.

Non-invasive Prenatal Testing

At the turn of the 19th century, it was discovered that fetal cells reach the maternal circulation, but confirmation that **cell-free fetal DNA** (cffDNA), derived from placental trophoblast tissue, is present in the plasma of pregnant women did not take place until 1997 (Fig. 20.17). This fact was initially exploited in clinical practice as early as 6 to 7 weeks of pregnancy to determine fetal sex by detection of Y-chromosome DNA sequences and the fetal Rhesus D gene. Early determination of fetal sex is clinically useful in a pregnancy at risk of an X-linked recessive disorder and enables a 50% reduction in the requirement for invasive testing. The problem with analysing cffDNA is that of isolation because maternal cell-free DNA constitutes 80% to 90% of all cell-free DNA in the maternal circulation. The absence of Y-chromosome DNA might indicate that the fetus is female, or that the quantity of fetal DNA

• BOX 20.2 Assisted Conception Treatments Requiring a License From the Human Fertilization and Embryology Authority

In vitro fertilization
Intracytoplasmic sperm injection
Preimplantation genetic diagnosis
Mitochondrial donation treatment
Sperm donation
Egg donation
Embryo donation
Surrogacy

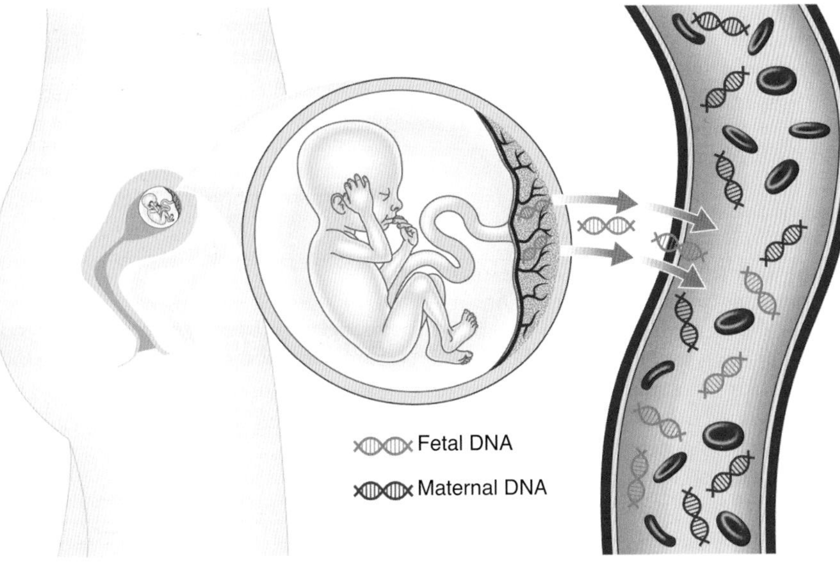

• **Fig. 20.17** Minute quantities of cell-free fetal DNA reach the maternal circulation from the trophoblasts of the placenta and can be accessed for genetic analysis.

is very low. This is resolved by using real-time PCR to quantify the amount of fetal or total DNA present in plasma.

Development of the technology to detect Down syndrome and other common trisomies in the fetus has been rapid. In this case the challenge lay in discriminating between a DNA sample in which the fetal component constitutes three copies of chromosome 21 as opposed to the two copies of the maternal plasma cell free DNA. This has been achieved using massive parallel "shotgun" sequencing technology combined with sophisticated sequencing data analysis. Essentially, millions of small fragments of cffDNA (both random and specific to chromosomes of interest) from maternal plasma (containing both fetal and maternal cell-free DNA) are amplified and sequenced. The fragments are then mapped to the human genome and analyzed for their frequency, or density, along each chromosome, enabling detection of Down syndrome in the fetus where chromosome 21 fragments are overrepresented, and likewise for the other common aneuploidies. Studies have shown an accuracy of 99% for trisomy 21, 96% for trisomy 18 and 91% for trisomy 13. As discussed previously (p. 328), replacing current early pregnancy screening solely with NIPT would be costly and at the expense of the benefits of current screening methodologies. However, NIPT will undoubtedly become an essential part of routine screening, in combination with those tests already available, and has been calculated to be cost-effective when used to replace CVS/amniocentesis following a high-risk first-trimester combined test result (≥1:150 trisomy risk). It is important to remember that NIPT remains a screening test and should not be relied upon to confirm a trisomy diagnosis. A high-risk NIPT result still requires confirmation with invasive testing.

Some companies offering NIPT also include assessment of common chromosomal CNVs, for example 22q11 deletions. The evidence and accuracy of NIPT for this purpose is less clear, and in the United Kingdom any such testing would only be available via research studies, or when self-funded.

Non-invasive Prenatal Diagnosis

The attraction of a very accurate prenatal test that avoids an invasive procedure carrying a risk of fetal loss is obvious. As a result, the non-invasive assessment of cffDNA has expanded allowing testing of a range of genetic conditions. In the United Kingdom, this is available for CF (p. 303), Apert syndrome (*FGFR2*-p. 118), *FGFR3*-related skeletal dysplasia (p. 117), DMD and Becker muscular dystrophy (p. 299), spinal muscular atrophy (p. 294), congenital adrenal hyperplasia (p. 277), and some of the craniosynostosis conditions secondary to variants in *FGFR2* (p. 117). Furthermore, bespoke non-invasive prenatal diagnosis is also possible with testing individually designed for the condition, and specific gene variants, affecting a family. For recessive conditions, this will generally involve looking for evidence of the paternal pathogenic gene variant, which, if absent, would be reassuring, as the baby could be no more than a carrier of the condition. Where the paternal variant is identified, couples would be offered invasive testing to confirm whether the fetus is merely a carrier or affected with the condition. The use of NIPD will reduce the need for invasive prenatal testing in a similar way to fetal sexing for X-linked disorders. Although there are inevitable concerns that the technology will make it possible to test the fetus for non-medical characteristics or features, this is extremely unlikely given the bespoke nature of each individual assay. It does, however, dramatically change the face of prenatal testing and screening for the foreseeable future.

Prenatal Rapid Exome Sequencing

One of the difficulties of prenatal genetics is making a diagnosis in a limited period of time, with limited phenotypic details. As extensive genetic testing, for example a large gene panel, can take many months to complete, much prenatal counseling will be based on scan findings and potential genetic diagnoses, perhaps only managing to confirm the diagnosis later in pregnancy, when termination may no longer be an option, or following completion of the pregnancy. For those pregnancies presenting with a complex picture of congenital abnormalities, with normal chromosome testing and where a genetic diagnosis is thought to be likely, exome sequencing is becoming a key part of the diagnostic pathway. Rapid testing, providing a result within a couple of weeks, can be hugely beneficial to a couple in providing information about the prognosis for their unborn child. In some cases, for example certain metabolic conditions, results have allowed rapid treatment in the newborn. In the years to come, whole-genome sequencing will inevitably have a role in the prenatal setting as well, and whilst many issues surround the use and interpretation of such complex data, the benefits could be significant in this field of genetics.

Prenatal Treatment

This chapter has focused mainly on prenatal screening and testing for abnormalities, and this inevitably means that the option of TOP is a possible outcome. For the future there is cautious optimism that prenatal testing will, in time, lead to the possibility of effective treatment *in utero*, at least for some conditions.

There have been a couple of reported cases of prenatal stem cell transplant in fetuses diagnosed with osteogenesis imperfecta which suggested that treatment led to a reduction in the expected number of fractures. Treatment of a fetus affected with severe combined immunodeficiency (p. 180) has also been reported. The immunological tolerance of the fetus to foreign antigens introduced *in utero* means that the transfused stem cells are recognized as "self," with the prospect of good long-term results.

When gene therapy (p. 218) proves to be both safe and effective, the immunological tolerance of the fetus should make it easier to commence such therapy before birth rather than afterward. This will have the added advantage of reducing the period in which irreversible damage can occur in organs such as the central nervous system, which can be affected by progressive neurodegenerative disorders.

ELEMENTS

1. Prenatal screening can be carried out by non-invasive methods such as the first trimester combined screen for Down, Edwards, and Patau syndromes, which combines biochemical markers, nuchal translucency measurement, and maternal age. Detailed ultrasonography for structural abnormalities is a vital part of prenatal screening.
2. Specific prenatal testing of chromosome and single-gene disorders traditionally relied upon invasive techniques, such as amniocentesis or chorionic villus sampling, to obtain material of fetal origin for analysis. Whilst these remain frequently requested tests, non-invasive approaches are becoming increasingly available.
3. Invasive prenatal testing procedures convey small risks for causing miscarriage (e.g., amniocentesis 0.5% to 1%, chorionic villus sampling 1%, cordocentesis 1% to 2%, fetoscopy 3% to 5%).
4. Common indications for invasive prenatal testing include: an increased combined risk or raised nuchal translucency, a previous, or family, history of a chromosomal or single-gene disorder or structural abnormalities identified on ultrasound.
5. Although the significance of many prenatal diagnostic findings is clear, situations frequently arise in which the implications for the fetus are very difficult to predict, in which case the couple should be offered specialized genetic counseling.
6. Non-invasive prenatal testing is changing the approach to prenatal screening and provides increased accuracy for testing of the common trisomies but is not considered confirmatory of the diagnosis.
7. Non-invasive prenatal diagnosis is increasingly available for a spectrum of single-gene disorders, thereby reducing the need for invasive testing.
8. Whole-exome and whole-genome sequencing are beginning to play a role in prenatal diagnosis of presumed genetic disorders and are likely to have a significant impact in the years to come.
9. Technology has not only advanced in terms of testing during a pregnancy, but increasing success of preimplantation genetic diagnosis is making this a popular choice for many couples who wish to avoid prenatal testing.

CLINICAL SCENARIO 1

A 36-year-old nulliparous female is given a high-risk combined screening result on the basis of maternal age and a low pregnancy-associated plasma protein-A measurement (<0.4 multiples of the median) at 12 weeks' gestation. No other scan abnormalities are detected.

What are the management options available? How would the outcomes of further testing impact the management of the pregnancy?

CLINICAL SCENARIO 2

A couple are referred to the genetics clinic on the basis of the family history of cystic fibrosis. They are expecting their first child, currently at 6 weeks' gestation.

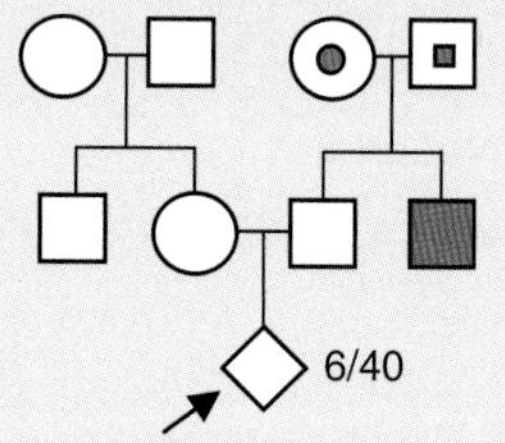

How would you counsel them about the risk to their unborn child, what further testing can you offer, and what testing is available in the pregnancy should both parents be carriers?

Further Reading

Allyse M, Minear MA, Berson E, et al. Non-invasive prenatal testing: a review of international implementation and challenges. *Int J Womens Health*. 2015;7:113–126.

A review of the international introduction of NIPT and the challenges of implementing its use across the world.

Best S, Wou K, Vora N, et al. Promises, pitfalls and practicalities of prenatal whole exome sequencing. *Prenat Diagn*. 2018;38(1):10–19.

A review of prenatal whole exome sequencing studies: the diagnostic rates, challenges, and limitations.

Evans M. *Prenatal Diagnosis*. McGraw-Hill Professional; 2006.

A comprehensive reference on diagnosis and evaluation of reproductive risks and genetically related high-risk pregnancies.

Ghi T, Sotiriadis A, Calda P, et al. ISUOG Practice Guidelines: invasive procedures for prenatal diagnosis. *Ultrasound Obstet Gynecol*. 2016;48(2):256–268.

A guideline summarizing when, how, and why to perform invasive procedures for prenatal diagnosis.

Gil MM, Quezada MS, Revello R, Akolekar R, Nicolaides KH. Analysis of cell-free DNA in maternal blood in screening for fetal aneuploidies: updated meta-analysis. *Ultrasound Obstet Gynecol*. 2015;45:249–266.

A meta-analysis of the performance of cfDNA testing in screening for fetal trisomies 21, 18, 13 and sex chromosome aneuploidies.

Human Fertilisation and Embryology Authority. *Conditions Approved for PGD*. Available at: https://www.hfea.gov.uk/pgd-conditions/.

A list of approved conditions, and those awaiting HFEA approval, for preimplantation genetic diagnosis.

Joint Committee on Genomics in Medicine. *Recommendations for the Use of Chromosome Microarray in Pregnancy*. London: The Royal College of Pathologists;; 2015. Available at: https://www.rcpath.org/uploads/assets/06664c28-0f90-4230-86158c91fea14be6/Recommendations-for-the-use-of-chromosome-microarray-in-pregnancy.pdf.

UK recommendations on the indications and reporting of array-CGH in the prentatal setting.

Lord J, McMullan DJ, Eberhardt RY, et al. Prenatal exome sequencing analysis in fetal structural anomalies detected by ultrasonography (PAGE): a cohort study. *Lancet*. 2019;393(10173):747–757.

A cohort study evaluating the use of whole-exome sequencing to detect the presence of variants in developmental disorder genes in fetuses with structural anomalies.

Odibo A, Krantz D. *Prenatal Screening and Diagnosis, An Issue of Clinics in Laboratory Medicine*. Saunders; 2010.

A comprehensive text covering prenatal screening and diagnosis of genetic disease in pregnancy.

Pereira E, Soria J, eds. *Handbook of Prenatal Diagnosis. Methods, Issues and Health Impacts*. Nova Science Publishers Inc; 2010.

A reference text on prenatal diagnosis.

Santorum M, Wright D, Syngelaki A, et al. Accuracy of first-trimester combined test in screening for trisomies 21, 18 and 13. *Ultrasound Obstet Gynecol*. 2017;49(6):714–720.

A prospective validation study of screening for trisomies 21, 18, and 13 using the first-trimester combined test.

21 Genetic Counseling

Q. What's the difference between... a doctor... and God?

A. God doesn't think He's a doctor.

Anon.

Any couple that has had a child with a serious abnormality must inevitably reflect on why this happened and whether any child (ren) they choose to have in the future might be similarly affected. Similarly, individuals with a family history of a serious disorder are likely to be concerned that they could either develop the disorder or transmit it to future generations. They are also very concerned about the risk that their seemingly unaffected children might transmit the condition to their offspring. For all those affected by a genetic condition that is serious to them, great sensitivity is needed in communication. Just a few words spoken with genuine caring concern can put patients at ease and allow a meaningful session to proceed; just a few careless words that make light of a serious situation can damage communication irrevocably. The importance of confidence and trust in the relationship between patient and health professional must never be underestimated, just as confidence is crucial to contractual business in the commercial world.

Realization of the needs of individuals and couples, together with awareness of the importance of providing them with accurate and appropriate information, have been key factors in the establishment of clinical genetics and genetic counseling.

Definition

Since the first introduction of genetic counseling services approximately 50 years ago, many attempts have been made to devise a satisfactory and all-embracing definition. All can agree that it is a process of communication and education that addresses concerns relating to the development and/or transmission of a hereditary disorder.

An individual who seeks genetic counseling is known as a **consultand**. During the genetic counseling process, it is widely agreed that the counselor should try to ensure that the consultand is provided with information that enables him or her to understand:

1. The medical diagnosis and its implications in terms of prognosis and possible treatment
2. The mode of inheritance of the disorder and the risk of developing and/or transmitting it
3. The choices or options available for dealing with the risks.

It is also agreed that genetic counseling should include a strong communicative and supportive element, so that those who seek information are able to reach their own fully informed decisions without undue pressure or stress (Box 21.1).

Establishing the Diagnosis

Establishing a diagnosis is central to the genetic consultation. If incorrect, inappropriate and totally misleading information could be given, with potentially tragic consequences. However, counseling skills may be greatly tested when both the diagnosis and risk are uncertain.

Reaching a diagnosis in clinical genetics usually involves the three steps fundamental to any medical consultation: taking a history, carrying out an examination, and undertaking appropriate investigations. Often, detailed information about the consultand's family history will have been obtained by a dedicated family history team skilled in confirming relevant information from the family history, or through prior consultation with a genetic counselor. A full and accurate family history is a cornerstone in the whole genetic assessment and counseling process. Further information about the family and personal medical history often emerges at the clinic, when a full examination can be undertaken and appropriate investigations initiated. Some patients may have had limited genetic testing before attendance, for example an array-comparative genomic hybridization (CGH) requested via their pediatrician, requiring a detailed discussion of results. Others will be offered appropriate genetic testing that may include anything from single-gene tests, to gene panels, to whole-exome sequencing, all of which require skilled counseling to gain informed consent. Referral to specialists in other fields, such as neurology, cardiology, and ophthalmology, may also be indicated. Good-quality genetic counseling usually depends on multidisciplinary input to help reach an accurate diagnosis.

Many disorders show **etiological heterogeneity**; for example, hearing loss and nonspecific intellectual disability could both be environmental or genetic in causation. If routine genetic tests and the family history are uninformative, counseling often relies on empirical risks (p. 102), although these are rarely as satisfactory as risks based on a precise and specific diagnosis.

• BOX 21.1 Steps in Genetic Counseling

Diagnosis—based on accurate family history, medical history, examination, and investigations
Risk assessment
Communication
Discussion of options
Long-term contact and support

A disorder shows **genetic heterogeneity** if it can be caused by more than one genetic mechanism (p. 103). Many such disorders are recognized, and counseling can be extremely difficult if the heterogeneity extends to different modes of inheritance. Common examples include sensorineural hearing impairment, retinitis pigmentosa, Charcot-Marie-Tooth disease (p. 292), and connective tissue conditions including the various forms of Ehlers-Danlos syndrome (Fig. 21.1). All can show autosomal dominant (AD), autosomal recessive (AR), and X-linked recessive inheritance, and in some cases mitochondrial inheritance (Table 21.1). Increasingly, gene panel tests for specific groups of genetic conditions, for example, inherited eye disease such as retinitis pigmentosa (Fig. 21.2), provide genetic diagnoses, although may also generate confusion if a variant of uncertain significance (VUS) is identified. These findings pose counseling challenges, both before taking a sample at the stage of explaining the test and when giving results. The challenge may relate to both the risk assessment and to communication of risk if there is a lack of certainty.

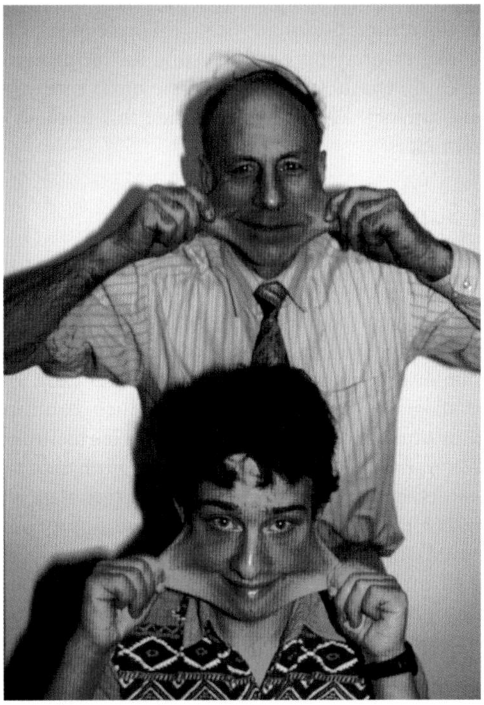

• **Fig. 21.1** Ehlers-Danlos syndrome. The inheritance pattern in this case is autosomal dominant because father and son are affected.

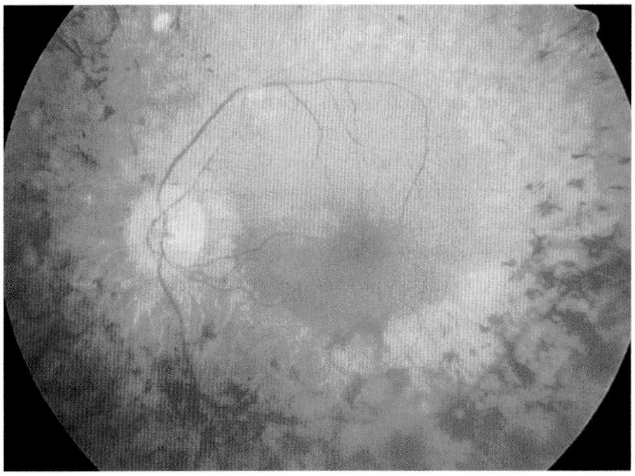

• **Fig. 21.2** Fundus showing typical pigmentary changes of retinitis pigmentosa. (From Yanoff M, Duker JS. *Ophthalmology*. 4th ed. Elsevier; 2014. With permission.)

TABLE 21.1 Hereditary disorders that can show different patterns of inheritance

Disorder	Inheritance Patterns
Cerebellar ataxia	AD, AR
Charcot-Marie-Tooth disease	AD, AR, XR
Congenital cataract	AD, AR, XR
Ehlers-Danlos syndrome	AD, AR, XR
Ichthyosis	AD, AR, XR
Microcephaly	AD, AR, XR
Polycystic kidney disease	AD, AR
Retinitis pigmentosa	AD, AR, XR, M
Sensorineural hearing loss	AD, AR, XR, M

AD, Autosomal dominant; AR, autosomal recessive; M, mitochondrial; XR, X-linked recessive.

Calculating and Presenting the Risk

Calculating and communicating recurrence risk may be straightforward if the pedigree information is very clear, even if the precise diagnosis is not. However, factors such as variable age of onset, reduced penetrance, the finding of a VUS, and conditions demonstrating digenic inheritance can make risk calculation more complex. But communicating risk is far more than simply conveying a numerical figure or percentage. Decision-making in the face of a risk is usually a multifaceted process, so as a working rule of thumb recurrence risks should be quantified, qualified, and placed in context.

Quantification—The Numerical Value of a Risk

Many people struggle to understand the basic concepts of risk, especially different ways of expressing it, such as a form of odds or as a percentage. Thus, a risk of 1 in 4 for AR disease can be presented as an odds ratio of 3 to 1 against, or numerically as 25%. Consistency and clarity are important to avoid confusion, and it is essential to emphasize that the risk applies to *each* pregnancy and that chance has no memory. For parents who have just had a child with an AR disorder, this does not mean their next three children will be unaffected. A tossed coin has no memory of whether it landed heads or tails at the last throw!

It is also important that genetic counselors are not seen as prophets of doom. The flip side of risk can be emphasized, so that if the empiric recurrence risk for bilateral cleft lip and palate is approximately 4%, it follows that there is a 96% chance that the problem will not occur next time.

Qualification—The Nature of a Risk

In making risk-based decisions, studies have shown that the numerical risk value is a less important factor than the nature, or burden, of health issues associated with the diagnosis. Thus a "high" risk of 1 in

2 for a trivial problem such as partial cutaneous syndactyly of toes 2 to 3 will not deter parents. However, a 1% germline mosaicism risk for a condition such as tuberous sclerosis will often be sufficient for parents to request prenatal testing. Other factors, such as whether a condition can be treated successfully, whether it is associated with pain or is life limiting, whether there was experience of bullying in childhood for an affected parent, and a person's own experience of the condition, for example if they nursed a relative through the illness, may all be relevant to decision-making.

Placing Risks in Context

Prospective parents seen at a genetic counseling clinic should be provided with information that enables them to put the risk in context so as to be able to decide for themselves whether it is "high" or "low." For example, it can be helpful (but also alarming) to point out that approximately 1 in 40 of all babies has a congenital malformation (often treatable) or disabling disorder. Therefore, an additional quoted risk of 1 in 50, although initially alarming, might on reflection be perceived as relatively low. As an arbitrary guide, risks of 1 in 10 or greater tend to be regarded as high, 1 in 20 or less as low, and intermediate values as moderate.

Discussing the Options

Having established the diagnosis and discussed the occurrence/recurrence risk, the counselor should provide all relevant information necessary for the individual/couple to make informed decisions of their own. If relevant, the availability of prenatal diagnosis should be discussed, together with details of the procedures, timing, limitations, and associated risks (see Chapter 20). If appropriate, assisted reproductive options should be mentioned, including gamete donation and preimplantation genetic diagnosis (p. 322–333). These techniques can be used when one partner is infertile, for example, for Klinefelter or Turner syndromes (see Chapter 17), or to prevent transmission of a genetic problem in one or both partners.

These issues should be presented very sensitively. For some, the prospect of prenatal diagnosis followed by selective termination of pregnancy is unacceptable, whereas others see this as their way of having healthy children. With wider accessibility of preimplantation genetic diagnosis, many couples, particularly those to whom termination is unacceptable, are choosing this path, but it is vitally important that couples are counseled on the lengthy treatment process, success rate, and associated risks. Whatever the personal views of the counselor, patients are entitled to full information about the prenatal options and procedures that are technically feasible and legally permissible.

Communication and Support

The ability to communicate is essential in genetic counseling and is a two-way process. Apart from providing information, the counselor should seek to be receptive to patients' fears and aspirations, expressed or unexpressed. Good listening skills are vital to the consultation, as well as an ability to present information in a clear, sympathetic, and appropriate manner, with cultural sensitivity.

Often an individual or couple will be emotional and upset when a genetic diagnosis is made, and guilty feelings may ensue. It is normal for patients to look back and scrutinize every event and happening, for example during a pregnancy. The presentation of potentially difficult information must therefore take into account the complex psychology and emotion that may affect the session. The setting should be peaceful and comfortable, with adequate time for discussion and questions. Where possible, technical terms should be avoided or carefully explained. Questions should be answered openly and honestly, including areas of uncertainty relating to the diagnosis and results. Most patients understand that there are limitations, and some parents of children without a diagnosis can accept that their child is special and has bamboozled the medical profession (unfortunately, this is not particularly difficult).

Despite every effort, a counseling session may be intense and the weight of information overwhelming. For this reason, patients should receive a letter, and sometimes additional written material, following the session. They may also be contacted later by a counselor, which provides an opportunity to clarify difficult or confusing issues. Patients and couples who have received complex and sometimes distressing information, for example in relation to prenatal diagnosis or presymptomatic testing for Huntington disease (HD; p. 289–290), should be offered the opportunity for further contact and support. Most centers provide this through a team of genetic counselors.

Patient Support Groups

Lay-led disease-specific support organizations are usually established by highly motivated and well-informed parents or affected families, and play an enormously valuable role. Many have links to experts in the field and provide accurate, understandable information for families. Some nonspecific groups also exist for families where the diagnosis remains unknown. When confronted by a new, rare, or unnamed diagnosis, many families feel very isolated, especially as most health professionals know little about their particular disorder, and these families greatly value contact with others having similar experiences. Information on appropriate support groups should be offered as a routine, although motivated individuals quickly make progress through the internet and social media. Many well-organized groups successfully fund research and help to initiate new services.

Genetic Counseling—Directive or Non-directive?

Genetic counseling is a process of communication that provides information, the goal being to ensure that an individual or couple reach their own decisions with full knowledge of risks and options. There is overwhelming agreement that genetic counseling should be non-directive, with no attempt being made to steer the consultand along a particular course of action. In the same spirit the genetic counselor should be non-judgmental, even if a decision reached seems ill-advised or is contrary to the counselor's own beliefs. The counselor therefore facilitates and enhances autonomy rather than prescribing a particular course of action. This person-centered approach conforms most closely to the model of counseling theory developed by the American Carl Rogers (1902–1987), rather than the psychodynamic approach of Sigmund Freud (1856–1939). If counselors are asked what they would do if facing the patient's situation, it is generally preferable to avoid being drawn into expressing an opinion. Instead, the counselor can help the consultand to imagine the consequences, and how they might feel, if different options were pursued. This is "scenario-based decision counseling" and encourages careful reflection, which is particularly important when decisions have irreversible consequences. It is the patients and their families who have to live with the consequences of their decisions, and they should be encouraged to make the decision that they can best live with—the one they are least likely to regret.

Outcomes in Genetic Counseling

The issue of defining outcomes in genetic counseling is difficult and contentious, partly because of its rather nebulous nature and the difficulty in defining quantifiable end points, but also because of the pressure on healthcare funding. Despite this, the importance of counseling expertise is increasingly recognized in relation to explaining the complexities of whole-exome or -genome sequencing, consenting for testing, and the explanation of genetic test results.

In general, the three main outcome measures that have been assessed are recall, impact on subsequent reproductive behavior, and patient satisfaction. Most studies have shown that the majority of individuals who have attended a genetic counseling clinic have a reasonable recall of the information given, particularly if this was reinforced by a personal letter or follow-up visit. Nevertheless, confusion can arise, and as many as 30% of counselees have difficulty in remembering a precise risk figure. Studies that have focused on the subsequent reproductive behavior of couples that have attended a genetic counseling clinic have shown that approximately 50% have been influenced to some extent, particularly in relation to the severity of the disorder, the desire of parents to have children, and whether prenatal diagnosis and/or treatment are available. Finally, studies that have attempted to assess patient satisfaction have struggled to address the problem of how this should best be defined. For example, an individual could be very satisfied with the way in which they were counseled but remain very dissatisfied by lack of a precise diagnosis or the availability of a definitive prenatal diagnostic test.

During times when there is little or no money for expansion of healthcare services, whether private or state funded, the "value" and "effectiveness" of genetics services, particularly genetic counseling, may be questioned. Health economics has often focused on the prevention of seriously disabling (and expensive) genetic diseases, but this always carries undertones of a eugenics philosophy. Patient autonomy has always been the guiding ethical principle for genetics healthcare professionals, and there is now a very significant profile for rare diseases at a political level. As mentioned, whole-exome and whole-genome sequencing are changing the landscape with respect to data interpretation, which in turn requires genetic counseling skills at the patient interface. Inevitably this will require upskilling within other specialties in order for testing to be delivered in the mainstream setting. The other development that may impact on future genetic counseling practice is the rise of direct-to-consumer testing, whereby individuals choose to pay for a range of genetic tests without the involvement of genetics professionals. This may prove to be a significant component of "personalized healthcare," which will lead to novel studies of outcome measures and patient satisfaction.

Special Issues in Genetic Counseling

There are a number of special issues that can arise in genetic counseling.

Consanguinity

A consanguineous relationship is one between blood relatives who have at least one common ancestor no more remote than a great-great-grandparent. Consanguineous marriage is widespread in many parts of the world (Table 21.2). In Arab populations, the most common type of consanguineous marriage occurs between first cousins who are the children of two brothers, whereas in the Indian subcontinent uncle–niece marriages are the most commonly encountered form of consanguineous relationship. Although there is in these communities some recognition of the potential disadvantageous genetic effects of consanguinity, there is also a strongly held view that these are greatly outweighed by social advantages such as greater family support and marital stability.

TABLE 21.2 Worldwide incidence of consanguineous marriage

Country	Incidence (%)
Kuwait	54
Saudi Arabia	54
Jordan	50
Pakistan	40–50
India	5–60
Syria	33
Egypt	28
Lebanon	25
Algeria	23
Japan	2–4
France, United Kingdom, United States	2

(Modified from various sources including Jaber L, Halpern GJ, Shohat M. The impact of consanguinity worldwide. *Commun Genet.* 1998;1:12–17.)

Many studies have shown that among the offspring of consanguineous marriages there is an increased incidence of both congenital malformations and other conditions that will present later, such as hearing loss and mental retardation. For the offspring of first cousins, the incidence of congenital malformations is increased to nearly twice that seen in the offspring of unrelated parents, attributed mainly to homozygosity for AR disorders.

On the basis of studies of children born to consanguineous parents, it has been estimated that the average human carries no more than one harmful AR disease gene. Most prospective consanguineous parents are concerned primarily with the risk that they will have a disabled child, and fortunately the overall risks are usually relatively small. When estimating a risk for a particular consanguineous relationship, it is generally assumed that each common ancestor carried one deleterious recessive pathogenic variant. Therefore, for first cousins, the probability that their first child will be homozygous for their common grandfather's deleterious gene will be 1 in 64 (Fig. 21.3). Similarly, the risk that this child will be homozygous for the common grandmother's recessive gene will also be 1 in 64. This gives a total probability that the child will be homozygous for one of the grandparent's deleterious genes of 1 in 32. This risk should be added to the general population risk of 1 in 40 that any baby will have a major congenital abnormality (p. 227), to give an overall risk of approximately 1 in 20 that a child born to first-cousin parents will have a significant medical problem. Risks arising from consanguinity for more distant relatives are much lower, although in consanguinity there is also a slightly

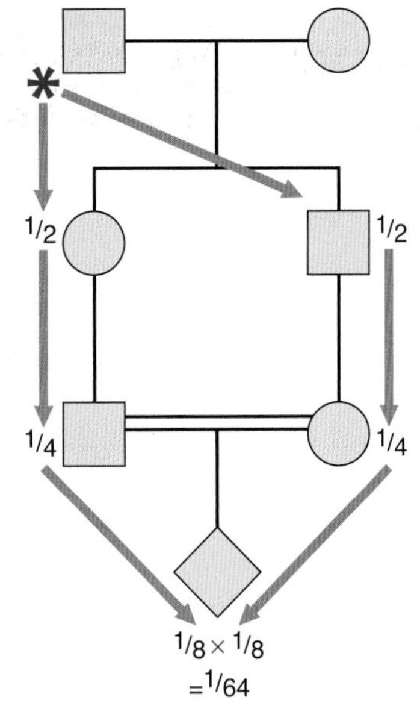

• **Fig. 21.3** Probability that the first child of first cousins will be homozygous for the deleterious allele (*) carried by the common great-grandfather. A similar risk of 1 in 64 will apply to the deleterious allele belonging to the common great-grandmother, giving a total risk of 1 in 32.

increased risk that a child will have a polygenic disorder. In practice this risk is usually very small. In contrast, a close family history of an AR disorder can convey a relatively high risk that a consanguineous couple will have an affected child. For example, if the sibling of someone with an AR disorder marries a first cousin, the risk that their first baby will be affected equals 1 in 24 (p. 99).

Incest

Incestuous relationships are those that occur between first-degree relatives—in other words, brother–sister or parent–child (Table 21.3). Marriage between first-degree relatives is forbidden, both on religious grounds and by legislation, in almost every culture. Incestuous relationships are associated with a very high risk of abnormality in offspring, with less than half the children of such unions being entirely healthy (Table 21.4).

TABLE 21.3 Genetic relationship between relatives and risk of abnormality in their offspring

Genetic Relationship	Proportion of Shared Genes	Risk of Abnormality in Offspring (%)
First Degree	½	50
Parent–child		
Brother–sister		
Second Degree	¼	5–10
Uncle–niece		
Aunt–nephew		
Double first cousins		
Third Degree	1/8	3–5
First cousins		

TABLE 21.4 Frequency of the three main types of abnormality in the children of incestuous relationships

Abnormality	Frequency (%)
Intellectual Impairment	
Severe	25
Mild	35
Autosomal recessive disorder	10–15
Congenital malformation	10

Adoption and Genetic Disorders

The issue of adoption can arise in several situations relating to genetics. First, parents at high risk of having a child with a serious abnormality sometimes express interest in adopting rather than running the risk of having an affected baby. In genetic terms, this is a perfectly reasonable option, although in practice the number of couples wishing to adopt usually far exceeds the number of babies and children available for adoption.

Secondly, geneticists are increasingly being asked to assess children who are available for placement, and these are frequently children whose parents have a history of learning disability and/or prenatal exposure to recreational drugs and alcohol. This can in itself pose great difficulties in the interpretation of genetic results. For example, a copy number variant of uncertain pathogenicity identified on array-CGH in a child with learning difficulties when neither parent is unavailable for follow-up testing. In some cases children are the offspring of an incestuous union, or there is a known family history of a hereditary disorder. This may raise the difficult ethical dilemma of predictive testing in childhood for late-onset conditions (p. 348–349), although most believe that adoption is not a reason to make exceptions to the normal conventions. This can lead to a complex counseling situation in adopted adults requesting testing for late-onset conditions if confirmation of the diagnosis in the family is not possible. Equally, if only part of a family history is known, for example a history of breast cancer, thresholds for offering genetic testing may need to be carefully considering and potentially lowered.

Concern about the possible misuse of genetic testing in neonates and young children who are up for adoption prompted the American Society of Human Genetics and the American College of Medical Genetics to issue joint recommendations. These are based on the best interests of the child and can be summarized as supporting genetic testing only when it would be appropriate for any child of that age, for disorders that manifest during childhood, and for which the application of preventive measures or screening is appropriate in childhood. The joint statement does not support testing for untreatable disorders of adult onset or for detecting predispositions to "physical, mental, or behavioral traits within the normal range."

Nonpaternity

Until the 1980s, blood group studies were the mainstay of trying to contest paternity, but the identity of the father could not be

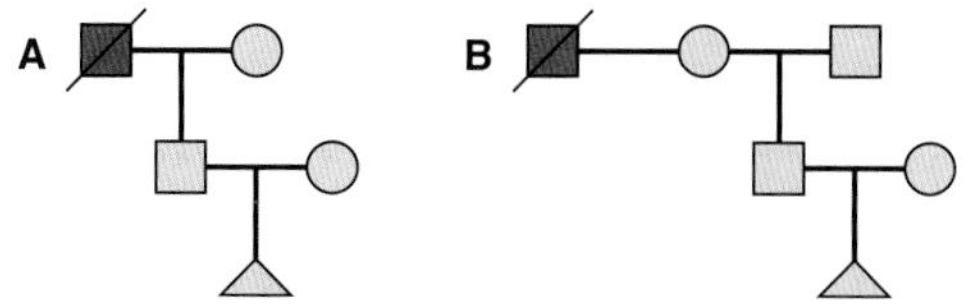

• **Fig. 21.4** Nonpaternity identified in (A) through haplotype analysis (not shown) to provide a couple with a genetic "exclusion" test for Huntington disease, from which the man's father died. The relationships are in fact as shown in (B). Prenatal testing was therefore not indicated, but it was necessary to explain the reason to the couple, which presented a significant counseling challenge.

proved with certainty. If a child possessed a blood group not present in either the mother or putative father, then paternity could be confidently excluded. Similarly, if a child lacked a marker that the putative father would have had to transmit to all of his children, then paternity could be excluded (e.g., a putative father with blood group AB could not have a child with blood group O).

This has now been superseded by DNA fingerprinting, which was first conceived of and developed by Alec Jeffreys in the 1980s and is based on highly variable (or polymorphic) repeat sequences of DNA—variable number tandem repeats, particularly short tandem repeats. In fact, establishing paternity in court cases seldom involves clinical geneticists or genetic counselors. However, very difficult situations may arise when routine genetic testing, mainly using polymorphic markers and haplotype patterns, unexpectedly uncovers nonpaternity. Where this has no medical consequences, genetic counselors will usually not disclose the full results because the impact on family relationships may be devastating. However, take, for example, a couple who request HD exclusion testing for a pregnancy (Fig. 21.4). The man believes he is at 50% risk of developing HD because his deceased father was affected (Fig. 21.4A), and he does not want to undergo predictive testing for himself. Exclusion testing uses polymorphic markers to establish a haplotype pattern, to exclude whether the pregnancy is at 50% risk of having inherited HD. The analysis shows that the man was not fathered by the deceased individual with HD (Fig. 21.4B), and is therefore extremely unlikely to be at risk of HD himself. In this case the results need to be sensitively disclosed because prenatal testing is no longer indicated, and this requires very careful approaches with good counseling skills.

ELEMENTS

1. Genetic counseling may be defined as a communication process that deals with the risk of developing or transmitting a genetic disorder.
2. The most important steps in genetic counseling are the establishment of a diagnosis, estimation of a recurrence risk, communication of relevant information, and provision of appropriate support.
3. The pertinent counseling theory is person-centered, non-directive, and non-judgmental. The goal of genetic counseling is to provide accurate information that enables counselees to make their own fully informed decisions and to help guide people through the process of making those decisions.
4. Marriage between blood relatives conveys an increased risk for an autosomal recessive (AR) disorder in future offspring. The probability that first cousins will have a child with an AR condition is approximately 3%, although this risk can be greater if there is a family history of a specific genetic disorder.
5. Some situations pose very significant genetic counseling challenges, particularly if the information is complex and unexpected disclosures become necessary (e.g., in cases of nonpaternity discovered through routine genetic analysis). Other situations demanding skilled counseling include cross-cultural communication, severe emotional stress in the family, and when facing pressure to perform predictive tests inappropriately.
6. Widespread use of next-generation sequencing poses counseling challenges not only in terms of the potential complexity, or uncertainty, of results but also requires significant involvement of mainstream medical specialists who, until now, may have had little experience discussing genetic testing as part of their role.

CLINICAL SCENARIO 1

A couple come to see you in clinic to discuss the risk of their baby being affected with adenosine deaminase deficiency—an autosomal recessive condition that leads to severe combined immunodeficiency. They are from a consanguineous family and are themselves first cousins.

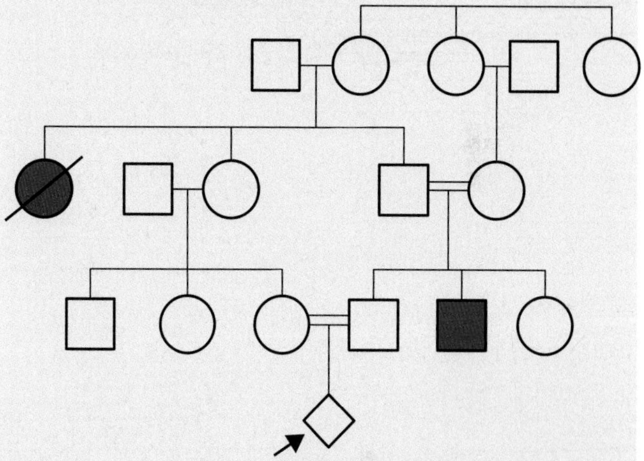

To counsel the couple effectively you need to understand the condition, calculate the risk of them having an affected child, and discuss the options available to further delineate the risk to their unborn child.

CLINICAL SCENARIO 2

A patient comes to clinic to discuss predictive testing for the pathogenic *BRCA1* variant that has been identified in his daughter. His wife has already had a negative predictive test result, so he is assumed likely to be an obligate carrier.

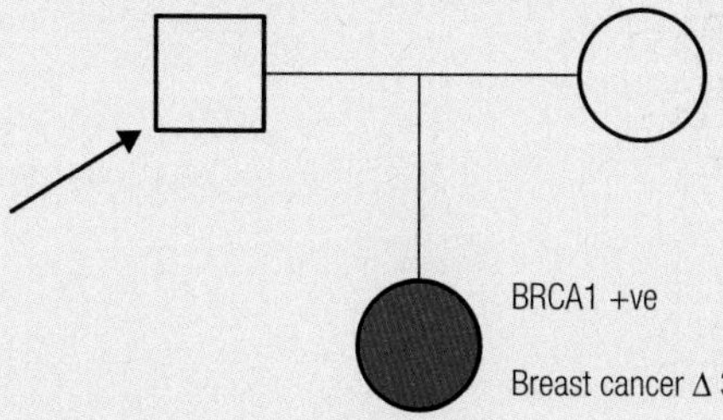

His predictive testing is also negative.
What are the potential explanations for this, and what will you do next?

Further Reading

ASHG/ACMG: Statement. Genetic testing in adoption. *Am J Hum Genet*. 2000;66:761–767.

The joint recommendations of the American Society of Human Genetics and the American College of Medical Genetics on genetic testing in young children who are being placed for adoption.

Clarke A, ed. *Genetic Counseling. Practice and Principles*. London: Routledge; 1994.

A thoughtful and provocative multiauthor text that addresses difficult issues such as predictive testing, screening, prenatal diagnosis, and confidentiality.

Clarke A, Parsons E, Williams A. Outcomes and process in genetic counseling. *Clin Genet*. 1996;50:462–469.

A critical review of previous studies of the outcomes of genetic counseling.

Frets PG, Niermeijer MF. Reproductive planning after genetic counseling: a perspective from the last decade. *Clin Genet*. 1990;38: 295–306.

A review of studies undertaken between 1980 and 1989 to determine which factors are most important in influencing reproductive decisions.

Harper PS. *Practical Genetic Counseling*. 5th ed. Oxford: Butterworth-Heinemann; 1998.

An extremely useful practical guide to all aspects of genetic counseling.

Jaber L, Halpern GJ, Shohat M. The impact of consanguinity worldwide. *Community Genet*. 1998;1:12–17.

A review of the incidence and consequences of consanguinity in various parts of the world.

Jeffreys AJ, Brookfield JFY, Semeonoff R. Positive identification of an immigration test-case using human DNA fingerprints. *Nature*. 1985;317:818–819.

A clever demonstration of the value of genetic fingerprinting in analyzing alleged family relationships.

Turnpenny P. *Parenting a Child with, or at Risk of, Genetic Disorders*. London: British Agencies for Adoption and Fostering; 2014.

A basic text targeting a lay readership, particularly those involved with or affected by adoption.

22 Ethical and Legal Issues in Medical Genetics

The mere existence of the complete reference map and DNA sequence down to the last nucleotide may lead to the absurdity of reductionism—the misconception that we know everything it means to be human; or to the absurdity of determinism—that what we are is a direct and inevitable consequence of what our genome is.

Victor McKusick (1991)

Ethics is the branch of knowledge that deals with moral principles, which in turn relate to principles of right and wrong, justice, and standards of behavior. Traditionally, the reference points are based on a synthesis of the philosophical and religious views of well-informed, respected, thinking members of society. In this way, a code of practice evolves that is seen as reasonable and acceptable by a majority, which often forms the basis for professional guidelines or regulations. It might be argued that there are no "absolutes" in ethical and moral debates. In complex scenarios, in which there may be competing and conflicting claims to an ethical principle, practical decisions and actions often have to be based on a balancing of duties, responsibilities, and rights. Ethics, like science, is not static but moves on, and in fact the development of the two disciplines is closely intertwined.

Ethical issues arise in all branches of medicine, but human genetics poses particular challenges because genetic identity impinges not just on an individual but also on close relatives and the extended family, and beyond kindreds to society in general. In the minds of the general public, clinical genetics and genetic counseling can easily be confused with eugenics—which may be defined as the science of "improving" a species through breeding, or "improving the gene pool." Crucially, modern clinical genetics bears no relationship with the appalling eugenic philosophies practiced in Nazi Germany and, to a much lesser extent, elsewhere in Europe and the United States between the two world wars. Eugenics was very fashionable for a period. The term was coined by Francis Galton in 1883, a year after the death of Charles Darwin, to whom Galton was related as a half-cousin. Three International Congresses of Eugenics took place between 1912 and 1932, the first in London, and the great and good of the day in science, politics, and social planning attended. In the United States a Eugenics Records Office was established in 1910 with funding from the Carnegie Institution, and conducted research until discredited in the mid-1930s. The site eventually became the Cold Spring Harbor Laboratory in 1962.

Emphasis has already been placed on the fundamental principle that genetic counseling is a non-directive and non-judgmental communication process whereby factual knowledge is imparted to facilitate informed personal choice (see Chapter 21). Indeed, clinical geneticists have been pioneers in practicing and promoting nonpaternalism in medicine, and 5% of the original budget for the Human Genome Project was set aside for funding studies into the ethical, legal, and social implications of the knowledge gained from the project. This was in recognition of the challenges generated by discoveries and new technologies in molecular genetics. Keen awareness and debate continues, as reflected in the controversy surrounding policies and practice in disclosing "incidental findings" from whole-exome or whole-genome sequencing, not to mention the complexities surrounding consent for such testing. As these technologies enter medicine's mainstream, there is a need for guidelines and some protections enshrined in law, and clinical geneticists will often be well placed to offer advice. Here we explore some of the controversial and difficult areas, although often there is no clear right or wrong approach, and individual views vary widely. Sometimes in a clinical setting the best that can be hoped for is to arrive at a mutually acceptable compromise, with an explicit agreement that opposing views are respected and, personal conscience permitting, patient needs are met, or at least fully addressed.

General Principles

The time-honored four principles of medical ethics that command wide consensus are listed in Box 22.1. Developed and championed by the American ethicists Tom Beauchamp and James Childress, these principles provide an acceptable framework, although close scrutiny of many difficult dilemmas highlights limitations in these principles and apparent conflicts between them. Everyone involved in clinical genetics will sooner or later be confronted by complex and challenging ethical situations, some of which pose

• BOX 22.1 Fundamental Ethical Principles

- **Autonomy**—incorporating respect for the individual, privacy, the importance of informed consent and confidentiality
- **Beneficence**—the principle of seeking to do good and therefore acting in the best interests of the patient
- **Non-maleficence**—the principle of seeking, overall, not to harm (i.e., not to leave the patient in a worse condition than before treatment)
- **Justice**—incorporating fairness for the patient in the context of the resources available, equity of access and opportunity

particularly difficult problems with no obvious solution, and certainly no perfect one. Just as patients need to balance risks when planning about a treatment option, so the clinician/counselor may need to balance these principles one against the other. A particular difficulty in medical genetics can be the principle of autonomy, given that genes are shared with biological relatives. Individual autonomy needs sometimes to be weighed against the principle of doing good and doing no harm, to close family members.

The **Beauchamp and Childress framework** of ethical principles is, unsurprisingly, not the only one in use, and others have developed them into practical approaches. These include the Jonsen framework (Box 22.2) and the more detailed scheme developed by Mike Parker of Oxford's Ethox Centre (Box 22.3), which builds on previous proposals. Taken together, these provide a practical approach to clinical ethics, which is an expanding discipline in healthcare.

In practice, the issues that commonly arise in the genetics clinic during any patient contact are outlined here.

Autonomy

It is the patient who should be empowered and in charge when it comes to decisions that have to be made. The degree to which this is possible is a function of the quality of information given. Sometimes patients are still seeking some form of guidance to give them confidence in the decision they reach, and it will require the judgment of the clinician/counselor as to how much guidance is appropriate in a given situation. The patient should feel comfortable to proceed no further and opt out freely at any stage of the process; this applies particularly in the context of predictive genetic testing and reproductive decisions.

Informed Choice

The patient is entitled to full information about all options available in a given situation, including the option of not participating. Potential consequences of each option should be discussed. No duress should be applied, and the clinician/counselor should not have a vested interest in the patient pursuing any particular course of action.

Informed Consent

A patient is entitled to an honest and full explanation before any procedure or test is undertaken. Information should include details of the risks, limitations, implications, and possible outcomes of each intervention. In the current climate, with respect to full information and the doctor–patient contract, some form of signed consent is generally obtained for every action that exposes the patient—access to medical records, clinical photography, genetic testing, and storage of DNA. In fact, there is no legal requirement to obtain signed consent for taking a blood test from which DNA is extracted and stored. The issue was addressed by the UK Human Tissue Act 2004. According to the act, DNA does not constitute "human tissue" in the same way as biopsy samples or cellular material, for which formal consent *is* required, whether the tissue is from the living or the dead. The act does require that consent is formally obtained where cellular material is used to obtain genetic information for another person. In a clinical setting, this must be clearly discussed and documented.

In clinical genetics, many patients who are candidates for clinical examination and genetic testing are children or adults with learning difficulties who may lack capacity to grant informed consent. Furthermore, the result of any examination or test may have only a small chance of directly benefiting the patient but is potentially very important for family members. Here the law is important. In England and Wales, the Mental Capacity Act of 2005 came into effect in 2007 and applies to adults aged 16 and older. It replaced case law for health (and social) care, and there is a legal duty to use the legislation and apply the "Test for Capacity" (Box 22.4) for any relevant decision in people who lack capacity. Decisions must take into account the "best interests" of the patient but can also embrace the wider interests that relate to the family. In England and Wales, the law allows for an appropriate person

• BOX 22.2 The Jonsen Framework: A Practical Approach to Clinical Ethics

- Indications for medical intervention—Establish a diagnosis. Determine the options for treatment and the prognoses for each of the options.
- Preferences of patient—Is the patient competent? If so, what does he or she want? If not competent, what is in the patient's best interest?
- Quality of life—Will the proposed treatment improve the patient's quality of life?
- Contextual features—Do religious, cultural, or legal factors have an impact on the decision?

• BOX 22.3 The Ethox Centre Clinical Ethics Framework (Mike Parker)

1. What are the relevant clinical and other facts (e.g., family dynamics, general practitioner support)?
2. What would constitute an appropriate decision-making process?
   - Who is to be held responsible?
   - When does the decision have to be made?
   - Who should be involved?
   - What are the procedural rules (e.g., confidentiality)?
3. List the available options.
4. What are the morally significant features of each option? For example:
   - What does the patient want to happen?
   - Is the patient competent?
   - If the patient is not competent, what is in his or her "best interests"?
   - What are the foreseeable consequences of each option?
5. What does the law/guidance say about each of these options?
6. For each realistic option, identify the moral arguments in favor and against.
7. Choose an option based on judgment of the relative merits of these arguments:
   - How does this case compare with others?
   - Are there any key terms for which the meaning needs to be agreed (e.g., "best interest," "person")?
   - Are the arguments "valid"?
   - Consider the foreseeable consequences (local and more broad).
   - Do the options "respect persons"?
   - What would be the implications of this decision applied as a general rule?
8. Identify the strongest counterargument to the option you have chosen.
9. Can you rebut this argument? What are your reasons?
10. Make a decision.
11. Review this decision in the light of what actually happens and learn from it.

• BOX 22.4 Mental Capacity Act, 2005, England and Wales (Outline)—Principles, Definition, and Test for Capacity

Principles
- A person must be assumed to have capacity unless proved otherwise
- A decision taken for someone lacking capacity must be in the person's best interests
- Practical steps must be taken to help someone make a decision
- If the test of capacity is passed, the decision taken must be respected

Definition of Capacity

'. . . a person lacks capacity in relation to a matter if at the material time he is unable to make a decision for himself in relation to the matter because of an impairment of, or a disturbance in the functioning of, the mind or brain.'
- In relation to any decision, it is therefore:
- Time-specific (a person's capacity may change)
- Decision-specific (capacity varies, depending on the decision)

Test for Capacity:

At a specific time and for a specific decision, the person should:
- Understand the information relevant to the decision
- Retain the information
- Weigh the information as part of decision-making
- Communicate the decision

appointed by the Court of Protection to act on their behalf, whereas in Scotland it is legally permitted for certain designated adults, including family members, to give consent (or refuse) on behalf of a person lacking capacity.

The United Kingdom, like many other countries, is beginning to see the more widespread use of genomic technology that will become commonplace within mainstream medicine in the near future. This poses significant challenges to the process of informed consent, as clinicians will not only be expected to provide detailed information on clinical testing and its possible outcomes but also discuss consent to the use of a person's genomic data by third-party research groups. This is a significant addition to the workload of busy mainstream clinicians who may have had little prior experience of discussing genetic testing, and it is therefore critical that appropriate training, guidance, and support are available.

Confidentiality

A patient has a right to complete confidentiality, and there are clearly many issues relating to genetic disease that a patient, or a couple, would wish to keep totally private. Stigmatization and guilt may still accompany the concept of hereditary illness. Historically, genetic services have tended to keep family files separate from a patient's hospital record, not only because of the sensitive nature of the information, but because there is likely to be significant detail of people other than the proband. The advent of electronic records systems challenges the concept of confidentiality in genetics, as these are generally accessible to all healthcare staff. Detailed information about family members should clearly not be available in an individual's record, without the appropriate consent, and there may be certain things that patients would not wish to be visible, for example a predictive Huntington disease (HD) result. Careful consideration of the design of such systems is therefore important.

Traditionally, confidentiality should be breached only under extreme circumstances; for example, when it is deemed that an individual's behavior could convey a high risk of harm to self or to others. In trying to help some patients in the genetics clinic, however, it may be desirable to have a sample of DNA from a key family member, necessitating at least some disclosure of detail. There is also the difficult area of sharing information and results between different regional genetic services. This is a complex and much-debated area in the context of genetic and hereditary disease, but the principle of patient consent for release and/or sharing of information should be the norm.

Universality

Much of traditional medical ethical thinking has upheld the autonomy of the individual as paramount. Growing appreciation of the ethical challenges posed by genetics has led to calls for a new pragmatism in bioethics, built on the concept that the human genome is fundamentally common to all humankind, and can—and indeed should—be considered a shared resource because we have a shared identity at this level. What we learn from one individual's genome, a family's genome, or a population's genome carries potential benefits far beyond the immediate relevance and impact for that individual or family. From this it is a direct and natural step to consider how best the genetic information is exchanged, for the medical benefits may be far-reaching. This ethical attitude therefore leads on to a realization of mutual respect, reciprocity, and world citizenry in the context of human genetics. It prompts the individual to consider his or her responsibility toward others, as well as to society, both in the present and in the future.

Meanwhile, however, very real ethical problems have to be faced and dealt with in some way, and it is to a few of these that we now turn.

Ethical Dilemmas in the Genetics Clinic

Prenatal Diagnosis

Many methods are now widely available for diagnosing structural abnormalities and genetic disorders during the first and second trimesters (see Chapter 20). The availability of tests to make these diagnoses, along with the Abortion Act of 1967, have lead to the first real availability of choice in the context of pregnancy in human history. Not surprisingly, the issue of prenatal diagnosis and subsequent offer of termination of pregnancy raises many difficult issues for those directly involved and raises serious questions about the way in which society views and cares for individuals with disability. In the United Kingdom, termination of pregnancy is permitted up to and beyond 24 weeks' gestation if the fetus has a lethal condition such as anencephaly, or if there is a serious risk of major physical or mental disability. For good reason, terms such as "serious" are not defined in the relevant legislation, but this can inevitably lead to controversy over interpretation.

The difficulties surrounding prenatal diagnosis can be illustrated by considering some of the general principles that have already been discussed. At the top of the list comes informed consent. In the United Kingdom, all pregnant women are offered maternal serum screening for Down syndrome, Edwards syndrome, and Patau syndrome in the first trimester. This combined screen includes blood tests alongside estimation of nuchal translucency by ultrasound at 12 weeks' gestation (p. 321). In addition, a 20-week fetal anomaly scan is routine and has replaced the 16-week assay of maternal serum α-fetoprotein to look for neural tube defects. For fully informed consent to be obtained in these situations, it is essential that pregnant women have access to detailed counseling by unhurried professionals who are knowledgeable, experienced, and sympathetic. All pregnant women in the United Kingdom are supplied with a pregnancy pack during their midwife booking appointment, which includes detailed written information on the screening tests offered in pregnancy, which should also be discussed by the midwife, with further time put aside before testing to answer questions.

The most difficult problems in prenatal diagnosis are those involving autonomy and individual choice relating to disease severity and the decision that termination is justified. Consider the following. First, parents whose first child, a boy, has autism, are expecting another baby. They have read that autism is more common in boys than girls, so they request sexing of the fetus with a view to terminating a male but continuing if female. However, the risk of having another child with autism is roughly 5%. Such a request presents the clinician and counselor with a challenge. Sex selection for purely social reasons is illegal in the United Kingdom as grounds for termination of pregnancy as well as embryo selection by preimplantation genetic diagnosis (PGD; supported overwhelmingly by a public consultation exercise)—children should be considered gifts, not consumer commodities. In the United States and elsewhere, however, it is permissible to perform sex selection by PGD for "family balancing." But when the risk of a second child having autism is low, and it cannot be guaranteed that a daughter would not be affected, clinicians would resist sex selection and termination. Second, consider the unusual request of parents with congenital deafness who indicate they wish to continue a pregnancy only if tests show that their unborn baby is also affected. Should the autonomy and choice of the couple, who live in a non-hearing world, be respected? Again, most clinicians would decline the request, but the scenario challenges perceptions and definitions of what it means to be normal. Third, when a fetus is found to have cleft lip and palate, for which surgical correction usually achieves an excellent outcome, if one of the parents themselves had an unhappy childhood because of stigmatization for the same problem, they may wish to exercise choice and legally could do so up until 24 weeks' gestation.

The subject of pregnancy termination frequently generates controversy. Proponents of choice argue that selective termination should be available, particularly if the alternative involves a lifetime of pain and suffering. But prenatal tests often provide reassurance, and without the availability of diagnostic techniques, couples might decide against trying to have (more) children at all. In the context of abortion in general, termination on grounds of fetal abnormality accounted for less than 2% of the over 200,000 abortions carried out in the United Kingdom in 2018.

Those who hold opposing views argue on religious, moral, or ethical grounds that termination of pregnancy is little less than legalized infanticide. Key to the ethical issue here are views on the status and rights of the embryo and fetus. For those who believe that the fertilized egg constitutes full human status, PGD and embryo research are unacceptable, as well as most in vitro fertilization (IVF) as practiced by virtue of generating spare frozen human embryos, most never to be used. There is also concern that prenatal diagnostic screening programs could lead to a devaluing of the "disabled" and "abnormal" in society (notwithstanding that these terms are difficult to define and all too often used pejoratively), with a possible shift of resources away from their care to the funding of programs aimed at "preventing" their birth. This ethical debate was fueled anew as array-comparative genomic hybridization (CGH) technology moved firmly into the prenatal setting. The Joint Committee on Genomics in Medicine, in 2015, published recommendations for the use of chromosome array in pregnancy, which gives clear guidance on the indications for use of array testing, reporting in pregnancy, and variants or incidental findings that should not be routinely reported, for example, low penetrance neurosusceptibility loci. This guidance should ensure that only certain pathogenic findings relevant to a pregnancy, or family, are reported. As we move into the era of next-generation sequencing, the debate continues with regard to whole-exome, or -genome, sequencing in the prenatal setting. Although not routinely used across all genetics centers in the United Kingdom, some have reported excellent diagnostic yields from rapid prenatal exome sequencing, which has been of huge benefit to families when making decisions about whether to continue a pregnancy. Of course, the complexities of interpreting exome data with the limited phenotype information available in the prenatal setting must not be underestimated, and while there are clear guidelines for managing this data in the postnatal setting, similar guidelines will be needed for prenatal cases. It is quite conceivable that a large range of tests will be technically possible on cell-free fetal DNA (p. 334) in the maternal circulation—without the risk of provoking a miscarriage from an invasive procedure. At the moment, this is available, as a standard test, for a limited list of conditions in the United Kingdom. However, patients can opt to have a privately funded bespoke non-invasive test designed for a particular genetic condition. How will these new genetic technologies affect the scope of prenatal tests that may be offered, and who will decide? And will anyone be so bold as to offer selection for "desirable characteristics," for example, hair color, musical ability, athleticism?

The results of public consultation exercises conducted by the Advisory Committee on Genetic Testing (subsumed into the Human Genetics Commission—abolished in 2010) and the Human Fertilisation and Embryology Act are reasonably reassuring. The views expressed support for the applications of genetic technologies in prenatal testing for serious disorders but demonstrated concern over wider applications. Similarly, research published by the British Social Attitudes survey suggested that the public supports these activities in general, but expressed deep reservations for application of the technologies for **genetic enhancement**. Enhancement of embryos or gametes strikes at the very heart of what it means to have one's own genetic identity through laws of chance. This seems to be a powerful undercurrent in the understanding of who we are as individuals and as a species but has been tested in the area of "mitochondrial donation" through nuclear transfer to prevent serious life-shortening mitochondrial disease. After much parliamentary debate, this became legal in the United Kingdom in 2015, with opponents and the media inappropriately branding the development "three-parent babies." One site in the United Kingdom is licensed by the Human Fertilisation and Embryology Authority to perform mitochondrial donation, and the first patient license for treatment was granted in 2018.

Predictive Testing in Childhood

Understandably, parents sometimes wish to know whether or not a child has inherited the gene for an adult-onset autosomal dominant disorder that runs in the family. It could be argued that this knowledge will help them guide their child toward the most appropriate support through education, and that to refuse their request is a denial of their rights as parents. Similarly, parents may request testing to clarify the status of young healthy children at risk of being carriers of a recessive disorder such as cystic fibrosis (CF; sometimes this information will have become available as a result of prenatal diagnostic testing).

The problem with agreeing to such a request is that it infringes the child's own future autonomy, so most geneticists recommend that testing be delayed until the child reaches an age at which an informed decision is possible. There is also concern for the child about the possible psychological harm of growing up with certain knowledge of developing a serious adult-onset hereditary disorder, or being a carrier of a recessive disorder, particularly if the tests have proved negative in the child's siblings. However, although there is consensus among geneticists that children should not be tested for carrier status, the evidence that such testing causes emotional or psychological harm is weak. The situation is of course very different if predictive testing could directly benefit the child by identifying the need for a medical or surgical intervention in childhood. This applies to conditions such as familial hypercholesterolemia (p. 277) and some of the familial cancer-predisposing syndromes when there is an associated risk of childhood cancer for which screening can be offered (Table 14.9). Generally in these situations, genetic testing is recommended around the time when screening tests or preventive measures would be initiated.

One of the arguments for not testing children for adult-onset disorders is that parents might view their child differently, or even prejudicially. This type of argument has been voiced in relation to the PGD cases that have selected embryos not only for their negative affection status for Fanconi anemia but also to be a potential stem-cell donor for an affected child—so-called "savior siblings," first successful in the United States in 2000. Those objecting to this use of technology cite a utilitarian, or instrumental, attitude toward the child created in this way. Furthermore, the child so created has no choice about whether to be a tissue-matched donor for the sick sibling. Will the child eventually feel "used" by the parents, and how might he or she feel if the treatment fails and the sick sibling dies? At present these questions are imponderables because most children created for this purpose are still young.

Implications for the Immediate Family (Inadvertent Testing or Testing by "Proxy")

A positive test result in an individual can have major implications for close antecedent relatives who themselves may not wish to be informed of their disease status. Consider HD, for example. A young man age 20 years requests predictive testing before starting his family, knowing that his 65-year-old paternal grandfather has a confirmed diagnosis. Predictive testing would be relatively straightforward were it not for the fact that his father, who is obviously at a prior risk of 1 in 2, specifically does not wish to know whether he will develop the disease. Thus the young man has raised the difficult question of how to honor his request without inadvertently carrying out a predictive test on his father. A negative result in the young man leaves the situation unchanged for his father, but a positive result might be difficult to conceal from an observant father. The son knows that his father will develop the disease if he has not done so already.

Although this can be a difficult scenario, guidelines drawn up in 1994 concluded that "every effort should be made by the counselors and the persons concerned to come to a satisfactory solution." Most geneticists follow the rider that, "if no consensus can be reached the right of the adult child to know should have priority over the right of the parent not to know."

Implications for the Extended Family

It is generally agreed that the diagnosis of a condition that could have implications for other family members should lead to the offer of tests for the extended family (e.g., balanced translocations and serious X-linked recessive disorders).

The main ethical problem that may arise here is one of confidentiality. A carrier of a translocation or serious X-linked recessive disorder is usually urged to alert close family relatives to the possibility that they could also be carriers and therefore at risk of having affected children. Alternatively, permission can be sought for members of the genetics team to make these approaches. Occasionally a patient, for whatever reason, will refuse to allow this information to be disseminated.

Faced with this situation, what should the clinical geneticist do? In practice most would try to convince their patient of the importance of offering information and tests to relatives by providing an explanation of the consequences and future ill-feeling that could ensue if a relative was to have an affected child whose birth could have been avoided. In most cases, skilled and sensitive counseling will lead to a satisfactory solution. Ultimately, however, some clinical geneticists would opt to respect their patient's confidentiality rather than break the trust that forms a cornerstone of the traditional doctor–patient relationship. Not all would agree, and therefore some clinicians will actively seek a sensitive way to disclose the medical/genetic information that may include involving others such as the patients' general practitioner. This view is backed up by the statements of authoritative working parties, such as the Nuffield Council on Bioethics. A recent legal case in the United Kingdom regarding a patient with HD and his family (*ABC vs. St George's Healthcare NHS Trust*) perfectly exemplifies the question over confidentiality and the rights of family members to be given relevant information about risks to their health. Until this case, UK law recognized a legal duty to protect individual patient confidentiality, and while professional guidance encouraged consideration of those who may be at risk of serious harm, there was no legal protection for breaching confidentiality when a patient refused consent to disclosure of information. Following a High Court trial, it was concluded that healthcare professionals do owe a legal duty to balance the rights and interests of third parties in these circumstances but only where there is an already established relationship between healthcare professionals and the at-risk family member(s). As genomic testing takes its place in mainstream medicine, this novel legal duty is likely to have implications for clinicians both within clinical genetics and the wider medical community.

Informed Consent in Genetic Research

Any offer of genetic testing should be accompanied by a full and clear explanation of what the test involves and how the results could have implications for the individual and family members. This applies equally to informed consent when participating in genetic research. Many people are perfectly willing to hold out their arm for a blood test which might "help others," particularly if they have personal experience of a serious disorder in their own family. However, their simple act of altruism may have unforeseen consequences. For example, it is unlikely that they will ever have considered whether their sample will be tested anonymously, who will be informed of the result, or whether other tests will be carried out on stored DNA in the future as new techniques are developed. The issues listed in Box 22.5 help to emphasise that all aspects of informed consent should be addressed when samples are collected for genetic research. Just as signed consent for genetic testing and storage of DNA has become routine in the service setting in the United Kingdom (although not a legal requirement under the Human Tissue Act 2004), similar rigor should be adhered to in a

• BOX 22.5 Issues of Disclosure and Consent in Genetic Research—The Nature of the Study

- Who is doing the study, and where is it being carried out?
- Availability of results and their implications for the individual and extended family regarding health, employment, and insurance
- Anonymity of testing and confidentiality of results
- Long-term storage of DNA and its possible use in other research projects
- Potential commercial applications and profit

research setting. As mentioned previously, this is of the utmost importance as genomic testing moves into mainstream medicine.

Secondary or Incidental Findings

The advent of whole-exome and whole-genome sequencing in research, and increasingly in service testing, has brought to the fore a debate regarding the handling and disclosure of so-called secondary, or incidental, findings. This should not be a problem where the analysis is restricted to genes of interest that are relevant to the phenotype, but may occur where there is no such restriction, and the issue is of particular concern for conditions where a presymptomatic medical or surgical intervention, or screening modality, would normally be offered. Looking at the 100,000 Genomes Project as an example, part of the consent process included discussion of additional, or secondary, findings for example the discovery of a pathogenic variant in a highly penetrant mendelian cancer condition. This may bear no relation to the reason for offering genome sequencing, but it has serious implications. A defined list of serious or life-threatening genetic conditions was looked for during the project, with the appropriate patient consent, although none of these results have yet been released. Incidental findings are not restricted to exome, or genome, sequencing; however, with more basic testing, such as array-CGH, having the potential to reveal such findings, for example, identifying Duchenne muscular dystrophy (DMD) carrier status on a prenatal test requested for a raised nuchal translucency, or a *PMP22* duplication (p. 293) in a child with developmental delay. Neither explains the phenotype, but both have potential clinical relevance. The dilemma is which incidental findings should be disclosed to the patients being tested, whether the circumstances of the test alter what ought to be disclosed, and whether results should only be disclosed if they are interpretable as definitely pathogenic. In addition, it is fair to question to what extent most people can understand the implications for a broad range of possible diseases, especially when testing may have been offered at a time of already great stress. How much time can realistically be devoted to counseling in this consent process, and do the complexities of the medical and genetic issues fundamentally undermine the very concept, and therefore legality, of "fully informed consent"? To this can be added the evolution of knowledge that will inevitably take place regarding the significance of certain findings, as well as the range of conditions for which a presymptomatic intervention becomes available, which has led to a separate debate regarding professionals' responsibilities to recontact patients when new information comes to light.

The American College of Genetics and Genomics previously issued a policy on secondary findings and settled on 56 genes that met the criteria for disclosure, if tested. The key points of the policy are summarized in Box 22.6.

Ethical Dilemmas and the Public Interest

Advances in genetics attract great media interest, and this has brought the ethical debate to a wide public arena. Topics such as insurance, forensic science and DNA databases, patenting, gene therapy, population screening, cloning, stem-cell research, and hybrids are seen as being of major societal, commercial, and political importance, and therefore impact clinical and laboratory practice in medical genetics.

Genetics and Insurance

Predictive genetic testing for adult-onset disorders that may give rise to chronic ill health and/or reduced life expectancy has led to concern about the extent to which the results of tests should be revealed to outside agencies, especially insurance companies providing life cover, private health care, and critical illness and disability income. Insurance arranged through an employer might, in theory, compromise career prospects.

The life insurance industry is competitive and profit driven. Private insurance is based on "mutuality," whereby risks are pooled for individuals in similar circumstances. In contrast, public health services are based on the principle of "solidarity," whereby health provision for everyone is funded from general taxation. It is understandable that the life insurance industry is concerned that individuals who receive a positive predictive test result will take out large policies without revealing their true risk status. On the other hand, the genetics community is concerned that individuals who test positive will become victims of discrimination, and perhaps uninsurable. This concern extends to those with a family history of a late-onset disorder, who might be refused insurance unless they undergo predictive testing.

The possibility that DNA testing will create an uninsurable "genetic underclass" led to the introduction of legislation in parts of the United States aimed at limiting the use of genetic information by health insurers. In 1996 this culminated in President Clinton signing The Health Insurance Portability and Accountability Act, which expressly prevented employer-based health plans from refusing coverage on genetic grounds when a person changes employment. In the United Kingdom, this whole arena was considered in 1995 by the House of Commons Science and Technology Committee, which recommended that a Human Genetics Advisory Commission be established to overview

• BOX 22.6 Key Points of the Policy of the American College of Genetics and Genomics Regarding Secondary (Incidental) Findings

- When clinical genome-scale sequencing is performed, written informed consent should be obtained by a qualified genetics healthcare professional regarding all aspects of the nature of the test, including the routine analysis of a set of genes deemed to be highly medically actionable.
- Patients may opt out of the analysis of this set of genes but should be made aware of the potential ramifications of doing so.
- The same policy should apply to children as well as adults, with parents being able to opt out of the analysis.
- It is not feasible for patients to be offered the option of choosing a subset of medically actionable genes for analysis, and the decision regarding routine analysis should apply to the entire set of genes deemed actionable by the American College of Medical Genetics and Genomics.

developments in human genetics. In 1997, this Advisory Commission recommended that applicants for life insurance should not have to disclose the results of any genetic test to a prospective insurer, and that a moratorium on disclosure of results should last for at least 2 years until genetic testing had been carefully evaluated.

Fortunately, the Association of British Insurers has negotiated amicably over the years, and the moratorium has been renewed several times, most recently in 2018, when it was extended indefinitely. The essential aspects of the agreement, in the joint document entitled "The Code on Genetic Testing and Insurance," are listed in Box 22.7.

These issues are likely to come under repeated scrutiny in the future. Clinical genome sequencing is now a reality, and there are many direct-to-consumer offers to discover one's genetic susceptibilities upon payment of a fee and production of a suitable saliva sample. Consequently, a large amount of individual genome data is being stored in the commercially driven private sector. The medical genetics community therefore has an advocacy role to ensure that the genetically disadvantaged, through no fault of their own, do not face discrimination when seeking healthcare or long-term life insurance, which are powerful arguments in favor of publicly funded healthcare systems.

• BOX 22.7 Key Points in the 'Code on Genetic Testing and Insurance' Negotiated Between the UK Government and the Association of British Insurers (ABI), 2018

- Applicants must not be asked to undergo predictive or diagnostic genetic testing in order to obtain insurance.
- The classes of insurance, and financial limits above which predictive test results may become relevant:
  1. Life insurance policies up to £500,000 (per person)
  2. Critical illness insurance up to £300,000 (per person)
  3. Income protection insurance up to £30,000 per annum
- There is no requirement for a customer to reveal:
  1. A predictive genetic test result from a test taken after the insurance cover has started, for as long as that cover is in force
  2. The test result of another person, such as a blood relative
  3. A genetic result acquired as part of clinical research
- Disclosure of a predictive genetic test result is only required if all of the following apply:
  1. The customer is seeking insurance cover above the financial limits set out in the Moratorium
  2. The test has been assessed by a panel of experts and approved by Government; the only test this applies to (in 2018) is Huntington disease when an application for life insurance surpasses £500,000
- Where insurers ask an applicant to disclose a result, under the limited accepted circumstances, they will not impose disproportionate terms, conditions or exclusions related to that result.
- An applicant may disclose a positive result from a predictive genetic test if they wish the result to be considered in the underwriting decision, and insurers must provide detail of how this may affect the insurance decision.

Forensic Science and DNA Databases

Similar themes relating to personal privacy apply to the existence of the police-controlled **National DNA Database**. The use of DNA fingerprinting in criminal investigations, to the tune of approximately 25,000 cases per annum, is now so sophisticated that there is a natural desire on the part of law enforcers to be able to identify the DNA fingerprint for anyone in the general population. Currently, nearly 6 million samples are stored, although one in seven of these are estimated to be duplicates, but that is still approaching 10% of the population (including an estimated 1 million with no criminal conviction), which is the largest of any country. For certain types of crime, whole communities are invited to come forward to give a sample of DNA so that they can be eliminated from enquiries. In 2009, the police came under political pressure to scrap "innocent" profiles after the European Court of Human Rights declared that to hold the profiles of innocents indefinitely was a breach of privacy. This led to the removal of nearly 2 million profiles of innocent individuals, including children, in 2012 to 2013 under the Protection of Freedoms Act 2012.

The National DNA Database is huge, but so too are the collections for big population studies, such as the Avon Longitudinal Study of Parents and Children, the UK Biobank, the UK10K, and the 100,000 Genomes Project. As research, these samples will have been rigorously consented, but it is essential for safeguards to be in place.

Gene Patenting and the Human Genome Project

Naturally occurring human DNA sequences have been the subject of some bitter and prolonged legal disputes over patenting, encapsulating the conflict between commercial goals and altruistic academia. During the 1990s, Myriad Genetics in the United States sought to impose their exclusive license for genetic testing for *BRCA1* and *BRCA2* (p. 201). In fact, in 2004, the European Patent Office revoked the patent, denying Myriad a license fee from every *BRCA* test undertaken in Europe, and thereby setting a precedent for other contentious cases. However, the rights to one gene associated with obesity were sold in 1995 for $70 million, and in 1997 DeCODE, the Icelandic genomics company at the center of the controversy regarding national assent, sold the potential rights to 12 genes associated with common complex diseases to Hoffman–La Roche for $200 million. Logically, commercial developments using human DNA sequences are based on "discovery" rather than "invention," whereas the engineering of a new sequencing platform would fall into the latter category. It is clearly acceptable for biotechnology companies that have invested heavily in molecular research to recover their costs and make a fair return, but our genome represents humankind's "common heritage," and the case is overwhelmingly persuasive that the information gained through the Human Genome and Human Variome Projects should be freely available for all to benefit. To this end an "International Charter" for sharing biospecimens and data has recently been proposed. There are examples, however, of patients and whole communities who have donated their blood samples for research, little realizing that their generosity could be exploited for financial gain, resulting in some high-profile court cases, particularly in the United States. The legal issues can be complex, especially in an international context, but we believe strongly in promoting equity of access, transparency, and scientific rigor toward the goal of evidence-based medicine available to as many as possible.

Gene Therapy

The prospect of successful gene therapy (p. 218) to treat genetic disease is one of the most exciting developments of the modern era. However, apart from a handful of notable examples, the potential has not yet been realized. As the furor over genetically modified foods has shown, the general public is seriously concerned about the safety and potential abuse of gene therapy. The "slippery slope" argument is frequently invoked, whereby to take the first step leads incrementally and inevitably to uncontrolled experimentation. The strongest advocates of new approaches, understandably, are the families affected by extremely unpleasant conditions, but their yearning for solutions should rightly be set into a societal context, and special advisory committees and working parties were set up in response. In the United Kingdom, the Gene Therapy Advisory Committee (GTAC) was established in 1993 to review all proposals to conduct gene therapy in humans and to monitor ongoing trials, thus safeguarding patients' rights and confidentiality. Significantly, the GTAC recommended that genetic modification involving the germline be prohibited and limited to somatic cells to prevent the possibility of newly modified genes being transmitted to future generations. Furthermore, modification of somatic cells should be restricted to the treatment of serious diseases, and not to the alteration human characteristics, such as intelligence or athletic prowess, for example. In 2011, the work of the GTAC was subsumed into the Health Research Authority.

Newborn and Population Screening

Newborn screening programs offering detection of common autosomal recessive disorders have been available for many years (p. 156), and in some countries the range of diseases tested has been greatly extended in recent years. These programs have generally been very well received (e.g., thalassemia and Tay-Sachs disease), although this was not the case for α1-antitrypsin deficiency screening in Scandinavia, which was abandoned because it proved stressful. Similarly, pilot studies to diagnose DMD soon after birth—essentially to inform and prevent the birth of a second affected son before a diagnosis is made in the first—have not resulted in widespread implementation of a population screening program.

As mentioned, the advent of clinical exome sequencing raises fresh ethical concerns about how the technology might be applied. This is particularly so in the field of prenatal genetics and screening. Analysis of DNA from chorionic villus tissue, for example, could theoretically be subjected to whole-exome sequencing in conjunction with parental samples, quite apart from a condition for which the fetus is at high risk. Although there is little interest in this at present, and the costs would be prohibitive for a public screening program, when the price of testing decreases, there may be strong pressure to offer this choice in some form.

With respect to screening programs that detect carrier status for disease, the issues are slightly different. Early efforts to introduce sickle-cell carrier detection in North America were largely unsuccessful because of misinformation, discrimination, and stigmatization. Also, pilot studies assessing the responses to CF carrier screening in Europeans yielded conflicting results (p. 159). These experiences illustrate the importance of informed consent and the difficulties of ensuring both autonomy and informed choice. Neonatal CF screening in the United Kingdom is aimed at identifying babies with CF, but the screening detects a roughly equal number who are simply carriers, who have obviously not made an informed choice. This is considered justifiable when weighed against the benefits of early diagnosis of CF. In general, however, well-intended programs of carrier detection should ensure that participation is entirely voluntary, with adequate counseling, and it is also essential to minimize the risk of conferring any sense of stigmatization or genetic inferiority. Furthermore, confidentiality is important. This may be difficult, however, for individuals found to be genetically susceptible to a medical problem from environmental industrial hazards, which could lead to employment discrimination. Legal protections should be in place for these individuals.

Cloning and Stem Cell Research

Dolly the sheep, born in July 1996 at Roslin, near Edinburgh, was the first mammal to be cloned from an adult cell, and when her existence was announced about 6 months later, the world suddenly became intensely interested in cloning. Dolly was "conceived" by fusing individual mammary gland cells with unfertilized eggs from which the nucleus had been removed; 277 attempts failed before a successful pregnancy ensued. It was immediately assumed that the technology would sooner or later lead to a cloned human being, and there have been some unsubstantiated, bogus claims to this effect. However, there has been widespread rejection of any move toward human reproductive cloning. Experiments with animals have continued to highlight a very poor success rate, and in some cloned animals the features have suggested possible defects in genomic imprinting. Dolly died prematurely from lung disease and other problems in 2003, but it is notable that her identical cloned siblings have not suffered the same fate.

Nevertheless, the lessons learned from Dolly shifted the focus to therapeutic cloning using stem cells, and this has begun to yield some impressive results with respect to treating human disease (p. 222).

The main ethical difficulty in this field relates to the source of stem cells. There is no serious ethical difficulty relating to stem cells harvested from the fully formed person, whether taken from the umbilical cord or the mature adult. But a strong school of scientific opinion maintains that there is no substitute for studying embryonic stem cells (ESCs) to understand how cells differentiate from primitive into more complex types. In 2005, the UK Parliament moved swiftly to approve an extension to research on early human embryos for this purpose. Research on human embryos up to 14 days of age was already permitted under the Human Fertilisation and Embryology Act 1990. The United Kingdom therefore became one of the most attractive places to work in stem-cell research because, although regulated, it is legal. Publicly funded research of this kind was not permitted in the United States until a change of political direction in 2009. Progress has been painfully slow for those engaged in this work, and the focus shifted to the creation of animal–human ("human-admixed") hybrids and chimeras because of the poor supply and quality of human oocytes (usually "leftovers" from infertility treatment) for use in nuclear cell transfer. In the United Kingdom, Newcastle University was granted a license to collect fresh eggs for stem-cell research from egg donors in return for a reduction in the cost of IVF treatment, a decision greeted with alarm in some quarters. This group was also the first, in 2005, to create a human blastocyst after nuclear transfer.

Those who object to the use of ESCs believe it is not only treating the human embryo with disrespect and tampering with the sanctity of life but also could lead eventually to reproductive cloning. The Human Fertilisation and Embryology Act 1990 permits the creation of human embryos for research, but very few have been created. This Act was reviewed and updated to

• BOX 22.8 The Key 2008 Amendments to the Human Fertilisation and Embryology Act (HFE) 1990

- Ensure that all human embryos outside the body—whatever the process used in their creation—are subject to regulation.
- Ensure regulation of 'human-admixed' embryos created from a combination of human and animal genetic material for research.
- Ban sex selection of offspring for non-medical reasons. This puts into statute a ban on non-medical sex selection currently in place as a matter of HFEA policy. Sex selection is allowed for medical reasons—for example, to avoid a serious disease that affects only boys.
- Recognise same-sex couples as legal parents of children conceived through the use of donated sperm, eggs or embryos. These provisions enable, for example, the civil partner of a woman who carries a child via *in vitro* fertilisation to be recognised as the child's legal parent.
- Retain a duty to take account of the welfare of the child in providing fertility treatment but replace the reference to 'the need for a father' with 'the need for supportive parenting'—hence valuing the role of all parents.
- Alter the restrictions on the use of HFEA-collected data to help enable follow-up research of infertility treatment.

accommodate new developments, and the revised Act came into effect in 2009. The main provisions are listed in Box 22.8, and the ethical debate continues.

Conclusion

Each new discovery in human molecular genetics and cell biology brings new challenges and raises new dilemmas for which there are often no easy answers. On a global scale it is essential that safeguards are in place to ensure that fundamental principles such as privacy, confidentiality, and respect for human life at all stages and ages are upheld. The medical genetics community can, and should, continue to play a pivotal role in trying to balance the needs of their patients and families with the ethical issues and tensions outlined here. That role will no doubt extend to support, and training, of non–genetics specialists as next-generation sequencing technology takes a more prominent role across all medical specialties. This is an important advocacy role, and toward that end it is hoped that this chapter, and indeed the rest of this book, can make a positive contribution.

ELEMENTS

1. Ethical considerations impinge on almost every aspect of clinical genetics. In a wider context, developments in molecular genetics have important ethical implications for society at large.
2. Particularly difficult problems in clinical genetics include prenatal diagnosis and screening, predictive testing in childhood, genetic testing in the extended family, confidentiality, consent, privacy, and disclosure of information.
3. Ethical issues on a wider scale, in relation to the possible applications of genetic technologies, include population screening, the handling of secondary (incidental) findings, the electronic storage of large amounts of genetic information, the use of genetic test results by the insurance industry and commercial sector, gene patenting, gene therapy, and cloning.
4. There are no easy or correct solutions for many of the difficult ethical problems that arise in medical genetics. Guidelines, codes of practice, and sometimes regulations have an important role in establishing and maintaining standards, as well as preserving respect for the individual, the family, and wider societal needs.

CLINICAL SCENARIO 1

A patient attends your clinic with an extensive family history of breast cancer. She has been diagnosed with a grade 3, triple negative, ductal carcinoma at the age of 38. You discuss *BRCA* gene testing, to which she consents. Testing identifies a pathogenic *BRCA1* variant.

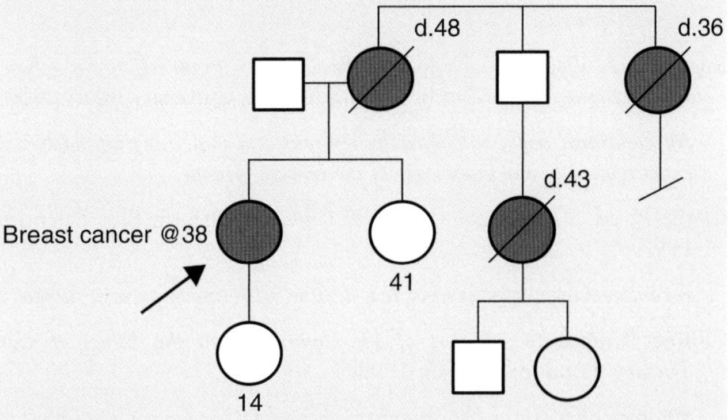

Before her follow-up appointment, the patient contacts you explaining that she no longer wishes to know her result. She understands that her result may have implications for family members, one of whom is known to you, but does not wish her result to be shared with them.

What considerations need to be made in this case, and how would you proceed?

CLINICAL SCENARIO 2

A 13-year-old girl is referred to your clinic to discuss testing for Friedreich ataxia, with which her brother is affected. Her brother was diagnosed at the age of 8, has since developed hypertrophic cardiomyopathy, and is largely wheelchair-bound at the age of 17.

How will you approach this case in clinic, and what are the key points to consider?

Further Reading

ACMG Board of Directors. ACMG policy statement: Updated recommendations regarding analysis and reporting of secondary findings in clinical genome-scale sequencing. *Genet Med.* 2015;17:68–69.

Recommendations from the American College of Genetics and Genomics on the use of whole-exome and whole-genome sequencing including analysis/reporting of looked for secondary findings.

American Society of Human Genetics Report. Statement on informed consent for genetic research. *Am J Hum Genet.* 1996;59:471–474.

The statement of the American Society of Human Genetics Board of Directors on the issues relating to informed consent in genetic research.

Baily MA, Murray TH, eds. *Ethics and Newborn Genetic Screening: New Technologies, New Challenges.* Baltimore, MD: Johns Hopkins University Press; 2009.

A multiauthor volume with a focus on the health economics of newborn screening and distributive justice.

British Medical Association. *Human genetics. Choice and responsibility.* Oxford: Oxford University Press; 1998.

A comprehensive, wide-ranging report produced by a British Medical Association medical ethics committee steering group on the ethical issues raised by genetics in clinical practice.

Bryant J, Baggott la Velle L, Searle J, eds. *Bioethics for Scientists.* Chichester: John Wiley; 2002.

A multiauthor text of wide scope with many contributions relevant to medical genetics.

Buchanan A, Daniels N, Wikler D, Brock DW. *From Chance to Choice: Genetics and Justice.* Cambridge: Cambridge University Press; 2000.

An acclaimed book, intellectually rigorous and wide-ranging, addressing issues related to our knowledge of the human genome.

Clarke A, ed. *The Genetic Testing of Children.* Oxford: Bios Scientific; 1997.

A comprehensive multiauthor text dealing with this important subject.

Clothier Committee. *Report of the Committee on the Ethics of Gene Therapy.* London: HMSO; 1992.

Recommendations of the committee chaired by Sir Cecil Clothier on the ethical aspects of somatic cell and germline gene therapy.

Collins FS. Shattuck lecture—medical and societal consequences of the human genome project. *N Engl J Med.* 1999;341:28–37.

A contemporary overview of the Human Genome Project with emphasis on its possible ethical and social implications.

Green RC, Berg JS, Grody WW, et al. ACMG recommendations for reporting of incidental findings in clinical exome and genome sequencing. *Genet Med.* 2013;15:565–574.

Recommendations for the management of incidental findings in exome or genome sequencing.

Harper PS, Clarke AJ. *Genetics: Society and Clinical Practice.* Oxford: Bios Scientific; 1997.

A thoughtful account of the important ethical and social aspects of recent developments in clinical genetics.

HM Government. Association of British Insurers. *Code on Genetic Testing and Insurance.* 2018. Available at: https://www.abi.org.uk/globalassets/files/publications/public/genetics/code-on-genetic-testing-and-insurance_embargoed.pdf.

The 6th iteration of an agreement between the Association of British Insurers and the UK government on how insurers use genetic information.

Human Genetics Commission. *Inside Information: Balancing Interests in the Use of Personal Genetic Data.* London: Department of Health; 2002.

A detailed working party report by the Human Genetics Commission covering the use and abuse of personal genetic information.

Joint Committee on Genomics in Medicine (JCGM). *Recommendations for the Use of Chromosome Microarray in Pregnancy.* London: The Royal College of Pathologists; 2015. Available at: https://www.rcpath.org/uploads/assets/06664c28-0f90-4230-86158c91fea14be6/Recommendations-for-the-use-of-chromosome-microarray-in-pregnancy.pdf.

UK recommendations for the use, interpretation, and reporting of array variants in pregnancy.

Jonsen AR, Siegler M, Winslade WJ. *Clinical Ethics: A Practical Approach to Ethical Decisions in Clinical Medicine.* 3rd ed. New York, NY: McGraw-Hill; 1992.

The key reference that outlines the Jonsen framework for decision-making in clinical ethics.

Knoppers BM. Status, sale and patenting of human genetic material: an international survey. *Nat Genet.* 1999;22:23–26.

An article written in the light of a landmark legal and social policy document "Directive on the Legal Protection of Biotechnology Inventions" from the European Parliament, 1998.

Knoppers BM, Chadwick R. Human genetic research: Emerging trends in ethics. *Nat Rev Genet.* 2005;6:75–79.

An overview of international policies on gene patenting.

Mascalzoni D, Dove ES, Rubinstein Y, et al. International charter of principles for sharing bio-specimens and data. *Eur J Hum Genet.* 2015;23:721–728.

Firm proposals to stimulate open access of information in the genomic era.

McInnis MG. The assent of a nation: genetics and Iceland. *Clin Genet.* 1999;55:234–239.

A critical review of the complex ethical issues raised by the decision of the Icelandic government to collaborate in genetic research with a biotechnology company.

Nuffield Council on Bioethics. *Genetic Screening: Ethical Issues.* London: Nuffield Council on Bioethics; 1993.

A very helpful document for professional guidance.

Nuffield Council on Bioethics. *Mental Disorders and Genetics: The Ethical Context.* London: Nuffield Council on Bioethics; 1998.

A further detailed document dealing with genetic issues in the context of mental health.

Pokorski RJ. Insurance underwriting in the genetic era. *Am J Hum Genet.* 1997;60:205–216.

A detailed account of the issues surrounding the use of genetic tests by the insurance industry.

Royal College of Physicians. Royal College of Pathologists and British Society for Genetic Medicine. *Consent and Confidentiality in Genomic Medicine: Guidance on the use of Genetic and Genomic Information in The clinic.* Report of the Joint Committee on Genomics in Medicine. 3rd ed. London: RCP, RCPath and BSGM; 2019.

A detailed report aimed to provide practical support for professionals in interpreting the law, regulatory guidance, and expectations of public ethics with regard to genetic and genomic information.

Glossary

A. Abbreviation for adenine.

Acentric. Lacking a centromere.

Acetylation. The introduction of an acetyl group into a molecule; often used by the body to help eliminate substances by the liver.

Acoustic neuromas. Tumors of the VIIIth cranial (hearing) nerve that occur in neurofibromatosis type 2, now known as "vestibular schwannomas."

Acquired. In genetics, refers to any medical condition not predetermined in the genetic make-up at fertilization (i.e., germline).

Acquired somatic genetic disease. Genetic disease caused by gene or chromosomal variants that may occur any time postfertilization.

Acrocentric. Term used to describe a chromosome where the centromere is near one end and the short arm usually consists of satellite material.

Activation. In genetics and molecular biology, any event leading to biologically active molecules acquiring the ability to perform their biological function.

Acute-phase proteins. Proteins involved in innate immunity produced in reaction to infection, including C-reactive protein, mannose-binding protein, and serum amyloid P component.

Adaptive immunity. The ability of the immune system to create immunological memory after an initial response to a specific pathogen.

Additive. Relating to genetic risk, the sum of individual effects.

Adenine. A purine base in DNA and RNA.

Adenomatous polyposis coli (APC). See *Familial adenomatous polyposis.*

Adenylate residue. Pertaining to the nucleic acid purine base "adenine."

Adult stem cell. Undifferentiated cell found in the body after early development (i.e., not embryonic).

AIDS. Acquired immune deficiency syndrome.

Allele (=allelomorph). Alternative form of a gene found at the same locus on homologous chromosomes.

Allelic association. Next to, or close to, a particular allele of interest.

Allograft. A tissue graft between nonidentical individuals.

Allotypes. Genetically determined variants of antibodies.

Alpha (α)-thalassemia. Inherited disorder of hemoglobin involving underproduction of the α-globin chains, occurring most commonly in people from Southeast Asia.

Alternative pathway. One of the two pathways of the activation of complement that, in this instance, involves cell membranes of microorganisms.

Alternative polyadenylation. Different mRNA transcripts generated by the addition of varying number(s) of adenine residues.

Alternative splicing. The process whereby particular exons of a gene may be included, or excluded, from the final, processed mRNA, so that one gene can encode for multiple different proteins.

Alu repeat. Short repeated DNA sequences that appear to have homology with transposable elements in other organisms.

Am. The group of genetic variants associated with the immunoglobulin A heavy chain.

Amino acid. An organic compound containing both carboxyl ($-COOH$) and amino ($-NH_2$) groups.

Amniocentesis. Procedure for obtaining amniotic fluid and cells for prenatal diagnosis.

Amorph. A mutation that leads to complete loss of function.

Amplicon. A section of DNA or RNA that may be either the source or product of natural or artificial amplification or replication events.

Amplimer. An alternative term for "amplicon."

Anaphase. The stage of cell division when the chromosomes leave the equatorial plate and migrate to opposite poles of the spindle.

Anaphase lag. Loss of a chromosome as it moves to the pole of the cell during anaphase; can lead to monosomy.

Aneuploid. A chromosome number that is not an exact multiple of the haploid number (e.g., $2\text{ N} - 1$ or $2\text{ N} + 1$, where N is the haploid number of chromosomes).

Anterior information. Information previously known that leads to the prior probability.

Antibody (=immunoglobulin). A serum protein formed in response to an antigenic stimulus that reacts specifically with that antigen.

Anticipation. The tendency for some autosomal dominant diseases to manifest at an earlier age and/or to increase in severity with each succeeding generation.

Anticodon. The complementary triplet of the transfer RNA molecule that binds to it with a particular amino acid.

Anti-D. Refers to the Rhesus immunoglobulin given to Rhesus-negative mothers who have been pregnant with a Rhesus-positive infant, to prevent sensitization to the D antigen.

Antigen. A substance that elicits the synthesis of antibody with which it specifically reacts.

Antigen-binding fragment (Fab). The fragment of the antibody molecule produced by papain digestion that is responsible for antigen binding.

Antiparallel. Opposite orientation of the two strands of a DNA duplex; one runs in the 3′ to 5′ direction, the other in the 5′ to 3′ direction.

Antisense oligonucleotide. A short oligonucleotide synthesized to bind to a particular RNA or DNA sequence to block its expression.

Antisense strand. The template strand of DNA.

Apical ectodermal ridge (AER). Area of ectoderm in the developing limb bud that produces growth factors.

Apolipoproteins. Proteins involved in lipid transportation in the circulation.

Apoptosis. Programmed involution or cell death of a developing tissue or organ of the body.

Artificial insemination by donor (AID). Use of semen from a male donor as a reproductive option for couples at high risk of transmitting a genetic disorder.

ARMS. Amplification-refractory mutation system, a form of allele-specific PCR using primers specific for the normal and variant sequences.

Ascertainment. The finding and selection of families with a hereditary disorder.

Association. The occurrence of a particular allele in a group of patients more often than can be accounted for by chance.

Assortative mating (= nonrandom mating). The preferential selection of a spouse with a particular phenotype.

Atherosclerosis. Fatty degenerative plaque that accumulates in the intimal wall of blood vessels.

Autoimmune diseases. Diseases believed to be caused by the body not recognizing its own antigens.

Autonomous replication sequences. DNA sequences that are necessary for accurate replication within yeast.

Autonomy. In medical ethics, the principle of a rational individual making an informed, uncoerced decision.

Autoradiography. Detection of radioactively labeled molecules on an X-ray film.

Autosomal dominant. A gene on one of the nonsex chromosomes that manifests in the heterozygous state.

Autosomal inheritance. The pattern of inheritance shown by a disorder or trait determined by a gene on one of the nonsex chromosomes.

Autosomal recessive. A gene located on one of the nonsex chromosomes that manifests in the homozygous state.

Autosome. Any of the 22 nonsex chromosomes.

Autozygosity. Homozygosity as a result of identity by descent from a common ancestor.

Autozygosity mapping. The technique used to identify a disease locus based on the principle of homozygosity by descent from a common ancestor.

Axonal. Relates to the axon—the long slender projection of a nerve cell (neuron).

Azoospermia. Absence of sperm in semen.

B lymphocytes. Antibody-producing lymphocytes involved in humoral immunity.

Bacterial artificial chromosome (BAC). An artificial chromosome created from modification of the fertility factor of plasmids that allows incorporation of up to 330 kilobases of foreign DNA.

Bacteriophage (= phage). A virus that infects bacteria.

Balanced polymorphism. Two different genetic variants that are stably present in a population (i.e., selective advantages and disadvantages cancel each other out).

Balanced translocation. See *Reciprocal translocation.*

BAM (binary alignment map) file. (*.bam) A compressed binary version of a sequence alignment map (SAM) file that is used to represent aligned genomic sequences up to 128 megabases.

Bare lymphocyte syndrome. A rare autosomal recessive form of severe combined immunodeficiency resulting from absence of the class II molecules of the major histocompatibility complex.

Barr body. The condensation of the inactive X chromosome seen in the nucleus of certain types of cells from females. See *Sex chromatin.*

Base. Short for the nitrogenous bases in nucleic acid molecules (A, adenine; T, thymine; U, uracil; C, cytosine; G, guanine).

Base excision repair. One of the cellular mechanisms that repairs damaged DNA throughout the cell cycle.

Base pair (bp). A pair of complementary bases in DNA (A with T, G with C).

Bayes' theorem. Combining the prior and conditional probabilities of certain events or the results of specific tests to give a joint probability to derive the posterior or relative probability.

Beauchamp and Childress framework. The universally acknowledged principles of medical ethics.

Bence Jones protein. The monoclonal antibody produced in large amounts by a person with multiple myeloma, a tumor of antibody-producing plasma cells.

Beneficence. The principle of doing good in medical ethics.

Beta (β)-thalassemia. Inherited disorder of hemoglobin involving underproduction of the β-globin chain, occurring most commonly in people from the Mediterranean region and the Indian subcontinent.

Bias of ascertainment. An artifact that must be taken into account in family studies when looking at segregation ratios, caused by families coming to attention because they have affected individual(s).

Bilaminar. Two-layered—in cell biology referring to two layers of cells.

Biochemical disorder. An inherited disorder involving a metabolic pathway (i.e., an inborn error of metabolism).

Biochemical genetics. In general, the discipline that concentrates on the diagnosis and management of inborn errors of metabolism.

Bioinformatics. The science of interpreting the significance of data generated by molecular genetics and DNA sequencing.

Biological or genetic determinism. The premise that our genetic makeup is the only factor determining all aspects of our health and disease.

Biosynthesis. Use of recombinant DNA techniques to produce molecules of biological and medical importance in the laboratory or commercially.

Bivalent. A pair of synapsed homologous chromosomes.

Blastocyst. Early embryo consisting of embryoblast and trophoblast.

Blastomere. A single cell of the early fertilized conceptus.

Blighted ovum. The fertilization of an egg (ovum) by a sperm that leads to a nonviable embryo.

Blood chimera. A mixture of cells of different genetic origin present in non-identical twins *in utero* as a result of an exchange of cells via the placenta.

Boundary elements. Short sequences of DNA, usually from 500 base pairs to 3 kilobases in size, that block or inhibit the influence of regulatory elements of adjacent genes.

Break-point cluster (bcr). Region of chromosome 22 involved in the translocation seen in the majority of people with chronic myeloid leukemia.

C. Abbreviation for cytosine.

CAAT box. A conserved, noncoding, so-called promoter sequence about 80 base pairs upstream from the start of transcription.

Café-au-lait (CAL). Refers to coffee-colored patches of skin.

Cancer family syndrome. Clustering in certain families of particular types of cancers, in which it has been proposed that the different types of malignancy could be caused by a single dominant gene, specifically Lynch type II.

Cancer genetics. The study of the genetic basis of cancer.

Candidate gene. A gene whose function or location suggests that it is likely to be responsible for a particular genetic disease or disorder.

5′ Cap. Modification of the nascent mRNA by the addition of a methylated guanine nucleotide to the 5′ end of the molecule by an unusual 5′ to 5′ triphosphate linkage.

CA repeat. A short dinucleotide sequence present as tandem repeats at multiple sites in the human genome, producing microsatellite polymorphisms.

Carrier. Person heterozygous for a recessive gene; male or female for autosomal genes or female for X-linked genes.

Cascade screening. Identification within a family of carriers for an autosomal recessive disorder or people with an autosomal dominant gene after ascertainment of an index case.

Case control study. A form of observational research; in medicine, a cohort of patients with a defined condition is compared with a group matched for other characteristics.

Cell-free fetal DNA. DNA from the fetus (derived from placental trophoblast tissue) that reaches the maternal circulation.

Cell-mediated immunity. Immunity that involves the T lymphocytes in fighting intracellular infection; is also involved in transplantation rejection and delayed hypersensitivity.

Cellular oncogene. See *Protooncogene.*

Centimorgan (cM). Unit used to measure map distances, equivalent to a 1% chance of recombination (crossing over).

Central dogma. The concept that genetic information is usually transmitted only from DNA to RNA to protein.

Centric fusion. The fusion of the centromeres of two acrocentric chromosomes to form a Robertsonian translocation.

Centriole. The cellular structure from which microtubules radiate in the mitotic spindle involved in the separation of chromosomes in mitosis.

Centromere (= kinetochore). The point at which the two chromatids of a chromosome are joined, and the region of the chromosome that becomes attached to the spindle during cell division.

Chain termination mutation. A coding DNA variant that converts an amino acid codon into a termination codon.

Chemotaxis. The attraction of phagocytes to the site of infection by components of complement.

Chiasmata. Crossovers between chromosomes in meiosis.

Chimera. An individual composed of two populations of cells with different genotypes.

Chimeric gene. A novel gene composed of two coding regions fused together, often caused by a replication error or translocation, that encodes a chimeric protein.

Chorion. Layer of cells covering a fertilized ovum, some of which (the chorion frondosum) will later form the placenta.

Chorionic villus sampling (CVS). Procedure using ultrasonographic guidance to obtain chorionic villi from the chorion frondosum for prenatal diagnosis.

Chromatid. During cell division, each chromosome divides longitudinally into two strands, or chromatids, which are held together by the centromere.

Chromatin. The tertiary coiling of the nucleosomes of the chromosomes with associated proteins.

Chromatin fiber. A "beads on a string" structure 30 nanometers in diameter consisting of nucleosome (DNA and histone protein) arrays in their most compact form.

Chromatin fiber fluorescence in situ hybridization. Use of extended chromatin or DNA fibers with fluorescence in situ hybridization to physically map DNA clones or sequences.

Chromosomal analysis. The process of counting and analyzing the banding pattern of an individual's chromosomes.

Chromosomal fragments. Acentric chromosomes that can arise as a result of segregation of a paracentric inversion and that are usually incapable of replication.

Chromosome. Thread-like, darkly staining body within the nucleus, composed of DNA and chromatin, that carries genetic information.

Chromosome instability. The presence of breaks and gaps in chromosomes from people with a number of disorders, associated with an increased risk of neoplasia.

Chromosome mapping. Assigning a gene or DNA sequence to a specific chromosome or a particular region of a chromosome.

Chromosome-mediated gene transfer. The technique of transferring chromosomes or parts of chromosomes to somatic cell hybrids to enable more detailed chromosome mapping.

Chromosome (or chromosomal) microarray (CMA). See *Microarray-comparative genomic hybridization.*

Chromosome painting. The *in situ* hybridization of fluorescently labeled probes to a chromosome preparation to allow identification of a particular chromosome(s).

Chromosome walking. Using an ordered assembly of clones to extend from a known start point.

Circos plot. A method of presenting genomic data in a circular diagram that demonstrates different variant types across all chromosomes and their relationship to each other.

***Cis*-acting.** Regulatory elements in the promoter region that act on genes on the same chromosome.

Class switching. The normal change in antibody class from IgM to IgG in the immune response.

Classic gene families. Multigene families that show a high degree of sequence homology.

Classic pathway. One of the two ways of activation of complement, in this instance involving antigen-antibody complexes.

ClinVar. A website hosted by the National Institutes of Health that aggregates information about human genomic variation.

Clone. A group of cells, all of which are derived from a single cell by repeated mitoses and all of which have the same genetic information.

Clone contigs. Assembly of clones that have been mapped and ordered to produce an overlapping array.

Cloning in silico. The use of a number of computer programs that can search genomic DNA sequence databases for sequence homology to known genes, as well as DNA sequences specific to all genes such as conserved intron/exon splice junctions, promoter sequences, polyadenylation sites, and stretches of open-reading frames, to identify novel genes.

cM. Abbreviation for centimorgan.

CNV. See *Copy number variation.*

Codominance. When both alleles are expressed in the heterozygote.

Codon. A sequence of three adjacent nucleotides that codes for one amino acid or chain termination.

Combined test. The test routinely offered in the first trimester of pregnancy to estimate risk of trisomy 13, 18, and 21. Combines measurement of nuchal translucency, maternal age, PAPP-A (pregnancy-associated plasma protein-A), and beta-hcg (human chorionic gonadotropin).

Common cancers. The cancers that occur commonly in humans, such as bowel and breast cancer.

Common diseases. The diseases that occur commonly in humans (e.g., cancer, coronary artery disease, diabetes).

Community genetics. The branch of medical genetics concerned with screening and the prevention of genetic diseases on a population basis.

Comparative genomic hybridization. A method of analyzing genomic material by comparing the genome of interest with a reference sample to identify copy number variation.

Comparative genomics. The identification of orthologous genes in different species.

Competent. Making bacterial cell membrane permeable to DNA by a variety of different methods, including exposure to certain salts or high voltage.

Complement. A series of at least 10 serum proteins in humans (and other vertebrates) that can be activated by either the "classic" or the "alternative" pathway and that interact in sequence to bring about the destruction of cellular antigens.

Complementary DNA (cDNA). DNA synthesized from mRNA by the enzyme reverse transcriptase.

Complementary strands. DNA strands whose sequences specifically pair together, adenine to thymine and guanine to cytosine.

Complete ascertainment. A term used in segregation analysis for a type of study that identifies all affected individuals in a population.

Complex trait. A genetic disease or characteristic that is not associated with a single gene (i.e., mendelian) but caused by multiple DNA variants.

Compound heterozygote. An individual who is affected by an autosomal recessive disorder having two different genetic variants in homologous genes.

Concordance. When both members of a pair of twins exhibit the same trait, they are said to be concordant. If only one twin has the trait, the twins are said to be discordant.

Conditional knockout. A mutation that is expressed only under certain conditions (e.g., raised temperature).

Conditional probability. Observations or tests that can be used to modify prior probabilities using Bayesian calculation in risk estimations.

Conditionally toxic or suicide gene. Genes that are introduced in gene therapy and that, under certain conditions or after the introduction of a certain substance, will kill the cell.

Confined placental mosaicism. The occurrence of a chromosomal abnormality in chorionic villus samples obtained for first-trimester prenatal diagnosis in which the fetus has a normal chromosomal complement.

Congenital. Any abnormality, whether genetic or not, that is present at birth.

Congenital hypertrophy of the retinal pigment epithelium (CHRPE). Abnormal retinal pigmentation that, when present in people at risk for familial adenomatous polyposis, is evidence of heterozygosity for the disease-associated variant.

Conjugation. A chemical process in which two molecules are joined, often used to describe the process by which certain drugs or chemicals can then be excreted by the body (e.g., acetylation of isoniazid by the liver).

Consanguineous. The union (mating) between two people descended from a common ancestor. In genetics this refers to the union between two people who are no further removed than a second-cousin relationship.

Consensus sequence. A GGGCGGG sequence promoter element to the 5′ end of genes in eukaryotes involved in the control of gene expression.

Conservative substitution. Single base pair substitution that, although resulting in the replacement by a different amino acid, if chemically similar, has no functional effect.

Constant (C). An unchanging value.

Constant region. The portion of the light and heavy chains of antibodies in which the amino acid sequence is relatively constant from molecule to molecule.

Constitutional. Present in the fertilized gamete.

Constitutional heterozygosity. The presence in an individual at the time of conception of obligate heterozygosity at a locus when the parents are homozygous at that locus for different alleles.

Consultand. The person presenting for genetic advice.

Contigs. Contiguous or overlapping DNA clones.

Contiguous gene syndrome. Disorder resulting from deletion of adjacent genes.

Continuous trait. A trait, such as height, for which there is a range of observations or findings, in contrast to traits that are all or none (see *Discontinuous trait*), such as cleft lip and palate.

Control gene. A gene that can turn other genes on or off (i.e., regulate).

Copy number variation (CNV). Refers to sections of the genome that are repeated and the number of copies varies between individuals. Copy number variants may account for 5% to 10% of the human genome.

Cor pulmonale. Right-sided heart failure that occurs secondary to serious lung disease, such as in people with cystic fibrosis.

Cordocentesis. The procedure of obtaining fetal blood samples for prenatal diagnosis.

Corona radiata. Cellular layer surrounding the mature oocyte.

Correlation. Statistical measure of the degree of association or resemblance between two parameters.

Cosmid. A plasmid that has had the maximum DNA removed to allow the largest possible insert for cloning but still has the DNA sequences necessary for *in vitro* packaging into an infective phage particle.

Cotwins. Both members of a twin pair, whether dizygotic or monozygotic.

Counselee. Person receiving genetic counseling.

Couple screening. The practice of conducting genetic screening for both members of a mating partnership at the same time.

Coupling. When a certain allele at a particular locus is on the same chromosome with a specific allele at a closely linked locus.

CpG dinucleotides. The occurrence of the nucleotides cytosine and guanine together in genomic DNA; frequently methylated and associated with spontaneous deamination of cytosine, converting it to thymine as a mechanism of mutation.

CpG islands. Clusters of unmethylated CpGs occur near the transcription sites of many genes.

CRISPR-Cas9. A technique of gene editing enabling investigation of DNA variants and potential for treating genetic disease (**c**lustered **r**egularly **i**nterspaced **s**hort **p**alindromic **r**epeats/CRISPR-associated protein 9).

Crossover (=recombination). The exchange of genetic material between homologous chromosomes in meiosis.

Cross-reacting material (CRM). Immunologically detected protein or enzyme that is functionally inactive.

Cryptic splice site. A pathogenic variant in a gene leading to the creation of the sequence of a splice site that results in abnormal splicing of the mRNA.

Culture artifact. In genetics, a chromosome aberration that arises *in vitro*, thus misrepresenting the situation *in vivo*.

Cycling gene. In development, a gene that is expressed in oscillatory, or periodic cycles.

Cystic fibrosis transmembrane conductance regulator (CFTR). The gene product of the cystic fibrosis gene responsible for chloride transport and mucin secretion.

Cytogenetics. The branch of genetics concerned principally with the study of chromosomes.

Cytokinesis. Division of the cytoplasm to form two daughter cells in meiosis and mitosis.

Cytoplasm. The ground substance of the cell, in which are situated the nucleus, endoplasmic reticulum, and mitochondria.

Cytoplasmic inheritance. See *Mitochondrial inheritance*.

Cytosine. A pyrimidine base in DNA and RNA.

Cytosol. The semi-soluble contents of the cytoplasm.

Cytotoxic T cells. A subclass of T lymphocytes sensitized to destroy cells bearing certain antigens.

Cytotoxic T lymphocytes (= killer T cells). A group of T cells that specifically kill foreign or virus-infected vertebrate cells.

Daltonism. A term given formerly to X-linked inheritance, after John Dalton, who noted this pattern of inheritance in color blindness.

deCODE. An Icelandic company founded in 1996 with the aim of studying population genetics and variations to understand and treat common diseases.

Deformation. A birth defect that results from an abnormal mechanical force which distorts an otherwise normal structure.

Degeneracy. Certain amino acids being coded for by more than one triplet codon of the genetic code.

Deleted in colorectal carcinoma (DCC). A region on the long arm of chromosome 18 often found to be deleted in colorectal carcinomas.

Deletion. A type of chromosomal aberration or mutation at the DNA level in which there is loss of part of a chromosome or of one or more nucleotides.

Delta–beta (δβ)-thalassemia. A form of thalassemia in which there is reduced production of both the δ- and β-globin chains.

Demyelinating. The process of a nerve fiber (neuron) losing its insulating myelin sheath.

***De novo*.** Literally "from new," as opposed to inherited. *De novo* pathogenic variant: DNM.

Deoxyribonucleic acid. See *DNA*.

Desert hedgehog. One of three mammalian homologs of the segment polarity hedgehog genes.

Dicentric. Possessing two centromeres.

Dictyotene. The stage in meiosis I in which primary oocytes are arrested in females until the time of ovulation.

Digenic inheritance. An inheritance mechanism resulting from the interaction of two nonhomologous genes.

Diploid. The condition in which the cell contains two sets of chromosomes. Normal state of somatic cells in humans where the diploid number (2 N) is 46.

Discontinuous trait. A trait that is all or none (e.g., cleft lip and palate), in contrast to continuous traits such as height.

Discordant. Differing phenotypic features between individuals, classically used in twin pairs.

Disease allele. A pathogenic variant in one copy of a DNA sequence.

Disomy. The normal state of an individual having two homologous chromosomes.

Dispermic chimera. Two separate sperm fertilize two separate ova, and the resulting two zygotes fuse to form one embryo.

Dispermy. Fertilization of an oocyte by two sperm.

Disruption. An abnormal structure of an organ or tissue as a result of external factors disturbing the normal developmental process.

Diversity (D). In genetics, the total number of characteristics in the genetic make-up (of a species).

Diversity region. DNA sequences coding for the segments of the hypervariable regions of antibodies.

Dizygotic twins (=fraternal). Twins produced by fertilization of two ova by two sperm.

DMRs. Differentially methylated regions.

DNA (=deoxyribonucleic acid). The nucleic acid in chromosomes in which genetic information is coded.

DNA chip. DNA microarrays that, with the appropriate computerized software, allow rapid, automated, high-throughput DNA sequencing and variant detection.

DNA fingerprint. Pattern of hypervariable tandem DNA repeats of a core sequence that is unique to an individual.

DNA haplotype. The pattern of DNA sequence polymorphisms flanking a DNA sequence or gene of interest.

DNA library. A collection of recombinant DNA molecules from a particular source, such as genomic or cDNA.

DNA ligase. An enzyme that catalyses the formation of a phosphodiester bond between a 3′-hydroxyl and a 5′-phosphate group in DNA, thereby joining two DNA fragments.

DNA mapping. The physical relationships of flanking DNA sequences, polymorphisms, and the detailed structure of a gene.

DNA polymorphisms. Inherited variation in the nucleotide sequence, usually of noncoding DNA.

DNA probes. A DNA sequence that is labeled, usually radioactively or fluorescently, and used to identify a gene or DNA sequence (e.g., a cDNA or genomic probe).

DNA repair. DNA damaged through a variety of mechanisms can be removed and repaired by a complex set of processes.

DNA replication. The process of copying the nucleotide sequence of the genome from one generation to the next.

DNA sequence amplification. See *Polymerase chain reaction.*

DNA sequence variants. See *DNA polymorphisms.*

DNA sequencing. Analysis of the nucleotide sequence of a gene or DNA fragment.

DNM. *De novo* mutation.

Dominant. A trait expressed in individuals who are heterozygous for a particular allele.

Dominant-negative mutation. A mutant allele in the heterozygous state that results in the loss of activity or function of its mutant gene product, as well as interfering with the function of the normal gene product of the corresponding allele.

Donor insemination (DI). In seeking to achieve a pregnancy, the use of sperm from a donor.

Dosage compensation. The phenomenon in women who have two copies of genes on the X chromosome having the same level of the products of those genes as males who have a single X chromosome.

Dosimetry. The measurement of radiation exposure.

Double heterozygote. An individual who is heterozygous at two different loci.

Double-minute chromosomes. Amplified sequences of DNA in tumor cells that can occur as small extra chromosomes, as in neuroblastoma.

Downstream. Relating to DNA and RNA, in the direction of the 3′ end (finish) of the molecule.

Drift (=random genetic drift). Fluctuations in gene frequencies that tend to occur in small isolated populations.

DSDs. Disorders of sex development.

Duplication. In genetics, the presence of an extra copy of DNA or chromosome material.

Dynamic mutation. See *Unstable mutation.*

Dysmorphology. The study of the definition, recognition, and etiology of multiple malformation syndromes.

Dysplasia. An abnormal organization of cells into tissue.

Ecogenetics. The study of genetically determined differences in susceptibility to the action of physical, chemical, and infectious agents in the environment.

Ectoderm. The outer layer of the three layers of cells in the early embryo; from this layer is formed the skin, hair, nails, teeth, sweat glands, and nervous system.

EGF(R). Epidermal growth factor (receptor).

Em. The group of genetic variants of the IgE heavy chain of immunoglobulins.

Embryoblast. Cell layer of the blastocyst which forms the embryo.

Embryonic stem cell (ESC). A cell in the early embryo that is totipotent in terms of cellular fate.

Empiric risks. Advice given in recurrence risk counseling for multifactorially determined disorders based on observation and experience, in which the inherited contribution is caused by a number of genes (i.e., polygenic).

Endoderm. The innermost layer of the three layers of cells in the early embryo; from this layer is formed the gut, the respiratory and urinary systems, the endocrine organs, and the auditory system.

Endoplasmic reticulum. A system of minute tubules within the cell involved in the biosynthesis of macromolecules.

Endoreduplication. Duplication of a haploid sperm chromosome set.

Enhancer. DNA sequence that increases transcription of a related gene.

Ensembl. A European-based genome database project providing a resource relating to human genomes, other vertebrates, and model organisms.

Enzyme. A protein that acts as a catalyst in biological systems.

Epigenetic. Heritable changes to gene expression that are *not* caused by differences in the genetic code.

Epistasis. Interaction between nonallelic genes.

Erythroblastosis fetalis. See *Hemolytic disease of the newborn.*

Etiological heterogeneity. In medicine, refers to a variety of different causes for a condition.

Euchromatin. Genetically active regions of the chromosomes.

Eugenics. The "science" that promotes the improvement of the hereditary qualities of a race or a species.

Eukaryote. Higher organism with a well-defined nucleus.

Exome. That part of the genome formed by exons (i.e., coding regions of genes [comprises ~1% of the total genome]).

Exon (=expressed sequence). Region of a gene that is not excised during transcription, forming part of the mature mRNA and therefore specifying part of the primary structure of the gene product.

Exon splicing enhancer (ESE). A DNA sequence consisting of six bases within an exon, which directs or enhances accurate splicing of nuclear RNA into messenger RNA.

Exon trapping. A process by which a recombinant DNA vector that contains the DNA sequences of the splice-site junctions is used to clone coding sequences or exons.

Expansion. Refers to the increase in the number of triplet repeat sequences in the various disorders caused by dynamic or unstable mutations.

Expressed sequence tags. Sequence-specific primers from cDNA clones designed to identify sequences of expressed genes in the genome.

Expressivity. Variation in the severity of the phenotypic features of a particular gene.

Extinguished. Loss of one allelic variant at a locus resulting from random genetic drift.

Extrinsic malformation. Term previously used for disruption.

Fab. The two antigen-binding fragments of an antibody molecule produced by digestion with the proteolytic enzyme papain.

False negative. Affected cases missed by a diagnostic or screening test.

False positive. Unaffected cases incorrectly diagnosed as affected by a screening or diagnostic test.

Familial cancer syndrome. One of a number of syndromes in which people are at risk of developing one or more types of cancer.

Favism. A hemolytic crisis resulting from glucose 6-phosphate dehydrogenase deficiency occurring after eating fava beans.

Fc. The complement binding fragment of an antibody molecule produced by digestion with the proteolytic enzyme papain.

Fetoscopy. Procedure used to visualize the fetus and often to take skin and/or blood samples from the fetus for prenatal diagnosis.

Fetus. Unborn infant during *in utero* development, usually from 12 weeks' gestation to term.

FGF(R). Fibroblast growth factor (receptor).

Filial. Relating to offspring.

First-degree relative (FDR). A close relative (parent, offspring, sibling), sharing on average 50% of genes.

Fitness (=biological fitness). The number of offspring who reach reproductive age.

Five-prime (5′) end. The end of a DNA or RNA strand with a free 5′ phosphate group.

Fixed. The establishment of a single allelic variant at a locus from random genetic drift.

Fixed mutation. See *Stable mutation.*

Flanking DNA. Nucleotide sequence adjacent to the DNA sequence being considered.

Flanking markers. Polymorphic markers that are located adjacent to a gene or DNA sequence of interest.

Flow cytometry. See *Fluorescence-activated cell sorting.*

Flow karyotype. A distribution histogram of chromosome size obtained using a fluorescence-activated cell sorter.

Fluorescence-activated cell sorting (FACS). A technique in which chromosomes are stained with a fluorescent dye that binds selectively to DNA; the differences in fluorescence of the various chromosomes allow them to be physically separated by a special laser.

Fluorescence in situ hybridization (FISH). Use of a single-stranded DNA sequence with a fluorescent label to hybridize with its complementary target sequence in the chromosomes, allowing it to be visualized under ultraviolet light.

Foreign DNA. A source of DNA incorporated into a vector in producing recombinant DNA molecules.

Founder effect. Certain genetic disorders can be relatively common in particular populations through all individuals being descended from a relatively small number of ancestors, one or a few of whom had a particular disorder.

Founder haplotype. A pattern of DNA variation, usually relating to a locus of interest, that traces unchanged back to an ancestor who was the first individual in a population with a particular disease.

Fragile site. A nonstaining gap in a chromatid where breakage is liable to occur.

Frameshift mutations. Mutations, such as insertions or deletions, that change the reading frame of the codon triplets.

Framework map. A set of markers distributed at defined approximately evenly spaced intervals along the chromosomes in the human genome.

Framework region. Parts of the variable regions of antibodies that are not hypervariable.

Fraternal twins. Nonidentical twins (see *Dizygotic twins*).

Freemartin. A chromosomally female twin calf with ambiguous genitalia resulting from gonadal chimerism.

Frequency. The number of times an event occurs in a period (e.g., 1000 cases per year).

Full ascertainment. See *Complete ascertainment.*

Functional cloning. Identification of a gene through its function (e.g., isolation of cDNAs expressed in a particular tissue in which a disease or disorder is manifest).

Functional genomics. The normal pattern of expression of genes in development and differentiation and the function of their protein products in normal development, as well as their dysfunction in inherited disorders.

Fusion polypeptide. Genes that are physically near to one another and have DNA sequence homology can undergo a crossover, leading to formation of a protein that has an amino acid sequence derived from both of the genes involved.

Fusion polypeptide. A protein that results from a fusion (chimeric) gene.

Fusion protein. Same as *Fusion polypeptide.*

G. Abbreviation for the nucleotide guanine.

Gain-of-function. DNA variants that, in the heterozygote, result in new functions.

Gain of methylation. The principle mechanism of epigenetics whereby DNA is methylated to alter its expression.

Gamete. A cell that fuses with another to bring about fertilization, or sexual reproduction (i.e., egg or sperm cells).

Gap mutant. Developmental genes identified in *Drosophila* that delete groups of adjacent segments.

Gastrulation. The formation of the bi- then trilaminar disc of the inner cell mass that becomes the early embryo.

Gene. A part of the DNA molecule of a chromosome that directs the synthesis of a specific polypeptide chain.

Gene amplification. Process in tumor cells of the production of multiple copies of certain genes, the visible evidence of which includes homogeneously staining regions and double-minute chromosomes.

Gene flow. Differences in allele frequencies between populations that reflect migration or contact between them.

Gene superfamilies. Multigene families that have limited sequence homology but are functionally related.

Gene targeting. The introduction of specific mutations into genes by homologous recombination in embryonic stem cells.

Gene therapy. Treatment of inherited disease by addition, insertion, or replacement of a normal gene or genes.

Genetic code. The triplets of DNA nucleotides that code for the various amino acids of proteins.

Genetic counseling. The process of providing information about a genetic disorder that includes details about the diagnosis, cause, risk of recurrence, and options available for prevention.

Genetic enhancement. The controversial concept of modifying DNA to bring about "improvement," which encompasses elimination of a genetic disease as well as alteration of characteristics.

Genetic heterogeneity. The phenomenon that a disorder can be caused by different allelic or nonallelic variants.

Genetic isolates. Groups isolated for geographical, religious, or ethnic reasons that often show differences in allele frequencies.

Genetic load. The total of all kinds of harmful alleles in a population.

Genetic register. A list of families and individuals who are either affected by or at risk of developing a serious hereditary disorder.

Genetic susceptibility. An inherited predisposition to a disease or disorder that is not as a result of a single-gene cause but is usually the result of a complex interaction of the effects of multiple different genes (i.e., polygenic inheritance).

Genocopy. The same phenotype but from different genetic causes.

Genome. The entire genetic material of a cell, including coding and noncoding DNA.

Genome-wide association study (GWAS). An examination of genetic variants across the entire genome, usually comparing a cohort of subjects with a defined phenotype or disease.

Genome-wide scan. Usually refers to a mapping study using probes across the entire genome (e.g., in a large family with a mendelian disorder).

Genomic DNA. The total DNA content of the chromosomes.

Genomic imprinting. Differing expression of genetic material dependent on the sex of the transmitting parent.

Genotype. The genetic constitution of an individual.

Genotype–phenotype correlation. Correlation of certain mutations with particular phenotypic features.

Germ cells. The cells of the body that transmit genetic information to the next generation.

Germline. The population of the body's cells so differentiated that in the usual processes of reproduction they may pass on their genetic material to the offspring.

Germline gene therapy. The alteration or insertion of genetic material in the gametes.

Germline mosaicism. The presence in the germline or gonadal tissue of two populations of cells that differ genetically.

Germline variant. A pathogenic variant in a gamete.

Gestational. Pertaining to events during pregnancy.

Ghent criteria. A system, devised by an expert working party that met in Ghent, Belgium, for scoring physical characteristics in assessing a patient for possible Marfan syndrome.

Gm. Genetic variants of the heavy chain of IgG immunoglobulins.

Goldberg–Hogness box. See *Hogness box.*

Gonad dose. Radiation dosimetry term that describes the radiation exposure of an individual to a particular radiological investigation or exposure.

Gonadal mosaicism. See *Germline mosaicism.*

Gonadal tissue. Cells and tissue of the organs producing sex cells (i.e., ovaries and testes).

gnomAD. The Genome Aggregation Database hosted by the Broad Institute which aggregates exome and genome sequencing data from different sources.

Gray (Gy). Equivalent to 100 rad.

Growth factor. A substance that must be present in culture medium to permit cell multiplication, or involved in promoting the growth of certain cell types, tissues, or parts of the body in development (e.g., fibroblast growth factor).

Guanine. A purine base in DNA and RNA.

Hamartoma. A benign, nonmalignant, focal malformation resembling a neoplasm in the tissue from which it originates and growing in a disorganized mass.

Haploid. The condition in which the cell contains one set of chromosomes (i.e., 23). This is the chromosome number in a normal gamete.

Haploinsufficiency. Mutations in the heterozygous state that result in half normal levels of the gene product leading to phenotypic effects (i.e., sensitive to gene dosage).

Haplotype. Conventionally used to refer to the particular alleles present at the four genes of the human leukocyte antigen complex on chromosome 6. The term is also used to describe DNA sequence variants on a particular chromosome adjacent to or closely flanking a locus of interest.

Hardy–Weinberg equilibrium. The maintenance of allele frequencies in a population with random mating and absence of selection.

Hardy–Weinberg formula. A simple binomial equation in population genetics that can be used to determine the frequency of the different genotypes from one of the phenotypes.

Hardy–Weinberg principle. The relative proportions of the different genotypes remain constant from one generation to the next.

Hb Barts. The tetramer of γ-globin chains found in the severe form of α-thalassemia, which causes hydrops fetalis.

HbH. Tetramer of the β-globin chains found in the less severe form of thalassemia.

Hedgehog. A group of morphogens produced by segment polarity genes.

Helix-loop-helix (HLH). A form of DNA-binding motif sometimes known as basic HLH (bHLH). Collectively they constitute a large family of transcriptional regulatory proteins.

Helix-turn-helix proteins. Proteins made up of two α-helices connected by a short chain of amino acids that make up a "turn."

Helper lymphocytes. A subclass of T lymphocytes necessary for the production of antibodies by B lymphocytes.

Helper virus. A retroviral provirus engineered to remove all but the sequences necessary to produce copies of the viral RNA sequences along with the sequences necessary for packaging of the viral genomic RNA in retrovirus-mediated gene therapy.

Heme. The iron-containing group of hemoglobin.

Hemizygous. A term used when describing the genotype of a male with regard to an X-linked trait, as males have only one set of X-linked genes.

Hemoglobin electrophoresis. The technique that separates different hemoglobin molecules to diagnose specific inherited blood disorders.

Hemoglobinopathy. An inherited disorder of hemoglobin.

Hemolytic disease of the newborn. Anemia resulting from an antibody produced by a Rhesus-negative mother to the Rhesus-positive blood group of the fetus crossing the placenta and causing hemolysis. If this hemolytic process is severe, it can cause death of the fetus from heart failure because of the anemia, or what is known as hemolytic disease of the newborn.

Hereditary persistence of fetal hemoglobin (HPFH). Persistence of the production of fetal hemoglobin into childhood and adult life.

Heritability. The proportion of the total variation of a character attributable to genetic as opposed to environmental factors.

Hermaphrodite. An individual with both male and female gonads, often in association with ambiguous external genitalia (this term is now out of favor, with disorders of sex development preferred).

Heterochromatin. Genetically inert or inactive regions of the chromosomes.

Heterogeneity. The phenomenon of there being more than a single cause for what appears to be a single entity. See *Genetic heterogeneity.*

Heteromorphism. An inherited structural polymorphism of a chromosome.

Heteroplasmy. The mitochondria of an individual consisting of more than one population.

Heteropyknotic. Condensed darkly staining chromosomal material (e.g., the inactivated X chromosome in females).

Heterozygote (=carrier). An individual who possesses two different alleles at one particular locus on a pair of homologous chromosomes.

Heterozygote advantage. An increase in biological fitness seen in unaffected heterozygotes compared with unaffected homozygotes (e.g., sickle cell trait and resistance to infection by the malarial parasite).

Heterozygous. The state of having different alleles at a locus on homologous chromosomes.

HGMD. Human Genome Mutation Database. A website dedicated to collating all known (published) gene variants responsible for human inherited disease, maintained in Cardiff.

HGVS. Human Genome Variation Society. HGVS nomenclature is a clinical standard for reporting DNA sequence variants.

High-resolution DNA mapping. Detailed physical mapping at the level of restriction site polymorphisms, expressed sequence tags, and so on.

Histocompatibility. Antigenic similarity of donor and recipient in organ transplantation.

Histone. Type of protein rich in lysine and arginine found in association with DNA in chromosomes.

HIV. Human immunodeficiency virus.

HLA (human leukocyte antigen). Antigens present on the cell surfaces of various tissues, including leukocytes.

HLA complex. The genes on chromosome 6 responsible for determining the cell-surface antigens important in organ transplantation and regulation of the immune system.

Hogness box (= TATA box). A conserved, noncoding, so-called promoter sequence about 30 base pairs upstream from the transcriptional start site. Also known as Goldberg-Hogness box.

Holandric inheritance. The pattern of inheritance of genes on the Y chromosome; only males are affected, and the trait is transmitted by affected males to their sons but to none of their daughters.

Homeobox. A stretch of approximately 180 base pairs conserved in different homeotic genes.

Homeotic gene. Genes that are involved in controlling the development of a region or compartment of an organism producing proteins or factors that regulate gene expression by binding particular DNA sequences.

Homogeneously staining regions (HSRs). Amplification of DNA sequences in tumor cells that can appear as extra or expanded areas of the chromosomes, which stain evenly.

Homograft. Graft between individuals of the same species but with different genotypes.

Homologous chromosomes. Chromosomes that pair during meiosis and contain identical loci.

Homologous recombination. The process by which a DNA sequence can be replaced by one with a similar sequence to determine the effect of changes in DNA sequence in the process of site-directed mutagenesis.

Homology. Genes or DNA sequences related by common ancestry.

Homoplasmy. The mitochondria of an individual consisting of a single population.

Homozygote. An individual who possesses two identical alleles at one particular locus on a pair of homologous chromosomes.

Homozygous. The presence of two identical alleles at a particular locus on a pair of homologous chromosomes.

Hormone nuclear receptors. Intracellular receptors involved in the control of transcription.

Housekeeping genes. Genes that express proteins common to all cells (e.g., ribosomal, chromosomal, and cytoskeletal proteins).

HPO. The Human Phenotype Ontology is a standardized set of terms, or vocabulary, describing phenotypic abnormalities encountered in dysmorphology and human disease.

HTF islands. Methylation-free clusters of CpG dinucleotides found near transcription initiation sites at the 5′ end of many eukaryotic genes; can be detected by cutting with the restriction enzyme *Hpa*II, producing *t*iny DNA *f*ragments.

Human Genome Project (HUGO). A major international collaborative effort to map and sequence the entire human genome.

Human Variome Project (HVP). A global initiative to study and document human genomic variation across all population groups, to be shared freely and openly.

Humoral immunity. Immunity that is caused by circulating antibodies in the blood and other bodily fluids.

Huntingtin. The protein product of the Huntington disease gene.

H-Y antigen. A histocompatibility antigen originally detected in the mouse and thought to be located on the Y chromosome.

Hydatidiform mole. An abnormal conceptus that consists of abnormal tissues. A complete mole contains no fetus, but can undergo malignant change and receives both sets of chromosomes from the father; a partial mole contains a chromosomally abnormal fetus with triploidy.

Hydrops fetalis. Hemolysis leads to severe fetal anemia and the accumulation of abnormal levels of fluid in multiple fetal body compartments. The condition can have both immune (Rhesus incompatibility) and nonimmune causes (for example, the most severe form of α-thalassemia and congenital infections). Untreated, the condition will lead to death of the fetus *in utero* from heart failure.

Hypervariable DNA length polymorphisms. Different types of variation in DNA sequence that are highly polymorphic (e.g., variable number tandem repeats, mini- and microsatellites).

Hypervariable minisatellite DNA. Highly polymorphic DNA consisting of a 9- to 24–base pair sequence often located near the telomeres.

Hypervariable region. Small regions present in the variable regions of the light and heavy chains of antibodies in which the majority of the variability in antibody sequence occurs.

Hypomorph. Loss-of-function mutations that result in a partial loss of reduced activity or decreased stability of the gene product.

ICRs. Imprinting control regions.

ID. Intellectual disability (a preferred term to MR—mental retardation).

Identical twins. See *Monozygotic twins.*

Idiogram. An idealized representation of an object (e.g., an idiogram of a karyotype).

Idiotype. In immunology, a shared characteristic between immunoglobulin or T-cell receptor molecules, according to antigen binding specificity, and thus structure of their variable region.

IGV (Integrative Genomics Viewer). The IGV app is a powerful genome browser for performing complex variant analysis from displays of alignments and variants from multiple samples.

Immunoglobulin. See *Antibody.*

Immunoglobulin allotypes. Genetically determined variants of the various antibody classes (e.g., the Gm system associated with the heavy chain of IgG).

Immunoglobulin superfamily. The multigene families primarily involved in the immune response with structural and DNA sequence homology.

Immunohistochemistry (IHC). The technique of detecting antigens in a tissue section using specific antibodies.

Immunological memory. The ability of the immune system to 'remember' previous exposure to a foreign antigen or infectious agents, leading to the enhanced secondary immune response on re-exposure.

Imprinting. The phenomenon of a gene or region of a chromosome showing different expression depending on the parent of origin.

Imputation. In genetic studies, the concept of inferring genotypes or haplotypes to avoid full sequencing of all individual genomes.

Inborn error of metabolism (IEM). An inherited metabolic defect that results in deficient production or synthesis of an abnormal enzyme.

Incest. Union between first-degree relatives.

Incestuous. Description of a relationship between first-degree relatives.

Incidence. The rate at which new cases occur; for example, two in 1000 births are affected by neural tube defects.

Incompatibility. A donor and host are incompatible if the latter rejects a graft from the former.

Incomplete ascertainment. A term used in segregation analysis to describe family studies in which complete ascertainment is not possible.

Indels. Insertion–deletion mutations, referring to insertion and/or deletion of nucleotides into genomic DNA, including events less than 1 kilobase in length.

Index case. See *Proband.*

Index map. See *Framework map.*

Indian hedgehog. One of three mammalian homologs of the segment polarity hedgehog genes.

Induced pluripotent stem cell (iPSC). A form of pluripotent stem cell that can be generated directly from adult cells.

Inducer. Small molecule that interacts with a regulator protein and triggers gene transcription.

Informative. Variation in a marker system in a family that enables a gene or inherited disease to be followed in that family.

Innate immunity. A number of nonspecific systems involved in immunity that do not require or involve prior contact with the infectious agent.

Insertion. Addition of chromosomal material or DNA sequence of one or more nucleotides within the genome.

Insertional mutagenesis. The introduction of mutations at specific sites to determine the effects of these changes.

***In situ* hybridization.** Hybridization with a DNA probe carried out directly on a chromosome preparation or histological section.

Insulin-dependent diabetes mellitus. Diabetes requiring the use of insulin, usually of juvenile onset, now known as type 1 diabetes.

INS VNTR. Refers to variable number of tandem repeats in the insulin gene.

Interferon. A type of cytokine signalling protein released by host cells in response to the presence of pathogens (e.g., viruses, bacteria, and parasites, but also tumor cells).

Intermediate inheritance. See *Codominance.*

Interphase. The stage between two successive cell divisions during which DNA replication occurs.

Interphase cytogenetics. The study of chromosomes during interphase, usually by FISH.

Intersex. An individual with external genitalia not clearly male or female.

Interval cancer. Developing cancer in the interval between repeated screening procedures.

Intracellular signal transduction. As part of cell signalling in general, the process whereby molecular events on the cell surface bring about change (e.g., nuclear gene expression).

Intrachromosomal. Usually referring to gene conversion events between different members of a gene family sited on the same chromosome.

Intracytoplasmic sperm injection (ICSI). A technique whereby a secondary spermatocyte or spermatozoon is removed from the testis and used to fertilize an egg.

Intrinsic malformation. A malformation resulting from an inherent abnormality in development.

Intron (=intervening sequence). Region of DNA that generates the part of precursor RNA that is spliced out during transcription and does not form mature mRNA and therefore does not specify the primary structure of the gene product.

Inv. Genetic variants of the κ light chains of immunoglobulins.

Inversion. A type of chromosomal aberration or mutation in which part of a chromosome or sequence of DNA is reversed in its order.

Inversion loop. The structure formed in meiosis I by a chromosome with either a paracentric or pericentric inversion.

***In vitro*.** In the laboratory—literally "in glass."

***In vitro* fertilization (IVF).** The techniques to bring about penetration of an ovum by a sperm in the laboratory.

***In vivo*.** In the normal cell—literally "in the living organism."

Ionizing radiation. Electromagnetic waves of very short wavelength (X-rays and γ-rays) and high-energy particles (α particles, β particles, and neutrons).

Ion channelopathy. A genetically determined abnormality of a pore-forming membrane protein which normally contributes to establishing a resting membrane potential.

Ion semiconductor sequencing. A method of DNA sequencing based on detecting hydrogen ions released during the polymerization of DNA.

Isochromosome. A type of chromosomal aberration in which one of the arms of a particular chromosome is duplicated because the centromere divides transversely and not longitudinally as normal during cell division. The two arms of an isochromosome are therefore of equal length and contain the same set of genes.

Isolated. A term used to describe a population or group of individuals that for geographical, cultural, or religious reasons has remained separate from other groups of people.

Isotype. Any of the related proteins or genes from a particular gene family.

Isozymes. Enzymes that exist in multiple molecular forms which can be distinguished by biochemical methods.

Joining (J) region. Short, conserved sequence of nucleotides involved in somatic recombinational events in the production of antibody diversity.

Joint probability. The product of the prior and conditional probability for two events.

Junk DNA. A loose term referring to the vast amount (proportionately) of noncoding DNA in the genome.

Justice. The principle in medical ethics of health care resources being equitably distributed.

Karyogram. Photomicrograph of chromosomes arranged in descending order of size.

Karyotype. The number, size, and shape of the chromosomes of an individual. Also used for the photomicrograph of an individual's chromosomes arranged in a standard manner.

Kb. Abbreviation for kilobase.

Killer lymphocytes. See *Cytotoxic T lymphocytes.*

Kilobase. 1000 base pairs (bp).

Km. Genetic variants of the κ light chain of immunoglobulins.

Knockout mutation. Complete loss of function of a gene.

Lagging strand. One of the two strands created in DNA replication which is synthesized in the 3′ to 5′ direction made up of pieces synthesized in the 5′ to 3′ direction, which are then joined together as a continuous strand by the enzyme DNA ligase.

Law of addition. If two or more events are mutually exclusive, then the probability that either one or the other will occur equals the sum of their individual probabilities.

Law of independent assortment. Members of different gene pairs segregate to offspring independently of one another.

Law of multiplication. If two or more events or outcomes are independent, the probability that both the first and the second will occur equals the product of their individual probabilities.

Law of segregation. Each individual possesses two genes for a particular characteristic, only one of which can be transmitted at any one time.

Law of uniformity. When two homozygotes with different alleles are crossed, all of the offspring in the F1 generation are identical and heterozygous (i.e., the characteristics do not blend and can reappear in later generations).

Leading strand. The synthesis of one of the DNA strands created in DNA replication; occurs in the 5′ to 3′ direction as a continuous process.

Lethal mutation. A mutation that leads to the premature death of an individual or organism.

Leucine zipper. A DNA-binding motif controlling gene expression.

Liability. A concept used in disorders that are determined multifactorially to take into account all possible causative factors.

Library. Set of cloned DNA fragments derived from a particular DNA source (e.g., a cDNA library from the transcript of particular tissue, or a genomic library.)

Ligase. Enzyme used to join DNA molecules.

Ligation. Formation of phosphodiester bonds to link two nucleic acid molecules.

Limbal stem cell (LSC). A stem cell located in the basal epithelial layer of the corneal limbus.

Linkage. Two loci situated close together on the same chromosome, the alleles at which are usually transmitted together in meiosis during gamete formation.

Linkage disequilibrium. The occurrence together of two or more alleles at closely linked loci more frequently than would be expected by chance.

Linkage phase. The arrangement of alleles that are transmitted together across generations.

Liposomes. Artificially prepared cell-like structures in which one or more bimolecular layers of phospholipid enclose one or more aqueous compartments, which can include proteins.

Localization sequences. Certain short amino acid sequences in newly synthesized proteins that result in their transport to specific cellular locations, such as the nucleus, or their secretion.

Location score. Diagrammatic representation of likelihood ratios used in multipoint linkage analysis.

Locus. The site of a gene on a chromosome.

Locus control region (LCR). A region near the β-like globin genes involved in the timing and tissue specificity of their expression in development.

Locus heterogeneity. The phenomenon of a disorder being caused by pathogenic variants in more than one gene or locus.

LOD score. Logarithm of the odds: a mathematical score of the relative likelihood of two loci being linked.

Long interspersed nuclear elements (LINEs). 50,000 to 100,000 copies of a DNA sequence of approximately 6000 base pairs that occurs approximately once every 50 kilobases and encodes a reverse transcriptase.

Long terminal repeat (LTR). One of two long sections of double-stranded DNA synthesized by reverse transcriptase from the RNA of a retrovirus involved in regulating viral expression.

Loss of constitutional heterozygosity (LOCH). Loss of an allele inherited from a parent; frequently seen as evidence of a 'second hit' in tumorigenesis.

Loss-of-function mutation. Reduced or absent activity of a gene, often leading to phenotypic features of a disorder.

Loss of heterozygosity (LOH). A chromosomal event that results in loss of one copy of a gene and the surrounding chromosomal region.

Loss of imprinting (LOI). In epigenetics, removal of the methylation of DNA, thus allowing gene expression.

Low-copy repeats (LCRs). Homologous sequences of DNA (more than 95% sequence identity) interspersed throughout the genome, predisposing to unequal recombination.

Low-resolution mapping. See *Chromosome mapping*.

Lymphokines. Glycoproteins released from T lymphocytes after contact with an antigen that act on other cells of the host immune system.

Lyonization. The process of inactivation of one of the X chromosomes in females, originally proposed by the geneticist Mary Lyon.

Lysosome. An intracellular membrane-bound organelle that acts as a waste disposal system by digesting unwanted materials.

Major histocompatibility complex (MHC). A multigene locus that codes for the histocompatibility antigens involved immune responses and important in organ transplantation.

Malformation. A primary structural defect of an organ or part of an organ that results from an inherent abnormality in development.

Manifesting heterozygote, or carrier. The phenomenon of a female carrier for an X-linked disorder having symptoms or signs of that disorder because of nonrandom X-inactivation (e.g., muscular weakness in a carrier for Duchenne muscular dystrophy).

Map unit. See *Centimorgan*.

Marker. A loose term used for a blood group, biochemical, or DNA polymorphism that, if shown to be linked to a disease locus of interest, can be used in presymptomatic diagnosis, carrier status determination, and prenatal diagnosis.

Marker chromosome. A small, extra, structurally abnormal chromosome.

Massively parallel sequencing. High-throughput DNA sequencing based on the assembly of multiple fragment reads that overlap, using DNA synthesis as opposed to the separation of chain termination products.

Maternal (matrilineal) inheritance. Transmission of a disorder through females.

Maximum likelihood method. The calculation of the LOD score for various values of the recombination fraction (θ—'theta') to determine the best estimate of the recombination fraction.

Meiosis. The type of cell division that occurs in gamete formation with halving of the somatic number of chromosomes, with the result that each gamete is haploid.

Meiotic drive. Preferential transmission of one of a pair of alleles during meiosis.

Membrane attack complex (MAC). A structure formed on the surface of pathogenic bacterial cells as a result of the activation of the host's immune pathways.

Mendelian inheritance. Inheritance that follows the laws of segregation and independent assortment, as proposed by Mendel.

Mesoderm. One of the three layers of cells in the early embryo; from this layer is formed muscle, the pharyngeal arches, connective tissue, bone and cartilage, endothelium of blood vessels, red and white blood cells, and kidneys.

Messenger RNA (mRNA). A single-stranded molecule complementary to one of the strands of double-stranded DNA that is synthesized during transcription and transmits the genetic information in the DNA to the ribosomes for protein synthesis.

Metabolic disorder. An inherited disorder involving a biochemical pathway (i.e., an inborn error of metabolism).

Metabolomics. The scientific study of processes involving chemical metabolites.

Metacentric. Term used to describe chromosomes in which the centromere is central with both arms being of approximately equal length.

Metaphase. The stage of cell division at which the chromosomes line up on the equatorial plate and the nuclear membrane disappears.

Metaphase spreads. The preparation of chromosomes during the metaphase stage of mitosis in which they are condensed.

Methylation. The chemical imprint applied to certain DNA sequences in their passage through gametogenesis (applying to a small proportion of the human genome).

Microarray-comparative genomic hybridization (microarray-CGH). Also known as chromosome microarray (CMA) or array-CGH; based on the two-dimensional plating, on a chip, of thousands of short sequences of DNA.

Microdeletion. A small chromosomal deletion detectable by high-resolution prometaphase chromosomal analysis or FISH.

Microdeletion syndrome. The pattern of abnormalities caused by a chromosome microdeletion.

Microsatellite DNA. Polymorphic variation in DNA sequences resulting from a variable number of tandem repeats of the dinucleotide CA, trinucleotides, or tetranucleotides.

Microsatellite instability (MSI). The alteration of the size of microsatellite polymorphic markers compared with the constitutional markers, indicative of defective DNA mismatch repair as seen in Lynch syndrome.

Microtubules. Long cylindrical tubes composed of bundles of small filaments that are an important part of the cytoskeleton.

Minichromosomes. Artificially constructed chromosomes containing centromeric and telomeric elements that allow replication of foreign DNA as a separate entity.

Minidystrophin. A modified dystrophin gene in which a large amount of the gene has been deleted, but that still has relatively normal function.

Minigene. A construct of a gene with the majority of the sequence removed that still remains functional (e.g., a dystrophin minigene).

Minisatellite. Polymorphic variation in DNA sequences from a variable number of tandem repeats of a short DNA sequence.

Mismatch repair. A molecular system for recognizing and repairing erroneous insertions and deletions that may arise during DNA replication, and the repair of some forms of DNA damage.

Mismatch repair genes. Those genes which, when mutated, lead to defects in the efficiency of correcting DNA errors, typically associated with Lynch syndrome.

Missense mutation. A point mutation that results in a change in an amino acid-specifying codon.

Missing heritability. A term applied to the notion that single genetic variants cannot account for much of the heritability of diseases, behaviors, and various phenotypes.

Mitochondria. Minute structures situated within the cytoplasm that are concerned with cell respiration.

Mitochondrial DNA (mtDNA). Mitochondria possess their own genetic material that codes for enzymes involved in energy-yielding reactions, pathogenic variants in which are associated with certain diseases in humans.

Mitochondrial inheritance. Transmission of a mitochondrial trait exclusively through maternal relatives.

Mitosis. The type of cell division that occurs in replication of somatic cells.

Mixoploidy. The presence of cell lines with a different genetic constitution in an individual.

Modifier gene. Phenotypic variability from the consequence of interactions with other genes.

Molecular genetics. The science that studies the structure and function of genes, disease and biological inheritance at a molecular level.

Monogenic. Refers to a genetically determined condition or trait that is caused by a DNA variant in a single gene (= mendelian).

Monosomy. Loss of one member of a homologous pair of chromosomes so that there is one less than the diploid number of chromosomes ($2N - 1$).

Monozygotic twins (= identical). Type of twins derived from a single fertilized ovum.

Morphogen. A chemical or substance that determines a developmental process.

Morpholino. An oligomer (oligo) molecule used to modify gene expression, mainly used in research to knock down gene function.

Morphogenesis. The evolution and development of form and shape.

Morula. The 12- to 16-cell stage of the early embryo at 3 days after conception.

Mosaicism. The presence of two or more cell lines in an individual or tissue, either at the chromosomal or gene level.

mRNA splicing. The excision of intervening noncoding sequences or introns in the primary mRNA resulting in the noncontiguous exons being spliced together to form a shorter mature mRNA before its transportation to the ribosomes in the cytoplasm for translation.

Multifactorial. In genetics, causation that is not monogenic but may be caused by multiple genetic variants ± environmental influences.

Multifactorial inheritance. Inheritance controlled by many genes with small additive effects (polygenic) plus the effects of the environment.

Multigene families. Genes with functional and/or sequence similarity.

Multiple alleles. The existence of more than two alleles at a particular locus in a population.

Multiple displacement amplification. A non–PCR-based DNA amplification technique that can rapidly amplify minute amounts of DNA, generating larger sized products than conventional PCR.

Multiple myeloma. A cancer of antibody-producing B cells that leads to the production of a single species of an antibody in large quantities.

Multipoint linkage analysis. Analysis of the segregation of alleles at a number of closely adjacent loci.

Mutable. In genetics, DNA that is capable of being altered.

Mutagen. Natural or artificial ionizing radiation, chemical agent, or physical agent that can induce alterations in DNA.

Mutant. A gene that has undergone a change or mutation.

Mutation. A change in genetic material, either of a single gene or in the number or structure of the chromosomes. A mutation that occurs in the gametes is inherited; a mutation in the somatic cells (somatic mutation) is not inherited. Used interchangeably with "pathogenic variant."

Mutation rate. The number of mutations at any one particular locus that occur per gamete per generation.

Mutational heterogeneity. The occurrence of more than one mutation in a particular single-gene disorder.

Mutational signature. In cancer genetics, a unique pattern of mutations seen in somatic cells, which occurs as a consequence of different mutational processes in the course of cancer development.

Mutator genes. The equivalent in yeast to the DNA proofreading enzymes that cause Lynch syndrome.

Natural killer (NK) cells. Large granular lymphocytes with carbohydrate-binding receptors on their cell surface that recognize high-molecular-weight glycoproteins expressed on the cell surface of the infected cell as a result of the virus taking over the cellular replicative functions.

NDD. Neurodevelopmental disorder.

Neural crest. Transient group of cells in vertebrate development arising from the embryonic ectoderm, eventually giving rise to melanocytes, craniofacial cartilage and bone, smooth muscle, and some nerve cells.

Neurocristopathy. A pathology arising from a defect in the cells and tissues derived from the neural crest.

Neutral gene. A gene that appears to have no obvious effect on the likelihood of an individual's ability to survive.

Neutropenias. Any condition with an abnormally low number of white blood cells.

New mutation. The occurrence of a change in a gene arising as a new event. Also known as *de novo* mutation.

Next generation sequencing (NGS). High-throughput DNA sequencing technologies that facilitate rapid whole-genome or whole-exome analysis.

Nonconservative substitution. A mutation that codes for an amino acid which is chemically dissimilar (e.g., has a different charge) and will result in a protein with an altered structure.

Nondisjunction. The failure of two members of a homologous chromosome pair to separate during cell division so that both pass to the same daughter cell.

Nonidentical twins. See *Dizygotic twins*.

Noninvasive prenatal diagnosis (NIPD). The technique of analysing cell-free fetal DNA in the circulation of the mother to achieve a fetal diagnosis whilst avoiding the risks of invasive methods (amniocentesis, chorionic villous sampling).

Noninvasive prenatal testing (NIPT). Analysis of cell-free fetal DNA in the maternal circulation used as a screening test for the common trisomies and fetal sexing.

Nonmaleficence. The principle in medical ethics of "first do no harm" (*primum non nocere*).

Nonmaternity. The biological mother is not as stated or believed.

Nonpaternity. The biological father is not as stated or believed.

Nonpenetrance. The occurrence of an individual being heterozygous for an autosomal dominant gene but showing no signs of it.

Nonrandom mating. See *Assortative mating*.

Nonsense-mediated decay (NMD). A pathway in eukaryotes that functions to reduce errors in gene expression by eliminating mRNA transcripts that contain premature stop codons.

Nonsense mutation. A mutation that results in one of the termination codons, thereby leading to premature termination of translation of a protein.

Nonsynonymous mutation. A mutation that leads to an alteration in the encoded polypeptide.

Normal allele. The nonmutated version of a gene or DNA sequence of interest.

Northern blotting. Electrophoretic separation of mRNA with subsequent transfer to a filter and localization with a radiolabeled probe.

Nuchal translucency. Refers to an assessment of the quantity of fluid collecting within the nape of the fetal neck, usually from an ultrasound scan around the end of the first trimester.

Nuclear envelope. The membrane around the nucleus, separating it from the cytoplasm.

Nuclear pores. Gaps in the nuclear envelope that allow substances to pass from the nucleus to the cytoplasm and vice versa.

Nucleolus. A structure within the nucleus that contains high levels of RNA.

Nucleosome. DNA–histone subunit of a chromosome.

Nucleotide. Nucleic acid is made up of many nucleotides, each of which consists of a nitrogenous base, a pentose sugar and a phosphate group.

Nucleotide excision repair. One of three excision repair pathways to repair single stranded DNA, particularly from damage caused by ultraviolet light.

Nucleus. A structure within the cell that contains the chromosomes and nucleolus.

Null allele. See *Amorph.*

Nullisomy. Loss of both members of a homologous pair of chromosomes.

Obligate carrier. An individual who, by pedigree analysis, must carry a particular gene variant (e.g., parents of a child with an autosomal recessive disorder).

Odds ratio (OR). A statistical way to quantify the strength of association of a property or characteristic; an OR of 1 means equal likelihood.

Oligogene. One of a relatively small number of genes that contribute to a disease phenotype.

Oligogenic. Pertaining to causation by a small number of gene variants.

Oligonucleotide. A chain of, literally, a few nucleotides.

Oncogene. A gene affecting cell growth or development that can cause cancer.

Oncogenic. Literally "cancer-causing."

One gene–one enzyme (or protein). The concept that each gene is the blueprint for a single enzyme, which in turn affects a single step in a metabolic pathway—now recognized to be a gross oversimplification.

Opsonization. The "making ready" of an infectious agent in the production of an immune response.

Origins of replication. The points at which DNA replication commences.

Orthologous. Conserved genes or sequences between species.

Ova. Mature haploid female gametes.

Oz. The group of genetic variants of the λ light-chain immunoglobulins.

P1-derived artificial chromosomes (PACs). Combination of the P1- and F-factor systems to incorporate foreign DNA inserts up to 150 kilobases.

Pachytene quadrivalent. The arrangement adopted by the two pairs of chromosomes involved in a reciprocal translocation when undergoing segregation in meiosis I.

Packaging cell line. A cell line that has been infected with a retrovirus in which the provirus is genetically engineered to lack the packaging sequence of the proviral DNA necessary to produce infectious viruses.

Packaging sequence. The DNA sequence of the proviral DNA of a retrovirus necessary for packaging of the retroviral RNA into an infectious virus.

Paint. Use of fluorescently labeled probes derived from a chromosome or region of a chromosome to hybridize with a chromosome in a metaphase spread.

Pair-rule mutant. Developmental genes identified in *Drosophila* that cause pattern deletions in alternating segments.

Panmixis. See *Random mating.*

Paracentric inversion. A chromosomal inversion that does not include the centromere.

Paralogous. Close resemblance of genes from different clusters (e.g., *HOXA13* and *HOXD13*).

Paraprotein. An abnormal immunoglobulin (Ig) fragment or Ig light chain produced in excess by an aberrant monoclonal proliferation of plasma cells.

Parthenogenesis. The development of an organism from an unfertilized oocyte.

Partial sex-linkage. A term used to describe genes on the homologous or pseudoautosomal portion of the X and Y chromosomes.

Pathogenic variant. See *Mutation.*

Penetrance. The proportion of heterozygotes for a dominant gene who express a trait, even if mildly.

Peptide. An amino acid, a portion of a protein.

Pericentric inversion. A chromosomal inversion that includes the centromere.

Peroxisome. An intracellular organelle found in nearly all eukaryotes, involved in catabolism of very long chain fatty acids, among other chemicals.

Permissible dose. An arbitrary safety limit that is probably much lower than that which would cause any significant effect on the frequency of harmful mutations within the population.

Phage. Abbreviation for bacteriophage.

Pharmacodynamics. The study of the biochemical and physiological effects of (mainly) pharmaceutically produced drugs.

Pharmacogenetics. The study of inherited genetic differences in drug metabolism, which can affect individual drug responsiveness.

Pharmacogenomics. Similar to Pharmacogenetics: the study of the role of the genome in drug responsiveness and the difference between individuals.

Pharmacokinetics. Similar to Pharmacodynamics: the study of the fate of drugs and substances administered to a living organism.

Phase. The relation of two or more alleles (DNA "markers") at two linked genetic loci. If the alleles are located on the same physical chromosome they are "in phase" or "coupled."

Phenocopy. A condition that is caused by environmental factors but resembles one that is genetic.

Phenol-enhanced reassociation technique (pERT). Use of the chemical phenol to facilitate rehybridization of slightly differing sources of double-stranded DNA to enable isolation of sequences that are absent from one of the two sources.

Phenotype. The appearance (physical, biochemical, and physiological) of an individual that results from the interaction of the environment and the genotype.

Philadelphia chromosome (Ph1). The shortened form of chromosome 22 arising from a translocation and containing a fusion gene called *BCR-ABL1*, seen particularly in chronic myeloid leukemia.

PI type. Abbreviation of "protease inhibitor" type, relating to alpha-1 antitrypsin deficiency.

Plasmid. Small, circular DNA duplex capable of autonomous replication within a bacterium.

Pleiotropy. The multiple effects of a gene.

Plexiform. Relating to, or resembling, a plexus; most often used in relation to a large and/or deep-seated neurofibroma.

Point mutation. A single nucleotide base substitution, insertion, or deletion in DNA ("mutation" implies pathogenic, usually in a coding region of a gene).

Polar body. The daughter cell of gamete division in the female in meiosis I and II that does not go on to become a mature gamete.

Polarity. In biochemistry, refers to molecules demonstrating a separation of positive and negative electrical charges within their structure. In developmental biology, refers to the establishment of an axis in early structures.

Polyadenylation signal mutation. A mutation affecting a poly(A) sequence which has a signaling function.

Poly(A) tail. A sequence of 20 to 200 adenylic acid residues that is added to the 3′ end of most eukaryotic mRNAs, increasing their stability by making them resistant to nuclease digestion.

Polygenes. Genes that make a small additive contribution to a polygenic trait.

Polygenic inheritance. The genetic contribution to the etiology of disorders in which there are both environmental and genetic causative factors.

Polygenic risk score (PRS). The sum of trait-associated single nucleotide variants, weighted according to their effect, providing an overall measure of an individual's liability to develop disease.

Polymerase chain reaction (PCR). The repeated serial reaction involving the use of oligonucleotide primers and DNA polymerase that is used to amplify a particular DNA sequence of interest.

Polymorphic information content (PIC). The amount of variation at a particular site in the DNA.

Polymorphism. The occurrence in a population of two or more genetically determined forms in such frequencies that the rarest of them could not be maintained by mutation alone.

Polypeptide. An organic compound consisting of three or more amino acids.

Polyploid. Any multiple of the haploid number of chromosomes (3N, 4N, etc.).

Polysome (= polyribosome). A group of ribosomes associated with the same molecule of mRNA.

Population genetics. The study of the distribution of alleles in populations.

Positional candidate gene. A gene located within a chromosome region believed to harbor the gene responsible for a disease or phenotype under study. It is a candidate because it is positioned within the critical chromosomal region.

Positional cloning. The mapping of a disorder to a particular region of a chromosome, leading to identification of the gene responsible.

Positive predictive value. In statistics, the number of true positives divided by the total number of positive results (the latter includes false positives).

Posterior information. Information available for risk calculation from the results of tests or analysis of offspring in pedigrees.

Posterior probability. The joint probability for a particular event divided by the sum of all possible joint probabilities.

Postreplication repair. Repair to damaged DNA that takes place after replication.

Posttranslational modification (or processing). The modification of polypeptide chains into mature proteins that occurs after their synthesis by ribosomal translation of mRNA.

Precision medicine. The use of genomic information, for example from pharmacogenetics or somatic tumor sequencing, to deliver tailor-made treatments (e.g., in cancer; an alternative term to personalized medicine).

Predictive testing. Presymptomatic testing (e.g., in relation to testing of people at risk for Huntington disease).

Preimplantation genetic diagnosis (PGD). The ability to detect the presence of an inherited disorder in an *in vitro* fertilized conceptus before reimplantation.

Preimplantation genetic haplotyping. The use of linked markers (rather than mutation analysis) to determine the genetic status of the early embryo in preimplantation genetic diagnosis.

Premutation. The existence of a gene in an unstable form that can undergo a further mutational event to cause a disease.

Prenatal diagnosis. The use of tests during a pregnancy to determine whether an unborn child is affected by a particular disorder.

Presymptomatic. In genetic disease with a late age of onset (i.e., not congenital, usually adult-onset), the period before symptoms and signs of the disorder are present.

Presymptomatic diagnosis. The use of tests to determine whether a person has inherited a gene for a disorder before he or she has any symptoms or signs.

Presymptomatic testing. An alternative term for "Predictive testing."

Prevalence. At a point in time, the proportion of people in a given population with a disorder or trait.

Primary response. The response to an infectious agent with an initial production of IgM, then subsequently IgG.

Prion. A proteinaceous infectious particle implicated in the cause of several rare neurodegenerative diseases.

Prior probability. The initial probability of an event.

Probability. The proportion of times an outcome occurs in a large series of events.

Proband (=index case). An affected individual (irrespective of sex) through whom a family comes to the attention of an investigator. Propositus if male; proposita if female.

Probe. A labeled, single-stranded DNA fragment that hybridizes with, and thereby detects and locates, complementary sequences among DNA fragments on, for example, a nitrocellulose filter.

Processing. Alterations of mRNA that occur during transcription including splicing, capping, and polyadenylation.

Progress zone. The area of growth beneath the apical ectodermal ridge in the developing limb bud.

Prokaryotes. Lower organisms with no well-defined nucleus (e.g., bacteria).

Prometaphase. The stage of cell division when the nuclear membrane begins to disintegrate, allowing the chromosomes to spread, with each chromosome attached at its centromere to a microtubule of the mitotic spindle.

Promoter. Recognition sequence for the binding of RNA polymerase.

Promoter elements. DNA sequences that include the GGGCGGG consensus sequence, the AT-rich TATA or Hogness box, and the CAAT box, in a 100- to 300—base pair region located 5′ or upstream to the coding sequence of many structural genes in eukaryotic organisms, which control gene expression.

Pronuclei. The stage just after fertilization of the oocyte with the nucleus of the oocyte and sperm present.

Prophase. The first visible stage of cell division when the chromosomes are contracted.

Proposita/propositus. A female/male individual as the presenting person (proband) in a family.

Protein. A complex organic compound composed of hundreds or thousands of amino acids.

Proteomics. The large scale of an organism's proteins (term first coined in 1997).

Protooncogene. A gene that can be converted to an oncogene by an activating mutation. The term 'oncogene' is now commonly used for both the normal and activated gene forms. The DNA genomic sequence shows homology to viral oncogenes.

Pseudoautosomal. Genes that behave like autosomal genes as a result of being located on the homologous portions of the X and Y chromosomes.

Pseudodominance. The apparent dominant transmission of a disorder when an individual homozygous for a recessive gene has affected offspring through having children with an individual who is also a carrier.

Pseudogene. DNA sequence homologous with a known gene but usually nonfunctional.

Pseudohermaphrodite. An individual with ambiguous genitalia or external genitalia opposite to the chromosomal sex in which there is gonadal tissue of only one type.

Pseudohypertrophy. Literally, false enlargement (e.g., seen in the calf muscles of boys with Duchenne muscular dystrophy).

Pseudomosaicism. False mosaicism seen occasionally as an artifact with cells in culture.

Pulsed-field gel electrophoresis (PFGE). A technique of DNA analysis using electrophoretic methods to separate large DNA fragments, up to 2 million base pairs in size, produced by digesting DNA with restriction enzymes with relatively long DNA recognition sequences that, as a consequence, cut DNA relatively infrequently.

Purine. A nitrogenous base with fused five- and six-member rings (adenine and guanine).

Pyrimidine. A nitrogenous base with a six-membered ring (cytosine, uracil, thymine).

Quantitative inheritance. See *Polygenic inheritance*.

Radiation absorbed dose (rad). A measure of the amount of any ionizing radiation that is absorbed by the tissues; 1 rad is equivalent to 100 erg of energy absorbed per gram of tissue.

Radiation hybrid. An abnormal cell containing numerous small fragments of human chromosomes, brought about by fusion with a lethally irradiated human cell. These cells have a very useful role in physical gene mapping.

Random genetic drift. The chance variation of allele frequencies from one generation to the next.

Random mating (= panmixis). Selection of a sexual partner regardless of the partner's genotype.

Reading frame. The order of the triplets of nucleotides in the codons of a gene that are translated into the amino acids of the protein.

Recessive. A trait expressed in individuals who are homozygous for a particular allele but not in those who are heterozygous.

Reciprocal translocation. A structural rearrangement of the chromosomes in which material is exchanged between one homolog of each of two pairs of chromosomes. The rearrangement is balanced if there is no loss or gain of chromosome material.

Recombinant DNA molecule. A union of two different DNA sequences from two different sources (e.g., a vector containing a 'foreign' DNA sequence).

Recombination. Cross-over between two linked loci.

Recombination fraction (θ—theta). A measure of the distance separating two loci determined by the likelihood that a crossover will occur between them.

Reduced penetrance. A dominant gene or allele that is not manifested in a proportion of heterozygotes.

Regression coefficient. In data presented graphically as a linear relationship, this coefficient is the constant that represents the rate of change of one variable as a function of changes in the other (i.e., it is the slope of the regression line).

Regression to the mean. In statistics, the phenomenon that a variable that is extreme on first measurement will tend to be closer to the average on the second measurement—and if extreme on the second measurement is likely to have been closer to the average on the first.

Regulome. Refers to the entire set of regulatory components in a cell and their interplay, including their dependence on variables.

Relative. The connection of one person with another by circumstances of birth.

Relative probability. See *Posterior probability*.

Relative risk. The frequency with which a disease occurs in an individual with a specific marker compared with that in those without the marker in the general population.

Repetitive DNA. DNA sequences of variable length that are repeated up to 100,000 (middle repetitive) or more than 100,000 (highly repetitive) copies per genome.

Replication. The process of copying double-stranded chromosomal DNA.

Replication bubble. The structure formed by coalescence of two adjacent replication forks in copying the DNA molecule of a chromosome.

Replication error. A mistake in the DNA replication process resulting in mismatched nucleotide bases, small insertions, or deletions. Many errors are corrected via proofreading, with mismatch repair and other DNA repair processes correcting those missed. Errors in the systems of repair are important in the pathogenesis of cancer.

Replication fork. The structure formed at the site(s) of origin of replication of the double-stranded DNA molecule of chromosomes.

Replication units. Clusters of 20 to 80 sites of origin of DNA replication.

Replicons. A generic term for DNA vectors such as plasmids, phages, and cosmids that replicate in host bacterial cells.

Repressor. The product of the regulator gene of an operon that inhibits the operator gene.

Repulsion. When a particular allele at a locus is on the homologous chromosome for a specific allele at a closely linked locus.

Repurposing. The process whereby any entity with one intended use is transformed or redeployed as something with an alternative use.

Response elements. Regulatory sequences in the DNA to which signaling molecules bind, resulting in control of transcription.

Restriction endonucleases or enzymes. Group of enzymes each of which cleaves double-stranded DNA at a specific nucleotide sequence and so produces fragments of DNA of different lengths.

Restriction enzyme. An enzyme (a protein-endonuclease) that has the property to cut DNA at or near a specific recognition nucleotide sequence (restriction site).

Restriction fragment. DNA fragment produced by a restriction endonuclease.

Restriction fragment length polymorphism (RFLP). Polymorphism resulting from the presence or absence of a particular restriction site.

Restriction map. Linear arrangement of restriction enzyme sites.

Restriction site. Base sequence recognized by a restriction endonuclease.

Reticulocytes. Immature red blood cells that still contain mRNA.

Retrovirus. A virus that uses its own reverse transcriptase to produce DNA in a host cell from its RNA genome (i.e., the reverse of the usual pattern); the host cell then treats the viral DNA as part of its own genome.

Reverse genetics. The process of identifying a protein or enzyme through its gene product.

Reverse painting. Amplification using PCR of an unidentified portion of chromosomal material, such as a small duplication or marker chromosome, which is then used as a probe for hybridization to a normal metaphase spread to identify its source of origin.

Reverse transcriptase. An enzyme that catalyses the synthesis of DNA from RNA.

Reverse transcriptase–PCR (RT-PCR). Using a special primer that contains a promoter and translation initiator from mRNA (for PCR) to make cDNA.

Ribonucleic acid (RNA). See *RNA*.

Ribosomal RNA (rRNA). The RNA component of ribosomes, essential for protein synthesis.

Ribosomes. Minute spherical structures in the cytoplasm, rich in RNA; the location of protein synthesis.

Ring chromosome. An abnormal chromosome caused by a break in both arms of the chromosome, the ends of which unite leading to the formation of a ring.

RNA (=ribonucleic acid). The nucleic acid found mainly in the nucleolus and ribosomes. Messenger RNA transfers genetic information from the nucleus to the ribosomes in the cytoplasm and also acts as a template for the synthesis of polypeptides.

RNA-directed DNA synthesis. An exception to the central dogma—a process used by many RNA viruses to produce DNA that can integrate with the host genome.

RNA modification mutation. A DNA variant in a nuclear gene that results in modulating the phenotypic manifestation of an RNA mutation.

Robertsonian translocation. A translocation between two acrocentric chromosomes with loss of satellite material from their short arms. Named after the American zoologist/cytogeneticist William Rees Robertson (1881–1941), who first described the phenomenon in grasshoppers in 1916.

Roentgen equivalent for man (rem). The dose of any radiation that has the same biological effect as 1 rad of x-rays.

SAM (Sequence Alignment Map) file. A text-based file format for storing short reads of nucleotide sequence data mapped against reference sequences, generated by next-generation sequencing technologies.

Sanger sequencing. Developed by Fred Sanger in 1997, a DNA sequencing technique based on the selective incorporation of chain-terminating dideoxynucleotides by DNA polymerase during *in vitro* DNA replication.

Satellite. A distal portion of the chromosome separated from the remainder of the chromosome by a narrowed segment or stalk.

Satellite DNA. A class of DNA sequences that separates out on density gradient centrifugation as a shoulder or "satellite" to the main peak of DNA and corresponds to 10% to 15% of the DNA of the human genome, consisting of short, tandemly repeated DNA sequences that code for ribosomal and transfer RNAs.

Screening. The identification of people from a population with a particular disorder, or who carry a gene for a particular disorder.

Secondary hypertension. Increased blood pressure that occurs as a result of another primary cause.

Secondary oocyte or spermatocyte. The intermediate stage of a female or male gamete in which the homologous duplicated chromosome pairs have separated.

Secondary response. The enhanced immune response seen after repeated exposure to an infectious organism or foreign antigen.

Secretor locus. A gene in humans that results in the secretion of the ABO blood group antigens in saliva and other body fluids.

Secretor status. The presence or absence of excretion of the ABO blood group antigens into various body fluids (e.g., saliva).

Segment polarity mutants. Developmental genes identified in *Drosophila* that cause pattern deletions in every segment.

Segmental. Limited area of involvement (e.g., a somatic mutation limited to one area of embryonic development).

Segregation. The separation of alleles during meiosis so that each gamete contains only one member of each pair of alleles.

Segregation analysis. Study of the way in which a disorder is transmitted in families to establish the mode of inheritance.

Segregation ratio. The proportion of affected to unaffected individuals in family studies.

Selection. The forces that affect biological fitness and therefore the frequency of a particular condition within a given population.

Selfish DNA. DNA sequences that appear to have little function and that, it has been proposed, preserve themselves as a result of selection within the genome.

Semiconservative. The process in DNA replication by which only one strand of each resultant daughter molecule is newly synthesized.

Sense strand. Strand of genomic DNA to which the mRNA is identical.

Sensitivity. Refers to the proportion of cases that are detected. A measure of sensitivity can be made by determining the proportion of false-negative results (i.e., how many cases are missed).

Sequence. A stretch of DNA nucleotides. Also used in relation to birth defects or congenital abnormalities that occur as a consequence of a cascade of events initiated by a single primary factor (e.g., Potter's sequence, which occurs as a consequence of renal agenesis).

Sequencing. The process of determining the order of nucleotides of a given DNA fragment.

Sequencing by synthesis. A sequencing method based on reversible dye-terminators that enable the identification of single bases as they are introduced into DNA strands; the technology facilitates massively parallel sequencing.

Sex chromatin (=Barr body). A darkly staining mass situated at the periphery of the nucleus during interphase which represents a single, inactive, condensed X chromosome. The number of sex chromatin masses is one less than the number of X chromosomes (e.g., none in normal males and 45,X females, one in normal females and XXY males).

Sex chromosomes. The chromosomes responsible for sex determination (XX in women, XY in men).

Sex-determining region of the Y chromosome (SRY). The part of the Y chromosome that contains the testis-determining gene.

Sex influence. When a genetic trait is expressed more frequently in one sex than another. In the extreme, when only one sex is affected, this is called sex limitation.

Sex limitation. When a trait is manifest only in individuals of one sex.

Sex linkage. The pattern of inheritance shown by genes carried on the sex chromosomes. Because there are very few mendelizing genes on the Y chromosome, the term is often used synonymously for X-linkage.

Sex-linked inheritance. A disorder determined by a gene on one of the sex chromosomes.

Sex ratio. The number of male births divided by the number of female births.

Short interspersed nuclear elements (SINEs). Five percent of the human genome consists of some 750,000 copies of DNA sequences of approximately 300 base pairs that have sequence similarity to a signal recognition particle involved in protein synthesis.

Siamese twins. Conjoined monozygotic twins.

Sib (=sibling). Brother or sister.

Sibship. A group of offspring having the same two parents.

Sievert (Sv). Equivalent to 100 rem.

Signal transduction. A complex multistep pathway from the cell membrane, through the cytoplasm to the nucleus, with positive and negative feedback loops for accurate cell proliferation and differentiation.

Silencers. A negative "enhancer," the normal action of which is to repress gene expression.

Silent mutation. A point mutation in a codon that, because of the degeneracy of the genetic code, still results in the same amino acid in the protein.

Single-nucleotide polymorphism (SNP). Single-nucleotide DNA sequence variation that is polymorphic, occurring every 1/500 to 1/2000 base pairs, present at a level of 0.5% in the population.

Single-nucleotide variant (SNV). Similar to SNP, but the variation in a single nucleotide occurs without limitations of frequency and may arise in somatic cells.

Single-stranded conformational polymorphism (SSCP). A mutation detection system in which differences in the three-dimensional structure of single-stranded DNA result in differential gel electrophoresis mobility under special conditions.

Sister chromatids. Identical daughter chromatids derived from a single chromosome.

Sister chromatid exchange (SCE). Exchange (crossing over) of genetic material between two chromatids of any particular chromosome in mitosis.

Site-directed mutagenesis. The ability to alter or modify DNA sequences or genes in a directed fashion by processes such as insertional mutagenesis or homologous recombination to determine the effect of these changes on their function.

Skeleton map. See *Framework map*.

Skewed X-inactivation. A nonrandom pattern of inactivation of one of the X chromosomes in a female that can arise through a variety of mechanisms (e.g., an X-autosome translocation).

Slippage. A type of mutation leading to either a trinucleotide or dinucleotide expansion, or contraction, during DNA replication.

Slipped strand mispairing. Incorrect pairing of the tandem repeats of the two complementary DNA strands during DNA replication that is thought to lead to variation in DNA microsatellite repeat number.

Small nuclear RNA molecules. RNA molecules involved in RNA splicing.

Soft markers. Minor structural ultrasound findings associated with the possibility of fetal abnormality.

Solenoid model. The complex model of the quaternary structure of chromosomes.

Somatic. Pertaining to body cells (as opposed to germ cells).

Somatic cell gene therapy. The alteration or replacement of a gene limited to the nongerm cells.

Somatic cell hybrid. A technique involving the fusion of cells from two different species that results in the loss of chromosomes from one of the cell types and is used in assigning genes to particular chromosomes.

Somatic cells. The nongermline cells of the body.

Somatic mosaicism. The occurrence of two different cell lines in a particular tissue or tissues that differ genetically.

Somatic mutation. A mutation limited to the nongerm cells.

Sonic hedgehog. One of three mammalian homologs of the segment polarity hedgehog genes.

Southern blot. Technique for transferring DNA fragments from an agarose gel to a nitrocellulose filter on which they can be hybridized to a radiolabeled single-stranded complementary DNA sequence or probe.

Specific acquired or adaptive immunity. A tailor-made immune response that occurs after exposure to an infectious agent.

Specificity. The extent to which a test detects only affected individuals. If unaffected people are detected as being affected, these are referred to as false positives.

Spermatid. Mature haploid male gamete.

Spindle. A structure responsible for the movement of the chromosomes during cell division.

Splicing. The removal of the introns and joining of exons in RNA during transcription, with introns being spliced out and exons being spliced together.

Splicing branch site. Intronic sequence involved in splicing of mRNA.

Splicing consensus sequences. DNA sequences surrounding splice sites.

Spontaneous mutation. A mutation that arises *de novo*, apparently not from environmental factors such as mutagens.

Sporadic. When a disorder affects a single individual in a family.

Stable mutation. A mutation that is transmitted unchanged.

Stop codons. One of three codons (UAG, UAA, and UGA) that cause termination of protein synthesis.

Stratified medicine. In genetics/genomics, the process of separating patients into groups according to their risk or predicted response to treatment; similar to personalized or precision medicine.

Subchromosomal mapping. Mapping of a gene or DNA sequence of interest to a region of a chromosome.

Submetacentric. Chromosomes in which the centromere is slightly off centre.

Substitution. A single base pair replaced by another nucleotide.

SV. Sequence variation. The nomenclature of SVs is collated by the Human Genome Variation Society.

Switching. Change in the type of β- or α-like globin chains produced in embryonic and fetal development.

Synapsis. The pairing of homologous chromosomes during meiosis.

Synaptonemal complex. A complex protein structure that forms between two homologous chromosomes that pair during meiosis.

Syndrome. The complex of symptoms and signs that occur together in any particular disorder.

Synonymous mutation. See *Silent mutation.*

Syntenic genes. Two genes at different loci on the same chromosome.

Synteny. The comparison of two sets of chromosomes and their conserved blocks of DNA sequence (across species).

T. Abbreviation for thymine.

Topographically associated domain (TAD). Any genomic region within which the DNA sequences physically interact with each other more frequently than with sequences outside the TAD.

TATA (Hogness) box. See *Hogness box.*

T cell. Also T lymphocyte: a type of lymphocyte that matures in the thymus gland, with a T-cell receptor on its surface.

T-cell surface antigen receptor. Antigenic receptor on the cell surface of T lymphocytes.

T helper cell. A cell that aids the activity of other immune cells by releasing T-cell cytokines helping to suppress or regulate immune responses.

Tandemly repeated DNA sequences. DNA consisting of blocks of tandem repeats of noncoding DNA that can be either highly dispersed or restricted in their location in the genome.

Target DNA. The carrier or vector DNA to which foreign DNA is incorporated or attached to produce recombinant DNA.

Telomere. The distal portion of a chromosome arm.

Telomeric DNA. The terminal portion of the telomeres of the chromosomes contains 10 to 15 kilobases of tandem repeats of a 6–base pair DNA sequence.

Telophase. The stage of cell division when the chromosomes have separated completely into two groups and each group has become invested in a nuclear membrane.

Template strand. The strand of the DNA double helix that is transcribed into mRNA.

Teratogen. An agent that causes congenital abnormalities in the developing embryo or fetus.

Teratogene. A gene that can mutate to form a developmental abnormality.

Termination codon. See *Stop codons.*

Terminator. A sequence of nucleotides in DNA that codes for the termination of translation of mRNA.

Tertiary trisomy. The outcome when three to one segregation of a balanced reciprocal translocation results in the presence of an additional derivative chromosome.

Tetraploidy. Twice the normal diploid number of chromosomes (4 N).

Three-prime (3′) end. The end of a DNA or RNA strand with a free 3′ hydroxyl group.

Threshold. A concept used in disorders that exhibit multifactorial inheritance to explain a discontinuous phenotype in a process or trait that is continuous (e.g., cleft lip as a result of disturbances in the process of facial development).

Thymine. A pyrimidine base in DNA.

Tissue typing. Cellular, serological, and DNA testing to determine histocompatibility for organ transplantation.

Toll-like receptor (TLR). A membrane-spanning protein that plays a key role in the innate immune system, recognizing conserved microbial molecules.

Trait. Any detectable phenotypic property or character.

***Trans*-acting.** Transcription factors that act on genes at a distance, usually on both copies of a gene on each chromosome.

Transcription. The process whereby genetic information is transmitted from the DNA in the chromosomes to mRNA.

Transcription factors. Genes, including the *Hox, Pax*, and zinc finger-containing genes, that control RNA transcription by binding to specific DNA regulatory sequences and forming complexes that initiate transcription by RNA polymerase.

Transcription mutation. A DNA variant that occurs within a transcription factor, and thus affects gene expression.

Transcriptomics. The study of all messenger RNA molecules in a cell or population of cells.

Transfection. The transformation of bacterial cells by infection with phage to produce infectious phage particles. Also the introduction of foreign DNA into eukaryotic cells in culture.

Transfer RNA (tRNA). RNA molecule involved in transfer of amino acids in the process of translation.

Transformation. Genetic recombination in bacteria in which foreign DNA introduced into the bacterium is incorporated into the chromosome of the recipient bacterium. Also, the change of a normal cell into a malignant cell (e.g., as results from infection of normal cells by oncogenic viruses).

Transforming principle. The observation, through experiments in the 1920s, that bacteria are capable of transferring genetic information, which led to the discovery that DNA is the chemical of inheritance.

Transgenic animal model. Use of techniques such as targeted gene replacement to introduce mutations into a particular gene in another animal species to study an inherited disorder in humans.

Transient polymorphism. Two different allelic variants present in a population whose relative frequencies are altering as a result of either selective advantage or disadvantage of one or the other.

Transition. A substitution involving replacement by the same type of nucleotide (i.e., a pyrimidine for a pyrimidine [C for T, or vice versa] or a purine for a purine [A for G, or vice versa]).

Translation. The process whereby genetic information from mRNA is translated into protein.

Translesion DNA synthesis. A process of DNA damage tolerance that allows the DNA replication machinery to replicate past lesions in DNA.

Translocation. The transfer of genetic material from one chromosome to another chromosome. If there is an exchange of genetic material between two chromosomes, then this is referred to as a reciprocal translocation. A translocation between two acrocentric chromosomes by fusion at the centromeres is referred to as a Robertsonian translocation.

Transmission disequilibrium test (TDT). In statistics, a family-based association test for the presence of genetic linkage between a genetic marker and a clinical trait.

Transposon. Mobile genetic element able to replicate and insert a copy of itself at a new location in the genome.

Transversion. Substitution of a pyrimidine by a purine, or vice versa.

Trilaminar. In embryology, refers to the three cell layers of the blastocyst.

Triple test. A test available in the second trimester that gives a risk for having a fetus with Down syndrome as a function of age, serum α-fetoprotein, estriol, and human chorionic gonadotropin levels. Becomes the quad test when combined with inhibin-A. Both less commonly used due to availability of first trimester combined screening.

Triplet amplification or expansion. Increase in the number of copies of triplet repeat sequences responsible for a number of single-gene disorders.

Triplet code. A series of three bases in the DNA or RNA molecule that codes for a specific amino acid.

Triploid. A cell with three times the haploid number of chromosomes (i.e., 3 N).

Trisomy. The presence of a chromosome additional to the normal complement (i.e., 2 N + 1), so that in each somatic nucleus one particular chromosome is represented three times rather than twice.

Trophoblast. The outer cell mass of the early embryo that gives rise to the placenta.

True fetal mosaicism. Chromosomal mosaicism that is genuinely present in the body of the fetus as opposed to "confined placental mosaicism" identified by chorionic villous biopsy.

Truncate ascertainment. See *Incomplete ascertainment.*

Tumor suppressor gene. A gene (also known as an antioncogene) that protects a cell from a step on the cancer pathway, and when mutated, loss of its function contributes to cancer progression.

Tyrosinase-negative albinism. Form of oculocutaneous albinism with no melanin production that can be tested for *in vitro.*

Tyrosinase-positive albinism. Form of oculocutaneous albinism with some melanin production that can be tested for *in vitro.*

U. Abbreviation for uracil.

UCSC Genome Browser. An online resource offering access to genome sequence data from various vertebrate and invertebrate species, and model organisms, hosted by the University of California, Santa Cruz.

Ultrasonography. Use of ultrasonic sound waves to image objects at a distance (e.g., the developing fetus *in utero*).

Unbalanced translocation. A translocation in which there is an overall loss or gain of chromosomal material (e.g., partial monosomy of one of the portions involved and partial trisomy of the other portion involved).

Unifactorial (=mendelizing). Inheritance controlled by a single locus.

Uniparental disomy (UPD). When an individual inherits both chromosomes of a homologous pair (or parts of chromosomes) from one parent.

Uniparental heterodisomy. Uniparental disomy resulting from inheritance of the two different homologs from one parent.

Uniparental isodisomy. Uniparental disomy resulting from inheritance of two copies of a single chromosome of a homologous pair from one parent.

Unstable mutation. A mutation that, when transmitted, can be passed on in altered form (e.g., triplet repeat mutations).

Upstream. Relating to DNA and RNA, in the direction of the 5′ end (start) of the molecule.

Uracil. A pyrimidine base in RNA.

Variable (V). In immunology, refers to the hypervariable regions of the large Y-shaped protein that is the immunoglobulin heavy chain antibody.

Variable expressivity. The variation in the severity of phenotypic features seen in people with autosomal dominant disorders (e.g., variable number of café-au-lait spots or neurofibromata in neurofibromatosis type I).

Variable region. The portion of the light and heavy chains of immunoglobulins that differs between molecules and helps to determine antibody specificity.

Variants. Alleles that occur less frequently than in 1% of the population.

VCF (variant call format). This specifies the format of a text file used in bioinformatics for storing gene sequence variations, developed to aid large-scale genotyping.

Vector. A plasmid, phage or cosmid into which foreign DNA can be inserted for cloning.

Virions. Infectious viral particles.

Virus. A protein-covered DNA- or RNA-containing organism that is capable of replication only within bacterial or eukaryotic cells.

Whole-exome sequencing (WES). A technique for sequencing all the expressed genes in a genome.

Whole-genome sequencing (WGS). A technique or process determining the entire sequence of an organism's genome, including noncoding DNA.

Wingless. A group of morphogens produced by segment polarity genes.

X-chromatin. See *Barr body or Sex chromatin.*

X-inactivation. See *Lyonization.*

X-inactivation centre. The part of the X chromosome responsible for the process of X-inactivation.

X-linkage. Genes carried on the X chromosome.

X-linked dominant. Genes on the X chromosome that manifest in heterozygous females.

X-linked dominant lethal. A disorder seen only in females as it is almost always incompatible with survival in hemizygous males (e.g., incontinentia pigmenti).

X-linked recessive. Genes that are carried by females and expressed in hemizygous males.

Yeast artificial chromosome (YAC). A plasmid-cloning vector that contains the DNA sequences for the centromere, telomere and autonomous chromosome replication sites that enable cloning of large DNA fragments up to 2 to 3 million base pairs in length.

Y-linked inheritance. See *Holandric inheritance.*

Zinc finger. A finger-like projection formed by amino acids, positioned between two separated cysteine residues, which is stabilized by forming a complex with a zinc ion and can then bind specifically to DNA sequences; commonly found in transcription factors.

Zona pellucida. Cellular layer surrounding the mature unfertilized oocyte.

Zone of polarizing activity. An area on the posterior margin of the developing limb bud that determines the anteroposterior axis.

Zoo blot. A Southern blot of DNA from a number of different species used to look for evidence of DNA sequences conserved during evolution.

Zygote. The fertilized ovum.

Appendix: Websites and Clinical Databases

The exponential rate of generation of information about human, medical, and clinical genetics means that access to current information is vital to both the student and the doctor, particularly as patients and families often come to the clinic armed with the same information!

There are a large number of general websites that students may find useful as entry points, with a wealth of links to other sites. Many educational websites are also now available with a wealth of illustrative material.

Clinical geneticists regularly use a number of expert databases to assist in the diagnosis of genetic disorders and diseases, some of which are listed. Other specialized websites include those that provide information regarding chromosome disorders, mutations, and nucleotide and protein sequences. Some additional websites have been listed under *Further Reading* at the end of individual chapters.

Students may find it helpful to look at professional societies' websites because they contain many useful links.

General Genetic Websites

Online Mendelian Inheritance in Man (OMIM)
http://www.ncbi.nlm.nih.gov/omim/
Online access to McKusick's catalog, an invaluable resource for clinical genetic information with a wealth of links to many other resources.

ClinVar
https://www.ncbi.nlm.nih.gov/clinvar/
ClinVar aggregates information about human genomic variation and its relationship to human health.

GeneReviews
http://www.ncbi.nlm.nih.gov/books/NBK1116/
Up-to-date reviews of many genetic and inherited conditions, each written by renowned experts in the field.

PubMed
http://www.ncbi.nlm.nih.gov/pubmed
The single most useful source to access any published paper in the biomedical literature.

Genetic Alliance UK
http://www.geneticalliance.org.uk/
Website for alliance of organizations supporting people affected by genetic disorders.

Orphanet
http://www.orpha.net/
A website with information about rare diseases, including many genetic disorders.

Unique: The Rare Chromosome Support Group
http://www.rarechromo.co.uk/html/home.asp
Unique produces excellent downloadable guides for many chromosomal disorders.

Contact a Family
http://www.cafamily.org.uk/
An umbrella organization for patient support groups for rare disorders.

Human Genome Websites

Database of Genomic Variants
http://dgv.tcag.ca/dgv/app/home
A curated catalog of human genomic structural variation.

Policy, Legal, and Ethical Issues in Genetic Research
https://www.genome.gov/about-genomics/policy-issues
A site providing areas of discussion for the responsible use of genomics in society.

Ensembl Genome Browser
http://www.ensembl.org/
Joint project between the European Bioinformatics Society and the Wellcome Trust Sanger Institute to provide annotated eukaryotic genomes.

UCSC Genome Bioinformatics
http://genome.ucsc.edu/
University of California at Santa Cruz genome browser.

Human Genome Organization
http://www.hugo-international.org/
The website for the Human Genome Organization, which was set up as a "United Nations for the human genome."

International HapMap Project
ftp://ftp.ncbi.nlm.nih.gov/hapmap/
The website of the project to map common DNA variants.

Genomics England and The 100,000 Genomes Project
https://www.genomicsengland.co.uk/
http://www.genomicsengland.co.uk/the-100000-genomes-project/
Run by Genomics England, this government-funded initiative in the United Kingdom aims to bring a genomic medicine service into the National Health Service.

1000 Genomes Project
http://1000genomes.org/
A deep catalog of human genetic variation.

Genome Aggregation Database (gnomAD)
https://gnomad.broadinstitute.org/
gnomAD is the successor to "exac" and aggregates exome and genome sequencing data from large-scale sequencing projects.

Exome Variant Server (EVS)
http://evs.gs.washington.edu/EVS/
This website is designed to disseminate exome sequencing data aimed at identifying novel genes and mechanisms, particularly contributing to heart, lung, and blood disorders.

GeneMatcher
https://genematcher.org/
A freely accessible website designed to enable connections between clinicians and researchers globally who share an interest in the same gene(s).

Molecular Genetics Websites

Human Gene Mutation Database
http://www.hgmd.cf.ac.uk/ac/index.php
A database of the reported mutations in human genes.

BROAD Institute
http://www.broad.mit.edu/
Human gene map, sequencing, and software programs.

***In silico* tools for variant prediction**
VEP: http://www.ensembl.org/info/docs/tools/vep/
SIFT: http://sift.jcvi.org/
POLYPHEN2: http://genetics.bwh.harvard.edu/pph2/
ALIGNGVGD: http://agvgd.hci.utah.edu/agvgd_input.php

Mammalian Genetics Unit and Mouse Genome Centre
http://www.har.mrc.ac.uk/
Mouse genome site.

***Drosophila melanogaster* Genome Database**
http://flybase.org/
A comprehensive database for information on the genetics and molecular biology of D. melanogaster, *including the genome sequence.*

***Caenorhabditis elegans* Genetics and Genomics**
http://www.wormbase.org/#012–34-5
C. elegans *genome project information.*

Yeast Genome Project
http://www.yeastgenome.org
Yeast genome project information.

Cytogenetics Websites

Decipher Website
http://decipher.sanger.ac.uk/
A database of submicroscopic chromosome imbalances that includes phenotypic data.

Educational Human Genetics Websites

Health Education England Genomics Education Programme
https://hee.nhs.uk/work-programmes/genomics/
https://www.genomicseducation.hee.nhs.uk/
Supporting education in genetics and genomics for health.

Dolan DNA Learning Center at Cold Spring Harbor Laboratory
http://www.dnalc.org/
Information about genes in education.

University of Kansas Medical Center
http://www.kumc.edu/gec/
For educators interested in human genetics and the Human Genome Project.

Human Genetics Societies

American Society of Human Genetics
http://www.ashg.org/

British Society for Genetic Medicine
http://www.bsgm.org.uk/

European Society of Human Genetics
http://www.eshg.org/

Human Genetics Society of Australasia
http://www.hgsa.org.au/

UK Genetic Testing Network
http://ukgtn.nhs.uk/
An advisory organization that provides commissioning support to the National Health Service; genetic tests available in National Health Service laboratories are listed here.

EDDNAL—European Directory of DNA Diagnostic Laboratories
http://www.eddnal.com/
A European-wide directory—sometimes very useful for unusual test requests.

Clinical Databases

London Medical Databases Online
http://www.fdna.com/london-medical-databases-online/
London Medical Databases have partnered with Face2Gene to make the databases available online. Includes the Winter–Baraitser Dysmorphology Database, the Baraitser–Winter Neurogenetics Database, and the London Ophthalmic Genetics Database.

Other Resources

UKBiobank
https://www.ukbiobank.ac.uk/
A national/international health resource, based on 500,000 volunteer participants, open to all bona fide *health researchers.*

Avon Longitudinal Study of Parents and Children (ALSPAC)
http://www.bristol.ac.uk/alspac/
Also known as ***Children of the 90s****, ALSPAC is a birth cohort study based on 14,000 pregnant women recruited in 1991–1992 in Bristol.*

Multiple-Choice Questions

TRUE or FALSE. There may be more than one correct answer per question.

CHAPTER 2: The Cellular and Molecular Basis of Inheritance

1. **Base substitutions:**
   a. May result in nonsense mutations
   b. Can affect splicing
   c. Are always pathogenic
   d. Can affect gene expression
   e. Result in frameshift mutations
2. **Transcription:**
   a. Describes the production of polypeptides from the mRNA template
   b. Occurs in the nucleus
   c. Produces single-stranded mRNA using the antisense DNA strand as a template
   d. Is regulated by transcription factors that bind to the 3′ UTR
   e. Precedes 5′ capping and polyadenylation
3. **The following are directly involved in DNA repair:**
   a. Glycosylases
   b. DNA polymerases
   c. Ligases
   d. Splicing
   e. Ribosomes
4. **During DNA replication:**
   a. DNA helicase separates the double-stranded DNA
   b. DNA is synthesized in one direction
   c. Okazaki fragments are synthesized
   d. DNA is synthesized in a conservative manner
   e. Uracil is inserted to pair with adenine

CHAPTER 3: Chromosomes and Cell Division

1. **Meiosis differs from mitosis in the following ways:**
   a. Daughter cells are haploid, not diploid
   b. Meiosis is restricted to the gametes, and mitosis occurs only in somatic cells
   c. In mitosis, there is only one division
   d. Meiosis generates genetic diversity
   e. The prophase stage of mitosis is one step; in meiosis I, there are four stages
2. **Chromosome abnormalities reliably detected by light microscopy include:**
   a. Trisomy
   b. Monosomy
   c. Reciprocal translocation
   d. Interstitial deletion
   e. Robertsonian translocation
3. **Fluorescence *in situ* hybridization using whole-chromosome (painting) or specific-locus probes enables routine detection of:**
   a. Gene amplification
   b. Subtelomeric deletion
   c. Trisomy
   d. Supernumerary marker chromosomes
   e. Reciprocal translocation
4. **In Robertsonian translocations:**
   a. The risk of Down syndrome is higher in the offspring of male carriers compared with female carriers
   b. For carriers of 21q21q the risk of Down syndrome in offspring is 25%
   c. Only acrocentric chromosomes are involved
   d. Chromosome 18 is frequently involved
   e. 10% of translocation Down syndrome cases occur *de novo*

CHAPTER 4: Finding the Cause of Monogenic Disorders by Identifying Disease Genes

1. **Positional cloning uses:**
   a. Genetic databases
   b. Knowledge of orthologous genes
   c. Patients with chromosomal abnormalities
   d. Candidate genes selected by biological knowledge
   e. Microsatellite markers
2. **A candidate gene is likely to be a disease-associated gene if:**
   a. A loss-of-function mutation causes the phenotype
   b. An animal model with a mutation in the orthologous gene has the same phenotype
   c. Multiple different mutations cause the phenotype
   d. The pattern of expression of the gene is consistent with the phenotype
   e. It is a pseudogene
3. **Achievements of the Human Genome Project include:**
   a. Draft sequence published in 2000
   b. Sequencing completed in 2003
   c. Development of bioinformatics tools
   d. Identification of all disease-causing genes
   e. Studies of ethical, legal, and social issues

CHAPTER 5: Laboratory Techniques for Diagnosis of Monogenic Disorders

1. **The following statements apply to restriction enzymes:**
   a. They can generate DNA fragments with "sticky" ends

b. They are viral in origin
c. They are used to detect point mutations
d. They are used in Southern blotting
e. They are also called restriction exonucleases

2. **The following describe the polymerase chain reaction:**
a. A type of cell-free cloning
b. A process that uses a heat-labile DNA polymerase
c. A very sensitive method of amplifying DNA that can be prone to contamination
d. A technique that can routinely amplify up to 100 kilobases of DNA
e. A method of amplifying genes that requires no prior sequence knowledge

3. **Types of nucleic acid hybridization include:**
a. Southern blotting
b. Microarray
c. Western blotting
d. Northern blotting
e. DNA fingerprinting

CHAPTER 6: Patterns of Inheritance

1. **Concerning autosomal recessive inheritance:**
a. Females are more likely to be affected than males
b. If both parents are carriers, the risk at conception that any child might be a carrier is 3/4
c. Diseases following this pattern of inheritance are more prevalent in societies where cousin marriages are common
d. Usually only a single generation has affected individuals
e. Angelman syndrome follows this pattern

2. **Concerning X-linked inheritance:**
a. The condition cannot be passed from an affected father to his son
b. When recessive, an affected man will not see the condition in his children, but it may appear in his grandchildren
c. When dominant, females are usually as severely affected as males
d. When dominant, there are usually more affected females than affected males in a family
e. The risk of germline mosaicism does not need to be considered

3. **In mitochondrial genetics:**
a. Heteroplasmy refers to the presence of more than one mutation in mitochondria
b. Mitochondrial genes mutate less often than nuclear genes
c. Mitochondrial conditions affect only muscle and nerve tissue
d. The risk of passing on a mitochondrial condition to the next generation may be as high as 100%
e. Mitochondrial diseases have nothing to do with nuclear genes

4. **Concerning terminology:**
a. Locus heterogeneity means that the same disease can be caused by different genes on different chromosomes
b. Pseudodominance refers to the risk to the offspring when both parents have the same dominantly inherited condition
c. If a condition demonstrates reduced penetrance, its phenotypic effects may skip generations
d. Variable expression characterizes diseases that demonstrate anticipation
e. Pleiotropy is simply a more technical term for variable expression

5. **In inheritance:**
a. An autosomal recessive condition can occasionally arise through uniparental disomy
b. Imprinted genes can be unmasked through uniparental disomy
c. Digenic inheritance is simply another way of referring to uniparental disomy
d. Hormonal factors may account for conditions demonstrating sex influence
e. Most of the human genome is subject to imprinting

CHAPTER 7: Population and Mathematical Genetics

1. **In applying the Hardy–Weinberg equilibrium, the following assumptions are made:**
a. The population is small
b. There is no consanguinity
c. New mutations do not occur
d. No babies are born by donor insemination where the sperm from one donor is used multiple times
e. There is no significant population migration

2. **If the population incidence of a recessive disease is 1 in 10,000, the carrier frequency in the population is:**
a. 1 in 100
b. 1 in 200
c. 1 in 25
d. 1 in 50
e. 1 in 500

3. **Heterozygote advantage:**
a. May lead to an increased incidence of autosomal dominant disorders
b. Does not mean that biological fitness is increased in the homozygous state
c. May explain the worldwide distribution of sickle cell disease and malaria
d. May lead to distortion of the Hardy–Weinberg equilibrium
e. Is very unlikely to be traced to a founder effect

4. **Polymorphic loci:**
a. Are defined as those loci at which there are at least two alleles, each with frequencies greater than 10%
b. Have been crucial to gene discoveries
c. Can be helpful in determining someone's genetic status in a family
d. Have nothing to do with calculating logarithm of the odds scores
e. By themselves have no consequence for genetically determined disease

5. **In population genetics:**
a. To calculate the mutation rate for a disorder, it is necessary only to know the biological fitness for the condition
b. If medical treatment can improve biological fitness, the frequency of an autosomal dominant condition will increase far more rapidly than that of an autosomal recessive condition
c. Even when a large number of families is studied, the calculated segregation ratio for a disorder might not yield the expected figures for a given pattern of inheritance
d. Founder effects seldom explain the high frequency of some alleles in genetic isolates
e. Autozygosity mapping is a useful strategy to look for the gene in any autosomal recessive condition

CHAPTER 8: Risk Calculation

1. **Probabilities:**
   a. A probability of 0.5 is the same as a 50% risk
   b. The probability of an event never exceeds unity
   c. In a dizygotic twin pregnancy, the probability that the babies will be the same sex equals 0.5
   d. Bayes' theorem takes account of both prior probability and conditional information
   e. In an autosomal dominant condition, a penetrance of 0.7 means that 30% of heterozygotes will not manifest the disorder
2. **For an autosomal recessive condition, the chance that the first cousin of an affected individual is a carrier is:**
   a. 1 in 8
   b. 1 in 2
   c. 1 in 4
   d. 1 in 10
   e. 1 in 6
3. **In X-linked recessive inheritance:**
   a. The sons of a female carrier have a 1 in 4 chance of being affected
   b. The mother of an affected male is an obligate carrier
   c. The gonadal mosaicism risk in Duchenne muscular dystrophy may be as high as 15%
   d. For a woman who has an affected son, her chance of being a carrier is reduced if she goes on to have three unaffected sons
   e. A dummy consultant refers to an individual in a pedigree who is ignored when it comes to calculating risk
4. **In autosomal recessive inheritance, the carrier risk to the nephew of an affected individual, that is, born to the affected individual's healthy sibling, is:**
   a. 1 in 2
   b. 1 in 4
   c. 2 in 3
   d. 1 in 3
   e. 1 in 6
5. **Risk-modifying information:**
   a. In calculating risk, conditional information can include negative DNA data
   b. In late-onset dominantly inherited conditions, calculation of heterozygote risk requires clinical expression data
   c. Calculating odds ratios does not require information about prior probabilities
   d. Empiric risks derived from epidemiological studies have limited application to a particular situation
   e. When using DNA marker data to predict risk, the recombination fraction does not really matter

CHAPTER 9: Developmental Genetics

1. **In development, *HOX* genes:**
   a. Function as transcription factors
   b. When mutated have been shown to be associated with numerous malformation syndromes
   c. Show very divergent structures across different species
   d. Are functionally redundant in postnatal life
   e. Individually can be important in the normal development of widely different body systems
2. **In the embryo and fetus:**
   a. Gastrulation is the process leading to the formation of the 16-cell early embryo 3 days after fertilization
   b. Organogenesis takes place at between 8 and 12 weeks' gestation
   c. The Notch signaling and Sonic hedgehog pathways are important for ensuring normal development in diverse organs and tissues
   d. Somites form in a caudo-rostral direction from the presomitic mesoderm
   e. *TBX* genes appear to be crucial to normal limb development
3. **Concerning developmental pathways and processes:**
   a. In mammalian development, the jaw is formed from the second pharyngeal arch
   b. Pharyngeal arch arteries ultimately become the great vessels around the heart
   c. *TBX1* is a key gene in the defects associated with DiGeorge syndrome (deletion 22q11.2)
   d. Achondroplasia can be caused by a wide variety of mutations in the *FGFR3* gene
   e. Loss-of-function mutations and gain-of-function mutations usually cause similar defects
4. **Regarding the X-chromosome:**
   a. In most phenotypic males with a karyotype of 46,XX the *SRY* gene is present and found on one of the X chromosomes
   b. In lyonization, or X-chromosome inactivation, all the genes of one X chromosome are switched off
   c. All females with lyonization are X-chromosome mosaics
   d. Male fetal development is solely dependent on the *SRY* gene functioning normally
   e. X-chromosome inactivation may be linked in some way to the monozygotic twinning process
5. **Transcription factors:**
   a. Are RNA sequences that interfere with translation in the ribosomes
   b. Their only function is to switch off genes in development
   c. When mutated in *Drosophila*, body segments may be completely reorganized
   d. Are not involved in defects of laterality
   e. Include genes that have a zinc finger motif

CHAPTER 10: Common Disease, Polygenic, and Multifactorial Genetics

1. **Concerning autism:**
   a. It is best classified as an inborn error of metabolism
   b. The concordance rate in dizygotic twins is approximately 50%
   c. Fragile X syndrome is a major cause
   d. The risk to the siblings of an affected person is approximately 5%
   e. Girls are more frequently affected than boys
2. **Linkage analysis is more difficult in multifactorial conditions than in single-gene disorders because:**
   a. Variants in more than one gene are likely to contribute to the disorder
   b. The number of affected persons within a family is likely to be fewer than for a single-gene disorder

c. The mode of inheritance is usually uncertain
d. Some multifactorial disorders are likely to have more than one etiology
e. Many multifactorial conditions have a late age of onset

3. **Association studies:**
a. Can give false-positive results because of population stratification
b. May include the transmission disequilibrium test
c. Positive association studies should be replicated
d. Are used to map genes in multifactorial disorders
e. Require closely matched control and patient groups

4. **Variants in genes that confer susceptibility to type 2 diabetes have been found:**
a. By linkage analysis using affected sibling pairs
b. Using animal models
c. By candidate gene studies from monogenic subtypes of diabetes
d. Through the study of biological candidates
e. In isolated populations

5. **Variants in the *NOD2/CARD15* gene:**
a. Are associated with Crohn disease and ulcerative colitis
b. Can result in a 40-fold increased risk of disease
c. Were identified after the gene was mapped to chromosome 16p12 by positional cloning
d. Has led to novel therapies
e. Are very rare in the general population

CHAPTER 11: Screening for Genetic Disease

1.
a. X-inactivation studies provide a useful means of identifying female carriers of some X-linked disorders
b. Reliable clinical signs to detect most carriers of X-linked disorders are lacking
c. DNA sequence variants are useful in targeted screening as long as they are not polymorphic
d. Hearing screening normally commences at 12 months of age
e. For the purposes of screening family members, opportunities should be taken for the banking of DNA from probands with lethal conditions

2.
a. Patients with presymptomatic tuberous sclerosis always have a characteristic facial rash
b. It is always possible to diagnose neurofibromatosis type 1 by age 2 years because it is a fully penetrant condition
c. Biochemical tests should not be considered as diagnostic genetic tests
d. Magnetic resonance imaging of the lumbar spine may be useful in diagnosing Marfan syndrome
e. Predictive genetic testing must always be done by direct gene analysis

3.
a. Population screening programs should be legally enforced
b. Population screening programs should be offered if some form of treatment or prevention is available
c. The sensitivity of a test refers to the extent to which the test detects only affected individuals
d. The positive predictive value of a screening test refers to the proportion of positive tests that are true positives
e. If there is no effective treatment for a late-onset condition, predictive genetic testing should be undertaken with great care

4.
a. A high proportion of people who undergo carrier testing cannot remember their result properly
b. Carrier screening for cystic fibrosis is the most useful program among Greek Cypriots
c. The possibility of a screening test leading to employment discrimination is not a major concern
d. Neonatal screening for Duchenne muscular dystrophy improves life expectancy
e. Neonatal screening for cystic fibrosis is a DNA-based test

5.
a. Newborn screening for hemochromatosis, the most common condition associated with an inherited gene mutation in European populations, is a nationally managed program in the United Kingdom
b. The presymptomatic screening of children for adult-onset genetic disease is a decision made by the parents
c. Neonatal screening for phenylketonuria and for congenital hypothyroidism are the longest-running screening programs
d. Screening for medium-chain acyl-CoA dehydrogenase deficiency is part of the newborn bloodspot screening program
e. Genetic registers are mainly for research

CHAPTER 12: Hemoglobin and the Hemoglobinopathies

1. **For different hemoglobins (Hbs):**
a. The fetal Hb chain, γ, differs markedly from the adult β chain
b. The Hb chains α, β, and γ are all expressed throughout fetal life
c. In α-thalassemia, there are too many α chains
d. Hb Barts is a form of β-thalassemia
e. Carriers of β-thalassemia frequently suffer from symptomatic anemia

2. **Regarding sickle cell disease:**
a. The sickling effect of red blood corpuscles is the result of abnormal hemoglobin binding with the red blood cell membrane
b. Life-threatening thromboses can occur
c. HbS differs from normal HbA by a single amino-acid substitution
d. Splenic infarction may occur, but this has little clinical consequence
e. Point (missense) mutations are the usual cause of abnormal hemoglobin in the sickling disorders

3. **Concerning hemoglobin (Hb) variants:**
a. Many Hb variants are harmless
b. The types of mutation occurring in the hemoglobinopathies are very limited
c. In the thalassemias, hypoplasia of the bone marrow occurs
d. In the thalassemias, Hb demonstrates abnormal oxygen affinity
e. In some thalassemias, increased red cell hemolysis occurs

4. **Regarding hemoglobins (Hbs) during life:**
a. Persistence of fetal Hb into adult life is an acquired, rather than inherited, disorder

b. Throughout fetal life, it is the liver that produces most of the body's Hb
c. The bone marrow is not involved in Hb production before birth
d. The liver continues to produce Hb into the second year of postnatal life
e. Persistence of fetal Hb into adult life is a benign condition

CHAPTER 13: Immunogenetics

1. **Concerning complement:**
   a. The complement cascade can be activated only by the binding of antibody and antigen
   b. C1-inhibitor deficiency can result in complement activation through the classic pathway
   c. C3 levels are reduced in hereditary angioneurotic edema
   d. Complement helps directly in the attack on microorganisms
   e. Complement is found mainly in the intracellular matrix
2. **In immunology:**
   a. The immunoglobulin molecule is made up of six polypeptide chains
   b. The genes for the various light and heavy immunoglobulin chains are found close together in the human genome
   c. Close relatives make the best organ donors because they are likely to share the same complement haplotypes
   d. The DNA encoding the κ light chain contains four distinct regions
   e. The diversity of T-cell surface antigen receptor can be compared with the process of immunoglobulin diversity
3. **In immunity and immunological disease:**
   a. Maternal transplacental mobility of antibodies gives infants protection for approximately 12 months
   b. X-linked severe combined immunodeficiency (SCID) accounts for approximately 5% to 10% of all SCID cases
   c. SCID, despite its name, is not always a severe condition
   d. There is always a T-cell abnormality in the different forms of SCID
   e. Chronic granulomatous disease is a disorder of humoral immunity
4. **In common immunological conditions:**
   a. DiGeorge/Sedláčková syndrome is a primary disorder of immune function
   b. Severe opportunistic bacterial infections are uncommon in DiGeorge syndrome
   c. Genetic prenatal diagnosis is possible for common variable immunodeficiency
   d. Autoimmune disorders follow autosomal dominant inheritance
   e. Investigation of immune function should be considered in any child with failure to thrive

CHAPTER 14: The Genetics of Cancer . . . and Cancer Genetics

1. **Relating to genetic mechanisms leading to cancer:**
   a. Chromosome translocations can lead to cancer through modification of oncogene activity
   b. Oncogenes are the most common form of genes predisposing to hereditary cancer syndromes
   c. Defective apoptosis may lead to tumorigenesis
   d. Loss of heterozygosity is another term for a mutational event in an oncogene
   e. A pathogenic variant in the *APC* gene is sufficient to cause colorectal cancer
2. **In familial cancer syndromes:**
   a. The two-hit hypothesis predicted that a tumor would develop when both copies of a critical gene are mutated
   b. *TP53* mutations are found only in Li-Fraumeni syndrome
   c. The *RET* protooncogene is implicated in all forms of multiple endocrine neoplasia
   d. Individuals with familial adenomatous polyposis should have screening of the upper gastrointestinal tract
   e. Endometrial cancer is a feature of Lynch syndrome
3. **In familial cancer syndromes:**
   a. Thyroid cancer is a risk in Bannayan–Riley–Ruvalcaba syndrome
   b. Men with a germline mutation in *BRCA2* are at increased risk of prostate cancer
   c. The genetic basis of all familial breast cancer is now well established
   d. Familial breast cancer is usually fully penetrant
   e. For men with prostate cancer, 3% of male first-degree relatives are similarly affected
4. **In familial cancer syndromes:**
   a. Medulloblastoma is a common tumor in von Hippel–Lindau disease
   b. Pheochromocytoma is frequently seen in Gorlin syndrome
   c. There is a risk of ovarian cancer in Peutz-Jeghers syndrome and Lynch syndrome
   d. Cutaneous manifestations occur in Peutz-Jeghers syndrome, Gorlin syndrome, and Lynch syndrome
   e. In two-thirds of Lynch syndrome cases the predisposing gene is unknown
5. **In cancer prevention and screening:**
   a. Screening for renal cancer in von Hippel–Lindau disease is recommended
   b. Mammography detects breast cancer more easily in premenopausal than postmenopausal women
   c. Screening for retinoblastoma should begin in the second year of life
   d. Colonoscopy screening is indicated only when the Amsterdam criteria are fulfilled in relatives with colorectal cancer
   e. Preventive surgery is strongly indicated in familial adenomatous polyposis and women positive for *BRCA1* mutations

CHAPTER 15: Pharmacogenomics, Precision Medicine, and the Treatment of Genetic Disease

1. **Thiopurine drugs used to treat leukemia:**
   a. Include 6-mercaptopurine, 6-thioguanine, and azathioprine
   b. Are also used to suppress the immune system
   c. May be toxic in 1% to 2% of patients
   d. Can have serious side effects
   e. Are metabolised by thiopurine methyltransferase
2. **Liver enzymes that show genetic variation of expression and hence influence the response to drugs include:**
   a. UDP-glucuronosyltransferase
   b. O-acetyltransferase

c. Alcohol dehydrogenase
d. CYP2D6
e. CYP2C9

3. **Examples of diseases in which treatment may be influenced by pharmacogenomics include:**
   a. Maturity-onset diabetes of the young (MODY), subtype glucokinase
   b. MODY, subtype HNF-1α
   c. Human immunodeficiency virus infection
   d. Epilepsy
   e. Tuberculosis
4. **Methods currently used to treat genetic disease include:**
   a. Germ-cell gene therapy
   b. Stem-cell transplantation
   c. Enzyme/protein replacement
   d. Dietary restriction
   e. *In situ* repair of mutations by cellular DNA repair mechanisms
5. **Gene therapy may be delivered by:**
   a. Liposomes
   b. Adeno-associated viruses
   c. Antisense oligonucleotides
   d. Lentiviruses
   e. Injection of plasmid DNA
6. **Gene therapy has been used successfully to treat patients with the following diseases:**
   a. Cystic fibrosis
   b. X-linked severe combined immunodeficiency
   c. Sickle cell disease
   d. Hemophilia
   e. Adenosine deaminase deficiency
7. **Potential gene therapy methods for cancer include:**
   a. Inhibition of fusion proteins
   b. Stimulation of the immune system
   c. Increased expression of the angiogenic factors
   d. RNA interference
   e. Antisense oligonucleotides

CHAPTER 16: Congenital Abnormalities, Dysmorphic Syndromes, and Learning Disability

1.
   a. Approximately 5% of all infant deaths are caused by congenital abnormalities
   b. At least half of all spontaneous miscarriages have a genetic basis
   c. A major congenital abnormality affects approximately 1 newborn baby in every 200
   d. Positional talipes is an example of a disruption to normal intrauterine development
   e. Multiple abnormalities are sometimes the result of a sequence
2.
   a. Down syndrome should more accurately be termed 'Down association'
   b. Sotos syndrome, as with Down syndrome, is caused by a chromosomal abnormality
   c. Spina bifida affects approximately 2 per 1000 births
   d. Infantile polycystic kidney disease is an example of a condition with different patterns of inheritance
   e. Holoprosencephaly is an example of a condition with different patterns of inheritance
3.
   a. Thalidomide embryopathy is an example of a disruption to normal intrauterine development
   b. Talipes may be a consequence of renal agenesis
   c. Limb defects are not a feature of fetal valproate syndrome
   d. Symmetrical abnormalities tend to feature in a dysplasia
   e. Birth defects are unexplained in 10% of cases
4. **Relating to maternal influences on fetal development:**
   a. Congenital infection could lead to someone being both blind and deaf
   b. The second trimester is the most dangerous time for a fetus to be exposed to a maternal infection
   c. Vertebral body defects can be a consequence of poorly treated diabetes mellitus in the first trimester
   d. A polymorphism in the methylenetetrahydrofolate reductase gene is always associated with an increased risk of neural tube defect
   e. Pulmonary stenosis is a feature of Noonan syndrome and congenital rubella
5. **In conditions that are often non-mendelian:**
   a. Cleft lip–palate occurs more frequently than 1 in 1000 births
   b. Associations generally have a high recurrence risk
   c. The recurrence risk for a multifactorial condition can usually be determined by looking at the patient's family pedigree
   d. One cause of holoprosencephaly is a metabolic defect
   e. Congenital heart disease affects 1 in 1000 babies

CHAPTER 17: Chromosome Disorders

1. **Relating to aneuploidies:**
   a. The chromosome number in humans was discovered after the discovery of the structure of DNA
   b. The Turner syndrome karyotype is the most common single chromosome abnormality in spontaneous abortuses
   c. The rate of miscarriage in Down syndrome is similar to the rate in karyotypically normal fetuses
   d. Most babies with Down syndrome are born to mothers who are less than 30 years of age
   e. All children with Down syndrome have to go to special school
2. **Relating to common chromosomal disorders:**
   a. The life expectancy of children with trisomy 18 (Edwards syndrome) is about 2 years
   b. 47,XYY males are fertile
   c. The origin of Turner syndrome (45,X) can be in paternal meiosis
   d. All persons with Angelman syndrome have a deletion on chromosome 15q that can be detected by microarray-comparative genomic hybridization analysis
   e. DiGeorge syndrome results from misaligned homologous recombination between flanking repeat DNA sequences
3. **In microdeletion conditions:**
   a. Premature vascular problems occur in adults with Williams syndrome
   b. Congenital heart disease is a feature of Prader–Willi and Smith–Magenis syndromes
   c. The Wilms tumor locus is on chromosome 13
   d. Aniridia may be caused by either a gene mutation or a chromosome microdeletion
   e. A child's behavior may help to make a diagnosis of a malformation syndrome

4.
   a. Klinefelter syndrome affects approximately 1 in 10,000 male live births
   b. Intellectual disability is common in Klinefelter syndrome
   c. Chromosome mosaicism is commonly seen in Turner syndrome
   d. Females with a karyotype 47,XXX are infertile
   e. Chromosome breakage syndromes can cause cancer

5.
   a. In fragile X syndrome, the triplet repeat does not change in size significantly when passed from father to daughter
   b. Fragile X syndrome is a single, well-defined condition
   c. Girls with bilateral inguinal hernia should have their chromosomes tested
   d. Normal karyotyping is a good way of diagnosing fragile X syndrome in girls
   e. Microarray–comparative genomic hybridization analysis will detect genetic imbalances in approximately 50% of children with neurodevelopmental disorders

CHAPTER 18: Inborn Errors of Metabolism

1. **In congenital adrenal hyperplasia:**
   a. Females may show virilization and ambiguous genitalia
   b. Males may show undermasculinization and ambiguous genitalia
   c. Mineralocorticoid deficiency can be life threatening
   d. Treatment is required during childhood but not usually in adult life
   e. In affected females, fertility is basically unaffected
2. **Phenylketonuria:**
   a. Is the only cause of a raised phenylalanine level in the neonatal period
   b. Requires lifelong treatment
   c. Is a cause of epilepsy and eczema
   d. Results in reduced levels of melanin
   e. Is part of the same pathway as cholesterol production
3. **Hepatomegaly is an important feature of:**
   a. Hurler syndrome
   b. Glycogen storage disorders
   c. Abnormalities of porphyrin metabolism
   d. Niemann–Pick disease
   e. Galactosemia
4. **Concerning mitochondrial disorders:**
   a. All follow matrilinear inheritance
   b. Retinal pigmentation and diabetes can both be features
   c. There are fewer than 50 gene products from the mitochondrial genome
   d. Leigh disease is always caused by the same point mutation
   e. The gene for Barth syndrome is known but the metabolic pathway is uncertain
5. **Regarding metabolic conditions:**
   a. The carnitine cycle and long-chain fatty acids are linked
   b. A single point mutation explains most cases of medium-chain acyl-CoA dehydrogenase deficiency
   c. Peroxisomal disorders include Menkes disease and Wilson disease
   d. Inborn errors of metabolism may present with hypotonia and acidosis alone
   e. X-rays are of no value in making a diagnosis of inborn errors of metabolism

CHAPTER 19: Mainstream Monogenic Disorders

1. **Huntington disease (HD):**
   a. In HD an earlier age of onset in the offspring is more likely if the gene is passed from an affected mother than an affected father
   b. In HD, those homozygous for the mutation are no more severely affected than those who are heterozygous
   c. From the onset of HD, the average duration of the illness until a terminal event is 35 years
   d. In HD, non-penetrance of the disease may be associated with low triplet repeat abnormal alleles
   e. Cognitive impairment and dementia are early features of symptomatic HD
2. **Myotonic dystrophy:**
   a. Insomnia is a feature of myotonic dystrophy
   b. Myotonic dystrophy is a cause of neonatal hypertonia
   c. The clinical effects of myotonic dystrophy are mediated through RNA
   d. Cardiac conduction defects are a feature of both myotonic dystrophy and ion channelopathies
   e. In myotonic dystrophy type 2, as in myotonic dystrophy type 1, the disease is primarily caused by the expansion of a DNA trinucleotide repeating sequence

3.
   a. In cystic fibrosis R117H is the most common mutation in northern Europe
   b. In the *CFTR* gene a modifying intragenic polymorphism affects the phenotype
   c. Hypertrophic cardiomyopathies are mostly caused by mutations in genes encoding ion channels
   d. Many different inherited muscular dystrophies can be linked to the complex that includes dystrophin (mutated in Duchenne and Becker muscular dystrophies)
   e. Learning difficulties are part of spinal muscular atrophy

4.
   a. Cystic fibrosis and hemophilia are unlikely candidates for gene therapy
   b. An abnormal span:height ratio alone is a major feature of Marfan syndrome
   c. Neurofibromatosis type 1 (NF1) often "skips generations"
   d. Scoliosis can be a feature of both NF1 and Marfan syndrome
   e. Cataracts can be a feature of NF1 but not of neurofibromatosis type 2

5. **In neuromuscular conditions:**
   a. Hereditary motor and sensory neuropathy (HMSN) types I and II refer to a genetic classification
   b. HMSN can follow all major patterns of inheritance
   c. It is the nerve sheath, rather than the nerve itself, that is altered in the most common form of HMSN
   d. Estimation of the creatine kinase level and the factor VIII level is good for identifying carriers of Duchenne dystrophy and hemophilia A, respectively
   e. Brugada syndrome is one of the varieties of spinal muscular atrophy

CHAPTER 20: Prenatal Testing and Reproductive Genetics

1. **In prenatal testing:**
   a. Amniocentesis is being routinely practiced earlier and earlier in pregnancy
   b. The cells grown from amniocentesis originate purely from fetal skin
   c. Chorionic villus sampling is a safe procedure at 9 weeks' gestation
   d. The karyotype from chorionic villus tissue will always be a true reflection of the karyotype in the unborn baby
   e. Fetal anomaly scanning by ultrasound is reliable at 15 weeks' gestation
2. **Regarding prenatal markers:**
   a. In Down syndrome pregnancies, maternal serum human chorionic gonadotropin (hCG) levels are usually raised
   b. In Down syndrome pregnancies, maternal serum α-fetoprotein (αFP) concentration is usually reduced
   c. In trisomy 18 pregnancies, maternal serum markers behave in the same way as in Down syndrome pregnancies
   d. About 95% of Down syndrome pregnancies are picked up by determining maternal age, serum αFP and hCG levels, and fetal nuchal translucency
   e. Twin pregnancy is a cause of increased maternal serum αFP levels
3.
   a. The accuracy of fetal sexing by non-invasive prenatal testing of cell-free fetal DNA in the maternal circulation is less than 90%
   b. Chromosome disorders are the main cause of abnormal nuchal translucency
   c. Echogenic fetal bowel on ultrasonography is a risk factor for cystic fibrosis
   d. For a couple who have had one child with Down syndrome, the risk in the next pregnancy is usually not greatly increased
   e. Familial marker chromosomes are usually not clinically significant
4. **In assisted reproduction:**
   a. Donor insemination is a procedure that does not require a license from the Human Fertilisation and Embryology Authority (in the UK)
   b. Surrogacy is illegal in the United Kingdom
   c. For preimplantation genetic diagnosis, fertilization of the egg is achieved by intracytoplasmic sperm injection
   d. The success rate from a single cycle of in vitro fertilization, in terms of taking home a baby, is ~60%
   e. Spinal muscular atrophy can be diagnosed by non-invasive prenatal diagnosis
5.
   a. There is an increased risk of genetic conditions in the fathers of children conceived by intracytoplasmic sperm injection
   b. The sperm of one donor may be used up to 25 times
   c. Children conceived by donor insemination are entitled to as much information as adopted children about their biological parents
   d. Non-invasive prenatal diagnosis based on cell-free fetal DNA in the maternal circulation is set to replace all other forms of prenatal testing and screening
   e. Infertility affects about 1 in 20 couples

CHAPTER 21: Genetic Counseling

1.
   a. The individual who seeks genetic counseling is the proband
   b. Retinitis pigmentosa mainly follows one pattern of inheritance
   c. Genetic counseling is all about recurrence risks
   d. The counsellor's own opinion about a difficult choice is always helpful
   e. Good counseling should not be measured by the patient's ability to remember genetic risks
2.
   a. First-cousin partnerships are 10 times more likely to have babies with congenital abnormalities than the general population
   b. On average, a grandparent and grandchild share 1/4 of their genes
   c. Incestuous relationships virtually always result in severe learning difficulties in the offspring
   d. Consanguinity should be regarded as extremely abnormal
   e. Consanguinity refers exclusively to cousin marriages/partnerships
3.
   a. Genetic disorders are accidents of nature, so guilty feelings are rare
   b. Clear genetic counseling changes patients' reproductive decisions in virtually all cases
   c. The chance of the first child born to first cousins being affected with an autosomal recessive condition caused by a deleterious gene inherited from a grandparent is 1 in 32
   d. Far more genetic testing of children for adoption takes place than for children reared by their birth parents
   e. Patient support groups have little value, given that modern medical genetics is so technically complex

Case-Based Questions

CHAPTER 6: Patterns of Inheritance

Case 1

A 34-year-old man has developed spasticity of his legs in the past few years, and his family has noted some memory problems and alteration in behavior. He has very brisk peripheral reflexes. He is seen with his mother in the genetic clinic, and she is found to have significantly brisk peripheral reflexes on examination but has no health complaints. It emerges that her own father may have had similar problems to her son's when he was a young adult, but he died in a road traffic accident aged 25.

1. *Which patterns of inheritance need to be considered in this scenario?*
2. *What diagnostic possibilities should be considered?*

Case 2

A couple attend for genetic counseling before starting a family. *Both* have moderately severe congenital sensorineural hearing loss; *he* is the only affected individual in his family, with one sister who has normal hearing, and *she* has two siblings, including one brother, with a similar deafness diagnosis and no other affected family members.

1. *What other information might be helpful before discussing possible genetic risks?*
2. *If all the additional enquiries and investigations are normal, what patterns of inheritance, and therefore risks to future offspring, need to be considered?*

Case 3

A couple has a child who suffers a number of bone fractures during early childhood after minor trauma and is told that this is probably a mild form of osteogenesis imperfecta. The parents did not suffer childhood fractures themselves, and when they have another child who also develops fractures, they are told the inheritance is autosomal recessive. This includes an explanation that the affected children would be very unlikely to have affected offspring themselves in the future.

1. *Is the information given to the parents correct?*
2. *If not, what is the most likely pattern of inheritance and explanation for the sibling recurrence of fractures?*

CHAPTER 7: Population and Mathematical Genetics

Case 1

The incidence of a certain autosomal recessive disorder in population A is well established at approximately 1 in 10,000, whereas in population B the incidence of the same disorder is much higher at approximately 1 in 900. A man from population group A and a woman from population group B are planning to marry and start a family. Being aware of the relatively high incidence of the disorder in population B, they seek genetic counseling.

1. *What essential question must be asked of each individual?*
2. *What is the risk of the disorder occurring in their first pregnancy, based on application of the Hardy–Weinberg equilibrium?*

Case 2

Neurofibromatosis type 1 is a relatively common mendelian condition. In a population survey of 50,000 people in one town, 12 cases are identified, of which 8 all belong to one large affected family.

1. *Based on these figures, what is the mutation rate in the neurofibromin gene?*
2. *Name some limitations to the validity of calculating the mutation rate from a survey such as this.*

CHAPTER 8: Risk Calculation

Case 1

In the pedigree shown, two cousins have married and would like to start a family. However, their uncle died many years ago from Hurler syndrome, one of the mucopolysaccharidoses, an inborn error of metabolism following autosomal recessive inheritance. No tissue samples are available for genetic studies.

1. *What is the risk that the couple's first child will be affected by Hurler syndrome?*
2. *Can the couple be offered anything more than a risk figure?*

Case 2

A woman has a brother and a maternal uncle affected by hemophilia A. She herself has had two unaffected sons and would like more children. She is referred to a genetics clinic to discuss the risk and the options.

1. *Purely on the basis of the information given, what is the woman's carrier risk for hemophilia A?*
2. *Can anything be done to modify her risk?*

CHAPTER 9: Developmental Genetics

Case 1

A 2-year-old child is referred to geneticists because of a large head circumference above the 97th centile, although it is growing parallel to the centile lines. The parents would like to have another child and are asking about the recurrence risk. The cerebral ventricles are dilated, and there has been much discussion with the neurosurgeons about possible ventriculoperitoneal shunting. On taking a full family history, it emerges that the paternal grandmother is under review by dermatologists for skin lesions, some of which have been removed, and a paternal uncle has had teeth cysts removed by a hospital dentist.

1. *Is there a diagnosis that embraces the various features in these different family members?*
2. *What investigations would be appropriate for the child's father, and what is the answer to the couple's question about recurrence risk?*

Case 2

On prenatal ultrasound at 20 weeks' gestation a fetus appears to have a narrow chest with short ribs, cystic changes in one kidney, and possibly an extra digit on both hands. The parents deny consanguinity but want as much information as possible about the diagnosis and prognosis.

1. *What group of disorders should be considered with these ultrasound findings, and which pattern of inheritance do they normally follow?*
2. *What additional anomalies might the ultrasonographer look for to help provide more prognostic information?*

Case 3

A 4-year-old girl is brought to a pediatrician because of behavioral difficulties, including problems with potty training. The pediatrician decides to test the child's chromosomes by microarray-comparative genomic hybridization because he has previously seen a case of 47, XXX (triple X) syndrome in which the girl had oppositional behavior. Somewhat to his surprise, the chromosome result is 47,XY—that is, the "girl" is genetically "male."

1. *What are the most important causes of sex reversal in a 4-year-old child who is phenotypically female and otherwise physically healthy?*
2. *What should the pediatrician tell the parents, and which investigations should be performed?*

CHAPTER 10: Common Disease, Polygenic, and Multifactorial Genetics

Case 1

A 16-year-old requests oral contraceptives from her general practitioner. On taking a family history, it emerges that her mother had a deep vein thrombosis at the age of 40 years and died after a pulmonary embolism at age 55 years. There is no other relevant family history.

1. *What genetic testing is appropriate?*
2. *What are the limitations of testing in this situation?*

Case 2

A 35-year-old woman is diagnosed with diabetes and started on insulin treatment. She and her 29-year-old brother were adopted and have no contact with their birth parents. Her brother has no symptoms of hyperglycemia. Both have normal hearing and no other significant findings.

1. *What possible subtypes of diabetes might she have, and what are the modes of inheritance of these subtypes?*
2. *For each of these subtypes, what is the risk of her brother developing diabetes?*

Case 3

A 2-year-old girl presents with partial seizures. The episode is brief and unaccompanied by fever. Because the child is well with no neurological deficit, a decision is made not to treat with an anticonvulsant drug. A year later she suffers a generalized seizure, again without fever. On this occasion, her 30-year-old mother asks whether this might have anything to do with her own seizures that began at the age of 15 years, although she has had only two episodes since. She had undergone computed tomography of the brain, and the doctors mentioned a condition whose name she could not remember. Magnetic resonance imaging of the child's brain shows uncalcified nodules on the lateral ventricular walls.

1. *The mother asks whether the epilepsy is genetic and whether it could happen again if she has another child. What can she be told?*
2. *What diagnoses should be considered, and can genetic testing be offered?*

Case 4

A 5-year-old boy is admitted to hospital with an unexplained fever and found to have a raised blood glucose level. He makes a good recovery, but 2 weeks later his fasting blood glucose level is shown to be increased at 7 mmol/L. There is a strong family history of diabetes on his mother's side, with his mother, maternal uncle, and maternal grandfather all affected. His father has no symptoms of diabetes, but his father's sister had gestational diabetes during her recent pregnancy. Molecular genetic testing identifies a heterozygous glucokinase gene mutation in the child.

1. *The parents believe that their son's hyperglycemia is inherited from the mother's side of the family. Is this correct?*
2. *What are the consequences of finding a glucokinase gene variant for this family?*

CHAPTER 11: Screening for Genetic Disease

Case 1

A 32-year-old man is tall and thin and has a normal echocardiogram, and 20 years ago his father died suddenly at age 50 years, having been suspected of having a thoracic aortic aneurysm. The general practitioner wonders whether his patient has Marfan syndrome and refers him to the local genetics service. He has some features of Marfan syndrome but, strictly speaking, would meet the accepted criteria only if the family history was definitely positive for the disorder. He has a brother of average height and three young children who are in good health.

1. *In terms of genetic testing, what are the limitations to screening if the diagnosis is Marfan syndrome?*
2. *What are the screening issues for the family?*

Case 2

A screening test for cystic fibrosis (CF) is being evaluated on a population of 100,000 newborn babies. The test is positive in 805 babies, of whom 45 are eventually shown to have CF by a combination of DNA analysis and sweat testing. Of those babies whose screening test is negative, five subsequently develop symptoms and are diagnosed with CF.

1. *What are the sensitivity and specificity of this screening test?*
2. *What is the positive predictive value of the screening test?*

CHAPTER 12: Hemoglobin and the Hemoglobinopathies

Case 1

A Chinese couple now residing in the United Kingdom had two pregnancies while living in Asia, and the outcome in both was a stillborn edematous baby (hydrops fetalis). They have no living children. They seek some genetic advice about the chances of this happening again, but no medical records are available for the pregnancies.

1. *What diagnostic possibilities should be considered?*
2. *What investigations are appropriate to this situation?*

Case 2

A young adolescent whose parents are of West Indian origin is admitted from accident and emergency after presenting with severe abdominal pain and some fever. An acute abdomen is suspected, and the patient undergoes laparotomy for possible appendicitis. However, no surgical pathology is identified. Subsequently the urine appears dark.

1. *What other investigations might be appropriate at this stage?*
2. *What form of follow-up is appropriate?*

CHAPTER 13: Immunogenetics

Case 1

A 32-year-old man has had low back pain and stiffness for 2 years and recently developed some irritation in his eyes. Radiography is performed, and a diagnosis of ankylosing spondylitis is made. He remembers his maternal grandfather having similar back problems, as well as arthritis in other joints. He has three young children.

1. *Is it likely that his grandfather also had ankylosing spondylitis?*
2. *What is the risk of passing the condition to his three children?*

Case 2

A 4-year-old girl suffers frequent upper respiratory infections with chest involvement, and each episode lasts longer compared with her preschool peers. Doctors have always assumed this is somehow a consequence of her stormy early months when she had major heart surgery for tetralogy of Fallot. She also has nasal speech, and in her neonatal record she had low calcium levels for a few days.

1. *Is there an underlying diagnosis that could explain her frequent and prolonged upper respiratory infections?*
2. *What further management of the family is indicated?*

CHAPTER 14: The Genetics of Cancer . . . and Cancer Genetics

Case 1

A 38-year-old woman, who recently had a mastectomy for breast cancer, requests a referral to the genetic service. Her father had some bowel polyps removed in his 50s, and a cousin on the same side of the family had some form of thyroid cancer in her 40s. The general practitioner consults a set of guidelines that suggest a familial form of breast cancer is unlikely because she is the only one affected, even though she is quite young. He is reluctant to refer her.

1. *Could the history suggest another familial condition? If so, which one?*
2. *What other clinical features might give a clue to the diagnosis?*

Case 2

A 30-year-old is referred for genetic counseling because she is concerned about her risk of developing breast cancer. The consultand's mother has recently been diagnosed with breast cancer at age 55 years. Her maternal uncle's daughter (the consultand's cousin) had bilateral breast cancer diagnosed at age 38 years and died 5 years ago from metastatic disease. The cousin had participated in a research study that identified a pathogenic *BRCA2* gene variant. The clinical geneticist suggests that the consultand's mother should be tested before predictive testing is offered to her, the consultand. They are surprised when a negative result is reported by the laboratory.

1. *What are the possible explanations for this result?*
2. *What is the risk of the consultand's uncle developing breast cancer?*

Case 3

A 58-year-old man has been diagnosed with a colorectal adenocarcinoma affecting the ascending colon. His paternal grandmother is believed to have died of renal cancer, while a female cousin on the same side of the family was diagnosed with endometrial cancer at the age of 50 years. The proband has three children in their mid-late 30s.

1. *Does this pattern of malignancies suggest a known family cancer syndrome, and if so, how might it be investigated?*
2. *Without any further information, what screening advice might be suggested for the proband's three children?*

CHAPTER 16: Congenital Abnormalities, Dysmorphic Syndromes, and Learning Disability

Case 1

A young couple has just lost their first pregnancy through fetal abnormality. Polyhydramnios was diagnosed on ultrasonography, as well as a small fetal kidney on one side. Amniocentesis was performed, and the karyotype showed a normal 46,XY pattern. The couple was unsure what to do, but eventually elected for a termination of pregnancy at 21 weeks. They were very upset and did not want any further investigations performed, including an autopsy. They did agree to whole-body radiography of the fetus, and some of the upper thoracic vertebrae were misshapen.

1. *The couple asks whether such a problem could recur—they do not feel they can go through this again. What can they be told?*
2. *What further investigations might have helped to inform the genetic risk?*

Case 2

On routine neonatal examination on the second day, a baby is found to have a cleft palate. The pregnancy was uneventful with no exposure to potential teratogens, and the family history is negative. The pediatric registrar also wonders whether the limbs are slightly short. The baby's birth weight is on the 25th centile, with length on the 2nd centile.

1. *What diagnoses might be considered?*
2. *What are the management issues in a case like this?*

Case 3

A couple have a 10-year-old daughter with severe intellectual disability, a history of hypotonia and feeding difficulties, occasional seizures but normal brain magnetic resonance imaging, almost no spoken language, growth parameters within the normal range, and some soft dysmorphic features. They have put off trying to extend their family because of concern that they might have another affected child and ask if anything further can be done.

1. *Without more information or investigations, what general comments can be made about the recurrence risk if they decide to try for another baby?*
2. *What investigative options are available to help the couple further?*

CHAPTER 17: Chromosome Disorders

Case 1

A newborn baby girl looks somewhat dysmorphic and is diagnosed with an atrioventricular septal defect, and the pediatricians think this may be Down syndrome. This is discussed with the parents, and microarray-comparative genomic hybridization is performed. The result comes back as normal. The baby is very "good" during infancy, with very little crying, and no further investigations are done. Subsequently the child shows moderate-severe global developmental delay and head-banging, wakes every night for about 4 hours, tends to hug people excessively, and has mild brachydactyly. The pediatricians refer her to a geneticist for an opinion.

1. *Does the history suggest a diagnosis?*
2. *What investigation should be requested?*

Case 2

A 45-year-old mother has two children but different partners. One is a 20-year-old son with normal stature, mild dysmorphic features, and mild intellectual disability; the other is an 18-year-old daughter with short stature, small head circumference, obesity, and mild intellectual disability. They both had normal karyotypes about 15 years ago. The mother tells you that her sister in Australia has a daughter who closely resembles her own daughter, and she also had a maternal uncle who was very similar to her son.

1. *Is there a way of explaining this family history?*
2. *What further tests should be considered?*

Case 3

A pediatrician arranges a microarray-comparative genomic hybridization test for an 8-year-old boy whose school performance is poor and requires additional support. He also has behavioral problems with social communication difficulties, and there is much discussion as to whether he should be assessed for possible autism. The professionals are inclined toward the view that poor parenting and difficult circumstances contribute to the overall problem because the mother looks after him and three other children on her own, and she was a low achiever at school herself. The microarray-comparative genomic hybridization result reveals a small deletion of 15q11.2, and the child is referred to a clinical geneticist.

1. *How might the microarray-comparative genomic hybridization finding help explain the situation at school and at home?*
2. *What further investigations are indicated?*

CHAPTER 18: Inborn Errors of Metabolism

Case 1

A 2-year-old boy, who has a baby sister age 4 months, is admitted to hospital with a vomiting illness and drowsiness. Despite vomiting, his symptoms improve quickly with intravenous fluid support, but his blood glucose remains low, and intravenous fluids are required longer than might normally be expected. The parents say that something like this happened before, although he recovered without seeing a doctor.

1. *What does this history suggest?*
2. *What investigations are appropriate?*

Case 2

A 1-year-old boy presents with tachypnoea, especially on feeding, and motor milestones are slightly delayed. His mother says that she had a maternal great-aunt who was believed to have had two sons who both died in late childhood from some "heart and muscle weakness" problem. On investigation the boy is found to have a dilated cardiomyopathy and mild general muscle weakness.

1. *What condition is suggested by the combination of clinical features and family history?*
2. *What further investigations are indicated?*

Case 3

A 28-year-old woman has become aware over several years that she does not have the same energy as she did at the age of 20. She tires relatively easily on exertion, and family members have noticed that she has developed slightly droopy eyelids, and they also think her hearing is deteriorating, which she vigorously denies.

1. *How might a detailed family history help toward a diagnosis in this case?*
2. *What investigations should be performed?*

CHAPTER 19: Mainstream Monogenic Disorders

Case 1

A 31-year-old woman would like to start a family but is worried because her 39-year-old brother was diagnosed as having Becker muscular dystrophy nearly 30 years ago, and she remembers having being told that the condition affects boys but that women pass it on. Her brother is still living but is now quite disabled by his condition. There is no wider family history of muscular dystrophy.

1. *Is the original diagnosis reliable—could there be other possibilities?*
2. *What are the next steps in investigating this situation?*

Case 2

A middle-aged couple is devastated when their 21-year-old daughter collapses at a dance and cannot be resuscitated. At postmortem examination all toxicology tests are negative, and no cause of death is found. The mother recalls that her father died suddenly in his 50s from what was presumed at the time to be a myocardial infarction, and her sister has had some dizzy spells but has not seen her doctor. The couple has three other children who are young, sport-loving adults, and they are very worried that this might happen again.

1. *What investigations are appropriate?*
2. *What advice should the family be given?*

Case 3

A young man of 21 years has suffered a spontaneous pneumothorax, which is resolving well. He is found to have some joint laxity and a high palate with a history of dental crowding. The physicians suggest he may have Marfan syndrome and perform an echocardiogram, which highlights mild mitral valve regurgitation. He mentions that his maternal grandfather suffered an aortic aneurysm aged 60 and died. The physicians refer him to clinical genetics with a diagnosis of probable Marfan syndrome.

1. *What steps can be taken to confirm or refute a diagnosis of Marfan syndrome?*
2. *If the diagnosis is not Marfan syndrome, what other conditions might be considered?*

CHAPTER 20: Prenatal Testing and Reproductive Genetics

Case 1

A 36-year-old pregnant woman elects to undergo prenatal testing by chorionic villus biopsy after the finding of increased nuchal translucency on ultrasonography. The initial result, using quantitative fluorescence-polymerase chain reaction, is good news—there is no evidence for trisomy 21—and the woman is greatly relieved. However, on the cultured cells more than 2 weeks later, it emerges that there is mosaicism for trisomy 20. She undergoes amniocentesis a week later, and 3 weeks after that the result also shows some cells with trisomy 20.

1. *Why was an amniocentesis performed in addition to the chorionic villus biopsy?*
2. *What else can be done following the amniocentesis result?*

Case 2

A couple has two sons with autism and would very much like to have another child. They are prepared to do anything to ensure that the problem does not recur. They acquire a lot of information from the internet and learn that boys are more commonly affected—the male: female sex ratio is approximately 4:1. As they see it, the simple solution to their problem is sex selection by preimplantation genetic diagnosis (PGD).

1. *What investigations might be performed on the autistic sons?*
2. *If tests on the sons fail to identify a diagnosis, can the request of the couple for sex selection by PGD be supported by the geneticist?*

Case 3

A 37-year-old woman whose father had hemophilia A has just learned that she is pregnant for the first time, and is at 6 weeks' gestation. She requests prenatal testing as her father suffered significantly during his life and she does not want to see the problem recur. She is also worried about Down syndrome on account of her age. She is first of all offered a blood test 2 weeks later and told it may not be necessary to perform chorionic villus sampling or amniocentesis.

1. *What blood test is this, and how might it avoid the need for an invasive prenatal test?*
2. *What statistical information should she have been given about the sensitivity of the test?*

CHAPTER 21: Genetic Counseling

Case 1

A couple has a son with dysmorphic features, short stature, and moderately severe developmental delay. Microarray-comparative genomic hybridization analysis identifies a subtle genetic imbalance that was not detected on a standard karyotype, and the father is found to have a balanced translocation that is predisposed to this. His family has always blamed the mother for the child's condition because of her history of drug abuse, with the result that the couple no longer talk to his wider family. If they try and explain the issues to his wider family, they believe a lot of derogatory and inaccurate information will be posted on social media. However, through friends he has learned that his sister is trying to start a family.

1. *What are the important genetic issues?*
2. *What other issues does this case raise?*

Case 2

A couple has a child who is diagnosed with cystic fibrosis (CF) through neonatal screening. The child is homozygous for the common p.Phe508del mutation. They request prenatal diagnosis in the next pregnancy, but DNA analysis shows that the father is not a carrier of p.Phe508del. It must be assumed he is not the biological father of the child with CF, and this is confirmed when further analysis shows that the child does not have a haplotype in common with him.

1. *What medical issue does this information raise?*
2. *What counseling issues are raised by these results?*

Multiple-Choice Answers

CHAPTER 2: The Cellular and Molecular Basis of Inheritance

1. **Base substitutions:**
   a. **True**. When a stop codon replaces an amino acid
   b. **True**. For example, by mutation of conserved splice donor and acceptor sites
   c. **False**. Silent mutations or substitutions in non-coding regions may not be pathogenic
   d. **True**. For example, promoter mutations may affect binding of transcription factors
   e. **False**. Frameshifts are caused by the insertion or deletion of nucleotides
2. **Transcription:**
   a. **False**. During transcription mRNA is produced from the DNA template
   b. **True**. The mRNA product is then translocated to the cytoplasm
   c. **True**. The mRNA is complementary to the antisense strand
   d. **False**. Transcription factors bind to regulatory sequences within the promoter
   e. **True**. The addition of the 5′ cap and 3′ poly(A) tail facilitates transport to the cytoplasm
3. **The following are directly involved in DNA repair:**
   a. **True**. The DNA glycosylase MYH is involved in base excision repair
   b. **True**. They incorporate the correct bases
   c. **True**. They seal gaps after abnormal base excision and correct base insertion
   d. **False**. Splicing removes introns during mRNA production
   e. **False**. Ribosomes are involved in translation
4. **During DNA replication:**
   a. **True**. It unwinds the DNA helix
   b. **False**. Replication occurs in both directions
   c. **True**. These fragments are joined by DNA ligase to form the lagging strand
   d. **False**. DNA replication is semiconservative, as only one strand is newly synthesized
   e. **False**. Uracil is incorporated in mRNA, thymine in DNA

CHAPTER 3: Chromosomes and Cell Division

1. **Meiosis differs from mitosis in the following ways:**
   a. **True**. During human meiosis, the number of chromosomes is reduced from 46 to 23
   b. **False**. Early cell divisions in gametogenesis are mitotic; meiosis occurs only at the final division
   c. **True**. In meiosis, the two divisions are known as meiosis I and II
   d. **True**. The bivalents separate independently during meiosis I, and crossovers (chiasmata) occur between homologous chromosomes
   e. **False**. The five stages of meiosis I prophase are leptotene, zygotene, pachytene, diplotene, and diakinesis
2. **Chromosome abnormalities reliably detected by light microscopy include:**
   a. **True**. An extra chromosome (e.g., chromosome 21 in Down syndrome) is easily seen
   b. **True**. A missing chromosome (e.g., Turner syndrome in females with a single X) is easily seen
   c. **False**. A subtle translocation may not be visible
   d. **False**. A small deletion may not be visible
   e. **True**. Centric fusion of the long arms of two acrocentric chromosomes is readily detected
3. **Fluorescence *in situ* hybridization using whole-chromosome (painting) or specific-locus probes enables routine detection of:**
   a. **False**. Changes in gene dosage may be identified by comparative genomic hybridization
   b. **True**. Subtelomeric probes are useful in the investigation of nonspecific learning difficulties
   c. **True**. Trisomies can be detected in interphase cells
   d. **True**. The origin of marker chromosomes can be determined by chromosome painting
   e. **True**. Subtle rearrangements can be detected by chromosome painting
4. **In Robertsonian translocations:**
   a. **False**. The opposite—the risk for male carriers is around 1% to 3%, and for female carriers around 10%
   b. **False**. The risk for Down syndrome in liveborn offspring is 100%
   c. **True**. The acrocentric chromosomes 13, 14, 15, 21, and 22
   d. **False**. Chromosome 18 is not an acrocentric chromosome
   e. **False**. Approximately two-thirds of translocation Down syndrome cases occur *de novo*

CHAPTER 4: Finding the Cause of Monogenic Disorders by Identifying Disease Genes

1. **Positional cloning uses:**
   a. **True**. Now that the human genome sequence is complete, it is possible to identify a disease-associated gene *in silico*
   b. **True**. After a gene has been mapped to a region, it can be helpful to check for syntenic regions in animal models
   c. **True**. Many genes have been identified through mapping of translocation or deletion breakpoints

d. **False.** Positional cloning describes the search for genes based on their chromosomal location
e. **True.** A genome-wide scan uses microsatellite markers located throughout the genome for linkage mapping

2. **A candidate gene is likely to be a disease associated gene if:**
a. **True.** This implies causality
b. **True.** This is strong evidence
c. **True.** This excludes the possibility that a single variant is a marker in linkage disequilibrium rather than a pathogenic variant
d. **True.** For example, a gene associated with blindness might be expected to be expressed in the eye
e. **False.** A pseudogene does not encode a functional protein, and variants are therefore unlikely to be pathogenic

3. **Achievements of the Human Genome Project include:**
a. **False.** The draft sequence was completed in 2000, but its publication date was February 2001
b. **True.** Sequencing was finished 2 years ahead of the original schedule
c. **True.** Annotation tools such as Ensembl were developed to assist users
d. **False.** More than 5500 have been identified to date, but the number is increasing rapidly
e. **True.** Around 5% of the US budget for the Human Genome Project was devoted to studying these issues

CHAPTER 5: Laboratory Techniques for Diagnosis of Monogenic Disorders

1. **The following statements apply to restriction enzymes:**
a. **True.** Double-stranded DNA can be digested to give overhanging (sticky) ends or blunt ends
b. **False.** More than 300 restriction enzymes have been isolated from various bacteria
c. **True.** If the mutation creates or destroys a recognition site
d. **True.** DNA digestion by a restriction enzyme is the first step in Southern blotting
e. **False.** They are endonucleases, as they digest DNA fragments internally, as opposed to exonuclease digestion from the 5′ or 3′ ends of DNA fragments

2. **The following describe polymerase chain reaction (PCR):**
a. **True.** Millions of copies of DNA can be produced from one template without using cloning vectors
b. **False.** PCR uses the heat-stable Taq polymerase (and others), because a high denaturing temperature (around 95° C) is required to separate double-stranded products at the start of each cycle
c. **True.** PCR may be used to amplify DNA from single cells (e.g., in preimplantation genetic diagnosis); therefore, appropriate control measures are important to avoid contamination
d. **False.** PCR routinely amplifies targets of up to 1 kilobases (kb), and long-range PCR is limited to around 40 kb
e. **False.** Knowledge of the sequence is required to design primers to flank the region of interest

3. **Types of nucleic acid hybridisation include:**
a. **True.** Southern blotting describes the hybridization of a radioactively labeled probe with DNA fragments separated by electrophoresis
b. **True.** Hybridization between the target and probe DNA takes place on a glass slide
c. **False.** Western blotting is used to analyze protein expression using antibody detection methods
d. **True.** Northern blotting is used to examine RNA expression
e. **True.** DNA fingerprinting employs a minisatellite DNA probe to hybridize to hypervariable DNA fragments

CHAPTER 6: Patterns of Inheritance

1. **Concerning autosomal recessive inheritance:**
a. **False.** Sex ratio is equal
b. **False.** The risk at the time of conception is 1/2 (50%)
c. **True.** All people carry pathogenic variants; consanguineous couples are more likely to have the same pathogenic variant inherited from a common ancestor
d. **True.** Affected individuals would have to partner with a carrier or another affected person for their offspring to be affected
e. **False.** The mechanisms causing Angelman syndrome are varied, but autosomal recessive inheritance is not one of them

2. **Concerning X-linked inheritance:**
a. **True.** A father passes his Y chromosome to his son
b. **True.** He might have affected grandsons through his daughters, who are obligate carriers
c. **False.** Although the condition affects females, in most diseases inherited in this way the males are more severely affected because the female has a normal copy of the gene on her other X chromosome, and X-inactivation means that the normal copy is expressed in about half of her tissues
d. **True.** All daughters of an affected man will be affected, but none of his sons
e. **False.** Germline mosaicism always needs to be considered when an isolated case of an X-linked condition occurs

3. **In mitochondrial genetics:**
a. **False.** This refers to two populations of mitochondrial DNA, one normal and one mutated
b. **False.** The opposite, probably because they replicate more frequently
c. **False.** Any tissue with mitochondria can be affected
d. **True.** If the affected woman's oocytes contain only mutated mitochondria
e. **False.** Many mitochondrial proteins of the respiratory chain and its complexes are encoded by nuclear genes

4. **Concerning terminology:**
a. **False.** The same disease caused by different genes—but not necessarily on different chromosomes
b. **False.** The basic pattern of inheritance in pseudodominance is autosomal recessive
c. **True.** A proportion of individuals with the mutated gene show no signs or symptoms
d. **True.** Diseases showing anticipation demonstrate increased severity, and earlier age of onset, with succeeding generations
e. **False.** Not a variation in severity (or variable expression), but two or more apparently unrelated effects from the same gene

5. **In inheritance:**
a. **True.** Both copies of a mutated gene can be passed to a child this way
b. **True.** This explains a proportion of cases of Prader-Willi and Angelman syndromes

c. **False**. Digenic inheritance refers to a phenotype that results from heterozygosity for two different genes
d. **True**. This explains presenile baldness and gout
e. **False**. Only a small proportion

CHAPTER 7: Population and Mathematical Genetics

1. **In applying the Hardy–Weinberg equilibrium, the following assumptions are made:**
   a. **False**. The population should be large to increase the likelihood of non-random mating
   b. **True**. Consanguinity is a form of non-random mating
   c. **True**. The introduction of new alleles introduces variables
   d. **True**. In theory, if sperm donors are used many times, this could introduce a form of non-random mating
   e. **True**. Migration introduces new alleles
2. **If the population incidence of a recessive disease is 1 in 10,000, the carrier frequency in the population is:**
   a. **False**.
   b. **False**.
   c. **False**.
   d. **True**. The carrier frequency is 2 times the square root of the incidence
   e. **False**.
3. **Heterozygote advantage:**
   a. **False**. It refers to conditions that follow autosomal recessive inheritance
   b. **True**. The homozygote may show markedly reduced biological fitness (e.g., cystic fibrosis)
   c. **True**. People with sickle-cell trait are more able to remove parasitized cells from the circulation
   d. **True**. A process of selective advantage may be at work
   e. **False**. The presence of the allele in a population may be a founder effect
4. **Polymorphic loci:**
   a. **False**. The alleles usually have low frequencies, for example, 1%
   b. **True**. They may be crucial to gene mapping by virtue of their cosegregation with disease
   c. **True**. Although direct variant analysis is usual nowadays, in some circumstances linkage analysis using polymorphic loci may be the only way to determine genetic status in presymptomatic diagnosis and prenatal testing
   d. **False**. The association of polymorphic loci with disease segregation is key to calculating a logarithm of the odds (LOD) score
   e. **False**. They may be important (e.g., blood groups)
5. **In population genetics:**
   a. **False**. The incidence of the disease must also be known
   b. **True**. In autosomal recessive disease most of the genes in the population are present in unaffected heterozygotes
   c. **True**. In recessive conditions sibships without any affected individual(s) will not be ascertained
   d. **False**. Founder effects are the main reason for the high frequency of certain alleles in population groups where consanguinity rates are often high; this applies particularly to autosomal recessive conditions
   e. **False**. It is useful only when there is a common ancestor from both sides of the family (i.e., inbreeding)

CHAPTER 8: Risk Calculation

1. **Probabilities:**
   a. **True**. These are two ways of expressing the same likelihood
   b. **True**. A probability of 1 means that the event will happen 100% of the time
   c. **True**. The probability that both will be boys is $1/2 \times 1/2 = 1/4$, for girls the same; therefore the chance of being the same sex is $1/4 + 1/4 = 1/2$ (0.5)
   d. **True**. These two approaches to a probability calculation are essential
   e. **True**. Some 70% of heterozygotes will manifest the condition
2. **For an autosomal recessive condition, the chance that the first cousin of an affected individual is a carrier is:**
   a. **False**.
   b. **False**.
   c. **True**. The affected individual's parents are obligate carriers, aunts and uncles have a 1 in 2 risk, cousins a 1 in 4 risk
   d. **False**.
   e. **False**.
3. **In X-linked recessive inheritance:**
   a. **False**. The risk is 1 in 2 if the sex of the fetus is known to be male
   b. **False**. The male might be affected because a *de novo* mutation has occurred
   c. **True**. This is significant and has to be allowed for in risk calculation and counseling
   d. **True**. This is conditional information that can be built into a Bayes' calculation
   e. **False**. This is a key individual whose risk must be calculated before the consultand's risk
4. **In autosomal recessive inheritance the risk that the nephew of an affected individual, born to the affected individual's healthy sibling, is a carrier is:**
   a. **False**.
   b. **False**.
   c. **False**.
   d. **True**. The healthy sibling of the affected individual has a 2 in 3 chance of being a carrier; this person's son has a risk that is half of that
   e. **False**.
5. **Risk-modifying information:**
   a. **True**. For example, negative mutation findings when testing for cystic fibrosis
   b. **True**. Age of onset (clinical expression) data must be derived from large family studies
   c. **False**. Without this information huge errors will be made
   d. **True**. An empiric risk is really a compromise figure and may not apply to a particular situation
   e. **False**. It may matter a lot because it is a measure of the likelihood that a meiotic recombination event will take place between the marker and the gene mutation causing the disease

CHAPTER 9: Developmental Genetics

1. **In development, *HOX* genes:**
   a. **True**. They are important in spatial determination and patterning

b. **False**. Relatively few malformation syndromes are known to be directly attributed to *HOX* gene variants, probably because of paralogous compensation
c. **False**. They contain an important conserved homeobox of 180 base pairs
d. **True**. They are probably important only in early development
e. **True**. Where malformation-causing variants have been identified, different organ systems may be involved, for example, hand–foot–genital syndrome (*HOXA13*)

2. **In the embryo and fetus:**
a. **False**. This occurs later and is the process of laying down the primary body axis in the second and third weeks
b. **False**. Organogenesis takes places mainly between 4 and 18 weeks' gestation
c. **True**. The genes in these pathways are expressed widely throughout the body
d. **False**. Somites form in a rostro-caudal direction
e. **True**. When mutated, the *TBX3* and *TBX5* genes lead to the ulnar–mammary and Holt-Oram syndromes, respectively

3. **Concerning development pathways and processes:**
a. **False**. It is formed from the first pharyngeal (branchial) arch
b. **True**. Remodeling occurs so that these vessels become the great arteries
c. **True**. This has been established in animals and is proving to be highly likely in humans
d. **False**. Most cases of achondroplasia are attributed to one particular variant, G380R, encoded by a point mutation at nucleotide 1138 of the *FGFR3* gene; only occasionally do other variants affect the membrane-bound part of the protein
e. **False**. These different types of DNA variant usually cause widely differing phenotypes (e.g., the *RET* gene)

4. **Regarding the X-chromosome:**
a. **True**. Sometimes the *SRY* gene is involved in recombination with the pseudoautosomal regions of X and Y
b. **False**. Not all regions of the X are switched off; otherwise there would presumably be no phenotypic effects in Turner syndrome
c. **True**. However, only when there is a pathogenic variant on one X chromosome does this have any consequences
d. **False**. *SRY* has an important initiating function, but other genes are very important
e. **True**. Some unusual phenomena occur in twins, leading to the conclusion that these processes may be linked

5. **Transcription factors:**
a. **False**. They are usually proteins that bind to specific regulatory DNA sequences
b. **False**. They also switch genes on
c. **True**. For example, a leg might develop in place of an antenna
d. **False**. Transcription factors are crucial to normal laterality
e. **True**. The zinc finger motif encodes a finger-like projection of amino acids that forms a complex with a zinc ion

CHAPTER 10: Common Disease, Polygenic, and Multifactorial Genetics

1. **Concerning autism:**
a. **False**. It is a neurodevelopmental disorder, and no metabolic abnormalities are found
b. **False**. This would imply autosomal dominant inheritance; the rate is about 20%
c. **False**. Although autism occurs in fragile-X syndrome, the vast majority of affected individuals do not have this condition
d. **True**. The figure is nearly 3% for full-blown autism and a further 3% for milder features—autistic spectrum disorder
e. **False**. The male:female ratio is approximately 4:1

2. **Linkage analysis is more difficult in multifactorial conditions than in single-gene disorders because:**
a. **True**. Identifying multiple genes, each with small effect, is very difficult
b. **True**. In a fully penetrant single-gene disorder, it is easier to find families with sufficient informative meioses
c. **True**. Parametric linkage analysis requires that the mode of inheritance is known
d. **True**. Different genetic and environmental factors may be involved
e. **True**. The late age of onset means that affection status may be uncertain

3. **Association studies:**
a. **True**. The disease and variant tested may be common in a population subset, but there is no causal relationship
b. **True**. The transmission disequilibrium test (TDT) uses family controls and thus avoids population stratification effects
c. **True**. Replication of positive studies in different populations will increase the evidence for an association
d. **False**. Association studies are used to test variants identified by gene-mapping techniques, including affected sibling-pair analysis
e. **True**. Variants with small effects may be missed if the patients and controls are not closely matched

4. **Variants in genes that confer susceptibility to type 2 diabetes mellitus (T2DM) have been found:**
a. **True**. The gene encoding calpain-10 was identified by positional cloning in Mexican-American sibling pairs
b. **False**. No confirmed T2DM susceptibility genes have been identified by this approach
c. **True**. Examples include two subtypes of maturity-onset diabetes of the young
d. **True**. The genes encoding the potassium channel subunits in the pancreatic β-cell were biological candidates
e. **True**. For example, the HNF-1A variant G319S has been reported only in the Oji Cree population (a First Nation Canadian group)

5. **Variants in the *NOD2/CARD15* gene:**
a. **False**. Evidence to date supports a role in Crohn disease, but not ulcerative colitis
b. **True**. Increased risk is estimated at 40-fold for homozygotes and 2.5-fold for heterozygotes
c. **True**. A genome-wide scan for inflammatory bowel disease initially identified the 16p12 region
d. **False**. The *NOD2/CARD15* gene activates NF-κB, but this complex is already targeted by the most effective drugs used to treat Crohn disease
e. **False**. The three reported variants are found at a frequency of 5% in the general population, compared with 15% in patients with Crohn disease

CHAPTER 11: Screening for Genetic Disease

1.
a. **True**. By looking for evidence of two populations of cells

b. **True**. Firm clinical signs are the exception rather than the rule
c. **False**. DNA sequence variants must be polymorphic to be useful
d. **False**. Screening should be in the newborn period and treated early to help ensure good speech development
e. **True**. As a rule, this is highly desirable and sometimes crucial, and requires informed consent

2.
a. **False**. The facial rash of angiokeratoma (adenoma sebaceum) is often not present
b. **False**. There may not be sufficient numbers of café-au-lait spots until age 5 to 6 years
c. **False**. They may be fully informative of an individual's genetic status
d. **True**. Dural ectasia of the lumbar spine is an important feature
e. **False**. This is usually the method of analysis, but in some circumstances linked DNA markers are informative, and in some cases conventional investigations (e.g., magnetic resonance imaging, ultrasonography) are sufficiently sensitive and specific

3.
a. **False**. Participation should, in principle, be voluntary
b. **True**. The outcome of population screening programs should be an improvement in health benefit
c. **False**. This is the specificity of a test
d. **True**. This is different from the sensitivity, which refers to the proportion of affected cases that are detected (i.e., there may be some false negatives)
e. **True**. Adequate expert counseling should be part of the predictive test program

4.
a. **True**. Recall of the result itself, or the interpretation, is frequently inaccurate
b. **False**. The highest incidence for a serious disease is that in β-thalassemia: 1 in 8 are carriers
c. **False**. This has happened before and should be a major concern
d. **False**. The benefit lies in informing the family for subsequent reproductive decisions
e. **False**. The first assay is biochemical, a measure of immunoreactive trypsin

5.
a. **False**. Although the carrier frequency is about 1 in 10, no population screening is undertaken in the United Kingdom
b. **False**. In general, unless a beneficial medical intervention can be offered, such testing should be deferred until the child is old enough to make the decision
c. **True**. They have been operational since the 1960s to 1970s
d. **True**. This is one of the newer tests introduced to the program
e. **False**. Their prime function in a service department is for clinical management of patients and families

CHAPTER 12: Hemoglobin and the Hemoglobinopathies

1. **For different hemoglobins:**
a. **False**. The γ chain of HbF bears a close resemblance to the adult β chain, differing by 39 amino acids
b. **False**. This is true for the α and γ chains only; the β chain appears toward the end of fetal life
c. **False**. There are too few α chains, which are replaced by β chains
d. **False**. It is a form of α-thalassemia
e. **False**. They have a mild anemia, and clinical symptoms are rare

2. **Regarding sickle-cell disease:**
a. **False**. The effect is attributed to reduced solubility and polymerization
b. **True**. Obstruction of arteries can be the result of sickling crises
c. **True**. A valine residue is substituted for a glutamic acid residue
d. **False**. Life-threatening sepsis can result from splenic infarction
e. **True**. These mutations give rise to an amino acid substitution

3. **Concerning hemoglobin variants:**
a. **True**. This applies to the majority of those known
b. **False**. All types of mutation are known
c. **False**. Bone marrow hyperplasia occurs, which leads to physical changes such as a thickened calvarium
d. **True**. Oxygen is not released so readily to tissues
e. **True**. HbH, for example, is unstable

4. **Regarding hemoglobins (Hbs) during life:**
a. **False**. It is a hereditary condition
b. **False**. This is true only between 2 and 7 months' gestation
c. **False**. The bone marrow starts producing Hb from 6 to 7 months of fetal life
d. **False**. Production ceases from 2 to 3 months of postnatal life
e. **True**. It gives rise to no symptoms—the Hb chains produced are normal

CHAPTER 13: Immunogenetics

1. **Concerning complement:**
a. **False**. The cascade can also be activated by the alternative pathway
b. **True**. C4 levels are reduced, and production of C2b is uncontrolled
c. **False**. C3 levels are normal, C4 levels are reduced
d. **True**. C3b adheres to the surface of microorganisms
e. **False**. Complement is a series of at least 20 interacting plasma proteins

2. **In immunology:**
a. **False**. It is made up of four polypeptide chains—two "light" and two "heavy"
b. **False**. They are distributed on different chromosomes
c. **False**. Donors are likely to share human leukocyte antigen haplotypes, which are crucial to tissue compatibility
d. **True**. These are: variable, diversity, junctional, and constant regions
e. **True**. Antigen receptors contain two immunoglobulin-like domains

3. **In immunity and immunological disease:**
a. **False**. They are protected for only 3 to 6 months
b. **False**. X-linked severe combined immunodeficiency (SCID) is 50% to 60% of the total
c. **True**. B-cell–positive SCID because of JAK3 deficiency can be subclinical
d. **True**. A defect in either T-cell function or development
e. **False**. Chronic granulomatous disease is an X-linked disorder of cell-mediated immunity

4. **In common immunological conditions:**
   a. **False.** It is classed as a secondary or associated immunodeficiency
   b. **True.** Immunodeficiency is usually mild, and the immune system improves with age as the thymus grows; there is a proneness to viral infections in childhood
   c. **False.** The causes of common variable immunodeficiency are poorly understood, and it is often a disorder of adult life
   d. **False.** The risk to first-degree relatives is increased, but the pedigree pattern is more suggestive of multifactorial inheritance
   e. **True.** Failure to thrive may be the only clue to an immunodeficiency disorder

CHAPTER 14: The Genetics of Cancer ... and Cancer Genetics

1. **Relating to genetic mechanisms leading to cancer:**
   a. **True.** The best-known example is chronic myeloid leukemia and the Philadelphia chromosome
   b. **False.** Tumor suppressor genes are more common than oncogenes
   c. **True.** Apoptosis is normal programmed cell death
   d. **False.** Loss of heterozygosity refers to the presence of two defective alleles in a tumor suppressor gene
   e. **False.** Although important, pathogenic *APC* variants are part of a sequence of genetic changes leading to colorectal cancer
2. **In familial cancer syndromes:**
   a. **True.** The paradigm was retinoblastoma, and the hypothesis (proposed by Knudson, 1971) was subsequently proved to be correct
   b. **False.** Mutations in *TP53* are found in many cancers, but are *germline* in Li-Fraumeni syndrome
   c. **False.** It is implicated in multiple endocrine neoplasia (MEN) type 2, but not multiple endocrine neoplasia type 1
   d. **True.** There is a significant risk of small bowel polyps and duodenal cancer
   e. **True.** Women with this condition have a lifetime risk of up to 50%
3. **In familial cancer syndromes:**
   a. **True.** This syndrome is allelic with Cowden disease, in which follicular thyroid cancer can occur
   b. **True.** The lifetime risk may be in the region of 16%
   c. **False.** The *BRCA1* and *BRCA2* genes do not account for all familial breast cancer
   d. **False.** The lifetime risk of breast cancer for female *BRCA1* or *BRCA2* carriers is 60% to 85%
   e. **False.** The figure is approximately 15%
4. **In familial cancer syndromes:**
   a. **False.** Cerebellar hemangioblastoma is a common tumor in von Hippel–Lindau (VHL) disease
   b. **False.** This tumor is seen in multiple endocrine neoplasia (MEN) type 2 and VHL disease
   c. **True.** There is also an increased risk in familial breast cancer
   d. **True.** Melanin spots in Peutz–Jeghers syndrome, basal cell carcinomas in Gorlin syndrome, and skin tumors in the Muir–Torré form of Lynch syndrome
   e. **False.** The figure is approximately one-third
5. **In cancer prevention and screening:**
   a. **True.** Clear cell renal carcinoma is a significant risk in VHL disease
   b. **False.** It is easier to detect breast cancer by mammography in postmenopausal women
   c. **False.** It should begin soon after birth
   d. **False.** Screening is advised in several family history scenarios that do not meet the Amsterdam criteria
   e. **False.** It is strongly indicated in familial adenomatous polyposis (FAP), but not in women positive for *BRCA1* mutations

CHAPTER 15: Pharmacogenomics, Precision Medicine, and the Treatment of Genetic Disease

1. **Thiopurine drugs used to treat leukemia:**
   a. **True.**
   b. **True.** They are used to treat autoimmune disorders and to prevent rejection of organ transplants
   c. **False.** They can be toxic in 10% to 15% of patients
   d. **True.** These include leukopenia and severe liver damage
   e. **True.** Variants in the *TPMT* gene are associated with thiopurine toxicity
2. **Liver enzymes that show genetic variation of expression and hence influence the response to drugs include:**
   a. **True.** Complete deficiency of this enzyme causes type 1 Crigler–Najjar disease
   b. **False.** N-acetyltransferase variation influences the metabolism of isoniazid
   c. **False.** Absence of acetaldehyde dehydrogenase is associated with an acute flushing response to alcohol
   d. **True.** Approximately 5% to 10% of the European population are poor metabolizers of debrisoquine because of a homozygous variant in the *CYP2D6* gene
   e. **True.** *CYP2C9* variants are associated with decreased metabolism of warfarin
3. **Examples of diseases in which treatment may be influenced by pharmacogenomics include:**
   a. **False.** Patients with glucokinase mutations are usually treated with diet alone
   b. **True.** Patients with *HNF-1A* mutations are sensitive to sulfonylureas
   c. **True.** Abacavir is an effective drug, but approximately 5% of patients show potentially fatal hypersensitivity
   d. **True.** Some patients show adverse reactions to the drug felbamate
   e. **True.** Slow inactivators of isoniazid are more likely to suffer side effects
4. **Methods currently used to treat genetic disease include:**
   a. **False.** Germ-cell gene therapy is considered unacceptable because of safety concerns and the risk of transmitting genetic changes to future generations
   b. **True.** For example, bone marrow transplantation is used to treat various inherited immunodeficiencies
   c. **True.** Examples include the replacement of factor VIII or IX in patients with hemophilia
   d. **True.** For example, restricted phenylalanine in patients with phenylketonuria
   e. **False.** This potential treatment has been tested in animal models

5. **Gene therapy may be delivered by:**
   a. **True.** Liposomes are widely used, as they are safe and can facilitate transfer of large genes
   b. **True.** *CFTR* gene therapy trials have used adeno-associated viral vectors
   c. **False.** Antisense oligonucleotides need to be delivered to the target cells
   d. **True.** Lentiviruses may be useful for delivery of genes to non-dividing cells
   e. **True.** An example is the injection of plasmid-borne factor IX into fibroblasts from patients with hemophilia B
6. **Gene therapy has been used successfully to treat patients with the following diseases:**
   a. **False.** Trials have shown safe delivery of the *CFTR* gene to the nasal passages, but truly effective treatment of cystic fibrosis by this means has not yet been demonstrated
   b. **True.** A number of patients have been treated successfully, although concern was raised when two boys developed leukemia
   c. **False.** This will be difficult because the number of α- and β-globin chains must be equal or a thalassemia phenotype might result
   d. **True.** Some patients have been able to reduce their exogenous clotting factors
   e. **True.** Although early attempts were unsuccessful, some patients have now been treated successfully by *ex vivo* gene transfer
7. **Potential gene therapy methods for cancer include:**
   a. **True.** An example is the protein kinase inhibitor used to treat chronic myeloid leukemia
   b. **True.** Perhaps through overexpression of interleukins
   c. **False.** Antiangiogenic factors might be used to reduce blood supply to tumors
   d. **True.** RNA interference is a promising new technique that can be used to target overexpressed genes associated with cancers
   e. **True.** A number of trials are ongoing to determine the utility of this technique

CHAPTER 16: Congenital Abnormalities, Dysmorphic Syndromes, and Learning Disability

1.
   a. **False.** The figure is approximately 25%
   b. **True.** This is the figure from chromosome studies. It might be higher if all lethal single-gene abnormalities could be included
   c. **False.** The figure is 2% to 3%
   d. **False.** This is an example of deformation
   e. **True.** "Sequence" implies a cascade of events traced to a single abnormality
2.
   a. **False.** Syndrome is correct because of the highly recognizable nature of the condition
   b. **False.** It has been found to be caused by mutations in a single gene, *NSD1*
   c. **True.** The figure varies between populations and is lowered by periconceptional folic acid intake
   d. **False.** This well-defined entity is an autosomal recessive condition
   e. **True.** It may be chromosomal, autosomal dominant, or autosomal recessive
3.
   a. **True.** A teratogen represents a chemical or toxic disruption
   b. **True.** Renal agenesis causes oligohydramnios, which leads to talipes through deformation
   c. **False.** A significant increase in various limb defects occurs
   d. **True.** There is a generalized effect on a particular tissue, such as bone or skin
   e. **False.** The figure is much higher, approximately 50%
4. **Relating to maternal influences on fetal development:**
   a. **True.** Deafness and various visual defects are features
   b. **False.** The first trimester is much more dangerous
   c. **True.** Vertebral defects at any level are possible, including sacral agenesis
   d. **False.** This is true for some populations, not all
   e. **True.** Peripheral pulmonary artery stenosis in the case of congenital rubella
5. **In conditions that are often non-mendelian:**
   a. **True.** The incidence is between 1 in 500 and 1 in 1000
   b. **False.** Low recurrence risk because they are thought not to be genetic in many cases
   c. **False.** Large studies of many families are required
   d. **True.** Smith–Lemli–Opitz syndrome is a defect of cholesterol metabolism, affecting the Sonic hedgehog pathway
   e. **False.** The figure is up to 10 cases per 1000

CHAPTER 17: Chromosome Disorders

1. **Relating to aneuploidies:**
   a. **True.** Chromosome number was confirmed in 1956, DNA structure in 1953
   b. **True.** A wide variety of abnormal karyotypes occur in spontaneous abortuses, but 45,X is the single most common one
   c. **False.** It is estimated that 80% of all Down syndrome fetuses are lost spontaneously
   d. **True.** Although the risk of Down syndrome increases with maternal age, the high proportion of younger mothers means that most Down syndrome babies are born to this group
   e. **False.** A small proportion has an intelligence quotient at the lower end of the normal range
2. **Relating to common chromosomal disorders:**
   a. **False.** Such children usually die within days or weeks of birth
   b. **False.** Males with Klinefelter syndrome (47,XXY) are usually infertile
   c. **True.** This accounts for a substantial proportion of cases
   d. **False.** This is not seen in either uniparental disomy or imprinting centre defect cases
   e. **True.** The deletion on 22q11.2 is an approximately 3-megabase region flanked by very similar DNA sequences
3. **In microdeletion conditions:**
   a. **True.** Probably because of haploinsufficiency for elastin
   b. **False.** Congenital heart disease is not a recognized feature of Prader–Willi syndrome
   c. **False.** Chromosome 11p13, and may be a feature of Wilms tumor, anirida, genitourinary anomalies, and intellectual disability (WAGR) syndrome and Beckwith–Wiedemann syndrome
   d. **True.** A mutation in *PAX6* or a deletion encompassing this locus at 11p15

e. **True**. Behavioral phenotypes can be very informative (e.g., Smith–Magenis syndrome)

4.
a. **False**. The figure is approximately 1 in 1000
b. **False**. Intelligence quotient is reduced by 10 to 20 points, but intellectual disability is not a feature
c. **True**. The other cell line may be normal but could also contain Y-chromosome material
d. **False**. They have normal fertility
e. **True**. This occurs because of DNA instability

5.
a. **True**. The mutation passes from a normal transmitting male to his daughters essentially unchanged
b. **False**. In addition to FRAXA, there is also FRAXE and FRAXF, although they are rare
c. **True**. Androgen insensitivity syndrome can present in this way
d. **False**. This is unreliable; DNA analysis is necessary
e. **False**. The figure is around 10% to 15%

CHAPTER 18: Inborn Errors of Metabolism

1. **In congenital adrenal hyperplasia (CAH):**
a. **True**. The most common enzyme defect is 21-hydroxylase deficiency
b. **True**. This occurs in the rare forms: 3β-dehydrogenase, 5α-reductase, and desmolase deficiencies
c. **True**. Hyponatremia and hyperkalemia may be severe and lead to circulatory collapse
d. **False**. Cortisol and fludrocortisone are required lifelong in salt-losing CAH
e. **False**. Fertility is reduced in the salt-losing form

2. **Phenylketonuria:**
a. **False**. There is a benign form, as well as abnormalities of cofactor synthesis
b. **False**. Dietary restriction of phenylalanine is necessary only during childhood and pregnancy
c. **True**. These are features if untreated
d. **True**. Affected individuals have reduced pigment and are fair
e. **False**. A different pathway

3. **Hepatomegaly is an important feature of:**
a. **True**. Hepatomegaly is a feature of most of the mucopolysaccharidoses
b. **True**. Hepatomegaly is a feature of most of the glycogen storage disorders, although not all
c. **False**. This is not a feature, even in the so-called hepatic porphyrias
d. **True**. This is one of the sphingolipidoses—lipid storage diseases
e. **False**. Cirrhosis can occur in the untreated

4. **Concerning mitochondrial disorders:**
a. **False**. The main patterns of inheritance also apply where mitochondrial proteins are encoded by nuclear genes
b. **True**. Especially in neuropathy, ataxia, and retinitis pigmentosa and maternally inherited diabetes and deafness (MIDD), respectively
c. **True**. There are 37 gene products
d. **False**. Leigh disease is genetically heterogeneous
e. **True**. The *G4.5* gene is mutated and urinary 3-methyglutaconic acid is raised, but the link remains to be elucidated

5. **Regarding metabolic conditions:**
a. **True**. The carnitine cycle is important for long-chain fatty acid transport into mitochondria
b. **True**. Some 90% of alleles are caused by the same mutation, and neonatal population screening has been suggested
c. **False**. These are inborn errors of copper transport metabolism
d. **True**. These features should prompt investigation for organic acidurias and mitochondrial disorders, among others
e. **False**. Important radiological features may be seen in peroxisomal and storage disorders

CHAPTER 19: Mainstream Monogenic Disorders

1. **Huntington disease (HD):**
a. **False**. Meiotic instability is greater in spermatogenesis than in oogenesis
b. **True**. This has been shown from studies in Venezuela
c. **False**. The duration is approximately 15 to 20 years
d. **True**. This is so for the reduced penetrance alleles containing 36 to 39 repeats
e. **False**. Some degree of cognitive impairment may be part of the early symptomatic phase of HD, but dementia is a later development

2. **Myotonic dystrophy:**
a. **False**. Somnolence is common
b. **False**. Neonatal hypotonia
c. **True**. Through a CUG RNA-binding protein, which interferes with a variety of genes
d. **True**. An important feature of myotonic dystrophy and the defining abnormality of many channelopathies
e. **False**. Myotonic dystrophy type 2 is due to the 4–base pair repeating element $(CCTG)_n$

3.
a. **False**. The Phe508del mutation is the most common
b. **True**. The polythymidine tract—5 T, 7 T, and 9 T—can be correlated with different cystic fibrosis phenotypes
c. **False**. This is true for most of the inherited cardiac arrhythmias; cardiomyopathies are often from defects in sarcomeric muscle proteins
d. **True**. This glycoprotein complex in the muscle membrane contains a variety of units; defects in these cause various limb-girdle dystrophies, for example
e. **False**. These patients have normal intelligence

4.
a. **False**. They are good candidates according to current thinking
b. **False**. It is only a component of the skeletal system criteria
c. **False**. It is thought to be a fully penetrant disorder
d. **True**. This is not usually severe, but is a recognized feature
e. **False**. The opposite is the case

5. **In neuromuscular conditions:**
a. **False**. This is a neurophysiological classification
b. **True**. Autosomal dominant, autosomal recessive, and X-linked
c. **True**. Mutations in the peripheral myelin protein affect Schwann cells
d. **False**. They are not good discriminatory tests, and DNA analysis should be performed
e. **False**. It is an inherited cardiac arrhythmia

CHAPTER 20: Prenatal Testing and Reproductive Genetics

1. **In prenatal testing:**
   a. **False.** It is still mainly performed around 16 weeks' gestation
   b. **False.** They also derive from the amnion and fetal urinary tract epithelium
   c. **False.** There is a small risk of causing limb abnormalities; chorionic villus sampling should not be performed before 11 weeks' gestation
   d. **False.** There is a small but significant risk of a different karyotype caused by confined placental mosaicism
   e. **False.** Fetal anomaly scanning is normally performed around 20 weeks' gestation because earlier scanning is not sufficiently sensitive
2. **Regarding prenatal markers:**
   a. **True.** This forms part of the combined (triple) test
   b. **True.** This forms part of the combined (triple) test
   c. **False.** In trisomy 18 all maternal serum markers are low
   d. **False.** The best figure achieved is approximately 86%
   e. **True.** There are two fetuses rather than one
3.
   a. **False.** The accuracy is greater than 99%
   b. **True.** Especially aneuploidies
   c. **True.** Probably because of the presence of inspissated meconium
   d. **True.** Most cases of Down syndrome are caused by meiotic nondisjunction
   e. **True.** They are unlikely to have different clinical effects in different members of the same family
4. **In assisted reproduction:**
   a. **False.** A license from the Human Fertilisation and Embryology Authority (HFEA) is required
   b. **False.** It is not illegal but does require an HFEA license in the UK
   c. **True.** This is undertaken to avoid the presence of extraneous sperm
   d. **False.** The figure is lower, at ~25% to 30%
   e. **True.** An increasing number of single-gene disorders can be diagnosed prenatally by non-invasive prenatal diagnosis
5.
   a. **True.** Subtle chromosome abnormalities are present in 10% to 12% of men with azoospermia or severe oligospermia, some of them heritable
   b. **False.** The rule is that no more than 10 pregnancies may result from one donor
   c. **False.** They are entitled to know the identity of their donor parent, but only when they reach the age of 18
   d. **False.** Non-invasive prenatal testing will have increasing applications but will not totally replace other methods, e.g., ultrasonography
   e. **False.** The figure is approximately 1 in 7

CHAPTER 21: Genetic Counseling

1.
   a. **False.** This is the consultand, the proband is the affected individual
   b. **False.** Retinitis pigmentosa can follow all the main patterns of inheritance
   c. **False.** It is far more—transfer of relevant information, presentation of options, and facilitation of decision-making in the face of difficult choices
   d. **False.** Non-directive counseling is the aim because patients/clients should be making their own decisions
   e. **True.** Patients do not remember risk information accurately, and there are other important measures of patient satisfaction
2.
   a. **False.** The risk is approximately twice the background risk
   b. **True.** This is a second-degree relationship
   c. **False.** The risk is roughly 25%
   d. **False.** It is perfectly normal in many societies
   e. **False.** It refers to anything from, for example, uncle–niece partnerships (second degree) to third cousins (seventh degree)
3.
   a. **False.** Guilty feelings from parents and grandparents are common when a genetic disease is first diagnosed in a child
   b. **False.** Many patients make the choice they would have made before genetic counseling—but after the counseling they should be much better informed
   c. **True.** The risk from each grandparent is 1 in 64, so the combined risk is $1/64 + 1/64 = 1/32$
   d. **False.** Such a practice is strongly discouraged, and the indications for genetic testing should be the same, although pressure is sometimes applied from agencies or even courts
   e. **False.** Good patient support groups have a huge role, and the patients/families themselves become the experts for their condition

Case-Based Answers and Discussion

CHAPTER 6: Patterns of Inheritance

Case 1

1. It is possible that the problems described in family members are unrelated, but this is unlikely. If the condition has passed from the maternal grandfather, it is either autosomal dominant with variability or X-linked. It is necessary to consider both possibilities, because this will affect genetic counseling and may determine which genetic tests are undertaken.
2. The spinocerebellar ataxias are a genetically heterogeneous group of conditions that usually follow autosomal dominant inheritance and could present in this way. A form of hereditary spastic paraparesis is possible, which is also genetically heterogeneous but usually follows autosomal dominant inheritance, although recessive and X-linked forms are described. Apart from these, X-linked adrenoleukodystrophy must be considered, especially because the man has signs of cognitive difficulties and behavioral problems. This is very important, not only because it can present early in life, but also because of the potential for adrenal insufficiency.

Case 2

1. Apart from detailed family history information, it is routine in cases of congenital sensorineural hearing loss (SNHL) to explore the possibility of congenital infection (which may be impossible in adults after this passage of time), undertake eye (Usher syndrome) and cardiac (Jervell and Lange–Nielsen syndrome) investigations, perform a magnetic resonance imaging scan of the inner ear (Pendred syndrome), and conduct parental audiograms.
2. It is likely that she has autosomal recessive sensorineural hearing loss (SNHL), given that she has an affected brother; he may also have autosomal recessive SNHL, in which case their children may have a 100% chance of inheriting SNHL, or a very low chance because their deafness is the result of pathogenic variants in different genes. However, it is also possible that he has X-linked recessive deafness with the associated risks to grandsons through any daughter(s) (obligate carrier(s)).

Case 3

1. The information may be correct, but given the clinical diagnosis of osteogenesis imperfecta, it is probably not, and other possibilities must be considered and explained to them.
2. Most forms of osteogenesis imperfecta (brittle bone disease) follow autosomal dominant inheritance, although there are rare forms that follow autosomal recessive inheritance. Sibling recurrence, when neither parent has signs or symptoms, can be explained by somatic and/or germline mosaicism in one of the parents, or possibly non-penetrance. The risk to the offspring of those affected would then be 50% (i.e., high). It is also important in such cases to consider the possibility of a non-genetic diagnosis, namely non-accidental injury. Confirmation of the diagnosis is therefore important.

CHAPTER 7: Population and Mathematical Genetics

Case 1

1. Clearly, it is essential to know whether the condition in question has ever knowingly occurred in the wider families of either of the two consultands. If this had occurred, it would potentially modify the carrier risk for one of the consultands regardless of the frequency of the disease in their population.
2. Assuming the disorder in question has not occurred previously in the family, the carrier frequency in population A is 1 in 50, and in population B 1 in 15. The risk in the first pregnancy is therefore $1/50 \times 1/15 \times 1/4 = 1/3000$.

Case 2

1. From the figures given, four cases in the town appear to be new mutations, that is, four new mutations per 100,000 genes inherited. The mutation rate is therefore 1 per 25,000 gametes.
2. New mutation rates should be based on birth incidence rather than population *prevalence*. The population sample is relatively small, and there may be ascertainment bias. For example, if there is bias toward an older, retired population, the proportion that is reproductively active may be small and the figures distorted by the migration of younger people away from the town. In addition, the four "new mutation" cases should be verified by proper examination of the parents.

CHAPTER 8: Risk Calculation

Case 1

1. Each of the siblings of the affected aunt has a chance of being a carrier (2/3); therefore, each of the cousins has a chance of being a carrier. The chance of the couple's first baby being affected is $1/3 \times 1/3 \times 1/4 = 1/36$.
2. Even though genetic studies cannot be performed directly on the deceased individual, DNA analysis can be offered to other family members in an attempt to identify the pathogenic variants for Hurler syndrome. If there is any doubt about the original diagnosis, it might also be worth looking for the

TABLE 1

Probability	Is a Carrier	Is Not a Carrier
Prior	1/2	1/2
Conditional (2 normal sons)	1/2 × 1/2	1
Joint	1/8	1/2
Posterior	1/8/(1/8 + 1/2) = 1/5	

mutations of Hunter syndrome, which closely resembles Hurler syndrome and is X-linked. If there are uncertainties about the results, biochemical prenatal testing for Hurler syndrome can be offered for their pregnancies (unnecessary for Hunter syndrome because this family structure means the fetus is not at risk of this X-linked condition).

Case 2

1. A simple Bayes calculation can be performed, taking into account that she has had two normal sons (Table 1). She therefore has a 1/5, or 20%, chance of being a carrier.
2. There is a good chance of identifying the factor VIII gene variant in either her brother or uncle, assuming at least one of them is available. If so, it should then be possible to determine her carrier status definitively. If not, mutation analysis can be offered to her, as well as tests of factor VIII levels and factor VIII–related antigen, although the latter tests are not always discriminatory. DNA linkage analysis could also be attempted if appropriate DNA samples are available, including those of her unaffected sons.

CHAPTER 9: Developmental Genetics

Case 1

1. The combination of macrocephaly, odontogenic keratocysts, and basal cell carcinomas occurs in Gorlin (basal cell nevoid carcinoma) syndrome. It is understandable that hydrocephalus would be the main concern, but true hydrocephalus is unusual in Gorlin syndrome. This condition should be in the differential diagnosis of a child with macrocephaly, with appropriate exploration of the family history. Other macrocephaly conditions to consider are Sotos and Cowden syndromes, but neither of these includes odontogenic keratocysts.
2. The child's father is an obligate carrier for the *PTCH* gene mutation causing Gorlin syndrome in the family. He should be screened regularly (at least annually) by radiography for odontogenic keratocysts and be under regular surveillance by a dermatologist for basal cell carcinomas. Assuming a pathogenic *PTCH* gene variant is identified, predictive testing should be offered to at-risk family members who wish to clarify their status.

Case 2

1. This combination of anomalies strongly suggests one of the ciliopathy conditions in the short-rib polydactyly group. They arise because of defective cilia, which are ubiquitous on cell surfaces and crucial for normal development. They almost all follow autosomal recessive inheritance.
2. The findings on ultrasound do not necessarily distinguish one of the more severe short-rib polydactyly syndromes from Jeune asphyxiating thoracic dystrophy or Ellis–van Crefeld syndrome. Detailed ultrasound examination of the fetal heart is indicated, as well as serial measurements of the chest size, because of the postnatal risk of respiratory insufficiency. Urogenital structures should be carefully evaluated.

Case 3

1. The two most likely causes of sex reversal in a young "girl" are androgen insensitivity syndrome, which is X-linked and results from pathogenic variants in the androgen receptor (*AR*) gene, and variants in the *SRY* gene on the Y chromosome.
2. Sequencing of both the *AR* and *SRY* genes can be performed to determine the genetic basis of the sex reversal. It is very important to investigate and locate, if present, remnants of gonadal tissue, because this should be removed to avoid the risk of malignant change. The parents should be given a full explanation, but the phenotypic sex of the child should be affirmed as female.

CHAPTER 10: Common Disease, Polygenic, and Multifactorial Genetics

Case 1

1. Testing for factor V Leiden and the prothrombin G20210A variant is appropriate. A positive result would provide a more accurate risk of her developing thromboembolism and would inform her choice of contraception. Heterozygosity for factor V Leiden or the prothrombin G20210A variant would increase her risk by four- to five-fold. Homozygosity or compound heterozygosity would increase her risk by up to 80-fold.
2. Negative results for factor V Leiden and the prothrombin G20210A variant in the consultand should be interpreted with caution because up to 50% of cases of venous thrombosis are not associated with these genetic risk factors.

Case 2

1. The proband might have type 1 diabetes mellitus (T1DM), type 2 diabetes mellitus (T2DM), or maturity-onset diabetes of the young (MODY). Because both have normal hearing, a diagnosis of maternally inherited diabetes and deafness (mitochondrial, MIDD) is unlikely. T1DM and T2DM show multifactorial inheritance, with environmental factors playing a role in addition to predisposing genetic susceptibility factors. MODY shows autosomal dominant inheritance.
2. The brother's risk of developing T1DM, T2DM, or MODY, is 6%, 35%, or 50%, respectively. If his sister is found to have a pathogenic variant in one of the genes causing MODY, he could then opt for predictive genetic testing. A negative test would reduce his risk relative to that of the population. A positive test would allow regular monitoring to make an early diagnosis of diabetes and reduce the risks of diabetic complications from long-standing undiagnosed/uncontrolled diabetes.

Case 3

1. Generally, the risk of epilepsy to first-degree relatives is around 4%. However, mother and daughter are affected here, which suggests the possibility of a mendelian form of epilepsy. Furthermore, it seems that both have an abnormal finding on brain imaging, and the mother's computed tomograms should be located and reviewed by an expert neuroradiologist, if possible. At this stage, an explanation of both autosomal dominant and X-linked inheritance is appropriate, as well as the possibility that the two cases of epilepsy are coincidental.
2. The condition that the mother's doctors mentioned would almost certainly have been tuberous sclerosis (TS), which follows autosomal dominant inheritance. Further evaluation of both mother and daughter, looking for clinical features of TS, is indicated and, if present, genetic testing has a high chance of finding a pathogenic variant. However, the nodules on the lateral ventricle walls may be pathognomonic of bilateral periventricular nodular heterotopia (BPVNH), and the images should be reviewed by someone who can recognise this. BPVNH is an abnormality of neuronal migration and is inherited as an X-linked dominant condition, caused by variants in the filamin-A (*FLNA*) gene, for which testing can be offered. In general, mendelian forms of epilepsy are rare apart from the genetically heterogeneous early infantile epileptic encephalopathies. Genetic testing for epilepsy often involves sequencing of a large panel of susceptibility genes.

Case 4

1. Not necessarily. Many people with glucokinase gene variants are asymptomatic, and their mild hyperglycemia is detected only upon screening (routine medicals, during pregnancy or intercurrent illness). Gestational diabetes in the father's sister raises the definite possibility that the DNA variant could have been inherited from his side of the family.
2. Identification of a glucokinase gene variant is 'good news' because the mild hyperglycemia is likely to be stable throughout life, can be treated by diet alone (except during pregnancy), and is unlikely to result in diabetic complications. Cascade testing can be offered to other relatives. If the variant has been inherited from the father, his father's sister and her child may be tested. The sister might avoid the anxiety of having a young child diagnosed with unexplained hyperglycemia.

CHAPTER 11: Screening for Genetic Disease

Case 1

1. Variant analysis of the fibrillin-1 (*FBN1*) gene, for Marfan syndrome, is possible for the consultand but not guaranteed to identify a pathogenic variant even if the clinical diagnosis is confident—variants of uncertain significance are commonly reported. In reality, if the family history is negative and the patient does not meet the clinical criteria for a diagnosis, most geneticists would not perform this test. If DNA from the deceased father is available, it may be possible to analyze this for a range of known "aortopathy" genes, but the positive yield is low. Genetic testing in this scenario is unlikely to be helpful.
2. The important life-threatening complication of Marfan syndrome is progressive aortic root dilatation carrying a risk of dissection. Those with a firm diagnosis must be followed until at least the age of 30 years. If there is doubt about the diagnosis, regular cardiac screening is a sensible precaution for all those at risk until at least their mid-20s.

Case 2

1. The sensitivity is the proportion of true positives detected by the test, that is, 45/50 (i.e., 45 + 5) = 90%. The specificity is the proportion of true negatives detected by the test, that is, 99,190 (the unaffected cases who test negative)/(99,190 + 760) (760 = the unaffected cases who test positive) = 99.2%.
2. The positive predictive value is the proportion of cases with a positive test who truly have the disease, that is, 45/805 = 5.6%.

CHAPTER 12: Hemoglobin and the Hemoglobinopathies

Case 1

1. The ethnic origin of the couple and the limited information should suggest the possibility of a hematological disorder. α-Thalassemia is the likely cause of stillbirth, hydrops being secondary to heart failure, which in turn is secondary to anemia. Rhesus isoimmunization and glucose-6-phosphate dehydrogenase deficiency are other possibilities. Severe forms of congenital heart disease (CHD) are frequently associated with hydrops, but the chance of a sibling recurrence of CHD is low (unless there was a recurrence of multiple abnormalities as a result of an unbalanced reciprocal translocation for which one of the parents is a balanced carrier). There are many other causes of recurrent hydrops, and these would need to be considered, including rare, lethal skeletal dysplasias and a wide range of metabolic diseases.
2. A full blood count, blood groups, hemoglobin electrophoresis, and maternal autoantibody and glucose-6-phosphate dehydrogenase deficiency screens should be performed for the couple. DNA analysis may detect the common mutation seen in Southeast Asia, which would then make it possible to offer genetic prenatal diagnosis by chorionic villus sampling. If no disorder is identified by these investigations, it is unlikely that further diagnostic progress will be made unless the couple has another affected pregnancy that can be fully investigated by examination of the fetus, including genetic testing.

Case 2

1. This presentation is consistent with acute intermittent porphyria and hemolytic uremic syndrome. However, the ethnic origin should also suggest the possibility of sickle-cell disease. The contents of the dark urine, as well as specific tests for porphyria, will help to differentiate these, and a sickle-cell test should be performed.
2. If the diagnosis is sickle-cell disease, there are various agents that can be tried to reduce the frequency of sickling crises—hydroxyurea in particular. Prophylactic penicillin is important for reducing the risk of serious pneumococcal infections, and the family should be offered genetic counseling and cascade screening of relatives.

CHAPTER 13: Immunogenetics

Case 1

1. The nature of his grandfather's symptoms are rather nonspecific—back pain and arthritis are both very common in the general population. However, it is certainly possible that he also had ankylosing spondylitis, a form of enthesitis (inflammation at the site of insertion of a ligament or tendon into bone) with involvement of synovial joints, as the heritability is greater than 90%.
2. Approximately 95% of patients with ankylosing spondylitis are positive for the HLA-B27 antigen; however, in the general population this test has only a low positive predictive value. His children have a 50% chance of being HLA-B27 positive; if positive, the risk of developing clinical ankylosing spondylitis is approximately 9%; if negative, the risk is less than 1%.

Case 2

1. This history, with tetralogy of Fallot, nasal speech (attributed to a short palate), and neonatal hypocalcemia, points strongly toward a diagnosis of deletion 22q11 (DiGeorge/Sedláčková) syndrome, which can easily be confirmed by microarray-comparative genomic hybridization analysis. Immunity is impaired, but gradual improvement usually occurs through childhood and adolescence.
2. Deletion 22q11 syndrome can be familial and does not always give rise to congenital heart disease. If confirmed in the child, both parents should be tested for the deletion, and other family members as appropriate. Genetic counseling for the child will be important when she is older.

CHAPTER 14: The Genetics of Cancer . . . and Cancer Genetics

Case 1

1. The family history should first of all be confirmed with the consent of the affected individuals. If the thyroid cancer in the cousin was papillary in type, and the polyps in her father hamartomatos, the pattern would be very suspicious for Cowden disease. This is also known as PTEN hamartoma tumor syndrome, which is autosomal dominant and usually because of a variant in the *PTEN* gene; the risk of breast cancer is high—approximately 50% in females.
2. Macrocephaly (head circumference usually above the upper limit of the normal range), a cobblestone appearance of the oral mucosa, and generalized lipomas are other features to look for in patients with this unusual history.

Case 2

1. If the *BRCA2* variant has not been confirmed in another family member or by testing another sample from the deceased cousin (e.g., a tissue section embedded in paraffin), the possibility of a sample mix-up in the research laboratory cannot be excluded. If, however, the uncle tests positive for the pathogenic variant, the consultand's mother is a phenocopy. If the consultand's mother and uncle both test negative the variant was probably inherited from the cousin's mother, but a *de novo* mutation event is also a possibility.
2. If the uncle tests positive for the *BRCA2* variant, then his lifetime risk of developing breast cancer is approximately 6%, more than 100-fold higher than that in the general male population.

Case 3

1. The alleged malignancies in relatives should be confirmed in cancer registries if possible. The pattern is consistent with Lynch syndrome, but the affected individuals are not connected by first-degree relationships. Renal cancer affecting the pelvis is a transitional cell carcinoma. The logical first investigations are immunohistochemistry studies on tumor tissue and microsatellite instability in DNA from the proband and/or his cousin with endometrial cancer. Positive findings can be followed up by variant analysis of the Lynch syndrome mismatch repair genes.
2. Screening to the proband's three children depends on the results of the Lynch syndrome tests in the proband. If a pathogenic variant is found, they can be offered predictive genetic testing. If not, they would probably be offered a one-off colonoscopy at approximately 55 years of age. There is no reliable screening for endometrial cancer.

CHAPTER 16: Congenital Abnormalities, Dysmorphic Syndromes, and Learning Disability

Case 1

1. This is not an unusual scenario. The karyotype on amniocentesis was normal, and polyhydramnios suggests the possibility of a gastrointestinal obstruction such as esophageal atresia. The abnormalities are more likely to represent an "association," for example VACTERL, rather than a syndrome or mendelian condition. The empiric recurrence risk is low, and without fetal samples or detailed information that an autopsy may have provided, all that can be offered is ultrasonography in subsequent pregnancies.
2. A fetal autopsy is highly desirable in this situation to know the full extent of internal organ anomalies. Microarray-comparative genomic hybridization analysis on fetal skin may have shown something that was not detected on amniocentesis, and DNA should be stored for possible future use—in cases such as this, whole-exome sequencing is increasingly performed. Maternal diabetes should be excluded. Parental karyotypes can be analyzed for the possibility of a balanced reciprocal translocation, including telomere screens to look for the possibility of a cryptic translocation.

Case 2

1. Isolated, non-syndromic cleft palate is statistically the most likely diagnosis, but the mild short stature might be significant. Syndromic possibilities include spondyloepiphyseal dysplasia—although there are many rare syndromes with more severe short stature and other features. Mild short stature is a feature of hypochondroplasia, Russell–Silver syndrome, and *SHOX*-associated short stature, for all of which gene tests are available; however, clefting is not usually associated with these disorders.
2. The short stature appears mild; it is therefore important to try to determine whether this might be familial—the parents need to be assessed. Follow-up of the baby is indicated, including a

radiological skeletal survey to see whether there is an identifiable skeletal dysplasia. Spondyloepiphyseal dysplasia may be accompanied by myopia and sensorineural hearing impairment; therefore hearing and vision assessments are important. However, the child has a cleft palate and is at risk of conductive hearing problems as a result. The cleft palate team needs to be involved from the beginning.

Case 3

1. Assuming the 10-year-old girl is an isolated case in the family, it is most likely that she has a new pathogenic variant in an intellectual disability gene, and therefore a low recurrence risk. However, there is a small risk that the condition may be because of autosomal recessive inheritance, with a 1 in 4 (25%) recurrence risk. X-linked inheritance is very unlikely given her gender, although a new variant for an X-linked dominant condition is certainly possible.
2. Cases like this are commonly encountered in clinical practice and remain without a diagnosis on a long-term basis. Unless there are clear features of a recognizable syndrome, which would then lead to specific genetic testing, DNA from the child can be analyzed on intellectual disability gene panels, or possibly investigated by a trio exome/genome analysis.

CHAPTER 17: Chromosome Disorders

Case 1

1. Head-banging is not rare in early childhood, especially in children with developmental delay, and it is not necessarily a helpful feature in making a diagnosis. However, combined with the persistently disturbed sleep pattern and unusual hugging behavior, the diagnosis of Smith–Magenis syndrome should be considered. These children can be quiet as babies and have congenital heart disease; later they may develop scoliosis. Melatonin has proved a very effective treatment for sleep disturbance.
2. Smith–Magenis syndrome is usually caused by a microdeletion at 17p11.2, which would be detected by microarray-comparative genomic hybridization analysis. In cases where this test is negative and the clinical diagnosis is still considered likely, mutation analysis in the critical gene, *RAI1*, should be requested.

Case 2

1. The occurrence of two distinct syndromic conditions in the same family raises the possibility of the segregation of a subtle reciprocal chromosome translocation. If the translocation involves only the tips of two chromosomes, there may be two types of unbalanced outcome that are not lost as miscarriages but each giving rise to a distinct phenotype with intellectual disability. Several members of the family, including the mother, are balanced carriers of the reciprocal translocation.
2. The children should have microarray-comparative genomic hybridization tests and the subtle imbalances (monosomy for one chromosome tip and trisomy for the other) should yield the diagnosis. There may be a number of other family members who should be tested for carrier status of the translocation, especially if they plan to have children.

Case 3

1. The 15q11.2 microdeletion is recognized to be associated with neurodevelopmental problems including mild intellectual disability and behavior disorder. It may therefore be the explanation for the child's problems and possibly those in the household as well. Objectively, however, the finding does not necessarily prove a causal link, as some individuals with these microdeletions are entirely normal in terms of intellectual ability and social skills.
2. Testing other family members for the same microdeletion can be offered. By doing this the clinical geneticist investigates whether the microdeletion segregates with intellectual difficulties and behavior disorder in the family. Often, the situation is not as clear-cut as one would wish in order to draw conclusions; however, if on balance a causal link seems likely, then the child will often be more fully supported through the education system.

CHAPTER 18: Inborn Errors of Metabolism

Case 1

1. Hypoglycemia can be part of severe illness in young children, but in this case the intercurrent problem appears relatively minor, suggesting that the child's metabolic capacity to cope with stress is compromised. This history should prompt investigations for a possible inborn error of metabolism, and if a diagnosis is made, the younger sibling should be tested.
2. Hypoglycemia is a common consequence of a number of inborn errors of amino acid and organic acid metabolism. Investigation should begin with analysis of urinary organic acids, plasma amino acids, ammonia, and liver function tests. If a biochemical diagnosis is reached, mutation analysis of the relevant gene(s) should be undertaken.

Case 2

1. The combination of clinical features—dilated cardiomyopathy and generalised muscle weakness, together with two more distant males in the family with a similar history connected through the female line—could be one of several mitochondrial conditions following mitochondrial inheritance. However, as all affected individuals are male, suspicion should be high for Barth syndrome, following X-linked inheritance.
2. Biochemical testing would be likely to show a 5- to 20-fold increase in urinary 3-methylglutaconic acid; in addition, neutropenia is common and a cause of mouth ulcers, pneumonia, and sepsis. Mutation analysis of the *G4.5* (*TAZ*) gene can also be requested, either as the first line or follow-up investigation. If positive, testing can be extended to other family members, starting with the mother.

Case 3

1. If there is a family history of similar symptoms, it might demonstrate matrilinear inheritance (with all the offspring of affected males being normal). If this person is the only affected individual, a family history by itself will not be informative with respect to the diagnosis.
2. All causes of myopathy need to be considered, but the combination of features is suggestive of a mitochondrial

cytopathy. This would explain the muscular symptoms, ptosis, and hearing impairment—and there might also be evidence of cardiomyopathy, neurological disturbance, retinitis pigmentosa, and diabetes mellitus. Mitochondrial DNA analysis on peripheral lymphocytes might identify a pathogenic variant, although a negative result would not rule out the diagnosis. A muscle biopsy might show ragged red fibers, and DNA analysis on this tissue might be more informative than on lymphocytes. Weakness and ptosis would also be consistent with myotonic dystrophy, although hearing impairment would not be expected. The family history for myotonic dystrophy may show a pattern of autosomal dominant transmission with anticipation.

CHAPTER 19: Mainstream Monogenic Disorders

Case 1

1. The history in the brother is consistent with his having Becker muscular dystrophy (BMD), but is also consistent with other diagnostic possibilities, for example limb-girdle muscular dystrophy (LGMD). These two conditions have sometimes been difficult to distinguish, and the inheritance is different (X-linked for BMD and nearly always autosomal recessive for LGMD), with quite different genetic risk implications for the woman who wishes to start a family.
2. The medical records of the affected brother should be reviewed, and he should be reassessed if possible. Thirty years ago the tests for BMD were very basic (no direct gene tests), but now dystrophin gene sequencing is available, which should be the initial investigation, along with creatine kinase estimation. In the event that dystrophin sequencing is difficult to interpret, a muscle biopsy subjected to specific dystrophin staining may be diagnostic, but if this is negative, staining techniques for different forms of LGMD are available. If the diagnosis is one of the LGMD group, the woman can be reassured because these follow autosomal recessive inheritance and she has a two-thirds chance of being a carrier. If BMD, carrier testing for the consultand would be straightforward if a specific pathogenic variant has been found in her brother.

Case 2

1. The sudden, unexpected death of anyone, especially young adults when no cause can be identified, is extremely shocking for a family. The focus of attention becomes the inherited arrhythmias and cardiomyopathies—sometimes the latter show no obvious features at postmortem examination. All close family members are eligible for cardiac evaluation by echocardiography, electrocardiography, and provocation tests, looking for evidence of the long QT and Brugada syndromes. Genetic testing is available but is not guaranteed to identify a pathogenic variant. Some forms of inherited arrhythmia/cardiomyopathy are amenable to prophylactic treatment.
2. Management will depend on the outcome of investigations and genetic testing—usually gene-panel analysis of genes known to be linked to inherited arrhythmias and cardiomyopathies. However, if no positive findings are made, it is very difficult to know how to advise families like this. Very high-intensity sports and swimming should probably be avoided because such activities may be precipitating factors for a life-threatening arrhythmia.

Case 3

1. Clinical examination should rigorously apply the Ghent, or revised Ghent, criteria in looking for features of Marfan syndrome. The family history should be taken into account, but the grandfather may have suffered an aortic aneurysm as a consequence of high blood pressure and smoking rather than a genetic predisposition, and it is important to try to establish if the aortic aneurysm was thoracic or abdominal. With a high index of suspicion for Marfan syndrome it would be possible to undertake genetic testing of the fibrillin-1 (*FBN1*) gene, but this should not be done if the clinical criteria are not met, because there is a strong possibility that a variant of uncertain significance will be found.
2. Other conditions to be considered include a connective tissue disorder within the Ehlers–Danlos syndrome family, and Loeys–Dietz syndrome.

CHAPTER 20: Prenatal Testing and Reproductive Genetics

Case 1

1. The finding of mosaicism for trisomy 20 in chorionic villus tissue might have been a case of confined placental mosaicism (CPM). CPM is not a rare event for a wide variety of chromosome aberrations, but, when *confined*, there are no serious consequences for the pregnancy. The difficulty with amniocentesis is interpretation of the result. If no abnormal cells are found, this does not completely rule out chromosome mosaicism in the fetus. If abnormal cells are found, the clinical implications are very difficult, if not impossible, to predict.
2. This case illustrates the rollercoaster of emotions that some women and couples experience as a result of different forms of prenatal tests and their interpretation. In fact, trisomy 20 mosaicism is unlikely to be of great clinical significance—but it is very difficult to be sure. Renal abnormalities have been reported, and detailed fetal anomaly scanning can be offered for the remainder of the pregnancy. However, what might have been an enjoyable pregnancy will probably continue to be an anxious one.

Case 2

1. In the majority of autism cases, no specific diagnosis is reached. Microarray-comparative genomic hybridization, fragile-X syndrome testing, metabolic screen, and examination for neurocutaneous disorders should all be performed. Because there are two affected sons, trio exome/genome analysis may also be considered.
2. If no genetic diagnosis is made, this is a very difficult situation. There is no proof in this family that autism is either truly X-linked or showing a gender bias toward males—the statistics apply to large cohort studies. Therefore, there is no guarantee that any daughter will be unaffected. It would therefore not be possible to support this request in the United Kingdom, where preimplantation genetic diagnosis is regulated by the Human

Fertilisation and Embryology Authority, and sex selection for anything other than clearly X-linked conditions is not licensed. In other countries, where these techniques are not regulated, the couple might find clinicians who would acquiesce to their request.

Case 3

1. The test she has been offered is likely to be the non-invasive prenatal test for two investigations on cell-free fetal DNA: sexing of the fetus and Down syndrome analysis. She is an obligate carrier of hemophilia A if her father was affected, so she wishes to know if her fetus is male. If so, chorionic villus sampling could be performed to know whether she is carrying an *affected* boy.
2. Sexing of the fetus is highly accurate. Non-invasive prenatal testing for Down syndrome is also highly accurate in all studies undertaken, at greater than 99%. This form of testing presents a clear advantage regarding safety to the pregnancy, as well as potentially avoiding an expensive invasive procedure.

CHAPTER 21: Genetic Counseling

Case 1

1. The couple is at risk of having further affected children, and prenatal diagnosis can be offered. The father may have inherited the balanced translocation from one of his parents, and his sister may also be a carrier. Carrier testing should be offered to his family, especially as his sister is trying to get pregnant.
2. The father's wider family needs to be made aware of the child's diagnosis, but they have fixed misconceptions, and it might be very difficult for them to accept that the child's problems have their origin on their side of the family. There is a severe communication problem, but a way needs to be found to inform the father's wider family of the genetic risk. Involvement of general practitioners and other health professionals, that is, using an independent and well-informed third party, might help.

Case 2

1. There is now no need for the woman to undergo an invasive prenatal test in future pregnancies, assuming her partner is the biological father; this would be a waste of resources and place the pregnancy at a small but unnecessary risk of miscarriage.
2. There is the difficulty of communicating the fact that a prenatal test is not necessary, but disclosure of nonpaternity may have far-reaching consequences for the couple's relationship. The genetic counselors do not know whether the partner suspects nonpaternity, and the mother may believe he is the biological father of the child. In the first instance genetic counselors may try to create an opportunity for the mother to be counseled alone and sensitively confronted with the results and their implications.

Clinical Scenario Answers and Discussion

Chapter 6

Clinical Scenario 1

Autosomal recessive, that is, both parents are unaffected carriers of a gene variant

Sporadic event occurring twice by chance, that is, the children have different conditions

Multifactorial, that is, the scenario is not explained by simple mendelian inheritance but rather by a polygenic model or a low penetrance gene with environmental, non-genetic influences

Teratogenic drug or agent taken by the mother in the pregnancies for the affected children, for example, alcohol, sodium valproate (antiepileptic drug)

Autosomal dominant—this is possibly caused by one or more of the following:

- Variable expression—so parents and perhaps other family members should be assessed
- Reduced penetrance—parents may have very mild or subclinical features of the phenotype, so need to be assessed
- "Anticipation" may be involved, so parents need to be assessed
- Somatic or germline mosaicism may be present in one of the parents
- Nonpaternity needs to be considered

X-linked recessive—possible if the affected daughter is a manifesting female

X-linked dominant—possible if there is reduced penetrance in the mother or somatic/germline mosaicism in the mother

Mitochondrial—reduced penetrance or subclinical features in the mother is common in this scenario

Imprinting—a parent of origin effect for a heterozygous variant in an imprinting gene could explain non-penetrance in a parent

Clinical Scenario 2

Autosomal dominant inheritance with variable expression is a possible explanation.

It cannot be **X-linked** because the father of the arrowed siblings has transmitted the condition to a son.

It cannot be **mitochondrial** because the arrowed siblings have inherited the condition from a male.

In fact, precocious puberty in this family is attributed to a **pathogenic variant in the gene MKRN3**, which is located within the ***15q11.2* imprinted region**. The pedigree demonstrates that precocious puberty only occurs when the variant is transmitted by a male, and in this pedigree these males are all unaffected because they inherited the variant from their mothers. The pedigree is entirely consistent with a **parent of origin effect**.

Chapter 8

Clinical Scenario 1

Spinal muscular atrophy (SMA) type follows autosomal recessive inheritance, and by far the most common pathogenic variant is deletion of exons 7–8 in the *SMN1* gene.

If it has an incidence of around 1:10,000, by the principles of the Hardy–Weinberg equilibrium the carrier frequency in the population is around 1:50 (2pq).

The pregnant woman's mother has a carrier risk of 2/3, so the pregnant woman's carrier risk is half of that, that is, 1/3.

Thus, the risk of the unborn baby being affected by SMA type 1 is:

$$1/50 \times 1/3 \times 1/4 = 1/600$$

Genetic testing for carrier status can be offered to provide more accurate risk counseling.

Clinical Scenario 2

John's risk of harboring the Huntington disease (HD) triplet repeat cannot be calculated directly. It is necessary to make his deceased father the **dummy consultand**.

Using Bayes' theorem:

Probability	Father is a Carrier	Father is not a Carrier
Prior	20% (or 1/5)	80% (or 4/5)
Conditional		
Two unaffected daughters (John's sisters)	$(1/2)^2 = 1/4$	$(1)^2 = 1$
Joint	1/20	4/5
Expressed as odds	1 to	16
Posterior	1/20 / (1/20 + 4/5)	
	= 1/20 / 17/20	
	= 1/17	
John's risk	Half of his father's risk	
	= 1/34 = ~3%	

John can of course opt for predictive genetic testing for HD to further clarify this risk. However, he would be advised to undergo appropriate counseling because he must be prepared for a positive (bad news) result even though his bayesian risk is relatively low.

Chapter 9

Clinical Scenario 1

Discussion:

Polydactyly is a feature of numerous syndromes but can also be isolated, that is, non-syndromic. The genetic basis of most syndromes is known. The clinical approach should include the following:

1. **Family history:** Does one of the parents have a history of extra digits being surgically removed when very young, a minor abnormality of the digits, or any other unusual dysmorphic feature?
2. **Type of polydactyly:** Is the polydactyly postaxial, preaxial, mesoaxial, or a combination of these types? If postaxial, is the extra digit well formed with a metacarpal bone (type A), or a skin tag attached to the medial border of the fifth finger (type B)?
3. **Other skeletal anomalies:** Are the stature and body proportions normal within the context of the family? Is the chest shape normal? Are the skull shape, head circumference, and dentition normal?
4. **Other (non-skeletal) anomalies:** Have the heart and renal system been scanned by ultrasound to check for structural anomalies? Are there genital anomalies? Has brain magnetic resonance imaging been performed? Have the eyes been examined?
5. **Cognitive development:** Has neurodevelopment been normal?

Simple, non-syndromic, postaxial polydactyly (type B) is sometimes an autosomal dominant (AD) trait with variable expression and incomplete penetrance. It can also be a feature of the large range of ciliopathy conditions, from short-rib polydactyly syndromes to Bardet–Biedl syndrome (BBS). All of these follow autosomal recessive inheritance and usually have additional presenting features, although BBS might be mild at 3 years of age, without obvious obesity, retinitis pigmentosa, or intellectual disability. Some 50% of cases of Smith–Lemli–Opitz syndrome have postaxial polydactyly.

Postaxial polydactyly is occasionally seen in Gorlin and Rubenstein–Taybi syndromes (both AD), and Simpson–Golabi–Behmel syndrome (X-linked).

Preaxial polydactyly is less common than postaxial, but the associated syndromes may be easier to diagnose clinically. Greig cephalopolysyndactyly, with mild macrocephaly and fontal bossing, is allelic with Pallister–Hall syndrome and due to variants in *GLI3*. They may include mesoaxial and/or postaxial polydactyly. Individuals with Pfeiffer syndrome, which is caused by variants in *FGFR1/2*, may have broad thumbs and/or halluces as well as features of craniosynostosis.

Clinical Scenario 2

Discussion:

The initial problem is whether this baby is a masculinized female or an under-masculinized male. Until this is resolved, neither the professionals nor the parents know the sex of the baby, which can be distressing.

The initial investigation is sex determination, which can be quickly achieved by quantitative fluorescence–polymerase chain reaction (QF-PCR) analysis. Ultrasound examination of the pelvis and abdomen to determine internal structures, particularly whether a uterus is present, should be performed. The scanning will also look for male gonads.

If the baby is genetically female, there is a possibility it has salt-losing congenital adrenal hyperplasia (CAH). If so, the baby is likely to develop a salt-losing crisis by the age of 10 to 20 days. Treatment and monitoring would then become crucial, and the baby would be raised as a female. Surgery at a later stage to normalise the genitalia may be indicated.

If the baby is female but does not have any form of CAH, the possibility of androgenic drugs or a maternal virilizing tumor needs to be considered.

If the baby is genetically male, the various disorders of androgen synthesis and androgen action need to be considered. Rare forms of CAH need to be investigated by biochemical and/or gene-panel analysis. Gene-panel testing should include a search for pathogenic variants in the androgen receptor (AR) gene, to take account of the possibility of partial androgen insensitivity syndrome (PAIS) due to the AR gene. However, AR gene variants are uncommon in PAIS, and, overall, this phenotype is often not currently explained through genetic testing.

Investigations:

Imaging—cardiac, renal/genitourinary, brain
Skeletal survey
7-dehydrocholesterol
Chromosome microarray analysis
Targeted gene analysis
Whole-exome sequencing

Chapter 11

Clinical Scenario 1

The tabulated data can be presented in this way.

AFFECTED		UNAFFECTED	
Positive	Negative	Positive	Negative
115	22	1312	460,364

Sensitivity (proportion of true positives):

$$115 / (115 + 22) = 84\%$$

Specificity (proportion of true negatives):

$$460{,}364 / (460{,}364 + 1312) = 99.8\%$$

Positive predictive value:

$$115 / (115 + 1312) = 8\%$$

For this test, the sensitivity (84%) is not as good as it should be for population screening because 16% with the diagnosis will not be picked up. However, the specificity is good (99.8%), because only a relatively small number of false positives are detected.

The ideal positive predictive value is 100%, that is, there are ***no*** false positives. However, this is very unlikely to be achieved in biochemical medical tests of this nature.

Clinical Scenario 2

The tabulated data can be presented in this way.

AFFECTED		UNAFFECTED	
Positive	Negative	Positive	Negative
115	22	1312	460,364

Sensitivity (proportion of true positives):

115 / (115 + 22) = 84%

Specificity (proportion of true negatives):

460,364 / (460,364 + 1,312) = 99.8%

Positive predictive value:

115 / (115 + 1312) = 8%

For this test, the sensitivity (84%) is not as good as it should be for population screening because 16% with the diagnosis will not be picked up. However, the specificity is good (99.8%) because only a relatively small number of false positives are detected.

The ideal positive predictive value is 100%, that is, there are ***no*** false positives. However, this is very unlikely to be achieved in biochemical medical tests of this nature.

Chapter 12

Clinical Scenario 1

Discussion:

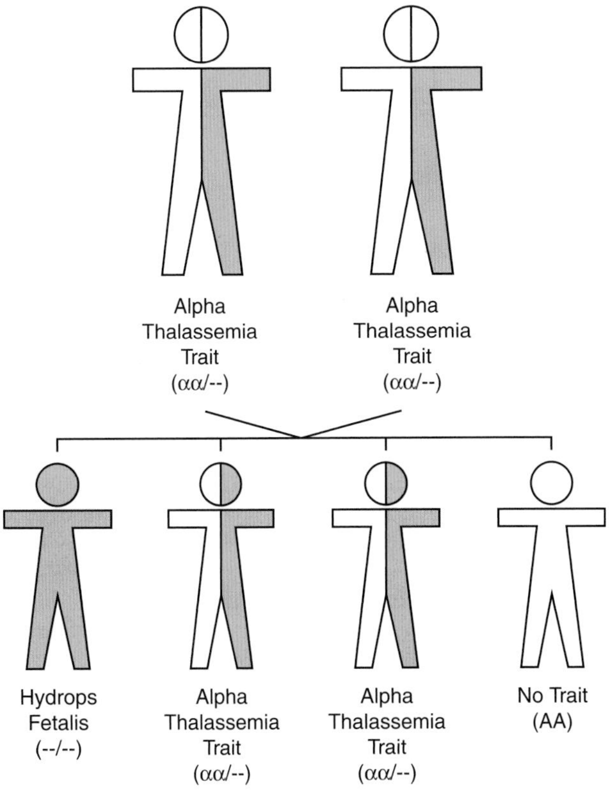

- There is a 1 in 4 chance of the fetus being affected with α-thalassemia major (hydrops fetalis).
- 1 in 2 children will be α^0 thalassemia trait, and in 1 in 4 will be unaffected.
- If the fetus is affected, a severe, life-threatening anemia is expected, which, without intervention, is not compatible with life.
- Hydrops is likely to present in the second trimester. Occasionally babies survive following intrauterine transfusion, but, if they do, there is a significant risk of disability after birth.
- A mother carrying a pregnancy affected with Bart's hydrops fetalis is also at risk of:
  - Preeclampsia
  - Antepartum hemorrhage
  - Retained placenta
  - Death (in up to 50%) if the condition is undiagnosed in the fetus
- Having received their screening results, the couple may opt for prenatal testing and termination of an affected pregnancy.
- The result provides information for future pregnancies, and for family members who may wish to consider screening before having children of their own.

Clinical Scenario 2

Principles of Management:

1. **Prophylactic penicillin** should be used to reduce the risk of sepsis from the age of 3 months. This should be considered on a life-long basis.
2. **Immunisations:** individuals with sickle-cell disease are susceptible to infection because of splenic hypofunction, which usually becomes apparent in the first year of life. Affected children should therefore receive all immunizations as per routine childhood immunization schedules. In addition, affected children should receive pneumococcus vaccination (at age 2 then 5-yearly boosters), annual influenza vaccine, and hepatitis B vaccine (from age 1), plus any relevant travel vaccines.
3. **Folic acid:** chronic hemolysis leads to an increase in folate turnover, and replacement should be considered to reduce the risk of bone marrow aplasia.
4. **Hydroxycarbamide (hydroxyurea):** works to increase HbF concentration, which, in turn, reduces the number of painful crises and the transfusion requirements of affected individuals. Importantly, patients need to be aware of possible teratogenic effects and given appropriate contraceptive advice. Currently recommended for use in:
   a. Patients with recurrent painful crises that impact on daily living
   b. Patients with more than three episodes of acute pain over a 12-month period
   c. Patients with two or more episodes of acute chest syndrome
5. **Stem cell transplant:** requires a matched donor and, in the United Kingdom, is considered in under-17s with sickle brain disease, or severe sickle cell–related complications that do not respond to hydroxycarbamide.

Counseling considerations:

Carrier status of parents/at risk relatives—a diagnosis in a child suggests carrier status of both parents, who may not have been aware of their status before embarking on a pregnancy. In addition, other family members of reproductive age, e.g., siblings, may be at risk of being carriers and could be offered testing.

1 in 4 risk to future pregnancies—couples should be carefully counseled about the risk to future children and the options available to them in future pregnancies.

Prenatal testing—couples may wish to consider testing in future pregnancies with chorionic villus sampling/amniocentesis. At the relevant time, they should be given details of the procedures, risks, and management of outcomes.

Preimplantation genetic diagnosis (PGD)—the Human Fertility and Embryology Authority (HFEA) has approved PGD for sickle-cell disease. In the United Kingdom, funding is currently available only for couples with affected children.

Preimplantation tissue typing (PTT) with PGD—PTT selects embryos that are an exact tissue match to their older, affected sibling. Using this technique alongside PGD allows a couple to have a child who can be a stem cell donor for their affected child, a so-called "savior sibling," but who is also born free of the disease. HFEA approval is in place for PTT in sickle-cell disease.

Chapter 13

Clinical Scenario 1

Discussion and answer:

There are several rare but important X-linked disorders of immune function, and the family history of a maternal uncle who succumbed to infection in his second year is highly suspicious for this group of conditions.

The presence of eczema in the patient and his deceased uncle, even though common in childhood, together with thrombocytopenia, suggests Wiskott–Aldrich syndrome (WAS). In this condition the platelets are small in size, and recurrent bacterial and viral infections occur, including ear infections.

WAS is caused by pathogenic variants in the *WAS* gene, which are also implicated in X-linked thrombocytopenia and X-linked congenital neutropenia.

Other important conditions to consider are:

- **X-linked severe combined immunodeficiency** presents in infancy with persistent infections—viral, bacterial, and fungal. Growth failure, thymic hypoplasia, and lymphocytopenia with near-complete absence of T and natural killer (NK) lymphocytes, as well as nonfunctional B lymphocytes, are features. It is caused by pathogenic variants in the *IL2RG* gene and is fatal within 2 years unless treated by bone marrow transplant or gene therapy.
- **X-linked hyper IgM syndrome** presents in infancy with recurrent bacterial infections—chest, ears, and sinuses—and males later develop autoimmune hematologic disorders including neutropenia, thrombocytopenia, and hemolytic anemia. It is caused by pathogenic variants in the *CD40LG* gene (also known as *TNFSF5*, encoding the CD40 ligand).
- **Chronic granulomatous disease (CGD)** is characterized by severe recurrent bacterial and fungal infections with granuloma formation and inflammatory disorders such as colitis. It may present between infancy and late adulthood, with the majority of individuals diagnosed before the age of 5 years. Diagnosis is by tests that assay neutrophil superoxide production via the nicotinamide adenine dinucleotide phosphate oxidase complex, and the *CYBB* gene is implicated in X-linked CGD (but there are autosomal recessive forms because of variants in *CYBA*, *NCF1*, *NCF2*, and *NCF4*).
- **X-linked agammaglobulinemia** males are usually healthy in early infancy because of protection from transplacentally acquired maternal immunoglobulin. Thereafter they are prone to developing recurrent bacterial infections and are usually recognized as having immunodeficiency by 5 years of age. Diagnosis is confirmed by sequencing of the *BTK* gene; in up to 5% of cases this is lost as part of a contiguous gene deletion.

Detailed tests of immune function and genetic testing using an appropriate gene panel will enable the diagnosis to be reached.

Clinical Scenario 2

Discussion and answer:

The combination of recurrent viral infections, dysmorphic features with a nasal quality to her speech, and low calcium in the neonatal period is highly suggestive of deletion 22q11.2 syndrome, also known as DiGeorge/Sedláčková syndrome.

Chromosome microarray is virtually guaranteed to yield the diagnosis and would be the first-line investigation. If confirmed, it is important to check immune function. T-cell production is impaired in two-thirds of cases, T-cell function is impaired in around one-fifth, and around a quarter of cases have defects of humoral immunity.

There are many complications of this well-characterized condition. It is important to investigate and consider the following:

- Check heart structures by echocardiogram
- Check calcium level
- Check the palate for a submucous cleft
- Check renal structures by ultrasound
- Check hearing by audiogram
- Examine the eyes
- Monitor growth
- Consider speech therapy and educational support
- Beware the development of autoimmune disorders such as rheumatoid arthritis
- Beware the development of mental health problems in adolescence and adult life

Chapter 14

Clinical Scenario 1

Discussion:

- **Germline *BRCA* analysis:** Although there is no family history of breast or ovarian cancer, the Manchester scoring system is significantly weighted for ovarian cancer. This patient would reach a score of 15 (8 + 5 + 2) and therefore meet the recognized 10% threshold for testing. In the United Kingdom all individuals with non-mucinous ovarian cancers would be offered *BRCA* gene testing regardless of age of diagnosis.
- **Somatic *BRCA* analysis:** If germline testing did not identify a pathogenic variant in *BRCA1* or *BRCA2*, it would be sensible to consider somatic *BRCA* analysis. Around 5% of cases will have a somatic variant in one of these genes, which may alter management.
- **PARP inhibitors:** In the United Kingdom, PARP inhibitors were previously licensed for use in *BRCA*-positive (germline or somatic), relapsed ovarian, fallopian tube, and primary peritoneal cancers following the third round of chemotherapy in which platinum sensitivity was demonstrated. Following

the success of its use, and the demonstration of longer progression-free survival, it is now approved as a first-line maintenance treatment. This emphasizes the importance of consideration of genetic testing at an early stage in the patient's cancer journey, and exemplifies the move toward personalized medicine.

Clinical Scenario 2

Discussion:

- **Familial renal cancer:** It is common for patients under the age of 45 with renal cancer of any type to be offered gene panel testing. This would generally include the following genes: *SDHB, FLCN, FH, VHL, MET*, and/or *BAP1*.
  Key points to note in the history include pheochromocytoma (*SDHB/VHL*), paraganglioma (*SDHB*), recurrent pneumothoraces (*FLCN*), women requiring hysterectomy (*FH*), and of course a history of any of the cancers or benign tumors known to be associated with these conditions.
  Renal cancer histology is also important and, in this case, is suggestive of Birt–Hogg–Dubé (BHD) syndrome.
  Further clues may be seen on skin examination for example, fibrofolliculomas in BHD and leiomyoma in hereditary leiomyomatosis and renal cell cancer.
  However, in this case, this would not identify the diagnosis.
- **Cowden syndrome (CS):** The clue in the history is the multinodular goiter, which is a common feature in CS. On further enquiry, a history of arteriovenous malformations is also present.
  When you examine the patient, she has macrocephaly, facial trichilemmomas, and papillomatous lesions of the oral mucosa.
  All types of renal cancer have been reported in CS.
  PTEN gene testing should be offered, and, where a pathogenic variant is identified, predictive testing can be arranged for relevant family members.
  There are a significant number of cancers associated with CS (breast, endometrial, thyroid, bowel, renal), so ongoing surveillance should be put in place, and risk-reducing hysterectomy should be considered.

Chapter 16

Clinical Scenario 1

Discussion and answer:

The two affected males are most likely to have variable manifestations of the same ectrodactyly, or split-hand/foot malformation, condition. It is important to assess them clinically for any evidence of syndromic associations, particularly ectrodactyly–ectodermal dysplasia–clefting syndrome.

The pedigree structure suggests X-linked inheritance, as the two males are connected by an unaffected female, II.3. Online Mendelian Inheritance in Man lists an X-linked locus for split-hand/foot malformation, but it is based on a huge inbred family from Pakistan in which there are several cases of male-to-male transmission—and a pathogenic variant does not seem to have been reported in the family. If the family in this scenario is manifesting an X-linked form of ectrodactyly, individual I.2 would be a carrier, with II.2 having a 50% risk of being a carrier, as well as the three female offspring of II.3, so the implications for other family members is significant.

In this scenario the laboratory sequenced the putative X-linked locus without finding a pathogenic variant. Later the laboratory undertook whole-genome sequencing on the family. This identified a small deletion in the *DYNC1I1* gene at chromosomal location 7q21.3. The function of the exons deleted is to regulate the expression of downstream *DLX5*, which is the ectrodactyly gene at this locus.

Thus, the family has an autosomal dominant form of ectrodactyly demonstrating variable expression, and for many individuals it is non-penetrant, including for individual I.3 who tested positive (individual I.2 tested negative). Later, individual II.5 fathered a very mildly affected daughter with his partner.

Clinical Scenario 2

Discussion and answer:

This young man has a multiple congenital abnormality syndrome, and the diagnosis may not be apparent from clinical evaluation.

Having had a normal chromosomal microarray analysis, the next step is whole-exome sequencing (WES). This could be undertaken purely on his DNA sample, followed up by testing the parents if a possible pathogenic variant is identified, or it could be a trio analysis if resources allow for this.

In fact, in this case a clinical diagnosis of Kabuki syndrome was made, and a *de novo* pathogenic variant in the *KMT2D* gene was subsequently identified without resorting to WES.

Anophthalmia/microphthalmia is an unusual presentation for Kabuki syndrome, but in fact all the other clinical features are reported in the syndrome.

The next step is to follow up the medical problems with appropriate investigations. Hypoglycemia may be due to hyperinsulinism, and this should be assayed. He should have tests of immune function because T-cell abnormalities have been reported in adolescents with Kabuki syndrome, and this may explain his proneness to infections. He should also have an echocardiogram and renal ultrasound performed if these have not been undertaken, and an assessment of his hearing if possible.

Kabuki syndrome attributed to *de novo* variants in *KMT2D* has been one of the more common conditions identified through studying large cohorts of patients with intellectual disability by WES, for example, the Deciphering Developmental Disorders project.

Chapter 17

Clinical Scenario 1

Discussion and answer:

The Rare Chromosome Disorder Support Group, Unique, has produced many excellent online booklets about microdeletion and microduplication disorders (www.rarechromo.org/). This is an easy place to start for a lot of helpful information about del15q11.2 syndrome.

The 6-year-old boy has severe intellectual disability (ID)—to a degree that is very rare in del15q11.2. These children may have mild speech delay, but not to this severe degree. They are also reported to be relatively contented children, even though short attention span and some autistic features are common—but this boy has extremely difficult behavior. Seizures may be part of del15q11.2, but they are severe in this boy, and hypogenitalism is not reported.

On balance it is therefore very unlikely that the chromosomal microarray analysis (CMA) finding is the explanation for the child's profound ID. However, his father had some mild educational difficulties, and these may well be explained by the finding.

Further investigation of the child's difficulties by genetic testing would best be conducted by whole-exome sequencing, preferably a "trio" approach incorporating DNA from both parents.

This scenario is not rare in clinical practice, that is, the finding of a microdeletion that may be the cause of mild ID but is also found in normal individuals. Some clinicians believe it is not helpful for these causes of "mild" ID to be reported because they change very little, if anything, for the family. Other clinicians may be happy to offer further testing of family members (on the father's side in this scenario) to identify who carries the deletion. For CMA used in prenatal testing there are many centers that would not report this finding because it is not regarded as significant enough.

Clinical Scenario 2

Discussion and answer:
The 10-year-old girl is not on the expected growth trajectory for 47,XXX syndrome, so a repeat chromosomal analysis is justified. This could be done on blood, but the previous result is reliable. Therefore, looking at chromosomes from another tissue is more likely to give additional information, and a full karyotype can be performed on fibroblasts from a skin biopsy.

It is certainly possible that the child may transpire to be 47, XXX/45,X mosaic—such cases occur, and this would explain her relatively short stature. Various forms of mosaicism with 45,X are common as varieties of Turner syndrome.

The presence of 45,X presents new clinical challenges in relation to growth, investigation of a possible heart abnormality (coarctation or the aorta), renal ultrasound (horseshoe kidney occurs in 45,X), and future fertility. She should therefore come under a pediatric endocrinologist for monitoring. There may be an indication to consider growth hormone treatment for the short stature besides the other potential endocrine issues.

Chapter 18

Clinical Scenario 1

Discussion and answer:
Q. 1: Metabolic diseases, or inborn errors of metabolism, can present in very subtle ways. This child is growing and developing normally, and there is nothing unusual to find on examination. For the more obvious and serious metabolic conditions a more significant history of illness and delayed development would be apparent.

The child does not have more infections that his peers, so this makes a disorder of immune function unlikely. The history of cot death, however, needs to be taken into account, and whether there is a connection to this boy's symptoms.

The fact that he has his symptoms in association with episodes when he is not eating properly, that is, during intercurrent illness, raises the specter of a disorder of fatty acid oxidation, of which the most common is medium-chain acyl-CoA dehydrogenase (MCAD) deficiency. This could also explain the earlier, tragic cot death. It is a variable disorder, and, although often presenting by 2 years of age, can present later. The fact that the parents had two healthy children following the cot death means they might have attributed that episode to a "one-off" tragedy, which was unlikely to be as a result of genetic causes.

Other disorders of fatty acid oxidation include:

- Very long-chain acyl-CoA dehydrogenase deficiency
- Long-chain 3-hydroxyacyl-CoA dehydrogenase deficiency

In these conditions the clinical presentation may be different, with features of liver dysfunction and cardiomyopathy.

- Short-chain acyl-CoA dehydrogenase deficiency

This condition is considered as clinically benign.

- Carnitine transport disorders

This group of rare disorders is also among the differential diagnosis and may present in a similar way.

MCAD deficiency is included in newborn bloodspot screening in many countries.

Q.2: It is likely that investigations will begin with a metabolic screen, that is, tests of liver and renal function, as well as straightforward biochemical tests. It is obviously helpful to investigate a child during an acute episode, as this may reveal hypoglycemia and disturbed liver function.

Testing should include **plasma acylcarnitine analysis** with expert interpretation—but acylcarnitine levels can normalize between acute episodes. **Urine organic acid analysis** and **urine acylglycine analysis** may provide supporting evidence for the identification of asymptomatic individuals and those with mild or intermittent biochemical phenotypes.

Molecular testing is now readily available and is likely to consist of a gene panel that includes *ACADM* and other genes of interest.

Targeted analysis for the common pathogenic variants found in northern Europe (c.985 A > G (p.Lys329Glu), c.199 T > C (p.Tyr67His)) may be performed first if appropriate. A different range of common variants will apply to other population groups.

Clinical Scenario 2

Discussion and answer:
There are many possible reasons for the 9-year-old child's history of increasing weakness, fatigue, and poor school performance. However, there are very strong clues in the family history—her mother and grandmother. Based on their history alone, that is, without the history in the 9-year-old girl, it is possible that a two-generation history of early strokes with early-onset dementia in the grandmother might suggest a diagnosis of cerebral autosomal dominant arteriopathy with subcortical infarcts and leukoencephalopathy (CADASIL, see p. 290), a late-onset autosomal dominant condition that usually includes headaches and migraines and is caused by pathogenic variants in *NOTCH3*.

The mother, like the 9-year-old child, is also complaining of weakness and fatigue. Again, this can have many causes—but she has had a premature stroke and is also losing her hearing prematurely. This, together with her daughter's history, suggests a mitochondrial disease, and in this three-generation family the inheritance is matrilinear.

Thus mitochondrial encephalomyopathy, lactic acidosis, and stroke-like episodes (MELAS), which is usually caused by the mt.3243 variant, is a strong possibility. It can be confirmed by targeted DNA analysis and will probably be present in blood DNA from the 9-year-old girl. However, the variant may not be present in every tissue, and one has to be aware of this when investigating possible pathogenic mitochondrial variants. For this reason muscle biopsy can be a crucial investigation, not only looking for "ragged-red fibers" but also performing DNA analysis on DNA from muscle.

Mitochondrial disease may also include diabetes mellitus, cardiomyopathy, and leukoencephalopathy.

Chapter 19

Clinical Scenario 1

Discussion and answer:

Q.1: On the face of it, the interpretation of the *DMD* gene analysis is straightforward. The boys' grandmother has tested negative for the *DMD* pathogenic variant. One therefore assumes that she has passed the variant to the mothers of the affected boys because she has *germline mosaicism*. This is not uncommon in Duchenne muscular dystrophy (DMD), and the chance of it occurring is surprisingly high. Without further analysis this is the information that would be given to the family.

Q.2: The genetics team has pursued haplotype studies in the family to check that the grandmother has germline mosaicism for the *DMD* variant.

The pathogenic allele is traveling with the pattern designated blue in this pedigree. The mothers of the boys have the "blue" haplotype, as expected. If this blue haplotype was inherited from the grandmother, then the other haplotype would be from the grandfather, which should be the same for both mothers. However, it is a different haplotype —"red" for one and "green" for the other. Thus, red and green must have been inherited from the mother and blue from the grandfather. These haplotype patterns were confirmed in the grandparents.

Therefore, the grandfather is a germline mosaic for the *DMD* pathogenic variant that has been passed on to his grandsons. This is a rare occurrence in DMD, but it highlights the value of studying haplotypes to clarify the transmission.

Clinical Scenario 2

Discussion and answer:

The young athlete appears to have suffered a sudden cardiac death, because no cause has been found. His death should certainly be viewed as likely resulting from cardiac causes.

With the heart looking normal on postmortem examination, there appears to be no evidence for a form of cardiomyopathy. This probably narrows the diagnosis to a form of inherited cardiac arrhythmia. If a sample of DNA had been stored, it would be reasonable for this to be analyzed on gene panels for long-QT syndrome (LQTS), Brugada syndrome, and catecholaminergic polymorphic ventricular tachycardia arrhythmia conditions.

In the absence of DNA being available for the deceased, there is the possibility of an inherited arrhythmia for which first-degree relatives (and members of the wider family) are at risk. The parents and their daughter should have conventional cardiac investigations in an attempt to identify a problem that might have been the underlying reason for the sudden death of the young man. The daughter has had two syncopal-like episodes, which may have been related to a cardiac problem, so her tests are potentially crucial.

The investigations to be considered are:

- Electrocardiogram
- Heart monitoring during a flecainide stimulation test
- Echocardiogram
- Cardiac magnetic resonance imaging scan

The object of these investigations is to see if there is any evidence of a first-degree relative having an abnormal cardiac rhythm, which might be heritable, and then offering genetic testing to that person using an appropriate gene panel, for example, for LQTS or another arrhythmia phenotype.

If a cardiac abnormality is found, followed by a positive genetic test, predictive testing can be offered to other family members at risk, which in turn would lead to appropriate intervention in the form of prophylactic treatment and ongoing surveillance.

Chapter 20

Clinical Scenario 1

Discussion:

1. Do nothing
   - Although this result may be suggestive of a risk of trisomy, the patient may decline further testing as she would not consider termination under any circumstance.
2. Non-invasive prenatal testing (NIPT)
   - Patient could be offered non-invasive testing to further assess the risk of trisomy.
   - If this was suggestive of a low trisomy risk, further invasive testing would not be indicated.
   - If a high-risk result, invasive testing should be offered.
3. Invasive testing
   - Where NIPT is unavailable, invasive testing should be offered which, at the current gestation, would involve chorionic villus sampling with quantitative fluorescent-polymerase chain reaction and array-comparative genomic hybridization testing.
   - This may confirm trisomy or another chromosome abnormality, in which case the patient may opt to end the pregnancy.
   - Testing may be normal, ruling out a chromosome abnormality as the cause of the raised combined risk.

In this case, NIPT suggested a low risk, and further invasive testing was not arranged.

Detailed anomaly scan at 20 weeks did not detect any structural abnormalities to suggest an underlying genetic disorder.

Is ongoing follow-up needed?

Yes. Pregnancy-associated plasma protein A (PAPP-A) is produced by the placenta, and low levels may be suggestive of reduced placental function. This can in turn be associated with pregnancy complications; for example, intrauterine growth restriction, premature delivery, late miscarriage, and an increased chance of preeclampsia.

Women with a low PAPP-A should, in addition to routine antenatal care, be offered:

- Daily aspirin
- Regular scans from 28 weeks to monitor the baby's growth, placental blood flow, and amniotic fluid levels
- Induction of labor at term with close monitoring during delivery

Clinical Scenario 2

Discussion:

1. Current risk to unborn child
   Carrier risk (father) = 2/3
   Carrier risk (mother) = population, or 1/25
   Risk of two carriers having an affected child = ¼
   Current risk to pregnancy = 2/3 × 1/25 × ¼ = 1/150
2. Delineating risk
   Confirm diagnosis in father's sibling and offer urgent testing for known pathogenic variants.

Offer urgent carrier screen to mother.

3. Both parents confirmed to be carriers—options for pregnancy:
   No testing—parents may not consider termination of an affected pregnancy but would consider testing of baby at birth so that pediatric input can begin from an early stage, which is thought to improve long-term outcome.
   Non-invasive prenatal diagnosis
   - can be offered from 9 weeks' gestation
   - uses relative haplotype dosage analysis by targeted next-generation sequencing
   - can be used when couples carry the same mutation
   - requires DNA from the proband
   - normally produces results within 5 days

   Invasive testing
   - chorionic villus sampling can be offered from 11 weeks' gestation.
4. Options for the future
   If the fetus is affected, and the couple decide to end the pregnancy, they may wish to discuss preimplantation genetic diagnosis as an option for future pregnancies.

Chapter 21

Clinical Scenario 1

Discussion:

Adenosine deaminase (ADA) deficiency: Individuals affected with ADA deficiency are prone to recurrent and persistent infections that may be life-threatening. These infections are normally caused by organisms that would not present any problem to people with a normal immune system, so-called "opportunistic" infections. Most are diagnosed in the first 6 months of life, with the main symptoms of: pneumonia, chronic diarrhea, and skin rashes. Growth may also be affected, and some children exhibit developmental delay. Without treatment, children are unlikely to live beyond the first 2 years of life. Treatment aims to restore normal immune function with bone marrow or stem cell transplant from a human leukocyte antigen–identical healthy sibling or relative. Where this is not possible, non-ideal donors or enzyme replacement therapy can be used. Gene therapy is currently being studied in this field.

Calculating risk to unborn baby: Father—has an affected sibling, therefore both of his parents must be carriers. His carrier risk = 2/3
Mother—has an affected maternal aunt, both grandparents must be carriers. She has half her mother's carrier risk (2/3), therefore her carrier risk = 1/3

Risk to unborn baby = 2/3 × 1/3x¼ = 1/18

Discussing the options:

- Carrier testing—if the pathogenic ADA variants are known in the family, the couple can be offered testing to better understand the risk to their unborn baby. This should be requested urgently in light of the ongoing pregnancy.
- Prenatal testing—if both parents are confirmed carriers, then chorionic villus sampling/amniocentesis could be offered, depending upon gestation and patient choice. The couple need to be counseled about associated miscarriage risk and options for management if unborn baby affected.
- ADA enzyme assays—if the ADA variants are unknown, ADA enzyme assays can be used on chorionic villus sampling fronds or cultured cells. Enzyme levels can be used as a guide to whether baby is affected, but are not as accurate as genetic analysis.

Clinical Scenario 2

Discussion:

- ***De novo* variant**
  The vast majority of pathogenic *BRCA1* variants are inherited from a parent. Although it is possible that this could be *de novo*, the chance of this happening is less than 5%.
- **Sample mix-up**
  Human error is unavoidable—it is possible that samples could have been mixed up in the lab, therefore leading to an inaccurate result. You could offer a repeat the test on a new blood sample.
- **Laboratory reporting error**
  Could the variant have been missed on analysis of the results? Definitely warrants a conversation with the reporting scientist to recheck the result.
- **Nonpaternity**
  Requires careful discussion with the patient/family, especially as, if true, there may be others at significant cancer risk.
  Whatever the explanation for this result, sensitive discussion and excellent communication skills are required to manage the potential impact that the result may have on the family.

Chapter 22

Clinical Scenario 1

Discussion:

Consider the basic ethical principles:

Autonomy—A clinician needs to respect an individual's decision, even if it is one that seems incorrect in their personal view. In the context of genetic testing, patients should be freely able to "opt out" at any point in the process. A patient's right to confidentiality sits within this principle, and while this is not absolute, any breach requires very careful consideration.

Beneficence—Why has the patient asked not to receive her results? Careful counseling may help in understanding the basis for this decision, and perhaps, at this time, it is in the patient's best interests not to know. However, the result confirms a high lifetime risk of ovarian cancer, and of further breast cancer—could it be argued that it is in her best interests to know? What about her relatives, one of whom is also your patient? Surely it is in their best interests to be told so that they can take appropriate action to reduce their cancer risk? In genetics, do you act in the best interests of the patient or the family?

Non-maleficence—Revealing a result that has been declined by the patient certainly has potential for harm. This may, for example, be psychological harm to the patient, or irreparable damage to the doctor–patient relationship.

Justice—Should this be considered for the patient or the family? Perhaps by not sharing this information we are denying opportunity and resources for screening to the family.

Consider the condition:

Pathogenic variants in *BRCA1* are associated with a significant lifetime risk of breast and ovarian cancer, for which screening and risk-reducing surgical options are available. If this were a condition with no available treatment, with 100% penetrance (e.g., Huntington disease), the argument may be slightly different. However, there are many "at-risk" female individuals in the family, and it is hard to argue that this information would not be beneficial to them. On the other hand, would they want to know?

Consider the process:

Complicated cases like this require multidisciplinary input. Certainly, discussions within the genetics team would be sensible, but if a breach in confidentiality is considered, involvement of the hospital legal team and ethics board would be appropriate.

Clinical Scenario 2

Discussion:

Friedreich ataxia (FA) is the most common autosomal recessive ataxia. Onset is usually in childhood or early adolescence (mean 10–15 years, and usually by 25 years), presenting with a slowly progressive ataxia. Other possible features include hypertrophic cardiomyopathy, diabetes, scoliosis, dysarthria, dysphagia, and optic nerve atrophy. FA is a life-shortening condition with the average age of death in the 40s, although this is variable, depending on the severity of features.

Is this a carrier test or predictive testing for a degenerative condition in a child?

At first glance, in an unaffected individual, this may appear as a carrier test. In actual fact, although FA often runs true in families, given the patient's age, testing could confirm that she will develop the condition.

Points to consider in the consultation:

- Who has requested testing—the parents or the child?
  Parents do sometimes request predictive testing in children. Generally, testing would only be arranged in childhood if symptoms of the condition were present, thereby allowing the child to make an informed decision about testing as an adult. If the child requests testing, very careful consideration of their understanding, and the impact of the result, is needed.
- The impact of a predictive positive test result on relationships
  How would this result affect the patient's relationship with her parents? Would they treat her differently? How would it impact her relationship with the affected sibling? Would there be an effect on this relationship if testing shows she is not affected, or is a carrier? Could it affect relationships with friends?
- Is there a risk of harm to the child?
  Can a 13-year-old truly understand the implications of predictive testing? Could the certainty of developing a serious condition lead to psychological harm? Might it stop her pursuing her dreams? Might it take away her childhood? Would she make the same decision if she were to consider testing in 5 or 10 years' time?
- How would she cope with a positive result?
  Does the patient have effective coping strategies to manage a positive result? Does she have the life experience to have developed these? Can she imagine what the future may look like and the difference the result may make?
- Timing
  Dealing with bad news is stressful and disruptive to everyday life. Is the potential disruption to schooling a reason not to test? Would it be more appropriate to wait until the patient is an adult, and perhaps considering her own children, when the results will have more relevance?
- Consent
  Given the patient's age, parental consent for testing would be needed. If the patient has requested testing, do the parents agree? Do they have any concerns?

This situation requires very careful counseling, and involvement of a genetic counselor would be advisable. There needs to be careful consideration of the ethical and legal issues, particularly thinking about consent and the best interests of the child.

Index

Page numbers followed by "*f*" indicate figures, "*t*" indicate tables, and "*b*" indicate boxes.

B

E

G

H

J

K

L

M

N

O

Q

R

S

U

V